Nursing Theorists
and Their Work

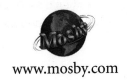

www.mosby.com

Nursing Theorists
and Their Work
Fifth Edition

Ann Marriner Tomey, PhD, RN, FAAN
Professor
Indiana State University
Terre Haute, Indiana

Martha Raile Alligood, PhD, RN
Professor and Chair, MSN Program
College of Nursing
University of Tennessee
Knoxville, Tennessee

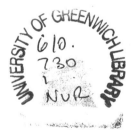 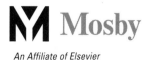

Mosby
An Affiliate of Elsevier

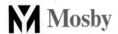

An Affiliate of Elsevier
Vice-President, Nursing Editorial Director: Sally Schrefer
Editor: Yvonne Alexopoulos
Developmental Editor: Melissa K. Boyle
Project Manager: Catherine Jackson
Production Editor: Jamie Lyn Thornton
Designer: Amy Buxton
Cover Design: Studio Montage

FIFTH EDITION

Mosby
11830 Westline Industrial Drive
St. Louis, Missouri 63146

Printed in the United States of America

Library of Congress Cataloging-in-Publication Data

Nuring theorists and thier work / [edited by] Ann Marriner and Martha Raile Alligood.-- 5th ed.
    p . cm.
Includes bibliographical references and index.
ISBN 0-323-01193-4
  1. Nuring--Philosophy. 2. Nursing models I. Marriner-Tomey, Ann 1943-II Alligood, Martha Raile

RT84.5 .N9 2001
610.73'01--dc21

2001044385

04   05   CL/FF   9   8   7   6   5   4   3

Contributors

Martha Raile Alligood, PhD, RN
Professor and Chair, MSN Program
College of Nursing
University of Tennessee
Knoxville, Tennessee

Donald E. Bailey, Jr, PhD(c)
Doctoral Candidate
School of Nursing
University of North Carolina
Chapel Hill, North Carolina

Sue Marquis Bishop, PhD, RN, FAAN
Dean
College of Nursing and Health Professions
University of North Carolina, Charlotte
Charlotte, North Carolina

Victoria M. Brown, RN, PhD, HNC
Professor of Nursing
Department of Adult and Gerontological Health
School of Health Sciences
Georgia College and State University
Milledgeville, Georgia

Karen A. Brykczynski, RN, CS, FNP, DNSc
Associate Professor
The University of Texas School of Nursing at
  Galveston
The University of Texas Medical Branch
Galveston, Texas

Thérèse Dowd, PhD, RN
Associate Professor
College of Nursing
The University of Akron
Akron, Ohio

Margaret E. Erickson, BSN, MSN, PhD
Holistic Healing Consultants
Executive Director, American Holistic Nurses
Certification Corporation
Austin, Texas

Carolyn H. Fakouri, DNS, RN
(Retired)

Julie M.B. Fine, PhD
Associate Professor
School of Nursing
Indiana State University
Terre Haute, Indiana

Barbara T. Freese, RN, EdD
Professor
School of Nursing
Lander University
Greenwood, South Carolina

Mary E. Gunther, RN, PhD
Instructor
College of Nursing
University of Tennessee
Knoxville, Tennessee

Chérie G. Howk, DNSc, RN, CS-FNP
Assistant Professor
Family Nurse Practitioner Program
Indiana State University
Terre Haute, Indiana

Mary M. (Molly) Meighan, RNC, PhD
Assistant Professor of Nursing
Carson-Newman College
Jefferson City, Tennessee

Gail Mitchell, PhD, RN
Chief Nursing Officer
Sunnybrook and Women's College Health Sciences
  Centre
Assistant Professor
University of Toronto
Toronto, Ontario, Canada

Ruth M. Neil, PhD, RN
Project Coordinator
National Resource Center for Health and Safety in
  Child Care
Associate Professor
University of Colorado School of Nursing
Aurora, Colorado

Susan A. Pfettscher, DNSc, RN
Associate Professor
Department of Nursing
California State University, Bakersfield
Bakersfield, California

Kenneth D. Phillips, PhD
Associate Professor
College of Nursing
University of South Carolina
Columbia, South Carolina

Teresa J. Sakraida, DNSc, RN
Coordinator
RN Options Program
School of Nursing
University of Pittsburgh
Pittsburgh, Pennsylvania

Karen Moore Schaefer, DNSc, RN
Assistant Professor
Department of Nursing
College of Allied Health Professions
Temple University
Philadelphia, Pennsylvania

Norma Jean Schmieding, EdD, RN
Professor
University of Rhode Island College of Nursing
Kingston, Rhode Island

Christina Leibold Sieloff, RN, PhD, CNA
Assistant Professor
School of Nursing
Oakland University
Rochester, Michigan

Janet L. Stewart, PhD(c)
Doctoral Student
University of North Carolina School of Nursing
Chapel Hill, North Carolina

Susan G. Taylor, RN, PhD, FAAN
Professor Emerita
Sinclair School of Nursing
University of Missouri, Columbia
Columbia, Missouri

Ann Marriner Tomey, PhD, RN, FAAN
Professor
Indiana State University
Terre Haute, Indiana

Alice Z. Welch, RN, PhD
(Retired)

Janet M. Witucki, RN, PhD
Assistant Professor
School of Nursing
University of Tennessee, Knoxville
Knoxville, Tennessee

Reviewers

Reviewed fourth edition in preparation for this fifth edition

Louise Selanders, RN, EdD
Associate Professor
College of Nursing
Michigan State University
East Lansing, Michigan

Mary Cipriano Silva, PhD, FAAN
Professor
George Mason University
Fairfax, Virginia

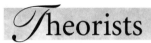

Theorists

Faye Glenn Abdellah
Dean and Professor
Uniformed Services University of the Health
  Sciences
Graduate School of Nursing
4301 Jones Bridge Road
Bethesda, MD 20814-4799
(301) 295-1933
fabdellah@usuhs.mil

Evelyn Adam
Professor Emeritus
University of Montreal
6950 Côte Saint-Lue
Montreal, Quebec H4V 2Z9
(514) 484-0217
evelyn.adam@sympatice.Ca

Kathryn E. Barnard
University of Washington
School of Nursing
T-303 H.S.B., SC-72
Seattle, WA 98195
(206) 543-4152

Patricia Benner
University of California, San Francisco
School of Nursing
San Francisco, CA 94143
(415) 476-4313

Helen C. Erickson
University of Texas
Austin, TX 78701
(512) 471-7311

Lydia E. Hall*

Virginia Henderson*

Dorothy E. Johnson*

* Deceased

Imogene King
(Retired)
7400 Sun Island Drive
South Pasadena, FL 32168
(904) 360-1943

Katharine Kolcaba
College of Nursing
The University of Akron
Akron, OH 44325-3701
Kolcaba@uakron.edu

Madeleine Leininger
1121 Woolworth Plaza
Omaha, NE 68144-1875
(402) 691-0791

Myra Estrin Levine*

Winifred W. Logan (Gordon)
108 Fernlea
The Spinney
Bearsden
Glasgow, Scotland
G6T-INB
UK

Ramona T. Mercer
(Retired)
1809 Ashton Avenue
Burlingame, CA 94010
(650) 697-2324

Merle Mishel
429 Carrington Hall
CB #7460
University of North Carolina, Chapel Hill
Chapel Hill, NC 27599
(919) 966-6610
mishel@email.unc.edu

Betty Neuman
P.O. Box 488
Beverly, OH 45715
(614) 749-3322

Margaret A. Newman
289 East Fifth #511
St. Paul, MN 55101
(651) 292-0437

Florence Nightingale*

Dorothea E. Orem
Savannah, GA

Rosemarie Rizzo Parse
Nursing Science Quarterly
320 Fort Duquesne Boulevard
Suite 251
Pittsburgh, PA 15222
(412) 391-8471

Ida Jean Orlando (Pelletier)
111 Waverly
Belmont, MA 02178
(401) 783-2442

Nola J. Pender
Associate Dean for Research
University of Michigan
School of Nursing
Grants and Research Office 4236
400 North Ingalls
Ann Arbor, MI 48108-0482
(734) 764-9555

Hildegard E. Peplau*

Martha E. Rogers*

Nancy Roper
70 Polwarth Gardens
Edinburgh, Scotland
United Kingdom EH11 1LL
0131-229-4748

*Deceased

Sister Callista Roy
Boston College
Cushing Hall
140 Commonwealth Avenue
Chestnut Hill, MA 02167
(617) 552-8811

Mary Ann P. Swain
Office of Academic Affairs
University of Michigan
Ann Arbor, MI 48109
(313) 764-0151

Alison J. Tierney
Department of Nursing Studies
University of Edinburgh
Adam Ferguson Building
40 George Square
Edinburgh, Scotland
United Kingdom, EH 8 9LL
0131-650-1000

Evelyn M. Tomlin
P.O. Box 128
Big Rock, IL 60511
(312) 556-3087

Joyce Travelbee*

Jean Watson
University of Colorado
Health Sciences Center
School of Nursing
4200 East Ninth Avenue
Denver, CO 80262
(303) 384-7754

Ernestine Wiedenbach*

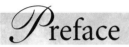

Preface

This book is a tribute to nursing theorists. It identifies major thinkers in nursing, reviews some of their important ideas, lists their publications, and lists what has been written about their publications and the major sources the theorists used. Chapter 1 presents a brief history of nursing theory, introduces theoretical terminology, and presents a framework for analysis of the theoretical works included in this volume. Chapter 2 discusses the significance of theory for nursing as a discipline and as a profession. The other chapters in Unit I discuss the history and philosophy of science, logical reasoning, and the theory development process.

The theorists are clustered into three categories. Nightingale, Wiedenbach, Henderson, Abellah, Hall, Watson, and Benner wrote philosophies. Orem; Levine; Rogers; Johnson; Roy; Neuman; King; and Roper, Logan, and Tierney designed conceptual models or grand theories. Peplau; Orlando; Travelbee; Kolcaba; Erickson, Tomlin, and Swain; Mercer; Barnard; Leininger; Parse; Mishel; Newman; Adam; and Pender wrote theories or middle-range theories.

The following are identified for each theorist: credentials and background, theoretical sources for theory development, use of empirical data, major concepts and definitions, major assumptions, theoretical assertions, logical form, acceptance by the nursing community, further development, and a critique of the work. The critical thinking activities and bibliographies are updated in this edition. Baccalaureate students may be most interested in the concepts, definitions, and theoretical assertions. Graduate students will be interested in logical form, acceptance by the nursing community, the theoretical sources for theory development, and the use of empirical data. The extensive bibliographies should be particularly useful to graduate students for locating primary and secondary sources.

These theorists have enriched our professional lives by providing theoretical works to guide our research and practice. It is now our responsibility to analyze and synthesize their work, generate new ideas, and continue theory development and application.

We would like to thank the theorists for critiquing the original and some subsequent chapters about themselves to keep the content current and accurate. So that their omission does not appear to have been an oversight, it must be noted that the work of Paterson and Zderad has not been included at their request.

We thank the librarians who have helped us obtain obscure information and all the other people working behind the scenes. Dr. Martha Raile Alligood reordered the chapters, served as a contributing author, and edited for consistency with the new organization in the third edition. After Dr. Alligood coedited *Nursing Theory: Utilization and Application* with Dr. Marriner Tomey, and based on her expertise in nursing science theory, she became a coeditor and a contributing author for the fourth and fifth editions.

We thank our loving husbands, Charlie K. Alligood and H. Keith Tomey, for enriching our private lives while supporting our professional activities.

Ann Marriner Tomey
Martha Raile Alligood

Contents

UNIT III
Conceptual Models and Grand Theories

UNIT IV
Theories and Middle-Range Theories

UNIT V

Future of Nursing Theory

Evolution of Nursing Theories

- *The evolution of nursing theories has been a search for nursing substance.*

- *Analysis includes such activities as examination, inquiry, investigation, study, appraisal, estimation, evaluation, and judgment.*

- *The purpose of analysis in education is to lead the student to new understanding through the process of organized review and critical thinking.*

- *Analysis of theoretical works uses knowledge of the theory development process, the history and philosophy of science, the nature of science within the discipline, the state of progress in the various theoretical endeavors, and logic.*

- *Theory is important to both nursing as a discipline (a branch of education) and as a profession (a specialized field of practice).*

Introduction to Nursing Theory: History, Terminology, and Analysis

Martha Raile Alligood and Ann Marriner Tomey

The literature has never been more replete with examples of nursing theory-based practice and research. The number of doctorally prepared nurse scholars with a commitment to nursing theories has never been higher. The challenge today is to translate the knowledge base nurtured and grown in the world of scholarship into practice in the worlds of nurses' direct experiences.[9:5]

This text is designed to introduce the reader to nursing theorists and their work. Nursing theory has been a prevalent theme in the nursing literature for the past 30 years and has stimulated phenomenal growth in the nursing profession. Selected nursing theorists are included to introduce the reader to nursing theory. Although many nurses of early eras delivered excellent care to patients, much of what was known about nursing was not written down and research to document the effectiveness of the care they delivered was not recorded. Therefore nurses began to move toward the goal of developing nursing knowledge upon which to base their practice. That goal served the nursing profession throughout the twentieth century as they worked toward the achievement of developing a substan-

Previous authors: Martha Raile Alligood, Elizabeth Chong Choi, Juanita Fogel Keck, and Ann Marriner Tomey.

tive body of nursing knowledge to guide nursing practice.[1]

In this chapter, the reader is introduced to nursing theory with a brief overview of the historical development of nursing, specifically, the search for nursing substance that led to this outstanding time in nursing history. In the first half of the twentieth century, nursing leaders began to understand that a knowledge base was required for professional nursing practice. Therefore nurses have worked toward developing a substantive body of nursing knowledge over the span of the last century, first with the goal of becoming a recognized profession and later with the goal of delivering care to patients as professionals. History provides a context for understanding nursing theory and establishes a rationale for why theory is essential for professional practice. Next, basic terminology specific to the reader's understanding of nursing theory is introduced in relation to a structure of nursing knowledge. Finally, this chapter discusses the analysis of nursing theory (an essential process for knowledge development), describes the criteria selected for use in this text to organize the analysis of each theoretical work, and concludes with reasons for theory.

HISTORY

The history of professional nursing begins with Florence Nightingale. It was Nightingale who envisioned nurses as a body of educated women when women were neither educated nor employed in public service. Following her years of service organizing and caring for the wounded in the Crimean War, her vision and her establishment of a school of nursing at St. Thomas' Hospital in London marked the birth of modern nursing. Nightingale's pioneer activities in nursing practice and her subsequent writings about nursing served as a guide for establishing nursing schools in the United States at the beginning of the twentieth century.[15,21]

In the last century, nursing began with a strong emphasis on practice. Throughout that century, nurses worked toward the development of the profession in what has been viewed as successive historical eras.[1]

The *curriculum era* addressed the question of what prospective nurses must study and learn to become a nurse. The emphasis was placed upon the courses nursing students needed to take with the goal of arriving at a standardized curriculum. Within this era, the idea of moving nursing education from hospital-based diploma programs into colleges and universities emerged, but it was mid-century before this goal began to be achieved in many states.[15]

As more and more nurses sought degrees in higher education, what is deemed the *research era* began to emerge. This era came about as more nurses embraced higher education and arrived at the common understanding of the scientific age: that research was the path to new knowledge. Nurses began to participate in research and research courses began to be included in the nursing curricula of developing graduate programs.

The research era was followed closely by the *graduate education era.* Masters programs in nursing emerged to meet the need for nurses with specialized education in nursing. Many of these programs included a course in nursing research in the curricula and, near the end of this era, most also included a course in nursing theory or nursing conceptual models that introduced students to the early nursing theorists and the theory development process.

The *theory era* was a natural outgrowth of the research era. With an increased understanding of research and knowledge development, it became obvious that research without theory produced isolated information; however, research and theory produced nursing science. Within the *contemporary phase,* there is an emphasis on theory use in theory-based nursing practice and continued theory development.*

Each of the eras emphasized nursing knowledge in a way that is evident in studying the history. Also, they all addressed the question of what knowledge was needed for the practice of nursing and did so according to the level of understanding they had in that era.[1]

Nightingale's[21] vision of nursing has been practiced for more than a century and theory development in nursing has evolved rapidly over the past four decades, which finally lead to the recognition of nursing as an academic discipline with a substantive body of knowledge.† In the mid1800s, Nightingale expressed her firm conviction that nursing knowledge was distinct from medical knowledge. She described a nurse's proper function as putting the patient in the best condition for nature to act upon him or her and set forth the idea that nursing was based on the knowledge of persons and their surroundings, which was a different knowledge base than physicians used in their practice.[21] Despite this early edict from Nightingale in the 1950s, it was before members of the nursing profession began serious discussion about the need to develop, articulate, and test nursing theory.[4,5,8,18,24] Until the emergence of nursing as a science in the 1950s, nursing practice was based on principles and traditions passed on through

---

*References 6, 8, 9, 13, 17, 18.
†References 1, 2, 5, 8, 13, 17, 25.

apprenticeship education and common-sense wisdom that came with years of experience.[1,15]

Although some nursing leaders aspired for nursing to develop as a profession and an academic discipline, nursing practice continued to reflect vocational heritage more than professional vision. The transition from vocation to profession included successive eras in the search for a body of substantive knowledge on which to base nursing practice. The curriculum era, which emphasized course selection and content for nursing programs, gave way to the research era, which focused on the research process and the goal of developing new knowledge. In the mid1970s, the evaluation of 25 years of nursing research revealed that nursing lacked conceptual connections and theoretical frameworks.[7] An awareness of the need for concept and theory development coincided with two other significant milestones in the evolution of nursing theory: the standardization of curricula for nursing master's education through the National League for Nursing accreditation criteria and the decision that doctoral education for nurses should be in nursing.[1]

The nursing theory era coupled with a new awareness of nursing as a profession and an academic discipline in its own right emerged from debates and discussions in the 1960s regarding the proper direction and appropriate discipline for nursing knowledge development. This new awareness was evidenced by an explosive proliferation of nursing doctoral programs and nursing theory literature.[19,20] The transition in the 1970s from vocation to profession was a major turning point for nursing because nurses asked the question, "Will nursing be other-discipline based or be nursing based?" and the answer was that nursing practice will be based on nursing science.[1:6-7,11] According to Meleis,[18] this progress in nursing theory is a most significant aspect of scholarly evolution and the cornerstone of the nursing discipline.

In the 1980s, developments in nursing theory characterized a transition from the preparadigm period to the paradigm period.[12,14] The prevailing paradigms (models) provided various perspectives for nursing practice, administration, education, research, and further theory development. The proposal for global nursing concepts as a metaparadigm in the 1980s introduced an organizational structure for nursing knowledge development to the nursing literature.[11,12,13] The classification of nursing models as paradigms, which address a metaparadigm with concepts of person, environment, health, and nursing, views nursing theoretical works in a systematic manner that improves the comprehension of knowledge development, imbeds the theorists' works in a larger context, and facilitates understanding of the growth of nursing science within these paradigm perspectives.[6,13] The body of nursing science and the methods for research, education, administration, and practice continues to expand through nursing scholarship. Papers are presented at national and international conferences; newsletters, journals, and books written by the community of scholars, who are associated with various nursing models and theories, describe the theoretical base of their practice and research with the selected model or theory (paradigm perspective).[5,13] These observations of nursing science development bring Kuhn's[16] ideas of normal science to life. Clearly his philosophy of science has furthered an understanding of the evolution of nursing theory through his concept of paradigm science.[16] It is important to remember that theory emerged through the individual efforts of various nursing leaders across the country and, in retrospect, they are viewed collectively in a process of knowledge development. Theory development emerged from scholarship that was a product of the professional growth process of nurse leaders, administrators, educators, and practitioners who sought higher education and saw the limitations of theory from other disciplines such as medicine to describe, explain, or predict nursing outcomes. These leaders labored to establish a sound scientific basis for nursing management, curricula, practice, and research. Theory's function to convey meaning as an organizing structure in these processes caused a convergence of ideas, which resulted in the emergence of what is referred to as the nursing theory era.[2,6,9,19,20]

The accomplishment of normal science ushers in the utilization phase of the theory era; that is, the time when the emphasis shifts from development to use and application of what is known.[6] For the discipline of nursing, the utilization phase restores the centrality of nursing practice and recognizes theory and research as tools of practice rather than ends in themselves. Refer to the second edition of Alligood and Marriner Tomey's text, *Nursing Theory: Utilization and Application*,[6] for a comprehensive discussion of this new phase of the theory era and for examples of applications of nursing theoretical works in nursing practice.

This brief history provides a context for the study of the nursing theorists and their work. In this new century, the theory era continues with an emphasis on the use of nursing knowledge to guide the critical thinking required for professional practice. Nursing theory guides the thought and action of nursing practice.[3,13] Therefore professional nurse preparation includes an introduction to the works of selected nursing theorists. This emphasis on the use of theory in practice takes place in concert with an emphasis on the development of new nursing knowledge as theory-based nursing research continues in this theory era.

TERMINOLOGY

Metaparadigm is the most abstract level of knowledge. It specifies the main concepts that encompass the subject matter and the scope of a discipline. Many years ago, person, environment, health, and nursing were proposed as both nursing phenomena and the first metaparadigm concepts of nursing and they continue to have utility as the main organizing concepts for the discipline and the profession.[3,13,16] Powers and Knapp[22:119] have noted, "There is general agreement that nursing's metaparadigm consists of the central concepts of person, environment, health and nursing."

Philosophy is the next knowledge level; it specifies the definitions of the metaparadigm concepts in each of the conceptual models of nursing.[13] There are other nursing theoretical works that may be considered philosophies; these are works that specify philosophical approaches to nursing.[5,15,17,18] Nightingale's work is an example of a philosophy of nursing. Theory may be formalized from these philosophies, such as the works of Watson and Benner (Chapters 11 and 12, respectively).

Conceptual models are frameworks or paradigms that provide "a broad frame of reference for systematic approaches to the phenomena with which the discipline is concerned."[6:223,13] Conceptual models provide different views of nursing according to the characteristics of the model. For example, Johnson (Chapter 16) focuses on behavior, King (Chapter 19) focuses on interaction, and Roy (Chapter 17) focuses on adaptation.

Theory is "a group of related concepts that propose actions that guide practice."[6:225]

Nursing theory is a group of related concepts that derive from the nursing models. Some nursing theories also derive from other disciplines such as Leininger's work (Chapter 28), which comes from anthropology, or Peplau's work (Chapter 21), which draws from psychiatric sources.

Middle-range theories are the least abstract level of theoretical knowledge because they include details specific to nursing practice. Middle-range theories include information indicating the situation or health condition, the patient population or age group, the location or area of practice, and the action of the nurse or the intervention (Chapters 26, 31, and 33).[3,4] Middle-range theories have also been developed from the themes of data in qualitative research (Chapters 24 and 30). The levels of theoretical works from metaparadigm to middle-range theory are illustrated in Table 1-1.

The range of theories is generally determined by the level of abstraction and by the content it specifies. Most of the conceptual models of nursing have a range of theories from which they have been derived.

Grand theories are nearly as broad as the nursing model they are derived from, but they are different from nursing models. Nursing models provide a view or perspective, but they do not propose testable truths. Therefore *grand theories* are *theories* because they do propose something that is true or testable, such as Roy's theory of the person as an adaptive system derived from the Roy Adaptation Model.

Theories may be broad but limited to the aspects of nursing they address, such as Leininger's Theory

Table 1-1

Knowledge Structure Levels with Examples

STRUCTURE LEVEL	EXAMPLE
Metaparadigm	Person, environment, health, and nursing
Philosophy	Nightingale
Conceptual Models	King's Systems Framework
Grand Theory	King's Theory of Goal Attainment
Theory	Goal attainment in hospital settings
Middle-Range Theory	Goal attainment in adolescent diabetic patients in the community

From Alligood, M.R. & Marriner Tomey, A. (2002). *Nursing theory: Utilization and application* (2nd ed.). St. Louis: Mosby. (Modified from Fawcett, J. [1995]. *Analysis and evaluation of conceptual models of nursing* [3rd ed.]. Philadelphia: F.A. Davis; Fawcett, J. [1993]. *Analysis and evaluation of nursing theories.* Philadelphia: F.A. Davis.)

of Cultural Care and Universality that is specific to culture, or Orlando's Theory of Nursing Process that is specific to the manner of the nurse-patient relationship. Theories may also be specific to a certain nursing approach or to a certain patient population, such as Mercer's Theory of Maternal Role Attainment.

Middle-range theory has a narrower focus than theory and specifies such things as the situation or health condition, the patient population or age group, the location or area of practice, and the action of the nurse or the intervention.[4,13]

In addition to the terminology associated with the structure of knowledge presented so far, other terms are found in broader discussions of knowledge and its development, which may contribute to the understanding of nursing theoretical works.

Science is performing the processes of observation, identification, description, experimental investigation, and theoretical explanation of natural phenomena. It is also a body of knowledge; therefore science is defined as both a unified body of knowledge concerned with specific subject matter and as the processes and methodologies necessary to provide such knowledge. Powers and Knapp[22:157] state that "science is best thought of as an activity that combines research (the advancement of knowledge) and theory (the explanation of knowledge)."

The term **knowledge** suggests an understanding acquired through learning or investigation of what is known about a discipline's subject matter. Knowledge may be based on fact or it may be theoretical-based knowledge that is more tentative and subject to change as theory is tested and developed.[23]

Phenomena are the subject matter of a discipline. In the midtwentieth century, American nurses identified their **phenomena of concern** as human beings and their environments.

A **concept** is "an idea or complex mental image of a phenomenon (object, property, or event). Concepts are the major components of theory."[22:24] Concepts are the labels used to identify phenomena.

Abstract concepts are independent of time or place and they are indirectly observable. Hope is an example of an abstract concept.

Concrete concepts are specific to time and place and are observable. A person's features, such as eye color, height, or weight, are examples of concrete concepts.

The term **model** is defined in several ways. *Verbal models* are worded statements, a form closely related to knowledge development. For example, conceptual models of nursing are word structures that provide a specific view on nursing through the interrelationship of concepts in the structure. A second form of model explains an idea by using schema, symbols, or physical visualization. *Schematic models* may be diagrams, drawings, graphs, or pictures that facilitate understanding.

A **paradigm** is another term for conceptual framework or conceptual model. It is a term used to denote the prevailing schema or approaches within a discipline, such as Roy's Adaptation Model or Neuman's Systems Model. These approaches include a worldview, a nursing model, the research methods and instruments, the outcomes specific to the model, and a community of scholars that contribute to the science.[16]

Theoretical definitions convey the meaning of a concept in a particular theory by specifying the empirical indicator.[13]

Operational definitions specify how a concept or variable (empirical indicator) is measured in a particular research project.

Assumptions are statements that the theorist or researcher holds as truth and excludes from measurement and testing.

Theoretical statements (also called *principles* or *propositions*) describe the relationship between two or more concepts.

Propositions are theoretical statements that specify the proposed relationships of the concepts of a theory. Proposition statements lead to the conclusive statement of the middle-range theory, which asserts what is proposed to be true and testable in the form of a hypothesis.

Hypothesis is a testable relationship statement.

Research is the application of systematic, scientific methods to study phenomena and generate knowledge. Research may generate theory when executed with an inductive approach or it may test theory when conducted with a deductive approach. Powers and Knapp[22:157] state that "science = research + theory."

Induction is a form of reasoning that is loosely described as moving from the specific to the general. In inductive logic, a series of particulars is combined into a larger whole, or set of things. In inductive research, particular events are observed and interpreted as a basis for formulating general theoretical statements such as in phenomenology or grounded theory.[22]

Deduction is a form of logical reasoning that is loosely described as progressing from the general to the specific. This process involves a sequence of theoretical statements derived from a conceptual model of nursing or a grand theory. Two or more relational statements are used to draw a conclusion (proposition). From the theoretical relationships, specific empirical hypotheses are derived.[22]

Retroduction combines induction and deduction to originate ideas. This form of reasoning uses analogy as a method of devising theory. (See Chapter 4 for more information on induction, deduction, and retroduction.)

This section has presented the terminology to facilitate understanding of the theoretical works presented in this textbook. Each of the works of the nursing theorists has been organized into one of three types of knowledge based on its predominant characteristics as a theoretical work in nursing. Classifying the works in this manner not only adds specificity to their discussion, but more importantly, it offers context to consider them in relation to a structure of nursing knowledge.[3,13]

Three general kinds of works are brought together in this text. The first type is nursing philosophy. Philosophy sets forth the meaning of nursing phenomena through analysis, reasoning, and logical argument. These include both early works, which predate or introduce the nursing theory era and have contributed to knowledge development in nursing by providing direction or forming a basis for subsequent developments, and later works, which reflect more recent expansion in the areas of human science and its methods.[2,18]

The second type, nursing conceptual models, is comprised of the works of the grand theorists or pioneers in nursing. As Fawcett[13:16] explains, "A conceptual model provides a distinct frame of reference for its adherents . . . that tells them how to observe and interpret the phenomena of interest to the discipline."

The works of the grand theorists are comprehensive nursing models that include their perspectives on human beings, their environment, and their health. Most nursing conceptual models have grand theories that the theorists derived from their own models. Grand theories differ from models because they provide propositional direction for members of the profession in a scientific field.[6] The nursing models have explicit and implicit grand theories within them. Examples of this may be observed in Roy's theory of the person as an adaptive system, derived from her Adaptation Model, or the Theory of Goal Attainment that King derived from her Interacting Systems Framework. The abstract level of grand theories facilitates the derivation of many middle-range theories that are very specific to nursing practice.[4]

The third type, nursing theories and middle-range theories, may have been derived from works in other disciplines and related to nursing from earlier nursing philosophies and theories, from nursing grand theories, or from nursing conceptual models.[3,13] Middle-range theory has a narrower focus and is much more concrete than grand theory in its level of abstraction.[2,4,8,13] Therefore middle-range theories are more precise and they focus on answering specific nursing practice questions. They specify such factors as the age group of the patient, the family situation, the health condition, the location of the patient, and most importantly, the action of the nurse.[3] Middle-range theories address the specifics of nursing situations within the perspective of the model or theory from which they are derived.[2,3,4,13]

ANALYSIS

The criteria for evaluating each theoretical work included in this text are clarity, simplicity, generality, empirical precision, and derivable consequences.[8] Analysis, critique, and evaluation are all methods of studying the nursing theoretical works critically. This process is useful in learning about the works and is very useful for nurse scientists who intend to test, expand, or extend the works. In addition, the areas in need of further development are discovered through the process of critique or analysis. Therefore analysis is an important process for learning, for developing research projects, and for developing the science associated with the theoretical works of nursing in the future.

Clarity

"How clear is this theory?"[8:100]

Consistency and semantic and structural clarity are important. To assess these, the major concepts, subconcepts, and their definitions are identified. Words often have multiple meanings within and across disciplines; therefore words should be defined carefully and specifically to the framework

(philosophy, conceptual model, or theory) from which it is derived. Diagrams and examples may facilitate clarity and should be consistent. The logical development should be clear and assumptions should be consistent with the theory's goals.[8,23,25]

Reynolds[23:13] refers to intersubjectivity when he states, "There must be shared agreement of the definitions of concepts and relationships between concepts within a theory." Hardy[14:106] refers to meaning and logical adequacy when she states, "Concepts and relationships between concepts must be clearly identified and valid." Ellis[10:221] refers to "the criterion of terminology" to evaluate theory and addresses "the danger of lost meaning when terms are borrowed from other disciplines and used in a different context." Walker and Avant[25] assert that the logical adequacy of a theory is the logical structure of the concepts and statements as proposed in the theory.

Simplicity

"How simple is this theory?"[8:100]

Simplicity is valued in theory development. Chinn and Kramer[8] suggest that nurses in practice need simple theory, such as middle-range theory, to guide practice. A theory should be sufficiently comprehensive and at a level of abstraction to provide guidance, but it should have as few concepts as possible with simplistic relations to aid clarity. Reynolds[23:135] contends that "the most useful theory provides the greatest sense of understanding." Walker and Avant[25:130] refer to parsimony as "elegant in its simplicity, even though it may be broad in content."

Generality

"How general is this theory?"[8:100]

To determine the generality of a theory, the scope of concepts and goals within the theory are examined. The more limited the concepts and goals, the less general the theory. Chinn and Kramer[8] believe that the situations the theory applies to should not be limited. Ellis[10:219] states, "The broader the scope, the greater the significance of the theory." This feature of scope is becoming better understood in recent years as more students have come to understand that the more abstract the work is, the more middle-range theories can be derived from the work. King's Theory of Goal Attainment and Rogers' Theory of Accelerating Change are examples of theories from which many middle-range theories may be derived.

Empirical Precision

"How accessible is this theory?"[8:100]

Empirical precision is linked to the testability and ultimate use of a theory and it refers to the "extent that the defined concepts are grounded in observable reality."[14:144] Hardy[14:105] states, "How well the evidence supports the theory is indicative of empirical adequacy" and she emphasizes that there "should be a match between theoretical claims and the empirical evidence." Reynolds refers to empirical relevance and the trait that "anyone be able to examine the correspondence between a particular theory and the objective empirical data."[23:18] He notes that other scientists should be able to evaluate and verify results by themselves. Walker and Avant[25] clarify that theory must generate hypotheses and be useful to scientists to add to the body of knowledge. Ellis[10] emphasizes that theories are tentative and subject to change.

Derivable Consequences

"How important is this theory?"[8:100]

Chinn and Kramer[8] propose that if research, theory, and practice are to be meaningfully related, then nursing theory should lend itself to research testing and research testing should lead to knowledge that guides practice. Further, they suggest that nursing theory guides research and practice, generates new ideas, and differentiates the focus of nursing from other professions.[8] Ellis[10:220] indicates that to be considered useful, "it is essential for theory to develop and guide practice . . . Theories should reveal what knowledge nurses must, and should, spend time pursuing."

These five analysis criteria—clarity, simplicity, generality, empirical precision, and derivable consequences—are used to review the theoretical work in each chapter of this text. They are sufficiently broad criteria to analyze nursing philosophies, conceptual models, and theories.

This chapter introduces the works of a large number of theorists. These works can be viewed in various ways for different purposes. To trace the evolution of theory development in nursing, the theorists and their works are presented chronologically in terms of their historical sequence and are classified as philosophies, conceptual models, and theories (Box 1-1). From nursing's theoretical works, the reader can trace the evolution of theory development in nursing. First, a philosophy for nursing evolved (Nightingale). Second, early nursing theories, with an emphasis on interpersonal relationships, were developed (Peplau, Orlando, Travelbee, Barnard, and Mercer). Next came more philosophies emphasizing the art of nursing (Henderson, Wiedenbach, and Hall), followed by the beginning of an emphasis on the scientific aspects of nursing (Abdellah). These philosophies were followed by the conceptual models of nursing, which reflect adaptation, behavioral field theory, systems approaches, and an emphasis on science (Johnson; Neuman; Rogers; King; Orem; Roy; Levine; and Roper, Logan, and Tierney). Finally, there is nursing theory derived from earlier philosophies and nursing models (Parse, Newman, and Adam). Along with these developments, nurses continue to synthesize theories from other disciplines into nursing applications (Erickson, Tomlin, and Swain; and Pender) as was accomplished earlier in nursing (Leininger). The late 1980s and early 1990s evidence the blending of theory and philosophy for a humanistic nursing approach that reemphasizes nursing practice (Watson, Parse, and Benner). More recent middle-range theories are emerging (Mishel and Kolcaba). The future of nursing is bright and hopeful. The theorists' different conceptualizations of nursing enrich the discipline and its knowledge. The task for the future is to test the theories in nursing practice and research and to derive new theories from the nursing conceptual models.

Kuhn[16:42] states, "Paradigms can guide research in the absence of rules," but "normal science cannot progress without paradigms." The same is true for nursing practice. As theory development gives way to theory utilization, the significance of nursing models and theories becomes even more obvious for professional practice and for nursing education.[6]

REASONS FOR THEORY

Theory gives meaning to knowledge to improve practice by describing, explaining, and predicting phenomena. A nurse's power is increased through theoretical knowledge because systematically developed methods guide critical thinking and decision making in professional practice and they are more likely to be successful. In addition, nurses will understand why they are doing what they are doing and be able to explain it clearly to other health professionals. Therefore theory leads to professional autonomy by guiding practice, education, and research within the profession. Furthermore, the study of theory develops analytical skills and critical thinking ability, clarifies values and assumptions, and directs the purposes of nursing practice, education, and research.*

Additionally, Kuhn[16:11] has said that the models or "paradigms of a scientific discipline primarily prepare students for practice as members of that professional community." The paradigm (model or framework) plays a vital role in practice because, "without a framework, all of the information that the professional encounters seems to be equally relevant."[16:15] Therefore students studying to enter a professional discipline are introduced to the models or paradigms as an orientation to the approaches used in the practice of that discipline. Following an introduction and survey of the models and theories, the students are ready to choose the ones they will use in their practice. For it is "by studying them and

*References 6, 8, 9, 13, 17, 18.

Box **1-1**

Evolution of Nursing Theory within Types of Works

PHILOSOPHIES
Nightingale
Wiedenbach
Henderson
Abdellah
Hall
Watson
Benner

CONCEPTUAL MODELS AND GRAND THEORIES
Orem
Levine
Rogers
Johnson
Roy
Neuman
King
Roper, Logan, and Tierney

THEORIES AND MIDDLE-RANGE NURSING THEORIES
Peplau
Orlando
Travelbee
Kolcaba
Erickson, Tomlin, and Swain
Mercer
Barnard
Leininger
Parse
Mishel
Newman
Adam
Pender

practicing with them, the members of their corresponding community learn their trade."[16:43]

Nurses are recognizing the rich heritage of the works of nursing theorists; that is, the philosophies, conceptual models, and theories of nursing. These contributions represent the status of nursing as a discipline and further developments continue to occur. Most importantly, models and theories guide the critical thinking of nurses and are becoming more accepted by the nursing community.[9] The debate should not be about what each model represents, but rather about how each model represents the diverse values that nurses are seeking. The direction is moving toward further clarification of the understanding of these works so they can be used as frameworks for structuring nursing practice with predictable outcomes and for deriving new middle-range theories to test in nursing research and practice.[4,6]

Recognition of the significance of normal science has occurred in this era. The scholarship of the past decade alone is a demonstration of that outcome, not only as nursing literature around the philosophies, models, and theories proliferates quantitatively, but also as the depth of the scientific scholarship improves qualitatively.[2,4] As the understanding of nursing models has expanded and their use has increased dramatically, their capacity for the development of nursing knowledge and the benefits for nursing practice has emerged. In fact, nursing models serve the purpose Kuhn's philosophy[16] of science would predict: as organizing structures for schools of thought or communities of scholars who share together in the work. Whether the individuals working within each community of scholars are focused on theory, research, administration, education, or nursing practice, they all work together and share their experiences in the development and use of nursing science through their work in the selected nursing model or theory. This is reflected in publications, organizations, and conferences (regional, national, and international) centered on the work of the nursing theorists.[5,17]

REFERENCES

1. Alligood, M.R. (1997). The nature of knowledge needed for nursing practice. In M.R. Alligood & A. Marriner-Tomey (Eds.), *Nursing theory: Utilization and application* (pp. 3-13). St. Louis: Mosby.
2. Alligood, M.R. (1997). Models and theories in nursing practice. In M.R. Alligood & A. Marriner-Tomey (Eds.), *Nursing theory: Utilization and application* (pp. 15-30). St. Louis: Mosby.
3. Alligood, M.R. (1997). Models and theories: Critical thinking structures. In M.R. Alligood & A. Marriner-Tomey (Eds.), *Nursing theory: Utilization and application* (pp. 31-45). St. Louis: Mosby.
4. Alligood, M.R. (1997). Areas for further development of theory-based nursing practice. In M.R. Alligood & A. Marriner-Tomey (Eds.), *Nursing theory: Utilization and application* (pp. 203-210). St. Louis: Mosby.
5. Alligood, M.R. (2000). Nursing theory: The basis for professional nursing. In K.K. Chitty (Ed.), *Professional nursing: Concepts and challenges* (3rd ed., pp. 246-274). Philadelphia: W.B. Saunders.
6. Alligood, M.R. & Marriner Tomey, A. (Eds.). (2002). *Nursing theory: Utilization and application* (2nd ed.). St. Louis: Mosby.
7. Batey, M.V. (1977). Conceptualization: Knowledge and logic guiding empirical research. *Nursing Research*, 26(5), 324-329.
8. Chinn, P. & Kramer, M. (1998). *Theory and nursing: A systematic approach* (5th ed.). St. Louis: Mosby.
9. Cody, W.K. (1997). Of tombstones, milestones, and gemstones: A retrospective and prospective on nursing theory. *Nursing Science Quarterly*, 10(1), 3-5.
10. Ellis, R. (1968). Characteristics of significant theories. *Nursing Research*, 17(5), 217-222.
11. Fawcett, J. (1978). The "what" of theory development. In National League for Nursing, *Theory development: What, why, how?* (pp.17-33). New York: National League for Nursing.
12. Fawcett, J. (1984). The metaparadigm of nursing: Current status and future refinements. *Image: The Journal of Nursing Scholarship*, 16, 84-87.
13. Fawcett, J. (2000). *Contemporary nursing knowledge: Conceptual models of nursing and nursing theories.* Philadelphia: F.A. Davis.
14. Hardy, M.E. (1978). Perspectives on nursing theory. *Advances in Nursing Science*, 1, 37-48.
15. Kalisch, P.A. & Kalisch, B.J. (1995). *The advance of American nursing* (3rd ed.). Philadelphia: J.B. Lippincott.
16. Kuhn, T.S. (1970). *The structure of scientific revolutions.* Chicago: University of Chicago Press.

17. Marriner Tomey, A. & Alligood, M.R. (1998). *Nursing theorists and their work* (4th ed.). St. Louis: Mosby.
18. Meleis, A. (1995). *Theoretical nursing: Development and progress* (3rd ed.). Philadelphia: J.B. Lippincott.
19. Nicoll, L. (1986). *Perspectives on nursing theory.* Boston: Little, Brown.
20. Nicoll, L. (1992). *Perspectives on nursing theory* (2nd ed.). Philadelphia: J.B. Lippincott.
21. Nightingale, F. (1969). *Notes on nursing: What it is and what it is not.* New York: Dover. (Originally published, 1859.)
22. Powers, B.A. & Knapp, T.R. (1995). *A dictionary of nursing theory and research* (2nd ed.). Thousand Oaks, CA: Sage.
23. Reynolds, P.D. (1971). *A primer for theory construction.* Indianapolis: Bobbs-Merrill.
24. Torres, G. & Yura, H. (1975). The meaning and functions of concepts and theories within education and nursing. In National League for Nursing, *Conceptual framework: Its meaning and function.* New York: National League for Nursing.
25. Walker, L.O. & Avant, K.C. (1995). *Strategies for theory construction in nursing.* Norwalk, CT: Appleton-Lange.

$\mathcal{S}$ignificance of Theory for Nursing As a Discipline and Profession

Martha Raile Alligood and Ann Marriner Tomey

$\mathcal{A}$t the beginning of the twentieth century, nursing was neither an academic discipline nor a profession. However, the accomplishments of the last century have led to the recognition of nursing in both areas. Although some nurses may have used these two words (discipline and profession) interchangeably, their meaning is not the same. As this chapter will illustrate, discipline and profession are definitely interrelated, but they each have specific meanings that are important to nursing.

- A **discipline** is specific to academia and refers to a branch of education, a department of learning, or a domain of knowledge.[20,60,84]
- A **profession** refers to a specialized field of practice, which is founded upon the theoretical structure of the science or knowledge of that discipline and the accompanying practice abilities.[82,114]

The achievements of nursing in the last century were highly relevant to nursing's development. These achievements did not come easily. History records the many nurses who pioneered the various causes and challenged the status quo with creative ideas for both the health of people and the forward development of nursing. Their achievements have ushered in this exciting time when nursing is recognized as both an academic discipline and a profession.[27,39,61] In this text, the pertinent question is: what is the significance of theoretical works for the discipline and the profession of nursing? *Nursing theoretical works* represent the most comprehensive ideas and systematic knowledge about nursing; therefore theory is vital to both the discipline and the profession.

SIGNIFICANCE OF THEORY FOR NURSING AS A DISCIPLINE

As nurses entered academia in larger numbers in the last half of the twentieth century, the goal to develop knowledge as a basis for nursing practice began to be realized. University baccalaureate programs proliferated, masters programs in nursing were developed, and the curricula began to be standardized through the accreditation process. As mentioned in Chapter 1, nursing went through gradual stages of development.[4] Nursing leaders presented several different perspectives for the development of nursing science. Some advocated nursing as an applied science and others proclaimed nursing as a basic science.[19,20,35,105] This debate gave way to a perspective they could all agree upon: nurses needed to learn the research process.[114]

In 1977, after 25 years of publishing *Nursing Research,* studies were comprehensively reviewed and the strengths and weaknesses of the research were noted. Batey[11,12] called attention to the importance of nursing conceptualizations for the research process and the role of a conceptual framework in the purpose and design of research for the production of science. This emphasis on the importance of conceptualization for nursing research projects and the development of conceptual frameworks for nursing curricula were precursors to the theory development era that moved nursing toward the goal of having nursing knowledge to guide nursing practice. At that time, nursing theoretical works also began to be published.* Fawcett[26] presented her double helix metaphor of the relationship of theory and research, which has become a classic reference on the topic. Also, at this time, some of the earlier works began to be recognized for their theoretical nature, such as Henderson, Nightingale, Orlando, Peplau, and Wiedenbach. Educators developed most of these works as frameworks to structure curriculum content or guide the teaching of nursing practice in nursing programs. Orlando's theory[85,86] was the outcome of a funded research project designed to study nursing practice.

When the Nurse Educator Nursing Theory Conference was held in New York City in 1978, the major theorists were brought together on the same stage for the first time. Most of them began their speeches by stating that they did not view themselves as theorists. An understanding of the significance of these works for nursing was limited at the time, but young masters and doctoral students in

the audience seemed to recognize the significance of the event. The audience laughed at the theorists' denials of being theorists and became silent and listened carefully to what each of the theorists had to share.

Also noteworthy, Donaldson and Crowley[20] presented the keynote address at the Western Commission of Higher Education in Nursing (WCHEN) Conference in 1977 as new nursing doctoral programs were beginning to open and they reopened the discussion of the nature of nursing science. The published version of the keynote address has become a classic reference for nursing as a discipline and for distinguishing between the discipline and the profession. The authors called for both basic and applied research and asserted that the use of this knowledge was vital to nursing as both a discipline and a profession. Critical topics were the nature of nursing knowledge and distinguishing between the discipline and the profession. The authors noted that, although the discipline and profession were inextricably linked, the failure to recognize the existence of the discipline as a body of knowledge and separate it from the activities of its practitioners contributed to the view that nursing was a vocation rather than a profession. Further, they raised the question of whether the discipline of nursing even existed. Soon after this period, nursing conceptual frameworks began to be noted as frameworks for curricula in nursing programs and as nursing conceptual models that addressed the major and most abstract concepts (metaparadigm) of nursing.[25] Fawcett's conceptualization of a nursing metaparadigm and a unifying conceptual-theoretical structure of knowledge recognized the works of the major nursing theorists as nursing conceptual frameworks and paradigms of nursing. This organization of nursing theoretical works introduced a cohesive understanding of the theoretical knowledge of nursing that theorists developed at different times and in different parts of the country. Each of the nursing conceptual models was judged to be so based on its performance in relation to a set of criteria for analysis and evaluation.

The significance of theory for the discipline of nursing is that the discipline is dependent upon theory.

---

*References 36, 37, 105, 40, 81, 109, 68, 54.

The theoretical works have taken nursing to a higher level. The emphasis has shifted from a focus on knowledge about how nurses function, which concentrated on the nursing process, to a focus on what nurses know and how they use knowledge to guide their thinking and decision making while concentrating on the patient.

Frameworks and theories are designed to provide the nurse with a perspective of the patient. This perspective is also characteristic of a profession. The professions provide a public service and the practice is focused on those served. The nursing process continues to take place, but it is no longer the primary focus. The fact that colleges and schools of nursing across the country award degrees in nursing is dependent upon the need for knowledge that is nursing. This knowledge forms the basis for nursing's recognition as a discipline; every discipline or field of knowledge includes theory.

Therefore nursing as an academic discipline is dependent upon the existence of nursing knowledge. This knowledge is transmitted to those entering the profession as a basis for their practice in the profession. Kuhn,[47:11] the philosopher of science, has stated, "The study of paradigms . . . is what mainly prepares the student for membership in the particular scientific community with which he [or she] will later practice." This is important to all nurses, but it is particularly important to those entering the profession because "in the absence of a paradigm . . . all of the facts that could possibly pertain to the development of a given science are likely to seem equally relevant."[47:15] Finally, with regard to the priority of paradigms, he states, "By studying them and by practicing with them, the members of their corresponding community learn their trade."[47:43]

In addition, masters-level nurses and students apply and test theoretical knowledge in their practice and test nursing knowledge in their theses. Doctoral-level students study to become nurse scientists to develop nursing theory, test theory, and contribute new nursing science through theory-based research studies.

SIGNIFICANCE OF THEORY FOR NURSING AS A PROFESSION

Not only is theory essential for the existence of nursing as an academic discipline, it is also vital to the practice of the profession. Although the topic of nursing as a profession became less urgent at the end of the twentieth century, it had been a primary topic throughout much of the century as nursing made consistent progress toward professional status. Clearly, nursing is recognized as a profession today. Throughout much of the twentieth century, the criteria for a profession served as a guide for the development of the profession. Nursing was the subject of a number of sociological studies regarding professional development and these studies used various sets of criteria. For example, Bixler and Bixler[18] published a set of criteria tailored to nursing in the *American Journal of Nursing* in 1959. They said that a profession:

1. Utilizes in its practice a well-defined and well-organized body of specialized knowledge [that] is on the intellectual level of the higher learning.
2. Constantly enlarges the body of knowledge it uses and improves its techniques of education and service by the use of the scientific method.
3. Entrusts the education of its practitioners to institutions of higher education.
4. Applies its body of knowledge in practical services [that] are vital to human and social welfare.
5. Functions autonomously in the formulation of professional policy and in the control of professional activity thereby.
6. Attracts individuals of intellectual and personal qualities who exalt service above personal gain and who recognize their chosen occupation as a life work.
7. Strives to compensate its practitioners by providing freedom of action, opportunity for continuous professional growth, and economic security.[18:1142-1146]

These criteria have historical value because they provide an understanding of the developmental path that nursing followed. For example, a knowledge that is well defined, organized, and specific to the discipline was formalized the last half of the last century, but this knowledge is not static. Rather, it continues to grow in relation to the profession's goals for the human and social welfare of the society that nurses serve. That is, although the body of knowledge is important, the theories and research are also vital to both the discipline and the profession as new knowledge is needed and continues to be generated. The application of nursing knowledge in practice is a criterion that is currently at the forefront with an emphasis on accountability for nursing practice, theory-based nursing practice, and growing recognition that middle-range theory is specific to nursing practice.[7]

In the last decades of the previous century, histories were written that presented specific goals and achievements of the profession. For example, Styles[115] developed a distinction between a *collective nursing profession* and the *individual nurse as a professional* and called for internal developments based on ideals and beliefs of nursing for a new endowment. Her premise was that the profession needed a new, positive approach for the future that was devoid of past problems, such as various levels of education for entry into the profession to progress in professional development. Fitzpatrick[27] presented a history that chronicled the achievements of the century leading to the professional status of nursing. These references are detailed and they give background and history specific to the development of nursing as a profession. This text recognizes that nursing has achieved the status of a profession and emphasizes the relationship of nursing theory to that achievement.

There are similarities and differences in the sets of criteria used to evaluate the status of professions; however, they all include the necessity of developing and using a body of knowledge that is foundational to the practice of the given profession.[115] In fact, the goal of developing such a body of knowledge served as a driving force for the developments of the nursing profession in the latter half of the last century.[4] As individual nurses grow in their professional status, the use of substantive knowledge as a basis for theory-based nursing is a characteristic of their practice.

Box **2-1**

Nursing Theory and the Practicing Nurse

Theory assists the practicing nurse to:
- Organize patient data.
- Understand patient data.
- Analyze patient data.
- Make decisions about nursing interventions.
- Plan patient care.
- Predict outcomes of care.
- Evaluate patient outcomes.

From Alligood, M.R. (2001). Nursing theory: The basis for professional nursing. In K.K. Chitty (Ed.), *Professional nursing: Concepts and challenges* (3rd ed.). Philadelphia: W.B. Saunders.

This commitment to theory-based practice is beneficial to the patient because it provides a systematic, knowledgeable approach to nursing practice. It also serves the profession of nursing because nurses are recognized for the contribution they make in the healthcare of society. That is, knowledge is desirable by its very nature. As we noted earlier in relation to the discipline of nursing, the development of knowledge is an important activity for nurse scholars to pursue. The activities of individual professional nurses also have an impact on the professional community of nurses. It is important that nursing is recognized and respected as a scholarly discipline that contributes to the health of society. Finally, and most importantly, nursing theory is a useful tool for reasoning, critical thinking, and decision making in nursing practice (Box 2-1).[6,5]

Nursing practice settings are complex, and the amount of data (information) confronting nurses is virtually endless. Nurses must analyze a vast amount of information about each patient and decide what to do. A theoretical approach helps practicing nurses not to be overwhelmed by the mass of information and to progress through the nursing process in an orderly manner. Theory enables them to organize and understand what happens in practice, to analyze critically patient situations for clinical decision making; to plan care and propose appropriate nursing interventions; and to predict patient outcomes from the care and evaluate its effectiveness.[6:247]

Professional practice requires a systematic approach that is focused on the patient. Nursing theoretical works provide a perspective of the patient. The philosophies of nursing, such as Nightingale's philosophy, guide the reader to a specific view of nursing and some of the philosophies, such as Benner and Watson's philosophy, also have formalized theories. The conceptual models of nursing are comprehensive and guide the reader to the specifics of practice. The nursing theories are more specific and they provide more direction for practice. Grand theories, such as Roy's Theory of the Person As an Adaptive System or King's Theory of Goal Attainment, are highly abstract. These theories are very useful in research and practice because many middle-range theories can be derived from them. Theories are less abstract than grand theories, but they are more comprehensive than middle-range theories. Middle-range theories contain the specifics of nursing practice such as "the age of the patients" if the theory is specific to a certain patient population, "the situation" and "the location" of the patient, "the health condition," and "the action of the nurse" or the proposed intervention.[5:32] To conclude this discussion of the significance of theory to the discipline of nursing and the profession of nursing, this chapter provides the reader with a brief overview of selected theoretical works classified as philosophies, nursing models, and theories.

OVERVIEW OF NURSING THEORETICAL WORKS

Philosophies

Florence Nightingale

Florence Nightingale's work is closely related to her philosophical orientation of the patient-environment interaction and the principles and rules on which nursing practice was founded. Nightingale's emphasis on surroundings reflected a predominant concern when sanitation was a major health problem in the late 1800s. Nightingale believed that disease was a reparative process and that the manipulation of the patient's surroundings—ventilation, warmth, light, diet, cleanliness, and noise—would contribute to the reparative process and the health of the patient. She recorded her directions regarding ventilation, warmth, light, diet, cleanliness, and noise in *Notes on Nursing: What It Is and What It Is Not.*[77-79] She did not subscribe to the germ theory that was being postulated during her lifetime. Nightingale's beliefs[78-80] regarding nursing formed the foundation for professional nursing and distinguished nursing from the work of domestic servants. She contributed to nursing theory by explicating a philosophical approach to nurs-ing with a focus on nursing and the patient-environment relationship. She is also renowned for pioneering statistical analysis, which she applied to health and professional nursing. Nightingale's writings represent a philosophy of nursing.

Ernestine Wiedenbach

Ernestine Wiedenbach concentrated on the art of nursing and focused on the needs of the patient. Wiedenbach's work grew from 40 years of experience, primarily in maternity nursing. Her definition of nursing reflects her background. She stated, "People may differ in their concept of nursing, but few would disagree that nursing is nurturing or caring for someone in a motherly fashion."[122:1] Wiedenbach's orientation is a philosophy of nursing. It guides the nurse's action in the art of nursing. Wiedenbach specified the following four elements: (1) philosophy, (2) purpose, (3) practice, and (4) art. She postulated that clinical nursing is directed toward meeting the patient's perceived need-for-help.[122:15] Wiedenbach's philosophy of practice is influenced by her conception of nursing as an art. Her vision of nursing reflects the period of nursing history when considerable emphasis was placed on the art of nursing. She follows Orlando's theory of deliberate rather than automatic nursing and incorporates the steps of the nursing process. In her book, *Clinical Nursing: A Helping Art,*[122] the concepts and subconcepts include patient, need-for-help, nurse, purpose, philosophy, practice (knowledge, judgment, and skills), ministration, validation, coordination (reporting, consulting, and conferring), and art (stimulus, preconception, interpretation, and actions [rational, reactionary, and deliberative]). She proposed that nurses identify patients' need-for-help by: (1) observing behaviors consistent or inconsistent with their comfort, (2) exploring the meaning of their behavior, (3) determining the cause of their discomfort or incapability, and (4) determining if they can resolve their problems or have a need-for-help. Following that, the nurse administers the help needed and validates that the need-for-help was met. Wiedenbach's work may be considered a philosophy of nursing.

Virginia Henderson

Virginia Henderson viewed the patient as an individual requiring help toward achieving independence. She envisioned the practice of nursing as independent from the practice of physicians and acknowledged her interpretation of the nurse's function as a synthesis of many influences. Her philosophy is based on Thorndike's work (an American psychologist), her experience in rehabilitation nursing, and Orlando's work regarding the conceptualization of deliberate nursing action.[2,3] Henderson emphasized the art of nursing and identified the 14 basic human needs on which nursing care is based. Her contributions include defining nursing, delineating autonomous nursing functions, stressing goals of interdependence for the patient, and creating self-help concepts. Her self-help concepts influenced the works of Abdellah and Adam.

Virginia Henderson made enormous contributions to nursing in more than 60 years of service as a nurse, teacher, author, and researcher and she published extensively throughout those years. Her definition of nursing first appeared in 1955 in the fifth edition of *Textbook of the Principles and Practice of Nursing*[31] by Harmer and Henderson. Henderson[33:7] stated, "The unique function of the nurse is to assist the individual, sick or well, in the performance of those activities contributing to health or its recovery (or to peaceful death) that he would perform unaided if he had the necessary strength, will, or knowledge and to do this in such a way as to help him gain independence as rapidly as possible."

In *The Nature of Nursing: A Definition and Its Implications for Practice, Research, and Education,*[33] she also identified the following 14 basic needs of patients that comprise the components of nursing care: (1) breathing, (2) eating and drinking, (3) elimination, (4) movement, (5) rest and sleep, (6) suitable clothing, (7) body temperature, (8) clean body and protected integument, (9) safe environment, (10) communication, (11) worship, (12) work, (13) play, and (14) learning.[33] She identified three levels of nurse-patient relationships in which the nurse is a: (1) substitute for the patient, (2) helper to the patient, and (3) partner with the patient.[33] She supports empathetic understanding and states that the nurse must "get inside the skin of each of her patients in order to know what he needs."[32:63] Although she believes the functions of nurses and physicians overlap, Henderson asserts that the nurse works in interdependence with other health professionals and compares the health team to wedges on a pie graph. The sizes of pie vary, depending upon the patient's needs, but the goal is to have the patient represented by the majority of the pie as he or she gains independence.[33] In *The Nature of Nursing: Reflections After 25 Years,*[34] Henderson added addendums to each chapter of the 1966 edition to present changes in her views and to explain her opinions.[33] Henderson's work may be viewed as a philosophy of nursing.

Faye Glenn Abdellah

Faye Glenn Abdellah's work is based on the problem-solving method and had a great impact on nursing curriculum development.[1] Problem solving was the vehicle for delineating nursing (patient) problems as the patient moved toward a healthy outcome. Abdellah[1] viewed nursing as both an art and a science that molds the attitude, intellectual competencies, and technical skills of the individual nurse into the desire and ability to help people cope with their health needs whether they are ill or well. Although she believed that nursing actions were carried out under general or specific medical direction, she formulated 21 nursing problems based on a review of nursing research studies. She used Henderson's 14 basic human needs and nursing research to establish the classification of nursing problems. Her work differs from Henderson; Abdellah's problems are formulated in terms of nursing-centered services, which are used to determine the patient's needs. Her contribution to nursing theory development was the systematic analysis of research reports to formulate the 21 nursing problems that served as an early guide for comprehensive nursing care. The typology of her 21 nursing problems first appeared in the 1960 edition of *Patient-Centered Approaches to Nursing.*[1] Abdellah's work is considered a philosophy of nursing.

Lydia E. Hall

Lydia E. Hall used her philosophy of nursing to design and develop the Loeb Center for Nursing at Montefiore Hospital in New York. She served as administrative director of the Loeb Center from its opening in 1963 until her death in 1969. Most of her work was published in the 1960s. In 1964, her work was presented in "Nursing: What Is It?" in *The Canadian Nurse.*[29] In 1969, it was discussed in "The Loeb Center for Nursing and Rehabilitation" in the *International Journal of Nursing Studies.*[30] She proposed that nursing functions differently by using three interlocking circles to represent aspects of the patient. She labeled the circles as the body (the care), the disease (the cure), and the person (the core). Nurses function in all three circles, but, to different degrees, they also share the circles with other providers. Hall believed that professional nursing care hastened recovery and, as less medical care was needed, more professional nursing care and teaching were necessary. Hall[29] stressed the autonomous function of nursing. Her conceptualization encompasses adult patients who have passed the acute stage of illness. The goal for the patient is rehabilitation and success in self-actualization and self-love. Her contribution to nursing theory was the development and use of her philosophy of nursing care at The Loeb Center in New York. She also recognized professional nurses and encouraged them to make a contribution to patient outcomes. Hall's work may be viewed as a philosophy of nursing.

Jean Watson

Jean Watson began publishing in the mid1970s. Her book, *Nursing: The Philosophy and Science of Caring,*[118] was published in 1979. She presented *Nursing: Human Science and Human Care*[119] in 1985, with another edition in 1988,[120] and published *Postmodern Nursing and Beyond*[121] in 1999. In an effort to reduce the dichotomy between theory and practice, Watson proposed a philosophy and science of caring. She identified the following 10 carative factors: (1) the formation of a humanistic-altruistic system of values; (2) the instillation of faith-hope; (3) the cultivation of sensitivity to self and to others; (4) the development of a helping-trust relationship; (5) the promotion and acceptance of the expression of positive and negative; (6) the systematic use of the scientific problem-solving method for decision making; (7) the promotion of interpersonal teaching-learning; (8) the provision for a supportive, protective, or corrective mental, physical, sociocultural, and spiritual environment; (9) assistance with the gratification of human needs; and (10) the allowance for existential-phenomenological forces. Watson proposes that nurses develop health promotion through preventive actions such as recognizing coping skills and adaptation to loss, teaching problem-solving methods, and providing situational support. Like Leininger's theory, Watson's work[118-121] emphasizes caring, but Watson borrows the existential phenomenologist view of psychology and the humanities and proposes nursing as a human science. In this work, nursing concerns itself with promoting and restoring health, preventing illness, and caring for the sick. Patients require holistic care that promotes humanism, health, and quality living. Caring is a universal, social phenomenon that is only effective when practiced interpersonally. Watson's work contributes to nursing by sensitizing individual practitioners to humanistic aspects and caring. Her work may be classified as a philosophy of nursing from which she formalized theory.

Patricia Benner

The Dreyfus Model of Skill Acquisition was developed in research about pilot's performance in emergency situations. Patricia Benner validated the Dreyfus Model of Skill Acquisition in nursing practice with her systematic description of the five stages (novice, advanced beginner, competent, proficient, and expert). In *From Novice to Expert: Excellence and Power in Clinical Nursing Practice*,[13] she provided exemplars and described nursing practice at each stage. Seven domains of nursing practice were derived from the descriptions of these cases and a list of 31 nursing competencies was generated. From Benner's description of nursing practice, a phenomenological theory describing caring evolved, which is presented in Benner and Wrubel's 1989 book, *The Primacy of Caring: Stress and Coping in Health and Illness*.[17] Further work was published in Benner's 1994 publication, *Interpretative Phenomenology: Embodiment, Caring, and Ethics in Health and Illness*,[14] and in Benner, Tanner, and Chesla's 1996 publication, *Expertise in Nursing Practice: Caring, Clinical Practice, and Ethics*.[16] In 1999, Benner, Hooper-Kyriakidis, and Stannard published *Clinical Wisdom and Intervention in Critical Care: A Thinking in Action Approach*.[15] This phenomenological work describes caring as a common bond of persons situated in meaning, which is a state of being that is essential to nursing. Benner's work may be classified as a philosophical theory of nursing.

Conceptual Models and Grand Theories of Nursing

Dorothea E. Orem

Dorothea E. Orem has been publishing about nursing practice and education since the 1950s. In 1958, she had an insight about the concept of nursing. Orem[81-84] explicated self-care as a human need and nursing as a human service; she emphasized nursing's special concern for a person's need for self-care actions on a continuous basis to sustain life and health or to recover from disease or injury. She formalized the Self-Care Deficit Theory of nursing as a general theory composed of the following three related theories: (1) the Theory of Self-Care, (2) the Theory of Self-Care Deficit, and (3) the Theory of Nursing Systems. Her work identifies three types of nursing systems: (1) wholly compensatory (doing for the patient), (2) partly compensatory (helping

the patient do for himself or herself), and (3) supportive-educative (helping the patient learn to do for himself or herself and emphasizing the important role of the nurse in designing nursing care). The theories are discussed more fully in her book, *Nursing: Concepts of Practice*,[81-84] which has been published in its sixth edition. She proposes that nurses share some functions with other healthcare providers. Orem's work is a conceptual model of nursing with three nursing theories.

Myra Estrin Levine

Myra Estrin Levine started publishing in the mid1960s. By contributing to the nursing literature, she facilitated the development of nursing. Without intending to develop a theory, she wrote *Introduction to Clinical Nursing*[55,57] as a textbook to teach medical-surgical nursing to beginning students. She published journal articles about holism and the four conservation principles of nursing including "Adaptation and Assessment: A Rationale for Nursing Intervention," "The Four Conservation Principles of Nursing," "For Lack of Love Alone," "The Pursuit of Wholeness," and "Holistic Nursing."[51-54,56] Wholism, holism, integrity, and conservation are major concepts. She proposed that nurses use the principles of conservation of: (1) energy, (2) structural integrity, (3) personal integrity, and (4) social integrity to keep the holism of the individual balanced. Levine specified four levels of organismic response: fear, inflammatory response, response to stress, and sensory response. She recommended trophicognosis, a scientific approach to determining nursing care, as an alternative to nursing diagnosis based on the lack of fit of the root meaning of diagnosis with nursing. Levine[58] updated her theory in her chapter, "The Conservation Principles: Twenty Years Later," in Riehl-Sisca's 1989 book, *Conceptual Models for Nursing Practice*.[104] She indicates that adaptation is the essence of conservation and elaborates on how redundancy characterizes the availability of adaptive responses when stability is threatened. Adaptation processes establish a body economy to safeguard the individual's stability. Levine recognizes that research must focus on discrete issues, but she stresses the importance of acknowledging all four conservation principles to sustain wholeness of a person, which she discusses in her chapter in *Levine's Conservation Model: A Framework for Nursing Practice,*[59] edited by Schaefer and Pond. Levine used the sciences, such as psychology, sociology, and physiology, to analyze various nursing practices and describe detailed nursing skills and activities.[51,55] Levine's nursing activity analysis resulted in the formulation of four conservation principles to help patients adapt to their environment. She proposed the person as holistic and the center of nursing activities. Her work has been shown to be relevant to the ill person in the healthcare setting and useful to the well person in health promotion. Levine's work[5] is categorized as a conceptual model of nursing with three theories: (1) conservation, (2) redundancy, and (3) therapeutic intention.

Martha E. Rogers

Martha E. Rogers has published widely since the early 1960s and is considered one of the most creative thinkers in nursing. Her work regarding unitary human beings appears in *An Introduction to the Theoretical Basis of Nursing.*[105] In 1986, Malinski's *Explorations on Martha Rogers' Science of Unitary Human Beings*[60] provided evidence of basic and applied research, which extended Rogers' conceptual system. In 1990, Barrett's *Visions of Rogers' Science-Based Nursing*[10] represented evolutionary development in Rogerian science. Rogers' Science of Unitary Human Beings[106] was influenced by general system theory and field theory. She clearly emphasized the science and art of nursing in her delineation of the unitary human being and environment as central to the discipline of nursing.[105] Over the years, Rogers was a clear voice proposing that nursing was a basic scientific discipline. Rogers' model continues to have significant influence on scientific inquiry and professional nursing practice. In addition, the model has served as a basis for the explication of other nursing theories including the theories of Newman and Parse. Rogers' model[10,60,105,106] promoted a body of research that influenced the scientific community of nursing scholars who investigated its utility in research, practice, education, and

administration. Rogers' work[5:38] is categorized as a conceptual model of nursing with "many theories."

Dorothy E. Johnson

Dorothy E. Johnson published from the mid1940s to the early 1970s. Most of her work published during the 1960s and many of her unpublished papers are housed at Vanderbilt University. Johnson presented the Behavioral System Model in Riehl and Roy's books, *Conceptual Models for Nursing Practice.*[102,103] Johnson developed the Behavioral System Model for nursing practice, education, and research. Ethological theory and general system theory influenced her model. Johnson[38] considered attachment, or the affiliative subsystem, as the cornerstone of social organizations. Her behavioral system also includes the subsystems of dependency, achievement, aggressive, ingestive, eliminative, and sexual. In Johnson's words,[38:214] "Nursing problems arise because there are disturbances in the structure or function of the subsystems of the system, or because the level of behavioral functioning is less than desirable."[38:214] Johnson[35-38] contributed to nursing theory through her writings related to philosophical issues and knowledge development and through her influences on students who have subsequently developed nursing theory, such as Roy, Neuman, and Adam. Johnson's work is a conceptual model of nursing with several theories.

Sister Callista Roy

Sister Callista Roy has been publishing consistently since the late 1960s. She developed her adaptation model after Johnson challenged her to develop a conceptual model for nursing. This is discussed in Roy's books, *An Introduction to Nursing: An Adaptation Model,*[110,111] *Essentials of the Roy Adaptation Model*[8] by Andrews and Roy, and *The Roy Adaptation Model: The Definitive Statement*[112,113] published in 1991 and 1998. Roy[110,111] based her work on Helson's Adaptation Theory. Roy's model is an excellent example of how borrowed knowledge becomes unique to nursing.[110] Roy synthesizes different (borrowed) theories, such as system, stress, and adaptation, into a collective view for explication of a person interacting with the environment. Roy proposed that humans are biopsychosocial beings who exist within an environment. Environment and self provide three classes of stimuli: (1) focal, (2) residual, and (3) contextual. Human stimuli create needs in one or more interrelated adaptation modes, such as physiological self-concept, role function, and interdependence. Through two adaptive mechanisms, regulator and cognator, an individual demonstrates adaptive responses or ineffective responses that require nursing intervention. Roy's Adaptation Model has been developed consistently. Although the model was developed for education, continued work in practice and research has led to broader use, testing, and numerous publica-tions.[110-113] Roy's work is a conceptual model of nursing with several theories.

Betty Neuman

Betty Neuman developed her first teaching-practice model for mental health consultation in the late 1960s. She designed the Systems Model in 1970 to help graduate students evaluate nursing problems. It was first published in *Nursing Research*[72] in 1972 and further refined in *The Neuman Systems Model*[69-71] in 1982, 1989, and 1995. Major concepts include: total persons approach, holism, open system, stressors, energy resources, lines of resistance, lines of defense, intervention, levels of prevention, and reconstitution. By 1989, the spiritual variable was explicitly added to the patient core (growth and development, psychological, sociocultural, and physiological) of the Neuman Systems Model and the created environment was added to the typology as a safety mechanism for the system. Neuman proposes that the nurse use purposeful interventions and a total person approach to help individuals, families, and groups reach and maintain wellness. Neuman's model[71] uses Gestalt theory, stress theory, system theory, and levels of prevention. Her conceptualization of the total-person approach to patient care helps individuals, families, and groups attain and maintain an optimal level of wellness by purposeful interventions. Nursing intervention is aimed at prevention through the reduction of stress factors and adverse conditions that potentially or actually impact on optimal patient functioning. Nurses and other health-related disciplines use Neuman's model in practice, education, and research. Her work is a conceptual model of nursing with two theories: optimal patient stability and prevention as intervention.[5]

Imogene King

Imogene King has been publishing since the mid1960s. *Toward a Theory for Nursing*[40] was published in 1971 and *A Theory for Nursing*[41] was published in 1981. Many of her publications have dealt with conceptual framework, models, theory, and, specifically, her Theory of Goal Attainment. King's conceptual framework specifies the following interacting systems: personal system, interpersonal system, and social system. The concepts of the personal system are perception, self, body image, growth and development, and time and space. The concepts of the interpersonal system are role, interaction, communication, and transaction and stress. The concepts of the social system are organization, power-authority status, and decision making and role. From her major concepts (interaction, perception, communication, transaction, role, stress, growth and development, and time and space), she derived her Theory of Goal Attainment. She proposes that the perceptions, judgments, and actions of the patient and the nurse lead to reaction, interaction, and transaction. King describes this as the process of nursing. The nurse and the patient perceive each other and judge the situation; then they act, react, interact, and transact. King[40] defines nursing as a process of human interaction between nurses and patients who communicate to set goals, explore means for achieving the goals, and agree on the means to attain the goals. King's work[41] is categorized as a conceptual model of nursing from which she derived the Theory of Goal Attainment.

Nancy Roper, Winifred W. Logan, and Alison J. Tierney

Logan and Tierney are European theorists who were new to the fourth edition of *The Elements of Nursing: A Model for Nursing Based on a Model for*

Living.[107] In the 1970s, research conducted to discover the core of nursing produced a Model of Living. This was in response to the use of qualifiers for naming nursing practice according to the ideas of medical practice. Three decades of study of the elements of nursing by Roper (and Logan, and Tierney who joined the efforts later) evolved into a Model of Living with five main components (concepts). The latest edition of their book, *The Elements of Nursing: A Model for Nursing Based on a Model for Living*[107] was published in 1996. Rather than revising the fourth edition of their textbook, the theorists prepared a monograph about the model, *The Roper-Logan-Tierney Model of Nursing: Based on Activities of Living,*[108] without the application of the model.

The 12 activities of living (ALs) include maintaining a safe environment, communicating, breathing, eating and drinking, eliminating, personal cleansing and dressing, controlling body temperature, mobilizing, working and playing, expressing sexuality, sleeping, and dying. Life span ranges from birth to death and the dependence-independence continuum ranges from total dependence to total independence. The five groups of factors influencing the ALs are biological, psychological, sociocultural, environmental, and politicoeconomic. The individuality of living is the way in which the individual attends to the ALs in regard to the individual's place on the life span and on the dependence-independence continuum and as influenced by biological, psychological, environmental, and politicoeconomic factors.

Twelve ALs describe the person (the central focus) in the complex process of living from the perspective of an amalgam of activities. Life span is the concept of continuous change from birth to death. The third conceptual component, the dependence-independence continuum, relates closely to the first two components and ranges from being incapacitated in ALs to having the capacity to achieve ALs. Both occur at anticipated points across the life span and at unanticipated times throughout life. The person experiences this complex process as an individual; therefore variances in the four conceptual components are both an expression and a reflection of the person's individuality. This model has been used as a guide for nursing practice, research, and education.

Theories and Middle-Range Nursing Theories

Hildegard E. Peplau

Hildegard E. Peplau's contributions to nursing in general and to the specialty of psychiatric nursing in particular have been enormous. Since the early 1950s, she published many texts beginning with her book, *Interpersonal Relations in Nursing.*[100] She taught psychodynamic nursing and stressed the importance of the nurse's ability to understand his or her own behavior to help others identify perceived difficulties. She identified four phases of the nurse-patient relationship: (1) orientation, (2) identification, (3) exploitation, and (4) resolution. Peplau proposed and described six nursing roles: (1) stranger, (2) resource person, (3) teacher, (4) leader, (5) surrogate, and (6) counselor. She discussed four psychobiological experiences that compel destructive or constructive responses: (1) needs, (2) frustrations, (3) conflicts, and (4) anxieties. Peplau's work[100] is a theory for the practice of nursing. She was influenced by Sullivan's interpersonal relationship theories and she reflects the view of the contemporaneous psychoanalytical model. Peplau is the first author to borrow theory from other scientific fields and synthesize a theory for nursing. Peplau's work is categorized as a theory of nursing.

Ida Jean Orlando (Pelletier)

In 1961, Ida Jean Orlando (Pelletier) first described her discipline's Professional Response Theory in *The Dynamic Nurse-Patient Relationship,*[85,87] which was reissued by the National League for Nursing in 1991. She reported related research in *The Discipline and Teaching of Nursing Process.*[86] Orlando[85,86] used the interpersonal nurse-patient relationship in response to the patient's needs as the basis for her work. She focused on the patient's verbal and nonverbal expressions of need and the nurse's reactions to the patient's behavior, emphasizing the meaning of the distress and what would alleviate the distress. Three elements comprise a nursing situation: (1) patient behaviors, (2) nurse reactions, and (3) nursing actions. Orlando differentiated automatic actions from deliberate actions. She stressed the importance of nurses testing their inferences about patients. Orlando used the nursing process to meet the patient's need with deliberate action and alleviated distress. Her contribution as a theorist advanced nursing beyond personal and automatic responses to a disciplined and professional response.[114] Orlando's work is categorized as a theory of nursing.

Joyce Travelbee

Joyce Travelbee published predominantly in the mid1960s. She died in 1973 at a relatively young age. Travelbee[116,117] proposed her Human-to-Human Relationship Theory in her book, *Interpersonal Aspects of Nursing.* She wrote about illness, suffering, pain, hope, communication, interaction, empathy, sympathy, rapport, and therapeutic use of self. She proposed that nursing was accomplished through human-to-human relationships that began with: (1) the original encounter and then progressed through stages of (2) emerging identities, (3) developing feelings of empathy and, later, (4) of sympathy, until (5) the nurse and patient attained rapport in the final stage. Travelbee's theory extended the interpersonal relationship theories of Peplau and Orlando, but her unique synthesis of their ideas differentiated her work in terms of the therapeutic human relationship between nurse and patient. Travelbee's emphasis[116,117] on caring stressed empathy, sympathy, rapport, and the emotional aspects of nursing. The work is categorized as a nursing theory.

Katharine Kolcaba

Katharine Kolcaba[42] defines healthcare needs as those needs for comfort including physical, psychospiritual, social, and environmental needs. Comfort measures include physiological, social, financial, psychological, spiritual, environmental, and physical measures. Intervening variables are interacting forces that influence the recipient's perception of comfort such as age, attitude, emotional support, experiences, finances, and prognosis. The types of comfort she proposes include relief when a specific need is fulfilled; a sense of ease, calm, or contentment; and transcendence when a person rises above problems of pain. Kolcaba uses Schlotfeldt's synthesis of health-seeking behaviors and applies her theory to institutional integrity. Kolcaba[42-46] did a concept analysis and diagrammed the aspects of comfort in 1991, she operationalized comfort as an outcome of care in 1992, she contextualized comfort in a midrange theory in 1994, and she has tested the theory in an online intervention study in 1999. This work is a middle-range theory of nursing.

Helen C. Erickson, Evelyn M. Tomlin, and Mary Ann P. Swain

Helen C. Erickson, Evelyn M. Tomlin, and Mary Ann P. Swain's work is a synthesis of the theories of Erikson, Maslow, Selye, Engel, and Piaget. Erickson, Tomlin, and Swain developed their Modeling and Role-Modeling Theory from the synthesis of multiple theories related to basic needs, developmental tasks, object attachment, and adaptive coping potential. Modeling and role modeling provides a framework for understanding how persons structure their world. Erickson, Tomlin, and Swain view nursing as self-care based on the person's perception of the world and adaptation to stressors. This is a theory that promotes the person's growth and development while recognizing individual differences according to the patient's worldview and inherent endowment. Their book, *Modeling and Role-Modeling: A Theory and Paradigm for Nursing,*[22,23] was published in 1983 and 1990. The sixth reprint edition published in 1998.[24] In 1990, Erickson and Kinney published *Modeling and Role-Modeling: Theory, Practice, and Research.*[21] Erickson, Tomlin, and Swain's work is categorized as a theory of nursing.

Ramona T. Mercer

Ramona T. Mercer has researched and published extensively since the 1970s. She systematically researched the field of maternal role attainment and developed a complex theory about factors influencing maternal role development over time. Mercer's work[62] culminates in her 1986 book, *First-Time*

Motherhood: Experiences from Teens to Forties. With Elizabeth G. Nichols and Glen Caspers Doyle, Mercer published a study of transitions in the life cycles of 80 women in *Transitions in a Woman's Life: Major Life Events in Developmental Context*[65] in 1989. Mercer's book,[63] *Parents at Risk,* was published in 1990 and *Becoming a Mother: Research on Maternal Role Identity Since Rubin*[64] was published in 1995. Mercer's theory[62] is focused on parenting and maternal role attainment in diverse populations. The Maternal Role Attainment Theory is a theory with close linkages between theory, research, and practice. This theory follows a traditional social science approach to theory development. Mercer's early research was based on Goffman's systems theory. Mercer systematically researched the area of maternal role attainment and developed a complex theory to explain the factors impacting the development of the maternal role over time. The application of Mercer's theory has predictable outcomes for nursing practice in women's health and maternal-child health. Mercer's work is categorized as a theory of nursing.

Kathryn E. Barnard

Kathryn E. Barnard[7] is an active researcher who has published extensively about infants and children since the mid1960s. She began by studying mentally and physically handicapped children and adults, then moved into studying the activities of the well child, and then expanded her work to include methods of evaluating the growth and development of children and mother-infant relationships. She was also concerned about disseminating research and, consequently, developed the Nursing Child Assessment Satellite Training Project. Although Barnard never intended to develop theory, the longitudinal nursing-child assessment study provided the basis for her Child Health Assessment Interaction Theory. Barnard[9] proposes that the individual characteristics of each member influence the parent-infant system and that adaptive behavior modifies those characteristics to meet the needs of the system. Barnard's theory borrows from psychology and human development and focuses on mother-infant interaction with the environment. Her theory is based on scales developed to measure feeding, teaching, and environment. With continuous research, she refined the theory and provided a close link to practice. She models the role of researcher in clinical practice as she engages in theory development in practice for the advancement of nursing science. Barnard's work is a theory of nursing.

Madeleine Leininger

Madeleine Leininger has published extensively about many nursing topics since 1960. Although she has written several books about transcultural nursing and caring, the most complete account of the Transcultural Care Theory is found in her 1984 book, *Care: The Essence of Nursing and Health.*[48] Some of the major concepts are care, caring, culture, cultural values, and cultural variations. Leininger has generated many hypotheses and hopes to stimulate further ethnoscience research by nurses in ethnonursing. Her more recent books are *Culture Care Diversity and Universality: A Theory of Nursing,*[49] *Transcultural Nursing: Concepts, Theories, Research and Practices,* second edition,[50] and *Caring: The Compassionate Healer*[28] with Gaut. Leininger[48-50] set forth caring as the central theme in nursing care, nursing knowledge, and nursing practice. Caring includes assistive, supportive, or facilitative acts toward an individual or a group with evident or anticipated needs. Caring serves to ameliorate or improve human conditions and life ways (life processes). She borrows her methodology from anthropology, but the concept of caring is synthesized as an essential characteristic of nursing practice. Leininger is credited with the foundation of transcultural nursing and the resultant nursing research, education, and practice in this subfield of nursing. Leininger's work is a theory of nursing.

Rosemarie Rizzo Parse

Rosemarie Rizzo Parse[89-95] derives her theory from Rogers' principles and concepts and from Heidegger, Ponty, and Sartre's existential phenomenology. Parse views nursing as a human science. Although Parse developed much of her work from Rogers, her subsequent work has explicated each concept existentially and in its relevance to nursing. The strength of Parse's theory may be a unique, humanistic approach as opposed to a physiological basis for nursing. Parse[89] published the first book of her theory, *Man-Living-Health: A Theory of Nursing* in 1981. Major concepts include imaging, valuing, languaging, revealing-concealing, enabling-limiting, connecting-separating, powering, originating, and transforming. Parse describes nursing as a human science that is not dependent on medicine or any discipline for its practice. She described research methods for studying her theory in *Nursing Research: Qualitative Methods*.[91] She presented her theory and others in *Nursing Science: Major Paradigms, Theories, and Critiques*.[90] She has also written *The Human Becoming School of Thought: A Perspective for Nurses and Other Health Professionals*,[92] *Hope: An International Human Becoming Perspective*,[93-94] and *Illumination: The Human Theory in Practice and Research*.[95] Parse's work is categorized as a theory of nursing derived from Rogers' conceptual model.

Merle Mishel

From her dissertation, Merle Mishel used qualitative and quantitative findings to conceptualize uncertainty in illness. Since the publication of her Uncertainty in Illness Scale in 1981, there has been extensive research into adults' experiences with uncertainty as it relates to chronic and life-threatening illness.[66] In 1990, she reconceptualized the Uncertainty Theory to accommodate the responses to uncertainty over time in people with chronic conditions who may not resolve the uncertainty.[67] The original theory included 11 major concepts in three themes. Several new concepts were added in the reconceptualization.

Margaret A. Newman

Margaret A. Newman began publishing in the mid1960s. She has drawn from several fields of inquiry and was influenced by Johnson and Rogers. Her model appeared in *Theory Development in Nursing*.[73] Subsequent chapters of various books and her 1986 book, *Health as Expanding Consciousness*,[74] further explained her model. More recently, she published a second edition of *Health as Expanding Consciousness*,[75] a third edition that is online,[77] and *A Developing Discipline: Selected Works of Margaret Newman*.[76] The major concepts in Newman's

model of health are movement, time, space, and consciousness. They are all interrelated. Newman[73:60] stated, "Movement is a reflection of consciousness. Time is a function of movement. Time is a measure of consciousness." Newman's theory of health is derived from Rogers' model. According to Newman, the goal of nursing is not to promote wellness or to prevent illness, but to help people use the power within them as they evolve toward a higher level of consciousness.[74] Her contributions to theory development are the replication of her earlier works; further expansion of her theory; and the methodology for research on the interaction of time, movement, space, and consciousness in maintaining life processes. Newman's theory text,[73] *Theory Development in Nursing,* has been, and continues to be, useful to numerous nurse scientists in their research. Newman's work is categorized as a theory of nursing derived from Rogers' conceptual model.

Evelyn Adam

Evelyn Adam is a Canadian nurse who started publishing in the mid1970s. Much of her work focuses on development models and theories on the concept of nursing. She uses a model she learned from Dorothy Johnson. In her book, *To Be a Nurse*,[2] she applies Virginia Henderson's definition of nursing to the theory and identifies the assumptions, beliefs and values, and major units. In the latter category, she includes the goal of the profession, the beneficiary of the professional service, the role of the professional, the source of the beneficiary's difficulty, the intervention of the professional, and the consequences. She expands her work in the second edition.[3] Adam's work is a good example of using a unique basis of nursing for further expansion.[2] She has contributed to theory development by clarification and explication of earlier work. Adam's work is a theory of nursing.

Nola J. Pender

Nola J. Pender defines the goal of nursing care as the optimal health of the individual. She began to build the foundation for studying how individuals make decisions about their own healthcare in her article, "A Conceptual Model for Preventive Health

Behavior."[96] In her book, *Health Promotion in Nursing Practice*,[97-99] she developed the idea that promoting optimal health supersedes disease prevention. Pender's theory identifies cognitive-perceptual factors in the individual, such as the importance of health-promoting behaviors and perceived barriers to health-promoting behaviors. According to Pender's theory, these factors are modified by demographical and biological characteristics, interpersonal influences, and situational and behavioral factors that help predict participation in health-promoting behavior. Pender's work is a theory of nursing.

CONCLUSION

Nursing has made phenomenal achievements in the last century that have led to the recognition of nursing as an academic discipline and a profession. Not only is the importance of using nursing theory for theory-based practice important for graduate nursing education, but it is also vital for the preparation of beginning nursing students who are learning the fundamentals of nursing. Potter and Perry[101:7] point this out in their textbook, *Fundamentals of Nursing: Concepts, Process, and Practice,* fourth edition, when they note that in the past, "nursing theories were studied in an isolated academic environment independent of nursing practice. There is, however, a contemporary move toward theory-based practice." They emphasize that nurses (present and future) need models of care on which to base their practice. "Conceptual and theoretical nursing models are used to provide knowledge to improve practice, guide research and curricula, and identify the goals of nursing practice."[101:7] In their discussion of nursing as a profession, they state that, "Trends in nursing as a profession include the growing emphasis on the aspects of nursing that characterize it as a profession, including education, theory, service, autonomy, and ethical codes."[101:30]

This chapter introduced the nursing discipline and the nursing profession with a conceptual and historical consideration of the two terms. The body of knowledge specific to nursing is vital to the recognition of nursing as a discipline and a profes-

sion. This chapter has reviewed nursing theoretical works that may be considered philosophies, conceptual models and grand theories, and theories and middle-range nursing theories. They provide the perspectives of nursing that guide the development and application of knowledge in research, education, administration, and nursing practice. These theoretical works of nursing have been reviewed to complete this introduction to the significance of theory for the discipline and profession of nursing.

REFERENCES

1. Abdellah, F.G., Beland, I.L., Martin, A., & Matheney, R.V. (1960). *Patient-centered approaches to nursing.* New York: Macmillan.
2. Adam, E. (1980). *To be a nurse.* Philadelphia: W.B. Saunders.
3. Adam, E. (1991). *To be a nurse* (2nd ed.). Montreal: W.B. Saunders Company Canada Ltd.
4. Alligood, M.R. (1997a). The nature of knowledge needed for nursing practice. In M.R. Alligood & A. Marriner Tomey (Eds.), *Nursing theory: Utilization and application* (pp. 3-13). St. Louis: Mosby.
5. Alligood, M.R. (1997b). Models and theories: Critical thinking structures. In M.R. Alligood & A. Marriner Tomey (Eds.), *Nursing theory: Utilization and application* (pp. 31-45). St. Louis: Mosby.
6. Alligood, M.R. (2000). Nursing theory: The basis for professional nursing. In K.K. Chitty, *Professional nursing: Concepts and challenges* (3rd ed., pp. 246-274). Philadelphia: W.B. Saunders.
7. Alligood, M.R. & Marriner Tomey, A. (2001). *Nursing theory: Utilization and application* (2nd ed.). St. Louis: Mosby.
8. Andrews, H. & Roy, C. (1986). *Essentials of the Roy adaptation model.* Norwalk, CT: Appleton-Century-Crofts.
9. Barnard, K.E. (1978). *Nursing child assessment and training: Learning resource manual.* Seattle: University of Washington.
10. Barrett, E.A.M. (Ed.). (1990). *Visions of Rogers' science-based nursing.* New York: National League for Nursing.
11. Batey, M.V. (1971). Conceptualizing the research process. *Nursing Research, 20,* 296-301.
12. Batey, M.V. (1977). Conceptualization: Knowledge and logic guiding empirical research. *Nursing Research, 26,* 324-329.
13. Benner, P. (1984). *From novice to expert: Excellence and power in clinical nursing practice.* Menlo Park, CA: Addison-Wesley.

14. Benner, P. (1994). *Interpretive phenomenology: Embodiment, caring and ethics in health and illness.* Thousand Oaks, CA: Sage.
15. Benner, P., Hooper-Kyriakidis, P.L., & Stannard, D. (1999). *Clinical wisdom and intervention in critical care: A thinking in action approach.* Philadelphia: W.B. Saunders.
16. Benner, P., Tanner, C., & Chesla, C. (1996). *Expertise in nursing practice: Caring, clinical practice, and ethics.* New York: Springer.
17. Benner, P. & Wrubel, J. (1989). *The primacy of caring: Stress and coping in health and illness.* Menlo Park, CA: Addison-Wesley.
18. Bixler, G.K. & Bixler, R.W. (1959). The professional status of nursing. *American Journal of Nursing,* 59(8), 1142-1146.
19. Dickoff, J., James, P., & Wiedenbach, E. (1968). Theory in a practice discipline, Part I. Practice oriented theory. *Nursing Research,* 17(5), 415-435.
20. Donaldson, S.K. & Crowley, D.M. (1978). The discipline of nursing. *Nursing Outlook,* 26(2), 1113-1120.
21. Erickson, H. & Kinney, C. (Eds.). (1990). *Modeling and role-modeling: Theory, practice and research.* Austin: Society for Advancement of Modeling and Role-Modeling.
22. Erickson, H.C., Tomlin, E.M., & Swain, M.A. (1983). *Modeling and role-modeling: A theory and paradigm for nursing.* Englewood Cliffs, NJ: Prentice-Hall.
23. Erickson, H.C., Tomlin, E.M., & Swain, M.A. (1990). *Modeling and role-modeling: A theory and paradigm for nursing.* Englewood Cliffs, NJ: Prentice-Hall. (EST Company original publication 1983.)
24. Erickson, H.C., Tomlin, E.M., & Swain, M.A. (1998). *Modeling and role-modeling: A theory and paradigm for nursing.* Englewood Cliffs, NJ: Prentice-Hall. (EST Company original publication 1983.)
25. Fawcett, J. (1984, June). The metaparadigm of nursing: Current status and future refinements. *Image: The Journal of Nursing Scholarship,* 16, 84-87.
26. Fawcett, J. (1999). *The relationship of theory and research* (2nd ed.). Philadelphia: F.A. Davis.
27. Fitzpatrick, M.L. (1983). *Prologue to professionalism.* Bowie, MD: Robert J. Brady.
28. Gaut, K. & Leininger, M. (1991). *Caring: The compassionate healer.* New York: National League for Nursing Press.
29. Hall, L.E. (1964, Feb.). Nursing: What is it? *The Canadian Nurse,* 60, 150-154.
30. Hall, L.E. (1969). The Loeb Center for nursing and rehabilitation. *International Journal of Nursing Studies,* 6, 81-95.
31. Hauner, B. & Henderson, V. (1955). *Textbook of the principles and practice of nursing.* New York: Macmillan.
32. Henderson, V. (1964, Aug.). The nature of nursing. *American Journal of Nursing,* 64, 62-68.
33. Henderson, V. (1966). *The nature of nursing: A definition and its implications for practice, research, and education.* New York: Macmillan.
34. Henderson, V.A. (1991). *The nature of nursing: Reflections after 25 years.* New York: National League for Nursing Press.
35. Johnson, D. (1959, May). The nature of a science of nursing. *Nursing Outlook,* 7, 291-294.
36. Johnson, D. (1968). *One conceptual model for nursing.* Unpublished paper presented at Vanderbilt University, Nashville, TN.
37. Johnson, D. (1974, Sept./Oct.). Development of theory: A requisite for nursing as a primary health profession. *Nursing Research,* 23, 372-377.
38. Johnson, D.E. (1980). The behavioral system model for nursing. In J.P. Riehl & C. Roy (Eds.), *Conceptual models for nursing practice* (2nd ed.). New York: Appleton-Century-Crofts.
39. Kalish, P.A. & Kalisch, B.J. (1995). *The advance of American nursing* (3rd ed.). Philadelphia: J.B. Lippincott.
40. King, I. (1971). *Toward a theory for nursing: General concepts of human behavior.* New York: John Wiley & Sons.
41. King, I. (1981). *A theory for nursing: Systems, concepts, process.* New York: John Wiley & Sons.
42. Kolcaba, K. (1991). A taxonomic structure for the concept comfort. *Image: Journal of Nursing Scholarship,* 23(4), 237-240.
43. Kolcaba, K. (1992). Holistic comfort: Operationalizing the construct as a nurse-sensitive outcome. *Advances in Nursing Science,* 12(1), 1-10.
44. Kolcaba, K. (1994). A theory of holistic comfort for nursing. *Journal of Advanced Nursing,* 19, 1178-1184.
45. Kolcaba, K. & Fox, C. (1999). The effects of guided imagery on comfort of women with early stage breast cancer undergoing radiation therapy. *Oncology Nursing Forum,* 26(1), 67-92.
46. Kolcaba, K. & Kolcaba, R. (1991). An analysis of the concept of comfort. *Journal of Advanced Nursing,* 16, 1301-1310.
47. Kuhn, T.S. (1970). *The structure of scientific revolutions* (2nd ed.). Chicago: The University of Chicago Press.
48. Leininger, M. (Ed.). (1984). *Care: The essence of nursing and health.* Thorofare, NJ: Charles B. Slack.
49. Leininger, M. (1991). *Culture care diversity and universality: A theory of nursing.* New York: National League for Nursing Press.
50. Leininger, M. (1995). *Transcultural nursing: Concepts, theories, research and practices* (2nd ed.). New York: McGraw-Hill.

51. Levine, M. (1967a). The four conservation principles of nursing. *Nursing Forum,* 6, 45.
52. Levine, M. (1967b, Dec.). For lack of love alone. *Minnesota Nursing Accent,* 39, 179.
53. Levine, M.E. (1966). Adaptation and assessment: A rationale for nursing intervention. *American Journal of Nursing,* 66(11), 2450-2453.
54. Levine, M.E. (1969, Jan.). The pursuit of wholeness. *American Journal of Nursing,* 69, 93.
55. Levine, M.E. (1969). *Introduction to clinical nursing.* Philadelphia: F.A. Davis.
56. Levine, M.E. (1971, June). Holistic nursing. *Nursing Clinics of North America,* 6, 253.
57. Levine, M.E. (1973). *Introduction to clinical nursing* (2nd ed.). Philadelphia: F.A. Davis.
58. Levine, M.E. (1989). The conservation principles: Twenty years later. In J.P. Reihl-Sisca (Ed.), *Conceptual models for nursing practice* (pp. 325-337). New York: Appleton-Century-Crofts.
59. Levine, M.E. (1991). The conservation principles: A model for health. In F.M. Schaefer & J.B. Pond (Eds.), *Levine's conservation model: A framework for nursing practice.* Philadelphia: F.A. Davis.
60. Malinski, V.M. (1986). *Explorations on Martha Rogers' science of unitary human beings.* Norwalk, CT: Appleton-Century-Crofts.
61. Meleis, A. (1997). *Theoretical nursing: Development and progress* (3rd ed.). Philadelphia: J.B. Lippincott.
62. Mercer, R.T. (1986). *First-time motherhood: Experiences from teens to forties.* New York: Springer.
63. Mercer, R.T. (1990). *Parents at risk.* New York: Springer.
64. Mercer, R.T. (1995). *Becoming a mother: Research on maternal role identity since Rubin.* New York: Springer.
65. Mercer, R.T., Nichols, E.G., & Doyle, G.C. (1989). *Transitions in a woman's life: Major life events in developmental context.* New York: Springer.
66. Mishel, M.H. (1981). The measurement of uncertainty in illness. *Nursing Research,* 30, 258-263.
67. Mishel, M.H. (1990). Reconceptualization of the uncertainty in illness theory. *Image Journal of Nursing Scholarship,* 22, 256-262.
68. Neuman, B. (1974). The Betty Newman health care systems model: A total person approach to patient problems. In J.P. Reihl & C. Roy (Eds.), *Conceptual models for nursing practice* (pp. 94-114). New York: Appleton-Century-Crofts.
69. Neuman, B. (1982). *The Neuman systems model: Application to nursing, education, and practice.* Norwalk, CT: Appleton-Century-Crofts.
70. Neuman, B. (1989). *The Neuman systems model: Application to nursing, education, and practice.* Norwalk, CT: Appleton-Century-Crofts.
71. Neuman, B. (1995). *The Neuman systems model* (3rd ed.). Norwalk, CT: Appleton-Lange.
72. Neuman, B.M. & Young, R.J. (1972, May/June). A model for teaching total person approach to patient problems. *Nursing Research,* 21, 264-269.
73. Newman, M.A. (1979). *Theory development in nursing.* Philadelphia: F.A. Davis.
74. Newman, M.A. (1986). *Health as expanding consciousness.* St. Louis: Mosby.
75. Newman, M.A. (1994). *Health as expanding consciousness* (2nd ed.). New York: National League for Nursing Press.
76. Newman, M.A. (1995). *A developing discipline: Selected works of Margaret Newman.* New York: National League for Nursing Press.
77. Newman, M.A. (1999). *Health as expanding consciousness* (3rd ed.). Universe Com Inc. (online.)
78. Nightingale, F. (1957). *Notes on nursing.* Philadelphia: J.B. Lippincott. (Originally published, 1859.)
79. Nightingale, F. (1969). *Notes on nursing: What it is and what it is not.* New York: Dover. (Originally published, 1859.)
80. Nightingale, F. (1992). *Notes on nursing: What it is and what it is not.* Philadelphia: J.B. Lippincott.
81. Orem, D. (1971). *Nursing: Concepts of practice.* Scarborough, Ontario: McGraw Hill.
82. Orem, D. (1985). *Nursing: Concepts of practice* (3rd ed.). New York: McGraw-Hill.
83. Orem, D. (1995). *Nursing: Concepts of practice* (5th ed.). St. Louis: Mosby.
84. Orem, D. (2001). *Nursing: Concepts of practice* (6th ed.). St. Louis: Mosby.
85. Orlando, I. (1961). *The dynamic nurse-patient relationship.* New York: G.P. Putnam's Sons.
86. Orlando, I. (1972). *The discipline and teaching of nursing process.* New York: G.P. Putnam's Sons.
87. Orlando, I.J. (reissued 1991). *The dynamic nurse-patient relationship.* New York: National League for Nursing.
88. Palmer, I.S. (1977). Florence Nightingale: Reformer, reactionary, researcher. *Nursing Research,* 26(2), 84-49.
89. Parse, R.R. (1981). *Man-living-health: A theory of nursing.* New York: John Wiley & Sons.
90. Parse, R.R. (1987). *Nursing science: Major paradigms, theories, and critiques.* Philadelphia: W.B. Saunders.
91. Parse, R.R., Coyne, A.B., & Smith, M.J. (1985). *Nursing research: Qualitative methods.* Bowie, MD: Robert J. Brady.
92. Parse, R.R. (1998). *Human becoming school of thought: A perspective for nurses and other health professionals.* Newbury Park: Sage.
93. Parse, R.R. (1998). *Hope: An international human becoming perspective.* New York: National League for Nursing.

94. Parse, R.R. (1999). *Hope: An international human becoming perspective.* Boston, MA: Jones & Bartlett.

95. Parse, R.R. (1999). *Illumination: The human theory in practice and research.* Boston, MA: Jones & Bartlett.

96. Pender, N.J. (1975). A conceptual model for preventive health behavior. *Nursing Outlook, 23*(6), 385-390.

97. Pender, N.J. (1982). *Health promotion in nursing practice.* New York: Appleton-Century-Crofts.

98. Pender, N.J. (1987). *Health promotion in nursing practice* (2nd ed.). New York: Appleton & Lange.

99. Pender, N.J. (1996). *Health promotion in nursing practice* (3rd ed.). Norwalk, CT: Appleton & Lange.

100. Peplau, H. (1952). *Interpersonal relations in nursing.* New York: G.P. Putnam's Sons.

101. Potter, P.A. & Perry, A.G. (1997). *Fundamentals of nursing: Concepts, process, and practice* (4th ed.). St. Louis: Mosby.

102. Riehl, J.P. & Roy, C. (Eds.). (1974). *Conceptual models for nursing practice.* Englewood Cliffs, NJ: Prentice Hall.

103. Riehl, J.P. & Roy, C. (Eds.). (1980). *Conceptual models for nursing practice* (2nd ed.). New York: Appleton-Century-Crofts.

104. Riehl-Sisca, J.P. (Ed.). (1989). *Conceptual models for nursing practice* (3rd ed.). New York: Appleton-Century-Crofts.

105. Rogers, M.E. (1970). *An introduction to the theoretical basis of nursing.* Philadelphia: F.A. Davis.

106. Rogers, M.E. (1994). The science of unitary human beings: Current perspectives. *Nursing Science Quarterly, 7,* 33-35.

107. Roper, N., Logan, W.W., & Tierney, A.J. (1996). *The elements of nursing: A model for nursing based on a model for living* (4th ed.). San Francisco: Churchill Livingstone.

108. Roper, N., Logan, W., & Tierney, A.J. (2000). *The Roper-Logan-Tierney model of nursing: Based on activities of living.* Edinburgh: Churchill Livingstone.

109. Roy, C. (1970). Adaptation: A conceptual framework for nursing. *Nursing Outlook,* 18(3), 42-45.

110. Roy, C. (1976). *An introduction to nursing: An adaptation model.* Englewood Cliffs, NJ: Prentice-Hall.

111. Roy, C. (1984). *An introduction to nursing: An adaptation model* (2nd ed.). Englewood Cliffs, NJ: Prentice-Hall.

112. Roy, C. & Andrews, H. (1991). *The Roy adaptation model: The definitive statement.* Norwalk, CT: Appleton & Lange.

113. Roy, C. & Heather, A.A. (1999). *The Roy adaptation model.* Upper Saddle River: Prentice Hall.

114. Schmeiding, N.J. (1983). An analysis of Orlando's nursing theory based on Kuhn's theory of science. In P. Chinn (Ed.), *Advances in nursing theory development.* Rockville, MD: Aspen Systems.

115. Styles, M.M. (1982). *On nursing: Toward a new endowment.* St. Louis: Mosby.

116. Travelbee, J. (1966). *Interpersonal aspects of nursing.* Philadelphia: F.A. Davis.

117. Travelbee, J. (1971). *Interpersonal aspects of nursing* (2nd ed.). Philadelphia: F.A. Davis.

118. Watson, J. (1979). *Nursing: The philosophy and science of caring.* Boston: Little, Brown.

119. Watson, J. (1985). *Nursing: Human science and human care.* Norwalk, CT: Appleton-Century-Crofts.

120. Watson, J. (1988). *Nursing: Human science and human care: A theory of nursing.* New York: National League for Nursing.

121. Watson, J. (1999). *Postmodern nursing and beyond.* New York: Churchill Livingstone.

122. Wiedenbach, E. (1964). *Clinical nursing: A helping art.* New York: Springer.

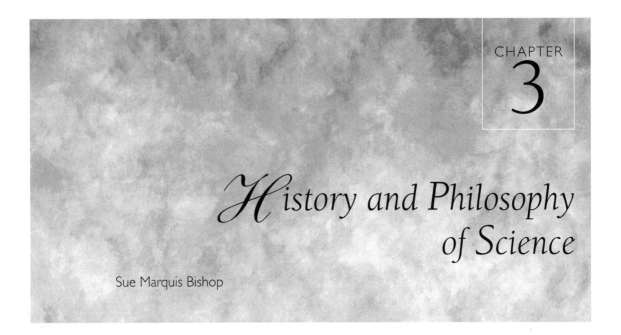

History and Philosophy of Science

Sue Marquis Bishop

Modern science is a relatively new intellectual activity. Established 400 years ago, modern science has occupied only a short time in the history of humankind.[4] Scientific activity has persisted because it has improved quality of life and has satisfied human needs for creative work, a sense of order, and the desire to understand the unknown.[4,15,31] The development of science requires the formalization of a given phenomena of interest and events concerning each science.[46] The construction of nursing theories is the formalization of attempts to describe, explain, predict, or control states of affairs in nursing (nursing phenomena).

HISTORICAL VIEWS OF THE NATURE OF SCIENCE

To formalize the science of nursing, basic questions much be considered, such as: What is science, knowledge, and truth?; What methods produce scientific knowledge? These are philosophical questions. The

Previous author: Sue Marquis Bishop.

term *epistemology* is concerned with the theory of knowledge in philosophical inquiry. The particular philosophical perspective selected to answer these questions will influence how scientists perform scientific activities, how they interpret outcomes, and what they regard as science and knowledge.[5] Although philosophy has been documented as an activity for 3000 years, formal science is a relatively new human pursuit.[13] Scientific activity has only recently become the object of investigation.[5]

Two competing theories of science, rationalism and empiricism, have evolved in the era of modern science with several variations.[15] Gale[15] labeled these alternative epistemologies as centrally concerned with the power of reason and the power of sensory experience. Gale noted some similarity in the divergent views of science in the time of the classical Greeks. For example, Aristotle believed advances in biological science would develop through systematic observation of objects and events in the natural world, whereas Pythagorus believed knowledge of the natural world would develop from mathematical reasoning.[5,15]

Rationalism

Rationalist epistemology emphasizes the importance of a priori reasoning as the appropriate method for advancing knowledge. The scientist in this tradition approaches the task of scientific inquiry by developing a systematic explanation (theory) of a given phenomenon.[15] This conceptual system is analyzed by addressing the logical structure of the theory and the logical reasoning involved in its development. Theoretical assertions derived by deductive reasoning are then subjected to experimental testing to corroborate the theory. Reynolds[34] labeled this approach the theory-then-research strategy. If the research findings fail to correspond with the theoretical assertions, additional research is conducted or modifications are made in the theory and further tests are devised; otherwise, the theory is discarded in favor of an alternative explanation.[15,48] Popper[32] argued that science would evolve more rapidly through the process of conjectures and refutations by devising research in an attempt to refute new ideas.

The rationalist view is most clearly evident in the work of Einstein, the theoretical physicist, who made extensive use of mathematical equations in developing his theories. The theories Einstein constructed offered an imaginative framework, which has directed research in numerous areas.[6] As Reynolds[34] noted, if someone believes that science is a process of inventing descriptions of phenomena, the appropriate strategy for theory construction is the theory-then-research strategy. In Reynolds's view, "As the continuous interplay between theory construction (invention) and testing with empirical research progresses, the theory becomes more precise and complete as a description of nature and, therefore, more useful for the goals of science."[34:145]

Empiricism

The empiricist view is based on the central idea that scientific knowledge can only be derived from sensory experience. Francis Bacon[15] received credit for popularizing the basis for the empiricist approach to inquiry. Bacon believed that scientific truth was discovered through the generalization of observed facts in the natural world. This approach, called the inductive method, is based on the idea that the collection of facts precedes attempts to formulate generalizations, called the research-then-theory approach.[34]

The strict empiricist view is reflected in the work of the behaviorists Watson and Skinner. In a 1950 paper, Skinner[38] asserted that advances in the science of psychology could be expected if scientists would focus on the collection of empirical data. He cautioned against drawing premature inferences and proposed a moratorium on theory building until further facts were collected. Skinner's approach to theory construction was clearly inductive. His view of science and the popularity of behaviorism have been credited with influencing psychology's shift in emphasis from theory construction to fact gathering between the 1950s and 1970s.[39] The difficulty with the inductive mode of inquiry is that the world presents an infinite number of possible observations.[41] Therefore the scientist must bring ideas to experiences to decide what to observe and what to exclude.[41] Although Skinner disclaimed to be developing a theory in his early writings, Bixenstine[2:465] noted, "Skinner is startlingly creative in applying the conceptual elements of his let's be frank theory to a wide variety of issues, ranging from training pigeons in the guidance of missiles, to developing teaching machines, to constructing a model society."

EARLY TWENTIETH-CENTURY VIEWS OF SCIENCE AND THEORY

During the first half of this century, philosophers focused on the analysis of theory structure, whereas scientists focused on empirical research.[5] There was minimal interest in the history of science, the nature of scientific discovery, or the similarities between the philosophical view of science and the scientific methods.[5] *Positivism,* a term first used by Comte, emerged as the dominant view of modern science.[15] Modern logical positivists believed empirical research and logical analysis were two approaches that would produce scientific knowledge. Logical positivists hailed the system of symbolic logic, published from 1910 to 1913 by Whitehead and Russell, as an appropriate approach to discovering truth.[5]

The logical empiricists offered a more lenient view of logical positivism and argued that theoretical propositions must be tested through observation and experimentation.[5] This perspective is rooted in the idea that empirical facts exist independently of theories and offer the only basis for objectivity in science.[5] Objective truth exists independently of the researcher. In this view, the task of science is to discover it. The empiricist view shares similarities with Aristotle's view of biological science and Bacon's inductive method as the true method of scientific inquiry.[15] Gale[15] argued that this view of science is often presented in methodology courses as the single orthodox view of the scientific enterprise. In his words, this view is taught in the following manner: "The scientist first sets up an experiment; observes what occurs . . .; reaches a preliminary hypothesis to describe the occurrence; runs further experiments to test the hypothesis [and] finally corrects or modifies the hypothesis in light of the results."[15:13]

The increasing use of computers, which permit the analysis of large data sets, may have contributed to the acceptance of the positivist approach to modern science.[39] However, in the 1950s, the literature began to reflect an increasing challenge to the positivist view, thereby ushering in a new view of science.[4]

EMERGENT VIEWS OF SCIENCE AND THEORY IN THE LATE TWENTIETH CENTURY

In the latter years of the twentieth century, several authors presented analyses challenging the positivist position, thus offering the basis for a new perspective of science.[13,17,21,43] Foucault[13] published his analysis (first published in French in 1966) of the epistemology of human sciences from the seventeenth to the nineteenth century. His major thesis stated that empirical knowledge was arranged in different patterns at a given time and in a given culture. Over time, he found changes in the focus of inquiry in what was regarded as scientific knowledge and in how knowledge was organized. Further, he concluded that humans only recently emerged as objects of study. Schutz,[36] in his Phenomenology of the Social World, argued that scientists seeking to understand the so-

cial world cannot cognitively know an external world that is independent of their own life experiences.

In 1977, Brown[5] argued that a new intellectual revolution in philosophy, which emphasized the history of science, replaced formal logic as the major analytical tool in the philosophy of science. One of the major perspectives in the new philosophy was the focus on science as a process of continuing research rather than the emphasis on accepted findings. In this emergent epistemology, the emphasis was on understanding scientific discovery and understanding the processes involved in changes in theories over time.

Empiricists argue that for science to maintain objectivity, data collection and analysis must be independent of theory.[5] This assertion is based on the position that objective truth exists in the world, just waiting to be discovered. Brown[5] argues that the new epistemology challenged the empiricist view of perception by acknowledging that theories play a significant role in determining what the scientist will observe and how it will be interpreted. The following story related to Marquis Bishop by her grandmother illustrates Brown's thesis that observations are concept-laden; that is, an observation is influenced by ideas in the mind of the observer.

A husband and wife are sitting by the fire silently watching their firstborn son asleep in the cradle. The mother looks at her infant son and imagines him learning to talk and then to walk. She continues her reverie by imagining him playing with friends, coming home from school, and then going to college. She ends her daydreaming by visualizing him elected president of the United States. She smiles and glances up at her husband, who also had been staring intently at their son. "What are you thinking, honey?"

The husband replies, "I was just thinking that I can't imagine how anyone could build a fine cradle like this, sell it for $12.98, and still make a profit."

Brown[5] presented the example of a chemist and a child walking together past a steel mill. The chemist perceived the odor of sulfur dioxide and the child smelled rotten eggs. They responded to the same observable data with distinctly different cognitive interpretations. In studying to become family therapists, students may analyze videotapes of family therapy sessions to learn the different approaches to family therapy. Novice student therapists tend to focus on the content of family interaction (what one member says to another) or the behavior of individual family members. After studying the system's view of families, which uses examples of patterned transactions among family members, students can recognize and describe transactions among family members that they did not perceive during the first viewing of the videotapes. For example, the son withdraws when his parents argue and the wife grits her teeth when her husband speaks. Concepts and theories create boundaries for selecting observable phenomena and for reasoning about specific patterns. For example, the social network concept may be more fruitful for studying social relations than the group concept because it focuses attention on a more complex set of relationships that are beyond the boundaries of any one setting.[1,19]

However, if scientists perceive patterns in the empirical world based on their presupposed theories, how can new patterns ever be perceived or new discoveries become formulated? Gale[15] answered this question by arguing that the scientist is able to perceive forceful intrusions from the environment that challenge his or her a priori mental set, thereby raising questions regarding the current theoretical perspective. Brown[5] maintained that, although a presupposed theoretical framework influences perception, theories are not the single determining factor of the scientist's perception. He identified three different views of the relationship between theories and observation:

1. Scientists are merely passive observers of occurrences in the empirical world. Observable data are objective truth waiting to be discovered.
2. Theories structure what the scientist perceives in the empirical world.
3. Presupposed theories and observable data interact in the process of scientific investigation.[5:298]

Brown's argument[5] for an interactionist's perspective coincides with the scientific consensus in the study of pattern recognition in human information processing. The following distinct minitheories have directed research efforts in this area: (1) the

Data-Driven, or Bottom-Up, Theory and (2) the Conceptually Driven, or Top-Down, Theory.[26] In the former, cognitive expectations (what is known or ways of organizing meaning) are used to select input and process incoming information from the environment. The second theory asserts that incoming data are perceived as unlabeled input and analyzed as raw data with increasing levels of complexity until all the data are classified. Current research evidence suggests that human pattern recognition progresses through an interaction of both data-driven and conceptually driven processes and it uses sources of information in both currently organized, cognitive categories and in stimuli from the sensory environment.[27]

The interactionist's perspective is clearly reflected in Piaget's Theory of Human Cognitive Functioning:

> Piagetian man actively selects and interprets environmental information in the construction of his own knowledge rather than passively copying the information just as it is presented to his senses. While paying attention to and taking account of the structure of the environment during knowledge seeking, Piagetian man reconstrues and reinterprets that environment [according to] his own mental framework. . . . The mind neither copies the world . . . nor does it ignore the world [by] creating a private mental conception of it out of whole cloth. . . . The mind meets the environment in an extremely active, self-directed way.[11:6]

If the thesis is accepted that objective truth does not exist and science is an interactive process between invented theories and empirical observations, how are scientists to determine truth and scientific knowledge? In the new epistemology, science is viewed as an ongoing process. Much importance is given to the idea of consensus among scientists. As Brown[5] concluded, it is a myth that science can establish final truths. Tentative consensus based on reasoned judgments about the available evidence is the most that can be expected.

In this view of science, scientific knowledge is what the community of scientists in any given historical era regard as scientific knowledge. Current consensus among scientists determines the truth of a given theoretical statement by concluding whether or not it presents an adequate description of reality.[5] This consensus is possible through the collaboration of many scientists as they make their work available for public review and debate and as they build upon previous inquiries.[33] "The individual (scientist) introduces ideas, the scientific community appraises them" by its objective criteria.[33:59]

In any given era and in any given discipline, science is structured by an accepted set of presuppositions that define the phenomena for study and define the appropriate methods for data collection and interpretation.[5] These presuppositions set the boundaries for the scientific enterprise in a particular field. In Brown's view[5:167] of the transactions between theory and empirical observation:

> Theory determines what observations are worth making and how they are to be understood, and observation provides challenges to accepted theoretical structures. The continuing attempt to produce a coherently organized body of theory and observation is the driving force of research, and the prolonged failure of specific research projects leads to scientific revolutions.

The presentation and acceptance of a revolutionary theory may alter the existing presuppositions and theories, thereby creating a different set of boundaries and procedures. The result is a new set of problems or a new way to interpret observations; that is, a new picture of the world.[21] In this view of science, the emphasis must be placed on ongoing research rather than established findings.

INTERDEPENDENCE OF THEORY AND RESEARCH

Traditionally, theory building and research have been presented to students in separate courses. Often, this separation has caused problems for students in understanding the nature of theories and in comprehending the relevance of research efforts.[47] The acceptance of the positivist view of science may have influenced the sharp distinction between theory and research methods.[15] Although theory and research can be viewed as distinct operations, they are regarded more appropriately as interdependent components of the scientific process.[9] In constructing a theory, the theorist must be knowledgeable about available empirical findings and be able to take these into account because theory is, in part, concerned with the formalization of available knowledge.[48] The theory is subject to revision if the hypotheses fail to correspond with empirical findings or the theory may be abandoned in favor of an alternative explanation that accounts for the new information.[5,9,21]

In contemporary theories of science, the scientific enterprise has been described as a series of phases with an emphasis on the discovery and verification (or acceptance) phases.[15,16] According to Gale,[15] these phases are primarily concerned with the presentation and testing of new ideas. New ways of thinking about phenomena or new data are introduced to the scientific community during the discovery phase. During this time, the focus is on presenting a persuasive argument to show that the new conceptions represent an improvement over previous conceptions.[15] Verification is characterized by the scientific community's efforts to critically analyze and test the new conceptions in an attempt to refute them. The new views are then subjected to testing and analyses.[15] However, Brown[5] argued that discovery and verification could not be viewed as distinct phases because the scientific community does not usually accept a new conception until it has been subjected to significant testing. Only then can it be accepted as a new discovery.

It should be clear that, in a scientific discipline, Randall[33] argued that it is not appropriate to judge a theory on the basis of authority, faith, or intuition. A theory should be judged on the basis of scientific consensus.[33] For example, if a specific nursing theory is determined acceptable, this judgment should not be made because a respected nursing leader advocates the theory. Personal feelings about the theory, such as "I like this theory" or "I don't like this theory," should not provide the basis for judgment either. The theory should only be judged acceptable on the basis of logical and conceptual or empirical grounds. The scientific community makes these judgments.[4]

The advancement of science is a collaborative endeavor in which many researchers evaluate and build on each other's work. Theories, procedures, and findings from empirical studies must be made available for critical review by scientists for evidence to be cumulative. The same procedures can be used to support or refute a given analysis or finding.[33] A theory is accepted when scientists agree that the theory provides a description of reality that captures the phenomenon of available research findings.[5] The acceptance of a scientific hypothesis depends on the appraisal of the coherence of theory, which involves questions of logic, and the correspondence of the theory, which involves efforts to relate the theory to observable phenomena through research.[42] Gale[15] labeled these criteria as epistemological and metaphysical concerns.

The consensus regarding the correspondence of the theory is not based on a single study. Repeated testing is crucial. The study must be replicated under the same conditions and the theoretical assertions must be explored under different conditions or with different measures. Consensus is therefore based on accumulated evidence.[16] When the theory does not appear to be supported by research, the scientific community does not necessarily reject it. Rather than agreeing that a problem exists with the theory itself, the community may make judgments about the validity or the reliability of the measures used in testing the theory or about the appropriateness of the research design. These possibilities are considered in critically evaluating the attempts to test a given theory.

Dubin[9,41,42] identified the following areas in which scientific consensus is necessary for any given theory: (1) agreement on the boundaries of the theory; that is, the phenomenon it addresses and the phenomena it excludes (criterion of coherence); (2) agreement on the logic used in constructing the theory to further understanding from a similar perspective (criterion of coherence); (3) agreement that the theory fits the data collected and analyzed through research (criterion of correspondence). Essentially, consensus in these three areas constitutes an agreement among scientists to "look at the same 'things,' to do so in the same way, and to have a level of confidence certified by an empirical test."[9:13] Therefore the theory must be capable of being operationalized for testing to check the theory against reality. Retroductive, deductive, and inductive forms of reasoning may be used as science progresses by building theoretical descriptions and explanations of reality, attempting to account for available findings, deriving testable hypotheses, and evaluating theories from the perspective of new empirical data.[42]

Most research may be considered within the category that Kuhn[21] called normal science. Scientific inquiry in normal science involves testing a given theory, developing new applications of a theory, or extending a given theory. Occasionally, a new theory with different assumptions is developed that could potentially replace previous theories. Kuhn[21] described this as revolutionary science and described the theory with different presuppositions as a revolutionary theory. A change in the accepted presuppositions creates a set of boundaries and procedures that suggest a new set of problems or a new way to interpret observations.[21]

In the social and behavioral sciences, there is some challenge to the assumptions underlying the accepted methods of experimental design, measurement, and statistical analysis that emphasize the search for universal laws and emphasize the use of procedures for the random assignment of subjects across contexts.[24] Mishler[24] argued that, in studying behavior, scientists should develop methods and procedures that are dependent on context for meaning rather than eliminate context by searching for laws that hold across contexts. This critique of the methods and assumptions of research is emerging from phenomenological and ethnomethodological theorists who view the scientific process from a very different paradigm.[3,18,24,29,44]

The proper focus of research is not the attempt to prove a theory or hypothesis, but the attempt to set up research to refute a given hypothesis.[32] Repeated failed attempts at refutation lends support to the theory and acceptance of the theory by the scientific community.[9] However, the emphasis is always placed on ongoing research rather than established findings.[5] In the future, new information or a new, compelling way to view the same evidence may lead to a reappraisal of the theory. One previously accepted theory may be abandoned for another theory if it fails to correspond with empirical findings or if it does not present clear directions for further research. The scientific community judges the selected alternative theory to account for available data and to suggest further lines of inquiry.[5]

Popper[31] observed that refutations of a given theory are frequently viewed as a failure of the theorist or the theory. In his view, "Every refutation should be regarded as a great success; not merely as a success of the scientist who refuted the theory, but also of the scientist who created the refuted theory and who thus . . . suggested, if only indirectly, the refutation experiment."[32:243]

There is neither a single science nor a single scientific method; there are several sciences, each with unique phenomena and structure and methods for inquiry.[40] The various sciences are at different stages of development. Physics, with the exception of mathematics, is considered the most exacting of the sciences; the life sciences, such as botany, are not as well developed scientifically; the social sciences are even less developed.[39] However, the commonality among sciences concerns the scientists' efforts to separate truth from speculation to advance knowledge.[39] In questions regarding the structure of knowledge in a given science, the consensus of scientists in the discipline decide what is to be regarded as scientific knowledge and the methods of inquiry.[5,15]

ISSUES IN NURSING PHILOSOPHY AND SCIENCE DEVELOPMENT

Compared with other developing sciences, nursing science is in the early stages of scientific development. Until the late 1950s, the use of the term *nursing science* in the literature was rare.[7] Consensus has emerged in the field of nursing, which concludes that the knowledge base for nursing practice is incomplete and the development of a scientific base for nursing practice is a high priority for the discipline.[35] In 1985, Meleis concluded, "Theory is no longer a luxury in nursing. There was a time when

theory use was equated with the development of a conceptual framework, to be used only as a guide to curriculum development. Theory now is part and parcel of the nursing lexicon in education, administration, and practice."[22:2]

Meleis[23] characterized the years of progress in the discipline of nursing in four stages: (1) practice, (2) education and administration, (3) research, and (4) the development of nursing theory. In 1952, Peplau developed the first theory for the nursing practice in her book, *Interpersonal Relations in Nursing*.[30] The journal *Nursing Research* was published the same year, providing a source for dissemination of research findings in nursing. During the 1950s and the early 1960s, other formulations of nursing were developed.

During the late 1960s and early 1970s, nurse theorists analyzed and debated a variety of metatheoretical issues. During this time, the first issue of the journal *Advances in Nursing Science* was published. Metatheoretical issues relate to theory-development issues or philosophy of science issues; that is, theories about theories. Nursing scholars questioned: What is a theory?; How should nursing theory be developed?; Should theories be borrowed from other fields?; How should theories be critiqued?; What is nursing knowledge? For example, in 1978, Carper[7] conceptualized four fundamental patterns of knowledge in nursing: (1) empirical knowledge (nursing science), (2) esthetic knowledge (nursing art), (3) moral knowledge (ethics in nursing), and (4) personal knowledge (therapeutic use of self). This period was characterized by nurse theorists' acceptance of the necessity to devise nursing theories and focus on developing directions for the field to continue the progress in theory development. (Refer to Meleis' text, *Theoretical Nursing: Development and Progress*,[23] for an analysis of the milestones in theory development in nursing from 1955 to 1995.)

During the 1980s, further acceptance of nursing theory was evidenced by continued theory development in nursing and increased incorporation of nursing theories into the nursing curricula. The nursing theory literature during this period increasingly addressed the analysis and use of nursing theories in clinical practice.[23] The number of nursing journals publishing articles on theory and research increased significantly. Consensus was achieved on the domain concepts of nursing (person, environment, health, and nursing) as defining the major concepts central to nursing.[10]

In the 1990s, philosophical debate continued in the literature over whether nursing science is a basic science, an applied science, or a practical science.[20] Further, although the numbers of educational and practice settings that adopt a single nursing theory approach to curriculum and nursing practice increased in the 1980s, the one theory approach has not achieved consensus in the field. A number of nursing scholars are emphasizing pluralism in nursing theories.[21] For example, Nagle and Mitchell[25] argued for theoretic diversity, which is the use of multiple theory approaches in the practice setting. Meleis[21,23] asserted that, in a discipline dealing with human beings, it is not feasible that only one theory should explain, describe, predict, and change all the discipline's phenomena. "This blanket acceptance of one (single theory) approach smothers creativity, scholarly inquiry and growth."[25:24]

In the early 1990s, the nursing literature continued to address the meaning of the domain concepts; in particular, the need to establish interconnections among these central nursing concepts. "Such unconnected concepts do not raise philosophic issues or scientific questions that stimulate inquiry."[26:2] Current nursing literature also reflects increasing concern with the methods of inquiry used in developing nursing knowledge; several scholars stress the importance of diversity in research methods and the use of both qualitative and quantitative methods.[3,8,29]

In the mid1990s, nursing scholars addressed the development of an epistemology of nursing therapeutics,[22] thereby enhancing the connectedness between nursing science and art (see "From Carper's Patterns of Knowing to Ways of Being: An Ontological Philosophical Shift in Nursing"[37]) and arguing for pluralism in nursing theories and research methods (see "Stories and Numbers: Coexistence Without Compromise"[12] and *In Search of Nursing Science*).[28] It may be that one theoretical perspective cannot capture the complexity of nursing knowledge or be the single driver to advance nursing

knowledge.[28] It has been argued that evolutionary changes associated with the information age are changing nurses' views of possible realities and are creating a philosophical shift in nursing.[37] This shift was viewed as transferring the focus from an exclusive, philosophical emphasis on epistemological questions about knowing to a focus on ontological questions about meaning, being, and reality.[37] Midrange and situation-specific theories evolved.[23] "How the nurse uses expert knowledge to administer complex chemotherapy treatments is as important as how the nurse uses artistry of being to help a young mother find meaning in her impending death. Often the two converge. . . . The gap between nursing science and art has begun to close, generating a creative synthesis of the two . . . the 'science-art' of nursing."[37:12,11]

The postpositivist and interpretive paradigms have achieved a current degree of acceptance in nursing as paradigms that guide knowledge development.[12] *Postpositivism* focuses on discovering patterns that may describe, explain, and predict phenomena. It rejects the older, traditional positivist views of an ultimate objective knowledge that is observable only through the senses (see "Stories and Numbers: Coexistence Without Compromise"[12] and "Contemporary Empiricism"[45] for more discussion).[12,45] The *interpretive* paradigm tends to promote understanding by addressing the meanings of the participants' social interaction that emphasize situation, context, and the multiple cognitive constructions that individuals create from everyday events.[12] The *critical* paradigm for knowledge development in nursing has been described as an emergent, postmodern paradigm that provides the framework for inquiring about the interaction between social, political, economic, gender, and cultural factors and the experiences of health and illness.[12] A broad conception of *postmodernism* includes the particular philosophies that challenge the "objectification of knowledge," such as phenomenology, hermeneutics, feminism, critical theory, and poststructuralism.[28:91]

The philosophy of nursing has been developing over a 150-year period.[14] However, in 1999, Fry[14] concluded that philosophical inquiry was only a recent development in nursing and it was not yet a well-defined field in nursing. She cited the following evidence of increasing interest and productivity in the philosophy of nursing as a field of inquiry: (1) the establishment of the Institute for Philosophical Nursing Research at the University of Alberta in the 1980s, (2) the increased publication of articles and books on nursing philosophy, and (3) the establishment of the journal, *The Philosophy of Nursing.*[14]

SCIENCE AS A SOCIAL ENTERPRISE

The process of scientific inquiry may be viewed as a social enterprise.[24] In Gale's words,[15:290] "Human beings do science." Therefore it might be anticipated that social, economic, or political factors may influence the scientific enterprise.[5] For example, the popularity of certain ideologies may influence how phenomena are viewed and what problems are selected for study.[18] In addition, the availability of funds for research in a specified area may increase research activity in that area. However, science does not depend on the personal characteristics or persuasions of any given scientist or group of scientists, but it is powerfully self-correcting within the community of scientists.[33] Science progresses by "reasoned judgments on the part of scientists and through debate within the scientific community."[5:167] This is evidenced by the fact that nursing scholars are fully engaged in this process to develop nursing science.

REFERENCES

1. Bishop, S.M. (1984). Perspectives on individual-family-social network interrelations. *Interrelational Journal of Family Therapy,* 6(2), 124-135.
2. Bixenstine, E. (1964). Empiricism in latter-day behavioral science. *Science,* 145, 465.
3. Bowers, L. (1992). Ethnomethodology I: An approach to nursing research. *International Journal of Nursing Studies,* 29(1), 59-67.
4. Bronowski, J. (1979). *The visionary eye: Essays in the arts, literature and science.* Cambridge, MA: The MIT Press.
5. Brown, H. (1977). *Perception, theory and commitment: The new philosophy of science.* Chicago: The University of Chicago Press.
6. Calder, N. (1979). *Einstein's universe.* New York: Viking.
7. Carper, B. (1978). Fundamental patterns of knowing in nursing. *Advances in Nursing Science,* 1(1), 13-23.
8. Cull-Wilby, B. & Pepin, J. (1987). Towards a coexistence of paradigms in nursing knowledge development. *Journal of Advanced Nursing,* 12, 515-521.
9. Dubin, R. (1978). *Theory building.* New York: The Free Press.
10. Fawcett, J. (1984). The metaparadigm of nursing: Present status and future refinements. *Image,* 16(3), 84-87.
11. Flavell, J.H. (1977). *Cognitive development.* Englewood Cliffs, NJ: Prentice-Hall.
12. Ford-Gilboe, M., Campbell, J., & Berman, H. (1995). Stories and numbers: Coexistence without compromise. *Advances in Nursing Science,* 18(1), 14-26.
13. Foucault, M. (1973). *The order of things: An archaeology of the human sciences.* New York: Vintage Books.
14. Fry, S. (1999). The philosophy of nursing. *Scholarly Inquiry for Nursing Practice: An International Journal,* 13(1), 5-15.
15. Gale, G. (1979). *Theory of science: An introduction to the history, logic and philosophy of science.* New York: McGraw-Hill.
16. Giere, R.N. (1979). *Understanding scientific reasoning.* New York: Holt, Rhinehart, & Winston.
17. Hanson, N.R. (1958). *Patterns of discovery.* Cambridge: Cambridge University Press.
18. Hudson, L. (1972). *The cult of the fact.* New York: Harper & Row.
19. Irving, H.W. (1977). Social networks in the modern city. *Social Forces,* 55, 867-880.
20. Johnson, J. (1991). Nursing science: Basic, applied, or practical? *Advances in Nursing Science,* 14(1), 7-16.
21. Kuhn, T.S. (1962). *The structure of scientific revolutions.* Chicago: The University of Chicago Press.
22. Liaschenko, J. (1995). Ethics in the work of acting for patients. *Advances in Nursing Sciences,* 18(2), 1-12.
23. Meleis, A. (1997). *Theoretical nursing: Development and progress.* Philadelphia: J.B. Lippincott.
24. Mishler, E.G. (1979). Meaning in context: Is there any other kind? *Harvard Educational Review,* 49, 1-19.
25. Nagle, L. & Mitchell, G. (1991). Theoretic diversity: Evolving paradigmatic issues in research and practice. *Advances in Nursing Science,* 14(1), 17-25.
26. Newman, M., Sime, A.M., & Cororan-Perry, S. (1991). The focus of the discipline of nursing. *Advances in Nursing Science,* 14(1), 1-6.
27. Norman, D.A. (1976). *Memory and attention: An introduction to human information processing.* New York: John Wiley & Sons.
28. Omery, A., Kasper, C.E., & Page, G.G. (1995). *In search of nursing science.* Thousand Oaks, CA: Sage.

29. Pallikkathayil, L. & Morgan, S. (1991). Phenomenology as a method for conducting clinical research. *Applied Nursing Research, 4*(4), 195-200.

30. Peplau, H. (1952). *Interpersonal relations in nursing.* New York: G.P. Putnam's Sons.

31. Piaget, J. (1970). *The place of the sciences of man in the system of sciences.* New York: Harper & Row.

32. Popper, K. (1962). *Conjectures and refutations.* New York: Basic Books.

33. Randall, J.H. (1964). *Philosophy: An introduction.* New York: Barnes & Noble.

34. Reynolds, P. (1971). *A primer in theory construction.* Indianapolis: Bobbs-Merrill.

35. Schlotfeldt, R. (1992). Why promote clinical nursing scholarship? *Clinical Nursing Research, 1*(1), 5-9.

36. Schutz, A. (1967). *The phenomenology of the social world.* Evanston, IL: Northwestern University Press.

37. Silva, M.C., Sorrell, J.M., & Sorrell, C.D. (1995). From Carper's patterns of knowing to ways of being: An ontological philosophical shift in nursing. *Advances in Nursing Science, 18*(1), 1-13.

38. Skinner, B.F. (1950). Are theories of learning necessary? *Psychological Review, 57,* 193-216.

39. Snelbecker, G. (1974). *Learning theory, instructional theory, and psychoeducational design.* New York: McGraw-Hill.

40. Springagesh, K. & Springagesh, S. (1986). Philosophy and scientific approach. *Contemporary Philosophy, 11*(6), 18-20.

41. Steiner, E. (1977). *Criteria for theory of art education [Monograph].* Presented at Seminar for Research in Art Education. Philadelphia: Unpublished.

42. Steiner, E. (1978). *Logical and conceptual analytic techniques for educational researchers.* Washington, DC: University Press.

43. Toulmin, S. (1961). *Foresight and understanding.* New York: Harper & Row.

44. Turner, J. (1978). *The structure of sociological theory.* Homewood, IL: The Dorsey Press.

45. Weiss, S.J. (1995). Contemporary empiricism. In A. Omery, C.E. Kasper, & G.G. Page (Eds.), *In search of nursing science.* Thousand Oaks, CA: Sage.

46. Werkmeister, W. (1959). Theory construction and the problem of objectivity. In L. Gross (Ed.), *Symposium of sociological theory.* Evanston, IL: Row, Peterson, & Co.

47. Winston, C. (1974). *Theory and measurement in sociology.* New York: John Wiley & Sons.

48. Zetterberg, H.L. (1966). *On theory and verification in sociology.* Totowa, NJ: The Bedminister Press.

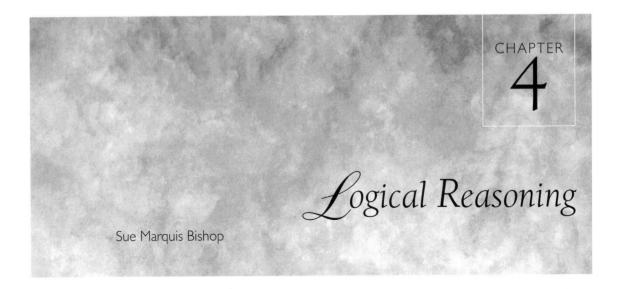

Logical Reasoning

Sue Marquis Bishop

A theory may be evaluated by using the criterion of logical development. This requires that the development of the series of theoretical statements follow a logical form of reasoning; that is, the premises must justify the conclusions. Logic is a branch of philosophy concerned with the analysis of inferences and arguments.[10] An inference involves forming a conclusion based on some evidence. Although the common meaning of argument implies a disagreement, in logic, an argument consists of a conclusion and its supportive evidence. The evidence supporting a conclusion may involve one or more theoretical statements, or premises. The tools of logic permit the analysis of reasoning from the premises to the conclusion.[8]

Theories can be developed and tested through deductive, inductive, or retroductive forms of reasoning. Traditionally, these approaches have been explicitly presented in the literature as systematic procedures for devising theory. An in-depth discussion of these forms is beyond the scope of this chapter. The reader is referred to Geach,[2] Giere,[3] Pospesel,[8] Salmon,[9,10] and Steiner[15] for further study. However, it is important to grasp the basic differences between these forms of reasoning to understand how a given theorist may choose to approach the task of theory building.

DEDUCTION

Deduction is a form of logical reasoning in which specific conclusions are inferred from more general premises or principles. Reasoning proceeds from the general to the particular.[14] The deductively developed theory usually involves a lengthy sequence of theoretical statements derived from relatively few broad axioms or general statements.[9] Derived conclusions may offer predictions that can be tested empirically. The deductive argument usually takes the form of a syllogism with general premises and a conclusion. In logical analysis, letters may be substituted for concepts because the emphasis on the analysis of the argument is focused on the form of the argument.[9] Example A presents a valid deductive argument with letter notation.

EXAMPLE A

Premise: All victims of abuse have low self-esteem. (**All S are M**)
Premise: Martha and Tom are victims of abuse. (**All P are S**)
Conclusion: Therefore Martha and Tom have low self-esteem. (**Ergo, all P are M**)

Previous author: Sue Marquis Bishop.

In Example A, the conclusion follows from, or was deduced from, the general premises. There may be a lengthy number of premises in a given argument preceding the conclusion. Note that in the above example, no new information is presented in the conclusion that is not at least implied in the premises. The deductive form of reasoning is defined as:

1. If A were true, then B would be true.
2. A is true.
3. Therefore B is true.[15]

In the nursing literature, arguments are not often presented in the form demonstrated in Example A with the premises and conclusions placed in order and clearly labeled. However, with practice, it is possible to sharpen skills in identifying the arguments and labeling the premises and conclusions from reading narrative text.[10] The conclusion may be presented at the beginning, end, or middle of an argument.[10] Salmon[10] suggests that certain words or phrases are clues that indicate specific statements are presented as premises or conclusions. Examples of terms that often precede a premise include "since," "for," and "because." Examples of terms that often precede a conclusion include "therefore," "consequently," "hence," "so," and "it follows that."[10]

Arguments may be evaluated in two different ways: (1) the validity of the argument may be assessed as to whether the conclusion logically follows the premises, and (2) the content of the premises may be assessed in terms of the truth or falsity of the statements.[8] The validity of a deductive argument refers to the logic involved in reasoning from the premises to the conclusion to ensure that, if the premises are true, the conclusion must be true.[8,10,15] A deductive argument may contain all true statements or one or more false statements and it may be considered either valid or invalid. This judgment is made on the basis of whether the conclusion is supported by the premises. For example:

EXAMPLE B

Premise: All victims of abuse have low self-esteem.
Premise: Martha has low self-esteem.
Conclusion: Therefore Martha is a victim of abuse.

Although Martha may be the victim of abuse, the truth or falsity of the conclusion or any of the statements is not an issue when evaluating the validity of an argument. In Example B, the supporting evidence in the premises does not establish the conclusion that Martha is a victim of abuse. The conclusion goes beyond the explicit and implicit information in the premises. This is not a valid argument. Compare the reasoning in Examples A and B.

Whereas validity refers to the forms of the deductive argument, truth refers to the content of a given theoretical statement. Therefore it is inappropriate to label a single theoretical statement as valid or label an argument as true.[10]

In a valid deductive argument, if the premises are true, the conclusion must be true. This combination is marked (R) in Figure 4-1. Therefore it is impossible for the conclusion to be false. This combination is marked (S) in Figure 4-1. *However, if one or more of the premises is false, two outcomes are possible: the conclusion may be either true or false.*

Example C presents a deductively valid argument that illustrates how false premises lead to a false conclusion. This combination is marked (X) in Figure 4-1.

		The conclusion is:	
		True	False
If the premises are:	All true	Necessary (R)	Impossible (S)
	Not all true	Possible (Y)	Possible (X)

(R) If the premises are true, it *necessarily follows* that the conclusion be true.
(S) If the premises are true, it is therefore *impossible* for the conclusion to be false.
(Y), (X) If one or more of the premises are false, it is *possible* the conclusion may be *either* true or false.

Figure **4-1** Potential outcomes of a valid deductive argument. (From *Understanding Scientific Reasoning, 1st edition,* by R.N. Giere © 1979. Reprinted with permission of Wadsworth, an imprint of Wadsworth Group, a division of Thomson Learning. Fax 800-730-2215.)

EXAMPLE C

Premise: The dime is larger than the nickel.
(**False**)
Premise: The nickel is larger than the silver dollar.
(**False**)
Conclusion: Therefore the dime is larger than the silver dollar. (**False**)

As Figure 4-1 suggests and Example D illustrates, it is also possible that a valid argument can lead to one or more false premises and a true conclusion. This combination is marked (Y) in Figure 4-1.

EXAMPLE D

Premise: The nickel is larger than the silver dollar. (**False**)
Premise: The silver dollar is larger than the dime. (**True**)
Conclusion: Therefore the nickel is larger than the dime. (**True**)

It may be helpful to study Examples C and D to understand how the conclusions are derived from the information given in the premises. (Note that in these examples, "larger than" refers to physical size, not the value of the coins.) In science, deductive arguments can be a powerful form of reasoning to derive new conclusions by making explicit implied information. Then these derived conclusions can be subjected to empirical testing.

INDUCTION

Induction is a form of logical reasoning in which a generalization is induced from a number of specific, observed instances. Inductive reasoning has not been as well developed as deductive reasoning.[8] The form of the inductive argument follows:

1. A is true of $b_1, b_2 \ldots b_n$.
2. $b_1, b_2 \ldots b_n$ are some members of class B.
3. Therefore A is true of all members of class B.[15]

The inductive form is based on the assumption that members of any given class share common characteristics. Therefore what is true for any randomly selected members of the class is accepted as true for all members of the class.[15] Suppose a sample of the population of abuse victims has been selected for study. Example E presents an argument in the in-

ductive form that may be developed based on this hypothetical study.

EXAMPLE E

Premise: Every victim of abuse that has been observed has low self-esteem.
Conclusion: All victims of abuse have low self-esteem.

The premise in Example E states observations from a number of instances; that is, a limited number of subjects. The conclusion states a generalization that extends beyond the observations to the entire class of abuse victims.

The inductive generalization may be stated in terms of a mathematical quantity.[10] For example, assume a researcher surveys a sample of 400 nurses to determine their opinions about whether nurses would establish independent private practices. Results indicate that 65% of nurses in the sample support independent private practice activities in nursing. The inductive statement may be stated as follows:

EXAMPLE F

Premise: Sixty-five percent of nurses in the sample support independent private practice activities in nursing.
Conclusion: Sixty-five percent of all nurses support independent private practice activities in nursing.

In a deductive argument, if the premises are true, the conclusion must be true. The inductive argument can have true premises and produce a false conclusion.

An inductive conclusion based on limited or biased evidence can clearly lead to a fallacious argument and perhaps a false conclusion.[10] Suppose the argument in Example E was developed through one nurse's experience in observing five victims of abuse. The conclusion that victims of abuse have low self-esteem may or may not be true. However, this conclusion is not warranted based on the number of observed instances. There is insufficient evidence in this case to justify the conclusion about all victims of abuse. Even if the sample size is appropriately sufficient (or based on several studies), the sample may be biased.

Assume that the sample of nurses in Example F was drawn from faculty in schools of nursing. The opinions of this select group of nurses may be expected to differ in some respects and may not reflect the opinions of all nurses. A larger proportion of nursing faculty members may be engaged in private practice activities compared with the proportion of all nurses. Considering a number of factors in selecting representative samples can help avoid introducing bias into observations. This reasoning is the basis for the random selection of subjects in research projects. Descriptive and inferential statistics are used to characterize the sample of the population and help with decisions about the strength of the evidence.[3] The inductive inference has been termed the *statistical inference.*[15,18]

In inductive arguments, the inferred conclusion goes beyond the implicit and explicit information in the premises. In Example E, not all victims of abuse have been observed. This conclusion is inferred on the basis of selected instances. In a deductive argument, the conclusion can be considered true if the argument is structured so implicit information in the premises is made explicit.[10] Conversely, the inductive argument goes beyond the information in the premises. The inductive argument expands upon the presented information. Giere[3] has argued that this characteristic permits the justification of scientific conclusions that may not be justifiable by deductive reasoning because they contain information beyond the premises. An example would be a scientific hypothesis about the future based on observations in the present.[3]

Whereas deductive arguments are considered either valid or invalid, the concept of validity does not apply to inductive arguments. The correctness of inductive arguments is not viewed in either/or terms; it is viewed on degrees of strength and measured in terms of the probability with which the premises lead to a given conclusion.[10] Then the inferred conclusion can be determined to have low, medium, or high probability.[10] Statistical procedures can be used in making these judgments.

In Example A, the conclusion can only be false if one or more of the premises are false; that is, if all victims of abuse do not have low self-esteem or if Martha and Tom are not victims of abuse. If these are true, the conclusion must be true. However, in Example E, the reasoning suggests that all victims of abuse have low self-esteem. The premises state that only selected victims of abuse have been observed. The premises may lend some support for the conclusion. The fact that victims of abuse without low self-esteem were not observed may be considered some evidence, but it will not preclude the possibility that a victim with high self-esteem will not be observed in the future.[10]

Deductive arguments are considered to preserve truth, whereas inductive arguments can be a source of new information.[3,10] Scientific generalizations about instances not observed in the present or projections about the future are examples. Although this form of reasoning is useful in advancing science, the very nature of induction may introduce error into the scientific process.[4] Even if the premises were accurate, the accuracy of the conclusion cannot be certain. In Giere's view,[3:37-38] if the premises are assumed to be true, then "the difference between a good inductive argument and a valid deductive argument is that the deductive argument guarantees the truth of its conclusion while the inductive argument guarantees only an appropriately high probability of its conclusion."

RETRODUCTION*

Whereas deduction and induction may explicate and evaluate ideas, retroduction originates ideas.[14] The retroductive form of reasoning is an approach to inquiry that uses analogy as a method for devising theory. In 1878, Pierce[15] described three kinds of reasoning as comprising the major steps of inquiry: (1) retroduction, (2) deduction, and (3) induction. Pierce viewed retroductive reasoning as the first stage in the search for understanding some surprising phenomenon in which a viewpoint offering a possible explanation is identified. Pierce stated that once a viewpoint was identified that held the promise of explaining observed phenomenon, de-

*The following discussion of retroduction has been adapted from the work of Elizabeth Steiner.[12,13,14,15] Copyright © Elizabeth Steiner. All rights reserved.

Table 4-1

Deduction, Induction, and Retroduction Summary		
TYPE	**QUESTION**	**TECHNIQUES**
DEDUCTION	Given that the premises are true, what other propositions may be inferred as necessary conclusions from the premises?[13]	Logical and conceptual analysis[13]
INDUCTION	Given that the premises are true, what is the strength of the link between them and the conclusion?[13]	Logical and conceptual analysis based on statistical analysis[12,16]
RETRODUCTION	Given a surprising observation, what explanation would result in the expectation that the observation would be a matter of course?[13]	Logical and conceptual analysis[12]

ductive reasoning was used to develop the explanation. Pierce considered the final stage of inquiry in terms of induction and focused on checking out the devised hypotheses in experience.[15] Steiner* further developed the theory models approach using retro-

ductive inference as a method for devising theory. The form of the retroductive inference follows:

1. The surprising fact, C, is observed.
2. If A were true, C would be a matter of course.
3. Therefore there is reason to suspect that A is true.[15]

An analysis of the preceding form reveals that the theory models (or retroductive) approach does

*Elizabeth Steiner's earlier work on theory models was published under her married name of Maccia.[4,5,12,13]

Table 4-1—cont'd

Deduction, Induction, and Retroduction Summary

DEFINITION	EXAMPLE	QUESTION
	Premises	*Explicates and derives further truths*[12]
1. If A were true, then B would be true.	All victims of abuse have low self-esteem. Marty and Tom are victims of abuse.	If premises are true, establishes truth of something else by derivation.[12]
2. A is true.	*Conclusion*	
3. Therefore B is true.[15]	Marty and Tom have low self-esteem.	
	Premise	*Evaluates and expands information*[3]
1. A is true of b_1, b_2 . . .b_n.	b_1, b_2 . . . b_n victims of abuse who have been observed have low self-esteem.	Based on probability of observed cases. Does not establish truth.
2. b_1, b_2 . . . b_n are some members of class B.	*Conclusion*	Establishes probability of certainty. New data
3. Therefore A is true of all members of class B.[15]	All victims of abuse have low self-esteem.	may change conclusion.[3,9,12]
	Proposition 1	*Originates ideas*[12]
1. The surprising fact, C, is observed.	The role of expecting *reward* determines a relation between *student* and *teacher* that establishes a path for influence of the teacher on the *student*.[5]	Does not establish truth. Suggests lines of thought worthy of exploration and testing.[12]
2. But if A were true, C would be a matter of course.	*Proposition 2*	
3. Therefore there is reason to suspect that A is true.[15]	The role of expecting *care* and *comfort* determines a relation between *patient* and *nurse* that establishes a path for influence of *nurse* on the *patient.*	

not establish truth. Its function is to originate ideas about selected phenomena that can be further developed and tested. The theory models approach is most useful as a strategy for devising theory in a field that has few available theories; innovation is indicated to advance the knowledge in describing and understanding selected observations.[15,17]

The retroductive theorist approaches the development of wanted theory by identifying a source theory in another field that may have the potential for developing the wanted theory. The theory models approach is based on the use of analogy and metaphor between two sets of phenomena. This requires that the theorist possess considerable creativity and an intuitive knowledge of the phenomena of interest.[13] The theory models approach is represented as follows:[14,15]

$$Theory_1 \longrightarrow \begin{array}{c} Theory \\ Model \end{array} \longrightarrow Theory_2$$

(Source theory)   (Wanted theory)

Therefore theory models are not *models of,* but are *models for* devising representations of selected phenomena.[13] The theory model is essentially a meta-model, which serves as a model to develop theory.[14]

To devise a theory using retroductive inference, the theorist seeks out a source theory to form a theory model. The wanted theory is devised from this theory model. The source theory is selected on the basis of a similarity in structure, form, or relationships between the two sets of phenomena.[15] The selected source theory is perceived to present ideas that may be useful for developing a theory about the observations of interest. These ideas are selected from theory 1 and formed into a point of view or theory model that will serve as the framework for developing theory 2. This approach is based on the assumption that new conjectures, or ideas, in a given field may be devised from other conjectures in theories in other fields.[4,5,15] The ideas selected from theory 1 for the theory model may involve any combination of concepts, hypothesized relationships, or theory structures. The viewpoint presented by the theory model is used to develop theory 2 by adding content to the theory model and by altering concepts and relationships to fit the phenomenon of interest for theory 2. It should be clear that this process of theory building is not simply borrowing a theory from one field and applying it unchanged to another.[12] The following components result in a new theory: the deliberate selection of aspects of theory 1 to form the theory model, the addition of new information, and the alteration of concepts and relationships for congruence with different phenomena in a new context. A theory devised by this method must meet the criteria for adequacy of a theory.[12] As Steiner (Maccia)[5,14,15] argued, the theory models approach cannot be considered reductive because theory 1 is not equivalent to theory 2.

To be reductive, the theorist would simply borrow concepts and hypotheses and use them, as formulated, in a new context. This approach cannot be considered deductive either, because theory 2 was not developed by deduction from theory 1. The hypotheses in theory 2 cannot be derived from theory 1.[14,15]

The use of analogy to develop theory has been a common occurrence in the development of many scientific fields. In Sigmund Freud's time, the machine model was a popular advanced model. Freud used the notion of machine operations to develop his theoretical assertions about psychological tension-reduction relationships in his theory of psychosexual development. Three or more decades ago, basic texts in human anatomy and physiology used the telephone switchboard as an analogy for explaining brain function. Currently, the computer is often used as a model for contemplating the brain and for developing theories of human information processing.[6,11] In nursing, general systems theory has been used as a model for developing nursing theory.[7] Steiner's development of the theory models approach provides guidelines for using this strategy in theory building.

Stevens[16] has argued that a large amount of nursing research has little impact on nursing practice because nursing research is often based on the categories and characteristics of borrowed theories. A borrowed theory tends to be used, unchanged, in the new context. Although theories in other fields may suggest a possible framework for addressing phenomena in the field of nursing, this framework may need to be contextualized within nursing. That is, aspects of the borrowed theory may need to be altered to reflect the appropriate categories and characteristics within nursing. Walker and Avant's derivation strategy for theory construction[17] draws from the theory models approach that Steiner developed. Walker and Avant[17] present many examples of using the derivation strategy to use and reformulate concepts, theoretical statements, and theories from other fields to the nursing field. The theory models approach permits the translation and expansion of ideas within the milieu of nursing and may result in the development of a new nursing theory. A nursing theory devised by this method can be further devel-

oped through the use of deductive strategies. Table 4-1 presents a summary of deducive, inductive, and retroductive forms of reasoning.

In contrast to the reasoning based on traditional logical assumptions presented in this chapter, scholarly work is also ongoing with other unconventional approaches to logic, such as fuzzy set theory and fuzzy logic theory, which provides a model for modes of reasoning that are approximate rather than exact. For example, Bosque[1] uses fuzzy logic in nursing to devise a theoretical perspective of nurse and machine symbiosis in the design of a new neonatal pulse oximeter alarm.

REFERENCES

1. Bosque, E.M. (1995). Symbiosis of nurse and machine through fuzzy logic: Improved specificity of neonatal pulse oximeter alarm. *Advances in Nursing Science,* 18(2), 67-75.
2. Geach, P.T. (1979). *Reason and argument.* Los Angeles: University of California Press.
3. Giere, R.N. (1979). *Understanding scientific reasoning.* New York: Holt, Rinehart, & Winston.
4. Maccia, E.S. & Maccia, G. (1966). *Construction of educational theory derived from three educational theory models* (Project No. 5-0638). Washington, DC: U.S. Department of Health, Education, and Welfare.
5. Maccia, E.S., Maccia, G., & Jewett, R. (1963). *Construction of educational theory models* (Cooperative Research Project No. 1632). Washington, DC: Office of Education, U.S. Department of Health, Education, and Welfare.
6. Norman, D.A. (1976). *Memory and attention: An introduction to human information processing.* New York: John Wiley & Sons.
7. Nursing Theories Conference Group. (1990). *Nursing theories: The base for professional nursing practice* (3rd ed.). Norwalk, CT: Appleton & Lange.
8. Pospesel, H. (1974). *Propositional logic.* Englewood Cliffs, NJ: Prentice Hall.
9. Salmon, W.C. (1967). *The foundations of scientific inference.* Pittsburgh: University of Pittsburgh Press.
10. Salmon, W.C. (1973). *Logic.* Englewood Cliffs, NJ: Prentice Hall.
11. Shepherd, G.M. (1974). *The synaptic organization of the brain.* New York: Oxford University Press.
12. Steiner, E. (1976). *Logical and conceptual analytic techniques for educational researchers.* Unpublished paper presented at the American Educational Research Association, San Francisco. Copyright © Elizabeth Steiner. All rights reserved.
13. Steiner, E. (1976). *The complete act of educational inquiry.* Unpublished. Copyright © Elizabeth Steiner. All rights reserved.
14. Steiner, E. (1977). *Criteria for theory of art education.* Unpublished paper presented at the Seminar for Research in Art Education, Philadelphia. Copyright © Elizabeth Steiner. All rights reserved.
15. Steiner, E. (1978). *Logical and conceptual analytic techniques for educational researchers.* Washington, DC: University Press.
16. Stevens, B. (1979). *Nursing theory: Analysis, application, evaluation.* Boston: Little, Brown.
17. Walker, L.O. & Avant, K.C. (1995). *Strategies for theory construction in nursing.* Norwalk, CT: Appleton & Lange.
18. Weiner, P. (1958). *Values in universe of chance.* New York: Doubleday.

$\mathcal{T}$heory Development Process

Sue Marquis Bishop

$\mathcal{N}$ursing theory development is not a mysterious, magical activity. Many nurses have been developing their own private ideas about the practice of nursing since their first day in the field (or perhaps before) and have continued to develop private assumptions based on their readings and experiences. These private notions may include such generalizations as a clean, smooth bed allows for greater rest and less need for pain medication for a patient, or encouraging the patient to have some say in his or her care leads to greater cooperation with treatment procedures. Nurses usually do not talk explicitly about their private theories, although these theories may influence the nursing activities they choose to implement and the manner in which they practice.

If in fact all nurses are evolving private theories of nursing, why all the fuss about studying published theories? The major reason is that nurses' private conceptions of nursing may be incomplete, inconsistent, or muddled.* This leads to considerable problems in using the private theory as a sound basis for practice. Further, an incomplete, inconsistent, or muddled the-

Previous author: Sue Marquis Bishop.
*I wish to acknowledge my indebtedness to Nicholas Mullins, one of my former teachers, for his discussion of private and public theories and for communicating both the complexity and creative playfulness in theoretical work.

ory may be difficult to use in studying clinical nursing situations that would advance nursing knowledge. If the availability of more systematic theories would provide a clearer understanding of nursing and would enable the exploration of whether this understanding corresponds with activities in nursing practice, then, as Hardy[13] notes, the rigorous development of nursing theory is a priority. The systematic development of scientific nursing theories has a better chance of advancing nursing and may lead to the basis for advancing nursing science.

It is important to grasp the concept of *systematic development*. Approaches to the construction of theory differ. However, one aspect they have in common is the agreement among scientists to approach theory development in a systematic fashion and to make the stages in development explicit so others can review the logical processes and test the presented hypotheses. The nurse who systematically devises a theory of nursing and presents it to the nursing community for public review is engaging in the process essential to advancing theory development.

THEORY COMPONENTS

Hage[12] identified six components of a complete theory and specified the contribution each makes to the

Table 5-1

Theory Components and Their Contributions to the Theory	
THEORY COMPONENTS	**CONTRIBUTIONS**
Concepts	Description and classification
Theoretical statements	Analysis
Definitions	
Theoretical	Meaning
Operational	Measurements
Linkages	
Theoretical	Plausibility
Operational	Testability
Ordering of concepts and definitions into primitive and derived terms	Elimination of overlap (tautology)
Ordering of statements and linkages into premises and equations	Elimination of inconsistency

Modified from Hage, J. (1972). *Techniques and problems in theory construction in sociology.* New York: John Wiley & Sons.

whole theory (Table 5-1). He argued that the failure to include one or more of the components resulted in the elimination of that particular contribution to the total theory. These six aspects of a theory are discussed as a basis for understanding the function of each element in the theory building process.

Concepts

Concepts, the building blocks of theories, classify the phenomena of interest.[12,16] In any separate discussion of concepts, it is crucial to recognize that concepts must not be considered separately from the theoretical system in which they are embedded and from which they derive their meaning.[5] Concepts may have completely different meanings in different theoretical systems. Scientific progress is based on the critical review and testing of a researcher's work by the scientific community; therefore consensus regarding the meaning of scientific concepts is important.[5,12]

Concepts may be classified as abstract or concrete. Abstract concepts are independent of a specific time or place, whereas concrete concepts relate to a particular time or place.[12,26]

Abstract Concepts	*Concrete Concepts*
Social system	The Jackson Family; University of North Carolina at Charlotte
Debate	Gore-Bush Debate

In the above example, the Jackson family is an example of the more general, abstract concept of social system.

Concepts may be classified as discrete or continuous. This system of labels differentiates the concepts that vary along a continuum from the concepts that specify categories of phenomena.

A *discrete concept* identifies categories or classes of phenomena, such as patient, nurse, or environment. A student can become a nurse or choose another discipline, but he or she cannot become a partial nurse. Therefore phenomena are identified as either belonging to or not belonging to a given class. For that reason, discrete concepts have been called nonvariable concepts.[9] Sorting phenomena into nonvariable, discrete categories carries the assumption that the reality associated with the given phenomenon is captured by the classification.[12] The amount or degree is not an issue. Max Weber devised the discrete concept of bureaucracy as an ideal type to characterize organizations.[20] Organizations can then be classified as *bureaucratic* or *nonbureaucratic.*

The definition of the discrete concept is critical in knowing how to classify the phenomenon. Theories may be developed using a series of nonvariable discrete concepts (and subconcepts) to build typologies.[26] Blegen and Tripp-Reimer[3] argued that the development of taxonomies of nursing diagnoses, nursing interventions, and nursing outcomes can facilitate theory building for nursing practice. *Typologies* consist of a systematic arrangement of the concepts. For example, a typology on marital status could be partitioned into marital statuses in which a population could be classified. These discrete categories could be further partitioned to permit the classification of an additional variable in this typology; for example, gender could be included and the typology could be used to classify subjects.

Typology of Marital Status

Married	Single/ Never Married	Divorced	Widowed
Male	Male	Male	Male·
Female	Female	Female	Female

A *continuous concept* permits the classification of dimensions or gradations of a phenomenon on a continuum, such as degree of marital conflict. For example, marital couples may be classified across a range representing the amount of marital conflict in their relationships.

Degree of Marital Conflict

0 ←—————————→ 120
Low   High

Other continuous concepts that may be used to classify couples could include degree of communication and number of shared activities. The use of variable concepts based on a range or a continuum tends to be focused on one dimension without assuming that a single dimension captures all the reality connected with the phenomenon.[9] Additional dimensions may be devised to measure further aspects of the phenomenon. In contrast to the nonvariable term *bureaucracy,* variable concepts, such as rate of conflict, ratio of professional to nonprofessional staff, and communication flow, may be used to characterize organizations.[12] Although nonvariable concepts are useful in classifying phenomena in theory development, Hage[12] has argued that major breakthroughs have occurred in several fields when the focus shifted from nonvariable to variable concepts. Variable concepts permit the scoring of the phenomenon's full range on a continuum.[12]

The development of theoretical concepts permits the description and classification of phenomena.[12] The labeled concept suggests boundaries for selecting phenomena to observe and for reasoning about the phenomena of interest. New concepts may focus attention on new phenomena or they may facilitate thinking about and classifying phenomena in a different way.[12]

Theoretical Statements

Although concepts are considered the building blocks of theory, they must be connected with a set of theoretical statements to devise theory.[2,5,9,20,28] The development of theoretical statements asserting a connection between two or more concepts introduces the possibility of analysis.[9]

Statements in a theory can be classified into three general categories: (1) existence statements, (2) definitions, and (3) relational statements.[26,35] Existence statements and definitions relate to specific concepts. Whereas definitions provide descriptions of the concept, existence statements simply assert that a given concept exists and is labeled with the concept name. Relational statements assert relationships between the properties of two or more concepts or variables. Various types of relational statements have been described in the literature.[23,26,35] Discussion in this chapter is limited to an introduction to probabilistic statements and necessary and sufficient conditional statements. These types of statements are important in understanding scientific reasoning.[11]

In the connections between variables, one variable may be assumed to influence a second variable. In this instance, the first variable may be labeled an antecedent (or determinant) variable and the second variable a consequent (or resultant) variable.[11,32,37] In this case, the first variable may be viewed as the independent variable and the second as the dependent variable.[11] On account of its complexity, nursing presents a situation in which multiple antecedents and consequences may be involved in studying a selected phenomenon. However, Zetterberg[37] concluded that the development of two-variate theoretical statements could be an important intermediate step in the development of a theory. These statements can be reformulated later as the theory evolves or as new information becomes available.

Relational statements may be expressed as either a necessary or sufficient condition, or both. These labels characterize the conditions that help explain the nature of the relationship between the two variables in the theoretical statements.

For example, a relational statement expressed as a sufficient condition could be: if nurses react with approval of patients' independent behaviors (NAPIB), patients increase their efforts in self-care activities (PSC). This is a type of compound statement linking antecedent and consequent variables. The statement does not assert the truth of the antecedent. Rather, the assertion is made that if the antecedent is true, then the consequent is true.[11] In addition, no assertion appears in the statement explaining why the antecedent is related to the consequent.[12] In symbolic notation form, the above statements can be expressed as:

$$NAPIB \longrightarrow PSC$$
$$(\text{Antecedent/determinant} \longrightarrow$$
$$\text{Consequent/resultant})$$

This statement asserts that nurse approval of a patient's independent behaviors is sufficient for the occurrence of the patient's self-care activities. However, patient assumption of self-care activities resulting from other factors, such as the patient's health status and personality variables, is not ruled out. There could be other antecedents that are sufficient conditions for the patient's assumption of self-care activities.

A statement in the form of a necessary condition asserts that one variable is required for the occurrence of another variable.[11,24,28] For example:

Without the motivation to get well (MGW), patients will not adhere strictly to their prescribed treatment regimen (PTR).

$$MGW \longrightarrow PTR$$

This means PTR never occurs when MGW does not occur.[11,24] No assertion is made that the patients' strict adherence to the PTRs comes from their MGW. However, it is asserted that if the MGW is absent, patients will not assume strict adherence to their PTR. The MGW is a necessary, but not a sufficient, condition for the occurrence of this consequent.

The term *if* is generally used to introduce a sufficient condition, whereas *only if* and *if . . . then* are used to introduce necessary conditions.[11] In most instances, conditional statements are not both necessary and sufficient.[11] However, it is possible for a statement to express both conditions. In such instances, the term *if* and *only if* is used to imply that the conditions are both necessary and sufficient for one another.[11] In this case, (1) the consequent never occurs in the absence of the antecedent and (2) the consequent always occurs when the antecedent occurs.[11,24]

Although causal statements (one variable causes another) may be expressed as a conditional statement, not all conditional statements are causal.[11] For example, the following statement, "If this month is March, then the next month is April," does not assert that March causes April to occur. Rather, the sequence of months suggests that April follows March.[8] (For an extensive discussion of conditional and unconditional causal statements, see Nowak.[24])

Probabilistic statements are generally derived from statistical data and express connections that do not always occur, but are likely to occur based on some estimate of probability.[35] Walker and Avant[35] used this example: regular inhaling of tobacco smoke may likely lead to cancer of the lung. It is clear that cigarette smoking (CS) does not always lead to lung cancer because some persons who smoke do not develop this disease. However, the probability of developing lung cancer (P LC) is increased for cigarette smokers. In symbolic notation:[26]

$$IF\ CS \longrightarrow P\ LC$$

The development of relational statements that assert connections between variables provides for analysis and establishes the basis for explanation and prediction.[12]

Definitions

The development of science is a collaborative endeavor in which the community of scientists critique, test, and build upon each other's work.[4] Therefore it is crucial that the concepts are as clearly defined as possible to reduce any ambiguity in understanding the given concept or set of concepts.

Although it is not possible to eliminate perceived differences in meaning entirely, offering explicit definitions can minimize these differences. In the development of a complete theory, both theoretical and operational definitions provide meaning for the concept and a basis for seeking empirical indicators.[9] Theoretical definitions also permit consideration of the relationship between a given concept and other theoretical ideas, but a clear meaning for concepts is not sufficient.

If theories are to be tested against reality, then concepts must be measurable.[12] Operational definitions relate the concepts to observable phenomena by specifying empirical indicators.[12] Hage[12] asserted that the concept name and the theoretical and operational definitions establish reference points for locating the concept; that is, viewing the concept as it is related to the theoretical systems and the observable environment.

Linkages

The specification of linkages is an important part of the development of theory.[12] Although the theoretical statements assert connections between concepts, the rationale for the stated connections must be developed. The development of theoretical linkages offers an explanation of why the variables in the theory may be connected in some manner; that is, the theoretical reasons for asserting particular interrelationships.[12] This rationale contributes plausibility to the theory.[12]

Operational linkages contribute the element of testability to the theory by specifying how variables are connected.[12] Although operational definitions provide for the measurability of the concepts, operational linkages provide for the testability of the assertions. The operational linkage contributes a perspective for understanding the nature of the relationship between concepts, such as whether the relationship between the concepts is negative or positive, linear or curvilinear.[12]

Ordering

Finally, Hage[12] concluded that a theory may be considered fairly complete if it presents the elements of

concepts, definitions, statements, and linkages. However, complete development of the theory requires organizing concepts and definitions into primitive and derived terms and organizing statements and linkages into premises and equations.[12] As the theory evolves, concepts and theoretical statements multiply and the need to establish some logical arrangement or ordering of the theoretical components arises to bring conceptual order to the theory.[12] Hage[12] stated that the concepts should be ordered if the theory contains more than two variables. He also recommended that concepts and definitions should be ordered into primitive and derived terms. Primitive terms are not defined within the theory. This process of ordering may identify any existing overlap between concepts and definitions.[12] The conceptual arrangement of statements and linkages into premises and equations may reveal areas of inconsistency.[12] Premises (or axioms) are regarded as the more general assertions from which the hypotheses are derived in the form of equations. Hage suggested that the ordering of statements and linkages is indicated when the theory contains a large number of theoretical statements.[12]

FORMS OF THEORY ORGANIZATIONS*

A formal theory is a systematically developed, conceptual system that addresses a given set of phenomena. There are different ideas about how this conceptual system should be organized to constitute a theory. Three forms for organizing theory are set-of-laws, axiomatic, and causal process.

Set-of-Laws Form

The set-of-laws approach attempts to organize findings from empirical research.[26] The theorist first reviews the research literature in an area of particular interest. Empirical findings from available research are identified and selected from the literature for evaluation. Findings are evaluated and sorted into categories based on the degree of empirical evidence

---

*This section is largely based on Reynolds' discussion[26] of these forms.

supporting each assertion.[19] The available categories are laws, empirical generalizations, and hypotheses.[26]

The construction of the set-of-laws form of theory requires the selection and evaluation of research findings in terms of the degree of empirical support; therefore several limitations emerge as a result of this approach to constructing theory. Reynolds[26] discussed these limitations as disadvantages to the set-of-laws approach to theory building.

First, the nature of research requires focusing on the relationships between a limited set of variables, which are often two variables. Therefore attempts to develop a set-of-laws theory from statements of findings may result in a lengthy number of statements that assert the relationships between two or more variables. This lengthy set of generalizations may be difficult to organize and interrelate.

Second, for research to be conducted, concepts must be operationally defined so they can be measurable. Therefore concepts in the statements of empirical findings are most likely to be measurable and operational. This procedure eliminates more highly abstract or theoretical concepts that might be useful in developing an understanding of the phenomenon of interest.

Reynolds[26] concluded that although the set-of-laws form may provide for the classification of phenomena or the predictions of relationships between selected variables, it does not permit understanding, which is crucial for the advancement of science. Finally, Reynolds[26] noted that each statement in the set-of-laws form is considered to be independent because the various statements have not been interrelated into a system of description and explanation (Figure 5-1). Therefore each statement must be tested. The statements are not interrelated; therefore research support for one statement does not provide support for any other statement. Research efforts must be more extensive.

The set-of-laws approach to theory building is consistent with the view that scientific knowledge consists of empirical findings and science is advanced by conducting research and searching for patterns in the data.[19] Patterns do not arise from empirical data of their own accord.[32] The theorist must bring ideas to experience to conceptualize and order theoretical relationships.[32] Reynolds[26] stated that this may be difficult to do with a lengthy list of empirical findings in the set-of-laws form.

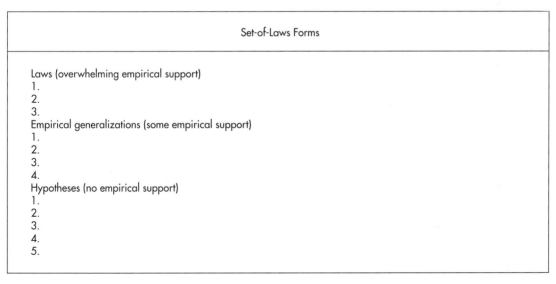

Set-of-Laws Forms

Laws (overwhelming empirical support)
1.
2.
3.
Empirical generalizations (some empirical support)
1.
2.
3.
4.
Hypotheses (no empirical support)
1.
2.
3.
4.
5.

Figure **5-1 Set-of-laws-forms.** (From P. Reynolds, A Primer in Theory Construction. Copyright © 1971 by Allyn & Bacon. Reprinted by permission.)

Axiomatic Form

In contrast to the set-of-laws forms, the axiomatic form of theory organization is an interrelated, logical system. Specifically, an axiomatic theory consists of explicit definitions, a set of concepts, a set of existence statements, and a set of relationship statements arranged in hierarchical order.[26,34,37] The concepts include highly abstract concepts, intermediate concepts, and more concrete concepts. The set of existence statements describes situations in which the theory is applicable.[26,34,35] Statements helping to delineate the boundaries of the theory are referred to as describing the scope conditions of the theory.[8,12,26] The relational statements consist of axioms and propositions. The highly abstract, theoretical statements, or axioms, are organized at the top of the hierarchy.[34] All other propositions are developed through logical deduction from the ax-ioms or from other more abstract propositions (Figure 5-2).[27]

The axiomatic theory is determined to be integrated when no propositions in Set B can be logically derived from Set A.[36] This results in a highly interrelated, explanatory system. An essential criterion for the axiomatic form is that the theoretical statements may not be contradictory.[36] A basic principle of logic asserts that when two statements are contradictory, one or both of the statements must be false.[28,36] Therefore axiomatic theorists seek to avoid this problem by developing a conceptual system with a few broad axioms from which a set of propositions can be derived.[29] As science progresses and new empirical data become known, the general axioms may be modified or extended. However, if these additions to the logical system produce contradictions in the theory, the theory must be rejected

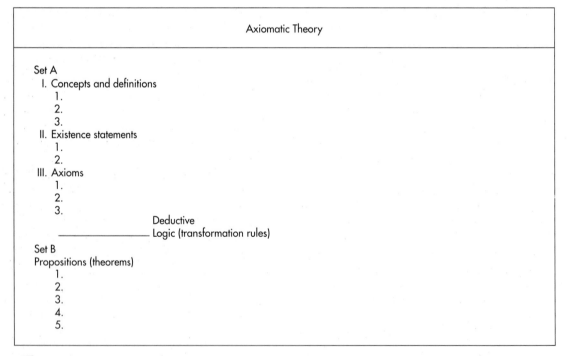

Figure 5-2 **Axiomatic theory represented in schematic form.** (Developed from Werkmeister, W. [1959]. Theory construction and the problem of objectivity. In L. Gross [Ed.], *Symposium of sociological theory.* Evanston, IL: Row, Peterson, & Co. [schemata]; and Reynolds, P. [1971]. *A primer in theory construction.* Indianapolis: Bobbs-Merrill [terminology].)

for a theory without contradictions.[29] New theories often subsume portions of previous theories as special cases.[5,36] For example, Einstein's Theory of Relativity incorporated Newton's Law of Gravitation as a special case within the theory.

Axiomatic theories are not common in the social and behavioral sciences, but they are clearly evident in the fields of physics and mathematics. For example, Euclidean geometry is an axiomatic theory.[36,37]

Developing theories in axiomatic form has several advantages.[26,28] First, because theory is a highly interrelated set of statements in which some statements are derived from others, all concepts do not need to be operationally defined.[26] This allows the theorist to incorporate some highly abstract concepts that may not be measurable, but provide explanation. The interrelated axiomatic system may also be more efficient for explanation than the lengthy number of theoretical statements in the set-of-laws form. In addition, empirical support for one theoretical statement may be judged to provide support for the theory, thereby permitting less extensive research than the requirement to test each statement in the set-of-laws form. Finally, Reynolds[26] concluded that, in certain instances, the axiomatic theory may be organized in a causal process form to increase understanding.

Causal Process Form

The distinguishing feature of the causal process form of theory is the development of theoretical statements that specify causal mechanisms between independent and dependent variables.[24,26] This form of theory organization consists of a set of concepts, a set of definitions, a set of existence statements, and a set of theoretical statements specifying causal process.[26] Concepts include abstract and concrete ideas. Existence statements function as they do in axiomatic theories to describe the scope conditions of the theory; that is, the situations to which the theory applies.[8,12,26] In contrast to the hierarchical arrangement in the axiomatic theory, causal process theories contain a set of statements describing the causal mechanisms or effects of one variable upon one or more other variables.[23,26] Causal

process theories may be limited to a few variables or they may be quite complex with several variables (Figure 5-3).

The causal statements specify the hypothesized effects of one variable upon one or more variables. In complex causal process theories, feedback loops and paths of influence through several variables may be hypothesized in the set of interrelated causal statements.[23,24] Reynolds[26] concluded that the causal process form of theory provides for an explanation of the process of how events happen. He identified several advantages of the causal process form of organization. First, like axiomatic theory, it provides for highly abstract, theoretical concepts. Second, like axiomatic theory, this form permits more efficient research testing with its interrelated theoretical statements. Finally, the causal process statements provide a sense of understanding in the phenomenon of interest that is not possible with other forms. However, Turner[34] observed that causal process theories might not include highly abstract concepts because a number of available theories simply contain descriptions of causal connections among events. This approach does permit the development of a causal explanation of the sequence of events that may affect the phenomenon of interest.[34]

CREATIVITY IN THEORY BUILDING

Although a number of strategies for developing theory have been presented in the literature, the theorist who attempts to approach theory construction in a mechanical way by applying structured procedures may have limited success. Theory building involves discovery and creativity. A scientific theory is clearly a creation of the human brain.[4] Bronowski[4] has written about the similarities in the processes of constructing theories and designing works of art; each requires a high level of imagination. In his view, "There is no difference in the use of such words as 'beauty' and 'truth' in the poem and such symbols as 'energy' and 'mass' in the equation."[4:21]

Although it is possible to teach specific techniques and content, it is not known how to facilitate creativity and originality in students. Rosenberg[27:2]

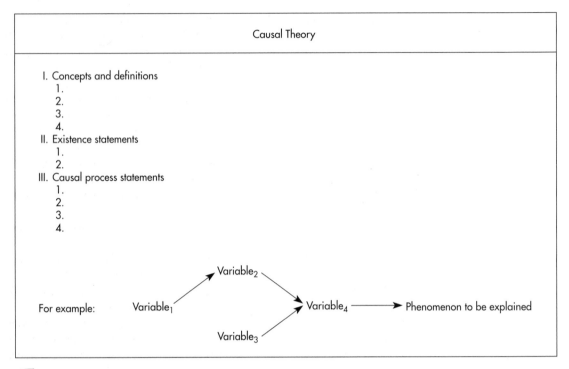

Figure 5-3 **Elements of causal theory.** (Developed from Reynolds, P. [1971]. *A primer in theory construction.* Indianapolis: Bobbs-Merrill; and Turner, J. [1978]. *The structure of sociological theory.* Homewood, IL: The Dorsey Press.)

stated, "You can teach someone how to look, but not how to see, how to search, but not how to find." Bronowski[4:22] suggests that a sense of "imagination, playfulness, and participation" is essential for the theorist and for the reader who seeks to understand theories. According to Bronowski,[4:22-23] "If science is a form of imagination, if all experiment is a form of play, then science cannot be dry-as-dust. Science, or art, every creative activity is fun. If a theorem in science seems dull to you, that is because you are not reading it with the same active sense of participation (and imagination) which you bring to the reading of a poem."

In addition to imagination, developing and presenting theories requires personal discipline. Innovative ideas tend to occur in an unconnected, ambiguous form.[21] Self-discipline is required to work with, develop, and express the idea in written form for others to review.[14] Rosenberg[27] stated that al-

though creativity cannot be taught, it can be nurtured and developed. The individual's role is to attain familiarity with the phenomenon of interest and continue to practice.[27]

NURSING THEORIES

During the 1960s and 1970s, the literature continued to address metatheoretical issues, such as the definition of nursing theory and whether or not nursing theories are merely frameworks. In 1980, Flaskerud and Halloran[9] noted that, although nurses identify formulations in nursing as only models or conceptual frameworks, they were not reluctant to label frameworks from other fields, such as psychology or sociology, as theories. They argued that this depreciated available efforts to systematize nursing. Meleis[19] characterized the early 1980s as the period of accepting the need to further develop nursing theory to advance the nursing discipline and as a time of lingering confusion in regard to the semantics of how theories were characterized. In 1985, Meleis asserted the view of several other nurse scholars. For example, in 1979, Stevens[33:28] stated:

> The differences between the different labels (theory, metaparadigm, conceptual frameworks, and so forth) are differences in emphasis rather than substance and are not worth the debate. . . . Why continue to unwittingly downgrade nursing theory by relegating it to a conceptual framework's status when other conceptualizations (in other fields) have been called theory. . . . A theory in process should not be considered a conceptual framework; it is simply in an expected stage in the process of development.

The use of rigorous criteria for a scientific theory to critique nursing formulations will surely result in nursing theories being found deficient because theory construction in nursing is still in the early stages. In efforts to prepare a new generation of nurse scholars to advance theory building in nursing, it may be more fruitful to give less attention to whether a given nursing formulation is a theory and concentrate on analyzing how much of a theory it is.[12]

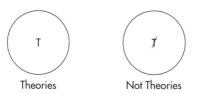

The major difficulty in discussing whether there is any (nursing) knowledge is that many individuals think about this issue in either-or terms. . . . We do not want an either-or conception of knowledge. Because we are used to reasoning in this way, we are prevented from perceiving that perhaps there is some knowledge in (nursing), albeit it is incomplete.[12:182*]

Once a nursing theory has been identified that fits an area of interest, several issues must be considered, such as the completeness of the theory, any missing components or relationships, the theory's internal consistency, the theory's correspondence with available empirical findings, and whether it is operationally defined for testing. Analyses of this nature logically lead to the consideration of the next steps in the development of this theory. The goal is to continue to direct attention and energies to the critical analysis of existing incomplete theories in terms of their potential for further development. In the 1990s, there was less preoccupation in nursing with the question of whether nursing formulations were really theories.

Scientific evidence can accumulate to support or refute theoretical assertions or provide the basis for suggesting modifications in a nursing theory only through repeated and rigorous research. Theory-testing research may lead to the decision to abandon one nursing theory in favor of another theory that explains available research data more adequately. However, in an analysis of 720 nursing practice studies in six research journals from 1977 to 1986, Moody and colleagues found that only three percent of the studies were designed to test theory from an explicit theoretical framework.[22] It is critical that theory-testing research in nursing continues to receive greater emphasis if nursing science is to advance. Current nursing literature reflects this need. Several nursing scholars have presented criteria for evaluating theory-testing research in nursing (for example, see Silva[30] and Acton, Irvin, and Hopkins[1]). These criteria emphasize the importance of using a nursing theory to design the purpose and focus of the study and to derive hypotheses and the necessity to relate the significance of the findings back to the nursing theory.

In recent years, the literature has given increasing attention to the appropriate methodology for the conduct of nursing inquiry and some authors

*Nursing has been substituted for sociology in Hage's statement[12] of conclusions about his field of sociology to illustrate relevance for states of affairs in nursing.

advocate for one method over another to advance the discipline of nursing. For example, some authors support quantitative or qualitative methods. Recent discussion is focusing on the effectiveness of using *methodological diversity,* or multiple methods, to advance nursing science.[2,10] It has been argued that the acceptance of multiple truths and the use of multiple methods in a research project builds several perspectives into the project and permits a richer and more fruitful exploration of the phenomena of interest. Further, multimethods may better ground the project in the context of clinical practice and lead to a more rapid development of the science of nursing. Acton and her colleagues suggested that "nurse scholars set aside methodological differences and avidly continue the pursuit of truth, in whatever form, using a variety of methodological approaches suited to scientific discovery and get on with advancing the discipline."[2:84]

In addition to the call for more rigorous theory-testing research in nursing, both nursing scholars and practitioners are arguing for the need for increased attention in the relationships between theory and practice (for example, see Chinn and Kramer,[6] Hoffman and Bertus,[14] Schlotfeldt,[29] Sparacino,[31] Liehr and Smith,[17] Lutz, Jones, and Kendall,[18] and Reed[25]). Recommendations include: (1) continued development of nursing theories that are relevant to nurses' specialty practice, (2) increased collaboration between scientists and practitioners, (3) increased encouragement of nurse researchers' efforts to communicate research findings to relevant practitioners, (4) increased effort to set a priority for using middle-range theories to devise linkages for research and practice in nursing, (5) increased emphasis on clinical research, and (6) increased use of nursing theories in clinical decision making. Regarding the use of nursing knowledge in clinical practice, Cody[7] asserted, "It is a professional nurse's ethical responsibility to utilize the knowledge base of her or his discipline."[7:4]

In 1992, in the first issue of the journal *Clinical Nursing Research,* Schlotfeldt[29:9] stated:

> It will be nursing's clinical scholars . . . that will identify the human phenomena that are central to nurses' practice . . . and that provoke consideration of the practice problems about which knowledge is needed but is not yet available. It is nursing's clinical scholarship that must be depended on to generate promising theories for testing that will advance nursing knowledge and ensure nursing's continued essential services to humankind.

Finally, the earlier focus on the development and refinement of grand nursing theories has evolved to an emphasis on the development of middle-range theories and focused situation-based theories and to an emphasis on the recent attention to situation-specific theories.[2,15,17,21,25] Contemporary nursing scholars are emphasizing: (1) pluralism in nursing theories, (2) continued development of philosophical inquiry, (3) methodological diversity in research, (4) emphasis on continued scholarship with middle-range theories and situation-specific theories, and (5) increased attention to developing stronger theory-research-practice linkages.

REFERENCES

1. Acton, G., Irvin, B., & Hopkins, B. (1991). Theory-testing research: Building the science. *Advances in Nursing Science, 14*(1), 52-61.
2. Acton, G., Irvin, B., Jensen, B., Hopkins, B., & Miller, E. (1997). Explicating middle-range theory through methodological diversity. *Advances in Nursing Science, 19*(3), 78-85.
3. Blegen, M. & Tripp-Reimer, T. (1997). Implications of nursing taxonomies for middle-range theory development. *Advances in Nursing Science, 19*(3), 37-49.
4. Bronowski, J. (1979). *The visionary age: Essay with arts, literature, and science.* Cambridge, MA: The MIT Press.
5. Brown, H. (1977). *Perception, theory and commitment: The new philosophy of science.* Chicago: The University of Chicago Press.
6. Chinn, P. & Kramer, M. (1991). *Theory and nursing: A systematic approach* (3rd ed.). St. Louis: Mosby.
7. Cody, W. (1997). Of tombstones, milestones, and gemstones: A retrospective and prospective on nursing theory. *Nursing Science Quarterly, 10*(1), 3-5
8. Dubin, R. (1978). *Theory building.* New York: The Free Press.
9. Flaskerud, J. & Halloran, E. (1980). Area of agreement in nursing theory development. *Advances in Nursing Science, 3,* 1-7.

10. Foster, L. (1997). Addressing epistemologic and practical issues in multimethod research: A procedure for conceptual triangulation. *Advances in Nursing Science,* 20(2), 1-12.

11. Giere, R.N. (1979). *Understanding scientific reasoning.* New York: Holt, Rhinehart, & Winston.

12. Hage, J. (1972). *Techniques and problems in theory construction in sociology.* New York: John Wiley & Sons.

13. Hardy, N. (1983). Metaparadigm and theory development. In N. Chaska (Ed.), *The nursing profession: A time to speak.* New York: McGraw-Hill.

14. Hoffman, A. & Bertus, P. (1991). Theory and practice: Bridging scientists' and practitioners' roles. *Archives of Psychiatric Nursing,* 7(1), 2-9.

15. Im, E. & Meleis, A. (1999). Situation-specific theories: Philosophical roots, properties and approach. *Advances in Nursing Science,* 22(2), 11-24.

16. Kaplan, A. (1964). *The conduct of inquiry: Methodology for behavioral science.* New York: Chandler.

17. Liehr, P. & Smith, M.J. (1999). Middle range theory: Spinning research and practice to create knowledge for the new millennium. *Advances in Nursing Science,* 21(4), 81-91.

18. Lutz, K., Jones, K., & Kendall, J. (1997). Expanding the praxis debate: Contributions to clinical inquiry. *Advances in Nursing Science,* 20(2), 13-22.

19. Meleis, A. (1985). *Theoretical nursing: Development and progress.* Philadelphia: J.B. Lippincott.

20. Merton, R.K. (Ed.). (1952). *Reader in bureaucracy.* New York: The Free Press.

21. Mills, C.W. (1959). On intellectual craftsmanship. In L. Gross (Ed.), *Symposium on sociological theory.* Evanston, IL: Row, Peterson, & Co.

22. Moody, L., Wilson, M., Smyth, K., Schwartz, R., Tittle, M., & VanCott, M.L. (1988). Analysis of a decade of nursing research: 1977-1986. *Nursing Research,* 27(6), 374-379.

23. Mullins, N. (1971). *The art of theory: Construction and use.* New York: Harper & Row.

24. Nowak, S. (1975). Causal interpretations of statistical relationships in social research. In H. Blalock (Ed.), *Quantitative sociology: International perspectives on mathematical and statistical modeling.* New York: Academic Press.

25. Reed, P. (2000). Nursing reformation: Historical reflections and philosophic foundations. *Nursing Science Quarterly,* 13(2), 129-136.

26. Reynolds, P. (1971). *A primer in theory construction.* Indianapolis: Bobbs-Merrill.

27. Rosenberg, J. (1978). *The practice of philosophy.* Englewood Cliffs, NJ: Prentice Hall.

28. Salmon, W.D. (1973). *Logic.* Englewood Cliffs, NJ: Prentice Hall.

29. Schlotfeldt, R. (1992). Why promote clinical nursing scholarship? *Clinical Nursing Research,* 1(1), 5-8.

30. Silva, M. (1986). Research testing nursing theory: State of the art. *Advances in Nursing Science,* 9(10), 1-11.

31. Sparacino, P. (1991). The reciprocal relationship between practice and theory. *Clinical Nurse Specialist,* 5(3), 138.

32. Steiner, E. (1978). *Logical and conceptual analytic techniques for educational researchers.* Washington, DC: University Press.

33. Stevens, B. (1979). *Nursing theory: Analysis, application and evaluation.* Boston: Little, Brown.

34. Turner, J. (1978). *The structure of sociological theory.* Homewood, IL: The Dorsey Press.

35. Walker, L. & Avant, K. (1983). *Strategies for theory construction in nursing.* Norwalk, CT: Appleton-Century-Crofts.

36. Werkmeister, W. (1959). Theory construction and the problem of objectivity. In L. Gross (Ed.), *Symposium of sociological theory.* Evanston, IL: Row, Peterson, & Co.

37. Zetterberg, H.L. (1966). *On theory and verification in sociology.* New York: John Wiley & Sons.

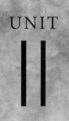

UNIT

II

Philosophies

- Nursing philosophy sets forth the meaning of nursing phenomena through analysis, reasoning, and logical argument.

- Philosophies contribute to nursing knowledge by providing direction for the discipline and forming a basis for professional scholarship, which leads to new theoretical understanding.

- Nursing philosophies represent early works that predate the theory era and later works of a philosophical nature.

- Philosophies are works that provide a broad understanding, which are used to further the discipline in its professional application.

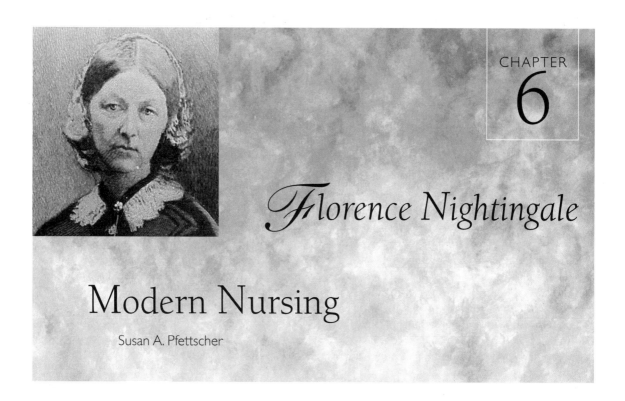

Florence Nightingale

Modern Nursing

Susan A. Pfettscher

CREDENTIALS AND BACKGROUND OF THE THEORIST

Florence Nightingale, the matriarch of modern nursing, was born on May 12, 1820. At the time of her birth, her parents were on an extended European tour. Her parents, Edward and Frances Nightingale, named their daughter after her birthplace, Florence, Italy. The Nightingales were a well-educated, affluent, aristocratic Victorian family who maintained residences in Derbyshire (Lea Hurst was their original home) and in Hampshire (Embley Park). This latter residence was near London, which allowed the family to participate in London's spring and autumn social seasons.

Although the extended Nightingale family was large, the immediate family included only Florence Nightingale and her elder sister, Parthenope. During her childhood, Nightingale's father educated her

Previous authors: Susan A. Pfettscher, Karen R. de Graff, Ann Marriner Tomey, Cynthia L. Mossman, and Maribeth Slebodnik.

much more broadly and rigorously than other young women of her time were educated. Nightingale was tutored in mathematics, languages, religion, and philosophy (subjects that later influenced the course of her work). Although she participated in the usual Victorian aristocratic activities and social events during her adolescence, Nightingale developed the sense that her life should become more useful.

In 1837, Nightingale[15:41] wrote about her *calling* in her diary; she wrote, "God spoke to me and called me to his service." Her calling was unclear to her for some time. After she understood that she was *called* to become a nurse, she was finally able to complete her training in 1851 when she was accepted for training at Kaiserworth, Germany, a Protestant religious community with a hospital facility. She stayed there for approximately three months and, at the end, her teachers declared her to be trained as a nurse.

Following her return to England, Nightingale began to examine hospital facilities, reformatories, and charitable institutions. Only two years after completing her training (in 1853), she became the superintendent of the Hospital for Invalid Gentlewomen in London.

During the Crimean War, Nightingale received a request from Sidney Herbert (a family friend and Secretary of War) to go to Scutari, Turkey to provide trained nurses to care for wounded soldiers. She arrived in November of 1854. To achieve her mission of providing nursing care, she needed to address the environmental problems that existed, including the lack of sanitation and the presence of filth (few chamber pots, contaminated water, contaminated sheets and blankets, and overflowing cesspools). In addition, the soldiers were faced with exposure, frostbite, lice infestations, and other opportunistic diseases during their recovery from battle wounds.[37]

Nightingale's work in improving these deplorable conditions made her a popular and revered person to the soldiers, but the support of physicians and military officers was less than enthusiastic. She was called "The Lady of the Lamp," as immortalized in the poem "Santa Filomena" by Henry Wadsworth Longfellow,[21] because she made ward rounds during the night. In Scutari, Nightingale became critically ill with Crimean fever, which might have been typhus or brucellosis.

Following the war, Nightingale returned to England to great accolades, particularly from the Royal family (Queen Victoria) and the soldiers who had served in the Crimean War. She was awarded funds in recognition of this work, which she used to establish a teaching institution for nurses at St. Thomas Hospital and King's College Hospital in London. Within a few years after it was founded, the Nightingale School began receiving requests to establish new schools at hospitals worldwide. Florence Nightingale's reputation as the founder of modern nursing was established.[20]

During her life, Nightingale devoted her energies to societal issues and causes in an attempt to create social change.[16] She continued to concentrate on army sanitation reform, the functions of army hospitals, sanitation in India, and sanitation and healthcare of the poor in England. Her writings, *Notes on Matters Affecting the Health, Efficiency, and Hospital Administration of the British Army,*[30] *Notes on Hospitals,*[31] and *Report on Measures Adopted for Sanitary Improvements in India from June 1869 to June 1870,*[32] reflect her continuing concerns about these issues, particularly for the military.

Shortly after her return to England, Nightingale confined herself to her residence, citing her continued ill health. However, she wrote between 15,000 and 20,000 letters to friends, acquaintances, allies, and opposition from this environment. Her written word was strong and clear and conveyed her beliefs, observations, and desire for changes in healthcare. Through this medium, her work was successfully achieved. In addition, she received the most powerful visitors in her home to maintain her dialogue with them, plot strategies to support causes, and carry out her work.

In her lifetime, Nightingale's work was recognized through the many awards she received from her own country and many other countries. She was able to work into her eighties and died in her sleep on August 13, 1910 at age 90.

Modern biographies and essays have attempted to analyze Nightingale's lifework through her family relationships (notably with her parents and sister) and film dramatizations have frequently and inaccurately focused on her personal relationships. Although her personal and public life holds great intrigue for many, often these retrospective analyses are either very negative and harshly critical or overly positive in their descriptions of this Victorian leader. Kalisch and Kalisch[17,18,19] have provided a critique of these multiple media portrayals that may assist the reader in better understanding the many portrayals of Florence Nightingale. The recently published book by Dossey,[8] *Florence Nightingale: Mystic, Visionary, Healer,* provides the reader with another in-depth history and interpretation of Nightingale's personal life and work. Using multiple quotes from Nightingale's own writings (her diaries and letters) and from those persons with whom she interacted and corresponded during her lifetime, Dossey[8] focuses on interpreting the spiritual nature of her being and her lifework, creating a new way of looking at Florence Nightingale.

THEORETICAL SOURCES FOR THEORY DEVELOPMENT

Many factors influenced the development of Nightingale's theory for nursing. Individual, societal, and professional values were all integral to the development of her work. She combined her individual resources with societal and professional resources to produce change.

Nightingale's education from her father was an unusual one for a Victorian girl. Her tutelage in subjects such as mathematics and philosophy from her well-educated, intellectual father provided her with the knowledge and conceptual thought that was unique for women of her time. Her Aunt Mai, a devoted relative and champion, described her as having a great mind; this was a description not used to describe Victorian women, but one totally accepted for Nightingale. It remains unknown whether or not Nightingale was a genius who developed her greatness through her unique, formal education; however, she would have likely been a leader in any century.

The Nightingale family's aristocratic social status provided her with access to persons of power and influence. Many were family friends, such as Stanley Herbert, who remained important to Nightingale throughout her life. She comprehended the political process of Victorian England through the experiences of her father in his short-lived political foray. Nightingale likely used this knowledge as she successfully waged political battles for her causes.

Nightingale also recognized the societal changes of her time and their impact on the health status of individuals. The industrial age had descended on England, which created new social classes, new diseases, and new social problems. Dickens' social commentaries and novels provided English society with scathing commentaries on healthcare and the need for both health and social reform in England. In particular, in his novel *Martin Chuzzlewit,*[7] his portrayal of Sarey Gamp, a drunken, untrained nurse provided society with an image of the horrors of Victorian untrained nursing. Nightingale's alliance with Dickens undoubtedly served as a factor in her definitions of nursing and healthcare and in her the-

ory for nursing and provided her with a forum to express her views about social and healthcare issues.[8,17,40]

Similar dialogues with many political leaders, intellectuals, and social reformers of the day (John Stuart Mill, Benjamin Jowett, Edwin Chadwick, and Harriet Marineau) developed Nightingale's philosophical and logical thinking, which is evident in her theory for nursing.[8,17,40] Most likely, these dialogues allowed her to continue to strive to change the things she viewed as unacceptable in the society in which she lived. No other nursing leader could better exemplify Chinn and Jacobs' statement[4:46] that "when individual or professional values are in conflict with and challenge societal values, there is potential for creating change in society."

Finally, Nightingale's religious affiliation and beliefs were especially strong sources for her nursing theory. Reared as a Unitarian, her religious belief that action for the benefit of others is a primary way of serving God is the foundation for her defining her nursing work as a religious calling. In addition, the Unitarian faith strongly supported the education of persons as a means of developing their divine potential and helping them move toward perfection in their lives and in their service to God. Nightingale's faith provided her with personal strength throughout her life and provided her with the belief that education was a critical factor in establishing the profession of nursing. Also, religious conflicts of the time (particularly Anglican-Catholic) may have provided her with the strongly held belief that nursing could and should be a *secular* profession.[8,14,27,40] Despite her strong religious beliefs and her acknowledgment of her *calling,* this was not a requirement for her nurses. Indeed, her opposition to the work of the nuns in Crimea (she reported that they were proselytizing) escalated the conflict to the level of the Pope's involvement.[8,40] As parish nursing has seen a resurgence in the United States and missionary work by nurses continues throughout the world, Nelson's review[27] of pastoral care in the nineteenth century provides an historical view of the role of religious service in nursing.

USE OF EMPIRICAL EVIDENCE

Nightingale's reports describing health and sanitary conditions in the Crimea and in England identify her as an outstanding scientist and empirical researcher. Her expertise as a statistician is also evident in the reports that she generated throughout her lifetime on the varied subjects of healthcare, nursing, and social reform.

Nightingale's carefully collected information that proved the efficacy of her hospital nursing system and organization during the Crimean War is perhaps her best known work. Her written report of her experiences and collected data in *Notes on Matters Affecting the Health, Efficiency, and Hospital Administration of the British Army*[30] was submitted to the British Royal Sanitary Commission. This commission had been organized in response to Nightingale's charges of poor sanitary conditions. The data in this report provided a strong argument in favor of her proposed reforms in the Crimean hospital barracks. According to Cohen,[5] she invented the polar-area diagram to dramatically represent the extent of needless death in the British military hospitals in the Crimea. In this article, Cohen[5:128] summarizes the work of Nightingale as both a researcher and a statistician by noting that "she helped to pioneer the revolutionary notion that social phenomena could be objectively measured and subjected to mathematical analysis." Palmer[33] identified Nightingale's research skills as including recording, communicating, ordering, coding, conceptualizing, inferring, analyzing, and synthesizing. The observation of social phenomena at both an individual and systems level was especially important to Nightingale and serves as the basis of her writings. Nightingale emphasized the concurrent use of observation and the performance of tasks in the education of nurses and expected them to continue to use these concurrent activities in their work.

MAJOR CONCEPTS & DEFINITIONS

Nightingale's theory focused on the environment. Murray and Zenther[26:149] define environment as "all the external conditions and influences affecting the life and development of an organism and capable of preventing, suppressing, or contributing to disease, accidents, or death." Although Nightingale never specifically used the term *environment* in her writing, she did define and describe in detail the concepts of ventilation, warmth, light, diet, cleanliness, and noise, which are components of the environment.

Although Nightingale often defined concepts precisely, she did not separate the patient's environment specifically into physical, emotional, or social aspects; she apparently assumed that all of these aspects were included in the environment. In reading *Notes on Nursing*[28] and her other writings, it is easy to identify her emphasis on the *physical* environment. In the context of the specific issues that she had identified and struggled to improve and correct in various settings (war-torn environment and workhouses) and within the context of the time, this emphasis appears to be most appropriate.[10] Her concern about healthy surroundings included not only the hospital settings in both the Crimea and England, but it also extended to the private homes of patients and to the physical living conditions of the poor. She believed that healthy surroundings were necessary for proper nursing care. Her theory of the five essential components of environmental health (pure air, pure water, efficient drainage, cleanliness, and light) are as essential today as they were 150 years ago.

Proper ventilation for the patient seemed to be of greatest concern to Nightingale; her charge to nurses was to "keep the air he breathes as pure as the external air, without chilling him."[28:12]

MAJOR CONCEPTS & DEFINITIONS—cont'd

Notwithstanding her rejection of the germ theory (newly developed at the time), Nightingale's emphasis on proper ventilation seemed to recognize this environmental component as a source of disease and recovery.

The concept of light was also of importance in Nightingale's theory.[28] In particular, she identified direct sunlight as a particular need of patients. She specifically noted that "light has quite as real and tangible effects upon the human body. . . . Who has not observed the purifying effect of light, and especially of direct sunlight, upon the air of a room?"[28:84-85] To achieve the beneficial effects of sunlight, nurses were instructed to move and position patients to expose them to sunlight.

Cleanliness as a concept is another critical component of Nightingale's environmental theory.[28] In regard to this concept, she specifically addressed the patient, the nurse, and the physical environment. She noted that a dirty environment (floors, carpets, walls, and bed linens) was a source of infection through the organic matter it contained. Even if the environment was well ventilated, the presence of organic material created a dirty area; therefore the appropriate handling and disposal of bodily excretions and sewage was required to prevent contamination of the environment. Finally, Nightingale advocated the bathing of patients on a frequent, even daily, basis at a time when this practice was not the norm. In addition, she required that nurses also bathe daily, that their clothing was clean, and that they washed their hands frequently.[28] This concept held special significance not only for individual patient care, but it was also critically important in improving the health status of the poor living in crowded, environmentally inferior conditions with inadequate sewage and limited access to pure water.[28]

Nightingale included the concepts of warmth, quiet, and diet in her environmental theory. In addition to discussing the ventilation in the room or home, Nightingale provided a description for measuring the patient's body temperature through palpation of extremities to assess for heat loss.[28] The nurse was instructed to continually manipulate the environment to maintain both ventilation and patient warmth by using a good fire, opening windows, and properly positioning the patient in the room.

Unnecessary noise and the need for quiet was also a concept that required assessment and intervention by the nurse.[28] Noise created by physical activities in the environment (room) was to be avoided by the nurse because it could harm the patient.

Nightingale was also concerned with the patient's diet.[28] She instructed nurses not only to assess dietary intake, but also to assess both the meal schedule and its effect on the patient. She believed that patients with chronic illnesses could be starved to death and that intelligent nurses were those who were successful in meeting a patient's nutritional needs.

Another component of Nightingale's theory was that of a definition or description of *petty management*.[28] The nurse was in control of the environment both physically and administratively. The nurse had to control the environment to protect the patient from both physical and psychological harm; for example, the nurse protected the patient from receiving upsetting news, from seeing visitors who could negatively affect recovery, and from experiencing sudden disruptions in sleep. In addition, Nightingale recognized that the visiting of pets (small animals) might be of comfort to the patient. Nightingale also believed that the nurse remained in charge of the environment even when she was not physically present because she was to oversee others who worked in her absence.

MAJOR ASSUMPTIONS
Nursing

Nightingale believed that every woman, at one time in her life, would be a nurse in the sense that nursing is having the responsibility for someone else's health. Nightingale[28:4] wrote *Notes on Nursing* to provide women with guidelines for providing nursing care and to give advice on how to "think like a nurse."

Person

In most of her writings, Nightingale referred to the person as a patient. Nurses performed tasks to and for the patient and controlled the patient's environment to enhance recovery. For the most part, Nightingale described a passive patient in this relationship. However, there are specific references to the patient performing self-care when possible and being involved in the timing and substance of meals. The nurse was specifically instructed to ask the patient about his or her preferences; however, Nightingale emphasized that the nurse was in control of the patient's environment.[28]

Health

Nightingale defined health as being well and using every power that the person has to the fullest extent. Additionally, she saw disease as a reparative process that nature instituted from a want of attention. Nightingale envisioned the maintenance of health through the prevention of disease via environmental control; what she described is modern public health nursing and the more modern concept of health promotion. She distinguished these concepts of nursing as different from nursing a sick patient to enhance recovery or from living better until death.

Environment

Fitzpatrick and Whall[9:16-17] describe Nightingale's concept of environment as "those elements external to and which affect the health of the sick and healthy person" and included "everything from the patient's food and flowers to the patient's verbal and nonverbal interactions with the patient." Little, if anything, in the patient's world is excluded from her definition of environment.

Nightingale's assumptions about societal conditions are also relevant to her theory. She believed that the sick, poor people would benefit from environmental improvements that addressed both their bodies and minds. She believed that nurses could be instrumental in changing the social status of the poor by improving their living conditions.

THEORETICAL ASSERTIONS

Nightingale believed that disease was a reparative process; disease was nature's effort to remedy a process of poisoning or decay, or a reaction against the conditions in which a person was placed. Nightingale did not provide a definition of *nature.* In her writings, she often capitalized the word nature in her writings, thereby suggesting that it was synonymous with God. Her Unitarian religious beliefs would support this view of God as nature. However, when she used the word nature without capitalization, it is unclear whether or not the intended meaning is different and perhaps synonymous with an organic pathological process. Nightingale believed that nursing's role was to prevent an interruption of the reparative process and to provide optimal conditions for its enhancement.

Nightingale was totally committed to nursing education (training). Although she wrote *Notes on Nursing*[28] for all women, her primary treatise was that women were to be specifically trained to provide care for the sick person and that nurses providing preventive healthcare (public health nursing) required even more training. Nightingale[28] also felt that nurses needed to be excellent at the observation of their patients and the environment; this was an ongoing activity for trained nurses. In addition, she believed that nurses needed to use common sense in their nursing practice, coupled with their observation, perseverance, and ingenuity. Finally, Nightingale believed that persons desired good health and that they would cooperate with the nurse and nature to allow the reparative process to occur or alter their environment to prevent disease.

Although Nightingale has often been maligned or ridiculed for not embracing the germ theory, she very clearly understood the concept of contagion and contamination through organic materials from the patient and/or the environment. Many of her observations are consistent with the concepts of infection and the germ theory; for example, she embraced the concept of vaccination against various diseases. Nightingale also strongly believed that appropriate manipulations of the environment would prevent disease; this concept underlies modern sanitation activities.

Nightingale did not explicitly discuss the *caring behaviors* of nurses. She wrote very little about interpersonal relationships except as they influenced the patient's reparative processes. She did describe the phenomenon of being *called* to nursing and the need for commitment to nursing work. From the perspectives of Victorian England and her religious beliefs, these descriptions may describe a caring component of her nursing theory.

Finally, Nightingale believed that nurses should be moral agents. She addressed their *professional* relationship with their patients; she instructed them on the principle of confidentiality and advocated for care to the poor to improve their health and social situation. In addition, she commented on patient decision making (a relevant modern ethical concept). Nightingale[28] called for concise and clear decision making regarding the patient, noting that indecision *(irresolution)* or changing the mind is more harmful to the patient than the patient having to make a decision.

LOGICAL FORM

Nightingale used inductive reasoning to extract laws of health, disease, and nursing from her observations and experiences. Her childhood education, particularly in philosophy and mathematics, may have contributed to her logical thinking and inductive reasoning abilities. For example, her observations of the conditions in the Scutari hospital led her to conclude that the contaminated, dirty, dark environment led to disease. Not only could she prevent disease from flourishing in such an environment, but she also recognized that disease prevention would be achieved through environmental controls. From her own nursing training, her brief experience as a superintendent in London, and from her experiences in the Crimea, she was able to make observations and form the principles for her nursing training and patient care.[28]

ACCEPTANCE BY THE NURSING COMMUNITY
Practice

Nightingale's nursing principles remain applicable today. The environmental aspects of her theory (ventilation, warmth, quiet, diet, and cleanliness) remain integral components of current nursing care. As nurses begin practice in the twenty-first century, these concepts continue to be relevant; in fact, they have increased relevance as the global society faces new issues of disease control. For example, modern sanitation and water treatment have controlled traditional sources of disease fairly successfully, but contaminated water has become a health issue again for many communities in the United States as global travel has dramatically altered the actual and potential spread of diseases more rapidly than ever anticipated.

Other new environmental concerns are created by modern architecture (for example, sick building syndrome); nurses need to ask whether modern, environmentally controlled buildings meet Nightingale's principle of good ventilation. Disposal of waste, including toxic waste, and the use of chemicals in this modern society also challenge healthcare professionals to reassess the concept of a healthy environment.[3,10,24,35,36]

In healthcare facilities, the ability to control room temperature for an individual patient is increasingly difficult. That same environment may create great noise through multiple activities and the technology (equipment) used to assist the patient's reparative process. Nurses are looking at these problems in a scholarly way as they continue to affect patients and the healthcare system.[22,23,34]

Monteiro[25] provided the American public health community with a comprehensive review of Nightingale's work as a sanitarian and social reformer, again reminding the healthcare community of the extent of Nightingale's impact on healthcare in various settings and her concern about poverty and sanitation issues. Although other disciplines in the United States have increasingly addressed such issues, it is clear that there is an active role for nurses and nursing both in providing direct patient care and in the social and political arena to assure healthy environments for all citizens.

Although some of Nightingale's rationales have been modified or disproved by medical advances and scientific discovery, many of her concepts and portions of her theory have endured both time and technological advances. In reading and interpreting Nightingale's Victorian writings, remembering the uniqueness of her early life, and considering the sociopolitical nature of the era, it is clear that much of her theory remains relevant for nursing today. Concepts from Nightingale's writings continue to be cited in the nursing literature, from political commentary to scholarly research.

Multiple authors have recently analyzed Nightingale's *petty management* concepts and actions, again identifying some of the timelessness and universality of her management style.[6,13,25,28]

Finally, several writers have analyzed Nightingale's role in the suffrage movement, especially in the context of feminist theory development. Although she has been criticized for not actively participating in this movement, in a letter to John Stuart Mill, Nightingale indicated that she could do work for women in other ways.[40] Although she supported the principle of political power for women, she did not feel she had time to actively participate in this movement. Her essay entitled *Cassandra*[29] appears to reflect a great support for the concept that is now known as feminism. Nightingale's other writings also support her belief that upper social-class women should be useful, contributing members of society and should not be active in more idle, social roles.[40] Scholars continue to assess and analyze her role and position in the feminist movement of this modern era.[8,12,15,39]

Education

Nightingale's principles of nursing training (instruction in scientific principles and practical experience for the mastery of skills) provided a universal template for early nurse training schools beginning with St. Thomas Hospital and King's College Hospital in London. Using the Nightingale model of nursing training, three experimental schools were established in the United States in 1873: (1) Bellevue Hospital in New York, (2) New Haven Hospital in Connecticut, and (3) Massachusetts Hospital in Boston.[2] The influence of this training system and many of its principles is still evident in today's nursing programs.

Although Nightingale advocated the nursing school's independence from a hospital to ensure that students would not be involved in the hospital's labor pool as part of their training, American nursing schools were unable to achieve such independence for many years.[2] Nightingale[6] believed that the measurement of the *art of nursing* could not be accomplished through licensing examinations, but she used testing methods, including case studies (notes), for nursing probationers at St. Thomas Hospital.

Clearly, Nightingale understood that good practice could result only from good education (training). This message resounds throughout her writings on nursing. Nightingale historian Joanne Farley[6:13] responds to a modern nursing student by noting that "Training is to teach a nurse to know her business. . . . Training is to enable the nurse to act for the best . . . like an intelligent and responsible being." It is difficult to imagine what the care of sick human beings would be like if Nightingale had not defined the educational needs of nurses and established these first schools.

Research

Nightingale's interest in scientific inquiry and statistics continues to define the scientific inquiry used in nursing research. She was exceptionally efficient and resourceful in her ability to gather and analyze data; her ability to graphically represent data was first identified in the polar diagrams (the graphic illustration style that she invented).[1,5] Her empirical approach to solving problems of healthcare delivery is obvious in the data she often included in her numerous letters.

If Nightingale's writings are defined and analyzed as theory, they do lack the complexity and testability found in modern nursing theories. Therefore her theory cannot generate the nursing research that is employed to test modern theories. However, concepts that Nightingale identified have served as the basis for current research, which adds to modern nursing science and practice. A review of the current nursing literature suggests that controversy regarding Nightingale's place as the matriarch or icon of nursing has escalated throughout the international nursing community; however, her concepts continue to serve as the basis of continued analysis and nursing research throughout the world.

Finally, it is interesting to note that Nightingale used brief case studies, possible exemplars, to illustrate a number of the concepts she discussed in *Notes on Nursing*.[28] Scholarly nurses have refined this technique for inclusion in texts and research studies; such a style has an auspicious history in nursing literature.

FURTHER DEVELOPMENT

Nightingale's theory for nursing is stated clearly and concisely; *Notes on Nursing*[28] is Nightingale's most widely known work. The text's content seems most amenable to theory analysis. Nightingale organized the chapters of this text by concept; however, continued discussion of other concepts may appear in a specific chapter as it relates to the discussion. Fitzpatrick and Whall[9] refer to this approach as a set-of-laws theory; they define laws as theoretical statements with overwhelming empirical support.

Hardy[11] proposed that Nightingale formulated a grand theory, which explains the totality of behavior. Grand theories tend to be somewhat vague without specific definition of terms and concepts and without full development of relationships between concepts; they often provide untestable formulations. This type of theory is an early development that relies on anecdotal situations to illustrate its meaning and support its claims. Although her work can be

classified as lower-level theory, Nightingale provided the foundation for the development of both nursing practice and current nursing theories.

CRITIQUE
Simplicity

Nightingale's theory contains three major relationships: (1) environment to patient, (2) nurse to environment, and (3) nurse to patient. She believed that the environment was the main factor creating illness in a patient; she regarded disease as "the reactions of kindly nature against the conditions in which we have placed ourselves."[28:56] Nightingale recognized not only the harmfulness of an environment, but she also emphasized the benefit of good environments in preventing disease.

The nurse's practice includes the manipulation of the environment in a number of ways to enhance patient recovery. Elimination of contamination and contagion and the exposure to fresh air, light, warmth, and quiet were all identified as elements to be controlled or manipulated in the environment. Nightingale began to develop relationships between some of these elements in her discussions of contamination and ventilation, light and patient position in the room, cleanliness and darkness, and noise and patient stimulation. She also described the relationship between the sickroom and the rest of the house and the relationship between the house and the surrounding neighborhood. In addition, Nightingale recognized the need to manipulate the environment to prevent disease, as evidenced by her discussion of the homes of the poor, the workhouses, and preventing exposure of children to measles.

The nurse-patient relationship may be the least well defined in Nightingale's writings. Yet there are suggestions of cooperation and collaboration between the nurse and patient in her discussions of a patient's eating patterns and preferences, the comfort a loved pet to the patient, the protection of the patient from emotional distress, and the conservation of energy while allowing the patient to participate in self-care. Finally, it is interesting to note that Nightingale discussed the concept of observation extensively, including the use of those observations to guide the care of patients and to measure improvement or lack of response to nursing interventions. This aspect of training and practice would suggest the origins of the nursing process.[38]

Combining the concepts that Nightingale identified does not aid in increasing their simplicity; her original statements are expressed in an economical form. Diagrams of these concepts and their relationships have been proposed, thereby supporting their logic and simplicity.[9]

Nightingale provided a descriptive, explanatory theory rather than one of prediction. However, its environmental focus with its epidemiological components had predictive potential, but Nightingale never tested the theory in that manner. It is unclear whether Nightingale intended to develop a theory of nursing. She did intend to define the science and art of nursing and provide general rules with explanations that would result in good nursing care for patients. Thus, her objective of setting forth general rules for the practice and development of nursing was met through this simple theory.

Generality

Nightingale's theory has been used to provide general guidelines for all nurses for the last 150 years. Although specific activities are no longer relevant, the universality and timelessness of her concepts remain pertinent. The relation concepts (nurse, patient, and environment) are applicable in all nursing settings today. To address her audience of women who may provide care to another (not only professional nurses), the theory she proposed remains relevant. Therefore it meets the criterion of generality.

Empirical Precision

Concepts and relationships within Nightingale's theory are frequently stated implicitly and are presented as truths rather than tentative, testable statements. In contrast to her quantitative research on mortality performed in the Crimea, Nightingale advised nurses that their practice should be based on their observations and experiences rather than systematic, empirical research. If she were addressing the development of the *art of nursing*, her admonition would suggest a role for qualitative and/or phenomenological research methodology in nursing.

Derivable Consequences

To an extraordinary degree, Nightingale's writings direct the nurse to action on behalf of the patient and the nurse. These directives encompass the areas of practice, research, and education. Her principles that attempt to shape nursing practice are the most specific. She urges nurses to provide physicians with "not your opinion, however respectfully given, but your facts."[28:122] Similarly, she advised that "if you cannot get the habit of observation one way or other, you had better give up the being a nurse, for it is not your calling, however kind and anxious you may be."[28:113] Her encouragement for a measure of independence and precision previously unknown in nursing may still guide and motivate nurses today as the profession continues to evolve.

Nightingale's view of humanity was consistent with her theories of nursing. She believed in a creative, universal humanity with the potential and ability for growth and change.[8,12,33] Deeply religious, she viewed nursing as a means of doing the will of her God. Perhaps it is because she viewed nursing as a divine calling that she relegated the patient to a relatively passive role with his or her wants and needs provided by the nurse. The zeal and self-righteousness that comes from being a reformer might explain some of her beliefs and the practices that she advocated. Finally, the historical period (Victorian England) in which she lived must be considered to better understand her views.

Nightingale's basic principles of environmental manipulation and psychological care of the patient can be applied in contemporary nursing settings. Although her rejection of the germ theory and her inability to recognize a unified body of nursing knowledge that is testable (rather than relying only on personal observation and experience) have subjected her to some ridicule, other parts of her theory and her activities are relevant to nursing's professional identity and practice.

Lack of specificity has hindered the use of Nightingale's ideas for the generation of nursing research. However, her writings continue to stimulate productive thinking for the individual nurse and the nursing profession; her work gives food for thought that continues to nourish the profession nearly 150 years later. It is only right that Nightingale continues to be recognized as the brilliant and creative founder of modern nursing and its first nursing theorist.

CRITICAL THINKING *Activities*

1. Using Nightingale's concepts of ventilation, light, noise, and cleanliness, analyze the setting in which you are practicing nursing (working as an employee or student).

2. Using Nightingale's theory, evaluate the nursing interventions you have identified for an individual patient in your facility or practice.

3. Your hospital patient is an 82-year-old woman. She does not have immediate family and has been living alone in her own home. Her hospitalization was unanticipated; it followed a visit to the emergency room for a burn on her lower legs. The patient has been hospitalized for 14 days. She pleads with you to allow her friend to bring her dog, a 16-year-old Scotty Terrier, to the hospital. She tells you that none of the other nurses have listened to her when she asked them about such a visit. Based on Nightingale's work, what actions would you take for this patient?

REFERENCES

1. Agnew, L.R. (1958, May). Florence Nightingale, statistician. *American Journal of Nursing,* 58, 644.
2. Ashley, J.A. (1976). *Hospitals, paternalism, and the role of the nurse.* New York: Teachers College Press.
3. Butterfield, P. (1999). Integrating environmental health into clinical nursing. *Journal of the New York State Nurses Association,* 30(1), 24-27.
4. Chinn, P. & Jacobs, M. (1983). *Theory and nursing: A systematic approach.* St. Louis: Mosby.
5. Cohen, I.B. (1984, March). Florence Nightingale. *Scientific American,* 250(3), 128-137.
6. Decker, B. & Farley, J.K. (1991, May/June). What would Nightingale say? *Nurse Educator,* 16(3), 12-3.
7. Dickens, C. (1987). *Life and adventures of Martin Chuzzlewit.* London: New Oxford Press.
8. Dossey, B.M. (2000). *Florence Nightingale: Mystic, visionary, healer.* Springhouse, PA: Springhouse Corporation.
9. Fitzpatrick, J. & Whall, A. (1983). *Conceptual models of nursing.* Bowie, MD: Prentice Hall.
10. Gropper, E.I. (1990). Florence Nightingale: Nursing's first environmental theorist. *Nursing Forum,* 25(3), 30-33.
11. Hardy, M. (1978). Perspectives on nursing theory. *Advances in Nursing Science,* 1, 37-48.
12. Hektor, M. (1994, Nov.). Florence Nightingale and the women's movement: Friend or foe? *Nursing Inquiry,* 1(1), 38-45.
13. Henry, B., Woods, S., & Nagelkerk, J. (1990). Nightingale's perspective of nursing administration. *Nursing and Health Care,* 11(4), 200-206.
14. Helmstadter, C. (1997). Doctors and nurses in the London teaching hospitals: Class, gender, religion, and professional expertise, 1850-1890. *Nursing History Review,* 5, 161-167.
15. Holliday, M.E. & Parker, D.L. (1997). Florence Nightingale, feminism and nursing. *Journal of Advanced Nursing,* 28, 483-488.
16. Isler, C. (1970). *Florence Nightingale: Rebel with a cause.* Oradell, NY: Medical Economics.
17. Kalisch, B.J. & Kalisch, P.A. (1983, April). Heroine out of focus: Media images of Florence Nightingale. Part I: Popular biographies and stage productions. *Nursing and Health Care,* 4(4), 181-7.
18. Kalisch, B.J. & Kalisch, P.A. (1983, May). Heroine out of focus: Media images of Florence Nightingale. Part II: Film, radio, and television dramatizations. *Nursing and Health Care,* 4(5), 270-8.
19. Kalisch, P.A. & Kalisch B.J. (1987). *The changing image of the nurse.* Menlo Park, CA: Addison-Wesley.
20. Lobo, M.L. (1995). Florence Nightingale. In J.B. George (Ed.), *Nursing theories: The base for professional nursing practice.* Norwalk, CT: Appleton & Lange.
21. Longfellow, H.W. (1857). Santa filomena. *Atlantic Monthly,* 1(1), 22-23.
22. McCarthy, D.O., Ouimet, M.E., & Daun, J.M. (1991, May). Shades of Florence Nightingale: Potential impact of noise stress on wound healing. *Holistic Nursing Practice,* 5(4), 39-48.
23. McLaughlin, A., McLaughlin, B., Elliott, J., & Campalani, G. (1996). Noise levels in a cardiac surgical intensive care unit: A preliminary study conducted in secret. *Intensive and Critical Care Nursing,* 12(4), 226-230.

24. Michigan Nurses Association. (1999). Nursing practice: Moving toward environmentally responsible health care. *Michigan Nurse,* 72(1), 8-9.
25. Monteiro, L.A. (1985, Feb.). Florence Nightingale on public health nursing. *American Journal of Public Health,* 75, 181-6.
26. Murray, R. & Zentner, J. (1975). *Nursing concepts in health promotion.* Englewood Cliffs, NJ: Prentice Hall.
27. Nelson, S. (1997). Pastoral care and moral government: Early nineteenth century nursing and solutions to the Irish question. *Journal of Advanced Nursing,* 26, 6-14.
28. Nightingale, F. (1969). *Notes on nursing: What it is and what it is not.* New York: Dover.
29. Nightingale, F. (1852). *Cassandra.* Unpublished essay.
30. Nightingale, F. (1858). *Notes on matters affecting the health, efficiency, and hospital administration of the British army founded chiefly on the experience of the late war. Presented by request to the secretary of state for war.* London: Harrison & Sons.
31. Nightingale, F. (1858). *Notes on hospitals: Being two papers read before the National Association for the Promotion of Social Science, at Liverpool, in October 1858. With evidence given to the Royal Commissioner on the state of the army in 1857.* London: John W. Park and Son.
32. Nightingale, F. (1870). *Report on measures adopted for sanitary improvements in India from June 1869 to June 1870: Together with abstracts.* London.
33. Palmer, I.S. (1977, March/April). Florence Nightingale: Reformer, reactionary, researcher. *Nursing Research,* 26, 84-9.
34. Pope, D.S. (1995, Winter). Music, noise, and the human voice in the nurse-patient environment. *Image: Journal of Nursing Scholarship,* 27, 291-5.
35. Sessler, A. (1999). Doing more than doing no harm: Nursing professionals turn their attention to the environment. *On-Call,* 2(4), 20-23.
36. Shaner, H. (1998). Pollution prevention for nurses: Minimizing the adverse environmental impact of healthcare delivery. *Vermont Registered Nurse,* 64(4), 9-11.
37. Thomas, S.P. (1993, April/June). The view from Scutari: A look at contemporary nursing. *Nursing Forum,* 28(2), 19-24.
38. Ulrich, B.T. (1992). *Leadership and management according to Florence Nightingale.* Norwalk, CT: Appleton & Lange.
39. Welch, M. (1990, June). Florence Nightingale: The social construction of a Victorian feminist. *Western Journal of Nursing Research,* 12, 404-7.
40. Woodham-Smith, C. (1951). *Florence Nightingale.* New York: McGraw-Hill.

BIBLIOGRAPHY
Primary Sources
Books

Nightingale, F. (1911). *Letters from Miss Florence Nightingale on health visiting in rural districts.* London: King.
Nightingale, F. (1954). *Selected writings. Compiled by Lucy R. Seymer.* New York: Macmillan.
Nightingale, F. (1956). *The institution of Kaiserwerth on the Rhine,* Dusseldorf, Germany: Anna Sticker.
Nightingale, F. (1957). *Notes on nursing.* Philadelphia: J.B. Lippincott. (Originally published, 1859.)
Nightingale, F. (1969). *Notes on nursing: What it is and what it is not.* New York: Dover.
Nightingale, F. (1974). *Letters of Florence Nightingale in the history of nursing archive.* Boston: Boston University Press.
Nightingale, F. (1976). *Notes on hospitals.* New York: Gordon.
Nightingale, F. (1978). *Notes on nursing.* London: Duckworth.
Nightingale, F. (1992). *Notes on nursing.* (Commemorative edition with commentaries by contemporary nursing leaders.) Philadelphia: J.B. Lippincott.

Journal Articles

Nightingale, F. (1930, July). Trained nursing for the sick poor. *International Nursing Review,* 5, 426-433.
Nightingale, F. (1954, May). Maternity hospital and midwifery school. *Nursing Mirror,* 99, ix-xi, 369.
Nightingale, F. (1954). The training of nurses. *Nursing Mirror,* 99, iv-xi.

Secondary Sources
Book Reviews

[Review of the article *Selected writings*]. (1955, April). *Royal Sanitary Institute Journal,* 75, 275-276.
[Review of the article *Selected writings*]. (1955, May). *American Journal of Nursing,* 55, 162.
[Review of the article *Selected writings*]. (1955, May). *Nursing Times,* 52, 502-503, 507.
[Review of the book *Notes on nursing: What it is and what it is not*]. (1970, June). *Nursing Times,* 66, 828.
[Review of the book *Notes on nursing: What it is and what it is not*]. (1970, Oct.). *Nursing Mirror,* 131, 47.
[Review of the book *What it is and what it is not, the science and art*]. (1980, Oct.). *Nursing Times,* 76, 187.
[Review of the book *What it is and what it is not, the science and art*]. (1980, Dec.). *Nursing Mirror,* 151, 41.
[Review of the book *What it is and what it is not, the science and art*]. (1981, Feb.) *Australian Nurses Journal,* 10, 29.
[Review of the book *Cassandra: An essay*]. (1981, May). *American Journal of Nursing,* 81, 1059-1061.

[Review of the book *Florence Nightingale*]. (1950, Nov.). *Nursing Mirror*, 92, 31.

[Review of the book *Florence Nightingale*]. (1950, Dec.). *Nursing Times*, 46, 1285, 16.

[Review of the book *Florence Nightingale*]. (1951, June). *Journal of the American Medical Association*, 146, 605.

[Review of the book *Florence Nightingale*]. (1951, Aug.). *Public Health Nursing*, 43, 459.

Books

Aiken, C.A. (1915). *Lessons from the life of Florence Nightingale.* New York: Lakeside.

Aldis, M. (1914). *Florence Nightingale.* New York: National Organization for Public Health Nursing.

Andrews, M.R. (1929). *A lost commander.* Garden City, NY: Doubleday.

Baly, M.E. (1986). *Florence Nightingale: The nursing legacy.* New York: Methuen.

Barth, R.J. (1945). *Fiery angel: The story of Florence Nightingale.* Coral Gables, FL: Glade House.

Bishop, W.J. (1962). *A bio-bibliography of Florence Nightingale.* London: Dawson's of Pall Mall.

Boyd, N. (1982). *Three Victorian women who changed their world.* New York: Oxford.

Bull, A. (1985). *Florence Nightingale.* North Pomfret, VT: David and Charles.

Bullough, V.L., Bullough, B., & Stanton, M.P. (Eds.). (1990). *Florence Nightingale and her era: A collection of new scholarship.* New York: Garland.

Calabria, M. & Macrae, J. (Eds.). (1994). *Suggestions for thought by Florence Nightingale: Selections and commentaries.* Philadelphia: University of Pennsylvania Press.

Collins, D. (1985). *Florence Nightingale.* Milford, MI: Mott Media.

Columbia University Faculty of Medicine and Department of Nursing. (1937). *Catalogue of the Florence Nightingale collection.* New York: The Author.

Cook, E.T. (1913). *The life of Florence Nightingale.* London: Macmillan.

Cook, E.T. (1941). *A short life of Florence Nightingale.* New York: Macmillan.

Cope, Z. (1958). *Florence Nightingale and the doctors.* Philadelphia: J.B. Lippincott.

Cope, Z. (1961). *Six disciples of Florence Nightingale.* New York: Pitman.

Davies, C. (1980). *Rewriting nursing history.* London: Croom Helm.

Dossey, B.M. (2000). *Florence Nightingale: Mystic, visionary, healer.* Springhouse, PA: Springhouse Corp.

Editors of *RN*. (1970). *Florence Nightingale: Rebel with a cause.* Oradell, NJ: Medical Economics.

French, Y. (1953). *Six great Englishwomen.* London: H. Hamilton.

Goldie, S. (1987). *I have done my duty: Florence Nightingale in the Crimea War, 1854-1856.* London: Manchester University Press.

Goldsmith, M.L. (1937). *Florence Nightingale: The woman and the legend.* London: Hodder and Stoughton.

Goldwater, S.S. (1947). *On hospitals.* New York: Macmillan.

Gordon, R. (1979). *The private life of Florence Nightingale.* New York: Atheneum.

Haldale, E. (1931). *Mrs. Gaskell and her friends.* New York: Appleton.

Hall, E.F. (1920). *Florence Nightingale.* New York: Macmillan.

Hallock, G.T. & Turner, C.E. (1928). *Florence Nightingale.* New York: Metropolitan Life Insurance Co.

Herbert, R.G. (1981). *Florence Nightingale: Saint, reformer, or rebel?* Melbourne, FL: Krieger.

Holmes, M. (n.d.). *Florence Nightingale: A cameo life-sketch.* London: Woman's Freedom League.

Huxley, E.J. (1975). *Florence Nightingale.* London: Putnam.

Hyndman, J.A. (1969). *Florence Nightingale: Nurse to the world.* Cleveland, OH: World Publishing.

Keele, J. (Ed.). (1981). *Florence Nightingale in Rome.* Philadelphia: American Philosophical Society.

Lammond, D. (1935). *Florence Nightingale.* London: Duckworth.

Miller, B.W. (1947). *Florence Nightingale: The lady with the lamp.* Grand Rapids, MI: Zondervan.

Miller, M. (1987). *Florence Nightingale.* Minneapolis: MN: Bethany House.

Mosby, C.V. (1938). *Little journey to the home of Florence Nightingale.* New York: C.V. Mosby.

Muir, D.E. (1946). *Florence Nightingale.* Glasgow: Blackie and Son.

Nash, R. (1937). *A sketch for the life of Florence Nightingale.* London: Society for Promoting Christian Knowledge.

Newton, M.E. (1949). *Florence Nightingale's philosophy of life and education.* Unpublished doctoral dissertation, Stanford, CA: Stanford University.

O'Malley, I.B. (1931). *Life of Florence Nightingale, 1820-1856.* London: Butterworth.

Pollard, E. (1902). *Florence Nightingale: The wounded soldiers' friend.* London: Partridge.

Presbyterian Hospital, School of Nursing. (1937). *Catalogue of the Florence Nightingale collection.* New York: The Author.

Quiller-Couch, A.T. (1927). *Victor of peace.* New York: Nelson.

Quinn, V. & Prest, J. (Eds.). (1987). *Dear Miss Nightingale: A selection of Benjamin Jowett's letters to Florence Nightingale, 1860-1893.* Oxford: Clarendon Press.

Rappe, E.C. (1977). *God bless you, my dear Miss Nightingale.* Stockholm: Almqvist och Wiksell.

Sabatini, R. (1934). *Heroic lives*. Boston: Houghton.

Saint Thomas's Hospital. (1960). *The Nightingale Training School: St. Thomas's Hospital, 1860-1960*. London: The Author.

Saleeby, C.W. (1912). *Surgery and society: A tribute to Listerism*. New York: Moffat, Yard & Co.

Schmidt, M.M. (1933). *400 Outstanding women of the world and costumology of their time*. Chicago: The Author.

Selanders, L.C. (1993). *Florence Nightingale: An environmental adaptation theory*. Newbury Park, CA: Sage Publications.

Seymer, L.R. (1951). *Florence Nightingale*. New York: Macmillan.

Shor, D. (1987). *Florence Nightingale*. Lexington, NH: Silver.

Smith, F.B. (1982). *Florence Nightingale: Reputation and power*. New York: St. Martin.

Stark, M. (1979). *Introduction to Cassandra: An essay by Florence Nightingale*. Old Westbury, NY: Feminist Press.

Stephenson, G.E. (1924). *Some pioneers in the medical and nursing world*. Shanghai: Nurses's Association of China.

Strachey, L. (1918). *Eminent Victorians*. London: Chatto & Windus.

Tabor, M.E. (1925). *Pioneer women*. London: Sheldon.

Tooley, S.A. (1905). *The life of Florence Nightingale*. New York: Macmillan.

Turner, D. (1986). *Florence Nightingale*. New York: Watts.

Vicinus, M. & Nergaard, B. (1990). *Ever yours, Florence Nightingale*. Cambridge, MA: Harvard University Press.

Wilson, W.G. (1940). *Soldier's heroine*. Edinburgh: Missionary Education Movement.

Woodman-Smith, C. (1983). *Florence Nightingale*. New York: Atheneum.

Woodham-Smith, C.B. (1951). *Florence Nightingale, 1820-1910*. New York: McGraw-Hill.

Woodham-Smith, C.B. (1951). *Lonely crusader: The life of Florence Nightingale, 1820-1910*. New York: Whittlesey House.

Woodham-Smith, C.B. (1956). *Lady-in-chief*. London: Methven.

Woodham-Smith, C.B. (1977). *Florence Nightingale, 1820-1910*. London: Collins.

Woodsey, A.H. (1950). *A century of nursing*. New York: Putnam.

World's Who's Who in Science. (1968). *Florence Nightingale (entry)*. Chicago: A.N. Marquis.

Wren, D. (1949). *They enriched humanity: Adventurers of the 19th century*. London: Skilton.

Book Chapters

Reed, P.G. & Zurakowski, T.L. (1983, 1989). Nightingale: A visionary model for nursing. In J. Fitzpatrick & A. Whall (Eds.), *Conceptual models of nursing: Analysis and application*. Bowie, MD: Robert J. Brady.

Torres, G.C. (1980, 1990). Florence Nightingale. In Nursing Theories Conference Group, J.B. George (Chairperson), *Nursing theories: The base for professional nursing practice*. Englewood Cliffs, NJ: Prentice Hall.

Unpublished Dissertations

Hektor, L.M. (1992). *Nursing, science, and gender: Florence Nightingale and Martha E. Rogers*. Unpublished doctoral dissertation, University of Miami.

Parker, E. (1994). *Of writing and nursing: A study of. . . .* Unpublished doctoral dissertation, University of Nevada, Reno.

Selanders, L.C. (1992). *An analysis of the utilization of power by Florence Nightingale*. Unpublished doctoral dissertation, Western Michigan University.

Tschirch, P. (1992). *The caring tradition: Nursing ethics in the United States, 1890-1915*. Unpublished doctoral dissertation, The University of Texas Graduate School of Biomedical Science at Galveston.

Journal Articles

A criticism of Miss Florence Nightingale. (1907, Feb.). *Nursing Times, 3*, 89.

Abbott, M.E. (1916, Sept. 14). Portraits of Florence Nightingale. *Boston Medical and Surgical Journal, 175*, 361-367.

Abbott, M.E. (1916, Sept. 21). Portraits of Florence Nightingale. *Boston Medical Surgery Journal, 175*, 413-422.

Abbott, M.E. (1916, Sept. 28). Portraits of Florence Nightingale. *Boston Medical Surgery Journal, 175*, 453-457.

Address by the Archbishop of York. (1970, May). Florence Nightingale. *Nursing Times, 66*, 670.

Address given at fiftieth anniversary of founding by Florence Nightingale of first training school for nurses at St. Thomas's Hospital, London, England. (1911, Feb.). *American Journal of Nursing, 11*, 331-361.

A passionate statistician. (1931, May). *American Journal of Nursing, 31*, 566.

At Embley Park and East Willow. (1937, July), *Nursing Times, 33*, 730-731.

Attewell, A. (1998). Florence Nightingale's relevance to nurses. *Journal of Holistic Nursing, 16*, 281-291.

Ball, O.F. (1952, May). Florence Nightingale. *Modern Hospital, 78*, 88-90, 144.

Baly, M. (1986, June). Shattering the Nightingale myth. *Nursing Times, 82*(24), 16-18.

Baly, M.E. (1969, Jan.). Florence Nightingale's influence on nursing today. *Nursing Times, 65*(Suppl.), 1-4.

Barber, E.M. (1935, July). A culinary campaign. *Journal of the American Dietetic Association, 11*, 89-98.

Barber, J.A. (1999). Concerning our national honour: Florence Nightingale and the welfare of Aboriginal Australians. *Collegian: Journal of the Royal College of Nursing Australia, 6*(1), 36-39.

Barker, E.R. (1989, Oct.). Caregivers as casualties . . . war experiences and the postwar consequences for both Nightingale- and Vietnam-era nurses. *Western Journal of Nursing Research,* 11, 628-631.

Barritt, E.R. (1973). Florence Nightingale's values and modern nursing education. *Nursing Forum,* 12, 7-47.

Berentson, L. (1982, April/May). Florence Nightingale: Change agent. *Registered Nurse,* 6(2), 3,7.

Berman, J.K. (1974, Aug.). Florentia and the Clarabellas: A tribute to nurses. *Journal of the Indiana State Medical Association,* 67, 717-719.

Bishop, W.J. (1957, Jan.). Florence Nightingale bibliography. *International Nursing Review,* 4, 64.

Bishop, W.J. (1957, May). Florence Nightingale's letters. *American Journal of Nursing,* 57, 607.

Bishop, W.J. (1960, May). Florence Nightingale's message for today. *Nursing Outlook,* 8, 246.

Black, B.W. (1939, July). A tribute to Florence Nightingale. *Pacific Coast Journal of Nursing,* 35, 408-409.

Blanc, E. (1980, May). Nightingale remembered: Reflections on times past. *California Nurse,* 75(10), 7.

Blanchard, J.R. (1939, June). Florence Nightingale: A study in vocation. *New Zealand Nursing Journal,* 32, 193-197.

Book reviews and digests. (1920, May). *Public Health Nursing,* 12, 442-448.

Boylen, J.O. (1974, April). The Florence Nightingale-Mary Stanley controversy: Some unpublished letters. *Medical History,* 18(2), 186-193.

Bridges, D.C. (1954, April). Florence Nightingale centenary. *International Nurses Review,* 1, 3.

Brow, E.J. (1954, April). Florence Nightingale and her international influence. *International Nursing Review,* 1, 17-19.

Brown, E. (2000). Nightingale's values live on. *Kai Tiaki: Nursing New Zealand,* 6(3), 31.

Carlisle, D. (1989, Dec.). A nightingale sings . . . Florence Nightingale . . . unknown details of her life story. *Nursing Times,* 85(50), 38-39.

Cartwright, F.F. (1976, March). President's address: Miss Nightingale's dearest friend. *Proceedings of the Royal Society of Medicine,* 69(3), 169-175.

Centenary [Editorial]. (1960, May). *Nursing Times,* 56, 587.

Centenary celebrations [Florence Nightingale]. (1954, Nov.). *Nursing Times,* 50, 1213-1214.

Charatan, F.B. (1990, Feb.). Florence Nightingale: The most famous nurse in the world. *Today's OR Nurse,* 12(2), 25-30.

Cherescavich, G. (1971, June). *Nursing Clinics of North America,* 6, 217-223.

Choa, G.H. (1971, May). Speech by Dr. the Hon. G.H. Choa at the Florence Nightingale Day Celebration on Wednesday, 12th May, 1971, at City Hall, Hong Kong. *Nursing Journal,* 10, 33-34.

Clayton, R.E. (1974, April). How men may live and not die in India: Florence Nightingale. *Australian Nurses Journal,* 2, 10-11.

Coakley, M.L. (1989, Winter). Florence Nightingale: A one-woman revolution. *Journal of Christian Nursing,* 6, 20-25.

Cohen, S. (1997). Miss Loane, Florence Nightingale, and district nursing in late Victorian Britain. *Nursing History Review,* 5, 83-103.

Collins, W.J. (1945, May 12). Florence Nightingale and district nursing. *Nursing Mirror,* 81, 74.

Cope, Z. (1960, May). Florence Nightingale and her nurses. *Nursing Times,* 56, 597.

Coxhead, E. (1973, May). Miss Nightingale's country hospital. *Nursing Times,* 65, 615-617.

Crowder, E.L. (1978, May). Florence Nightingale. *Texas Nursing,* 52(5), 6-7.

Cruse, P. (1980, Sept.). Florence Nightingale. *Surgery,* 88(3), 394-399.

Davidson, C. (1937, March). Jeanne Mance and Florence Nightingale. *Hospital Progress,* 18, 83-85.

de Guzman, G. (1935, July). Florence Nightingale. *Filipino Nurse,* 10, 10-14.

de Tornavay, R. (1976, Nov./Dec.). Past is prologue: Florence Nightingale, *Pulse,* 12(6), 9-11.

Dennis, K.E. & Prescott, P.A. (1985, Jan.). Florence Nightingale: Yesterday, today, and tomorrow. *Advances in Nursing Science,* 7(2), 66-81.

Draper, J.M. (1907, Jan.). A brief sketch of the life of Florence Nightingale. *Trained Nurse,* 38, 1-4.

Duggan, R. (1981, June). Florence Nightingale memorial service. *Australian Nurses Journal,* 10(6), 30.

Dunbar, V.M. (1954, Oct.). Florence Nightingale's influence on nursing education. *International Nursing Review,* 1, 17-23.

Dwyer, B.A. (1937, Jan.). The mother of our modern nursing system. *Filipino Nurse,* 12, 8-10.

Echos of the past. (1907, Nov.). *British Journal of Nursing,* 39, 396-397.

Echos of the past. (1907, Dec.). *British Journal of Nursing,* 39, 497-498.

Ellett, E.C. (1904, May). Florence Nightingale. *Trained Nurse,* 32, 305-310.

Extracts from letters from the Crimea. (1932, May). *American Journal of Nursing,* 32, 537-538.

Fink, L.G. (1934, Dec.). Catholic influences in the life of Florence Nightingale. *Hospital Progress,* 15, 482-489.

Florence Nightingale [Editorial]. (1903, July). *Medical Dial,* 5, 122-124.

Florence Nightingale [Editorial]. (1964, May). *Nursing Mirror,* 118, 131.

Florence Nightingale as a leader in the religious and civic thought of her time. (1936, July). *Hospitals,* 10, 78-84.

The Florence Nightingale bibliography. (1956, April). *South African Nursing Journal,* 22, 16.

Florence Nightingale bibliography. (1956, Oct.). *Nursing Research*, 5, 87.

Florence Nightingale bibliography is compiled. (1931, May). *Modern Hospital*, 36, 126.

Florence Nightingale: Looking back . . . notes on hospitals. (1979, Sept.). *Lamp*, 36, 39-43.

Florence Nightingale O.M. (1910, Aug.). *British Journal of Nursing*, 45, 141-147.

Florence Nightingale: The original geriatric nurse. (1980, May). Oklahoma Nurse, 25(4), 6.

Florence Nightingale: Rebel with a cause. (1970, May). *Registered Nurse*, 33, 39-55.

Florence Nightingale's influence on nursing today. (1969, Jan.). *Nursing Times*, 65, 1.

Florence Nightingale's letter. (1932, July 2). *Nursing Times*, 28, 699.

Florence Nightingale's letter of advice to Bellevue. (1911, Feb.). *American Journal of Nursing*, 11, 361-364.

Florence Nightingale's tomb. (1957, June). *Canadian Nurse*, 53, 529.

Florence Nightingale's work for public health [Editorial]. (1914, June). *American Journal of Public Health*, 4, 510-511.

Food for thought [Editorial]. (1958, Aug.). *Nursing Outlook*, 6, 437.

Footnote to a dedicated life. (1958, Aug.). *Registered Nurse*, 21, 53.

Fraga, M. & Tanenbaum, L. (1980, May). Florence Nightingale: Model for today's nurse. *Florida Nurse*, 29(5), 11.

Gibbon, C. (1997). The influence of Florence Nightingale's image on Liverpool nurses 1945-1995. *International History of Nursing Journal*, 2(3), 17-26.

Gordon, J.E. (1972, Oct.). Nurses and nursing in Britain. 21. The work of Florence Nightingale. I. For the health of the army. *Midwife Health Visitor and Community Nurse*, 8, 351-359.

Gordon, J.E. (1972, Nov.). Nurses and nursing in Britain. 22. The work of Florence Nightingale. II. The establishment of nurse training in Britain. *Midwife Health Visitor and Community Nurse*, 8, 391-396.

Gordon, J.E. (1973, Jan.). Nurses and nursing in Britain. 23. The work of Florence Nightingale. III. Her influence throughout the world. *Midwife Health Visitor and Community Nurse*, 9, 17-22.

Gottstein, W.K. (1956, May). Miss Nightingale's personality. *Registered Nurse*, 19, 58-60,80,82.

Gould, M.E. (1970, May). A woman of parts. *Nursing Times*, 66, 606.

Graham, S. (1980, Oct.). Notes on nursing, 1860-1980: Angels of plain speech. *Nursing Times*, 76(43), 1874.

Greatness in little things. (1954, May). *Nursing Times*, 50, 508-510.

Grier, B. & Grier, M. (1978, Oct.). Contributions of the passionate statistician (Florence Nightingale). *Research in Nursing and Health*, 1(3), 103-109.

Grier, M.R. (1978, Oct.). Florence Nightingale: Saint or scientist? [Editorial]. *Research in Nursing and Health*, 1(3), 91.

Hallowes, R. (1957, Sept.). Florence Nightingale. In distinguished British nurses. *Nursing Mirror*, 105, viii-x.

Hamash Dash, D.M. (1971, June). Florence Nightingale's writings. *Nursing Journal of India*, 62, 179.

Headberry, J.E. (1966, Jan.). Florence Nightingale and modern nursing. *Journal of the West Australian Nurses*, 32, 7-16.

Headberry, J.E. (1966, Feb.). Florence Nightingale and modern nursing. *Australian Nurses Journal*, 64, 32-36.

Headberry, J.E. (1966, March/April). Florence Nightingale and modern nursing. *UNA Nursing Journal*, 64, 80-87.

Headberry, J.E. (1966, Sept.). Florence Nightingale and modern nursing. *Nursing Mirrors*, 122, xiii.

Health as a personal and community asset. (1926, Dec.). *Journal of Education*, 104, 566.

Hearn, M.J. (1920, April). Florence Nightingale. *Quarterly Journal of Chinese Nurses*, 1, 12-14.

Her letters [Florence Nightingale]. (1955, June). *Nursing Journal of India*, 46, 210.

Her letters [Florence Nightingale]. (1955, July). *Nursing Journal of India*, 46, 236.

Her letters [Florence Nightingale]. (1955, Aug.). *Nursing Journal of India*, 46, 268.

Her letters [Florence Nightingale]. (1955, Oct.). *Nursing Journal of India*, 46, 326.

Holly, H. (1967, Winter). Wanted: A day's work for a day's pay. *Nevada Nurses Association Newsletter*, 1.

Hoole, L. (2000). Florence Nightingale must remain as nursing's icon. *British Journal of Nursing*, 4, 189.

Hurd, H.M. (1920, June). Florence Nightingale: A force in medicine. *Johns Hopkins Nurses Alumnae Magazine*, 9, 68-81.

Ifemesia, C.C. (1976, July/Sept.). Florence Nightingale (1820-1910). *Nigerian Nurse*, 8(3), 26-34.

In her memory. (1957, May). *Registered Nurse*, 20, 53.

Isler, C. (1970, May). Florence Nightingale, *Registered Nurse*, 33, 35-55.

Iu, S. (1971, May). President's address at Florence Nightingale Day Celebration 12th May 1971, City Hall Theatre. *Hong Kong Nursing Journal*, 10, 27-32.

Iveson-Iveson, J. (1983, May). Nurses in society: A legend in the breaking (Florence Nightingale). *Nursing Mirror*, 156(19), 26-27.

Jake, D.G. (1975, Nov.). Florence Nightingale: Mission impossible. *Arizona Medicine*, 32(11), 894-895.

Jamme, A.C. (1920, May). Florence Nightingale: The great teacher of nurses. *Pacific Coast Journal of Nursing*, 16, 282-285.

Jones, H.W. (1940, Nov.). Some unpublished letters of Florence Nightingale. *Bulletin of the History of Medicine*, 8, 1389-1396.

Jones, O.C. (1972, Aug.). A useful memorial (Florence Nightingale). *Canadian Nurse*, 68, 38-39.

Journey among women: Responsibility at the top. Part II. (1970, June 4). *Nursing Times,* 66, 77.

Kelly, L.Y. (1976, Oct.). Our nursing heritage: Have we renounced it? (Florence Nightingale). *Image,* 8(3), 43-48.

Kerling, N.J. (1976, July). Letters from Florence Nightingale. *Nursing Mirror,* 143(1), 68.

Kiereini, E.M. (1981, June). The way ahead: On the occasion of Florence Nightingale oration at the Perth Concert Hall, Australia, 24th October, 1979. *Kenya Nursing Journal,* 10(1), 5-8.

King, A.G. (1964, June). The changing role of the nurse. *Hospital Topics,* 42, 89.

King, F.A. (1954, Oct. 22). Miss Nightingale and her ladies in the Crimea. *Nursing Mirror,* 100, xi-xii.

King, F.A. (1954, Oct. 29). Miss Nightingale and her ladies in the Crimea. *Nursing Mirror,* 100, viii-ix.

King, F.A. (1954, Nov. 5). Miss Nightingale and her ladies in the Crimea. *Nursing Mirror,* 100, v-vi.

King, F.A. (1954, Nov. 12). Miss Nightingale and her ladies in the Crimea. *Nursing Mirror,* 100, x-xi.

Konderska, Z. (1971, Oct.) The birthday of nursing (Florence Nightingale). *Pielig Polozna,* 8, 12-13.

Konstatinova, M. (1923, Oct.). In the cradle of nursing. *American Journal of Nursing,* 24, 47-49.

Kopf, E.W. (1978, Oct.). Florence Nightingale as statistician. *Research in Nursing and Health,* 1(3), 93-102.

Kovacs, A.F. (1973, May/June). The personality of Florence Nightingale. *International Nursing Review,* 20, 78-79.

The lady with a lamp. (1929, Feb.). *Nursing Times,* 25, 154.

Large, J.T. (1985, May). Florence Nightingale: A multifaceted personality. *Nursing Journal of India,* 76(5), 110, 114.

Lee, C.A. (1987, Feb.). Thrusts of Florence Nightingale in the social context of the 19th century. *Kansas Nurse,* 62(2), 3-4.

Lee, C.A. (1987, May). Discussion/life of Florence Nightingale. *Kansas Nurse,* 63(5), 12-13.

LeVasseur, J. (1998). Student scholarship: Plato, Nightingale, and contemporary nursing. *Image: Journal of Nursing Scholarship,* 30, 281-285.

Levine, M.E. (1963, April). Florence Nightingale: The legend that lives. *Nursing Forum,* 2, 24.

Light, K.M. (1997). Florence Nightingale and holistic philosophy. *Journal of Holistic Nursing,* 15(1), 25-40.

Literature of Florence Nightingale. (1931, April). *Hospital Progress,* 12, 188.

Loane, S.F. (1911, Feb.). Florence Nightingale and district nursing. *American Journal of Nursing,* 11, 383-384.

McKee, E.S. (1909, Sept.). Florence Nightingale and her followers. *Nashville Journal of Medicine and Surgery,* 103, 385-392.

Mackie, T.T. (1942, Jan.). Florence Nightingale and tropical and military medicine. *American Journal of Tropical Medicine,* 22, 1-8.

Macmillan, K. (1994, April/May). Brilliant mind gave Florence her edge . . . Florence Nightingale. *Registered Nurse,* 6(2), 29-30.

Macrae, J. (1995, Spring). Nightingale's spiritual philosophy and its significance for modern nursing. *Image: Journal of Nursing Scholarship,* 27, 8-10.

Materials for the study of Florence Nightingale. (1931, May). *Trained Nurse and Hospital Review,* 86, 656-657.

The meaning of the lamp. (1956, May). *Registered Nurse,* 19, 61.

McDonald, L. (1998). Florence Nightingale: Passionate statistician. *Journal of Holistic Nursing,* 16, 267-277.

Menon, M. (1980, Aug.). The lamp she lit [Florence Nightingale]. *Nursing Journal of India,* 81(8), 214-215.

Miss Nightingale's book of the Crimea. (1954, May). *Nursing Journal of India,* 99, ii-iii.

Monteiro, L. (1972, Nov./Dec.). Research into things past: Tracking down one of Miss Nightingale's correspondents. *Nursing Research,* 21, 526-529.

Monteiro, L. (1973, Nov.). Letters to a friend. *Nursing Times,* 69, 1474-1476.

Monteiro, L.A. (1985, Nov.). Response in anger: Florence Nightingale on the importance of training for nurses. *Journal of Nursing History,* 1(1), 11-18.

The most beautiful old lady. (1951, May 11). *Nursing Journal of India,* 93, 101.

Nagpal, N. (1985, May). Florence Nightingale: A multifaceted personality. *Nursing Journal of India,* 76, 110-114.

Nauright, L. (1984). Politics and power: A new look at Florence Nightingale. *Nursing Forum,* 21, 5-8.

Nelson, J. (1976, May). Florence: The legend [Florence Nightingale]. *Nursing Mirror,* 142(2), 40-41.

Newton, M.E. (1951, Sept.). The power of statistics. *Public Health Nursing,* 43, 502-505.

Newton, M.E. (1952, May). Florence Nightingale's concept of clinical teaching. *Nursing World,* 126, 220-221.

Nightingale bibliography. (1957, May). *American Journal of Nursing,* 57, 585.

Nightingale letter to Alice Fisher in Philadelphia. (1976, Jan.). *American Nurse,* 8(2), 2.

The Nightingale saga (Vol. 1). (1962, Aug.). *Nursing Mirror,* 114, 425.

Ninan, R. (1982, June). The lady with the lamp: A profile. *Nursing Journal of India,* 73(6), 154-155.

No other earth. (1962, Nov.). *Today's Health,* 40, 63.

Noguchi, M. (1969, Oct.). Nightingale's philosophy and its limitations: My theory on Nightingale. *Japanese Journal of Nursing Art,* 10, 65-75.

Notting, M.A. (1927, May). Florence Nightingale as a statistician. *Public Health Nursing,* 19, 207-209.

Noyes, C.D. (1931, Jan.). Florence Nightingale: Sanitarian and Hygienist. *Red Cross Courier,* 10, 41-42.

Nuttall, P. (1983, Sept./Oct.). The passionate statistician . . . Florence Nightingale. *Nursing Times,* 79(30), 25-27.

O'Malley, I.B. (1935, May). Florence Nightingale after the Crimean War (1856-1861). *Trained Nurse, 94,* 401-407.

Oman, C. (1950, Nov.). Florence Nightingale as seen by two biographers. *Nursing Mirror, 92,* 30-31.

The other side of the coin [Editorial]. (1967, May). *New Zealand Nursing Journal, 60,* 40.

Palmer, I.S. (1976, Sept./Oct.). Florence Nightingale and the Salisbury incident. *Nursing Research, 25*(5), 370-377.

Palmer, I.S. (1981, June). Florence Nightingale and international origins of modern nursing. *Image, 13,* 28-31.

Palmer, I.S. (1983, July/Aug.). Nightingale revisited. *Nursing Outlook, 31*(4), 229-233.

Palmer, I.S. (1983, Aug.). Florence Nightingale: The myth and the reality. *Nursing Times, 79,* 40-42.

Parker, P. (1977, March). Florence Nightingale: First lady of administrative nursing. *Supervisor Nurse, 8,* 24-25.

Pearce, E.C. (1954, April). The influence of Florence Nightingale on the spirit of nursing. *International Nursing Review, 1,* 20-22.

Penner, S.J. (1987, May). The remarkable Miss Nightingale. *Kansas Nurse, 62*(5), 11.

Peter, M. (1936, May). A personal interview with Florence Nightingale. *Pacific Coast Journal of Nursing, 32,* 270-271.

Phillips, E.C. (1920, May). Florence Nightingale: A study. *Pacific Coast Journal of Nursing, 16,* 272-274.

Pickering, G. (1974, Dec.). Florence Nightingale's illness [Letter]. *British Medical Journal, 4*(5945), 656.

Public health nursing: Florence Nightingale as a consultant. (1920, May). *Pacific Coast Journal of Nursing, 16,* 299-300.

Rabstein, C. (2000). Patron saint or has-been? . . . Role models: Is Florence Nightingale holding us back? *Nursing, 30*(1), 8.

Rains, A.J. (1982, Feb.). Mitchiner memorial lecture: "The Nightingale touch." *Journal of the Royal Army Medical Corps, 128*(1), 4-17.

Rao, G.A. (1971, June). Florence Nightingale's writings. *Nursing Journal of India, 62,* 179.

Remembering Florence Nightingale. (1979, Sept.). *Nursing Focus, 1*(1), 34.

Rhynas, M. (1931, May). Intimate sketch of the life of Florence Nightingale. *Canadian Nurse, 27,* 229-233.

Richards, L. (1920, May). Recollections of Florence Nightingale. *American Journal of Nursing, 20,* 649.

Richards, L. (Ed.). (1934). Letters of Florence Nightingale. *Yale Review, 24,* 326-347.

Roberts, M.M. (1937, July). Florence Nightingale as a nurse educator. *American Journal of Nursing, 37,* 773-778.

Rogers, P. (1982, July). Florence Nightingale: The myth and the reality. *Nursing Focus, 3*(11), 10.

Ross, M. (1954, May). Miss Nightingale's letters. *American Journal of Nursing, 53,* 593-594.

Scovil, E.R. (1911, Feb.). Personal recollections of Florence Nightingale. *American Journal of Nursing, 11,* 365-368.

Scovil, E.R. (1913, Oct.). Florence Nightingale. *American Journal of Nursing, 14,* 28-33.

Scovil, E.R. (1914, Oct.). Florence Nightingale and her nurses. *American Journal of Nursing, 15,* 13-18.

Scovil, E.R. (1916, Dec.). The love story of Florence Nightingale. *American Journal of Nursing, 17,* 209-212.

Scovil, E.R. (1920, May). The later activities of Florence Nightingale. *American Journal of Nursing, 20,* 609-612.

Scovil, E.R. (1927, May). Florence Nightingale's notes on nursing. *American Journal of Nursing, 27,* 355-357.

Seden, F. (1947, July.). Florence Nightingale and Turkish education. *Public Health Nursing, 39,* 349.

Selanders, L.C. (1998). Florence Nightingale: The evolution and social impact of feminist values in nursing. *Journal of Holistic Nursing, 16*(2), 227-243.

Selanders, L.C. (1998). The power of environmental adaptation: Florence Nightingale's original theory for nursing practice. *Journal of Holistic Nursing, 16,* 247-263.

Sellman, D. (1977, Jan.). The virtues of moral education of nurses: Florence Nightingale revisited. *Nursing Ethics: An International Journal for Health Care Professionals, 4,* 3-11.

Seymer, L.R. (1947, Sept.). Florence Nightingale oration. *International Nursing Bulletin, 3,* 12-17.

Seymer, L.R. (1951, July). Florence Nightingale at Kaiserwerth. *American Journal of Nursing, 51,* 424-426.

Seymer, L.R. (1954, April). Florence Nightingale. *Nursing Mirror, 99,* 34-36.

Seymer, L.R. (1960, May). Nightingale Nursing School: 100 years ago. *American Journal of Nursing, 60,* 658.

Seymer, S. (1979, May). The writings of Florence Nightingale. *Nursing Journal of India, 70*(5), 121-128.

Skeet, M. (1980, Oct.). Nightingale's notes on nursing, 1860-1980 [Interview by Alison Dunn]. *Nursing Times, 76*(43), 1871-1873.

Slater, V.E. (1994, Feb.). The educational and philosophical influences on Florence Nightingale, an enlightened conductor. *Nursing History Review, 2,* 137-152.

Smith, F.T. (1981, May). Florence Nightingale: Early feminist. *American Journal of Nursing, 81,* 1059-1061.

Some letters from Florence Nightingale. (1935, Feb.). *Hospital, 31,* 50.

Sotejo, J.V. (1970, April/June). Florence Nightingale: Nurse for all seasons. *ANPHI Papers, 5,* 4.

Sparacino, P.S.A. (1994, March). Clinical practice: Florence Nightingale: A CNS role model. *Clinical Nurse Specialist, 8*(2), 64.

Stewart, I.M. (1939, Dec.). Florence Nightingale: Educator. *Teachers College Record, 41,* 208-223.

Stronk, K. (1997). Florence Nightingale: Mother of all nurses. *Journal of Nursing Jocularity, 7*(2), 14.

Swain, V. (1983, March). No plaster saint! *Nursing Times, 79*(11), 62-63.

That lamp. (1966, May 13). *Nursing Times, 62,* 631.

The call to war. (1970, May). *Registered Nurse, 33,* 42.

The death of Florence Nightingale [Editorial]. (1910, Sept.). *American Journal of Nursing, 10,* 919-920.

The passing of Florence Nightingale. (1910, Nov.). *Pacific Coast Journal of Nursing, 6,* 481-519.

The real Florence Nightingale. (1912, April 6). *British Journal of Nursing, 48,* 267.

The revolting revisionist historian perspective. (1979, Jan.). *Arizona Medicine, 36*(1), 65-66.

The romantic Florence Nightingale. (1968, May). *Canadian Nurse, 64,* 57.

The wider education of the nurse. (1951, Sept.). *Nursing Journal of India, 93,* 438.

The works of mercy window. (1956, May). *American Journal of Nursing, 56,* 574.

Thompson, J.D. (1980, May). The passionate humanist: From Nightingale to the new nurse. *Nursing Outlook, 28*(5), 290-295.

Tinkler, L.F. (1973, Aug.). The barracks at Scutari: Start of a nursing legend. *Nursing Times, 69,* 1006-1007.

Tobin, J. (1969, March). Observations on Florence Nightingale. *Tar Heel Nurse, 31,* 52-55.

Tracy, M.A. (1940, July). Florence Nightingale and her influence on hospitals. *Pacific Coast Journal of Nursing, 36,* 406-407.

Trautman, M.J. (1971, April). Nurses as poets. *American Journal of Nursing, 71,* 725-728.

Two unpublished letters. (1937, May). *Public Health Nursing, 29,* 307.

Ulrich, B.T. (1999). Continuing Education. Still so much to do: The legacy of Florence Nightingale. *NurseWeek, 12*(25), 10-12.

Verney, H. (1980, Spring). The perfect aunt: FN 1820-1910. *News Letter of the Florence Nightingale International Nurses Association, 70,* 13-16.

Walton, P. (1972, Jan./March). The lady with the lamp: Florence Nightingale. *Philippine Journal of Nursing, 41,* 11-12.

Walton, P. (1986, May). The lady with the lamp (Florence Nightingale). *Nursing Journal of India, 77*(5), 115-116.

Watkin, B. (1976, May). Notes on Nightingale. *Nursing Mirror, 142*(19), 42.

Watson, J. (1998). Reflections: Florence Nightingale and the enduring legacy of transpersonal human caring. *Journal of Holistic Nursing, 16,* 292-294.

Welch, M. (1986, April). Nineteenth-century philosophic influences on Nightingale's concept of the person. *Journal of Nursing History, 1*(2), 3-11.

Westminster Abbey Florence Nightingale Commemorative Service, May 12th, 1970. The 150th anniversary of her birth. (1970, Autumn). *News Letter of the Florence Nightingale International Nurses Association,* pp. 21-24.

Wheeler, W. & Walker, M. (1999, May). Florence: Death of an icon? . . . Florence Nightingale. *Nursing Times, 95*(19), 24-26.

White, F.S. (1923, June). At the gate of the temple. *Public Health Nursing, 15,* 279-283.

Whittaker, E. & Olesen, V.L. (1967, Nov.). Why Florence Nightingale? *American Journal of Nursing, 67,* 2338.

Widerquist, J.G. (1992, Jan./Feb.). The spirituality of Florence Nightingale. *Nursing Research, 41,* 49-55.

Widerquist, J.G. (1997). Sanitary reform and nursing: Edwin Chadwick and Florence Nightingale. *Nursing History Review, 5,* 149-160.

Williams, B. (2000). Florence Nightingale: A relevant heroine for nurses today? *California Nurse, 96*(1), 9, 27.

Williams, C.B. (1961, May). Stories from Scutari. *American Journal of Nursing, 61,* 88.

Winchester, J.H. (1967, May). Tough angel of the battlefield. *Today's Health, 45,* 30.

Winslow, C.E.A (1946, July). Florence Nightingale and public health nursing. *Public Health Nursing, 38,* 330-332.

Wolstenholme, G.E. (1980, Dec.). Florence Nightingale: New lamps for old. *Proceedings of the Royal Society of Medicine, 63,* 1282-1288.

Woodham-Smith, C. (1947, May). Florence Nightingale as a child. *Nursing Mirror, 85,* 91-92.

Woodham-Smith, C. (1952, May). Florence Nightingale revealed. *American Journal of Nursing, 52,* 570-572.

Woodham-Smith, C. (1954, July). The greatest Victorian. *Nursing Times, 50,* 737, 738-741.

Yeates, E.L. (1962, May). The prince consort and Florence Nightingale. *Nursing Mirror, 114,* iii-iv.

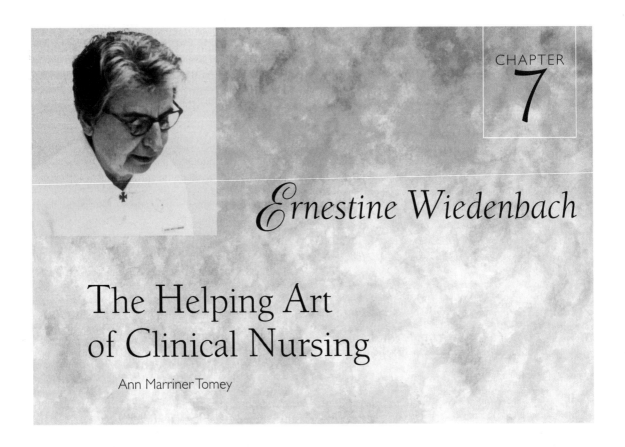

Ernestine Wiedenbach

The Helping Art
of Clinical Nursing

Ann Marriner Tomey

CREDENTIALS AND BACKGROUND OF THE THEORIST

Ernestine Wiedenbach's affluent family immigrated from Germany when she was a young girl. Her interest in nursing began with her childhood experiences with nurses. She greatly admired the private duty nurse who cared for her ailing grandmother. She later enjoyed hearing accounts of nurses' roles in the hospital experiences of a young intern her sister was dating. Captivated by the role of the nurse, Wiedenbach en-

Previous authors: Nancy J. McKee, Marguerite Danko, Terrence J. Heidenreiter, Nancy E. Hunt, Judith E. Marich, Ann Marriner Tomey, Cynthia A. McCreary, and Margery Stuart.
The authors wish to express appreciation to Catherine Martin, Janet Pezelle, and Nancy Preuss for their assistance with data collection and to Ernestine Wiedenbach for critiquing the original chapter.

rolled in the Johns Hopkins Hospital School of Nursing after graduating from Wellesley College in 1922 with a bachelor's degree in liberal arts. After completing her study at Johns Hopkins, she held a variety of positions in hospitals and public health nursing agencies in New York. She also continued her education by attending evening classes at Teachers College at Columbia University, where she received a master's degree and a Certificate in Public Health Nursing. During this period, Hazel Corbin, director of the Maternity Center Association of New York, persuaded Wiedenbach to enroll in the association's School for Nurse-Midwives. After completing the program, Wiedenbach practiced as a nurse-midwife in the home delivery service of the Maternity Center Association.

In addition to her practice, Wiedenbach also developed her academic career. She taught an evening course in advanced maternity nursing at Teachers

College, wrote several articles for professional publications, and remained active in professional nursing organizations. Then, in 1952, she moved from New York to Connecticut, where she was subsequently appointed to the faculty of the Yale University School of Nursing. She was the director of graduate programs in maternal-newborn health nursing, which began in 1956.[5] She wrote *Family-Centered Maternity Nursing*,[8] a text on clinical nursing that was published in 1958. She published classic articles about theory in practice with William Dickoff and Patricia James in 1968.[2]

Wiedenbach[9] developed her model from her vast practical experience and education and, after a long career at Yale, she retired and moved to Florida. She passed away in 1996.

THEORETICAL SOURCES

At Yale, Wiedenbach's theory development benefited from her contact with other faculty members. Ida

Jean Orlando Pelletier stimulated Wiedenbach's understanding of the use of self and the effect of a nurse's thoughts and feelings on the outcome of her actions. In addition, James and Dickoff, philosophy professors who taught classes for nursing faculty on theory related to research and philosophical concepts, reviewed the manuscript for Wiedenbach's book, *Clinical Nursing: A Helping Art*.[9] In her text, they identified elements of a prescriptive theory, which Wiedenbach developed more fully in *Meeting the Realities in Clinical Teaching*.[10]

USE OF EMPIRICAL EVIDENCE

Wiedenbach's model was developed on the basis of her years of experience in clinical practice and teaching. Gustafson[4] did an exploratory study using a naturalistic inquiry design that found a need-for-help in units of vocal and bodily communications in stage one labor.

MAJOR CONCEPTS & DEFINITIONS

PATIENT

To understand Ernestine Wiedenbach's theory, it is necessary to understand her concepts and how her definitions of common nursing terms may differ from or be similar to the current definitions of those words. She defines a patient as "any individual who is receiving help of some kind, be it care, instruction or advice, from a member of the health professions or from a worker in the field of health."[9:3] Therefore to be a patient, the individual does not necessarily have to be sick. Someone receiving preventive healthcare teaching would qualify as a patient.

NEED-FOR-HELP

Wiedenbach believed that every individual experiences needs as a normal part of living. A need is anything the individual may require "to maintain or sustain himself comfortably or capably in

his situation."[9:5] An attempt to meet the need is made by the intervention of help, which is "any measure or action that enables the individual to overcome whatever interferes with his ability to function capably in relation to his situation. . . . To be meaningful, help must be used by an individual and must succeed in enhancing or extending his capability."[9:5-6] Wiedenbach combines these two definitions into a more critical concept for her theory of a need-for-help.

A need-for-help is "any measure or action required and desired by the individual and which has potential for restoring or extending his ability to cope with the demands implicit in his situation."[9:6] It is crucial to the nursing profession that a need-for-help is based on the individual's perception of his own situation. If the individual does not perceive a need as a need-for-help, he or she may not take action to relieve or resolve it.

Continued

MAJOR CONCEPTS & DEFINITIONS—cont'd

NURSE

"The nurse is a functioning human being. As such she not only acts, but she thinks and feels as well. The thoughts she thinks and the feelings she feels as she goes about her nursing are important; they are intimately involved not only in what she does but also in how she does it. They underlie every action she takes, be it the form of a spoken word, a written communication, a gesture, or a deed of any kind. For the nurse whose action is directed toward achievement of a specific purpose, thoughts and feelings have a disciplined role to play."[9:8]

PURPOSE

"Purpose—that which the nurse wants to accomplish through what she does—is the overall goal toward which she is striving, and so is constant. It is her reason for being and for doing; it is the why of clinical nursing and transcends the immediate intent of her assignment or task by specifically directing her activities towards the 'good' of her patient."[9:13]

PHILOSOPHY

"Philosophy, an attitude toward life and reality that evolves from each nurse's beliefs and code of conduct, motivates the nurse to act, guides her thinking about what she is to do and influences her decisions. It stems from both her culture and sub-culture, and is an integral part of her. It is personal in character, unique to each nurse, and expressed in her way of nursing. Philosophy underlines purpose, and her purpose reflects philosophy."[9:13]

PRACTICE

"Overt action, directed by disciplined thoughts and feelings toward meeting the patient's need-for-help, constitutes the practice of clinical nursing. . . . [It] is goal-directed, deliberately carried out and patient-centered."[9:23]

Knowledge, judgment, and skills are three aspects that are necessary for effective practice.[9] Identification, ministration, and validation are three components of practice directly related to the patient's care. Coordination of resources is indirectly related to patient's care.[9]

KNOWLEDGE

"Knowledge encompasses all that has been perceived and grasped by the human mind; its scope and range are infinite. Knowledge may be acquired by the nurse, apart from judgment and skills, in a so-called ivory-tower setting. When acquired in this way, it has potentiality for use in directing, teaching, coordinating and planning care of the patient, but is not sufficient to meet his need-for-help. To be effective in meeting his need, such knowledge must be supplemented by opportunity for the nurse to function in a nurse-patient relationship with responsibility to exercise judgment and to implement skills for the benefit of the patient. Knowledge may be factual, speculative, or practical."[9:25]

Factual Knowledge

"Factual knowledge is something that may be accepted as existing or as being true."[9:25-26]

Speculative Knowledge

"Speculative knowledge, on the other hand, encompasses theories, general principles offered to explain phenomena, beliefs or concepts, and the context of such special subject areas as the natural sciences, the social sciences, and the humanities."[9:26]

Practical Knowledge

"Practical knowledge is knowing how to apply factual or speculative knowledge to the situation at hand."[9:26]

MAJOR CONCEPTS & DEFINITIONS—cont'd

JUDGMENT

[handwritten: evaluation]

[handwritten margin, vertical: her knowledge experience + how she interprets it.]

"Judgment represents the nurse's potentiality for making sound decisions. Judgment grows out of a cognitive process which involves weighing facts—both general and particular—against personal values derived from ideals, principles and convictions. It also involves differentiating facts from assumptions, and relating them to cause and effect. Judgment is personal in character; it will be exercised by the nurse according to how clearly she envisions the purpose to be served, how available relevant knowledge is to her at the time, and how she reacts to prevailing circumstances such as time, setting, and individuals. Decisions resulting from the exercise of judgment will be sound or unsound according to whether or not the nurse has disciplined the functioning of her emotions and of her mind. Uncontrollable emotions can blot out knowledge as well as purpose. Unfounded assumptions can distort facts. Although whatever decision the nurse may make represents her best judgment at the moment of making it, the broader her knowledge and the more available it is to her, and the greater her clarity of purpose, the firmer will be the foundation on which her decisions rest."[9:27]

SKILLS

[handwritten: nurses will ↑ overtime learn and must continually be attentive.]

"Skills represent the nurse's potentiality for achieving desired results. Skills comprise numerous and varied acts, characterized by harmony of movement, expression and intent, by precision, and by adroit use of self. These acts are always carried out with deliberation to achieve a specific purpose and are not goals in themselves. Deliberation and purpose, therefore, differentiate skills from nurses' actions, which, although they may be carried out with proficiency, are performed with the execution of the act as the end to be attained rather than the means by which it is reached."[9:27]

Skills may be classified as procedural skills or communication skills.

Procedural Skills

"Procedural skills are potentialities for implementing procedures that the nurse may need to initiate and carry out in order to identify and meet her patient's need-for-help."[9:27-28]

Communication Skills

"Communication skills are capacities for expression of thoughts and feelings that the nurse desires to convey to her patient and to others associated with his care. Both verbal and nonverbal expression may be used, singly or together, to deliver a message or to elicit a particular response."[9:28]

IDENTIFICATION

[handwritten: nurses must develop there communication skill.]

"Identification involves individualization of the patient, his experiences, and recognition of the patient's perception of his condition."[9:31-32]

"Activities in identification are directed toward ascertaining: (1) whether the patient has a need; (2) whether he recognizes that he has a need; (3) what is interfering with his ability to meet his need; and (4) whether the need represents a need-for-help, in other words, a need that the patient is unable to meet himself."[9:32]

MINISTRATION

Ministration is providing the needed help. It requires the identification of the need-for-help, the selection of a helping measure appropriate to that need, and the acceptability of the help to the patient.[9]

VALIDATION

Validation is evidence that the patient's functional ability was restored as a result of the help given.[9]

Continued

MAJOR CONCEPTS & DEFINITIONS—cont'd

COORDINATION

While striving for unity and continuity, the nurse coordinates all patient services to ensure that care will not be fragmented. Reporting, consulting, and conferring are functional elements of coordination.[9]

REPORTING

"Reporting is the act of presenting information in written or oral form and is important in keeping others informed not only about the patient's health and social history, but also about his current condition, reaction, progress, care and plan of care."[9:33-34]

CONSULTING

"Consulting, the act of seeking information or of asking advice, is a means of gaining, from others, an opinion or suggestion that may help the nurse to broaden her understanding before deciding on a course of action."[9:34]

CONFERRING

"Conferring, the act of exchanging and comparing ideas, is most often initiated to review the patient's response to the care he has so far received, and to plan his future care."[9:35]

ART

Art is "the application of knowledge and skill to bring about desired results. . . . Art is individualized action. Nursing art, then, is carried out by the nurse in a one-to-one relationship with the patient, and constitutes the nurse's conscious responses to specifics in the patient's immediate situation."[9:36]

"The art of clinical nursing is directed toward achievement of four main goals: (1) understanding of the patient and his condition, situation, and need; (2) enhancement of the patient's capability;

(3) improvement of his condition or situation within the framework of the medical plan for his care; and (4) prevention of the recurrence of his problem or development of a new one which may cause anxiety, disability or distress."[9:30-31] Nursing art involves three initial operations: stimulus, preconception, and interpretation.[9] The nurse reacts on the basis of those operations. "Her action may be rational, reactionary, or deliberative."[9:40]

STIMULUS

The helping process is triggered by a stimulus, which is the patient's presenting behavior.[9]

PRECONCEPTION

Preconception is an expectation of what the patient may be like. "The preconception is based on knowledge gained from a great variety of sources including the patient's chart, reports from other nurses, doctors or family members, what the nurse has read or heard of patients in similar condition, her own experiences with patients in similar condition, and, finally, her recollection of previous contacts with the patient."[9:38]

INTERPRETATION

Interpretation is the comparison of perception with expectation or hope. Perception is an interpretation of the stimulus and may misinterpret the patient's behavior.[9]

RATIONAL ACTION

"Rational action is an overt act taken in response solely or mainly to the doer's immediate perception of another's action—verbal or nonverbal—or situation. In a nurse-patient relationship, the nurse's action would be called rational if she responds in a way guided by only her immediate perception of the patient's behavior— what he says, what he does, or how he appears."[9:40]

REACTIONARY ACTION

"Reactionary action, in contrast with rational action, is an overt act taken spontaneously in response to strong feelings the doer experiences when he compares his perception of another's behavior or situation with his expectation or hope about that behavior. In nurse-patient relationship, the nurse's action is reactionary if it is taken solely or mainly in response to her reaction, to the feelings aroused in her by comparing what she perceived as the patient's behavior with what she hoped for or expected."[9:40]

DELIBERATIVE ACTION

"Deliberative action is in contrast with both rational action and reactionary action. A deliberative action is an overt act which, although not failing to take account of the doer's immediate perceptions and feeling-reactions, is, nonetheless, not based solely on these perceptions or feelings. Rather, deliberative action is interaction, directed toward fulfillment of an explicit purpose and carried out with judgment and understanding of how the other means the behavior, which he is manifesting either verbally or nonverbally. In a nurse-patient relationship, the nurse's action is deliberative if her overt action is based on the application—in the fulfillment of her nursing purpose—of principles of helping to gain understanding of how the patient means the behavior he is manifesting."[9:41]

Wiedenbach[9:42] concluded her consideration of the types of action by stating, "My thesis is that nursing art is not comprised of rational nor reactionary actions but rather of deliberative action."

FRAMEWORK OF NURSING

Limits, supports, and research provide a broad framework in which clinical nursing functions. Limits, or boundaries, in a professional service give the individual guidelines to follow in practicing that profession. The profession's code sets professional limits; legal limits are those found in state laws and licensing requirements; the hospital, agency, or individual the nurse works for sets local limits; and the nurse herself sets personal limits.[9]

Supportive facilities for the practicing nurse are nursing administration, nursing education, and nursing organizations. Although these are rarely found at the patient's bedside or in the one-to-one relationship between the nurse and the patient, they are nevertheless important to the nurse by maintaining standards of quality of nursing care for the profession.[9]

Although more nursing research was beginning to occur, Wiedenbach recognized that nursing research had not received a great deal of emphasis from the profession in the past. She acknowledged that such activity was essential to the growth of nursing and might even "prove to be crucial to the conservation of life and the promotion of health."[9:85]

MAJOR ASSUMPTIONS

Nursing

Nurses ascribe to an explicit philosophy. Basic to this philosophy of nursing are: "(1) reverence for the gift of life; (2) respect for the dignity, worth, autonomy, and individuality of each human being; (3) resolution to act dynamically in relation to one's beliefs."[9:16] The rationale for nursing is stated in

". . . the reason she has come into being is that there is a patient who needs her help."[9:3] Wiedenbach[9:2] identifies five essential attributes of a professional person:

1. Clarity of purpose.
2. Mastery of skill and knowledge essential for fulfilling the purpose.

3. Ability to establish and sustain purposeful working relationships with others (both professional and nonprofessional individuals).

4. Interest in advancing knowledge in the area of interest and in creating new knowledge.

5. Dedication to furthering the goal of humankind rather than supporting self-aggrandizement.

Person

Four explicit assumptions are stated in relation to human nature:

1. Each human being is endowed with the unique potential to develop—within self—resources that enable them to maintain and sustain himself.

2. The human being basically strives toward self-direction and relative independence and desires not only to make best use of his capabilities and potentialities, but to fulfill his responsibilities.

3. Self-awareness and self-acceptance are essential to the individual's sense of integrity and self-worth.

4. Whatever the individual does represents his or her best judgment at the moment of his doing.[9:17,11]

In relation to the patient's perception of his or her condition, Wiedenbach[9:14] wrote, "An individual should want to be healthy, comfortable, and capable, and . . . when unimpeded, he strives by his own efforts to achieve such states."

Health

The concept of health is neither defined nor discussed in Wiedenbach's model. The definitions of nursing, patient, and need-for-help, and the relationships among these concepts, imply health-related concerns in the nurse-patient situation.

Environment

Wiedenbach does not specifically address the concept of environment; however, she recognized the potential effects of the environment. In a statement of purpose for clinical nursing, she said, "To facilitate the efforts of the individual to overcome the obsta-cles which currently interfere with his ability to respond capably to demands made of him by this condition, environment, situation, and time."[9:14-15] It is implied that the environment may produce obstacles resulting in the person experiencing a need-for-help.

THEORETICAL ASSERTIONS

Identification of the patient's need-for-help involves four steps. First, the nurse uses powers of observation to look and listen for actual consistencies and inconsistencies in the patient's behavior compared with the nurse's expectations for patient behavior. Second, the nurse explores the meaning of the patient's behavior with the patient. Third, the nurse determines the cause of the patient's discomfort or incapability. Finally, the nurse determines whether the patient can resolve his or her problem or if the patient has a need-for-help (Figure 7-1).[9]

Ministration of needed help involves the nurse making a plan to meet patient needs and presenting it to the patient. If the patient concurs with the plan and accepts suggestions for implementing it, the nurse implements it and ministration of needed help occurs. If the patient does not concur with the plan or accept suggestions for implementation, the nurse needs to explore causes of the patient's nonacceptance. If the patient has an interfering problem, the nurse needs to explore the patient's ability to solve the problem. If the patient has a need-for-help, the nurse once again forms a plan to meet the need, presents the plan, and seeks patient concurrence and acceptance of suggestions for implementation (Figure 7-2).[9]

Validation that the need-for-help was met is important. The nurse perceives whether the patient's behavior is consistent with the nurse's concept of comfort and seeks clarification from the patient to determine whether he or she believes the need-for-help was met. Then the nurse needs to take appropriate action on the basis of the feedback (Figure 7-3).[9]

LOGICAL FORM

Wiedenbach developed this model through induction. The reasoning method in inductive logic begins with observation of specific instances and then com-

model.

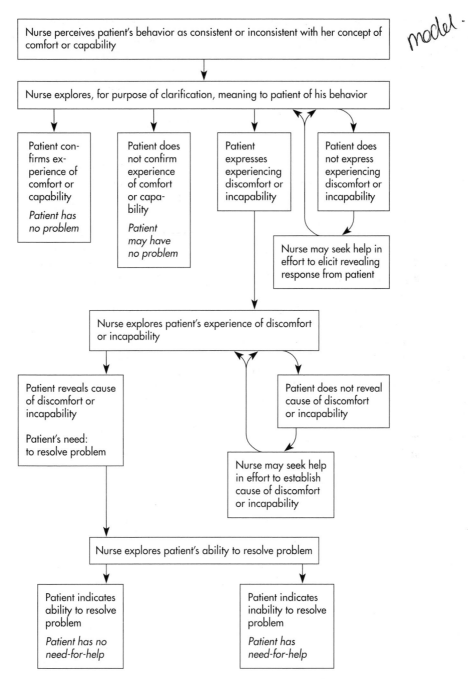

Figure **7-1** **Identification of a need-for-help.** (From Wiedenbach, E. [1964]. *Clinical nursing: A helping art* [p. 60]. New York: Springer. Used with permission.)

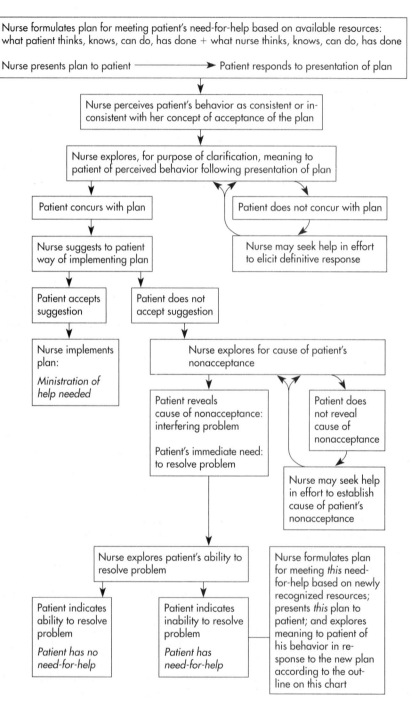

Figure **7-2 Ministration of help.** (From Wiedenbach, E. [1964]. *Clinical nursing: A helping art* [p. 61]. New York: Springer. Used with permission.)

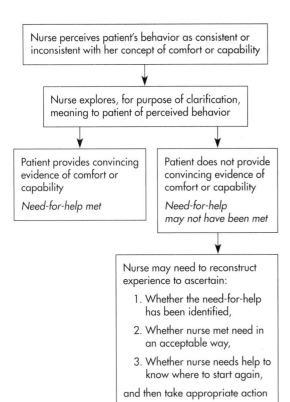

┌───┐
│ Nurse perceives patient's behavior as consistent or │
│ inconsistent with her concept of comfort or capability │
└───┘

┌───┐
│ Nurse explores, for purpose of clarification, │
│ meaning to patient of perceived behavior │
└───┘

┌──────────────────────┐ ┌──────────────────────┐
│ Patient provides convincing │ │ Patient does not provide │
│ evidence of comfort or │ │ convincing evidence of │
│ capability │ │ comfort or capability │
│ *Need-for-help met* │ │ *Need-for-help* │
│ │ │ *may not have been met* │
└──────────────────────┘ └──────────────────────┘

┌───┐
│ Nurse may need to reconstruct │
│ experience to ascertain: │
│ 　1. Whether the need-for-help │
│ 　　has been identified, │
│ 　2. Whether nurse met need in │
│ 　　an acceptable way, │
│ 　3. Whether nurse needs help to │
│ 　　know where to start again, │
│ and then take appropriate action │
└───┘

Figure **7-3** Validation that need-for-help was met. (From Wiedenbach, E. [1964]. *Clinical nursing: A helping art* [p. 62]. New York: Springer. Used with permission.)

bines the specifics into a more generalized whole. The common features of the specific instances enable the grouping of specifics into a larger set of phenomena.[1] An analysis of clinical experiences (specific nursing situations) leads to the interrelationships and development of concepts in Wiedenbach's model.[6]

Dickoff, James, and Wiedenbach[2] have identified four levels of theory development in a practice discipline. In order of increasing sophistication, these levels are factor-isolating, factor-relating, situation-relating, and situation-producing. Wiedenbach[11] considers her work a situation-producing prescriptive theory.

ACCEPTANCE BY THE NURSING COMMUNITY

Practice

Today, nurses are applying Wiedenbach's concepts to their clinical practice, more so than nurses in the 1950s and 1960s. According to Wiedenbach,[9:23] the practice of clinical nursing is an "overt action, directed by disciplined thoughts and feelings toward meeting the patient's need-for-help." Drawing from her many years of experience as a nurse-midwife, she published "Childbirth as Mothers Say They Like It."[7] In this article, Wiedenbach noted that mothers wanted childbirth to be as natural as possible. In addition, mothers wanted instruction on childbirth, father participation, full participation in the labor and delivery process, and rooming-in with their infant during the postpartum period.[7] However, some or most of these needs-for-help were not met until the 1970s. In the 1980s, the healthcare industry provided the supposedly unique concept of family-centered care, which Wiedenbach addressed some 20 years ago.

Education

Wiedenbach[9:75,11] proposed that nursing education serves the nursing practice in four major ways:

1. It is responsible for the preparation of future practitioners of nursing.
2. It arranges for nursing students to gain experience in clinical areas of the hospital or in the homes of patients.
3. Its representatives may function in the clinical area and work closely with the staff.
4. It offers educational opportunities to the nurse for special or advanced study.

The application of Wiedenbach's model to clinical practice requires the nurse to have a sound knowledge of the normal and pathological states, a thorough understanding of human psychology, competence in clinical skills, and the ability to initiate and maintain therapeutic communication with the patient and family. Also, the nurse must develop sound clinical judgment in making decisions about patient care and be able to interpret the patient's behavior. These skills require a general education for nurses.

Today, many nursing schools are meeting this need for general education. Students are prepared with two years of courses in the humanities, biological science, and the social sciences, which is followed by two years in nursing science. This curriculum prepares a generalist in professional nursing and serves as the basis for graduate study.

Wiedenbach[9] saw graduate study as a means for nurses to extend the personal limits of their practice and to realize, to a greater degree than before, their potential for creative and imaginative practice within the area of their responsibility in the total field of health. Today's focus on graduate education is much the same. It is directed toward preparing advanced practitioners who are competent, self-directed, and concerned with the exploration of practices, issues, and problems of healthcare in a selected area of nursing.

Research

Before the development of Wiedenbach's model, nursing research focused more on the medical model than on a nursing model. However, in Wiedenbach's model, the focus of nursing research is related to the patient's response to the healthcare experience. Her model would support research designed to promote family relationships, to control factors responsible for disabling conditions, and to foster sound healthcare practices. Although they are not specifically based on Wiedenbach's model, numerous nursing research studies have been carried out in those areas. The results of those studies have been reported in nursing periodicals such as *Nursing Research*. Nurses are better able to meet the patient's need for help because these nursing studies were conducted.

Wiedenbach's concept of need-for-help was used as a focus for doctoral research that was completed in 1988. The vocal and bodily behaviors of women in the first stage of labor were videotaped to determine when a need-for-help occurred. The women and the researcher reviewed these tapes the day after delivery. Findings indicated that care-eliciting be-

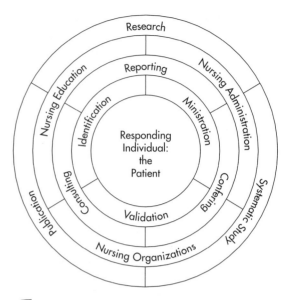

Figure **7-4 Clinical nursing: The relationship between its focus and its constituents.** (From Wiedenbach, E. [©1964]. *Clinical nursing: A helping art* [p. 108]. New York: Springer Publishing Company, Inc., New York 10012. Used by permission.)

haviors were influenced by a cognitively experienced need-for-help and that these behaviors were observable measures of nonverbalized need-for-help and decreased coping.[4]

In a graph, Wiedenbach displayed all the constituent parts of her clinical nursing model at the end of her 1964 treatise (Figure 7-4).[9]

FURTHER DEVELOPMENT

Wiedenbach is a pioneer in the writing of nursing theory. Her model of clinical nursing is one of the early attempts to systematically describe what nurses do and what nursing is about. Wiedenbach's model needs to be further developed by more clearly defining the concepts of health and environment. In addition, the component of nursing art needs to be identified in an operational way.

CRITIQUE

Wiedenbach's model evolved out of a desire to describe the practice of professional nursing. Pelletier influenced her theory, as did the philosophy of Dickoff and James, her colleagues at Yale University. Wiedenbach's theory was one of the earlier nursing theories developed.

Clarity

Wiedenbach's model meets the criterion of clarity because the concepts and definitions are clear, consistent, and intelligible.

Simplicity

There are too many relational statements for the theory to be classified as a simple theory. The concepts include need-for-help, nursing practice, and nursing art. All of these concepts are interrelated, equal in importance, and have no meaning aside from their interaction.[6] Relationships among the major components can be linked, but it is difficult to diagram some of the concepts in the model. In addition, the concepts describe or explain phenomena, but they do not predict.

Generality

The scope of the concepts of patient, nursing, and need-for-help are very broad and therefore possess generality. However, the concept of need-for-help is based on the patient's recognition of his or her need for help. This concept is not applicable to infants, comatose patients, or many other physiologically or psychologically incompetent persons. Also, the assumption that all nurses do not share a similar philosophy of nursing lessens the generality of the model.

Empirical Precision

Substantiation of a theory is accomplished through research; therefore the usefulness of the theory is determined. In Wiedenbach's model, the criterion is only partially met. The concepts of nursing practice and need-for-help are operationally defined and measurable. However, the concept of need-for-help is not always applicable. Also, within this theory, there is little attempt to operationally define

nursing art. Therefore it would be difficult to test this theory.

However, the potential exists for research to be done with this model. Fawcett believes three steps must be taken before the model can be tested. Fawcett[3:26] stated, "First, the model must be formulated; secondly, a theory must be derived from the model; and third, operational definitions must be given to the concepts, and hypothesis derived."

Derivable Consequences

Derivable consequences refer to the overall effect of the theory and its importance to nursing research, practice, and education. Wiedenbach's model fulfills the purpose for which it was developed; that is, to describe professional practice. The theory focuses on nurse-patient interactions and regards the patient from a holistic point of view. Wiedenbach's work influenced the work of other early scholars, including Orlando and Peplau. As one of the early nursing theorists, Wiedenbach made an important contribution to the nursing profession.

CRITICAL THINKING *Activities*

1. Compare Wiedenbach's identification of a need-for-help or no need-for-help to Virginia Henderson's definition of nursing (see Chapter 8).

2. Relate Wiedenbach's model to the nursing process. Determine similarities and differences.

3. Identify communication skills that are necessary to use Wiedenbach's model. Practice these skills with a patient, coworker, or friend.

4. Write definitions for health and environment as they are inferred in Wiedenbach's definitions of need-for-help and nursing art.

5. Differentiate skills and actions as described in the Wiedenbach model.

6. Compare and contrast deliberative action with rational and reactionary actions.

REFERENCES

1. Chinn, P.L. & Jacobs, M.K. (1983). *Theory and nursing: A systematic approach.* St. Louis: Mosby.
2. Dickoff, J.J., James, P.A., & Wiedenbach, E. (1968, Nov./Dec.). Theory in a practice discipline. II: Practice-oriented research. *Nursing Research,* 17, 545-554.
3. Fawcett, J. (1984). *Analysis and evaluation of conceptual models of nursing.* Philadelphia: F.A. Davis.
4. Gustafson, D.C. (1988). Signaling behavior in stage I labor to elicit care: A clinical referent for Wiedenbach's need-for-help (Doctoral dissertation, Texas Woman's University, 1988). *Dissertation Abstracts International*–B, 49/10, 4230.
5. Nickel, S., Gesse, T., & MacLaren, A. (1992). Ernestine Wiedenbach: Her professional legacy. *Journal of Nurse-Midwifery,* 37, 161-167.
6. Raleigh, E. (1983). Wiedenbach's model. In J. Fitzpatrick & A. Whall (Eds.), *Conceptual models of nursing: Analysis and application.* Bowie, MD: Robert J. Brady.
7. Wiedenbach, E. (1949, Aug.). Childbirth as mothers say they like it. *Public Health Nursing,* 41, 417-421.
8. Wiedenbach, E. (1958). *Family-centered maternity nursing.* New York: Putnam.
9. Wiedenbach, E. (©1964). *Clinical nursing: A helping art.* New York: Springer Publishing Company, Inc., New York 10012. Quotes used by permission.
10. Wiedenbach, E. (1969). *Meeting the realities in clinical teaching.* New York: Springer.
11. Wiedenbach, E. (1984, Spring). Written interview.

BIBLIOGRAPHY
Primary Sources
Books

Wiedenbach, E. (1958). *Family-centered maternity nursing.* New York: Putnam.

Wiedenbach, E. (1964). *Clinical nursing: A helping art.* New York: Springer.

Wiedenbach, E. (1967). *Family-centered maternity nursing* (2nd ed.). New York: Putnam.

Wiedenbach, E. (1969). *Meeting the realities in clinical teaching.* New York: Springer.

Wiedenbach, E. (1982). *Communication: Key to effective nursing.* New York: Tiresias.

Wiedenbach, E. & Falls, C.E. (1978). *Communication: Key to effective nursing.* New York: Tiresias.

Book Chapter

Wiedenbach, E. (1973). The nursing process in maternity nursing. In J.P. Clausen (Ed.), *Maternity nursing today.* New York: McGraw-Hill.

Journal Articles

Dickoff, J.J., James, P.A., & Wiedenbach, E. (1968, Sept./Oct.). Theory in a practice discipline. I: Practice-oriented theory. *Nursing Research,* 14, 415-435.

Dickoff, J.J., James, P.A., & Wiedenbach, E. (1968, Nov./Dec.). Theory in a practice discipline. II: Practice-oriented theory. *Nursing Research,* 17, 545-554.

Wiedenbach, E. (1940, Jan.). Toward educating 130 million people: A history of the nursing information bureau. *American Journal of Nursing,* 40, 13-18.

Wiedenbach, E. (1949, Aug.). Childbirth as mothers say they like it. *Public Health Nursing,* 41, 417-421.

Wiedenbach, E. (1951). Safeguarding the mother's breasts. *American Journal of Nursing,* 51, 544-548.

Wiedenbach, E. (1956). *Family-centered maternity nursing.* New York: Putnam.

Wiedenbach, E. (1960, May). Nurse-midwifery: Purpose, practice, and opportunity. *Nursing Outlook,* 8, 256.

Wiedenbach, E. (1963, Nov.). The helping art of nursing. *American Journal of Nursing,* 63, 54-57.

Wiedenbach, E. (1965, Dec.). Family nurse practitioner for maternal and child care. *Nursing Outlook,* 13, 50.

Wiedenbach, E. (1968, June). The nurse's role in family planning: A conceptual base for practice. *Nursing Clinics of North America,* 3, 355-365.

Wiedenbach, E. (1968, May). Genetics and the nurse. *Bulletin of the American College of Nurse Midwifery,* 13, 8-13.

Wiedenbach, E. (1970, May). Nurses' wisdom in nursing theory. *American Journal of Nursing,* 70, 1057-1062.

Secondary Sources
Journal Articles

Carrington, B.W., Loftman, P.O., Boucher, E., Irish, G., Piniaz, D.K., & Mitchell, J.L. (1994). Modifying a childbirth education curriculum for two specific populations: Inner-city adolescents and substance-using women. *Journal of Nurse-Midwifery,* 39, 312-320.

Dickoff, J. & James, P. (1970). Beliefs and values: Bases for curriculum design. *Nursing Research,* 19, 415-427.

Eisler, J., Wolfer, J.A., & Diers, D. (1972). Relationship between the need for social approval and postoperative recovery welfare. *Nursing Research,* 21, 520-525.

McCabe, P. (1994, Dec./1995, Jan.). Nursing, healing and natural therapies: Testing the waters. *The Lamp,* 35-36.

McKay, S. & Roberts, J. (1990). Obstetrics by ear: Maternal and caregiver perceptions of the meaning of maternal sounds during second stage labor. *Journal of Nurse-Midwifery,* 35, 266-273.

Nelson, M. (1988). Advocacy in nursing. *Nursing Outlook,* 36, 136-141.

Nickel, S., Gesse, T., & MacLaren, A. (1992, May/June). Ernestine Wiedenbach: Her professional legacy. *Journal of Nurse-Midwifery, 37*(3), 161-167.

Pranulis, M.F. (1986). Re: Toward a theory of nursing: Skills and competency in nurse-patient interaction [letter to the editor]. *Nursing Research, 35,* 329, 391.

Rickleman, B.L. (1971). Bio-psycho-social linguistics: A conceptual approach to nurse-patient interaction. *Nursing Research, 20,* 398-403.

Schmidt, J. (1972). Availability: A concept of nursing practice. *American Journal of Nursing, 72,* 1086-1089.

Shields, D. (1978). Nursing care in labor and patient satisfaction: A descriptive study. *Journal of Advanced Nursing, 3,* 535-550.

Thompson, J.B. (1981). Nurse midwives and health promotion during pregnancy. *Birth Defects, 17*(6), 29-57.

Tolley, K.A. (1995). Theory from practice for practice: Is this a reality? *Journal of Advanced Nursing, 21,* 184-190.

VandeVusse, L. (1997, Jan./Feb.). Education exchange: Sculpting a nurse-midwifery philosophy: Ernestine Wiedebach's influence. *Journal of Nurse-Midwifery, 42*(1), 43-48.

Wallace, C.L. & Appleton, C. (1995). Nursing as the promotion of well-being: The client's experience. *Journal of Advanced Nursing, 22,* 285-289.

Wolfer, J. (1993). Aspects of "reality" and ways of knowing in nursing: In search of an integrating paradigm. *Image Journal of Nursing Scholarship, 25*(2), 141-146.

Wolfer, J. & Visintainer, M. (1975). Pediatric surgical patients' and parents' stress responses and adjustment. *Nursing Research, 24,* 244-255.

Wooden, H.E. & Engel, E.L. (1965). Infection control in family-centered maternity care. *Obstetrics and Gynecology, 25,* 232-234.

Dissertation

Gustafson, D.C. (1988). Signaling behavior in stage I labor to elicit care: A clinical referent for Wiedenbach's need-for-help (Doctoral dissertation, Texas Woman's University, 1988). *Dissertation Abstracts International*–B, 49/10, 4230.

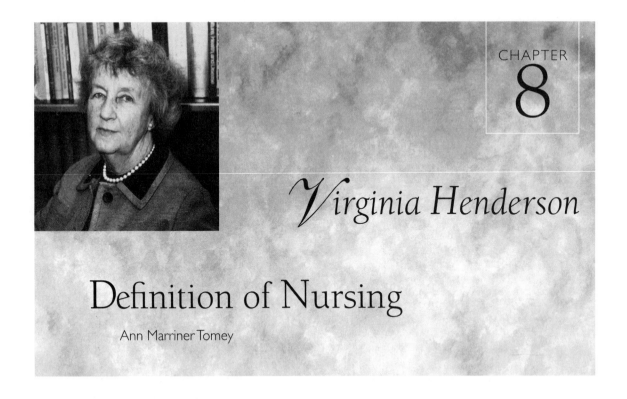

*V*irginia Henderson

Definition of Nursing

Ann Marriner Tomey

CREDENTIALS AND BACKGROUND OF THE THEORIST

Virginia Henderson, the fifth of eight children in her family, was born in 1897. A native of Kansas City, Missouri, Henderson spent her developmental years in Virginia because her father practiced law in Washington, DC.

During World War I, Henderson developed an interest in nursing. In 1918, she entered the Army School of Nursing in Washington, DC and graduated in 1921. She accepted a position as a staff nurse with the Henry Street Visiting Nurse Service in New York City. In 1922, Henderson began teaching nursing in Norfolk Protestant Hospital in Virginia. Five years later, she entered Teachers College at Columbia University where she subsequently earned her B.S. and

Previous authors: Sr. Judith E. Alexander, Deborah Wertman DeMeester, Tamara Lauer, Ann Marriner Tomey, Susan E. Neal, and Sandy Williams.
The authors wish to express appreciation to Virginia Henderson for critiquing the original chapter.

M.A. degrees in nursing education. In 1929, Henderson served as a teaching supervisor in the clinics of Strong Memorial Hospital in Rochester, New York. She returned to Teachers College in 1930 as a faculty member and, until 1948, she taught courses in the nursing analytical process and clinical practice.[4,32,33]

Henderson enjoyed a long career as an author and researcher. While on the Teachers College faculty, she rewrote the fourth edition of Bertha Harmer's 1939 *Textbook of the Principles and Practice of Nursing*.[9] The fifth edition of the textbook was published in 1955 and contained Henderson's own definition of nursing. Henderson was associated with Yale University from the early 1950s and did much to further nursing research through this association. From 1959 to 1971, Henderson directed the Yale-sponsored Nursing Studies Index Project. The Nursing Studies Index was developed into a four volume, annotated index to nursing's biographical, analytical, and historical literature from 1900 to 1959. Concurrently, Henderson authored or coauthored several other important works. Her pamphlet, *Basic Principles of Nursing Care*,[15] was published for the International Council of Nurses in 1960 and was translated into more than 20 languages. Henderson's five-year collaboration with Leo Simmons produced a national survey of nursing research that was published in 1964. Her book, *The Nature of Nursing*,[13] was published in 1966 and it described her concept of nursing's primary, unique function. The National League for Nursing reprinted it in 1991. The sixth edition of *The Principles and Practice of Nursing*,[28] published in 1978, was coauthored by Henderson and Gladys Nite and edited by Henderson. This textbook has been widely used in the curriculums of various nursing schools. Her classic textbooks have been translated into more than 25 languages. Henderson was cofounder of the Interagency Council on Information Resources for Nursing, which was created to address information issues in nursing. She was also the cofounder of the New England Regional Council on Library Resources for Nursing and the first chairperson of the International Nursing Index Editorial Advisory Committee. Throughout the 1980s, Henderson remained active as a research associate emeritus at Yale. Henderson's achievements and influence in the nursing profession have brought her more than nine honorary doctoral degrees and the first Christiane Reimann Award. Henderson was given the Mary Adelaide Nutting Award from the U.S. National League for Nursing, an honorary Fellowship in the American Academy of Nursing, an honorary membership in the London Association of Integrated and Degree Courses in Nursing, and an honorary Fellowship in the Royal College of Nursing in England. In 1983, she received Sigma Theta Tau International's Mary Tolle Wright Founders Award for Leadership, one of the honor society's highest honors.[25] At the 1988 American Nurses Association (ANA) Convention, she received a special citation of honor for her lifelong contributions to nursing research, education, and professionalism.

Henderson died in March of 1996 at the age of 98. Her definition of nursing is known around the world and her work continues to influence the practice of nursing, the education of nurses, and nursing research internationally. Henderson became a legend in her lifetime, which led to the naming of Sigma Theta Tau's International Nursing Library in her honor. It was fitting that the announcement of Henderson's death traveled through the nursing community on the Internet. Online, Halloran[6] wrote, "Miss Virginia Avenel Henderson was to the twentieth century as Florence Nightingale was to the nineteenth. Both wrote extensive works that have influenced the world."

THEORETICAL SOURCES

Henderson first published her definition of nursing in the 1955 revision of Harmer and Henderson's *The Principles and Practice of Nursing*.[8] There were three major influences on Henderson's decision to synthesize her own definition of nursing. First, she revised *Textbook of the Principles and Practice of Nursing*[9] in 1939. Henderson[32:119] identified her work for this text as the source that made her realize "the necessity of being clear about the function of nurses."

A second source was her involvement as a committee member in a regional conference of the National Nursing Council in 1946. Her committee work was incorporated into Esther Lucile Brown's 1948 report, *Nursing for the Future*.[2] Henderson[12:62] stated that this report represented her "point of view modified by the thinking of others in the group." Finally, the ANA's five-year investigation of the function of the nurse interested Henderson, who was not fully satisfied with the definition the ANA adopted in 1955.

Henderson labeled her work as a definition rather than a theory because theory was not in vogue at that time. She described her interpretation as the "synthesis of many influences, some positive and some negative."[10:64] In *The Nature of Nursing*,[13] she identified the following sources of influence during her early years of nursing.

Annie W. Goodrich

Goodrich was an inspiration to Henderson. She was the dean of the Army School of Nursing, where

Henderson achieved her basic nursing education. Henderson[13:7] recalled, "Whenever she visited our unit, she lifted our sights above techniques and routine." She also attributed Goodrich with "my early discontent with the regimentalized patient care in which I participated and the concept of nursing as merely ancillary to medicine."[13:7]

Caroline Stackpole

When Henderson was a graduate student, Stackpole was a philosophy professor at Teachers College at Columbia University. She impressed upon Henderson the importance of maintaining physiological balance.[13]

Jean Broadhurst

Broadhurst was a microbiology professor at Teachers College. The importance of hygiene and asepsis made an impact on Henderson.[13]

Dr. Edward Thorndike

Thorndike worked in psychology at Teachers College. He conducted investigational studies on the fundamental needs of humans. Henderson[13:11] realized that illness is "more than a state of disease" and that most fundamental needs are not met in hospitals.

Dr. George Deaver

Deaver was a physicist at the Institute for the Crippled and Disabled and, later, at Bellevue Hospital. Henderson[13] observed that the goal of rehabilitative efforts at the institute was rebuilding the patient's independence.

Bertha Harmer

Harmer, a Canadian nurse, was the original author of *Textbook of the Principles and Practice of Nursing*,[7] which Henderson revised. Henderson never met Harmer, but similarities of their respective definitions of nursing are obvious. Harmer's 1922 definition[7:54] begins, "Nursing is rooted in the needs of the humanity."

Ida Jean Orlando (Pelletier)

Henderson identified Orlando as an influence on her concept of the nurse-patient relationship. She stated, "Ida Orlando (Pelletier) made me realize how easily the nurse can act on misconceptions of the patient's needs if she does not check her interpretation of them with him."[13:14]

USE OF EMPIRICAL EVIDENCE

Henderson incorporated physiological and psychological principles into her personal concept of nursing. Her background in these areas stemmed from her association with Stackpole and Thorndike during her graduate studies at Teachers College.

Stackpole[13] based her physiology course on Claude Bernard's dictum that health depends on keeping lymph constant around the cell. From this, Henderson[13:11] surmised that "a definition of nursing should imply an appreciation of the principle of physiological balance." From Bernard's theory, Henderson also gained an appreciation for psychosomatic medicine and its implications for nursing. She stated her view in the following way: "It was obvious that emotional balance is inseparable from physiological balance once I realized that an emotion is actually our interpretation of cellular response to fluctuations in the chemical composition of the intercellular fluids."[13:11]

Henderson did not identify the precise theories that Thorndike supported; she only stated that they involved the fundamental needs of human beings. A correlation with Abraham Maslow's hierarchy of needs is seen in Henderson's 14 components of nursing care, which begin with physical needs and progress to the psychosocial components. Although she does not cite Maslow as an influence, she described his theory of human motivation in the sixth edition of *The Principles and Practice of Nursing* in 1978.[28]

MAJOR CONCEPTS & DEFINITIONS

NURSING

Henderson defined nursing in functional terms. She stated, "The unique function of the nurse is to assist the individual, sick or well, in the performance of those activities contributing to health or its recovery (or to peaceful death) that he would perform unaided if he had the necessary strength, will or knowledge. And to do this in such a way as to help him gain independence as rapidly as possible."[13:15]

HEALTH

Henderson did not state her own definition of health. But in her writing, she equated health with independence. In the sixth edition of *The Principles and Practice of Nursing*,[28] she cited several definitions of health from various sources, including the one from the charter of the World Health Organization. She viewed health in terms of the patient's ability to perform the 14 components of nursing care unaided. She said it is "the quality of health rather than life itself, that margin of mental/physical vigor that allows a person to work most effectively and to reach his highest potential level of satisfaction in life."[28:122]

ENVIRONMENT

Again, Henderson did not give her own definition of environment. Instead, she used *Webster's New Collegiate Dictionary*,[34] 1961, which defined environment as "the aggregate of all the external conditions and influences affecting the life and development of an organism."[28:829]

PERSON (PATIENT)

Henderson[12] viewed the patient as an individual who requires assistance to achieve health and independence or peaceful death. The mind and body are inseparable. The patient and his or her family are viewed as a unit.

NEEDS

No specific definition of a need is found, but Henderson identified 14 basic needs of the patient, which comprise the components of nursing care.* These include the following needs:

1. Breathe normally.
2. Eat and drink adequately.
3. Eliminate body wastes.
4. Move and maintain desirable postures.
5. Sleep and rest.
6. Select suitable clothes—dress and undress.
7. Maintain body temperature within normal range by adjusting clothing and modifying the environment.
8. Keep the body clean and well groomed and protect the integument.
9. Avoid dangers in the environment and avoid injuring others.
10. Communicate with others in expressing emotions, needs, fears, or opinions.
11. Worship according to one's faith.
12. Work in such a way that there is a sense of accomplishment.
13. Play or participate in various forms of recreation.
14. Learn, discover, or satisfy the curiosity that leads to normal development and health and use the available health facilities.

From Henderson, V.A. (1991). *The nature of nursing: Reflections after 25 years* (pp. 22-23). New York: National League for Nursing Press. Reprinted with permission from the National League for Nursing, New York, NY.

MAJOR ASSUMPTIONS

Henderson did not cite directly what she felt her underlying assumptions included. The following assumptions have been adapted from Henderson's publications.

Nursing

- The nurse has a unique function to help sick or well individuals.
- The nurse functions as a member of a medical team.
- The nurse functions independently of the physician, but promotes his or her plan if there is a physician in attendance. (For example, Henderson stressed that the nurse-midwife can and must function independently if he or she is the best-prepared health worker in the situation. The nurse can and must diagnose and treat the individual if the situation demands it. Henderson is especially emphatic on this point in the sixth edition of *The Principles and Practice of Nursing.*[28])
- The nurse is knowledgeable in both biological and social sciences.
- The nurse can assess basic human needs.
- The 14 components of nursing care encompass all possible functions of nursing.[12,13,28]

Person (Patient)

- The person must maintain physiological and emotional balance.
- The mind and body of the person are inseparable.
- The patient requires help toward independence.
- The patient and his or her family are a unit.
- The patient's needs are encompassed by the 14 components of nursing.[13]

Health

- Health is a quality of life.
- Health is basic to human functioning.
- Health requires independence and interdependence.

- Promotion of health is more important than care of the sick.
- Individuals will achieve or maintain health if they have the necessary strength, will, or knowledge.[13,17]

Environment

- Healthy individuals may be able to control their environment, but illness may interfere with that ability.
- Nurses should have safety education.
- Nurses should protect patients from mechanical injury.
- Nurses should minimize the chances of injury through recommendations regarding construction of buildings, purchase of equipment, and maintenance.
- Doctors use nurses' observations and judgments as the base of their prescriptions for protective devices.
- Nurses must know about social customs and religious practices to assess dangers.[11]

THEORETICAL ASSERTIONS
The Nurse-Patient Relationship

Three levels comprising the nurse-patient relationship can be identified, ranging from a very dependent to a quite independent relationship: (1) the nurse as a substitute for the patient, (2) the nurse as a helper to the patient, and (3) the nurse as a partner with the patient. In times of grave illness, the nurse is seen as a "substitute for what the patient lacks to make him 'complete,' 'whole,' or 'independent,' by the lack of physical strength, will, or knowledge."[12:63] Henderson[11:16] reflected this view in her statement that the nurse "is temporarily the consciousness of the unconscious, the love of life for the suicidal, the leg of the amputee, the eyes of the newly blind, a means of locomotion for the infant, knowledge and confidence for the young mother, the 'mouthpiece' for those too weak or withdrawn to speak and so on."

During conditions of convalescence, the nurse helps the patient acquire or regain his or her independence. Henderson[26:120] stated, "Independence is a relative term. None of us is independent of others, but we strive for a healthy interdependence, not a sick dependence."

As partners, the nurse and patient formulate the care plan together. Basic needs exist regardless of diagnosis, but they are modified by pathology and other conditions such as age, temperament, emotional state, social or cultural status, and physical and intellectual capacities.[11]

The nurse must be able to assess not only the patient's needs, but also those conditions and pathological states that alter them. Henderson[12:63] said the nurse must "get 'inside the skin' of each of her patients in order to know what he needs." Then the needs must be validated with the patient.

The nurse can alter the environment wherever he or she deems necessary. Henderson[28:831] believed that "in every situation nurses who know physiologic and psychologic reactions to temperature and humidity, light and color, gas pressures, odors, noise, chemical impurities, and microorganisms can organize and make the best use of the facilities available."

The nurse and the patient are always working toward a goal, whether it is independence or peaceful death. One goal of the nurse must be to keep the patient's day as "normal as possible."[12:67] Promotion of health is another important goal of the nurse. Henderson[17:33] stated, "There is more to be gained by helping every man learn how to be healthy than by preparing the most skilled therapists for service to those in crises."

The Nurse-Physician Relationship

Henderson insisted that the nurse have a unique function that is distinct from the physician's function. The care plan, formulated by both the nurse and patient, must be implemented in such a way as to promote the physician's prescribed therapeutic plan. Henderson[17:34] stressed that nurses do not follow doctor's orders because a nurse "questions a philosophy that allows a physician to give orders to patients or other health workers." She extended this to emphasize that nurses help patients with health management when physicians are unavailable.[28] She

also indicated that many nurse and physician functions overlap.[24]

The Nurse As a Member of the Healthcare Team

The nurse works in interdependence with other healthcare professionals. The nurse and other team members help each other carry out the total program of care, but they should not do each other's jobs. Henderson[12:63] stated, "No one of the team should make such heavy demands on another member that any one of them is unable to perform his or her unique function."

Henderson compared the entire medical team, including the patient and family, to wedges on a pie graph (Figure 8-1). The size of each member's section depends on the patient's current needs; therefore it changes as the patient progresses toward independence. In some situations, certain team members are not included in the pie. The goal is for the patient to have the largest wedge possible or to take the whole pie.

Just as the patient's needs change, so may the definition of nursing. Henderson[33:121] admitted, "This does not say that it is a definition that will stand for all time. I believe nursing is modified by the era in which it is practiced, and depends to a great extent on what other health workers do."

Henderson believed her sixth edition of *The Principles and Practice of Nursing*,[28] coauthored with Gladys Nite, expanded her definition to include nurse practitioners. In a telephone interview, she stated, "Nursing must not exist in a vacuum. Nursing must grow and learn to meet the new health needs of the public as we encounter them."[23]

LOGICAL FORM

Henderson appeared to use the deductive form of logical reasoning to develop her definition of nursing. She deduced her definition of nursing and 14 needs from physiological and psychological principles. The assumptions of Henderson's definition must be studied to assess logical adequacy. Many of the assumptions have validity because they have a

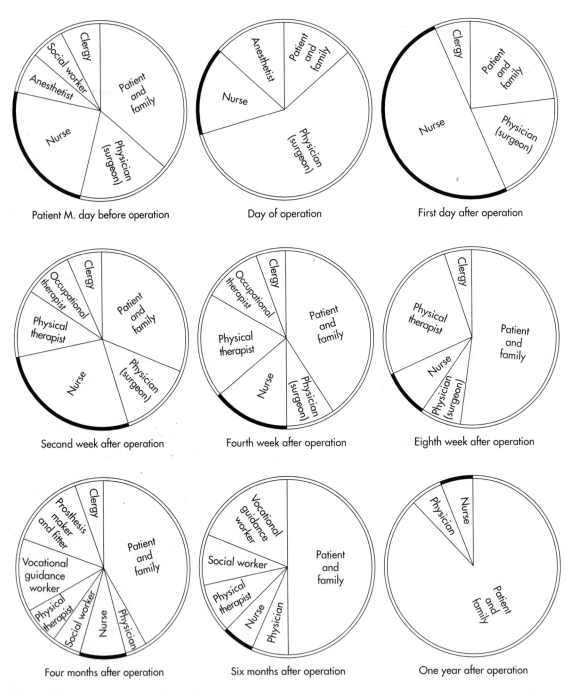

Figure 8-1 Showing how the nurse's role diminishes as rehabilitation progresses in the case of a young man having his leg amputated, for example. (From Henderson, V.A. (1991). *The nature of nursing: Reflections after 25 years* (pp. 29-30). New York: National League for Nursing Press. Reprinted with permission of the National League for Nursing, New York, NY.)

high level of agreement with the literature and research conclusions of scientists in other fields. For example, although Henderson's 14 basic needs were listed before she read Maslow's work, they correspond closely with Maslow's widely accepted human needs hierarchy.

In her book, *To Be a Nurse,*[1] Evelyn Adam analyzes Henderson's work using a framework she learned from Dorothy Johnson. Adam[1] identifies Henderson's assumptions and values, the goal of nursing, the patient, the role of the nurse, the source of difficulty, the intervention, and the desired consequences.

ACCEPTANCE BY THE NURSING COMMUNITY

Practice

Henderson's definition of nursing, as it relates to nursing practice, indicates that the nurse, who's primary function is being the direct caregiver to the patient, will find an immediate reward in the patient's progress from dependence to independence. The nurse must make every effort to understand the patient when he or she lacks will, knowledge, or strength. As Henderson[13:24] stated, the nurse will "get inside his skin." The nurse can help the patient move to an independent state by assessing, planning, implementing, and evaluating each of the 14 components of basic nursing care.

Henderson's approach to patient care was deliberative and involved decision making. Although she did not mention the steps in the nursing process specifically, it is clear how the concepts are interrelated. Henderson[22] believed that the nursing process is the problem-solving process and is not peculiar to nursing.

In the assessment phase, the nurse would assess the patient in all 14 components of basic nursing care. After the first component was completely assessed, the nurse would move on to the next component until all 14 areas were assessed. In gathering data, the nurse uses observation, smell, feeling, and hearing. To complete the assessment phase, the nurse must analyze the collected data. This requires knowledge of what is normal in health and disease.

Henderson[26] stated that as long as nursing is the only service available on a 24-hour, 7-day-a-week basis, the assessment function of nurses is indisputable. Nurses need to differentiate the normal from the abnormal in patient health.

According to Henderson,[28] the planning phase involves making the plan fit the individual's needs, updating the plan as necessary on the basis of the changes, using the plan as a record, and ensuring that it fits with the physician's prescribed plan. A good plan, in her opinion, integrates the work of all those on the health team.[23]

In the implementation phase, the nurse helps the patient perform activities to maintain health, to recover from illness, or to aid in peaceful death. Interventions are individualized, depending on physiological principles, age, cultural background, emotional balance, and physical and intellectual capacities. Henderson[13,18] would evaluate the patient according to the degree in which he or she performs independently. However, infants or the unconscious cannot be independent. In some phases of illness, nurses should accept the patient's desire to depend on others.

Education

Henderson[13:69] stated, "In order for a nurse to practice as an expert in her own right and to use the scientific approach to the improvement of practice, the nurse needs the kind of education available only in colleges and universities." The nurse's education demands universal understanding of diverse human beings. The statement supports the position taken in 1965 by the ANA.

In addition, Henderson believed that the value of education comes from the added confidence the individual develops in the institute of higher education environment and the knowledge that is gained. She thought nursing is a universal occupation and higher education allows the nurse to do it better.[30]

In her book, *The Nature of Nursing: A Definition and Its Implications for Practice, Research, and Education,*[13] Henderson designed three phases of curriculum development that students should progress through in their learning. The focus in all three phases remains the same—assisting the patient when he or she needs strength, will, or knowledge in performing daily activities or in carrying out prescribed therapy with the ultimate goal of independence.

In the first phase, emphasis is placed on the fundamental needs of the patient, the planning of the nursing care, and the unique function of the nurse in helping the patient perform his activities of daily living. In this phase, the curriculum plan does not emphasize pathological states or specific illnesses, but takes into account the ever-present conditions that affect basic needs.[13] In the second phase, emphasis is placed on helping patients meet their needs during marked body disturbances or pathological states that demand modifications in the nurse's plan of care. The patient presents the nursing student with problems of greater complexity. More medical science is involved and the student begins to understand the rationale of symptomatic treatment.[13] In the third phase, instruction is patient and family centered. The student becomes involved in the complete study of the patient and the patient's needs.[13]

Henderson[21] has stressed the importance of having nursing students develop a habit of inquiry; take courses in biological, physical, and social sciences and in the humanities; study with students in other fields; observe effective care; and give effective care in a variety of settings.

The textbook in which Henderson's definition of nursing is found, *The Principles and Practice of Nursing*,[28] is an excellent source for nursing students and practicing nurses. It provides the depth that is usually lacking in such texts. Kelly[29:59] states, "If only one nursing book can be saved when the bomb falls, *PPN* is that book. In it are the breadth and depth of nursing, framed within the accumulated wisdom of law, medicine, and religion, documented from the world literature, fascinatingly footnoted—and eminently practical."

Research

Henderson recommended library research and did a vast amount of it herself. She surveyed library resources and nursing research.[10] She supported developing nurses at the baccalaureate level and believed research was needed to evaluate and improve practice.[9]

Henderson[30] thought nurses should base their practice on research findings and acquire the habit of looking for research. She recommended that nurses make greater use of library resources and hoped that nurses would conduct research to improve practice rather than to merely gain academic respectability.[14-16,19,20]

In Henderson and Leo W. Simmons' 1964 survey and assessment of nursing research,[13:34] several reasons for the lack of research in clinical nursing were identified, including the following:

"1. Major energies of the profession have gone towards improving the preparation for nursing.

2. Learning how to recruit and hold sufficient numbers of nurses to meet the growing demand has taken considerable energy.

3. The need for administrators and educators has almost exhausted the supply of degree nurses.

4. A lack of support from administrators, nursing service administrators, and physicians has discouraged researchers."

Research questions arise from each of the 14 components of basic nursing care. It is the nurse's function to assume responsibility for identifying problems, continually validating his or her function, improving the methods he or she uses, and reassuring the effectiveness of nursing care.

Henderson[13:39] concluded, "No profession, occupation, or industry in this age can evaluate adequately or improve its practice without research." Research is the most reliable type of analysis.

Henderson[24] believed that nursing would not become a research-based profession until practicing nurses learn how to use library resources such as indexes from the National Library of Medicine.

FURTHER DEVELOPMENT

Henderson's last revision of her nursing definition[23] was in 1966. She continued to write and reflect on the practice of nursing throughout her life. In 1991, she stated that caring for patients was the "essential element of nurse's service."[27:58] Henderson[22,27] raised questions regarding nursing practice and the use of the nursing process. She stressed a continued assessment of the patient's needs as the patient's condition and goals change. Henderson[21] encouraged nurses to identify new needs beyond the 14 she enumerated. Henderson believed that nursing research is essential for nursing practice in the age of technological advances.

Halloran[5] has compiled the writings of Henderson in *A Virginia Henderson Reader: Excellence in Nursing*. Nurses unfamiliar with Henderson are introduced to this world-renowned nurse in her own words. The writings and reflections are excerpts from her most important publications and are presented and organized to enable the reader to appreciate Henderson's work in light of contemporary nursing issues.

CRITIQUE

Before Henderson's theory of nursing can be evaluated with respect to the generally accepted criteria of simplicity, generality, empirical precision, and derivable consequences, it is important to understand that she did not intend to develop a definitive nursing theory. Instead, she developed a personal concept or definition in an attempt to clarify what she considered to be the unique function of nursing. She stated, "My interpretation of the nurse's function is the synthesis of many influences, some positive and some negative. . . . I should first make clear that I do not expect everyone to agree with me. Rather, I would urge every nurse to develop her own concept."[12:64]

Henderson's definition can be considered a grand theory or philosophy within the preparadigm stage of theory development in nursing. Her concept is descriptive and easy to read. It is defined in common language terms. Her definitions of nursing and her enumeration of the 14 basic nursing functions present a perspective aimed at explaining a totality of nursing behavior. She had no intention of developing a theory; therefore Henderson did not develop the interrelated theoretical statements or operational definitions necessary to provide the theory testability. However, that can be done.

Simplicity

Henderson's concept of nursing is complex rather than simplistic. It contains many variables and several different descriptive and explanatory relationships. It is not associated with structural organizations within a framework or model form to enhance simplicity, but some work has been done in this area. Diagrams of Henderson and Orem's concepts of nursing from the Nursing Theories Conference Group's book, *Nursing Theories: The Base for Professional Nursing Practice*,[31] have been reproduced in Henderson and Nite's book. In addition, the 14 basic needs appear simple as stated, but they become complex when an alteration of a need occurs and all the parameters relating to that need are considered. The sixth edition of *The Principles and Practice of Nursing*[28] is extremely comprehensive and well illustrated to add clarity.

Generality

Generality is present in Henderson's definition because it is broad in scope. It attempts to include the function of all nurses and all patients in their various interrelationships and interdependencies.

Derivable Consequences

Henderson's perspective has been useful in promoting new ideas and furthering conceptual development of emerging theorists. In her many published works, she has discussed the importance of nursing's independence from, and interdependence with, other branches of the healthcare field. She has also influenced curriculum development and made a great contribution by promoting the importance of research in the clinical practice of nursing. She has made extensive use of other theorists' research in her work. Evans[3] stated that *The Principles and Practice of Nursing*[28] made a revolutionary change in the thinking about nursing research. He states that the revolutionary thesis of the book is "the habits of mind which inform the everyday tasks of a nurse are exactly the same as those which undergird the very finest published research; in this way, every nurse ought not just to do simple research tasks as part of her work, but she ought also always to be a researcher, whether or not she writes or speaks a word in print or public."[3:338-339]

Henderson's definition of the unique function of nursing has been widely read; therefore it has functioned as a major stepping stone in the emergence of nursing as a professional scientific discipline. She continues to be cited in current nursing literature and publications in all areas of nursing practice from holistic nursing to the nursing process.

CRITICAL THINKING *Activities*

1. Identify the philosophical beliefs that guided Henderson's definition of nursing.

2. Apply Henderson's definition of nursing to your nursing practice. How does the definition reflect your current nursing practice?

3. As you reread Henderson's definition of nursing, what nursing functions and actions are applicable today?

REFERENCES

1. Adam, E. (1980). *To be a nurse.* New York: W.B. Saunders.
2. Brown, L. (1948). *Nursing for the future.* New York: Russell Sage Foundation.
3. Evans, D.L. (1980). Every nurse as a researcher: An argumentative critique of principles and practice of nursing. *Nursing Forum, 19*(4), 335-349.
4. Furukawa, C.Y. & Howe, J.K. (1995). Virginia Henderson. In Nursing Theories Practice Group & J.B. George (Chairperson), *Nursing theories: The base for professional nursing practice.* Englewood Cliffs, NJ: Prentice Hall.
5. Halloran, E.J. (Ed.). (1995). *A Virginia Henderson reader: Excellence in nursing.* New York: Springer.
6. Halloran, E.J. (1996). Internet communication, March 21, 1996.
7. Harmer, B. (1922). *Textbook for the principles and practice of nursing.* New York: Macmillan.
8. Harmer, B. (1955). *Textbook of the principles and practice of nursing.* New York: Macmillan.
9. Harmer, B. & Henderson, V. (1939). *Textbook of the principles and practice of nursing* (4th ed.). New York: Macmillan.
10. Henderson, V. (1957, Oct.). An overview of nursing research. *Nursing Research,* 6, 61-71.
11. Henderson, V. (1958, May 9). The basic principles of nursing care. *Nursing Mirror,* 107, 337-338, 415-416, 497-498, 583-584, 651-652, 733-734, 803-804.
12. Henderson, V. (1964, Aug.). The nature of nursing. *American Journal of Nursing,* 64, 62-68.
13. Henderson, V. (1966). *The nature of nursing: A definition and its implications for practice, research, and education.* New York: Macmillan.
14. Henderson, V. (1968). Library resources in nursing: Their development and use. *International Nursing Review,* 15, 164-174, 236-246.
15. Henderson, V. (1960). *Basic principles of nursing care.* Geneva, Switzerland: International Council of Nurses.
16. Henderson, V. (1971, Jan.). Implications for nursing in the library activities of the regional medical programs. *Bulletin of the Medical Library Association,* 59, 53-64.
17. Henderson, V. (1971, March). Health is everybody's business. *Canadian Nurse,* 67, 31-34.
18. Henderson, V. (1973, June). On nursing care plans and their history. *Nursing Outlook,* 21, 378-379.
19. Henderson, V. (1977). Awareness of library resources: A characteristic of professional workers; an essential in research and continuing education. In ANA Staff, *Reference resources for research and continuing education in nursing.* Kansas City, MO: American Nurses Association.
20. Henderson, V. (1977, May/June). We've "come a long way," but what of the direction? *Nursing Research,* 26, 163-164.
21. Henderson, V. (1978, March). The concepts of nursing. *Journal of Advanced Nursing,* 3, 13-30.
22. Henderson, V. (1982, March). The nursing process: Is the title right? *Journal of Advanced Nursing,* 7, 103-109.
23. Henderson, V. (1984-1985). Telephone interviews.
24. Henderson, V. (1985, Summer). The essence of nursing in high technology. *Nursing Administration Quarterly,* 9(4), 1-9.
25. Henderson, V. (1985). Personal correspondence.
26. Henderson, V. (1987, May). Nursing process: a critique. *Holistic Nursing Practice,* 1(3), 7-18.
27. Henderson, V. (1991). *The nature of nursing—Reflections after 25 years.* New York: National League for Nursing.
28. Henderson, V. & Nite, G.A. (1978). *The principles and practice of nursing* (6th ed.). New York: Macmillan.
29. Henderson, V. & Watt, S. (1983). 70 plus and going strong: Virginia Henderson, a nurse for all ages. *Geriatric Nursing,* 4, 58-59.
30. Holmes, P. (1985, Aug.). Who's afraid of Virginia Henderson? *Nursing Times,* 81(32), 16-17.
31. The Nursing Theories Conference Group. (1980). *Nursing theories: The base for professional practice.* Englewood Cliffs, NJ: Prentice Hall, Inc.

32. Runk, J.A. & Muth Quillin, S.I. (1983). Henderson's definition of nursing. In J.J. Fitzpatrick & A.L. Whall (Eds.), *Conceptual models of nursing: An analysis and application.* Bowie, MD: Robert J. Brady.

33. Safier, G. (1977). Virginia Henderson: Practitioner. In G. Safier (Ed.), *Contemporary American leaders in nursing: An oral history.* New York: McGraw-Hill.

34. Webster, N. (1961). *Webster's new collegiate dictionary.* New York: The World Publishing Company.

BIBLIOGRAPHY
Primary Sources
Books

Harmer, B. & Henderson, V. (1939). *Textbook of the principles and practice of nursing* (4th ed.). New York: Macmillan.

Harmer, B. & Henderson, V. (1955). *Textbook of the principles and practice of nursing* (5th ed.). New York: Macmillan.

Henderson, V. (1960). *Basic principles of nursing care.* (Pamphlet prepared for International Council of Nurses.) Geneva, Switzerland: International Council of Nurses.

Henderson, V. (1966). *The nature of nursing: A definition and its implications for practice, research, and education.* New York: Macmillan.

Henderson, V. (1969). *ICN basic principles of nursing care.* Geneva: International Council of Nursing.

Henderson, V. (1991). *The nature of nursing: Reflections after 25 years.* New York: National League for Nursing.

Henderson, V. & Nite, G. (1978). *The principles and practice of nursing* (6th ed.). New York: Macmillan.

Henderson, V. & Simons, L.W. (1957). *The yearbook of modern nursing: 1956.* New York: G.P. Putnam's Sons.

Simmons, L.W. & Henderson, V. (1964). *Nursing research: A survey and assessment.* New York: Appleton-Century-Crofts.

Yale University School of Nursing Index Staff under the direction of Virginia Henderson. (1963-1972). *Nursing studies index* (4 vols.). Philadelphia: J.B. Lippincott.

Book Chapters

Henderson, V. (1974). On nursing care plans and their history. In American Journal of Nursing, *The nursing process in practice.* Kansas City, MO: American Nurses Association.

Henderson, V. (1977). Annie Warburton Goodrich. In J.A. Garraty (Ed.), *Dictionary of American biography: Supplement five, 1951-1955.* New York: Charles Scribner's Sons.

Henderson, V. (1977). Awareness of library resources: A characteristic of professional workers. In American Nurses Association, *Reference resources for research and continuing education.* Kansas City, MO: American Nurses Association.

Journal Articles

Henderson, V. (1937, Jan.). Paper and other substitutes for woven fabric. *American Journal of Nursing, 37,* 23-32.

Henderson, V. (1938, Nov.). Oxygen therapy: A study of some aspects of the operation of an oxygen tent. *American Journal of Nursing, 38,* 1203-1216.

Henderson, V. (1955, Dec.). Annie Warburton Goodrich. *American Journal of Nursing, 38,* 1203-1216.

Henderson, V. (1956, Feb.). Research in nursing practice—When? *Nursing Research, 4,* 99.

Henderson, V. (1957, Oct.). An overview of nursing research. *Nursing Research, 6,* 61-71.

Henderson, V. (1958, May 2). The basic principles of nursing care. *Nursing Mirror, 107,* 337-338.

Henderson, V. (1958, May 9). The basic principles of nursing care. *Nursing Mirror, 107,* 415-416.

Henderson, V. (1958, May 16). The basic principles of nursing care. *Nursing Mirror, 107,* 497-498.

Henderson, V. (1958, May 23). The basic principles of nursing care. *Nursing Mirror, 107,* 583-584.

Henderson, V. (1958, May 30). The basic principles of nursing care. *Nursing Mirror, 107,* 651-652.

Henderson, V. (1958, June 6). The basic principles of nursing care. *Nursing Mirror, 107,* 733-734.

Henderson, V. (1958, June 13). The basic principles of nursing care. *Nursing Mirror, 107,* 803-804.

Henderson, V. (1964, Aug.). The nature of nursing. *American Journal of Nursing, 64,* 63-68.

Henderson, V. (1965, Jan./Feb.). The nature of nursing. *International Nursing Review, 12(1),* 23-30.

Henderson, V. (1968, Spring). Some comments for nurses today. *The Alumnae Magazine* (Columbia University-Presbyterian Hospital School of Nursing Alumnae Association), 5-15.

Henderson, V. (1968, April). Library resources in nursing: Their development and use (Part I). *International Nursing Review, 15(2),* 164-182.

Henderson, V. (1968, July). Library resources in nursing: Their development and use (Part II). *International Nursing Review, 15(3),* 236-247.

Henderson, V. (1968, Oct.). Is the role of the nurse changing? *Weather Vane,* 12-43.

Henderson, V. (1968, Oct.). Library resources in nursing: Their development and use (Part III). *International Nursing Review, 15(4),* 348-358.

Henderson, V. (1969, Oct.). Excellence in nursing. *American Journal of Nursing, 69,* 2133, 2137.

Henderson, V. (1971, Jan.). Implications for nursing in the library activities in regional medical programs. *Bulletin of the Medical Library Association, 59(1),* 53-61.

Henderson, V. (1971, March). Health is everybody's business. *Canadian Nurse, 67,* 31-34.

Henderson, V. (1973, June). On nursing care plans and their history. *Nursing Outlook, 21,* 378-379.

Henderson, V. (1977, Jan./Feb.). We've "come a long way," but what of the direction? (Guest editorial). *Nursing Research, 26*, 163-164.

Henderson, V. (1978). The concept of nursing. *Journal of Advanced Nursing, 3*, 113-130.

Henderson, V. (1978, May 1). Professional writing. *Nursing Mirror and Midwives Journal*, 5-18.

Henderson, V. (1979, Nov. 22-23). Preserving the essence of nursing in a technological age. *Nursing Times, 75*, 2012.

Henderson, V. (1980, May). Preserving the essence of nursing in a technological age. *Journal of Advanced Nursing, 5*, 245-260.

Henderson, V. (1980, May 22). Nursing—Yesterday and tomorrow. *Nursing Times, 76*, 905-907.

Henderson, V. (1982, Spring). Is the study of history rewarding for nurses? *Society for Nursing History Gazette, 2*(1), 1-2.

Henderson, V. (1982, March). The nursing process—Is the title right? *Journal of Advanced Nursing, 7*, 103-109.

Henderson, V. (1985, Summer). The essence of nursing in high technology. *Nursing Administration Quarterly, 9*, 1-9.

Henderson, V. (1986, Jan.). Some observations on health care by health services or health industries. *Journal of Advanced Nursing, 11*(1), 1-2.

Henderson, V. (1987, Nov.). The nursing process in perspective [Editorial]. *Journal of Advanced Nursing, 12*(6), 657-658.

Henderson, V. (1989). Countdown to 2000: A major international conference for the primary health care team. *Journal of Advanced Nursing, 14*, 81-85.

Henderson, V. (1989, Nov./Dec.). Nursing information sources [Letter Comment]. *Nursing Outlet, 37*(6), 256.

Henderson, V. (1990, April). Excellence in nursing 1969 [Classic Article]. *American Journal of Nursing, 90*, 76-77.

Book Reviews

Henderson, V. (1969, Jan.). Review of "Edith Cavell: Pioneer and patriot" by A.E. Clark-Kennedy. *Journal of the History of Medicine and Allied Sciences, 24*(1), 100-101.

Henderson, V. (1969, March/April). Review of "A bibliography of nursing literature: 1859-1960" edited by Alice M.C. Thompson. *Nursing Research, 18*(2), 174-176.

Henderson, V. (1976, Aug.). Review of "Equity in health services: Empirical analysis in social policy" by Ronald Anderson. *American Journal of Nursing, 76*(1), 1339-1340.

Henderson, V. (1979, Aug.). Review of "The advance of American nursing" by Philip A. Kalish & Beatrice J. Kalish. *Nursing Outlook, 27*(8), 554.

Thesis

Henderson, V. (1935, June). *Medical and surgical asepsis: The development of asepsis and a study of current practice with recommendations in relation to certain aseptic nursing methods in hospitals.* Department of Nursing Education, Teachers College, Columbia University.

Correspondence

Henderson, V. (1984-1985). Telephone interviews.

Henderson, V. (1985). Personal correspondence.

Interviews

Anonymous. (1983). 70 plus and going strong: Virginia Henderson, a nurse for all ages. *Geriatric Nursing, 4*, 58-59.

Anonymous. (1984). Virginia Henderson: A nursing's treasure. *Focus on Critical Care, 11*(3), 60-61.

Darby C. (1997, May 11). Who's afraid of Virginia Henderson? *Nursing Mirror and Midwives Journal, 146*, 15-18.

Henderson, V. (1987, Oct.). A model for nursing (interview by Charlotte Alderman). *Nursing Times, 83*(41), 17-18.

Henderson, V. (1988, May 8). Song to today's and tomorrow's nurse (interview by Mette-Marie Davidson). *Sygeplejersken, 88*(20), 5-8.

Henderson, V. (1988, Nov. 26). An interview of Virginia Henderson (interview by Trevor Clay). *Nursing Standard, 3*(9), 18-9.

Shamansky, S.L. (1984). Community health nursing revisited: A conversation with Virginia Henderson. *Public Health Nursing, 1*(4), 193-201.

Videotapes

National League for Nursing. (1987). *Nursing theory: A circle of knowledge* [Videotape]. (Available from the author, 10 Columbus Circle, New York, NY 10019.)

National League for Nursing. (1989). *A conversation with Virginia Henderson* [Videotape]. (Available from the author, 10 Columbus Circle, New York, NY 10019.)

Studio III. (1988). *The nurse theorists: Portraits of excellence: Virginia Henderson* [Videotape]. (Available from Fuld Video Project, 370 Hawthorne Avenue, Oakland, CA 94609.)

The National Advisory Center. (1979). *A distinguished leader in nursing: Virginia Henderson* [Videotape]. (Available from National Institutes of Health, National Library of Medicine, and Sigma Theta Tau International, 1200 Waterway Blvd., Indianapolis, IN 46202.)

Secondary Sources
Books

Adam, E. (1980). *To be a nurse.* New York: W.B. Saunders.

Chinn, P.L. & Jacobs, M.K. (1983). *Theory and nursing: A systematic approach.* St. Louis: Mosby.

Herrmann, E.K. (1998). *Virginia Henderson: Signature for nursing.* Indianapolis: Center Nursing Press.

Walker, L.O. & Avant, K.C. (1983). *Strategies for theory construction in nursing.* Norwalk, CT: Appleton-Century-Crofts.

Book Chapters

Furukawa, C.Y. & Howe, J.K. (1980,1990). Virginia Henderson. In Nursing Theories Practice Group & J.B. George (Chairperson), *Nursing theories: The base for professional nursing practice.* Englewood Cliffs, NJ: Prentice Hall.

Furukawa, C.Y. & Howe, J.K. (1995). Virginia Henderson. In J.B. George (Ed.), *Nursing theories: The base for professional nursing practice* (4th ed.). Norwalk, CT: Appleton & Lange.

Runk, J.A. & Muth Quillin, S.I. (1983,1989). Henderson's definition of nursing. In J.J. Fitzpatrick & A.L. Whall (Eds.), *Conceptual models of nursing: Analysis and application.* Bowie, MD: Robert J. Brady.

Safier, G. (1977). Virginia Henderson: Practitioner. In G. Safier, *Contemporary American leaders in nursing: An oral history.* New York: McGraw-Hill.

Journal Articles

Anonymous. (1996). Virginia Avenel Henderson. The mother of modern nursing dies at age 98. *Canadian Journal of Cardiovascular Nursing, 7*(2), 2.

Anonymous. (1996, April 19). On March 19 at the Connecticut Hospice of Brandford, Virginia Henderson died. With her dies a great nurse and a great woman. *Revista de Enfermeria, 212,* 9.

Anonymous. (1996, April/June).Virginia Henderson, "the most loved nurse in the world" died at the age of 98 years. *Professional Inferministiche, 49*(2), 56-57.

Brodie, B. (1996, Nov.). A tribute to Virginia Avenel Henderson, RN: November 30, 1897-March 19, 1996. *Journal of Wound Ostomy Continence Nursing, 23*(6), 281-282.

Castledine, G. (1996, April 25-May 8). Virginia Henderson's legacy. *British Journal of Nursing, 5*(8), 517.

Coffman, S. (1996, 2nd Quarter). Virginia Henderson International Nursing Library, science on the loose. *Reflections, 22*(2), 30.

Ellis, R. (1968, May/June). Characteristics of significant theories. *Nursing Research, 17,* 217-222.

Flynn, K.T. (1997, Mar.). Janforum. I remember Virginia A. Henderson. *Journal of Advanced Nursing, 25*(3), 648-651.

Futton, J.S. (1987, Oct.). Virginia Henderson: Theorist, prophet, poet (biography). *Advances in Nursing Science, 10*(1), 1-9.

Gibbons, B.J. (1994). Venture into nursing cyberspace with the Virginia Henderson International Nursing Library. *Reflections, 20*(2), 14.

Gillett, V.A. (1996, Aug.). Applying nursing theory to perioperative nursing practice. *Association of Operating Room Nurses, 4*(2), 267-270.

Graves, J.R. (1997, Spring). The Virginia Henderson International Nursing Library: Resource for nurse administrators. *Nursing Administration Quarterly, 21*(3), 76-83.

Halamandaris, V.J. (1993). Virginia Henderson: First lady of nursing. *Caring People,* 44-54.

Hardy, M.E. (1978). Perspectives on nursing theory. *Advances in Nursing Science, 1,* 37-48.

Holloran, E.J. (1996, Jan.). Virginia Henderson and her timeless writings. *Journal of Advanced Nursing, 23*(1), 17-24.

Jezierski, M. (1997, Aug.). Virginia Henderson: Reflections on a twentieth century Florence Nightingale. *Journal of Emergency Nursing, 23*(4), 386-387.

Knollmueller, R.N. (1996, Aug.). Virginia Henderson: Her definition of nursing applies more than ever to home care practice. *Home Health Nurse, 14*(8), 625-629.

McBride, A.B. (1996). In celebration of Virginia Avenel Henderson. *Reflections, 22*(1), 22-23.

McCarty, P. (1987). How can nurses prepare for the year 2000? A response from Virginia Henderson. *The American Nurse, 19*(1), 3, 6.

O'Malley, J. (1996, Fall). A nursing legacy: Virginia Henderson. *Advanced Practice Nursing Quarterly, 2*(2), v-vii.

Roberts, K.L. (1996, Sept.). Virginia Henderson: A contemporary nurse 1987-1996. *Contemporary Nurse, 5*(3), 90-92.

Schmieding, N.J. (1990). An integrative theoretical framework. *Journal of Advanced Nursing, 15*(4), 463-467.

Schoolcraft, V. (1996, Spring). Portrait of a Virginia Henderson fellow: Victoria Schoolcraft. *Reflections, 22*(1), 40.

Schweer, K.D. (1996, 2nd Quarter). Profile of Virginia Henderson fellow: Kathryn D. Schweer. *Reflections, 22*(2), 48.

Shadbolt, Y. (1996, July). Miss Virginia Henderson. *Nursing Praxis in New Zealand, 11*(2), 46-47.

Sigma Theta Tau International. (1992). Virginia Henderson, RN: Humanitarian and scholar. *Reflections, 18*(1), 4-5.

Smith, J.P. (1997, Jan.). Virginia Avenelle Henderson, RN, MA, FAAN, FRCN: 1997-1996. *Journal of Advanced Nursing, 25*(1), 1.

Watkins, M. (1996, July). Virginia Henderson's contribution to nursing. *Journal of Clinical Nursing, 5*(4), 205.

Watson, M.J. (1996, May/June). President's message: In honor of Virginia Henderson. *Nursing Health Care Perspectives on Community, 17*(3), 142.

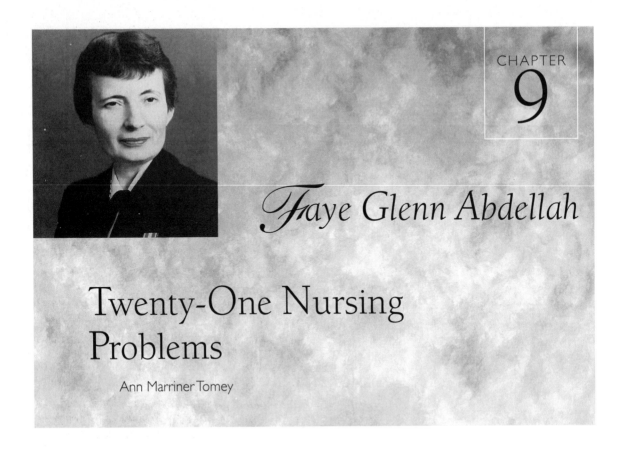

Faye Glenn Abdellah

Twenty-One Nursing Problems

Ann Marriner Tomey

CREDENTIALS AND BACKGROUND OF THE THEORIST

Faye Glenn Abdellah was born in New York City in 1919. She graduated magna cum laude from Fitkin Memorial Hospital School of Nursing (now Ann May School of Nursing) in 1942. Abdellah received her B.S. in 1945, her M.A. in 1947, and her Ed.D. in 1955 from Teachers College at Columbia University.

Recognized as "one of the country's leading and best known researchers in health and public policy" and as an "international expert of health problems," Abdellah has practiced in many settings.[7:ix] She has been a staff nurse, a head nurse, a faculty member at

Yale University and Columbia University, a public health nurse, a researcher, and an author of more than 150 articles and books, some of which have been translated into six languages. Since 1949, Abdellah has held various positions in the U.S. Public Health Service (USPHS) including nurse consultant to the states, chief of the nurse education branch, senior consultant of nursing research, principal investigator in the progressive patient care project that tested the first federal coronary care unit, chief of the research grants branch, director of nursing home affairs, and director of long-term care.

Abdellah was appointed Chief Nurse Officer of the USPHS in 1970 and served in that position for 17 years. Concurrently, in 1982, she was selected as Deputy Surgeon General, the first nurse and first woman to hold the post until her retirement in 1989. In this position, she was the focal point for

Previous authors: Tamara D. Halterman, Dorothy Kay Dycus, Elizabeth A. McClure, Donna N. Schmeiser, Flossie M. Taggart, and Roseanne Yancey.
The author wishes to thank Faye Glenn Abdellah for reviewing the chapter.

nursing and a chief advisor on long-term care policy within the Office of the Surgeon General. Abdellah represented the interests of health professionals in all categories in the USPHS. She was advisor on matters related to nursing, long-term care policy, mental retardation, the developmentally disabled, home health services, aging, hospice, and acquired immunodeficiency syndrome (AIDS). Her efforts were directed toward the improvement of healthcare quality for all Americans; therefore she supervised the activities in both health and nonhealth agencies. Abdellah is the recipient of more than 79 academic honors and professional awards. These include her selection as a charter fellow of the American Academy of Nursing where she later served as vice president and president; 11 honorary degrees including an honorary doctor of laws degree from Case Western Reserve University for pioneering nursing research and being responsible for the advent of the nurse-scientist scholar; an honorary degree from the University of Bridgeport for devoting her career to advancing the quality of healthcare through research and being an innovative and inspirational leader for nursing professionals; the Federal Nursing Service Award for the advancement of professional nursing; the Distinguished Service Honor Award of the U.S. Department of Health, Education, and Welfare for exceptional leadership and professional commitment; and the first presidential award of Sigma Theta Tau International. In 1989, Abdellah received the prestigious Allied-Signal Achievement Award for research in aging. In 1992, she received the Gustav O. Lienhard Award from the Institute of Medicine, National Academy of Sciences in recognition of her contributions to the betterment of the health of all Americans. In 1994, she was awarded the American Academy of Nursing Living Legend Award. In 1999, she was elected to the Columbia University Hall of Fame Distinguished Graduates and Scholars. In 2000, she was inducted into the National Women's Hall of Fame.

In 1988 and 1989, former Surgeon General C.E. Koop presented Abdellah with the Surgeon General's Medallion and Medal in recognition of her contributions as Chief Nurse Officer and Deputy Surgeon General for the USPHS and her exemplary service to the Surgeon General. Other military awards include two Distinguished Service Medals; a Uniformed Services of the Health Sciences Distinguished Service Medal; a Meritorious Service Medal; the Secretary of the Department of Health, Education, and Welfare Distinguished Service Award; and two Founders Medals from the Association of Military Surgeons of the United States.[10,12,14]

Abdellah's international involvement is extensive and includes her consultation to the Portuguese government in the development of programs for the care of the elderly and the disabled. While in the People's Republic of China, she studied the care of the elderly and the mentally retarded. She was assigned direct responsibility for developing a resolution to organize the World Assembly on the Elderly in 1982.

Abdellah was instrumental in the implementation of exchange programs for the United States and the Soviet Union and for the United States and France. She worked with U.S. scientists and health professionals and their counterparts in the Soviet Union and France and she worked with exchange programs for nurses in developing countries. Abdellah's leadership assistance in Yugoslavia resulted in the enactment of a law requiring the establishment of training programs for hospital managers. Her expertise and consultation led to the formation of nursing research programs at Tel Aviv University in Israel and the development of a prescreening examination for foreign nurses. She served as a consultant to the Japanese Nursing Association in setting up graduate programs in nursing education and research. Abdellah also participated in a seminar series for nursing home leaders in Australia and took part in nursing education and research meetings in New Zealand. She is the founding dean and professor of the first Uniformed Services Graduate School of Nursing at the Uniformed Services University of the Health Sciences at Bethesda, Maryland since 1993.*

Abdellah realized that for nursing to gain full professional status and autonomy, a strong knowledge base was imperative. Nursing also needed to move away from the control of medicine and toward a philosophy of comprehensive patient-centered

*References 3, 5, 8, 10, 12, 13, 14.

care. Abdellah and her colleagues conceptualized 21 nursing problems used to teach to students and used to evaluate students. The typology of 21 nursing problems first appeared in the 1960 edition of *Patient-Centered Approaches to Nursing*[15] and had a far-reaching impact on the profession and on the development of nursing theories (Box 9-1).* The 21 nursing problems have been reproduced in the various editions of this text[27-29] and further evolved in *Preparing for Nursing Research in the 21st Century: Evolution, Methodologies, Challenges.*[20]

*References 1, 8, 14, 15, 17, 21.

THEORETICAL SOURCES

A critique of Abdellah's work cannot be isolated from the background in which her typology of nursing problems was developed. In the 1950s, nursing practice and education were facing major problems resulting from technological advancement and social change. Old methods of educational preparation and practice based on functions and medical services were inadequate to meet the demands of rapid change. The definition of nursing was becoming clouded. In Abdellah's opinion, one of the greatest barriers that kept nursing from a professional status was the lack of a scientific body of knowledge

Box 9-1

Abdellah's Typology of 21 Nursing Problems

  1. To maintain good hygiene and physical comfort.
  2. To promote optimal activity: exercise, rest, sleep.
  3. To promote safety through prevention of accident, injury, or other trauma and through the prevention of the spread of infection.
  4. To maintain good body mechanics and prevent and correct deformity.
  5. To facilitate the maintenance of a supply of oxygen to all body cells.
  6. To facilitate the maintenance of nutrition of all body cells.
  7. To facilitate the maintenance of elimination.
  8. To facilitate the maintenance of fluid and electrolyte balance.
  9. To recognize the physiological responses of the body to disease conditions—pathological, physiological, and compensatory.
 10. To facilitate the maintenance of regulatory mechanisms and functions.
 11. To facilitate the maintenance of sensory function.
 12. To identify and accept positive and negative expressions, feelings, and reactions.
 13. To identify and accept interrelatedness of emotions and organic illness.
 14. To facilitate the maintenance of effective verbal and nonverbal communication.
 15. To promote the development of productive interpersonal relationships.
 16. To facilitate progress toward achievement and personal spiritual goals.
 17. To create or maintain a therapeutic environment.
 18. To facilitate awareness of self as an individual with varying physical, emotional, and developmental needs.
 19. To accept the optimum possible goals in the light of limitations, physical and emotional.
 20. To use community resources as an aid in resolving problems arising from illness.
 21. To understand the role of social problems as influencing factors in the cause of illness.

unique to nursing. The educational system was not providing students and practitioners with a means to cope with changing technology. The evaluation of students' clinical experiences based on a services approach provided no measure of the quality of the experience. The delivery of care to patients was organized around meeting the needs of the institution rather than the needs of the patient.

The problem-solving method is the basis for Abdellah's model. It was formulated as a remedy to the problems facing nursing. The typology of 21 nursing problems and skills was developed to constitute the unique body of knowledge that is nursing.

Abdellah[20] indicates that nursing is an art and a science that forms the attitude, intellectual competencies, and technical skills of the nurse into the ability and desire to help people, whether ill or not, cope with their health needs.

Abdellah[7] named Virginia Henderson as both an influence and mentor. Abdellah said her work is related to Henderson's 14 principles and to her own research studies to establish the classification of nursing problems.[6] Knowledge of the problem-solving approach to nursing problems would provide a method of change with the advancing technology. A qualitative assessment of student experiences could be made on the basis of the nursing problems encountered and alleviated while providing patients with patient-centered nursing care. Like many other theorists from Columbia University, Abdellah[31:252] was of the need school of thought "based on Maslow's hierarchy of needs and influenced by Erickson's stages of development."

USE OF EMPIRICAL EVIDENCE

The typology was developed from several studies conducted during the 1950s. In the study *Appraising the Clinical Resources in Small Hospitals*,[17] Abdellah and Levine classified medical diagnoses of more than 1700 patients into 58 categories thought to represent common nursing problems. Diagnostic groups identified the nursing problems that were presented. A similar analytical approach was followed in the development of the problem-oriented medical record more than a decade later and served as a basis for the development of diagnostic related groups (DRGs) in 1983.

Abdellah's dissertation, *Methods of Determining Covert and Overt Aspects of Nursing Problems As a Basis for Improved Clinical Teaching*,[1] reported findings from her study designed to identify what interview technique provided the most complete list of patients' problems. The study revealed that a free-answer method was the most productive for identifying nursing problems. When used with patients, this method elicited many more covert (emotional-social) problems than did a pictorial interview technique or direct questioning covert approach.[2] Also in 1955, the National League for Nursing (NLN) Committee on Records formed a subcommittee to develop a meaningful, clinical evaluation tool. The subcommittee members, with the assistance of faculties from 40 NLN-accredited collegiate schools of nursing, compressed the 58 patient categories into 21 common nursing problems and reported their development and use in *Patient-Centered Approaches to Nursing*[15] in 1960.

MAJOR CONCEPTS & DEFINITIONS

NURSING

In writing the typology of 21 nursing problems, which served as the basis of her nursing theory, Abdellah[6] was also creating a guide for nurses to use in identifying and solving patient problems. The concept of nursing was therefore a primary component of her writing. Abdellah[15:24] defined nursing as "service to individuals and families; therefore, to society. It is based upon art and science which mold the attitudes, intellectual competencies, and technical skills of the individual nurse into the desire and ability to help people sick or well cope with their health needs, and may be carried out under general or specific medical direction."

Continued

MAJOR CONCEPTS & DEFINITIONS—cont'd

Abdellah was clearly promoting the image of the nurse who was not only kind and caring, but also intelligent, competent, and technically well prepared to provide service to the patient.

NURSING PROBLEM

A second major concept in Abdellah's work was the nursing problem. The "nursing problem presented by the patient is a condition faced by the patient or family which the nurse can assist him or them to meet through the performance of her professional functions."[15:7] The problem can be either an overt or covert nursing problem.

Abdellah states that her present perception would be to change nursing problem to patient problem. An "overt nursing problem is an apparent condition faced by the patient or family which the nurse can assist him or them to meet through the performance of her professional functions."[2:4] The "covert nursing problem is a concealed or hidden condition faced by the patient or family which the nurse can assist him or them to meet through the performance of her professional functions."[2:4] Both types of nursing or patient problems can now be documented and measured by the use of outcome measures based on clinical practice guidelines.[11]

Although Abdellah spoke about the patient-centered approaches, she wrote about nurses identifying and solving specific problems. This identification and classification of problems was called the typology of 21 nursing problems (see Box 9-1). Abdellah's typology[15:11] was divided into three areas: "(1) physical, sociological, and emotional needs of the patient; (2) types of interpersonal relationships between the nurse and the patient; and (3) common elements of patient care." Abdellah and her colleagues thought the typology would provide a method to evaluate a student's experiences and also a method to evaluate a nurse's competency based on outcome measures.

PROBLEM SOLVING

The process of identifying overt and covert nursing problems and interpreting, analyzing, and selecting appropriate courses of action to solve these problems is problem solving, the final building block of Abdellah's writing.[15] Abdellah wrote that the nurse must be able to solve problems to give the best professional nursing care. This process, which closely resembles the steps of the nursing process, involves identifying the problem; selecting data; and formulating, testing, and revising hypotheses. According to Abdellah, the patient will not receive quality nursing care if the steps to problem solving are done incorrectly.

Abdellah identifies nursing diagnosis as a sub-concept of the problem-solving process and as an independent nursing function of determining the nature and extent of nursing problems presented by individual patients or families receiving care.[15]

MAJOR ASSUMPTIONS

Nursing

Nursing is a helping profession. In Abdellah's model, nursing care is doing something to or for the person or providing information to the person with the goal of meeting needs, increasing or restoring their self-help ability, or alleviating an impairment.

Determining the nursing care strategies to administer is based on the problem-solving approach. The nursing process is viewed as problem solving and the correct identification of nursing problems is of paramount concern. Direct observation of overt needs may be possible, but the determination of covert needs requires the mastery of communication skills and patient interaction. Deciding the best way to meet patient needs is the responsibility of hospital and public health personnel.

Abdellah[15:56] stated, "As long as self-help ability is developed and maintained at a level at which need satisfaction can take place without assistance, nursing care will not be required." The role of the nurse in health promotion is limited to circumstances of anticipated impairment. In 1960, Abdellah[15] stated that physicians need more knowledge about prevention and rehabilitation than do nurses. However, in correspondence in 1984, Abdellah[4] indicated that it is also important for nurses to know about prevention and rehabilitation.

In 1984, Abdellah[26:111] also stated, "It is hoped that preoccupation with illness-oriented assessment methods will not diminish concern with the promotion of wellness." Consideration is not given to the achievement of a level of wellness that is higher than the level present when only personal needs are met or when actual and anticipated impairments are absent.

Person

Abdellah describes people as having physical, emotional, and sociological needs. These needs may be overt, largely consisting of physical needs, or covert, consisting of emotional and social needs. According to Abdellah, the typology of nursing problems evolve from the recognition of a need for patient-centered approaches to nursing. She describes the patient as the only justification for the existence of nursing. However, as previously discussed, the patient is not the central focus of Abdellah's work.

People are helped by the identification and alleviation of the problems they are experiencing. The model implies that, by resolving each problem, the person returns to a healthy state or a state in which he or she can cope; therefore the ideal of holism is absent in this model. The whole, which is the patient, is not greater than the sum of its parts, which are the patient's problems.

In Abdellah's model, all persons have self-help ability and the capacity to learn, both of which vary from one individual to another. Identifying these qualities in a comatose patient or in an infant without family resources may be difficult; therefore omissions could result when organizing such patients' care with this model.

In 1991, Abdellah[8:24] addressed the i of self-help by stating, "There is increase tion that self-help groups can perform u valuable health services. Such groups sh come a part of the mainstream healthcare delivery system. Eventually, self-help will be the other healthcare delivery system in this country, and it will accept the burden of disease prevention and health promotion."

Health

Health, as discussed in *Patient-Centered Approaches to Nursing,*[15] is a state that is mutually exclusive of illness. Abdellah implicitly defined health as a state when the individual has no unmet needs and no anticipated or actual impairments. In the 1950s, much of nursing practice focused on remedial or illness care, so it is not surprising that health was not clearly defined. Several decades have passed since the book was published and Abdellah[3] now states that she "would certainly place greater emphasis today on health status as an important part of the wellness-sickness continuum." She also fully supports the holistic approach to patient-centered care and the need to lend greater attention to environmental factors.

Environment

The environment is the least-discussed concept in Abdellah's model. Nursing problem 17, from the typology, is "to create and/or maintain a therapeutic environment."[15:17] Abdellah also states that if the nurse's reaction to the patient is hostile or negative, the atmosphere in the room may be hostile or negative. This suggests that patients interact with and respond to their environment and the nurse is part of that environment.

The home and community that the patient comes from is also the environment. Although fleetingly discussed, Abdellah urges nurses not to limit the identification of nursing problems to those existing only in the hospital. She predicts a future community center that will extend beyond the four walls of the hospital into the community. Abdellah[6] stated that in 1988, she would "give greater emphasis to environment and health promotion."

THEORETICAL ASSERTIONS

Abdellah repeatedly stated several assertions, although they were not labeled assertions:

1. "The nursing problem and nursing treatment typologies are the principles of nursing practice and constitute the unique body of knowledge that is nursing."[15:12]
2. "Correct identification of the nursing problem influences the nurse's judgment in selecting steps in solving the patient's problem."[21:492]
3. The core of nursing is the patient/client problems that focus on the patient and his/her problems.[7]

According to Reynolds,[32] statements of assertion can either be existence or relational statements. Assertions one and three above are of the existence type, whereas assertion two above is relational.

Neither the major components of the nursing paradigm nor the central concepts are clearly linked with relational statements. Such structure cannot be diagrammed without imposing the critic's conclusions regarding the existence of relationships. The components of person, health, and environment were only implicitly defined; therefore no attempt will be made to propose relationships between them. The major concepts that Abdellah defines more clearly are thought to be associated in this manner. Through the identification of nursing problems and the usage of the problem-solving process, nursing helps the patient meet his or her needs. In 1972, Abdellah[3:234] stated, "The patient, his needs, and the nurse meeting his needs through nursing service is the only raison d'être for the nursing profession." Abdellah's statement exemplifies her major concerns and implied relationships.

LOGICAL FORM

The logical form is best described as an inductive approach that generalizes from particulars. Abdellah used her multiple observations from the previously mentioned studies as the basis for her typology.

Therefore the typology developed inductively from research toward theory.

ACCEPTANCE BY THE NURSING COMMUNITY

In discussing the acceptance by the nursing community, the individual must be aware of two distinct times within the history of nursing; that is, the mid1950s to the early 1960s and the present. When *Patient-Centered Approaches to Nursing*[15] was published in 1960, the profession of nursing was striving to clarify its practice area and to identify rationale for its actions on the basis of scientific knowledge. The introduction of the 21 nursing problems had profound effects on the areas of practice, education, and research. Now they are associated with nursing diagnosis. Abdellah's studies in research, practice, and education are extensively cited by nursing scholars today.

Practice

Abdellah's typology of 21 nursing problems helps nurses practice in an organized, systematic way. The use of this scientific base enabled the nurse to understand the reasons for his or her actions. Using the 21 nursing problems, the clinical practitioner could assess the patient, make a nursing diagnosis, and plan interventions. Through the problem-solving process, the nurse attempted to make the patient the central figure rather than his or her medical condition. By using the typology and the problem-solving process in the clinical setting, nurses gave their practice a scientific basis.

When asked to contrast the 21 nursing problems with the nursing diagnoses being promoted today, Abdellah[5] stated that 30 years ago it would have been heresy to use the term *diagnosis* in relation to nursing. Today she would describe them as being problems that patients present rather than nursing problems. However, she adds that there is much similarity between the 21 nursing problems and the established DRGs.[6] Both involve classification systems and the former could be used to provide the basis for determining the acuity of illness, nursing outcomes, and the costs of nursing services. This is particularly important as DRGs move into home care and ambulatory settings.[5]

Education

Barnum[23:288] stated, "Historically, Abdellah probably had more impact on nursing curriculum development than any other nurse theorist." Abdellah's 21 nursing problems had their most dramatic effect on the educational system within nursing. Nursing educators were aware that changes were needed if nurses were to become autonomous. They recognized that the greatest weakness in the profession was the lack of a scientific body of knowledge unique to nursing. The typology provided such a body of knowledge and an opportunity to move away from the medical model of educating nurses. The typology of 21 problems was widely accepted in the nursing community in two-, three-, and four-year programs.

Research

The typology of 21 nursing problems was created through research; therefore it is not surprising that more research followed its introduction. Function studies examined the amount of time the nurse spent with the patient. Was this typology necessary from an administrative point of view? Were hospitals not doing well without it? How could the patient receive comprehensive patient care in 18 minutes per eight-hour shift? Does the hospital administration serve the patient or does it serve someone else? To answer these questions, Abdellah and Strachan[22] extended the research and used the typology as the basis for developing the nursing care model used for planning staffing patterns in clinical settings. These staffing patterns were based on the patients' identified needs and, as Abdellah envisioned, they consisted of intensive care, intermediate care, long-term care, self-care, and home-care units. By grouping patients according to similar needs rather than by diagnoses, nursing service could provide the best staffing patterns to meet patients' needs.

In 1965, Abdellah and Levine published *Better Patient Care Through Nursing Research*,[19] the first major textbook in nursing research. In 1991, Abdellah[8:39] stated, "As nurse researchers, we need to be expedient and make a greater effort to let society know about the benefits of our research. This means translating research findings into practice that the patient/client can understand and see as a benefit." In 2000, Abdellah stated, "Evidence-based practice based on scientific data has come to the forefront as the basis for making medical and nursing decisions."[13]

Abdellah[8] specifically targeted members of Sigma Theta Tau to assist in meeting the goals and challenges of research in health and public policy as clearly outlined in her scholarly publication, *Nursing's Role in the Future: A Case for Health Policy Decision Making*. She continues to author articles on research and has coauthored *Preparing for Nursing Research in the 21st Century: Evolution, Methodologies, and Challenges*.[20]

FURTHER DEVELOPMENT

According to the categories of Dickoff and James,[24] Abdellah's typology may be recognized as a level one theory (categories or classifications). Currently, the nursing community's use of the 21 nursing problems has moved into a second generation of development, which includes patient problems and patient outcomes rather than nursing problems and nursing outcomes.

Abdellah[4] is pleased with the shift of emphasis from nursing problems to patient outcomes. She believes that 40 years ago the concept of nursing problems was used to identify a strong nursing role in patient care. If the initial emphasis had been on patient problems instead, the concept would not have been accepted and the medical model would have been perpetuated.

The concepts of problem solving and nursing diagnosis are still used in practice, education, and research settings. Critical thinking and theory validation in the practice area is needed within the profession. More sophisticated research tools might be designed to thoroughly study problem solving and how nurses apply this concept. The nursing diagnosis classification system may be considered an outgrowth of the typology. Currently, nursing diagnosis is a classification system describing patient signs and symptoms. Expanding this system to explain outcomes may be possible through additional research.

Abdellah served as Sigma Theta Tau's Distinguished Research Fellow (1990 to 1991) and she spoke with its members at all seven regional assemblies. There, and in her monograph published in 1991,[8] she addressed the relevance of nursing's role for policy decision making.

In *Nursing's Role in the Future: A Case for Health Policy Decision Making,*[8:ix] Abdellah has

> proposed health policy as a means for influencing legislation at local, state, and national levels for the purpose of making healthcare accessible to the 45 million persons who do not have it as of 2000. She has clearly identified nursing's role in policy issues, identified criteria to evaluate health policy decision making and outcomes, and has strongly made the case that more research of these issues by nurses is needed.

In addition, Abdellah[6,13] encourages nurses to read the *Federal Register,* which she calls the most influential document in Washington, DC.

CRITIQUE
Simplicity

The typology is very simple and it is descriptive of the nursing problems thought to be common among patients. The concepts of nursing, nursing problems, and the problem-solving process, which are central to this work, are defined explicitly. The concepts of person, health, and environment, which are associated with the nursing paradigm today, are implied. Relationships between Abdellah's major concepts or those of the nursing paradigm are not stated in her writing. This model has a limited number of concepts and its only structure is a list. A somewhat mixed approach to concept definition is present in this work. Nursing and nursing problems are connotatively defined, whereas the problem-solving process is defined denotatively. These approaches to definitions do not seem to detract from the clarity of

the definitions. The typology served as the basis for the patient classification system and the DRGs (both of which were based on outcome measures); therefore Abdellah[13] believes there is justification for a theory.

Generality

The 21 nursing problems are general and linked to neither time nor environment. Abdellah[5:33] "acknowledges that her list is neither exhaustive nor listed according to priorities." She also recognized that more emphasis should be placed on environment.[5,13] With the assumption that persons experience similar needs, nurses could use the nursing goals listed in the 21 problems in any time frame to meet patients' needs. However, according to this model, some persons do not need nursing.

Other service professions could use the typology of 21 nursing problems to focus on the psychosocial and emotional needs that patients present. The goals of this model vary in generality. The broadest goal is to affect nursing education positively, whereas subgoals are to provide a scientific basis for practice and to provide a method of qualitative evaluation of educational experiences for students. The goals are appropriate for nursing.

Empirical Precision

The concepts are very specific with empirical referents that are easily identifiable. The concepts are within the domain of nursing. Ready linkage of the concepts and the typology to reality is secondary to an inductive approach to theory development. The faculty of 40 collegiate schools of nursing validated the typology. Chapters 4, 5, and 6 of *Patient-Centered Approaches to Nursing*[15] describe different approaches to the implementation and use of the typology in three programs of nursing.

Derivable Consequences

The typology provided a general framework, but despite the title of the book (*Patient-Centered Approaches to Nursing*[15]), it neither continued specific nursing actions nor patient-centered outcomes. However, two subsequent publications did address outcome measures (effect variables) and suggested models for organizing curricula to emphasize patient-centered outcomes.[15,16] Except for stating the importance of nursing the whole patient, today's idea of holism is not apparent in this work.[25] The skills list includes skills thought necessary to meet patients' needs, but it was not prescriptive initially. The skills list became prescriptive in the 1980s and again in 1993 when Abdellah founded the Graduate School of Nursing where the curricula are prescriptive and based on outcomes measures.[13] Abdellah suggests nursing research as a method for validating treatments toward the resolution of patients' needs.

The emphasis on problem solving is not limited by time or space and therefore provides a means for continued growth and change in the provision of nursing care. The problem-solving process and the typology of the 21 nursing problems can be considered precursors of the nursing care process, classification of nursing diagnoses, and outcome measures in evidence today.

In Abdellah's *Patient-Centered Approaches to Nursing*,[15] she addressed nursing education problems that were linked to the use of the medical model before nursing models existed. Her typology provided a new way to qualitatively evaluate experiences and emphasized a practice based on outcome measures and sound rationales rather than rote.[13] Abdellah[4:33] "proposes that nurses could take a leadership role in making the public aware that quality nursing healthcare is available. Quality is defined as the care that the patient needs. Need is determined by a classification system that identifies the medical treatment and nursing care essential for that individual." Abdellah has made significant contributions to patient care, education, and research in nursing and healthcare in this country and throughout the world.[4]

CRITICAL THINKING *Activities*

1. Compare and contrast the 21 nursing problems with North American Nursing Diagnoses Association (NANDA) nursing diagnoses.

2. Select a patient in your practice setting. Use Abdellah's typology of 21 nursing problems to assess the patient, make a nursing diagnosis, plan appropriate interventions, and identify outcome measures.

3. You are working on a cardiopulmonary unit and are assigned to two thoracotomy patients. It is the first postoperative day for both patients. What nursing problems do you anticipate? Is it correct to assume that both patients will exhibit the same problems and needs?

REFERENCES

1. Abdellah, F.G. (1955). *Methods of determining covert and overt aspects of nursing problems as a basis for improved clinical teaching.* Doctoral dissertation, New York Teachers College, Columbia University.
2. Abdellah, F.G. (1957, June). Methods of identifying covert aspects of nursing problems. *Nursing Research,* 6, 4.
3. Abdellah, F.G. (1972). Evolution of nursing as a profession: Perspective on manpower development. *International Nursing Review,* 19, 3.
4. Abdellah, F.G. (1984, March 7). Personal correspondence.
5. Abdellah, F.G. (1986, Oct.). Faye G. Abdellah—Working to enrich the profession (interview). *Focus on Critical Care,* 13(5), 32-33.
6. Abdellah, F.G. (1988, April 28). Personal correspondence.
7. Abdellah, F.G. (1989, Nov. 13). *Plenary Session I: Scientific Session* [Audiocassette]. Indianapolis: Sigma Theta Tau International, Inc.
8. Abdellah, F.G. (1991). *Nursing's role in the future: A case for health policy decision making* [Monograph Series No. 91]. Indianapolis: Sigma Theta Tau International, Inc.
9. Abdellah, F.G. (1992, April). Telephone interview.
10. Abdellah, F.G. (1996, April). Vitae.
11. Abdellah, F.G. (1996, July). Telephone interview.
12. Abdellah, F.G. (2000, May). Telephone interview.
13. Abdellah, F.G. (2000, June). Personal correspondance.
14. Abdellah, F.G. (2000, June). Vitae.
15. Abdellah, F.G., Beland, I.L., Martin, A., & Matheny, R. (1960). *Patient-centered approaches to nursing.* New York: Macmillan.

16. Abdellah, F.G., Beland, I.L., Martin, A., & Matheny, R. (1973). *New directions in patient-centered nursing: Guidelines for systems of service, education, and research.* New York: Macmillan.
17. Abdellah, F.G. & Levine, E. (1954). *Appraising the clinical resources in small hospitals* (U.S. Public Health Service. Pub. No. 389). Washington, DC: U.S. Government Printing Office.
18. Abdellah, F. & Levine, E. (1958). *Effect of nurse staffing on satisfactions with nursing care.* Hospital Monograph Series No. 4. Chicago: American Hospital Association.
19. Abdellah, F.G. & Levine, E. (1965). *Better patient care through nursing research.* New York: Macmillan.
20. Abdellah, F.G. & Levine, E. (1994). *Preparing for nursing research in the 21st century: Evolution, methodologies, challenges.* New York: Springer.
21. Abdellah, F.G., Levine, E., & Levine, B.S. (1986). *Better patient care through nursing research* (3rd ed.). New York: Macmillan.
22. Abdellah, F.G. & Strachan, E.J. (1959, May). Progressive patient care. *American Journal of Nursing,* 59, 5.
23. Barnum, B.S. (1990). *Nursing theory* (3rd ed.). Glenview, IL: Scott, Foresman.
24. Dickoff, J. & James, P. (1968, March). A theory of theories: A position paper. *Nursing Research,* 17, 3.
25. Falco, S.M. (1980). Faye G. Abdellah. In Nursing Theories Conference Group & J.B. George (Chairperson), *Nursing theories: The base for professional practice.* Englewood Cliffs, NJ: Prentice Hall.
26. Levine, E. & Abdellah, F.G. (1984, Summer). DRGs: A recent refinement to an old method. *Inquiry,* 21: 105-112.
27. Marriner, A. (1986). *Nursing theorists and their work.* St. Louis: Mosby.
28. Marriner-Tomey, A. (1989, 1994). *Nursing theorists and their work* (2nd ed., 3rd ed.). St. Louis: Mosby.
29. Marriner Tomey, A. & Alligood, M.R. (1998). *Nursing theorists and their work* (4th ed.). St. Louis: Mosby.
30. Marriner Tomey, A. & Alligood, M.R. (2001). *Nursing theorists and their work* (5th ed.). St. Louis: Mosby.
31. Meleis, A.J. (1997). *Theoretical nursing: Development and progress* (3rd ed.). Philadelphia: J.B. Lippincott.
32. Reynolds, P.D. (1971). *A primer in theory construction.* Indianapolis: Bobbs-Merrill.

BIBLIOGRAPHY
Primary Sources
Books and Monographs

Abdellah, F.G. (1954). *For better nursing in Michigan: A survey.* Detroit: Cunningham Drug Company Foundation.
Abdellah, F.G. (1954, April). *Job guide for medical occupations.* Washington, DC: U.S. Department of Labor.

Abdellah, F.G. (1962, Sept.). *The elements of progressive patient care* (U.S. Public Health Service Publication No. 930-C-1). Washington, DC: U.S. Government Printing Office.
Abdellah, F.G. (1968). *An overview of nurse-scientist programs in the country* (National League for Nursing No. 15-1342). New York: National League for Nursing.
Abdellah, F.G. (1969). *Research in nursing: 1955-1968* (U.S. Public Health Service Publication No. 1356). Washington, DC: U.S. Government Printing Office.
Abdellah, F.G. (1971, Nov.). *Extending the scope of nursing practice: A report of the secretary's committee to study extended roles for nurses,* Washington, DC: U.S. Department of Health, Education, and Welfare.
Abdellah, F.G. (1972). *A career in nursing* (B'nai B'rith Career and Counseling Services Occupational Brief Series). Washington, DC: B'nai B'rith.
Abdellah, F.G. (1972). *Extending the scope of nursing practice* (National League for Nursing Pub. No. 16-1473). New York: National League for Nursing.
Abdellah, F.G. (1975). Models for health care systems. In *Models for health care delivery: Now and for the future,* pp. 3-19. Publication Code G-1192M5/75. (Papers presented at the annual meeting of the American Academy of Nursing held on January 20-21, 1975.) Kansas City: American Nurses Association.
Abdellah, F.G. (1976). *How to select a nursing home* (No. 017-022-00502-6 DHEW [OS] 76-50045). Washington, DC: U.S. Government Printing Office.
Abdellah, F.G. (1976, March). *Assessing health care needs in skilled nursing facilities: Health professional perspectives.* Long-term care facility improvement monograph No. 1. (DHEW Publication No. [OS] 76-50049.) Washington, DC: U.S. Government Printing Office.
Abdellah, F.G. (1976, June). *Physicians' drug prescribing patterns in skilled nursing facilities.* Monograph No. 2. (DHEW Publication No. [OS] 76-50050.) Washington, DC: U.S. Government Printing Office.
Abdellah, F.G. (1991). *Nursing's role in the future: The case for health policy decision making.* Monograph Series No. 91. Indianapolis: Sigma Theta Tau International, Inc.
Abdellah, F.G., Beland, I.L., Martin, A., & Matheney, R.V. (1960). *Patient-centered approaches to nursing.* New York: Macmillan.
Abdellah, F.G., Beland, I.L., Martin, A., & Matheney, R.V. (1968). *Patient-centered approaches to nursing* (2nd ed.). New York: Macmillan.
Abdellah, F.G., Beland, I.L., Martin, A., & Matheney, R.V. (1973). *New directions in patient-centered nursing.* New York: Macmillan.

Abdellah, F.G., Beland, I.L., Martin, A., & Matheney, R.V. (1982, Nov.). *Report on hospice care in the United States* (Publication No. HCFA-82-02152). Washington, DC: U.S. Department of Health and Human Services.

Abdellah, F.G. & Harper, B. (1981). *Fact sheet on Hospice Care in the U.S. Information for Health Professionals.* Washington, DC: U.S. Public Health Service, Department of Health and Human Service.

Abdellah, F.G. & Levine, E. (1954). *Appraising the clinical resources in small hospitals* (U.S. Public Health Service Pub. No. 389). Washington, DC: U.S. Government Printing Office.

Abdellah, F.G. & Levine, E. (1957). *Patients and personnel speak: A method of studying patient care in hospitals* (U.S. Public Health Service Publication No. 527). Washington, DC: U.S. Government Printing Office.

Abdellah, F.G. & Levine, E. (1958). *Effect of nurse staffing on satisfactions with nursing care: A study of how omissions in nursing services, as perceived by patients and personnel, are influenced by the number of nursing hours available.* Chicago: American Hospital Association.

Abdellah, F.G. & Levine, E. (1965). *Better patient care through nursing research.* New York: Macmillan.

Abdellah, F.G. & Levine, E. (1979). *Better patient care through nursing research* (2nd ed.). New York: Macmillan.

Abdellah, F.G. & Levine, E. (1994). *Preparing for nursing research in the twenty-first century: Evolution, methodologies, challenges.* New York: Springer.

Abdellah, F.G., Levine, E., & Levine, B.S. (1986). *Better patient care through nursing research* (3rd ed.). New York: Macmillan.

Abdellah, F.G., Meltzer, L.E., & Kitchell, J.R. (Eds.). (1969). *Concepts and practices of intensive care for nursing specialists.* Philadelphia: Charles Press.

Abdellah, F.G., Meltzer, L.E., & Kitchell, J.R. (Eds.). (1976). *Concepts and practices of intensive care for nursing specialists* (2nd ed.). Bowie, MD: Charles Press.

Abdellah, F.G. & Moore, S.R. (1988). *Surgeon General's workshop on health promotion and aging. Proceedings.* Washington, DC: Department of Health and Human Services, U.S. Public Health Service.

Abdellah, F.G., Moore, S., Moritsugu, K., & Wickizer, S. (1994). *Public Health Service flag officer's manual.* Washington, DC: Office of the Surgeon General, U.S. Public Health Service.

Abdellah, F.G., Schwartz, D.R., & Smoyak, S.A. (1975). *Models for health care delivery: Now and for the future* (American Nurses Association No. G119). Washington, DC: American Academy of Nursing.

Abdellah, F.G., Walsh, M.E., & Brown, E.L. (1979). *Health care in the 1980's: Who provides? Who plans? Who pays?* (Publication No. 52-1755). New York: National League for Nursing.

Meltzer, L., Abdellah, F.G., & Kitchell, J.R. (Eds.). (1973). *Intensive care een handleiding voor intensive verpleging.* Amsterdam: Excerpta Medica.

Dissertation

Abdellah, F.G. (1955). *Methods of determining covert aspects of nursing problems as basis for improved clinical teaching.* Unpublished doctoral dissertation, New York Teachers College, New York, Columbia University.

Book Chapters

Abdellah, F.G. (1959). Improving the teaching of nursing through research in patient care. In L.E. Heidgerkin (Ed.), *The improvement of nursing through research* (pp. 74-91). Washington, DC: The Catholic University Press.

Abdellah, F.G. (1968). An overview of nurse-scientist programs in the country. In *Extending the boundaries of nursing education: The preparation and role of the nurse scientist* (pp. 11-24). New York: National League for Nursing.

Abdellah, F.G. (1972). The nursing role in coronary care system. In L.E. Meltzer & A.J. Dunning (Eds.), *Textbook of coronary care* (pp. 35-51). Amsterdam: Excerpta Medica.

Abdellah, F.G. (1974). Overview of emerging health services delivery projects. In M. Leininger (Ed.), *Health care dimensions* (pp. 125-139). Health Care Issues Series. Philadelphia: F.A. Davis.

Abdellah, F.G. (1977). Criterion measures for research in nursing. In P.J. Verhonick (Ed.), *Nursing research II.* Boston: Little, Brown.

Abdellah, F.G. (1981). New directions in the care of the elderly. In L.A. Copp (Ed.), *Recent advances in nursing 2: Care of the aging.* New York: Churchill Livingstone.

Abdellah, F.G. (1981). The National Health Service Corps: Providing settings for nursing practice. In L.H. Aiken (Ed.), *Health policy and nursing practice.* New York: McGraw-Hill.

Abdellah, F.G. (1985). Public health aspects of rehabilitation of the aged. In S.J. Brody (Ed.), *Aging and rehabilitation.* New York: Springer.

Abdellah, F.G. (1985). The aging woman and the future of health care delivery. In M.R. Haug, A.B. Ford, & M. Scheafor (Eds.), *The physical and mental health of aged women.* New York: Springer.

Abdellah, F.G. (1986). Nurses as primary health care providers in the USA. In *The accountability of nurses in changing society.* Tokyo: International Nurses' Foundation of Japan.

Abdellah, F.G. (1986). The nature of nursing science. In L.H. Nicoll (Ed.), *Perspectives on nursing theory.* Boston: Little, Brown.

Abdellah, F.G. (1988). Future directions: Refining, implementing, testing, and evaluating the nursing minimum data set. In H.H. Werley & N.M. Lang (Eds.), *Identification of the nursing minimum set.* New York: Springer.

Abdellah, F.G. (1988, Jan.). Welcome and opening remarks from the Public Health Service. In Levine Associates (Eds.), *Evaluating the environmental health work force* (Publication No. HRP 0907160). Washington, DC: Department of Health and Human Services, U.S. Public Health Service.

Abdellah, F.G. (1991). Nursing research in the 21st century: An unfinished revolution. In S.R. Moore (Ed.), *The C. Everett Koop Honorary Lectures 1991-1996* (pp. 13-31). Rockville, MD: Anchor & Caduceus Society, Inc.

Abdellah, F.G. (1991). Public policy impacting on nursing care of older adults. In E.M. Baines (Ed.), *Perspectives on gerontological nursing.* Newbury, CA: Sage Publications.

McCormick, K.A. & Abdellah, F.G. (1984). Respiratory failure: Technological care in the home and hospital. In S.J. Reiser & M. Anbar (Eds.), *The machine at the bedside.* Cambridge, MA: Harvard University Press.

Journal Articles

Abdellah, F.G. (1952, June). State nursing surveys and community action. *Public Health Reports, 67,* 554-560.

Abdellah, F.G. (1953, July). Some trends in nursing education. *American Journal of Nursing, 53,* 841-843.

Abdellah, F.G. (1954, May). Surveys stimulate community action. *Nursing Outlook, 2,* 268-270.

Abdellah, F.G. (1955). Let the patients tell us where we fail. *Modern Hospital, 85*(2), 71-74.

Abdellah, F.G. (1955, March). Data from patients, nurses, and doctors on the needs for nursing service. *Military Medicine, 16,* 205-208.

Abdellah, F.G. (1957, June). Methods of identifying covert aspects of nursing problems. *Nursing Research, 6,* 4.

Abdellah, F.G. (1959, Jan.). Symposium on progressive patient care. *Hospitals, 33,* 42-46.

Abdellah, F.G. (1959, May). How we look at ourselves. *Nursing Outlook, 7,* 273.

Abdellah, F.G. (1960, June). Progressive patient care: A challenge for nursing. *Hospital Management, 89,* 102-106,135-137.

Abdellah, F.G. (1960, Aug.). Nursing patterns vary in progressive care. *Modern Hospital, 95,* 85.

Abdellah, F.G. (1961, April). The decision is yours. *Nursing Outlook, 9,* 223.

Abdellah, F.G. (1961, Winter). Criterion measures in nursing. *Nursing Research, 10,* 21.

Abdellah, F.G. (1965, Oct.). Search or research? An experiment to stimulate research. *Nursing Outlook, 13,* 65-67.

Abdellah, F.G. (1966). Doctoral preparation for nurses. *Nursing Forum, 5*(3), 44-53.

Abdellah, F.G. (1966). Frontiers in nursing research. *Nursing Forum, 5,* 28-38.

Abdellah, F.G. (1967, Fall). Approaches to protecting the rights of human subjects. *Nursing Research, 16,* 315-320.

Abdellah, F.G. (1969, Sept./Oct.). The nature of nursing science. *Nursing Research, 18,* 390-393.

Abdellah, F.G. (1969, Dec.). Nursing research in the health services [Editorial]. *Nursing Research Reports, 4,* 2.

Abdellah, F.G. (1970, Jan./Feb.). Overview of nursing research: 1955-1968 (Part I). *Nursing Research, 19,* 6-17.

Abdellah, F.G. (1970, March/April). Overview of nursing research: 1955-1968 (Part II). *Nursing Research, 19,* 151-162.

Abdellah, F.G. (1970, May). Training and development of the health care team. *AORN Journal, 11,* 86-91.

Abdellah, F.G. (1970, May/June). Overview of nursing research: 1955-1968 (Part III). *Nursing Research, 19,* 239-252.

Abdellah, F.G. (1970, Summer). Conference on the nature of science in nursing. The nature of nursing science. *Japanese Journal of Nursing Research, 3,* 248-252.

Abdellah, F.G. (1971, May). Problems, issues, challenges of nursing research. *Canadian Nurse, 67,* 44-46.

Abdellah, F.G. (1972). Evolution of nursing as a profession: Perspective on manpower development. *International Nursing Review, 19,* 219-238.

Abdellah, F.G. (1972, Sept.). The physician-nurse team approach to coronary care. In R. Pinneo (Ed.), *Symposium on Concepts in Cardiac Nursing. Nursing Clinics of North America, 7*(3), 423-430.

Abdellah, F.G. (1972, Oct.). No legal bars to expanded nursing practice. *Stat, 41,* 4.

Abdellah, F.G. (1973, Jan./Feb.). Criterios de avaliac as em enfermagem. *Revista Brasileira de Enfermagem, 26,* 17-32. (Portugal.)

Abdellah, F.G. (1973, May). Research on career development in the health professions: Nursing. *Occupational Health Nursing, 21,* 12-16.

Abdellah, F.G. (1973, June). School nurse practitioner: An expanded role for nurses. *Journal of the American College Health Association, 21,* 423-432.

Abdellah, F.G. (1973, Dec.). Nursing and health care in the USSR. *American Journal of Nursing, 73,* 2096-2099.

Abdellah, F.G. (1974). A national health strategy for the delivery of long-term health care: Implications for nursing. *Journal of New York State Nurses' Association, 5*(4), 7-13.

Abdellah, F.G. (1974, Spring). Long-term care: A top health priority [Guest editorial]. *Journal of Long-Term Care Administration, 2*(2), 1-3.

Abdellah, F.G. (1974, Fall). Health care issues: Overview of emerging health services delivery projects. *Health Care Dimensions,* 125-139.

Abdellah, F.G. (1975). A national health strategy for the delivery of long-term health care: Implication for nursing. *Nursing Digest,* 4(5), 15-17.

Abdellah, F.G. (1975). Campaign for improvement for long-term care [Editorial]. *Public Health Reports,* 90(6).

Abdellah, F.G. (1975). Nursing home infection control held 'essential.' *Hospital Infection Control,* 2(8), 103-104.

Abdellah, F.G. (1975, Jan./Feb.). National Library of Medicine is official nursing archives [Letter]. *Nursing Research,* 24(1), 64.

Abdellah, F.G. (1975, Sept./Oct.). The nursing archives at the National Library of Medicine [Letter]. *Nursing Research,* 24(5), 389.

Abdellah, F.G. (1975, Nov.). Three views. Patient assessment: Its potential and use (Part I). *American Health Care Association Journal,* 1, 69.

Abdellah, F.G. (1976). HEW task force examines ways to upgrade and expand home health care programs. *Geriatrics,* 12, 31-43, 46.

Abdellah, F.G. (1976, March). Nurse practitioners and nursing practice [Editorial]. *American Journal of Public Health,* 66(3), 245-246.

Abdellah, F.G. (1976, Aug.). Nursing's role in future health care. *AORN Journal,* 24(2), 236-240.

Abdellah, F.G. (1977, Jan./Feb.). A nationwide study to evaluate the care of patients in nursing homes. *Public Health Reports,* 92(1), 30-32.

Abdellah, F.G. (1977, July/Aug.). U.S. Public Health Service's contribution to nursing research: Past, present, future. *Nursing Research,* 27(4), 244-249.

Abdellah, F.G. (1978). The future of long-term care. *Bulletin of the New York Academy of Medicine,* 54(3), 261-270.

Abdellah, F.G. (1978, July). Long-term care policy issues: Alternatives to institutional care. *American Academy of Political and Social Science Annals,* 438, 28-29.

Abdellah, F.G. (1979). Cross-cultural comparison: Care of the elderly in China and U.S.S.R. *The Journal of Intercare,* 1(2), 1, 3, 8, 12-14.

Abdellah, F.G. (1981). Thirty-second world health assembly: Actions and implications for nursing. *The Journal of Intercare,* 1, 1,3,6,7,10-13.

Abdellah, F.G. (1981, Nov.). Nursing care of the aged in the United States of America. *Journal of Gerontological Nursing,* 7(11), 657-663.

Abdellah, F.G. (1982, Summer). The nurse practitioner 17 years later: Present and emerging issues. *Inquiry,* 19(2), 105-116.

Abdellah, F.G. (1982, Dec.). Keynote address, 75th anniversary of the West Virginia State Nurses' Association. *Weather Vane,* 51(6), 10-13, 15.

Abdellah, F.G. (1983, Feb./March). Future directions: Impact of the NSNA 1982 and 2012. *Imprint,* 30(1), 66-74.

Abdellah, F.G. (1983, March/April). 1983-2008: Nursing Practice. *Arizona Nurse,* 36(2), 6-7.

Abdellah, F.G. (1983, April/May). Future directions: Impact of the NSNA 1982 and 2012. *Imprint,* 30(2), 91-97.

Abdellah, F.G. (1984, Feb.). New roles in the Federal Nursing Services. *Today's OR Nurse,* 6(2), 6.

Abdellah, F.G. (1984, July). Nursing in the world: 35 years of development after World War II. Changes affecting nursing in the United States 1949-1984. *Kango Tenbo,* 36(3), 2-10.

Abdellah, F.G. (1984, Aug.). Changes affecting nursing in the United States 1949-1984. *Kango Tenbo,* 9(8), 2-10.

Abdellah, F.G. (1985, June 5-11). Standards of care: Hospitals mean business. *Nursing Times,* 81(23), 36-37.

Abdellah, F.G. (1987, Feb.). Practice mode of nursing the "Health for All." *Kango Tenbo,* 12(2), 164-169.

Abdellah, F.G. (1987, Sept./Oct.). The federal role in nursing education. *Nursing Outlook,* 35(5), 224-225.

Abdellah, F.G. (1988). Incontinence: Implications for health care policy. *Nursing Clinics of North America,* 231, 1, 291-297.

Abdellah, F.G. (1990). Agency for health care policy and research: A challenge for nurse researchers. *Journal for Professional Nursing,* 6(6), 325.

Abdellah, F.G. (1990). Management of clinical trials. *Journal of Professional Nursing,* 6, 4, 189.

Abdellah, F.G. (1990). Peer review: The only answer to high-quality research? *Journal of Professional Nursing,* 6, 2, 70.

Abdellah, F.G. (1990). Reflections of a recurring theme: Historical perspective of nursing shortage. *Nursing Clinics of North America,* 25, 509-516.

Abdellah, F.G. (1990). Scientific misconduct: Myth or reality? *Journal of Professional Nursing,* 6, 1, 6, 63.

Abdellah, F.G. (1990). Self-help groups offer prime areas for nurse researchers. *Journal of Professional Nursing,* 6(5), 257.

Abdellah, F.G. (1990). The National Library of Medicine: A treasure trove for nurse researchers [Editorial]. *Journal of Professional Nursing,* 6, 3, 134.

Abdellah, F.G. (1991). The funding crisis in biomedical research: Addressing the issue (Part 1). *Journal of Professional Nursing,* 7(1), 7.

Abdellah, F.G. (1991). The funding crisis in biomedical research: Options for action. (Part 2). *Journal of Professional Nursing,* 7(2), 75.

Abdellah, F.G. (1991). The human genome initiative: Implications for nurse researchers. *Journal of Professional Nursing,* 7(6), 332.

Abdellah, F.G. (1992). The politics of health and policy formation. *Reflections,* 18(1), 23.

Abdellah, F.G. (1993). Doctoral preparation and research productivity. *Journal of Professional Nursing,* 9(2), 71.

Abdellah, F.G. (1995). Management perspectives: "I'm the aspiring vice president of nursing at a university hospital, and I'm wondering how to avoid hitting the 'glass ceiling.'" *Nursing Spectrum of Washington DC,* 5(9), 7.

Abdellah, F.G., Burke, C., & Chall, C.L. (1956). A time study of nursing activities in psychiatric hospital. *Nursing Research,* 5(1), 27-35.

Abdellah, F.G., Chamberlain, J.G., & Levine, I.S. (1986, Sept./Oct.). Role of nurses in meeting needs of the homeless: Summary of a workshop for providers, researchers, and educators. *Public Health Reports,* 101(5), 494-498.

Abdellah, F.G. & Chow, R.K. (1976, Nov./Dec.). The long-term care facility improvement campaign: The PACE project. *Association of Rehabilitation Nurses' Journal,* 1(7), 3-4.

Abdellah, F.G. & Chow, R.K. (1976, Winter). Long-term care facility improvement: A nationwide research effort. *Journal of Long-Term Care Administration,* 4(1), 5-19.

Abdellah, F.G., Foerst, H.V., & Chow, R.K. (1979, June). PACE: An approach to improving the care of the elderly. *American Journal of Nursing,* 79(6), 1109-1110.

Abdellah, F.G. & Haldeman, J.C. (1959, May 16). The concept of progressive patient care (Part 1, Part 2). *Hospitals,* 33, 38-42, 142, 143.

Abdellah, F.G. & Levine E. (1952, Jan.). Survey shows only 19 percent of West Virginia workers covered by in-plant nursing services. *Occupational Health,* 12(1), 4-6.

Abdellah, F.G. & Levine, E. (1954, June). Why nurses leave home. *Hospitals,* 28, 80-81.

Abdellah, F.G. & Levine, E. (1954, June). Work sampling applied to the study of nursing personnel. *Nursing Research,* 3(1), 11-16.

Abdellah, F.G. & Levine, E. (1957, Feb.). Developing a measure of patient and personnel satisfaction with nursing care. *Nursing Research,* 5, 100.

Abdellah, F.G. & Levine, E. (1957, Nov. 1). Polling patients and personnel: What patients say about their nursing care (Part 1). *Hospitals,* 31, 44-48.

Abdellah, F.G. & Levine, E. (1957, Nov. 16). What factors affect patients' opinions of their nursing care? (Part 2). *Hospitals,* 31, 61-64.

Abdellah, F.G. & Levine, E. (1957, Dec. 1). What personnel say about nursing care (Part 3). *Hospitals,* 3, 53-57.

Abdellah, F.G. & Levine, E. (1957, Dec. 16). What hospitals have done to improve patient care (Part 4). *Hospitals,* 31, 43-44.

Abdellah, F.G. & Levine, E. (1965, April). Better patient care through nursing research. *International Journal of Nursing Studies,* 2, 1.

Abdellah, F.G. & Levine, E. (1965, Winter). The aims of nursing research. *Nursing Research,* 14, 27-32.

Abdellah, F.G. & Levine, E. (1966, Jan.). Future directions of research in nursing. *American Journal of Nursing,* 66, 112-116.

Abdellah, F.G. & Levine, E. (1968, Summer). The aims of nursing research. *Comprehensive Nursing Monthly,* 3, 12-31.

Abdellah, F.G. & Levine, E. (1982, Aug.). Better patient care through nursing research (Part 1). *Kango Tenbo,* 7(8), 714-719.

Abdellah, F.G. & Strachan, E.J. (1959, May). Progressive patient care. *American Journal of Nursing,* 59, 649.

Fuller, E.O., Hasselmeyer, E.G., Hunter, J.C., Abdellah, F.G., & Hinshaw, A.S. (1991). Summary statements of the NIH nursing research grant applications. *Nursing Research,* 40(6), 346-351.

Levine, E. & Abdellah, F.G. (1984, Summer). DRGs: A recent refinement to an old method. *Inquiry,* 21(2), 105-112.

Matarazzo, J.D. & Abdellah, F.G. (1971, Sept./Oct.). Doctoral education for nurses in the U.S. *Nursing Research,* 20, 404-414.

Muller, J.E., Abdellah, F.G., Billings, F.T., Hess, A.E., Petit, D., & Egeberg, R.D. (1972, March). The Soviet health system: Aspects of relevance for medicine in the U.S. *New England Journal of Medicine,* 286, 693-702.

Conferences

Abdellah, F.G. (1959, Feb./Mar.). *Criterion measures in nursing for experimental research. Report on Nursing Research Conference.* Washington, DC: Walter Reed Army Medical Center.

Abdellah, F.G. (1972, May 31). *An effective health care delivery system: Can it be achieved?* Commencement Address at the Cornell University Medical College and Cornell University-New York Hospital School of Nursing, New York City.

Abdellah, F.G. (1975, July 27-31). *Long term care facility improvement: A nationwide research effort.* Proceedings of the First North American Symposium on Long Term Care Administration (pp. 3-22). Toronto, Ontario, Canada: American College of Nursing Home Administrators.

Abdellah, F.G. (1976, June 4). A nursing issue: Administration of medications by unlicensed personnel. In *A Look to the Future* (pp. 17-18). Conference sponsored by American Nurses' Association, Council of State Boards of Nursing, Shelburne Hotel, Atlantic City, NJ.

Abdellah, F.G. (1978, Feb.). New nurse practitioners and care of the aging. In C. Spieler (Ed.), *Care of the Aging* (pp. 37-55). Conference report of Josiah Macy, Jr. Foundation.

Abdellah, F.G. (1986, Nov. 6-8). Elder abuse. In A.Z. Reed & J.C. Sullivan (Eds.), *Violence in America* (pp. 23-25). Proceedings of the Southern Regional Research Conference, Family Advocacy Program of USAF and LBJ School of Public Affairs, University of Texas, Austin.

Abdellah, F.G. (1987, Sept. 20-22). *Report of the Surgeon General's Workshop on Self-Help and Public Health. Proceedings.* Los Angeles, CA: Department of Health and Human Services, U.S. Public Health Service.

Abdellah, F.G. & Moore, S.R. (Eds.). (1988, March 20-23). *Surgeon General's Workshop on Health Promotion and Aging. Background Papers.* Washington, DC: Department of Health and Human Services, U.S. Public Health Service.

Chow, R.K. & Abdellah, F.G. (1974, Sept.). Intensive nursing care of the patient in myocardial failure: A videotaped case study. *Abstracts,* No. 399. Buenos Aires, Argentina: World Congress of Cardiology.

Hogness, J.R., Atkinson, H., Abdellah, F.G., Foster, J., Haley, R.W., & Patterson, R.A. (1984, March 29-30). *International conference on the reuse of disposable medical devices in the 1980's. Final report of the conference panel.* Conference proceedings also published by the Institute for Health Policy Analysis. Washington, DC: Institute for Health Policy Analysis, Georgetown University Medical Center.

Forewords

Abdellah, F.G. (1971). Foreword in J.F. Murphy (Ed.), *Theoretical issues in professional nursing* (p.196). New York: Meredith.

Department of Health, Education, and Welfare. (1975). Foreword in F.G. Abdellah (Ed.), *Long term care facility improvement study: Introductory report* (p. 137). Washington, DC: U.S. Government Printing Office.

Correspondence

Abdellah, F.G. (1984, March 7). Personal letter.
Abdellah, F.G. (1988, April 28). Personal letter.
Abdellah, F.G. (1992, March). Vitae.
Abdellah, F.G. (1992, April 4). Telephone interview.
Abdellah, F.G. (2000). Personal correspondence.

Secondary Sources
Book Reviews

Abdellah, F.G. (1972). [Review of the book *The physician's assistant: today and tomorrow*]. *The New England Journal of Medicine, 287*(24), 1257-1258.

Abdellah, F.G., Beland, I.L., Martin, A., & Matheney, R.V. (1963, Spring). [Review of the book *Patient-centered approaches to nursing*]. *Hospital Administration, 8,* 48.

Abdellah, F.G., Beland, I.L., Martin, A., & Matheny, R.V. (1973, Aug.). [Review of the book *New directions in patient-centered nursing*]. *American Journal of Nursing, 73,* 1439.

Abdellah, F.G., Beland, I.L., Martin, A., & Matheny, R.V. (1974, Sept.). [Review of the book *New directions in patient-centered nursing*]. *Nursing Outlook, 22,* 555.

Abdellah, F.G. & Levine, E. (1957, May). [Review of the book *Patients and personnel speak: A method of studying patient care in hospitals*]. *American Journal of Nursing, 59,* 634-635.

Abdellah, F.G. & Levine, E. (1965, Nov.). [Review of the book *Better patient care through nursing research*]. *Hospitals, 39,* 115.

[Review of the book *Better patient care through nursing research*]. (1965, Dec.). *Nursing Outlook, 13,* 18.

[Review of the book *Better patient care through nursing research*]. (1966, March). *Catholic Nurse, 14,* 63.

[Review of the book *Better patient care through nursing research*]. (1966, April). *American Journal of Nursing, 66,* 828.

[Review of the book *Better patient care through nursing research*]. (1966, Summer). *Nursing Research, 15,* 217.

[Review of the book *Better patient care through nursing research*]. (1967, June). *Nursing Research Reports, 2,* 6.

Abdellah, F.G. & Levine, E. (Jan. 1979). [Review of the book *Better patient care through nursing research* (2nd ed.)]. *American Journal of Nursing, 80,* 67-68.

Abdellah, F.G. & Levine, E. (1986). [Review of the book *Better patient care through nursing research* (3rd ed.)]. *Journal of Advanced Nursing, 12*(3), 400.

Interviews

Abdellah, F.G. (1984, Jan.). Interview with Faye Abdellah (interview by Judith Rodin). *American Psychologist, 39*(1), 67-70.

Abdellah, F.G. (1986, May). An interview with Faye G. Abdellah (interview by S. Senno). *Kango Tenbo,*11(6), 592-593.

News Releases

Appointments. (1971, Jan.). H.S.M.H.A. *Health Report, 36,* 27-38.

Department of Health, Education, and Welfare. (1971, Jan./Feb.). Faye G. Abdellah: A new appointment. *Journal of Continuing Education in Nursing, 2,* 9.

Public Health Service now has two lady admirals: Jessie Scott and Faye Abdellah. (1970, Nov.). *American Journal of Nursing, 70,* 2281.

Two named to top nurse rank in P.H.S. (1970, Nov.). *Nursing Outlook, 18,* 10.

Biographical Sources

Directory of nurses with doctoral degrees. (1980, Aug.). ANA Publication No. G-143. Washington, DC: American Nurses Association.

Faye Abdellah sees bright future for nurses. (1980, Sept.). *American Journal of Nursing, 80,* 1671-1672.

Laurence, K.E. (1982). *The national nursing directory.* Rockville, MD: Aspen Systems.

Who's who in America: 1982-1983 (42nd ed.). (1982). Chicago: Marquis.

Books

Dolan, J.A., Fitzpatrick, M.L., & Hermann, E.K. (1983). *Nursing in society: A historic perspective* (15th ed.). Philadelphia: W.B. Saunders.

Griffin, J.G. & Griffin, J.K. (1973). *History and trends of professional nursing.* St. Louis: Mosby.

Nursing Theories Conference Group, J.B. George (Chairperson). (1980). *Nursing theories: The base for professional practice.* Englewood Cliffs, NJ: Prentice Hall.

Orem, D.E. (Ed.). (1979). *Concept formalization in nursing, process and product.* Boston: Little, Brown.

Book Chapter

Falco, S.M. (1980). Faye Abdellah. Nursing theories: The base for professional nursing practice. In J.B. George (Ed.), *Nursing Theories Conference Group,* Englewood Cliffs, NJ: Prentice Hall.

Journal Articles

Abraham, I.L., Chalifoux, Z.L., Evers, G.C.M., & DeGeest, S. (1995). Conditions, interventions, and outcomes in nursing research: A comparative analysis of North American and European International journals. (1981-1990). *International Journal of Nursing Studies, 32*(2), 173-187.

Adebo, E.O., (1974). Identifying problems for nursing research. *International Nursing Review, 21*(2), 53.

Alward, R.R. (1983). Patient classification system. The ideal vs. reality. *Journal of Nursing Administration, 13*(2), 14-19.

Armiger, B. (1977). Ethics of nursing research: Profile, principles perspective. *Nursing Research, 26*(5), 330-336.

Auger, J.A. & Dee, V. (1983). A patient classification system based on the behavioral system model of nursing. *Journal of Nursing Administration, 13*(4), 38-43.

Auster, D. (1978). Occupational values of male and female nursing students. *Sociology of Work and Occupations, 5*(2), 209-233.

Avis, M. (1995). Valid arguments? A consideration of the concept of validity in establishing the credibility of research findings. *Journal of Advanced Nursing, 22*(6), 1203-1209.

Ballard, K.A., Gray, R.F., Knauf, R.A., & Uppal, P. (1993). Measuring variations in nursing care per DRG. *Nursing Management, 24*(4), 40-41.

Ballard, S. & McNamara, R. (1983). Qualifying nursing needs in home health care. *Nursing Research, 32*(4), 236-241.

Becker, G. & Kaufman, S. (1988). Old age, rehabilitation and research: A review of the issues. *Gerontologist, 28*(4), 459-468.

Bergman, R., Stocker, R.A., Shavit, N., Sharon, R., Feinberg, O., & Danon, A. (1981). Role, selection and preparation of unit head nurses (Part 1). *International Journal of Nursing Studies, 18*(2), 123-152.

Bergman, R., Stocker, R.A., Shavit, N., Sharon, R., Feinberg, O., & Danon, A. (1981). Role, selection and preparation of unit head nurses (Part 2). *International Journal of Nursing Studies, 18*(3), 191-211.

Bergman, R., Stocker, R.A., Shavit, N., Sharon, R., Feinberg, O., & Danon, A. (1981). Role, selection and preparation of unit head nurses (Part 3). *International Journal of Nursing Studies, 18*(4), 237-250.

Bernal, H., Church, O.M., Arevian, M., & Schensul, S.L. (1995). Community health nursing in a former Soviet Union Republic: A case study of change in Armenia. *Nursing Outlook, 43*(2), 78-83.

Bircumshaw, D. & Chapman, C.M. (1988). A study to compare the practice style of graduate and non-graduate nurses and midwives: The pilot study. *Journal of Advanced Nursing, 13*(5), 605-614.

Blancett, S.S. (1991). The ethics of writing and publishing. *The Journal of Nursing Administration, 21*(5), 31-36.

Boschma, G. (1994). The meaning of holism in nursing: Historical shifts in holistic nursing ideas. *Public Health Nursing, 11*(5), 324-330.

Brickhill, C.E. (1995). ICU for the '90s: The "intensive customer unit." *Nursing Management, 26*(1), 44-48.

Brown, G.D. (1995). Understanding barriers to basing nursing practice upon research: A communication model approach. *Journal of Advanced Nursing, 21*(1), 154-157.

Buttriss, G., Kuiper, R., & Newbold, B. (1995). The use of a homeless shelter as a clinical rotation for nursing students. *Journal of Nursing Education, 38*(8), 375-377.

Carnegie, M.E. (1975). Financial assistance for nursing research: Past and present. *Nursing Research, 24*(3), 163.

Carter, M.D. (1973). Identification of behaviors displayed by children experiencing prolonged hospitalization. *International Journal of Nursing Studies, 10*(2), 125-135.

Cateriniccho, R.P. & Davis, R.H. (1983). Developing a client focused allocation statistic of inpatient nursing resource use: An alternative to the patient day. *Social Science and Medicine, 17*(5), 259-272.

Chamorro, I.L., Davis, M.L., Green, D., & Kramer, M. (1973). Development of an instrument to measure premature infant behavior and caretaker activities: Time-sampling methodology. *Nursing Research, 22*(4), 300-309.

Chamorro, T. (1981). The role of a nurse clinician in joint practice with a gynecologic oncologist. *Cancer, 48*(2), 622-631.

Chandler, M.C. & Mason, W.H. (1995). Solution-focused therapy: An alternative approach to addictions in nursing. *Perspectives in Psychiatric Care, 31*(1), 8-13.

Chow, R.K. (1974). Significant research and future needs for improving patient care. *Military Medicine,* 139(4), 302-306.

Clay, T. (1986). Unity for change? *Journal of Advanced Nursing,* 11(1), 21-33.

Colaizzi, J. (1975). Proper object of nursing science. *International Journal of Nursing Studies,* 12(4), 197-200.

Conine, T.A. & Hopper, D.L. (1978). Work sampling: Tool in management. *American Journal of Occupational Therapy,* 32(5), 301-304.

Connelly, C.E. (1986). Replication research in nursing. *International Journal of Nursing Studies,* 23(1), 71-77.

Copp, L.A. (1973). Professional change: Which trends do nurses endorse? *International Journal of Nursing Studies,* 10(1), 55-63.

Copp, L.A. (1974). Critical concerns and commitments of a new department of nursing. *International Journal of Nursing Studies,* 11(4), 203-210.

Cornell, S.A. (1974). Development of an instrument for measuring quality of nursing care. *Nursing Research,* 23(1), 103-117.

Corner, J. (1991). In search of more complete answers to research questions. Quantitative versus qualitative methods: Is there a way forward? *Journal of Advanced Nursing,* 16(16), 718-727.

Craig, S.L. (1980). Theory development and its relevance for nursing. *Journal of Advanced Nursing,* 5(4), 349-355.

Cronenwett, L.R. (1983). Helping and nursing models. *Nursing Research,* 6(6), 342-346.

Crow, R.A. (1981). Research and the standards of nursing care: What is the relationship? *Journal of Advanced Nursing,* 6(6), 491-496.

Daeffler, R.J. (1977). Outcomes of primary nursing for the patient. *Military Medicine,* 142,(3), 204-208.

DeGroot, H.A. (1989). Patient classification system evaluation. Part I: Essential system elements. *The Journal of Nursing Administration,* 19(6), 30-35.

Delacuestra, C. (1983). The nursing process: From development to implementation. *Journal of Advanced Nursing,* 8(5), 365-371.

DeLeon, P.H., Kjervik, D.K., Kraut, A.G., & VandenBos, G.R. (1985). Psychology and nursing: A natural alliance. *American Psychologist,* 40(11), 1153-1164.

Denton, J.A. & Wisenbaker, V.B. (1977). Death experience and death anxiety among nurses and nursing students. *Nursing Research,* 26(1), 61-64.

Dickoff, J., James, P., & Semradek, J. (1975). Designing nursing research: Eight points to encounter. *Nursing Research,* 24(3), 164-176.

Dickoff, J., James, P., & Semradek, J. (1975). Stance for nursing research: Tenacity or inquiry? *Nursing Research,* 24(2), 84-88.

Dickson, W.M. (1978). Measuring pharmacist time use: Note on use of fixed interval work sampling. *American Journal of Hospital Pharmacy,* 35(10), 1241-1243.

DiMarco, N., Castels, M.R., Carter, J.H., & Corrigan, M.K. (1976). Nursing resources on nursing unit and quality of patient care. *International Journal of Nursing Studies,* 13(3), 139-152.

Doerr, B.C. & Jones, J.W. (1979). Effect of family preparation on the state anxiety level of the C.C.U. patient. *Nursing Research,* 28(5), 315-316.

Doessel, D.P. & Marshall, J.V. (1985). A rehabilitation of health outcome in quality assessment. *Social Science and Medicine,* 21(12), 1319-1328.

Duhart, J. & Chartonb, J. (1973). Hospital reform and health care in medical ordinance. *Revue Francaise De Sociologie,* 14, 77-101.

Dungy, C.I. & Mullins, R.G. (1981). School nurse practitioner: Analysis of questionnaire and time-motion data. *Journal of School Health,* 51(7), 475-478.

Dunning, T. (1995). Development of nursing care manual to improve the knowledge of nurses caring for hospitalized patients with diabetes. *Journal of Continuing Education in Nursing,* 26(6), 261-266.

Edwardson, S.R. (1988). Outcomes of coronary care in the acute care setting. *Research in Nursing and Health,* 11, 215-222.

Edwardson, S.R. & Giovannetti, P.B. (1994). Nursing workload measurement systems. *Annual Review of Nursing Research,* 12, 95-123.

Ellis, R. (1977). Fallibilities, fragments, and frames: Contemplation on 25 years of research in medical-surgical nursing. *Nursing Research,* 26(3), 177-182.

Elms, R.R. (1972). Recovery room behavior and postoperative convalescence. *Nursing Research,* 21(5), 390-397.

Eriksen, L.R. (1987, July). Patient satisfaction: An indicator of nursing care quality? *Nursing Management,* 18(7), 31-35.

Falcone, A.R. (1983). Comprehensive functional assessment as an administrative tool. *Journal of the American Geriatrics Society,* 31(11), 642-650.

Fiedler, J.L. (1981). A review of the literature on access and utilization of medical care with special emphasis on rural primary care, social science and medical (Part C). *Medical Economics,* 15(3c), 129-142.

Flook, E. (1973). Health services research and R and D in perspective. *American Journal of Public Health and the Nations Health,* 63(8), 681-686.

Fortinsky, R.H., Granger, C.F., & Seltzer, G.B. (1981). The use of functional assessment in understanding home care needs. *Medical Care,* 19(5), 489-497.

Foster, S.B. (1974). Adrenal measure for evaluating nursing effectiveness. *Nursing Research,* 23(2), 118-124.

Fowler, S.B. (1995). Hope: Implications for neuroscience nursing. *Journal of Neuroscience Nursing,* 27(5), 298-304.

Fox, R.N. & Ventura, M.R. (1983). Small scale administration of instruments procedures. *Nursing Research,* 32(2), 122-125.

Frelick, R.W. & Frelick, J.H. (1976). Coming to grips with main issues. *American Journal of Public Health,* 66(8), 795.

French, K. (1981). Methodological considerations in hospital patient opinion surveys. *International Journal of Nursing Studies,* 18(1), 7-32.

Fuhrer, M.J. (1983). Commentary: Communicating and utilizing research in medical rehabilitation. *Archives of Physical Medicine and Rehabilitation,* 64(12), 608-610.

Glover, T.L. (1995). Preliminary exploration of variables related to operating room staffing methods. *Surgical Services Management,* 1(4), 37-41.

Golden, A.S. (1975). Task analysis in health manpower development and utilization. *Medical Care,* 13(8), 704-710.

Goodwin, J.D. & Edwards, B.S. (1975). Developing a computer program to assist nursing process: Phase 1: From systems analysis to an expandable program. *Nursing Research,* 24(4), 299-305.

Gordon, M. (1980). Determining study topics. *Nursing Research,* 2, 83-87.

Gordon, M., Sweeney, M.A., & McKeehan, K. (1980). Development of nursing diagnoses. *American Journal of Nursing,* 4, 669.

Gortner, S.R. & Nahm, H. (1977). Overview of nursing research in the United States. *Nursing Research,* 26(1), 10-33.

Greaves, F. (1980). Objectively toward curriculum improvement in nursing: Education in England and Wales. *Journal of Advanced Nursing,* 5(6), 591-599.

Grier, M.R. & Schnitzler, C.P. (1979). Nurses' propensity to risk. *Nursing Research,* 28(3), 186-191.

Grobe, S.J. (1990). Nursing intervention lexicon and taxonomy study: Language and classification methods. *Advances in Nursing Science,* 13(2), 22-35.

Gunter, L.M. & Miller, J.C. (1977). Toward a nurse gerontology. *Nursing Research,* 26(3), 209-221.

Hagell, E.I. (1989). Nursing knowledge: Women's knowledge—a sociological perspective. *Journal of Advanced Nursing,* 14(3), 226-233.

Hall, J.A. & Dornan, M.C. (1988). What patients like about their medical care and how often they are asked: A meta-analysis of the satisfaction literature. *Social Science and Medicine,* 27(9), 935-939.

Halloran, E.J. (1985). Nursing workload, medical diagnosis related groups and nursing diagnosis. *Research in Nursing and Health,* 8(4), 421-433.

Halloran, E.J. & Kiley, M. (1985). The nurses' role and length of stay [Letter]. *Medical Care,* 23(9), 1122-1124.

Handa, A. (1995). Sex education for adolescents. *Nursing Journal of India,* 86(8), 173-177.

Hanucharurnkul, S. (1989). Comparative analysis of Orem's and King's theories. *Journal of Advanced Nursing,* 14(5), 365-372.

Hardy, L.K. (1982). Nursing models and nursing: A restrictive view. *Journal of Advanced Nursing,* 7(5), 447-451.

Harrington, A. (1995). Spiritual care: What does it mean to RNs? *Australian Journal of Advanced Nursing,* 12(4), 5-14.

Hawthorne, P.J. (1984). Measuring change in nursing practice. *Journal of Advanced Nursing,* 9(3), 239-247.

Hayesbautista, D.E. (1976). Classification of practitioners by urban Chicano patients: Aspects of sociology of lay knowledge. *American Journal of Optometry and Physiological Optics,* 53(3), 156-163.

Heagarty, M.C., Boehringer, J.R., Lavinge, P.A., Brooks, E.G., & Evans, M.E. (1973). Evaluation of activities of nurses and pediatricians in a university outpatient department. *Journal of Pediatrics,* 83(5), 875-879.

Hendrickson, G., Doddato, T.M., & Kovner, C.T. (1990). How do nurses use their time? *Journal of Nursing Administration,* 20(3), 31-38.

Hodgman, E.L. (1979). Closing the gap between research and practice: Changing the answer to the who, the where and the how of nursing research. *International Journal of Nursing Studies,* 16(1), 105-110.

Holmes, S. (1989). Use of a modified symptom distress scale in assessment of the cancer patient. *International Journal of Nursing Studies,* 26(1), 69-79.

Holmes, S. (1991). Preliminary investigations of symptom distress in two cancer patient populations: Evaluation of a measurement instrument. *Journal of Advanced Nursing,* 16(4), 439-446.

Holmes, S. & Eburn, E. (1989). Patients' and nurses' perceptions of symptom distress in cancer. *Journal of Advanced Nursing,* 14(10), 840-846.

Hooker, B.B. (1977). Diploma school of nursing: Option in post-secondary education. *Journal of Nursing Education,* 16(3), 36-42.

Horn, S.D. & Horn, R.A. (1986). Reliability and validity of the Severity of Illness Index. *Medical Care,* 24(2), 159-168.

Hubbard, S.M. & Donehower, M.G. (1980). The nurse in a cancer research setting. *Seminars in Oncology,* 1, 9-17.

Huckabay, L.M. & Roberts, S.L. (1984). Effect of verbal mediators on cognitive learning, transfer of learning, and effective behaviors of student nurses as they apply to the care of patients with myocardial infarctions. *Heart and Lung,* 13(3), 280-286.

Jackson, B.S. & Kinney, M.R. (1978). Energy-expenditure, heart rate, rhythm and blood pressure in normal female subjects engaged in common hospitalized patient positions and modes of patient transfer. *International Journal of Nursing Studies,* 15(3), 115-128.

Jacobsen, B.S. & Meininger, J.C. (1985). The designs and methods of published nursing research: 1956-1983. *Nursing Research,* 34(5), 306-312.

Jennings, B.M. (1988). Merging nursing research and practice: A case of multiple identities. *Journal of Advanced Nursing,* 13(6), 752-758.

Jennings, C.P. & Jennings, T.F. (1977). Containing costs through perspective reimbursement. *American Journal of Nursing,* 77(7), 1155-1159.

Ketefian, S. (1975). Application of selected nursing research findings into nursing practice. Pilot study. *Nursing Research,* 24(2), 89-92.

Ketefien, S. (1976). Curriculum change in nursing education: Sources of knowledge utilized. *International Nursing Review,* 23(4), 107-115.

Krueger, J.C. (1980). Establishing priorities for evaluation and evaluation research: Nursing perspective. *Nursing Research,* 2, 115-118.

Kuhn, B.G. (1980). Prediction of nursing requirements from patient characteristics. *International Journal of Nursing Studies,* 1, 5-15.

Lanara, V.A. (1976). Philosophy of nursing and current nursing problems. *International Nursing Review,* 23(2), 48-54.

Levow, J.L. (1974). Consumer assessments of quality of medical care. *Medical Care,* 12(4), 328-337.

Leininger, M. (1976). Doctoral trends for nurses: Trends, questions, and projected plans. Part I: Trends, questions and issues on doctoral programs. *Nursing Research,* 25(3), 201-210.

Levine, E. & Abdellah, F.G. (1984). DRGs: A recent refinement to an old method. *Inquiry,* 21(2), 105-112.

Lewandowski, L.A. & Kositsky, A.M. (1983). Research priorities for critical care nursing: A study by the American Association of Critical Care Nurses. *Heart and Lung,* 12(1), 35-44.

Leyden, D.R. (1983). Measuring patients attitudes in a comprehensive health care setting. *Computers in Biology and Medicine,* 13(2), 99-124.

Lindeman, C.A. (1975). Delphi survey of priorities in clinical nursing research. *Nursing Research,* 24(6), 434-441.

Lindquist, R.D., Tracy, M.F., Treat-Jacobson, D. (1995). Peer review of nursing research proposals. *American Journal of Critical Care,* 4(1), 59-65.

Linn, L.S., Brook, R.H., Clark, V.A., Davies, A.R., Fink, A., & Kosecoff, J. (1985). Physician and patient satisfaction as factors related to the organization of internal medicine group practices. *Medical Care,* 23(10), 1171-1178.

Loomis, M.E. (1985). Emerging content in nursing: An analysis of dissertation abstracts and titles: 1976-1982. *Nursing Research,* 34(2), 113-118.

Lynaugh, J. (1990). Moments in nursing history: Four hundred postcards. *Nursing Research,* 39(4), 254-256.

MacGuire, J.M. (1990). Putting nursing research findings into practice: Research utilization as an aspect of the management of change. *Journal of Advanced Nursing,* 15(5), 614-620.

Maddox, M.A. & Fishbein, E.G. (1994). Survey results: Academic courses of women's health across the life-span. *Journal of Gerontological Nursing,* 20(6), 43-47.

Majesky, S.J., Brester, M.H., & Nishio, K.T. (1978). Development of a research tool: Patient indications of nursing care. *Nursing Research,* 27(6), 365-371.

Martin, K. (1988). Research in home care. *Nursing Clinics of North America,* 23(2), 363-385.

McGee, D.C. (1995). The perinatal nurse practitioner: An innovative model of advanced practice. *Journal of Obstetric Gynecologic and Neonatal Nursing,* 24(7), 602-606.

McGilloway, F.A. (1980). The nursing process: A problem-solving approach to patient care. *International Journal of Nursing Studies,* 2, 79-90.

McKinnon, E.L. (1978). Circulation research: Exploring its potential in clinical nursing. *Nursing Research,* 21(6), 494-498.

McLane, A.M. (1978). Core competencies of masters-prepared nurses. *Nursing Research,* 27(1), 48-53.

McMillan, S.C. (1985). A comparison of professional performance examination scores of graduating associate and baccalaureate degree nursing students. *Research in Nursing and Health,* 8(2), 167-172.

Meleis, A.I. (1979). Development of a conceptually based nursing curriculum: International experiment. *Journal of Advanced Nursing,* 6, 659-671.

Mickely, B.B. (1974). Physiologic and psychologic responses of elective surgical patients: Early definite or late indefinite scheduling of surgical procedures. *Nursing Research,* 23(5), 392-401.

Miller, A. (1984). Nurse/patient dependency: A review of different approaches with particular reference to studies of the dependency of elderly patients. *Journal of Advanced Nursing,* 9(5), 479-486.

Minnick, A., Young, W.B., & Roberts, M.J. (1995). 2,000 patients relate their hospital experiences. *Nursing Management,* 26(12), 29-31.

Mitchell, D. & Hicks, M. (1995). Components of life model in practice. *Accident and Emergency Nursing,* 3(4), 190-200.

Molde, S. & Diers, D. (1985). Nurse practitioner research: Selected literature review and research agenda. *Nursing Research,* 34(6), 362-367.

Molzahn, A.E. (1993). An evaluation of the nephrology nursing research literature: 1979-1989 (including commentary by Abbink C. with author response. *ANNA Journal,* 20(4), 395-428.

Moores, B. & Thompson, A.G.H. (1986). What 1357 hospital inpatients think about aspects of their stay in British acute hospitals. *Journal of Advanced Nursing,* 11(1), 87-102.

Munro, C.L. & Pickler, R.H. (1994). The technology and use of blastomere analysis. *Journal of Obstetric Gynecologic and Neonatal Nursing,* 23(3), 229-234.

Newman, B. (1995). Enhancing patient care: Case management and critical pathways. *Australian Journal of Advanced Nursing,* 13(1), 16-24.

Newman, S.J. (1985). Housing and long-term care: The suitability of the elderly's housing to the provision of in-home services. *Gerontologist,* 25(1), 35-40.

Nunnally, D.M. (1974). Patients' evaluation of other prenatal and delivery care. *Nursing Research,* 23(6), 469-474.

Orr, J.A. (1979). Nursing and the process of scientific inquiry. *Journal of Advanced Nursing,* 6, 603-610.

Paradis, L.F. & Cummings, S.B. (1986). The evolution of hospice in America toward organizational homogeneity. *Journal of Health and Social Behavior,* 27(4), 370-386.

Penchansky, R. & Thomas, J.W. (1981). The concept of access: Definitions and relationship to consumer satisfaction. *Medical Care,* 19(2), 127-140.

Peters, D.A. (1988). Development of a community health intensity rating scale. *Nursing Research,* 37(4), 202-207.

Proudfoot, L.M., Farmer, E.S., & McIntosh, J.B. (1994). Testing incontinence pads using single-case research designs. *British Journal of Nursing,* 3(7), 316.

Rankin, M.A. (1974). Pienschke's theoretical framework for guardedness or openness on the cancer unit [Letter]. *Nursing Research,* 23(5), 434.

Razquin, M.I.S., Solis, M.H.N., Sastre, R.S., Izco, M.S., & Garchitorena, E.C. (1995). Health problems identified in patients in a cardiovascular surgery department [Spanish]. *Enfermeria Clinica,* 5(4), 150-156.

Risser, N.L. (1975). Development of an instrument to measure patient satisfaction with nurses and nursing care in primary care settings. *Nursing Research,* 24(1), 45-52.

Roberts, K.L (1985). Theory of nursing as curriculum content. *Journal of Advanced Nursing,* 10(3), 209-215.

Rodgers, M.W. (1986). Implementing faculty practice: A question of human and financial resources. *Journal of Advanced Nursing,* 11(6), 687-696.

Santus, G., Ranzenigo, A., Caregnato, R., & Inzoli, M.R. (1990). Social and family integration of hemiplegic elderly patients 1 year after stroke. *Stroke,* 21(7), 1019-1022.

Sarnecky, M.T. (1990). Historiography: A legitimate research methodology for nursing. *Advances in Nursing Science,* 12(4), 1-10.

Schlotfeldt, R.M. (1975). Research in nursing and research training for nurses: Retrospect and prospect. *Nursing Research,* 24(3), 177-183.

Schuster, C. (1995). Have we forgotten the older adults? An argument in support of more health promotion programs for and research directed toward people 65 years and older. *Journal of Health Education,* 26(6), 338-344.

Seither, F.G. (1974). Predictive validity study of screening measures used to select practical nursing students. *Nursing Research,* 23(1), 60-63.

Sheahan, J. (1980). Some aspects of the teaching and learning of nursing. *Journal of Advanced Nursing,* 5(5), 491-511.

Shopa, M.A. (1975). Historical materials in nursing. *Nursing Research,* 24(4), 308.

Shukla, R.K. & Turner, W.E. III (1984). Patients perception of care under primary and team nursing. *Research in Nursing and Health,* 7(2), 93-99.

Simms, L.M., Pfoutz, S.K., & Price, S.C. (1986). Caring for older people: A challenge for nurse administrators. *Nursing Outlook,* 34(3), 145-148.

Smoyak, S.A. (1976). Is practice responding to research? *American Journal of Nursing,* 76(7), 1146-1150.

Spiegel, A.D., Hyman, H.H., & Gary, L.R. (1980). Issues and opportunities in the regulation of home health care. *Health Policy and Education,* 1(3), 237-253.

Stevenson, J.S. (1987). Forging a research discipline. *Nursing Research,* 36(1), 60-64.

Stolte, K., Myers, S.T., & Owen, W.L. (1994). Changes in maternity care and the impact on nurses and nursing practice. *Journal of Obstetric Gynecologic and Neonatal Nursing,* 23(7), 603-608.

Stratton, T.D., Dunkin, J.W., & Juhl, N. (1995). Redefining the nursing shortage: A rural perspective. *Nursing Outlook,* 43(2), 71-77.

Sutcliffe, J. & Holmes, S. (1991). Quality of life: Verification and use of a self-assessment scale in two patient populations. *Journal of Advanced Nursing,* 16(4), 490-498.

Taylor, S.D. (1974). Development of a classification system for current nursing research. *Nursing Research,* 23(1), 63-68.

Taylor, S.D. (1975). Bibliography on nursing research: 1950-1974. *Milbank Memorial Fund Quarterly,* 24(3), 207-225.

Temkingreener, H. (1983). Interprofessional perspectives on teamwork in health care: A case study. *Milbank Memorial Fund Quarterly: Health and Society,* 61(4), 641-658.

Thompson, D.R. & Sutton, T.W. (1985). Nursing decision making in a coronary care unit. *International Journal of Nursing Studies,* 22(3), 259-266.

Thurston, N. (1995). Hospital research comes of age. *Canadian Nurse,* 91(4), 34-38.

Tiesinga, L.J., Halfens, R.J.G., Algera-Osinga, J.T., & Hasman, A. (1994). The application of a factor evaluation system for community nursing in the Netherlands. *Journal of Nursing Management,* 2(4), 175-179.

Tornary, R.D. (1977). Nursing research: Road ahead. *Nursing Research,* 26(6), 404-407.

Trivedi, V.M. & Hancock, W.J. (1975). Measurement of nursing workload using head nurses' perceptions. *Nursing Research,* 24(5), 371-376.

Trivedi, V.M. & Warner, D.M. (1976). Branch and bound algorithm for optimum allocation of float nurses. *Management Science, 22*(9), 972-981.

Turnbull, E.M. (1978). Effect of basic preventive health practices and mass-media on practice of breast self-examination. *Nursing Research, 27*(2), 98-102.

Ventura, M.R. & Waligoraserofur, B. (1981). Study priorities identified by nurses in mental health setting. *International Journal of Nursing Studies, 19*(1), 41-46.

Vredevoe, D.L. (1972). Nursing research involving physiological mechanisms: Definitions of variables. *Nursing Research, 21*(1), 68-72.

Wade, G.H. (1995). Is research in the patient setting feasible? *Journal of Continuing Education in Nursing, 26*(6), 253-256.

Wade, S. (1995). Partnership in care: A critical review. *Nursing Standard, 9*(48), 29-32.

Wagner, V.D., Kee, C.C., & Gray, D.P. (1995). A historical decline of educational perioperative clinical experiences. *AORN Journal, 62*(5), 771-772.

Ware, J.E. & Berwick, D.M. (1990). Conclusions and recommendations (of a Pilot-study: patient judgments of hospital quality). *Medical Care, 28*(9), S39-S44.

Warner, D.M. (1976). Nurse staffing, scheduling, reallocation in hospital. *Hospital and Health Services Administration, 21*(3), 77-90.

Webber, P.B. (1994). National response to the nursing shortage: Implications for nursing education. *Journal of Nursing Education, 33*(3), 107-111.

White, M.B. (1972). Importance of selected nursing activities. *Nursing Research, 21*(1), 4-14.

Wolfer, J.A. (1973). Definition and assessment of surgical patients' welfare and recovery. *Nursing Research, 22*(5), 394-401.

Wright, D. (1984). An introduction to the evaluation of nursing care: A review of the literature. *Journal of Advanced Nursing, 9*(5), 457-467.

Yurick, A., Burgio, L., & Paton, S.M. (1995). Assessing disruptive behaviors of nursing home residents: Use of microcomputer technology to promote objectivity in planning nursing interventions. *Journal of Gerontological Nursing, 21*(4), 29-34.

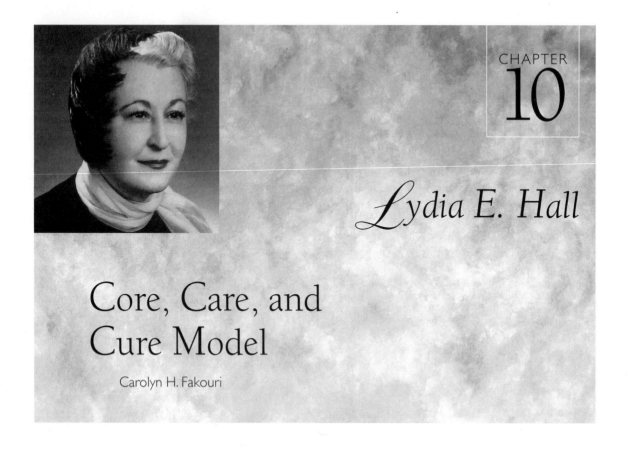

Lydia E. Hall

Core, Care, and Cure Model

Carolyn H. Fakouri

CREDENTIALS AND BACKGROUND OF THE THEORIST

Lydia Hall began her prestigious career in nursing as a graduate of the York Hospital School of Nursing in York, Pennsylvania. She then earned her B.S. and M.A. degrees from Teachers College, Columbia University, in New York.

Hall held faculty positions at the York Hospital School of Nursing and the Fordham Hospital School of Nursing and was a consultant in nursing education to the nursing faculty at State University of New York, Upstate Medical Center. She also was an instructor of nursing education at Teachers College.

Previous authors: Carolyn H. Fakouri, Marcy Grandstaff, S. Brook Gumm, Ann Marriner Tomey, and Kim Tippey Peskoe.

Hall's career interests revolved around public health nursing, cardiovascular nursing, pediatric cardiology, and nursing of long-term illnesses. She authored 21 publications and the bulk of the articles and addresses regarding her nursing theory were published in the early to middle 1960s. In 1967, she received the Award for Distinguished Achievement in Nursing Practice from Columbia University.

Perhaps Hall's greatest achievement in nursing was her design and development of the Loeb Center for Nursing at Montefiore Hospital in New York City. Established to apply her theory to nursing practice, the center opened in January of 1963. Hall designed the 80-bed Loeb Center for persons aged 16 years or older who were no longer having acute biological disturbances. Candidates for the Loeb Center were recommended by their physicians and had favorable potential for recovery and subsequent return to their community. Within the nondirective setting, patients demonstrated success and provided empirical evidence to support the major concepts in Hall's theory. Hall served as administrative director of the Loeb Center for Nursing from its opening until her death in February 1969.

In 2000, the 80-patient bed Loeb Center continued to be a vital part of Montefiore Medical Center.[13] The skilled nursing facility provided a team approach to assist hospital patients who had chronic disease or were recovering from an acute illness or surgical procedure. The range of conditions that patients at Loeb experience remains fairly consistent to the original patient population, which included diabetes, cerebrovascular accidents, postoperative heart surgery, hip fractures, amputations, and arthritis.[2] During the year 2000, several patients requiring wound care were admitted to Loeb. The patients were admitted for rehabilitation and remained for four to six weeks. Consistent with Hall's original model, nurses and the interdisciplinary rehabilitation staff worked together with the patient and family to assist the patient to make the transition from hospital to home. The professional nurse was the chief therapist. The unit was staffed with a physician's assistant around the clock. Practical nurses and nurse attendants assisted with patient care, but they were not a substitute for the nurse. The patient was viewed as an individual with goals. The treatment plan was designed to meet those goals that would help achieve eventual recovery and rehabilitation.

THEORETICAL SOURCES

Hall drew extensively from the schools of psychiatry and psychology in theorizing about the nurse-patient relationship. She was a proponent of Carl Rogers' philosophy of client-centered therapy. This method of therapy entails establishing a relationship of warmth and safety and conveying a sensitive empathy with the patient's feelings and communications.[17] A major premise Hall borrowed from Rogers[17] is that patients achieve their maximal potential through a learning process. Rogers[17:280-281] states that psychotherapy facilitates significant learning by:

(1) pointing out and labeling unsatisfying behaviors, (2) exploring objectively with the patient the reasons for the behaviors, and (3) establishing through reeducation more effective problem-solving habits. In client-centered therapy, changes occur when:

1. The person accepts himself and his feelings more fully.

2. He becomes more self-confident and self-directing.

3. He changes maladaptive behaviors.

4. He becomes more open to the evidence, both to what is going on outside of himself and to what is going on inside himself.

Extensive documentation indicates that physiological and psychological tensions are reduced and the change lasts as a result of this treatment.[17]

Hall also advocates the Rogerian therapeutic approach. This approach is the use of reflection, a nondirective method of helping the patient clarify, explore, and validate what he or she says. Rogers[17:43] states, "The therapist procedure which [clients] had found most helpful was that the therapist clarified and openly stated feelings which the client had been approaching hazily and hesitantly."

Hall derived her postulates regarding the nature of feeling-based behavior from Rogers, who repeatedly speaks to the interaction of known feelings and feelings-out-of-awareness. Rogers[17:36] hypothesizes that in a client-centered relationship, the patient "will reorganize himself at both the conscious and deeper levels of his personality in such a manner as to cope with life more constructively. . . . He shows . . . more of the characteristics of the healthy, well-functioning person. . . . He is less frustrated by stress, and recovers from stress more quickly."

Hall also adopted Rogers' theory on motivation for change. In this theory, Rogers asserts that, although the therapist does not motivate the patient, the patient does not supply the motivation either. Alternatively, motivation for change "springs from the self-actualizing tendency of life itself."[17:285] This tendency is released in the proper psychological climate.

In addition to using Rogers' theories, Hall also integrated educational and interpersonal theories into her theory. Hall developed her ideas regarding interpersonal behavior from Harry Stack Sullivan and also used teaching and learning ideas integrated from John Dewey. Hall did not use ideas of the contemporary nursing theorists. The influence of Dewey is evident in Hall's emphasis on the teaching-learning process with the nurse's primary responsibility as being the teacher. Sullivan's influence was evidenced in the role of the nurse as nurturer for the patient within the Core circle.[18]

USE OF EMPIRICAL EVIDENCE

Rogers' theories have received wide acclaim in the fields of psychiatry, psychology, and social work. His methods of therapy have been used in caring for patients and in the area of education, where a nondirective approach is less than common. In *On Becoming a Person*,[17] one of Rogers' students, Samuel Tenenbaum, discussed learning and teaching through a nondirective approach.

The application of client-centered therapy in play therapy for children is addressed by Elaine Dorfman in Rogers' book, *Client-Centered Therapy*.[16] In this specialized area, the therapist must work at the child's level of communication. Even with small children, reflection and clarification techniques are instrumental in helping children examine their feelings in leadership and administration situations.[16] Thomas Gordon has addressed Rogers' concepts as they relate to group dynamics and group-centered leadership.[17] Gordon believes a leader can strive to create a nonthreatening psychological climate by conveying warmth and acceptance; clarification statements can be used to link chains of thought.

The multiplicity of applications of Rogerian theory in everyday life is almost endless. Rogers[8:395] deserves his venerable title of the "founder of nondirective client-centered therapy." His writings would have constituted the most current literature on this topic in the 1960s, a time when Hall was building her theory of nursing.

Although Hall did not actually research her theory, Blue Cross Insurance[1] studies indicated that patients at Loeb recovered in half the time, at less than half the cost, and with fewer readmissions than patients who stayed in Montefiore Hospital. Twenty-two home-care programs in the New York area had a readmission rate five times higher than Loeb's rate.[1] On a follow-up questionnaire, 40 physicians indicated the hospital stay of patients at the Loeb Center ranged from 3 to 43 days shorter than at other hospitals, with the usual difference of one to three weeks. Patients and physicians were both pleased with the care.[1]

Not only did the studies conducted at Loeb show increased patient satisfaction and decreased length of stay, but they also indicated increased nurse satisfaction. A study conducted in 1968[18] recorded the perceptions of baccalaureate graduates hired at Loeb Center and compared them with the perceptions of nurses at similar educational levels working in a hospital setting. The researchers found that the philosophy at Loeb and the support of administration created a greater amount of satisfaction for nurses at Loeb compared with their hospital cohorts.[18]

Given recent interest in nursing-led inpatient units, especially in the United Kingdom (UK), Griffiths and Wilson-Barnett[3] conducted a literature search to determine the effectiveness of care in the Loeb Center and two UK centers. Griffiths and Wilson-Barnett[3] found improved patient independence, fewer readmissions, lower mortality, and cost saving in the nurse-managed centers. However, they also identified methodological limitations in identifying well-tested outcome measures.

MAJOR CONCEPTS & DEFINITIONS

BEHAVIOR

Hall broadly defines behavior as everything that is said or done. Behavior is dictated by feelings, both conscious and unconscious.[7]

REFLECTION

Reflection is a Rogerian method of communication in which selected verbalizations of patients are repeated back to them with different phraseology, to invite them to explore feelings further.[7]

MAJOR CONCEPTS & DEFINITIONS—cont'd

SELF-AWARENESS

Self-awareness refers to the state of being that nurses endeavor to help their patients achieve. The more self-awareness persons have of their feelings, the more control they have over their behavior.[7]

PHASES OF MEDICAL CARE

Hall divides medical care into two phases: biologically critical and evaluative follow-up. Biologically critical medicine lasts a few days to a week or more and is the period when physicians devise treatment plans that help the patient reach the second phase. During the first phase, the patient receives intensive medical care and multiple diagnostic tests.[7]

SECOND-STAGE ILLNESS

The patient enters the second phase of medical care once the doctors begin giving only follow-up care. Hall defines second-stage illness as the nonacute recovery phase of illness. This stage is conducive to learning and rehabilitation.[7] The need for medical care is minimal, although the need for nurturing and learning is great. Therefore this is the ideal time for wholly professional nursing care.

WHOLLY PROFESSIONAL NURSING

Wholly professional nursing implies nursing care given exclusively by professional registered nurses educated in the behavioral sciences who take the responsibility and opportunity to coordinate and deliver the total care of their patients.[7] This concept includes the roles of nurturing, teaching, and advocacy in the fostering of healing.

Nursing circles of Care, Core, and Cure are the central concepts of Hall's theory (Figure 10-1). Care alludes to the "hands-on," intimate bodily care of the patient and implies a comforting, nurturing relationship.[7:85] While intimate physical care is provided, the nurse and patient develop a close relationship representing the teaching-learning aspect of nursing. Core involves the therapeutic use of self in communicating with the patient. The nurse, through the use of reflective technique, helps the patient clarify motives and goals, facilitating the process of increasing the patient's self-awareness. Cure is the aspect of nursing involved with administration of medications and treatments. The nurse functions in this role as an investigator and potential cause of pain related to skills such as injections and dressing changes.[6]

MAJOR ASSUMPTIONS

The following assumptions are basic to Hall's theory of nursing. They are explicit and, for the most part, are adequately defined in her writings.

Nursing

Nursing can and should be professional.[5] Hall stipulated that patients should be cared for only by professional registered nurses who can take total responsibility for the care and teaching of their patients. The following interesting afternote appears in one of her articles on the Loeb Center:

> We hire from 3-year schools, community colleges, baccalaureate, and even master's degree pro-

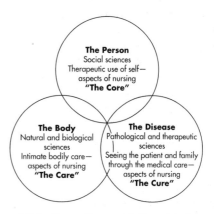

Figure **10-1** Core, Care, and Cure Model. (From Hall, L. [1964, Feb.]. Nursing: What is it? *The Canadian Nurse,* 60[2], 151.)

grammes. . . . Although all learn to master satisfactorily, those from the 2 and 3-year programmes reach a plateau. The baccalaureate graduates keep on learning and being and don't seem to stop growing in their ability to gain skills in the nurturing process.[7:95]

The professional nurse functions most therapeutically when patients have entered the second stage of their hospital stay.[7] The second stage is the recuperating, or nonacute, phase of illness. The first stage of illness is a time of biological crisis, with nursing being ancillary to medicine. After the crisis period, the patient is more able to benefit and learn from the teaching that nurses can offer.

Nursing is complex.[7] The patient is certainly complex. Not only is the patient a human being, bringing the influences of his or her culture and environment, but the patient may be suffering from an illness that medicine is still struggling to understand and treat. The nurse giving the care is also a unique human being, interacting with the patient in a complex process of teaching and learning.

Nursing expertise centers around the body.[7] This statement refers to Hall's theoretical model because she viewed the patient as composed of Body, Pathology, and Personality. The uniqueness of nursing lies not only in knowing bodily care, but also in knowing how to modify these processes in line with the pathological process and treatment and amend them in line with the personality of the patient.

Person

Patients achieve their maximal potential through a learning process; therefore the chief therapy they need is teaching.[7] Rehabilitation is a process of learning to live within limitations. Physical and mental skills must be learned, but a prerequisite is learning about oneself as a person, becoming aware of feelings and behaviors, and clarifying motivations. Hall believed that the professional nurse, educated in communication skills, could best facilitate the teaching-learning process.

People strive to reach their own goals, not goals that others set for them.[7] Hall declared that in the usual medical setting, the doctor defines the goals for the patient, but too often these goals do not coincide with the patient's goals. In this situation, effective teaching and learning cannot occur.

A patient is composed of three aspects: (1) Body, (2) Pathology, and (3) Person.[7] (These elements are discussed later.) This particular assumption is crucial to Hall's theory of nursing.

People behave on the basis of their feelings, not on the basis of their knowledge.[7] The evidence that learning has occurred is a resultant change in some behavior. Changes in behavior do not usually happen strictly from knowing information. Actions occur in conjunction with feelings and feelings are not influenced by rationality.

There are two types of feelings: (1) known feelings and (2) feelings-out-of-awareness.[7] When people act on the basis of known feelings, they are free and in control of their behavior. When they act on feelings-out-of-awareness, they have no choice as to their behavior and the feelings that cause them to act.

Health

According to Hall's definition of behavior,[7] becoming ill is a behavior. Illness is directed by feelings-out-of-awareness, which are the root of adjustment difficulties.

Healing may be hastened by helping people move in the direction of self-awareness.[7] Once people are brought to terms with their true feelings and motivations, they become free to release their own powers of healing.

Through the process of reflection, "the patient has a chance to move from the unlabeled threat of anxiety . . . through a mislabeled threat of 'phobia' or 'dis-ease' . . . to a properly labeled threat (fear) with which he can deal constructively."[7:91]

Environment

Hospital nursing services are organized to accomplish tasks efficiently.[7] Hall viewed these organizations as being an end unto themselves. She did not believe they had patient care and teaching as their goal, but she believed their goal was helping physicians and administrators get their work finished.

Hall was not pleased with the concept of team nursing. She said, "Any career that is defined around the work that has to be done, and how it is divided to get it done, is a trade."[7:83] She vehemently opposed the idea of anyone other than educated, professional nurses taking direct care of patients and she decried the fact that nursing has trained nonprofessionals to function as practical nurses so professional nurses can function as practical doctors.

There are two phases of medical care practiced in medical centers: (1) biological crisis and (2) evaluative medicine.[7] The biological crisis phase involves intensive medical and diagnostic treatment of the patient. The evaluative medicine phase follows and, generally, it is the time when the patient is observed to appraise whether he or she is meeting the doctor's goals.

THEORETICAL ASSERTIONS

Hall's theory consists of three major tenets. The first is that nursing functions differently in the three interlocking circles that constitute aspects of the patient.[7] These three circles are interrelated and are influenced by each other. The three circles are: (1) the patient's Body, (2) the Disease affecting the body, and (3) the Person of the patient, which is being affected by each of the other circles. Nursing operates in all three circles, but it shares them with other professions to different degrees. Pathological conditions are treated with medical care (Cure); therefore nursing shares this circle with physicians. The Person aspect (Core) is cared for by therapeutic use of the self. Therefore this arena is shared with psychiatry, psychology, social work, and religious ministry. The body of the patient is cared for exclusively by nursing (Care). The Care circle includes all intimate bodily care such as feeding, bathing, and toileting. The Care component is the exclusive domain of nursing.

Hall's second assertion[5] relates to the Core postulate of her theory. As the patient needs less medical care, he or she needs more professional nursing care and teaching. This inversely proportional relationship alters the ratio of nursing care in the three cir-

cles. Patients in the second stage of illness (nonacute phase) are primarily in need of rehabilitation through learning; therefore the Care and Core circles predominate the Cure circle. The Loeb Center was designed for the care of nonacute patients in need of teaching and rehabilitation; it is no surprise that Loeb is staffed and operated by nurses and physicians function as ancillaries.

The third assertion of the theory is that wholly professional nursing care will hasten recovery. Hall decried the concept of team nursing, which gives the care of less complicated cases to caregivers with less training. Nurses are complex people using a complex process of teaching and learning in caring for complex patients with complex diseases. Only professional nurses are inherently qualified to provide the teaching, counseling, and nurturing needed in the second stage of illness.[6,7] At the Loeb Center, secretaries and messenger-attendants were employed for indirect patient care. The professional nurse is the coordinator for all his or her patients' therapies and all disciplines act in a consulting capacity to nursing.[7]

LOGICAL FORM

Hall's theory is formulated using inductive logic, moving from specific observations to a generalized concept. For example:

- Nursing care shortens patient recovery time.
- Nursing care facilitates patient recovery.
- Professional nursing improves patient care.
- Therefore "wholly professional nursing will hasten recovery."[1:82]

ACCEPTANCE BY THE NURSING COMMUNITY
Practice

Hall's theory closely resembles the nursing model of primary care. Her emphasis on the professional nurse as the primary caregiver parallels primary care nursing to the extent that continuity and coordination of patient care are provided. In addition, Hall's concepts of nurses being accountable and responsible for their own practice are pertinent and applicable ideas. Concern for these concepts demonstrates support for her theory.

Education

Hall's theory delineates definite ideas regarding nursing care provided by a professional nursing staff. The acceptance of this philosophy is apparent in the shift toward professional staffing in some healthcare facilities and in the rationale for the BSN degree as the minimum entry-level requirement for professional practice. Hall[5] also emphasized the concept of nurses practicing nursing rather than practicing as practical doctors. Issues of narrowing the divide between nursing education and service and of using nursing diagnoses as a guide for patient care rather than medical diagnoses support Hall's concepts from her theory.

Research

Until the late 1980s, research testing Hall's theory had been conducted only at Loeb Center. Two different facilities in Europe used Hall's ideas to develop nursing care units. Pearson, Durand, and Punton[14] compared patients in an acute care hospital with patients receiving care at a nursing unit. All patients were over 65 years of age and had fractures of the femoral neck. The researchers compared length of acute stay, quality of nursing care, and satisfaction of life six months after discharge. Those patients who received care on the nursing unit spent less time in acute care, received more consistent quality of nursing care, and reported improvements in level of life satisfaction after six months.[14]

Pearson, Durand, and Punton[15] conducted a larger study similar to the 1988 study. They found the same results of increased satisfaction for patients who received care on a nursing unit. Hall's theory is also being implemented in Oxford, UK. No specific research studies were performed, but McMahon[9,10] wrote two articles detailing the use and success of the Oxford Nursing Development Unit. Implementation of Hall's theory in nursing units within the United States was not found outside the Loeb Cen-

ter. Given the changes in healthcare and current Medicare and Medicaid policies and procedures, it may be difficult to further test Hall's original assertion that wholly professional nursing care will hasten recovery.

FURTHER DEVELOPMENT

Much research and testing of Hall's theory is needed before it can be applicable and useful to areas of nursing other than long-term illnesses and rehabilitative nursing. In particular, the theory needs to be adapted to healthcare facilities that differ from the Loeb Center for Nursing before its true impact and contribution to nursing can be judged. This step would require flexibility and change in several of Hall's main concepts and relationships, particularly those relating to the age and illness orientation of the patient. It would be interesting to further develop the concept of increased nursing care as a means to hasten patient recovery in a variety of settings. This tenet has been highly successful at the Loeb Center in reducing both patient days and healthcare costs.

Home healthcare is one domain of nursing in which testing could be performed to verify whether or not using Hall's ideas could decrease readmissions to the hospital. With the installation of diagnostic-related groups, patients leave the hospital as soon as the acute phase of illness is resolved. Home health nurses could use Hall's ideas of teaching-learning by using reflection to increase self-awareness. The patient was ill while hospitalized; therefore the patient would not have learned all the information necessary for proper care at home. Home health nurses can intervene to ensure that the patient learns all the needed information for proper care.

CRITIQUE
Simplicity

Hall's theory is simple and easily understood. The major concepts and relationships are limited and clear. The three aspects of professional nursing are identified both individually and as they relate to each other in the total process of patient care. Hall designed basic models to represent the major concepts and relationships of her theory, using individual and interlocking circles to define the three aspects of the patient and their relationships to the three aspects of nursing. The language used to define and describe the theory is easily understood and is indigenous to nursing.

Generality

Perhaps the most serious flaw in Hall's theory of nursing is its limited generality. Hall's primary target[1] is the adult patient who has passed the acute phase of his or her illness and has a relatively good chance at rehabilitation. This concept limits application of the theory to a population of patients of specific age and stage of illness. Although the ideas of Core, Care, and Cure can be applied to patients in the acute phase of their illness, the theory would be most difficult to apply to infants, small children, and comatose patients. In addition, Hall[1] devotes her theory to adult individuals who are ill. The function of the nurse in preventive healthcare and health maintenance is not addressed, nor is the nurse's role in community health, but the model could be adapted.

Hall viewed the role of the nurse as heavily involved in the Care and Core aspects of patient care. Unfortunately, this concept provides for little interaction between the nurse and the family because her theory delineates the family aspect of patient care only in the Cure circle.[6,7]

The use of therapeutic communication to help patients look at and explore their feelings regarding their illnesses and the potential changes the illnesses might cause is discussed in the Core aspect of nursing care. Therapeutic communication is also thought to motivate patients by making them aware of their true feelings. However, reflection was the only communication technique that Hall[7] described in her theory as a means to assist the patient toward self-awareness. This is a very limited approach to therapeutic communication because not all nurses can effectively use the technique of reflection and it is not always the most effective and successful communication tool in dealing with patients.[4]

Empirical Precision

Hall's concept of professional nursing hastening patient recovery with increased care as the patient improves has been subjected to a great amount of testing at the Loeb Center for Nursing.[1] The fact that the theory is identified with empirical reality cannot be disputed. Evidence obtained through research at the Loeb Center demonstrates that Hall's theory[7] does obtain its goal of shortening patient recovery time through concentrated, professional nursing efforts. Currently, the available literature supports the results obtained at the Loeb Center in testing the theory. Although research support has been demonstrated by the success of the Center, a wider range of testing in various settings is necessary to allow for increased empirical precision of the theory.

Hall's theory has been tested at two other facilities and has been found successful. These two facilities only care for adults, mainly those over 65 years of age. Therefore empirical precision of Hall's theory continues to be limited; further testing in facilities not caring for adults will still be needed.

Derivable Consequences

The theory provides a general framework for nursing and the concepts are within the domain of nursing, although the aspects of Cure and Core are shared with other health professionals and family members. Although the theory does not provide for the resolution of specific issues and problems, it does address itself to the pertinent and contemporary issues of accountability, responsibility, and professionalism. Application of the theory in practice has produced valued outcomes in all three areas. In addition, the theory demonstrates a great impact on the educational preparation of nursing students. Hall[5:806] stated, "With early field experience in a center where nursing rather than medicine is emphasized, the student may emerge a nurse first." Hall believed that in nursing centers, the student would benefit from experiencing nursing as it is taught to them in the classroom.

Despite the shortcomings of Hall's theory of nursing, her contribution to nursing practice is significant. Her insight into the problems of nursing in the 1960s has provided a base for professional practice in the multidimensional modern domain of nursing.

CRITICAL THINKING *Activities*

1. Given the changes in healthcare, which settings lend themselves to the application of Hall's theory of nursing practice?[11] Are Hall's theoretical assertions applicable to subacute care?

2. Advanced practice nurses (nurse-practitioners, clinical nurse specialists, nurse-midwives, and nurse-anesthetists) include advocacy as an integral part of the nurse-patient relationship. Some nurse theorists refer to advocacy as an extension of the Care concept.[12] How can advanced practice nurses include advocacy while applying Hall's Core, Care, Cure Model in their clinical practice?

3. In the 1960s, Hall described the Cure concept in her model as helping the patient and family through the medical, surgical, and rehabilitation phases of a pathological process. The Cure concept was the physician's domain and it was shared with other members of the health team. Given nursing's knowledge of stress-related illness, could advanced practice nurses cure patients of stress-related symptoms such as anxiety, nausea, and pain? Under which situations can a nurse cure a stress-related illness?

REFERENCES

1. Alfano, G. (1964, June). Can nursing care hasten recovery? *American Journal of Nursing,* 64, 80-83.
2. Englert, B. (1971, June). How a staff nurse perceives her role in the Loeb Center. *Nursing Clinics of North America,* 6(2), 281-292.
3. Griffiths, P. & Wilson-Barnett, J. (1998, June). The effectiveness of "nursing beds": A review of the literature. *Journal of Advanced Nursing,* 27(6), 1184-1192.
4. Hale, K. & George, J. (1980). Lydia E. Hall. In Nursing Theories Conference Group, J.B. George (Chairperson), *Nursing theories: The base for professional practice.* Englewood Cliffs, NJ: Prentice Hall.
5. Hall, L.E. (1963, Nov.). Center for nursing. *Nursing Outlook,* 11, 805-806.
6. Hall, L.E. (1964, Feb.). Nursing: What is it? *Canadian Nurse,* 60, 150-154.
7. Hall, L.E. (1969). The Loeb Center for Nursing and Rehabilitation. *International Journal of Nursing Studies,* 6, 81-95.
8. Krech, D. (1976). *Psychology: A basic course.* New York: Alfred A. Knopf.
9. McMahon, R. (1989). Partners in care. *Nursing Times,* 85(8), 34-37.
10. McMahon, R. (1989). Primary nursing: One to one. *Nursing Times,* 85(2), 39-40.
11. Muxlow, J. (1995, Oct.). The relationship between nurse and patient. *Professional Nurse,* 11(1), 63-65.
12. Nelson, M.L. (1995). Client advocacy. In M. Snyder & M.P. Mirr (Eds.), *Advanced practice nursing: A guide to professional development.* New York: Springer.
13. Oodal, D. (2000, June 19). Telephone interview with the Secretary of the Loeb Center.
14. Pearson, A., Durand, I., & Punton, S. (1988, Nov. 23). The feasibility and effectiveness of nursing beds. *Nursing Times,* 84(47), 48-50.
15. Pearson, A., Durand, I., & Punton, S. (1989). Determining quality in a unit where nursing is the primary intervention. *Journal of Advanced Nursing,* 14, 269-273.
16. Rogers, C. (1951). *Client-centered therapy.* Boston: Houghton Mifflin.
17. Rogers, C. (1961). *On becoming a person.* Boston: Houghton Mifflin.
18. Wiggins, L.R. (1980). Lydia Hall's place in the development of theory in nursing. *Image,* 12 (1), 10-12.

BIBLIOGRAPHY
Primary Sources
Book Chapters

Hall, L. (1965). Nursing: What is it? In H. Baumgarten, Jr. (Ed.), *Concepts of nursing home administration.* New York: Macmillan.
Hall, L. (1966). Another view of nursing care and quality. In M.K. Straub (Ed.), *Continuity of patient care: The role of nursing.* Washington, DC: Catholic University of America Press.

Journal Articles

Hall, L. (1955, June). Quality of nursing care. *Public Health News,* 36 (6), 212-215.

Hall, L. (1963, Nov.). Center for nursing. *Nursing Outlook,* 11, 805-806.

Hall, L. (1964, Feb.). Nursing: What is it? *Canadian Nurse,* 60, 150-154.

Hall L. (1969). The Loeb Center for nursing and rehabilitation. *International Journal of Nursing Studies,* 6, 81-95.

Pamphlets

Hall, L. (1951). *What the classroom teacher should know and do about children with heart disease.* American Heart Association.

Hall, L., Hauck, M., & Rosenson, L. (1949, March). *The cardiac child in school and community.* New York: New York Heart Association Publication.

Reports

Hall, L. (1960). *Report of a work conference on nursing in long-term chronic disease and aging* (National League for Nursing as a League Exchange #50). New York: National League for Nursing.

Hall, L. (1963, June). *Report of Loeb Center for nursing and rehabilitation project report* (Congressional record hearings before the Special Subcommittee on Intermediate Care of the Committee on Veterans' Affairs). Washington, DC.

Secondary Sources
Book Chapters

Alfano, G.J. (1987). The Loeb Center for Nursing and Rehabilitation: A model for extended care. In B.C. Vladeck & G.J. Alfano (Eds.), *Medicare and extended care: Issues, problems and prospects.* Owings Mills, MD: Rynd Communications.

Chinn, P.L. & Jacobs, M.K. (1987). Theory in nursing: A current overview. In P.L. Chinn & M. K. Jacobs (Eds.), *Theory and nursing: A current overview* (2nd ed.). St. Louis: Mosby.

George, J.B. (1995). Lydia E. Hall. In J.B. George (Ed.), *Nursing theories: The base for professional nursing practice.* Norwalk, CT: Appleton & Lange.

Griffith, J. (1982). Other frameworks and models. In J. Griffith & P. Christenson (Eds.), *Nursing process: Application of theories, frameworks, and models.* St. Louis: Mosby.

Hale, K. & George, J. (1980). Lydia E. Hall. In Nursing Theories Group Conference, J.B. George, Chairperson, *Nursing theories: The base for professional practice.* Englewood Cliffs, NJ: Prentice Hall.

Journal Articles

Alfano, G. (1964, June). Administration means working with nurses. *American Journal of Nursing,* 64, 83-85.

Alfano, G. (1971, June). Healing or caretaking—which will it be? *Nursing Clinics of North America,* 6, 273-280.

Alfano, G.J. (1988, Jan./Feb.). A different kind of nursing. *Nursing Outlook,* 36, 34-37.

Anderson, N. (1971, June). Rehabilitative nursing practice. *Nursing Clinics of North America,* 6, 303-309.

Beasley, T., Gerbis, P., & Lyon, J. (1995, Feb.). Workplace advocacy: New roles for nurses. *Nevada-RNformation,* 4(1), 1-2.

Bernardin, E. (1964, June). Loeb Center: As the staff nurse sees it. *American Journal of Nursing,* 64, 85-86.

Berube, P.A. (1998). Revolution. *The Journal of Nurse Empowerment,* 8(2), 40-42.

Bowar, S. (1971, June). Enabling professional practice through leadership skills. *Nursing Clinics of North America,* 6, 293-301.

Bowar-Ferres, S. (1975, May). Loeb Center and its philosophy of nursing. *American Journal of Nursing,* 65, 810.

Bryan, C. (1995, Jan.). Practice nursing: A study of the role. *Nursing Standard,* 9, 25-29.

Cawley, N. (1997, Jan./Feb.). Towards defining spirituality. An exploration of the concept of spirituality. *International Journal of Palliative Nursing,* 3(1), 31-36.

Glasgow, G.M. (1990). Quality of care in occupational health through nursing diagnosis. *AAOHN Journal,* 38 (3), 105-109.

Griffiths, P. (1997, May). Practice. In search of the pioneers of nurse-led care...the Loeb Center. *Nursing Times,* 93(21), 46-48.

Griffiths, P. (1997, June/July). In search of therapeutic nursing: Subacute care. *Nursing Times,* 93(26), 54-55.

Henderson, C. (1964, June). Can nursing care hasten recovery? *American Journal of Nursing,* 64, 80-83.

Isler, C. (1964, June). New concepts in nursing therapy: More care as the patient improves. *RN,* 27, 58-70.

Kitson, A.L. (1987). Raising standards of clinical practice: The fundamental issue of effective nursing practice. *Journal of Advanced Nursing,* 12, 321-329.

McMahon, R. (1989, Jan. 11). Primary nursing: One to one. *Nursing Times,* 85(2), 39-40.

McMahon, R. (1989, Feb. 22). Partners in care. *Nursing Times,* 85(8), 34-37.

Pearson, A., Durand, I., & Punton, S. (1988, Nov. 23). The feasibility and effectiveness of nursing beds. *Nursing Times,* 84(47), 48-50.

Pearson, A., Durand, I., & Punton, S. (1989). Determining quality in a unit where nursing is the primary intervention. *Journal of Advanced Nursing,* 14, 269-273.

Pontin, D. (1999, March). Primary nursing: A mode of care or a philosophy of nursing? *Journal of Advanced Nursing,* 29(3), 584-591.

Tabak, N. & Ben-Or, T. (1994). The nurse's challenge in coping with ethical dilemmas in occupational health. *Nursing Ethics,* 1(4), 208-215.

Wiggins, L.R. (1980). Lydia Hall's place in the development of theory in nursing. *Image: Journal of Nursing Scholarship,* 12(1), 10-12.

Wilkinson, R.A. (1994, July). A more autonomous and independent role: Primary nursing versus patient allocation. *Professional Nurse,* 9, (10), 680-684.

Correspondence

Alfano, G.J. (1984, Jan. 26). Personal correspondence.

Alfano, G.J. (1984, Feb. 15). Personal correspondence.

Oodal, D. (1996, July 12). Telephone interview with the Secretary of the Loeb Center.

Oodal, D. (2000, June 19). Telephone interview with the Secretary of the Loeb Center.

Wender, B. (1984, Jan. 25). Telephone interview with the Secretary of the Loeb Center.

Other Sources

Chinn, P.L. & Jacobs, M.K. (1983). *Theory and nursing: A current overview* (2nd ed.). St. Louis: Mosby.

Rogers, C. (1951). *Client-centered therapy.* Boston: Houghton Mifflin.

Rogers, C. (1961). *On becoming a person.* Boston: Houghton Mifflin.

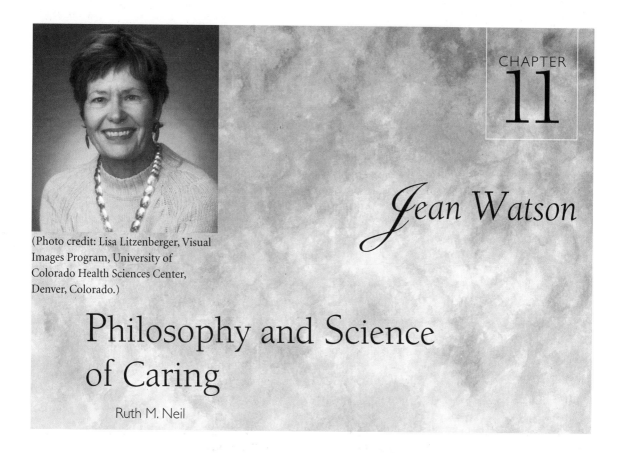

(Photo credit: Lisa Litzenberger, Visual Images Program, University of Colorado Health Sciences Center, Denver, Colorado.)

Jean Watson

Philosophy and Science of Caring

Ruth M. Neil

CREDENTIALS AND BACKGROUND OF THE THEORIST

Margaret Jean Harman Watson was born in southern West Virginia and grew up during the 1940s and 1950s in the small town of Welch, West Virginia in the Appalachian Mountains. As the youngest of eight children, she was surrounded by an extended family-community environment.

Watson attended high school in West Virginia and then attended the Lewis Gale School of Nursing in Roanoke, Virginia. After graduation in 1961, she married her husband, Douglas, and

Previous authors: Tracey J.F. Patton, Deborah A. Barnhart, Patricia M. Bennett, Beverly D. Porter, and Rebecca S. Sloan. The author wishes to thank Dr. Jean Watson for her ongoing inspiration and support. An additional thanks for her review of the content of this chapter and her assistance in updating the references and bibliography.

moved west to his native state of Colorado. Douglas, whom Watson describes not only as her physical and spiritual partner, but also as her best friend, died in 1998. She has two grown daughters, Jennifer (born in 1963) and Julie (born in 1967), and five grandchildren. She continues to live in Boulder, Colorado.

After moving to Colorado, Watson continued her nursing education and graduate studies at the University of Colorado. She earned a B.S. in nursing in 1964 at the Boulder campus; an M.S. in psychiatric-mental health nursing in 1966 at the Health Sciences campus; and a Ph.D. in educational psychology and counseling in 1973 at the Graduate School, Boulder campus. After Watson completed her Ph.D. degree, she joined the School of Nursing faculty of the University of Colorado Health Sciences Center in Denver, where she has served in both faculty and administrative positions. She has been chair and assistant dean of the undergraduate program and she was involved in early planning and implementation of the nursing Ph.D. program in Colorado, which was initiated in 1978. She was coordinator and director of the Ph.D. program between 1978 and 1981. In 1981 and 1982, she pursued sabbatical studies and, upon her return, was dean of the University of Colorado School of Nursing and Associate Director, Nursing Practice at University Hospital from 1983 to 1990. Currently, she is a professor of nursing and holds the Endowed Chair in Caring Science at the University of Colorado School of Nursing. She continues to offer her basic theory courses, which can be taken for credit or for continuing education twice a year. Information about these courses can be obtained by contacting Dr. Watson at the address listed in the front of this book. During her deanship, she was instrumental in the development of a postbaccalaureate nursing curriculum in human caring, health, and healing, which leads to a career professional clinical doctoral degree (ND). This pilot ND program was selected as a national demonstration program by the Helene Fuld Health Trust in New York and was funded by the Trust and Colorado clinical agencies. The program was implemented in 1990 as a partnership between nursing education and practice, whereby clinical and academic agencies in Colorado and beyond work jointly to simultaneously restructure nursing education and nursing practice for the future.

The Center for Human Caring at the University of Colorado was the nation's first interdisciplinary center with an overall commitment to develop and use knowledge of human caring and healing as the moral and scientific basis of clinical practice and nursing scholarship and as the foundation for efforts to transform the current healthcare system.[28] During its existence, the center developed and sponsored numerous clinical, educational, and community scholarship activities and projects in human caring, including participation of national and international scholars in residence. During her career, Watson has been active in community programs, having served as a founder and member of the Board of Boulder County Hospice and she has initiated numerous collaborations with area healthcare facilities. As the recipient of several research and advanced education federal grants and awards, Watson has also received numerous university and private grants and extramural funding for her faculty and administrative projects and scholarships in human caring.

Other honors include honorary doctoral degrees from Assumption College in Worcester, Massachusetts, the University of Akron, the University of West Virginia, Göteborg University in Sweden, and Luton University in London. Watson also received the high honor of Distinguished Professor of Nursing at the University of Colorado in 1992. In 1993, she was the recipient of the National League for Nursing (NLN) Martha E. Rogers Award, which recognizes a nurse scholar who has made significant contributions to nursing knowledge that advances the science of caring in nursing and health sciences. Between 1993 and 1996, Watson served as a member of the Executive Committee, the Governing Board, and as an officer for the NLN. She was president from 1995 to 1996. In 1997, she was given an Honorary Lifetime Certification as a holistic nurse. In 1998, she was recognized as a Distinguished Nurse Scholar by New York University and in 1999, she was honored with the Norman Cousins Award by the Fetzer Institute in recognition of her commitment to developing, maintaining, and exemplifying relationship-centered care practices.[36]

Watson's national and international work includes distinguished lectureships throughout the United States at well-known universities including Boston College, Catholic University, Adelphi University, Columbia University-Teachers College, State University of New York, and at universities and scholarly meetings in numerous foreign countries including Canada, England, Finland, Sweden, Germany, Australia, Nova Scotia, Micronesia, Portugal, Scotland, Korea, and Israel.

Her international activities also include an International Kellogg Fellowship in Australia (1982), a Fulbright Research and Lecture Award to Sweden and other parts of Scandinavia (1991), and a lecture tour in the United Kingdom (1993). She has also been involved in international projects and invitations in New Zealand, India, Thailand, Taiwan, Israel, and Japan.

Watson is featured in several national videos on nursing theory. These include "Circles of Knowledge" and "Conversations on Caring with Jean Watson and Janet Quinn" from the NLN; "Portraits of Excellence: Nursing Theorists and Their Work" from the Helene Fuld Health Trust; and "Theory in Practice" from the NLN, which features the Denver Nursing Project in Human Caring, a nurse-directed caring center for persons with acquired immunodeficiency syndrome (AIDS).[36] The Denver Nursing Project in Human Caring was a clinical (caring-theory based) demonstration project of the University of Colorado Center for Human Caring and School of Nursing and served patients from 1988 to 1996. More recent media productions include the NLN-produced video, "Applying the Art and Science of Human Caring, Parts I and II"; "A Meta-Reflection on Nursing's Present," an audiotape produced by the American Holistic Nurses Association; and "Private Psalm: A Mantra and Meditation for Healing," a compact disc set.[36]

Watson's publications reflect the evolution of her theory of caring. Her writings have been geared toward educating nursing students and providing them with the ontological and epistemological basis for their praxis and research directions. Much of her current work began with the 1979 publication, *Nursing: The Philosophy and Science of Caring,*[23] which she says began as class notes for a course she was developing. She says the book "emerged from her quest to bring new meaning and dignity to the world of nursing and patient care—care that seemed too limited in its scope at the time, largely defined by medicine's paradigm and traditional biomedical science models."[35:49]

Nursing: Human Science and Human Care—A Theory of Nursing,[26] published in 1985 and rereleased in 1988,[31] was her second major work. The purpose of this book was to address some of the conceptual and philosophical problems that still existed in nursing. She hoped that others would join her as she sought to "elucidate the human care process in nursing, preserve the concept of the person in our science, and better our contribution to society."[31:ix] This book has been translated into Chinese, German, Japanese, Korean, and Swedish.[36]

Postmodern Nursing and Beyond,[33] published in 1999, is Watson's most recent work. This work projects nursing and healthcare into the midtwenty-first century. It seeks to illuminate ". . .a model of caring and healing practices that take medicine, nursing, and the public beyond traditional Western medicine, beyond the 'cure at all costs' approach"[33:xii] and embeds caring and healing practices in a new paradigm that acknowledges the symbiotic relationship between humankind-technology-nature and the larger, expanding universe. "It offers a search for the spiritual aspects of our being and our approaches to health and healing."[33:xiv]

In the dedication section of *Postmodern Nursing and Beyond,*[33] Watson described recent traumatic personal experiences that contributed to her insights as expressed in the book. One of these was an accidental injury in 1997 that resulted in the loss of her left eye after many months of trying to save it. The other was her husband's death in 1998. Watson states that she is now "attempting to integrate these wounds into her life and work. One of the gifts through the suffering was the privilege of experiencing and receiving my own theory from the care from my husband and loving nurse friends and colleagues."[38]

In Watson's original philosophy and science of caring,[9] she referred to caring as the essence of nursing practice. Caring is a moral ideal rather than a task-oriented behavior and includes such characteristics as the actual caring occasion and the transpersonal caring moment, phenomena that occur when an authentic caring relationship exists between the nurse and the patient. One of her earliest written treatises on the caring model was presented at an American Nurses Association Division of Practice Meeting in 1979.[37] As her work evolved, Watson posited that caring is intrinsically related to healing. "Such an ethic and ethos of caring, healing, and health comprises nursing's professional context and mission—its *raison d'être* to society."[35:50]

THEORETICAL SOURCES

In addition to traditional nursing knowledge and the works of Nightingale, Henderson, Krueter, and

Hall, Watson acknowledges the work of Leininger, Gadow, and Peplau[26,35] as background for her work. In her more recent work, Watson refers to the works of others such as Maslow, Heidegger, Erickson, Selye, Lazarus, Whitehead, de Chardin, and Sarte. In addition, she acknowledges philosophical and intellectual guidance from feminist theory, quantum physics, wisdom traditions, and perennial philosophy.[33,34,35] To develop her framework, Watson drew heavily on the sciences and the humanities, providing a phenomenological, existential, and spiritual orientation.

Watson explains that the concepts she defined to bring new meaning to nursing's paradigm were "derived from clinically inducted, empirical experiences, combined with my philosophical, intellectual and experiential background; thus my early work emerged from my own values, beliefs, and perceptions about personhood, life, health, and healing . . ."[35:49]

Watson attributes her emphasis on the interpersonal and transpersonal qualities of congruence, empathy, and warmth to the views of Carl Rogers and more recent transpersonal psychology writers. Rogers described several incidents that led to the formulation of his thoughts on human behavior. One involved learning that "it is the client who knows what hurts and that the facilitator should allow the direction of the therapeutic process to come from the client."[17:11-12] Rogers[17:18-19] believed that "through understanding" the patient would come to accept himself, an initial step toward a positive outcome. The therapist, motivated by a warm interest in the patient, helps by clarifying and stating feelings about which the patient has been unclear. Together, the therapist and the patient understand the meaning of the patient's experience. Another crucial concept of Rogerian theory is that the therapist-patient relationship is more important to the outcome than adherence to traditional methods. Rogers[17:33] states, "In my early professional years I was asking the question, 'How can I treat, or cure, or change this person?' Now I phrase the question in this way: 'How can I provide a relationship which this person may use for his own personal growth?'" For additional information about Rogers, see Betz and Whitehorn[1] and Seeman.[19] Watson points out that Rogers' phenomenological approach, with his view that nurses are not here to manipulate and control others, but rather to understand, were profoundly influential at a time when "clinicalization" (therapeutic control and manipulation of the patient) was considered the norm.[38]

Watson believes a strong liberal arts background is also essential to the process of holistic care for patients. She believes the study of the humanities expands the mind and increases thinking skills and personal growth. Watson[24,35] compares the current status of nursing to the mythological Danaides, who attempted to fill a broken jar with water, only to see water flow through the cracks. Until nursing merges theory and practice through the combined study of the sciences and the humanities, she believes similar cracks will be evident in the scientific basis of nursing knowledge.

Yalom's 11 curative factors stimulated Watson's thinking[23] about the psychodynamic and human components that could apply to nursing and caring and, consequently, to her 10 carative factors in nursing.

Watson's work has been called a treatise, a conceptual model, a framework, and a theory. This chapter uses the terms *theory* and *framework* interchangeably. In addition, Watson states that, both retrospectively and prospectively, her work "can be read as philosophy, ethic, or even paradigm or worldview."[35:50]

USE OF EMPIRICAL EVIDENCE

Watson and her colleagues have attempted to study the concept of caring by collecting data to use in classifying caring behaviors, to describe the similarities and differences between what nurses consider care and what patients consider care, and to generate testable hypotheses around the concept of nursing care. They studied responses from registered nurses, nursing students, and patients to the same open-ended questionnaire covering a variety of aspects of (1) taking care of and (2) caring about patients. Their findings revealed a discrepancy in the values considered most important by patients, nursing students, and registered nurses. They stressed the need for further study to clarify what behaviors and values are important from each viewpoint. The study also raised a question about differences in values for persons in various situations and the question of meeting minimum care needs before the quality of care can be evaluated.[24]

Watson's research into caring incorporates empiricism, but emphasizes methodologies that begin with nursing phenomena rather than the natural sciences.[9] She has used human science, empirical phenomenology, and transcendent phenomenology in her latest work. More recently, she has been investigating new language, such as metaphor and poetry, to communicate, convey, and elucidate human caring and healing.[29] In her inquiry and writing, she increasingly incorporates her conviction that there is a sacred relationship between humankind and the universe.[35]

Major Concepts & Definitions

Watson[23] bases her theory for nursing practice on the following 10 carative factors. Each has a dynamic phenomenological component that is relative to the individuals involved in the relationship as encompassed by nursing. The first three interdependent factors serve as the "philosophical foundation for the science of caring."[23:9-10]

I. FORMATION OF A HUMANISTIC-ALTRUISTIC SYSTEM OF VALUES

Humanistic and altruistic values are learned early in life, but can be greatly influenced by nurse-educators. This factor can be defined as satisfaction through giving and extension of the sense of self.[23]

2. INSTILLATION OF FAITH-HOPE

This factor, incorporating humanistic and altruistic values, facilitates the promotion of holistic nursing care and positive health within the patient population. It also describes the nurse's role in developing effective nurse-patient interrelationships and in promoting wellness by helping the patient adopt health-seeking behaviors.[23]

3. CULTIVATION OF SENSITIVITY TO SELF AND TO OTHERS

The recognition of feelings leads to self-actualization through self-acceptance for both the nurse and the patient. As nurses acknowledge their sensitivity and feelings, they become more genuine, authentic, and sensitive to others.[23]

4. DEVELOPMENT OF A HELPING-TRUST RELATIONSHIP

The development of a helping-trust relationship between the nurse and patient is crucial for transpersonal caring. A trusting relationship promotes and accepts the expression of both positive and negative feelings. It involves congruence, empathy, nonpossessive warmth, and effective communication.[23] Congruence involves being real, honest, genuine, and authentic.[23] Empathy is the ability to experience and, thereby, understand the other person's perceptions and feelings and to communicate those understandings.[23] Nonpossessive warmth is demonstrated by a moderate speaking volume; a relaxed, open posture; and facial expressions that are congruent with other communications.[23] Effective communication has cognitive, affective, and behavior response components.[23]

5. PROMOTION AND ACCEPTANCE OF THE EXPRESSION OF POSITIVE AND NEGATIVE FEELINGS

The sharing of feelings is a risk-taking experience for both nurse and patient. The nurse must be prepared for either positive or negative feelings. The nurse must recognize that intellectual and emotional understandings of a situation differ.[23]

Continued

MAJOR CONCEPTS & DEFINITIONS—cont'd

6. SYSTEMATIC USE OF THE SCIENTIFIC PROBLEM-SOLVING METHOD FOR DECISION MAKING

Use of the nursing process brings a scientific problem-solving approach to nursing care, dispelling the traditional image of nurses as the doctor's handmaiden. The nursing process is similar to the research process in that it is systematic and organized.[23]

7. PROMOTION OF INTERPERSONAL TEACHING-LEARNING

This factor is an important concept for nursing in that it separates caring from curing. It allows the patient to be informed and shifts the responsibility for wellness and health to the patient. The nurse facilitates this process with teaching-learning techniques that are designed to enable patients to provide self-care, determine personal needs, and provide opportunities for their personal growth.[23]

8. PROVISION FOR SUPPORTIVE, PROTECTIVE, AND CORRECTIVE MENTAL, PHYSICAL, SOCIOCULTURAL, AND SPIRITUAL ENVIRONMENT

Nurses must recognize the influence that internal and external environments have on the health and illness of individuals. Concepts relevant to the internal environment include the mental and spiritual well being and sociocultural beliefs of an individual. In addition to epidemiological variables, other external variables include comfort, privacy, safety, and clean, aesthetic surroundings.[23]

9. ASSISTANCE WITH GRATIFICATION OF HUMAN NEEDS

The nurse recognizes the biophysical, psychophysical, psychosocial, and intrapersonal needs of self and patient. Patients must satisfy lower-order needs before attempting to attain higher-order needs. Food, elimination, and ventilation are examples of lower-order biophysical needs, whereas activity, inactivity, and sexuality are considered lower-order psychophysical needs. Achievement and affiliation are higher-order psychosocial needs. Self-actualization is a higher-order intrapersonal-interpersonal need.[23]

10. ALLOWANCE FOR EXISTENTIAL-PHENOMENOLOGICAL FORCES

Phenomenology describes data of the immediate situation that help people understand the phenomena in question.[23] Existential psychology is a science of human existence that uses phenomenological analysis.[23] Watson considers this factor to be difficult to understand. It is included to provide a thought-provoking experience leading to a better understanding of the self and others.[23]

Watson believes that nurses have the responsibility to go beyond the 10 carative factors and to facilitate patients' development in the area of health promotion through preventive health actions. This goal is accomplished by teaching patients personal changes to promote health, providing situational support, teaching problem-solving methods, and recognizing coping skills and adaptation to loss.[23]

MAJOR ASSUMPTIONS

In her first book, *Nursing: The Philosophy and Science of Caring*, Watson[23:8-9] states the major assumptions of the science of caring in nursing:

1. Caring can be only effectively demonstrated and practiced only interpersonally.

2. Caring consists of carative factors that result in the satisfaction of certain human needs.

3. Effective caring promotes health and individual or family growth.

4. Caring responses accept a person not only as he/she is now but as what he/she may become.

5. A caring environment offers the development of potential while allowing the person to

choose the best action for himself/herself at a given time.

6. Caring is more "healthogenic" than is curing. The practice of caring integrates biophysical knowledge with knowledge of human behavior to generate or promote health and to provide ministrations to those who are ill. A science of caring is therefore complementary to the science of curing.

7. The practice of caring is central to nursing.

Gaut identified three conditions necessary for caring. These include: "(1) an awareness and knowledge about one's need for care; (2) an intention to act, and actions based on knowledge; (3) a positive change as a result of caring, judged solely on the basis of welfare of others."[6:313-324] Watson[32:33] expanded Gaut's work by adding two additional conditions: "an underlying value and moral commitment to care; and a will to care."

In her second book, *Nursing: Human Science and Human Care,* Watson[26:33] states, ". . . both nursing education and the health care delivery system must be based on human values and concern for the welfare of others." To further define the social and ethical responsibilities of nursing and to explicate the human care concepts in nursing, Watson[31] proposes the following 11 assumptions related to human care values:

1. Care and love comprise the primal and universal psychic energy.
2. Care and love, often overlooked, are the cornerstones of humanness; nourishment of these needs fulfills humanity.
3. The ability to sustain the caring ideal and ideology in practice will affect the development of civilization and determine nursing's contribution to society.
4. Caring for the self is a prerequisite to caring for others.
5. Historically, nursing has held a human care and caring stance in regard to people with health-illness concerns.
6. Caring is the central unifying focus of nursing practice—the essence of nursing.
7. Caring, at the human level, has been increasingly deemphasized in the healthcare system.
8. Technological advancements and institutional constraints have sublimated nursing's caring foundation.
9. A significant issue for nursing today and in the future is the preservation and advancement of human care.
10. Only through interpersonal relationships can human care be effectively demonstrated and practiced.
11. Nursing's social, moral, and scientific contributions to humankind and society lie in its commitments to human care ideals in theory, practice, and research.

In *Postmodern Nursing and Beyond,*[33] Watson seeks to describe a more fundamental ontological shift in human consciousness that evokes a return to the sacred core of humankind and its relation with the universe, connecting with a sense of the divine and inviting awe and mystery back into life and work. Such thinking holds a sense of reverence and openness for the infinite possibilities contained within an individual's inner and outer space. It offers a search for the spiritual aspects of being and approaches to health and healing. This ontological shift invites practitioners to embark upon the following paths:

- Path of awareness, of awakening to the sacred feminine archetype/cosmology to rebalance the disorder of conventional modern medicine and the modern, cultural mindset.
- Path of cultivation of higher/deeper self and a higher consciousness: transpersonal self.
- Path of honoring the sacred within and without; open to deeper explorations of the mystery of the human body and life-healing processes: postmodern-transpersonal body.
- Path of acknowledging the metaphysical/spiritual level, attending to the non-physical, spiritual dimensions of existence.
- Path of acknowledging quantum concepts and phenomena such as caring-healing energy, intentionality and consciousness, as paths toward expanding

human existence and the evolving human consciousness.

- Path of honoring the connectedness of all; unitary consciousness; the eternal 'caring moment'; 'transpersonal caring-healing.'
- Path of honoring the unity of mind-bodyspirit; both immanence and transcendence of the human being and becoming.
- Path of reintegrating the caring-healing arts, as an artistry of being into healing practices: ontological competencies.
- Path of creating healing space: healing architecture.
- Path of a relational ontology, open to new epistemologies of existence.
- Path of moving beyond the modern-postmodern into the open, transpersonal space and the new thinking required for the next millennium.[33:xv]

THEORETICAL ASSERTIONS

According to Watson, nursing is interested in understanding health, illness, and the human experience. Within the philosophy and science of caring, she tries to define an outcome of scientific activity with regard to the humanistic aspects of life. She attempts to make nursing an interrelationship of quality of life, including death and the prolongation of life.[23]

Watson believes nursing is concerned with health promotion, restoration, and illness prevention. Health, more than the absence of illness, is an elusive concept because it has a subjective nature.[23] Health refers to "unity and harmony within the mind, body, and soul" and is associated with the "degree of congruence between the self as perceived and the self as experienced."[31:48]

According to Watson, caring is a nursing term representing the factors nurses use to deliver healthcare to patients.[26] She states that by responding to others as unique individuals, the caring person perceives the feelings of the other and recognizes the uniqueness of the other.[26]

Using the 10 carative factors, the nurse provides care to various patients.[23] Each carative factor describes the caring process of how a patient attains, or maintains, health or dies a peaceful death. Conversely, Watson describes curing as a medical term referring to the elimination of disease.[23]

In her initial work, *Nursing: The Philosophy and Science of Caring*, Watson[23:8] describes the basic premises of a science for nursing:

1. Caring (and nursing) has existed in every society. Every society has had some people who have cared for others. A caring attitude is transmitted by the culture of the profession as a unique way of coping with its environment. The opportunities for nurses to obtain advanced education and engage in higher level analyses of problems and concerns in their education and practice have allowed nursing to combine its humanistic orientation with the relevant science.

2. There is often a discrepancy between theory and practice or between the scientific and artistic aspects of caring, partly because of the disjunction between scientific values and humanistic values.

Expanding on her previous work, Watson[26:16] added the following components for the context of human science theory development:

1. A philosophy of human freedom, choice, and responsibility
2. A biology and psychology of holism (nonreducible persons interconnected with others and nature)
3. An epistemology that allows not only for empirics but also for advancement of esthetics, ethical values, intuition, and process discovery
4. An ontology of time and space
5. A context of interhuman events, processes, and relationships
6. A scientific world view that is open

As Watson's work evolved, she continued to focus more on the human care process and the transpersonal aspects of caring-healing. The basic premises Watson stated in *Nursing: Human Science and Human Care—A Theory of Nursing*[26] are a reflection of the interpersonal-transpersonal-spiritual aspects of her work.[30] These aspects represent an integration of her beliefs and values about human life and provide the foundation for further development of her theory.[26]

1. A person's mind and emotions are windows to the soul.
2. A person's body is confined in time and space, but the mind and soul are not confined to the physical universe.
3. Access to a person's body, mind, and soul is possible as long as the person is perceived as and treated as a whole.
4. The spirit, inner self, or soul (giest) of a person exists in and for itself.
5. People need each other in a caring, loving way.
6. To find solutions, it is necessary to find meanings.
7. The totality of experience at any given moment constitutes a phenomenal field.

Watson's evolving work continues to make it explicit that humans cannot be treated as objects and humans cannot be separated from self, other, nature, and the larger universe. The caring-healing paradigm is located within a cosmology that is both metaphysical and transcendent with the coevolving human in the universe. The context calls for a sense of reverence and sacredness with regard to life and all living things. It incorporates both art and science, as they are also being redefined, acknowledging a convergence between the two.[35]

LOGICAL FORM

The framework is presented in a logical form. It contains broad ideas and addresses many situations on the health-illness continuum. Watson's definition of caring as opposed to curing delineates nursing from medicine. This concept is helpful in classifying the body of nursing knowledge as a separate science.

Since 1979, the development of the theory has been toward clarifying the person of the nurse and the person of the patient. Another emphasis has been on existential-phenomenological and spiritual factors.

Watson's theory has foundational support from theorists in other disciplines, such as Rogers, Erikson, and Maslow. She is adamant in her support for nursing education that incorporates holistic knowledge from many disciplines and integrates the humanities, arts, and sciences. She believes the increasingly complex requirements of the healthcare system and patient needs require nurses to have a broad, liberal education. The ideals, content, and theory of liberal education must be integrated into professional nursing education.[18]

Watson has recently incorporated dimensions of a postmodern paradigm shift throughout her theory of transpersonal caring. Modern theoretical underpinnings have been associated with concepts such as steady state maintenance, adaptation, linear interactions, and problem-based nursing practice. The postmodern approach moves beyond this point; the redefining of such a nursing paradigm leads to a more holistic, humanistic, open system wherein harmony, interpretation, and self-transcendence are the emerging directions reflected in this epistemological shift. Watson[33] believes that nursing must be challenged to construct and coconstruct ancient and new knowledge toward an ever-evolving humanity of possibilities to further clarify nursing for a new era. "The theory evolution has tended to place greater emphasis on transpersonal caring, intentionality, caring consciousness, and the caring field."[38]

ACCEPTANCE BY THE NURSING COMMUNITY
Practice

Institutions that are seeking a holistic approach to nursing care are integrating many aspects of Watson's theoretical commitment to caring. For example, nursing journals that are concerned with the delivery of nursing care contain increasing numbers of articles that reference Watson and incorporate the importance of caring as an essential domain of nursing.[2]

Watson's theory is being clinically validated in a variety of settings and with various populations.

The clinical settings have included critical care units, neonatal intensive care units, and pediatric and gerontological care units.[3,5,15,20,21]

The populations have included women who have miscarried, women who have had newborns in intensive care units, and women identified as socially at risk;[22] postmyocardial infarction patients;[5] oncology patients;[8] persons with AIDS;[13] and the elderly.[4] The relationship of caring to nursing administration has also been examined.[10,14,16]

The acuity level of hospitalized individuals, the short length of hospital stays, and the increasing complexity of technology have been identified as possibly interfering with the implementation of the caring theory.

Education

Watson has been active in curriculum planning at the University of Colorado. Her framework is being taught in numerous baccalaureate nursing curricula, including Bellarmine College in Louisville, Kentucky; Assumption College in Worcester, Massachusetts; Indiana State University in Terre Haute, Indiana; and Florida Atlantic University in Boca Raton, Florida. In addition, these concepts are now widely used in nursing programs in Australia, Sweden, Finland, and the United Kingdom.

Critics of Watson's work have concentrated on the use of undefined terms, the incomplete treatment of subject matter when describing the 10 carative factors, and a lack of attention to the pathophysiological aspect of nursing. Watson[26] addresses these aspects in the preface of her second book, *Nursing: Human Science and Human Care—A Theory of Nursing,* where she defines her intent to describe the core of nursing (those aspects of the nurse-patient relationship resulting in a therapeutic outcome) rather than the trim of nursing (the procedures, tasks, and techniques used by various practice settings). With this focus, the framework is not limited to any nursing specialty. Although she emphasizes that both the core and the trim are necessary, she believes that the trim cannot be the center of a professional model of "nursing qua nursing."[35:50] Watson[26] hopes her work will help nurses develop a meaningful moral and philosophical base for practice. A study of Watson's framework leads the reader through a thought-provoking experience by emphasizing deep inner reflection and personal growth, communication skills, use of self-transpersonal growth, attention to both nurse and patient, and the human caring process that potentiates human health and healing.

Research

Watson and colleagues[7,11,12,27] are attempting to research the caring framework and to arrive at empirical data amenable to research techniques. However, this abstract framework is difficult to study concretely. Watson believes that a chasm often exists between the essential qualities and subject matter of nursing and the methods used for research. As with her concern for uniting the liberal arts with nursing education, she hopes that nursing research will incorporate and explore esthetic, metaphysical, empirical, and contextual methodologies.[9,29]

Morse, Bottorff, Neander, and Solberg[11,12] have analyzed the caring literature for themes related to conceptual and theoretical development. They conclude that the abstractness of the concept and the clinical reality in some situations (for example, the brief interactions with patients afforded by outpatient or office visits) has limited the development of a knowledge base in Watson's caring theory, whether caring exists in nursing situations that have yet to develop interpersonally and whether caring is unique to nursing. Patient outcomes in caring transactions need further study.

Research and practice must focus on both subjective and objective patient outcomes in determining whether caring is the essence of nursing. The development of behaviors and predictors of change is critical to further development of this work.

FURTHER DEVELOPMENT

Early nursing research traditionally followed the received view format in which single-factor methodology is compared with rigorous standards of truth, operational definitions, and observational criteria.[19,24] Watson writes about the inadequacy of this methodology for studying the multidimensional phenomena of nursing care. She proposes that, as nursing advances in its doctoral programs, the process of scientific development will be used on itself. Nursing research will adopt the received view, reject it, and synthesize new ideas, which will result in a new nursing model for the next century.

Watson has identified some critical issues for future research conditions that foster the person as an end and not a means in a highly technological society and identified conditions that promote caring when humanity is threatened.[26] This theory lends itself to creative research methodologies that assist nursing in formulating a philosophical base for professional human care concepts.

CRITIQUE
Clarity

Watson's theory uses nontechnical, yet sophisticated, language. At times, lengthy phrases (for example, "symbiotic relationship between humankind-technology-nature"[33:xiv]) and sentences need to be read more than once to gain meaning. Her increasing inclusion of metaphor, personal reflections, artwork, and poetry make her complex concepts more tangible and more aesthetically appealing.

Simplicity

Watson draws on a number of disciplines to formulate her theory. The reader does best by being familiar with a variety of subject matters to understand the theory as it is presented. It is viewed as complex when considering the existential-phenomenological nature of her work, which is partly because many nurses have a limited liberal arts background and baccalaureate-nursing curricula has a limited integration of liberal arts.

Generality

The theory seeks to provide a moral and philosophical basis for nursing. The scope of the framework encompasses all aspects of the health-illness continuum. In addition, the theory addresses aspects of preventing illness and experiencing a peaceful death, thereby increasing its generality. The carative factors that Watson described have provided important guidelines for nurse-patient interactions; however, some critics have stated that the generality is limited by the emphasis placed on the psychosocial aspects rather than the physiological aspects of caring.

Another characteristic of the theory is that it does not furnish explicit directions about what to *do* to achieve authentic caring-healing relationships. It is more about *being* than about *doing* and it must be thoroughly internalized by the nurse to be actualized in practice. Nurses who want concrete guidelines may not feel secure when trying to rely on this theory alone.

Empirical Precision

Although the framework is difficult to study empirically, Watson draws heavily on widely accepted work from other disciplines. This solid foundation strengthens her views. Watson describes her theory as descriptive and she acknowledges the evolving nature of the theory and welcomes input by others. The theory does not lend itself to research conducted with traditional scientific methodologies. In her second book, *Nursing: Human Science and Human Care—A Theory of Nursing*[26] Watson addresses the issue of methodology. The methodologies relevant to studying transpersonal caring and developing nursing as a human science and art can be classified as qualitative, naturalistic, or phenomenological. Watson does acknowledge that a combination of qualitative-quantitative inquiry may also be useful.

Derivable Consequences

Watson's theory continues to provide a useful and important metaphysical orientation for the delivery of nursing care. Watson's theoretical concepts, such as use of self, patient-identified needs, the caring process, and the spiritual sense of being human, may help nurses and their patients find meaning and harmony in a period of increasing complexity. Watson's rich and varied knowledge of philosophy, the arts, the human sciences, and traditional science and traditions, joined with her prolific ability to communicate, has enabled professionals in many disciplines to share and recognize her work.

CRITICAL THINKING *Activities*

Critical thinking with Watson's philosophy and science of caring offers a holistic and humanistic approach in the assessment, diagnosis, planning, implementation, and evaluation phases of the nursing process. On the basis of 10 carative assumptions, Watson's theory provides a framework on which nurses can establish a precedent of collaboration to assist the patient in gaining control, knowledge, and health. The following exercises demonstrate critical and reflective thinking from the perspective of Watson's theory.

1. Examine your own values and beliefs to ascertain how each of Watson's 10 carative assumptions would fit with your own personal philosophy of caring in relation to the patient, environment, health, and nursing.

2. Think of a time in your life when you felt someone truly cared for you. Then think of a time when you demonstrated care for another person. (These can be either health-care related or not.) Then identify what the major characteristics of those interactions were.

3. In her third book, *Postmodern Nursing and Beyond,*[33] Watson includes a chapter entitled "Exercises for Experiencing the Transpersonal Body." Her hope for the continued evolution of transpersonal caring-healing depends so strongly on the continuing spiritual evolution of each individual; therefore a brief description of her own approach to personal meditation follows.

She suggests that participants close their eyes, breathe deeply, and find a quiet place inside themselves. "Then allow yourself to be quiet and still . . . try to dwell there . . . feel the lovely sensation of just being still and quiet . . . and access a sense of inner peace."[33:171] She continues the discussion by describing how the meditation can lead to a reconnection for the participant between mind and body. Watson advises, "Feel yourself in your body; explore your body and gently note points of tension."[33:172] "Once you have explored the body and experienced the sensations, you can move to more focused breathing, concentrating on a given word, or a visual image that comforts and soothes you."[33:174]

The concluding words of the chapter are like a benediction. "In cultivating one's transpersonal self, one experiences the 'at-one-ment' of all. May you be graced on your spiritual journey and deepened through your contemplative practices, whatever they may be."[33:175]

REFERENCES

1. Betz, B.J. & Whitehorn, J.C. (1956). *The relationship of the therapist to the outcome of therapy in schizophrenia. Research techniques in schizophrenia. Psychiatric research reports #5.* Washington, DC: American Psychiatric Association.
2. Brenner, P., Boyd, C., Thompson, T., Cervantez, M., Buerhaus, P., & Leininger, M. (1986, Jan.). The care symposium: Considerations for nursing administrators. *JONA,* 16(1), 25-26.
3. Byrd, R. (1988). Positive therapeutic effects of intercessory prayer in a coronary care unit population. *Southern Medical Journal,* 81(7), 826-829.
4. Clayton, G. (1989). Research testing Watson's theory. In J. Riehl-Siska (Ed.), *Conceptual models for nursing practice* (pp. 245-252). Norwalk, CT: Appleton & Lange.
5. Cronin, S. & Harrison, B. (1988). Importance of nursing care behaviors as perceived by patient after myocardial infarction. *Heart and Lung,* 17(4), 374-380.
6. Gaut, D. (1983). Development of a theoretically adequate description of caring. *Western Journal of Nursing Research,* 5(4), 313-324.

7. Hester, N.O. & Ray, M.A. (1987). *Assessment of Watson's carative factors: A qualitative research study*. Paper presented at the International Nursing Research Congress, Edinburgh, Scotland.

8. Larson, P. (1987). Comparison of cancer patients' and professional nurses' perceptions of important nurse caring behaviors. *Heart and Lung,* 16(2), 187-193.

9. Leininger, M. (1979). Preface. In J. Watson (Ed.), *Nursing: The philosophy and science of caring.* Boston: Little, Brown.

10. Miller, K. (1987). The human care perspective in nursing administration. *Journal of Nursing Administration,* 17(2), 10-12.

11. Morse, J., Bottorff, J., Neander, W., & Solberg, S. (1991). Comparative analysis of conceptualizations and theories of caring. *Image: Journal of Nursing Scholarship,* 23(2), 119-126.

12. Morse, J., Solberg, S., Neander, W., Bottorff, J., & Johnson, J. (1990). Concepts of caring and caring as a concept. *Advances in Nursing Science,* 13(1), 1-14.

13. Neil, R. (1990). Watson's theory of caring in nursing: The rainbow of and for people living with AIDS. In M.E. Parker (Ed.), *Nursing theories in practice* (pp. 289-301). New York: National League for Nursing.

14. Nyberg, J. (1989). The element of caring in nursing administration. *Nursing Administration Quarterly,* 13(3), 9-16.

15. Ray, M. (1987). Technological caring: A new model in critical care. *Dimensions of Critical Care Nursing,* 6, 166-173.

16. Ray, M. (1989). The theory of bureaucratic caring in nursing practice in the organizational culture. *Nursing Administration Quarterly,* 13(2), 31-42.

17. Rogers, C.R. (1961). *On becoming a person: A therapist's view of psychology.* Boston: Houghton Mifflin.

18. Sakalys, J.A. & Watson, J. (1986). Professional education: Post-baccalaureate education for professional nursing. *Journal of Professional Nursing,* 2(2), 91-97.

19. Seeman, J. (1954). Counselor judgments of therapeutic process and outcome. In C.R. Rogers & R.F. Dymond (Eds.), *Psychotherapy and personality change* (pp. 272-299). Chicago: University of Chicago Press.

20. Sithichoke-Rattan, N. (1989). A clinical application of Watson's theory. *Pediatric Nursing,* 15(5), 458-462.

21. Swanson, K. (1990). Providing care in the NICU: Sometimes an act of love. *Advances in Nursing Science,* 13(1), 60-73.

22. Swanson, K. (1991). Empirical development of a middle range theory of caring. *Nursing Research,* 40(3), 161-166.

23. Watson, J. (1979). *Nursing: The philosophy and science of caring.* Boston: Little, Brown.

24. Watson, J. (1981, July). Nursing's scientific quest. *Nursing Outlook,* 29, 413-416.

25. Watson, J. (1984). Telephone interview.

26. Watson, J. (1985). *Nursing: Human science and human care—A theory of nursing.* Norwalk, CT: Appleton-Century-Crofts.

27. Watson, J. (1985). Reflections on new methodologies for study of human care. In M. Leininger (Ed.), *Qualitative research methods in nursing* (pp. 343-349). Orlando, FL: Grune & Stratton.

28. Watson, J. (1986, Dec.). The dean speaks out: Center for human caring established. *The University of Colorado School of Nursing News,* 1-6.

29. Watson, J. (1987). Nursing on the caring edge: Metaphorical vignettes. *Advances in Nursing Science,* 10(1), 10-17.

30. Watson, J. (1988). Telephone interview.

31. Watson, J. (1988). *Nursing: Human science and human care—A theory of nursing.* New York: National League for Nursing.

32. Watson, J. (1992). Personal communication, Aug. 3, 1992.

33. Watson, J. (1999). *Postmodern nursing and beyond.* Edinburgh: Churchill Livingstone.

34. Watson, J. (1995). Post modernism and knowledge development in nursing. *Nursing Science Quarterly,* 8(2), 60-64.

35. Watson, J. (1997). The theory of human caring: Retrospective and prospective. *Nursing Science Quarterly,* 10(1), 49-52.

36. Watson, J. (2000, Aug. 14). Personal communication.

37. Watson, J., Burckhardt, C., Brown, L., Block, D., & Hester, N. (1979). *A model of caring: An alternative health care model for nursing practice and research.* American Nurses Association NP-59 3W8179190, pp. 32-44. Kansas City, MO: Clinical and Scientific Sessions, Division of Practice.

38. Watson, J. (2000, Aug. 31). Personal communication.

BIBLIOGRAPHY (includes citations compiled by Dr. Watson that represent work based on her theory)

Books

Bevis, E.O. & Watson, J. (1989). *Toward a caring curriculum: A new pedagogy for nursing.* New York: National League for Nursing.

Brencick, J. & Webster, G. (1999). *Philosophy of Nursing.* Albany: State University of New York.

Chinn, P. & Watson, J. (Eds.). (1994). *Art and aesthetics of nursing.* New York: National League for Nursing.

Leininger, M. & Watson, J. (Eds.). (1990). *The caring imperative in education.* New York: National League for Nursing.

Montgomery, C. (1993). *Healing through communication: The practice of caring.* Newbury Park: Sage.

Nyberg, J. (1988). *A caring approach to nursing administration.* Boulder, CO: University of Colorado Press.

Taylor, R. & Watson, J. (Eds.). (1989). *They shall not hurt: Human suffering and human caring.* Boulder, CO: University Press of Colorado.

Watson, J. (1979). *Nursing: The philosophy and science of caring.* Boston: Little, Brown.

Watson, J. (1985). *Nursing: The philosophy and science of caring* [second printing]. Boulder, CO: University Press of Colorado.

Watson, J. (1985). *Nursing: Human science and human care.* Norwalk, CT: Appleton-Century-Crofts.

Watson, J. (1988). *Nursing: Human science and human care* [second printing]. New York: National League for Nursing. (Translated into Japanese, 1990.)

Watson, J. (1999). *Postmodern nursing and beyond.* Edinburgh, Scotland, UK: Churchill Livingstone, W.B. Saunders.

Watson, J. (2000). *Monograph of instruments for measuring and assessing caring* .New York: Springer Publishing.

Watson, J. (Ed.). (1994). *Applying the art and science of human caring.* New York: National League for Nursing.

Watson, J., Jones, W., & Levin, J. (Eds.). (1999). *Essentials of complementary alternative medicine.* Philadelphia: Lippincott, Williams, & Wilkins.

Watson, J. & Ray, M. (Eds.). (1988). *The ethics of care and the ethics of cure: Synthesis in chronicity.* New York: National League for Nursing.

Chapters and Monographs

Burns, P. (1991). Elements of spirituality and Watson's theory of transpersonal caring. Expansion of focus. In P.L. Chinn (Ed.), *Anthology of caring* (pp. 141-153). New York: National League for Nursing.

Clayton, G. (1989). Research testing Watson's theory: The phenomena of caring in an elderly population. In J.P. Riehl-Sisca (Ed.), *Conceptual models for nursing practice* (3rd Ed.) (pp. 245-252). Norwalk, CT: Appleton and Lange.

Duffy, J.R. (1992). The impact of nursing caring on patient outcomes. In D. Gaut, (Ed.), *The presence of caring in nursing* (pp. 113-136). New York: National League for Nursing.

Fawcett, J. (2000). Watson's theory of human caring. In J. Fawcett (Ed.), *Analysis and evaluation of contemporary nursing knowledge: Nursing models and theories* (pp. 657-687). Philadelphia: F.A. Davis.

Gray, D.P. (1992). A feminist critique of Jean Watson's theory of caring. In J.L. Thompson, D.G. Allen, & L. Rodrigues-Fisher (Eds.), *Critique, resistance, and action: Working papers in the politics of nursing* (pp. 85-96). New York: National League for Nursing.

Morris, D.L. (1998). Watson's human care model. In J.J. Fitzpatrick (Ed.), *Encyclopedia of Nursing Research* (pp. 593-595). New York: Springer.

Neil, R.M. (1990). Watson's theory of caring in nursing. The rainbow of and for people living with AIDS. In M.E. Parker (Ed.), *Nursing theories in practice* (pp. 289-301). New York: National League for Nursing.

Neil, R.M. (1995). Evidence in support of basing a nursing center on nursing theory: The Denver nursing project in human caring. In B. Murphy (Ed.), *Nursing centers: The time is now* (pp. 33-46). New York: National League for Nursing.

Nyberg, J. (1994). Implementing Watson's theory of caring. In J. Watson (Ed.), *Applying the art and science of human caring* (pp. 53-61). New York: National League for Nursing.

Schroeder, C. (1993). Cost effectiveness of a theory-based nurse-managed center for persons living with HIV/AIDS. In M.E. Parker (Ed.), *Patterns of nursing theories in practice* (pp. 159-179). New York: National League for Nursing.

Schroeder, C. & Astorino, G. (1996). The Denver nursing education project: Promoting the health of persons living with HIV/AIDS. In E.L. Cohen (Ed.), *Nurse case management in the 21st century* (pp. 63-67). St. Louis: Mosby.

Watson, J. (1980). Self losses. In F. Bower (Ed.), *Nursing and the concept of loss* (pp. 51-84). New York: Wiley.

Watson, J. (1981). Some issues related to a science of caring for nursing practice. In M. Leininger (Ed.), *Caring: An essential human need* (pp. 61-67). Proceedings from National Caring Conference, Universtiy of Utah. Thorofare, NJ: Charles B. Slack.

Watson, J. (1982). The nurse-client relationship. In L. Sonstegard, K. Kowalski, & B. Jennings (Eds.), *Women's health care* (pp. 45-56). New York: Grune & Stratton.

Watson, J. (1983). Delivery and assurance of quality health care: A rights based foundation. In R. Luke, J. Krueger, & R. Madrow (Eds.), *Organization and change in health care quality assurance* (pp. 13-19). Rockville, MD: Aspen Systems.

Watson, J. (1985). Reflection on different methodologies for the future of nursing. In M. Leininger (Ed.), *Qualitative research methods in nursing* (pp. 343-349). Orlando, FL: Grune & Stratton.

Watson, J. (1987). The dream curriculum. In National League for Nursing (Ed.), *Patterns in* nursing: Strategic planning for nursing education (pp. 91-104). New York: The Author.

Watson, J. (1988). A case study: Curriculum in transition. In National League for Nursing (Ed.), *Curriculum revolution: Mandate for change* (pp. 1-8). New York: The Author.

Watson, J. (1988). Introduction. In J. Watson & M. Ray (Eds.), *The ethics of care and the ethics of cure: Synthesis in chronicity* (pp. 1-3). New York: National League for Nursing.

Watson, J. (1988). The professional doctorate as an entry level into practice. In National League for Nursing (Ed.), *Perspectives* (p. 41-47). New York: The Author.

Watson, J. (1989). Human caring and suffering: A subjective model for health sciences. In R. Taylor & J. Watson (Eds.), *They shall not hurt* (pp. 125-135). Boulder, CO: University Press of Colorado.

Watson, J. (1989). Preface and introduction. In M. Krysl (Ed.), *Midwife and other poems on caring* (p. v, vii-viii). New York: National League for Nursing.

Watson, J. (1989). Watson's philosophy and theory of human caring in nursing. In J. Riehl-Sisca (Ed.), *Conceptual models for nursing practice* (3rd ed.) (pp. 219-236). Norwalk, CT: Appleton & Lange.

Watson, J. (1990). Foreword. In L. Hill & N. Smith (Eds.), *Self care nursing: Promotion of health* (pp. xi-xii). Norwalk, CT: Appleton & Lange.

Watson, J. (1990). Human caring: A public agenda. From revolution to renaissance. In J. Stevenson & T. Tripp-Reiner (Eds.), *Knowledge about care and caring: State of the art and future developments* (pp.41-48). Proceedings of a Wingspread Conference, Racine, Wisconsin, Feb. 1-3, 1989. St. Louis: American Academy of Nursing.

Watson, J. (1990). Informed moral passion. In *Proceedings for the 1989 National Forum of Doctoral Education in Nursing,* Indianapolis: Indiana University School of Nursing.

Watson, J. (1990). Preface. In G. Gaut & M. Leninger (Eds.), *Caring: The compassionate healer.* New York: National League for Nursing.

Watson, J. (1990). Preface. In M. Leininger & J. Watson (Eds.), *The caring imperative in education* (pp. xiii-xiv). New York: National League for Nursing.

Watson, J. (1990). Transformation in nursing: Bring care back to health care. In National League for Nursing (Ed.), *Curriculum revolution: Redefining the student-teacher relationship* (pp. 15-20). New York: National League for Nursing.

Watson, J. (1990). Transpersonal caring: A transcendent view of person, health, and healing. In M. Parker (Ed.), *Nursing theories in practice* (pp. 277-288). New York: National League for Nursing.

Watson, J. (1991). Foreword. In A. Pearson & R. McMahon (Eds.), *Nursing as therapy.* London & New York: Chapman and Hall.

Watson, J. (1991). Introduction. In M. Leininger (Ed.), *Theory of transcultural nursing.* New York: National League for Nursing.

Watson, J. (1991). Preface: The caring imperative on education. In R. Neil & R. Watts (Eds.), *Caring and nursing: Explorations in feminist perspectives* (pp. ix-x). New York: National League for Nursing.

Watson, J. (1992). Notes on nursing: Guidelines for caring then and now. In F. Nightingale (Ed.), *Notes on nursing.* Philadelphia: J.B. Lippincott.

Watson, J. (1992). Prelude. In E. Gee (Ed.), *The light around the dark.* New York: National League for Nursing.

Watson, J. (1993). Foreword. In N. Diekelman (Ed.), *Transforming nursing education.* New York: National League for Nursing.

Watson, J. (1994). A frog, a rock, a ritual: An eco-caring cosmology. In E. Schuster & C. Brown (Eds.), *Caring and environmental connection.* New York: National League for Nursing.

Watson, J. (1994). Foreword/chapter. In C. Johns (Ed.), *The Burford NDU model. Caring in practice.* Oxford: Blackwell Scientific.

Watson, J. (1994). Poeticizing as truth through language. In P.L. Chinn & J. Watson (Eds.), *Art and aesthetics in nursing* (pp. 3-17). New York: National League for Nursing.

Watson, J. (1996). Beyond art and science. In D. Marks-Mara (Ed.), *Reconstructing nursing: Beyond art and science.* London: Bailliere Tindall.

Watson, J. (1996). Poeticizing as truth on nursing inquiry. In J. Kikuchi, H. Simmons, & D. Romyn (Eds.), *Truth on nursing inquiry* (pp. 125-138). Thousand Oaks, CA: Sage.

Watson, J. (1996). Watson's theory of transpersonal caring. In P.J. Walker & B. Neuman (Eds.), *Blueprint for use of nursing models: Education, research, practice and administration* (pp. 141-184). New York: National League for Nursing Press.

Watson, J. (1997). Alternative therapies and nursing practice. In *Nurse's handbook of alternative and complementary therapies.* Springhouse, PA: Springhouse.

Watson, J. (1997). A meta-reflection of reflective practice. In C. Johns (Ed.), *Reflective practice.* Oxford, UK: Blackwell Science.

Watson, J. (1998). Foreword. In A. Pearson & R. McMahon (Eds.), *Nursing as therapy* [second printing]. Cheltenfam, UK: Stanley Thomas.

Watson, J. (1999). Foreword. In B.M. Dossey, L. Keegan, & C. Guzzetta (Eds.), *Holistic nursing: A handbook for practice* (3rd ed.). Gaithersburg, MD: Aspen Publishers.

Watson, J. (1999). Postmodern nursing and beyond. In N. Chaska (Ed.), *The nursing profession: Tomorrow's vision.* Thousand Oaks, CA: Sage.

Watson, J. (1999). Postscript. In C. Johns (Ed.), *Becoming a reflective practitioner.* Oxford, UK: Blackwell Science.

Watson, J. (2000). Postmodern nursing and beyond. In N.L. Chaska (Ed.), *The nursing profession: Tomorrow's vision and beyond.* Thousand Oaks, CA: Sage.

Watson, J. (2000). Theory of human caring. In J.M. Parker (Ed.), *Nursing theories in practice.* Philadelphia: F.A. Davis.

Watson, J. (1994). Overview of caring theory. In J. Watson (Ed.), *Applying the art and science of human caring.* New York: National League for Nursing.

Watson, J. & Bevis, E. (1990). Coming of age for a new age. In N.L. Chaska (Ed.), *The nursing profession: Turning points* (pp. 100-105). St. Louis: Mosby.

Watson, J. & Chinn, P.L. (1994). Art and aesthetics as passage between centuries. In P.L. Chinn & J. Watson (Eds.), *Art and aesthetics in nursing* (pp. xiii-xviii). New York: National League for Nursing.

Watson, J. & Chinn, P. (1994). Introduction to aesthetics and art of nursing. In P.L. Chinn & J. Watson (Eds.), *Anthology on art and aesthetics in nursing*. New York: National League for Nursing.

Journal Articles

Bent, K.N. (1999). The ecologies of community caring. *Advances in Nursing Science,* 21, 29-36.

Biley, A. (2000). Postmodern nursing and beyond (book review). *Journal of Clinical Nursing,* 9, 649-653.

Burchiel, R.N. (1995). The Watson theory of human care applied to ASPO/Lamaze perinatal education. *Journal of Perinatal Education,* 6, 1,43-47.

Carozza, V., Congdon, J.A., & Watson, J. (1978, Nov.). An experimental educationally sponsored pilot internship program. *Journal of Nursing Education,* 17, 14-20.

Carson, M.G. (1992). An application of Watson's theory to group work with the elderly. *Perspectives,* 16(4), 7-13.

Coates, C.J. (1997). The caring efficacy scale: Nurses' self-reports of caring in practice settings. *Advanced Practice Nursing Quarterly,* 3(1), 53-59.

Cohen, J.A. (1991). Two portraits of caring: A comparison of the artists, Leininger and Watson. *Journal of Advanced Nursing,* 16, 899-909.

Cronin, S.N. & Harrison, B. (1988). Importance of nurse caring behaviors as perceived by patients after myocardial infarction. *Heart and Lung,* 17, 374-380.

Eddins, B.B. & Riley-Eddins, E.A. (1997). Watson's theory of human caring: The twentieth century and beyond. *Journal of Multicultural Nursing and Health,* 3, 30-35.

Falk, R., & Adeline, R. (2000). Watson's philosophy, science and theory of human caring as a conceptual framework for guiding community health nursing practice. *Advances in Nursing Science,* 23(2): 34-50.

Fawcett, J., Watson, J., Neuman, B., & Hinton-Walker, P. (2001). On missing theories and evidence. *Journal of Nursing Scholarship,* 33(2), 115-119.

From, M.A. (1995). Utilizing the home setting to teach Watson's theory of human caring. *Nursing Forum,* 30, 5-11.

Gramling, L. & Nugent, K. (1988). Teaching caring within the context of health. *Nurse Educator,* 23(2): 47-51.

Gray, P. (1993). Perioperative nurse caring behaviors: Perceptions of surgical patients. *AORN Journal,* 57, 1106-1114.

Horrigan, B. (2000). Regions hospital opens holistic nursing unit. *Alternative Therapies,* 6(4), 92-93.

Jensen, K.P., Back-Pettersson, S.R., & Segesten, K.M. (1996). The caring moment and the green-thumb phenomenon among Swedish nurses. *Nursing Science Quarterly,* 6, 98-104.

Kilby, J.W. (1997). Case study: Transpersonal caring theory in perinatal loss. *Journal of Perinatal Education,* 6(2), 45-50.

Krysl, M. & Watson, J. (1988, Jan.). Poetry on caring and addendum on center for human caring. *Advances in Nursing Science,* 10(2), 12-17.

Lemmer, C.M. (1991). Parental perceptions of caring following perinatal bereavement. *Western Journal of Nursing Research,* 13, 475-494.

Maltby, H., Drury, J., & Fischer-Rasmussen, V. (1994). The roots of nursing: Teaching caring based on Watson. *Nursing Education Today,* 15, 44-46.

Marck, B.B. (1995). Watson's theory of caring: A model for implementation in practice. *Journal of Nursing Care Quality,* 9(4), 43-54.

McNamara, S.A. (1995). Perioperative nurses' perceptions of caring practices. *AORN Journal,* 61, 377, 380-385.

Mullaney, J.A. (June, 2000). The lived experience of using Watson's actual caring occasion to treat depressed women. *Journal of Holistic Nursing,* 18(2), 129-142.

Nelson-Marten, P., Hecomovich, K., & Pangle, M. (1998). Caring theory: A framework for advanced practice nursing. *Advanced Practice Nursing Quarterly,* 4, 70-77.

Norred, C. (2000). Minimizing preoperative anxiety with alternative caring-healing therapies. *AORN Journal,* 72(3), 1-4.

Nyman, C.S. & Lutzen, K. (1999). Caring needs of patients with rheumatoid arthritis. *Nursing Science Quarterly,* 12(2), 164-169.

Perry, B. (1997). Beliefs of eight exemplary nurses related to Watson's nursing theory. *Canadian Oncology Nursing Journal,* 8(2), 97-101.

Quinn, J. (1992). Holding sacred space. The nurse as healing environment. *Holistic Nursing Practice,* 6(4), 26-36.

Ray, M.A. (1997). Consciousness and the moral ideal: A transcultural analysis of Watson's theory of transpersonal caring. *Advanced Practice Nursing Quarterly,* 3, 25-31.

Saewyc, E. (2000, June). Nursing theories of caring. *Journal of Holistic Nursing,* 18(2), 109-113.

Sakalys, J. & Watson, J. (1985, Sept./Oct.). New directions in higher education. A review of trends. *Journal of Professional Nursing,* 1(5), 293-299.

Sakalys, J. & Watson, J. (1986, Mar./Apr.). Professional education: Post-baccalaureate education for professional nursing. *Journal of Professional Nursing,* 2(2), 91-97.

Schindel-Martin, L. (1991). Using Watson's theory to explore the dimensions of adult polycystic kidney disease. *American Nephrology Nurses' Association Journal,* 18, 493-496.

Schroeder, C. (1993). Nursing's response to the crisis of access, costs, and quality in health care. *Advances in Nursing Science,* 16(1), 1-20.

Schroeder, C. & Maéve, M.K. (1992). Nursing care partnerships at the Denver nursing project in human caring: An application and extension of caring theory in practice. *Advances in Nursing Science,* 15(2), 25-38.

Sithichoke-Rattan, N. (1989). A clinical application of Watson's theory. *Pediatric Nursing,* 15, 458-462.

Smith, M.C. (1997). Nursing theory-guided practice: Practice guided by Watson's theory. The Denver nursing project in human caring. *Nursing Science Quarterly,* 10, 56-58.

Swanson, K.M. (1991). Empirical development of a middle range theory of caring. *Nursing Research,* 40, 161-166.

Updike, P., Cleveland, M.J., & Nyberg, J. (2000). Complementary caring-healing practices of nurses caring for children with life-challenging illnesses and their families: A pilot project with case reports. *Alternative Therapies,* 6(4), 108-112.

Walker, C.A. (1996). Coalescing the theories of two nurse visionaries: Parse and Watson. *Journal of Advanced Nursing,* 24, 988-996.

Ward, S. (1998). Caring and healing in the 21st century. *MCN Journal,* 23(4), 210-215.

Watson, J. (1968, Feb.). Death—A necessary concern for nurses. *Nursing Outlook,* 15(1), 47-48.

Watson, J. (1972). Death—A necessary concern for nurses. In *The dying patient: A nursing perspective* (Contemporary Nursing Series, pp. 196-200). New York: American Journal of Nursing Publication Co.

Watson, J. (1973, May). Self examination—A necessary concern for counselors. *Awareness.*

Watson, J. (1976). Research and literature on children's responses to injections: Some general nursing implications. *Pediatric Nursing,* 2(1), 7-8.

Watson, J. (1976). Research: Question-answer. Creative approach to researchable questions. *Nursing Research,* 25(6), 438.

Watson, J. (1976, Jan./Feb.). The quasirational element in conflict: A review of selected conflict literature. *Nursing Research,* 25, 19-23.

Watson, J. (1977). Follow-up study of University of Colorado undergraduate nursing program. *Colorado Nurse,* 77(1), 6-19.

Watson, J. (1978). Conceptual systems of undergraduate nursing students compared with college students at large and practicing nurses. *Nursing Research,* 27(3), 151-155.

Watson, J. (1979). Research answer. Content analysis. *Western Journal of Nursing Research,* 1(3), 214-219.

Watson, J. (1980). [Review of the book *Nursing: Philosophy and science of caring*]. *Western Journal of Nursing Research,* 2(2), 514-515.

Watson, J. (1980). [Review of the book *Starting point: An introduction to the dialectic of existence*]. *Western Journal of Nursing Research,* 2(3), 637-638.

Watson, J. (1981). Conceptual systems of students and practicing nurses. *Western Journal of Nursing Research,* 3(2), 172-192.

Watson, J. (1981). Nursing's scientific quest. *Nursing Outlook,* 29(7), 413-416.

Watson, J. (1981). Response to Conceptual systems, students, practitioner. *Western Journal of Nursing Research,* 3(2), 197-198.

Watson, J. (1981). The lost art of nursing. *Nursing Forum,* 20(3), 244-249.

Watson, J. (1981, Aug.). Professional identity crisis—Is nursing finally growing up? *American Journal of Nursing,* 81, 1488-1490.

Watson, J. (1982, Aug.). Traditional v. tertiary: Ideological shifts in nursing education. *The Australian Nurses Journal,* 12(2), 44-46.

Watson, J. (1983, Fall). Commentary on instructor directed research model. *Western Journal of Nursing Research,* 5(4), 310-311.

Watson, J. (1987). Academic and clinical collaboration: Advancing the art and science of human caring (Communicating nursing research, vol. 20; Collaboration in nursing research: Advancing the science of human care, pp. 1-16). *Proceedings of the Western Society for Research in Nursing Conference,* Western Institute of Nursing, Tempe, AZ.

Watson, J. (1987). [Review of the book *Health as expanding consciousness*]. *Journal of Professional Nursing,* 3(5), 315.

Watson, J. (1987). Review of the book *Practical psychotherapy*]. *Journal of Psychosocial Nursing and Mental Health Services,* 25(3), 42.

Watson, J. (1987, Oct.). Nursing on the caring edge: Metaphorical vignettes. *Advances in Nursing Science,* 10-18.

Watson, J. (1988). Human caring as moral context for nursing education. *Nursing and Health Care,* 9(8), 422-425.

Watson, J. (1988). New dimensions of human caring theory. *Nursing Science Quarterly,* 1(4), 175-181.

Watson, J. (1988). Response to Caring and practice. Construction of the nurses' world. *Scholarly Inquiry for Nursing Practice: An International Journal,* 2(3), 217-221.

Watson, J. (1988, July). Of nurses, women, and the devaluation of caring. [Review of the book *Images of Nurses: Perspectives for history, art, and literature*]. *Medical Humanities Review,* 2(2), 60-62.

Watson, J. (1989, Oct.). Keynote address: Caring theory. *Journal of Japan Academy of Nursing Science,* 9(2), 9-37.

Watson, J. (1990). Caring knowledge and informed moral passion. *Advances in Nursing Science*, 13(1), 15-24.

Watson, J. (1990). Reconceptualizing nursing ethics: A response. *Scholarly Inquiry for Nursing Practice: An International Journal*, 4(3), 219-221.

Watson, J. (1990). The moral failure of the patriarchy. *Nursing Outlook*, 28(2), 62-66.

Watson, J. (1991). From revolution to renaissance. *Revolution: Journal of Nurse Empowerment*, 1(1), 94-100.

Watson, J. (1991). Robb, Dock, and Nutting: I wish I'd been there. *Nursing and Health Care*, 12(4), 210.

Watson, J. (1992). Response to caring, virtue, theory, and a foundation for nursing ethics. *Scholarly Inquiry for Nursing Practice: An International Journal*, 6(2), 169-171.

Watson, J. (1992, Summer). Caring, virtue through a foundation for nursing ethics. A response to Pamela Salsberry. *Scholarly Inquiry for Nursing Practice: An International Journal*, 6(2), 169-171.

Watson, J. & Phillips, S. (1992). A call for educational reform: Colorado nursing doctorate model as exemplar. *Nursing Outlook*, 40, 20-26.

Watson, J. (1993). Dr. Jean Watson with E. Henderson— An interview. *Alberta Association of Registered Nurses Newsletter*, 49(6), 10-12.

Watson, J. (1993). Should NPs, CNM, and CNAs, etc., add graduate credentials? *Open Mind*, 2(3), 2.

Watson, J. (1994). Guest editorial. *Nursing praxis in New Zealand*, 9(1), 2-5.

Watson, J. (1994). Have we arrived or are we on our way out? Promises, possibilities, and paradigms. (Invited editorial.) *Image: Journal of Nursing Scholarship*, 26(2), 86.

Watson, J. (1994). Postmodern crisis in science and method. *Proceedings of National Institutes of Health-Office of Alternative Medicine Conference*, Bethesda, MD.

Watson, J. (1995). Advanced nursing practice and what might be. *Journal of Nursing and Health Care*, 16(2), 78-83.

Watson, J. (1995). A Fulbright in Sweden: Runes, academics, archetypal motifs, and other things. *Image: Journal of Nursing Scholarship*, 27(1), 71-75.

Watson, J. (1995). Concerning the spiritual in caring. (A publication effort with the Scottish Highlands Center for Human Caring and the University of Colorado School of Nursing Center for Human Caring.) *British Journal of Nursing*.

Watson, J. (1995). Postmodernism and knowledge development in nursing. *Nursing Science Quarterly*, 8(2), 60-64.

Watson, J. (1995, July). Nursing's caring-healing model as exemplar for alternative medicine. *Journal of Alternative Therapies in Health and Medicine*, 1(3), 64-69.

Watson, J. (1995, Aug.). A yearning for new debates. *National League for Nursing Update*, 1(3), 6-8.

Watson, J. (1996). Nursing, caring-healing paradigm. In D. Pesat (Ed.), *Capsules of comments in psychiatric nursing*. St. Louis: Mosby.

Watson, J. (1996). United States of America: Can nursing theory and practice survive? *International Journal of Nursing Practice*, 2(4), 241-243.

Watson, J. (1996, May). The wait, the wonder, the watch: Caring in a transplant unit. *Journal of Clinical Nursing*, 5(3), 199-200.

Watson, J. (1997) Guest Editorial. From the mountaintop to the marsh/fens: Punting on the River Cam. *Journal of Clinical Nursing*, 6(1), 3-4.

Watson, J. (1997). The theory of human caring: Retrospective and prospective. *Nursing Science Quarterly*, 10(1), 49-52.

Watson, J. (1998). Nightingale and the enduring legacy of transpersonal human caring. *Journal of Holistic Nursing*, 16(2), 292.

Watson, J. (1999, Spring). Aesthetic expressions of caring: Private psalms—surrendering to the sacred. Personal professional reflections on caring and healing. *International Journal of Human Caring*, 3(3), 34.

Watson, J. (2000). Considering caring by way of non-caring. *Australian Journal of Holistic Nursing*, 7(1), 4-8.

Watson, J. (2000). Leading via caring-healing: The four-fold way toward transformative leadership. *Nursing Administration Quarterly*, 25(1): 1-6.

Watson, J. (2000). Philosophical perspectives in home care: Reconsidering caring. *Journal of Geriatric Nursing*, 21(6): 330-331.

Abstracts and Other Publications

Bevis, E. & Watson, J. (1989). *Coming of age for a new age.* (Abstract.) International Council of Nurses, 19th Quadrennial Congress. Seoul, Korea.

Watson, J. (1975, Dec.). Invitational farewell address to graduating class of 1975. *CU School of Nursing Commencement Exercise Bulletin*.

Watson, J. (1977, Feb.). Preparation of faculty for nurse practitioner role. The future of nurse practitioners. *Proceedings of WICHE Conference*, Boulder, CO: Western Interstate Commission for Higher Education.

Watson, J. (1978, Jan.). Integration of practitioner skills in an undergraduate nursing curriculum. *Proceedings of HEW, Division of Nursing Conference*, Denver, CO.

Watson, J. (1979, Dec.). *Terminal progress report, HEW research project, division of nursing research, conceptual systems, students, practitioners* (Report No. NU-000590).

Watson, J. (1981, Apr.). The need to clarify faculty governance. (University of Colorado publication.) *Silver and Gold Record*, 2.

Watson, J. (1982). A hospice home care program. *Kellogg Publication* (No. 2). Centre for Advanced Studies in Health Sciences, W.A.I.T.. Based on presentation at International Conference—Care of Dying in Australia and Third World, Perth, Western Australia.

Watson, J. (1982). Changing demands and perspectives in nursing education. *Kellogg Publication* (No. 4). Centre for Advanced Studies in Health Sciences, W.A.I.T., Western Australia.

Watson, J. (1982). Ethical issues in nursing and health sciences. *Kellogg Publication* (No. 6). Centre for Advanced Studies in Health Sciences, W.A.I.T., Western Australia.

Watson, J. (1982). *Final Report.* Visiting Kellogg Fellow Centre for Advanced Studies Division of Health Sciences. Western Australian Institute of Technology, Bentley, Western Australia.

Watson, J. (1982). Ideological shifts between traditional hospital training and tertiary nursing education. *Kellogg Publication* (No.7). Centre for Advanced Studies in Health Sciences, W.A.I.T., Western Australia.

Watson, J. (1982). Issues of interdisciplinary health education and practice. *Kellogg Publication* (No. 3). Centre for Advanced Studies in Health Sciences, W.A.I.T., Western Australia.

Watson, J. (1982). Nursing's "new" art and "new" science. *Kellogg Publication* (No. 5). Centre for Advanced Studies in Health Sciences, W.A.I.T., Western Australia.

Watson, J. (1982). Review of the misguided cell. *Kellogg Publication* (No. 8). Centre for Advanced Studies in Health Sciences, Sunderland, MA: Sinauer Associates.

Watson, J. (1982). Understanding loss and grief. *Kellogg Publication* (No. 1). Centre for Advanced Studies in Health Sciences, W.A.I.T., Western Australia. Based on presentation at International Conference—Care of Dying in Australia and Third World, Perth, Western Australia.

Watson, J. (1983-1984). University of Colorado planning directions for year 2000. *University of Colorado School of Nursing Newsletter,* 1.

Watson, J. (1984-1990). The Dean speaks out. *University of Colorado School of Nursing Newsletter.*

Watson, J. (1985, Jan.). *Nursing education and current trends—Needs and supply data.* Report to Colorado Commission on Higher Education.

Watson, J. (1989). *Humanitarian–human caring paradigm for nursing education.* (Abstract.) International Council of Nurses, 19th Quadrennial Congress. Seoul, Korea.

Watson, J. (1989, Sept.). Colorado shows leadership in solving the nursing crisis. (Guest editorial.) *Boulder Daily Camera.*

Watson, J. (1993). Poeticizing as truth. *Proceedings of 1993 Institute for Philosophical Nursing,* University of Alberta, Canada.

Watson, J. (1995). President's message: Challenges and summons from within and without. *Journal of Nursing and Health Care,* 16(6), 340.

Watson, J. (1995, Sept./Oct.). President's message: Visioning on: Toward action and transformation. *Journal of Nursing and Health Care,* 16(5), 290.

Watson, J. (1996, March/April). President's message: From discipline specific to "inter" to "multi" to "transdisciplinary" health care education and practice. *Journal of Nursing and Health Care,* 17(2), 0-91.

Watson, J. (1996, May). [Review of the book *Healing nutrition*]. *Journal Alternative Therapies Health and Medicine,* 2(3), 91.

Watson, J. [Review of the book *Healing power of aromatherapy*]. *Journal of Alternative Therapies in Health and Medicine.*

Watson, J. (1997) [Review of the book *Kitchen table wisdom*]. *Journal of Clinical Nursing.*

Watson, J. (1999). [Review of the book *Nursing and the experience of illness*]. *International Journal of Nursing Research.*

Unpublished Manuscript

Watson, J. (1973). *The effect of feelings and various forms of feedback upon conflict in a political group problem-solving situation.* Unpublished doctoral dissertation, University of Colorado.

Audiovisual or Media Productions

Watson, J. (1974). *Interview of patient with progressive-permanent threat to steady state maintenance—Mr. J.* [Audiotape]. Denver, CO: University of Colorado School of Nursing Learning Resource Laboratory.

Watson, J., Peterson, C., & Walsh, K. (1974, Nov.). *Surgical preparation of hospitalized child* [Videotape]. Denver, CO: University of Colorado Medical Center Educational Resources Production.

Watson, J. (1981, Fall). *A phenomenological approach to person* [Videotape]. Denver, CO: University of Colorado Health Sciences Center Educational Resources Production.

Watson, J. (1987, Feb.). *The balance between objectivity and caring* [Audiotape]. Denver, CO: The Value of Many Voices Conference, Rose Medical Center, The Center for Applied Biomedical Ethics.

Watson, J. (1988). *The power of caring: the power to make a difference* [Videotape]. Denver, CO: Center for Human Caring, University of Colorado Health Sciences Center, School of Nursing.

Watson, J. (1988). *It's nice to be loved* [Videotape]. Denver, CO: Ravenfilms.

Watson, J., Chinn, P., & Schroeder, C. (1992). *A dialogue with nursing theorists* [Videotape]. Denver, CO: University of Colorado Health Sciences Center Production.

Watson, J. (1989) *Theories at work* [Videotape]. New York: National League for Nursing.

Watson, J. (1989). *The nurse theorists: portraits of excellence* [Videotape]. New York: Helene Fuld Health Trust. Available: www.fitne.ev.net.

Watson, J. (1994). *A guide to applying the art and science of human caring* [Videotape]. Denver, CO: University of Colorado, Center for Human Caring.

Watson, J. (1999). *A meta-reflection on nursing's present* [Audiotape]. Boulder, CO: American Holistic Nurses Association. Sounds True Recording Studios.

Watson, J. (1999). *Private psalms. A mantra and meditation for healing* [CD]. Denver, CO: University of Colorado Health Sciences Center Bookstore. (Music by Dallas Smith and Susan Mazer.) Available: Michael.Klee@uchsc.edu.

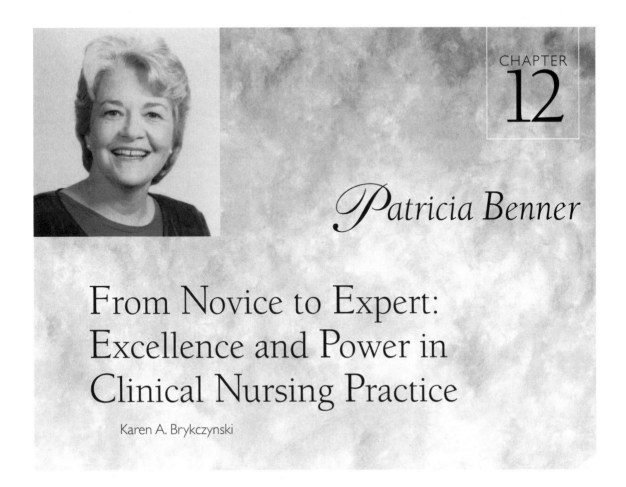

Patricia Benner

From Novice to Expert: Excellence and Power in Clinical Nursing Practice

Karen A. Brykczynski

CREDENTIALS AND BACKGROUND OF THE THEORIST

Patricia Benner was born in Hampton, Virginia and spent her childhood in California, where she received her early and professional education. Majoring in nursing, she obtained a Bachelor of Arts degree from Pasadena College in 1964. In 1970, she earned a master's degree in nursing, with her major emphasis in medical-surgical nursing from the University of California, San Francisco School of Nursing. She worked as a research assistant to Richard

Previous authors: Jullette C. Mitre, Sr. Judith E. Alexander, and Susan L. Keller.

The author wishes to express appreciation to Patricia Benner for critiquing this chapter.

Lazarus at the University of California, Berkeley, while working on her Ph.D. in stress, coping, and health, which was conferred in 1982.

Benner has a wide range of clinical experience including acute medical-surgical, critical care, and home healthcare. She has held staff and head nurse positions.

Benner has a rich background in research and began this part of her career in 1970 as a postgraduate nurse researcher in the School of Nursing at the University of California, San Francisco. In 1982, Benner achieved the position of associate professor in the Department of Physiological Nursing at the University of California, San Francisco and, in 1989, was tenured to professor, a position she currently holds.

165

She teaches at the doctoral and master's levels and serves on 8 to 10 dissertation committees per year.

Benner acknowledges that her thinking in nursing has been greatly influenced by Virginia Henderson. Henderson[50] writes that, as clinically focused research, Benner's *From Novice to Expert: Excellence and Power in Clinical Nursing Practice*[7] might materially affect practice and preparation of nurses for practice. Virginia Henderson wrote the foreword to Benner's work *The Primacy of Caring: Stress and Coping in Health and Illness.*[24]

The recent book by Benner, Tanner, and Chesla, *Expertise in Nursing Practice: Caring, Clinical Judgment, and Ethics,*[22] is a continuation and expansion of *From Novice to Expert.*[7] These authors provide several implications for nursing administration, practice, and education. Barbara Stevens Barnum wrote the foreword to this work. She writes,

> This work continues to challenge our traditional understanding of what it means to know, to be, and to act skillfully and ethically in nursing practice. Equally important, the book enables the reader to see how we might begin to shape our systems to better accommodate expert caring work. One of the truths of learning made clear by the work is that clinical learning is a dialogue between principles and practice. [4:vii-viii]

The most recent book by Benner, Hooper-Kyriakidis, and Stannard, *Clinical Wisdom in Critical Care: A Thinking-in-Action Approach,*[18] constitutes phase two of the articulation of critical care nursing practice begun in *Expertise in Nursing Practice: Caring, Clinical Judgment, and Ethics.*[22] In the first forward to *Clinical Wisdom in Critical Care: A Thinking-in-Action Approach,*[18] Joan Lynaugh writes,

> Perhaps the most important accomplishment of this text is its insistence on incorporating all the elements of critical care: clinical thinking and thinking ahead, caregiving to patients and families, ethical and moral issues, dealing with breakdown and technological hazard, communication and negotiation among all participants, teaching and coaching, and understanding the linkages between the larger systems and the individual patient. [58:vi]

In the second forward, Joyce Clifford[30:vii] writes that the work "provides the nurse administrator a wonderful understanding of the way organizational design can facilitate the caregiving process of clinical experts . . . [and] also provides guidance to those entrusted with the development of practice environments that promote the clinical learning and advancement of those just entering the profession."

Hubert Dreyfus, a philosophy professor at Berkeley, introduced Benner to phenomenology. Stuart Dreyfus, in operations research, and Herbert Dreyfus, in philosophy, developed the Dreyfus Model of Skill Acquisition, which Benner applied in her work *From Novice to Expert.*[7] She credits Jane Rubin's scholarship, teaching, and colleagueship[66] as sources of inspiration and influence, especially in relationship to the works of Heidegger and Kierkegaard.[49,52] R.S. Lazarus,[54,55] with whom she worked at Berkeley, has mentored her in the field of stress and coping. Judith Wrubel has been a participant and co-author with Benner for years, collaborating on the ontology of caring and caring practices.

Benner has published extensively and has been the recipient of numerous honors and awards, including the 1984, 1988, and 1999 *American Journal of Nursing* Book of the Year awards for *From Novice to Expert,*[7] *The Primacy of Caring,*[24] and *Clinical Wisdom in Critical Care: A Thinking-in-Action Approach,*[18] respectively.

The Crisis of Care: Affirming and Restoring Caring Practices in the Helping Professions,[64] edited by Susan S. Phillips and Patricia Benner, was selected for the CHOICE list of Outstanding Academic Books for 1995. Benner's books have been translated into 10 languages. Several of her articles have also been translated and read worldwide.

In 1985, Benner was inducted into the American Academy of Nurses; in 1989, she received the National League for Nursing's Linda Richards Award for Leadership in Education. In 1990, she received the Excellence in Nursing Research and Education Award from the Organization of Nurse Executives-California. She also received the Alumnus of the Year Award from Point Loma Nazarene College (formerly Pasadena College) in 1993. In 1994, Benner became an Honorary Fellow in the Royal College of Nursing, United Kingdom. In 1995, she was the faculty member recognized at the University of California, San Francisco for her contribution to nursing science and research. She was awarded The Helen Nahm Research Lecture Award. She is invited worldwide to lecture and lead workshops on health, stress and coping, skill acquisition, and ethics.

Benner expressed that nursing is a cultural paradox in a highly technical society, which is slow to value and articulate caring practices. She feels that the value of extreme individualism makes it difficult to perceive the brilliance of caring in expert nursing practice.

THEORETICAL SOURCES

Benner studied clinical nursing practice in an attempt to discover and describe the knowledge embedded in nursing practice; that is, knowledge that accrues over time in a practice discipline and the difference between practical and theoretical knowledge.[7] One of the first theoretical distinctions that Benner made was related to theory itself. Benner stated that knowledge development in a practice discipline "consists of extending practical knowledge (know-how) through theory-based scientific investigations and through the charting of the existent 'know-how' developed through clinical experience in the practice of that discipline."[7:3]

She believes that nurses have been delinquent in documenting their clinical learning and "this lack of charting of our practices and clinical observations deprives nursing theory of the uniqueness and richness of the knowledge embedded in expert clinical practice."[6:36] Benner has contributed to the description of the know-how of nursing practice.

Scientists have long distinguished interactional causal relationships as "knowing that" from "knowing how." Citing Kuhn[53] and Polanyi,[65] philosophers of science, Benner emphasized the difference in "knowing how," a practical knowledge that may elude formulations, and "knowing that," or theoretical explanations.[7] "Knowing that" is the way an individual comes to know by establishing causal relationships between events. "Knowing how" is skill acquisition that may defy "knowing that"; that is, an individual may know how before the development of a theoretical explanation. Benner[7] maintains that practical knowledge may extend theory or be developed before scientific formulas. Clinical situations are always more varied and complicated than theoretical accounts; therefore clinical practice is an area of inquiry and a source of knowledge development. Clinical practice embodies the notion of excellence; by studying practice, nurses can uncover new knowledge. Nursing must develop the knowledge base of its practice (know-how) and, through scientific investigation and observation, it must begin to record and develop the know-how of clinical expertise. Ideally, practice and theory set up a dialogue that creates new possibilities. Theory is derived from practice and practice is altered or extended by theory.

Benner adapted Dreyfus and Dreyfus' Model of Skill Acquisition and Skill Development[36,37] to clinical nursing practice. Stuart and Hubert Dreyfus, both professors at the University of California at Berkeley, developed the Dreyfus model. The model is situational and describes five levels of skill acquisition and development: (1) novice, (2) advanced beginner, (3) competent, (4) proficient, and (5) expert. The model posits that changes in four aspects of performance occur in movement through the levels of skill acquisition: (1) movement from a reliance on abstract principles and rules to use of past, concrete experience; (2) shift from reliance on analytical, rule-based thinking to intuition; (3) change in the learner's perception of the situation from viewing it as a compilation of equally relevant bits to viewing it as an increasingly complex whole in which certain parts stand out as more or less relevant; and (4) passage from a detached observer, standing outside the situation, to one of a position of involvement, fully engaged in the situation.[21] The performance level can be determined only by consensual validation of expert judges and the assessment of the outcomes of the situation.[7]

In subsequent research further explicating the Dreyfus model, Benner identified two interrelated aspects of practice that also distinguish the levels of practice from advanced beginner to expert. First, clinicians at different levels of practice live in different clinical worlds, recognizing and responding to different situated needs for action. Second, clinicians develop what Benner terms *agency,* or the sense of responsibility toward the patient, and evolve into becoming a member of the healthcare team.[21]

Benner attempted to highlight the growing edges of clinical knowledge rather than to describe a typical nurse's day. Benner's explanation of nursing practice[7:xx] goes beyond the rigid application of rules and theories and is based on "reasonable behavior that responds to the demands of a given situation." The skills acquired through nursing experience and the perceptual awareness that expert nurses develop as decision makers from the "gestalt of the situation" lead them to follow their hunches as they search for evidence to confirm the subtle changes they observe in patients.[7:xviii]

The concept of experience defined as the outcome when preconceived notions are challenged, refined, or refuted in the situation is based on Heidegger[49] and Gadamer.[44] As the nurse gains experience, clinical knowledge becomes a blend of practical and theoretical knowledge. Expertise develops as the clinician tests and modifies principle-based expectations in the actual situation. Heidegger's influence is evident in this and in Benner's subsequent writings on the primacy of caring. Benner refutes the dualistic Cartesian descriptions of mind-body person and espouses Heidegger's phenomenological description of person as a self-interpreting being who is defined by concerns, practices, and life experiences. Persons are always situated; that is, they are engaged meaningfully in the context of where they are. Persons come to situations with an understanding of the self in the world. Heidegger[49] termed practical knowledge as the kind of knowing that occurs when an individual is involved in the situation. Persons share background meanings, skills, and habits derived from their cultural practices. Benner and Wrubel[24:43] state, "Skilled activity, which is made possible by our embodied intelligence, has been long regarded as 'lower' than intellectual, reflective activity" but argue that intellectual, reflective capacities are dependent on embodied knowing. Embodied knowing and the meaning of being are premises for the capacity to care; things matter and "cause us to be involved in and defined by our concerns."[24:42]

While doing her doctoral studies at Berkeley, Benner[54,55] was a research assistant to Richard S. Lazarus, who is known for his development of stress and coping theory. As part of Lazarus' larger study, Benner conducted a study of midcareer male's meaning of work and coping, which was published as *Stress and Satisfaction on the Job: Work Meanings and Coping of Mid-Career Men.*[25] In this study, coping is defined as a form of practical knowledge and it was determined that work meanings influence what is experienced as stress and what coping options are available to the individual.

Lazarus' Theory of Stress and Coping is described as phenomenological; that is, the person is understood to constitute and be constituted by meanings. Stress is described as the disruption of meanings and coping is what the person does about the disruption. Both doing something and refraining from doing something about the stressful situation are ways of coping. Coping is bound by the meanings inherent in what the person interprets as stressful. The person must be understood as a "participant self" in a situation that is shaped by reflective and nonreflective meanings and concerns.[24:63] "The way the person is in the situation sets up different possibilities."[24:63] Benner uses this key concept to describe clinical nursing practice in terms of nurses making a positive difference by being in the situation in a caring way.

USE OF EMPIRICAL EVIDENCE

Benner's early work focused on the anticipatory socialization of nurses. Benner and Kramer[19] studied the differences between nurses who worked in special care units and those who worked in regular hospital units. She was a research consultant for a nursing activity study to determine the use and productivity of nursing personnel in 1974 and 1975. Concurrently, she was a consultant on a study of new nurse work-entry. Benner and Benner[16] conducted a systematic evaluation of the competencies, the job finding, and work-entry problems of new graduate nurses. Benner also studied methods of increasing teacher competencies through the use of a mobile microteaching laboratory.

From 1978 to 1981, Benner was the author and project director of a federally funded grant, Achieving Methods of Intraprofessional Consensus, Assessment and Evaluation, known as the AMICAE Project. This research led to the publication of *From Novice to Expert*[7] and numerous articles. Benner and Wrubel have further explained and developed the background to this study in *The Primacy of Caring: Stress and Coping in Health and Illness*, "an interpretive theory of nursing practice as it is concerned with helping patients cope with the stress of illness."[24:7] The primacy of caring is three-pronged "as the producer of both stress and coping in the lived experience of health and illness, . . . as the enabling condition of nursing practice (indeed any practice), and the ways that nursing practice based in such caring can positively affect the outcome of an illness."[24:7]

Benner directed the AMICAE Project to develop evaluation methods for participating schools of nursing and hospitals in the San Francisco area. It was an interpretive, descriptive study that led to the use of Dreyfus' five levels of competency to describe skill acquisition in clinical nursing practice. In describing the interpretive approach, Benner's approach seeks a rich description of nursing practice from observation and narrative accounts of actual nursing practice to provide the text for interpretation (hermeneutics).[7] The nurses' descriptions of patient care situations in which they made a positive difference "present the uniqueness of nursing as a discipline and an art."[7:xxvi] Over 1200 nurse participants completed questionnaires and interviews; of these, trained researchers observed 51 participants. Paired interviews with preceptors and preceptees were "aimed at discovering if there were distinguishable, characteristic differences in the novice's and expert's descriptions of the same clinical incident."[7:14] Further interviews and participant obser-

vations were conducted with 51 nurse-clinicians and other newly graduated nurses and senior nursing students to "describe characteristics of nurse performance at different stages of skill acquisition."[7:15] The purpose "of the inquiry has been to uncover meanings and knowledge embedded in skilled practice. By bringing these meanings, skills, and knowledge into public discourse, new knowledge and understandings are constituted."[7:218]

The Dreyfus Model of Skill Acquisition was developed by studying the performance of chess players and pilots in emergency situations.[36,37] In applying the model to nursing, Benner[7:xix] noted that "experience-based skill acquisition is safer and quicker when it rests upon a sound educational base." Skill and skilled practice, as Benner[7] defined, means implementing skilled nursing interventions and clinical judgment skills in actual clinical situations. In no case does this refer to context-free psychomotor skills or other demonstrable enabling skills outside the context of nursing practice.

Thirty-one competencies emerged from the analysis of the transcripts of interviews about nurses' detailed descriptions of patient care episodes, including their intentions and interpretations of the events. From these competencies identified from actual practice situations, the following seven domains were inductively derived on the basis of similarity of function and intent:

- The helping role
- The teaching-coaching function
- The diagnostic and patient-monitoring function
- Effective management of rapidly changing situations
- Administering and monitoring therapeutic interventions and regimens
- Monitoring and ensuring the quality of healthcare practices
- Organizational work-role competencies[7]

Each of these domains was described with the related competencies from the exemplars describing nursing practice. Benner presented the domains and competencies of nursing practice as an open-ended interpretive framework for enhancing the understanding of the knowledge embedded in nursing practice. As a result of the socially embedded, relational, and dialogical nature of clinical knowledge, the domains and competencies need to be adapted for use in each institution through the study of clinical practice at each specific locale.[17] Such adaptations have been implemented in many institutions for nursing staff in hospitals around the world.* The domains and competencies have also been useful for ongoing articulation of the knowledge embedded in advanced practice nursing.[27,42,43,56,59]

Benner extended her research presented in *From Novice to Expert: Excellence and Power in Clinical Nursing Practice*[7] and presents the work in *Expertise in Nursing Practice: Caring, Clinical Judgment, and Ethics.*[22] The book is based on a six-year study of 130 hospital nurses, primarily critical care nurses, examining the acquisition of clinical expertise and the nature of clinical knowledge, clinical inquiry, clinical judgment, and expert ethical comportment.[22] The key aims of the study were to:

1. Delineate the practical knowledge embedded in expert practice.
2. Describe the nature of skill acquisition in critical care nursing practice.
3. Identify institutional impediments and resources for the development of expertise in nursing practice.
4. Begin to identify educational strategies that encourage the development of expertise.[22]

Benner[22:xiii] states, "In the study we found that examining the nature of the nurse's agency, by which we mean the sense and possibilities for acting in particular clinical situations, gave new insights about how perception and action are both shaped by a practice community." As a result of the study, there was a clearer understanding of the distinctions between engagement with a problem or situation and the requisite nursing skills of interpersonal involvement. It appears that the requisite nursing skills of involvement with patients and families are learned over time experientially.[22] The skill of involvement with patients and families seems central in gaining nursing expertise. These researchers cite the interlinkage of clinical and ethical decision making; that is, how an individual's notions of good and poor outcomes and visions of excellence shape clinical judgments and actions.[22] This study represents phase one of the articulation project to describe the nature of critical care nursing practice. Articulation signifies "describing, illustrating, and giving language to taken-for-granted areas of practical wisdom, skilled know-how, and notions of good practice."[18:5]

Identification of clinical grasp and clinical forethought (two pervasive habits of thought linked with action in nursing practice in phase two of this articulation project) enriched the understanding of clinical judgment.[18] Benner[15:317] explains that clinical grasp is

> clinical inquiry in action that includes problem identification and clinical judgment across time about the particular transitions of particular patients and families. It has four components: making qualitative distinctions, engaging in detective work, recognizing changing clinical relevance, and developing clinical knowledge in specific patient populations.

She adds that clinical forethought, although playing a role in clinical grasp, "also plays an essential role in structuring the practical logic of clinicians. Clinical forethought refers to at least four habits of thought and action: future think, clinical forethought about specific diagnoses and injuries, anticipation of risks for particular patients, and seeing the unexpected."[15:317]

Nine domains of critical care nursing practice were identified as broad themes in phase two of this work. They are:

- Diagnosing and managing life-sustaining physiological functions in unstable patients.
- The skilled know-how of managing a crisis.
- Providing comfort measures for the critically ill.
- Caring for patients' families.
- Preventing hazards in a technological environment.
- Facing death: end-of-life care and decision making.
- Communicating and negotiating multiple perspectives.

---

*References 1, 2, 26, 33, 45, 47, 48, 57, 62, 66, 67.

- Monitoring quality and managing breakdown.
- The skilled know-how of clinical leadership and the coaching and mentoring of others.[18]

Phase two took place from 1996 to 1997 and included 76 nurses (32 were advanced practice nurses) from six different hospitals. The nine domains of critical care nursing practice were used as broad themes to interpret the data with the incorporation of the descriptions of six aspects of clinical judgment and skillful comportment. These aspects, (1) reasoning-in-transition; (2) skilled know-how; (3) response-based practice; (4) agency; (5) perceptual acuity and the skill of involvement; and (6) the links between clinical and ethical reasoning, provided a guide for actively reflecting on each of the domains of practice. This work is presented in the book by Benner, Hooper-Kyriakidis, and Stannard, *Clinical Wisdom in Critical Care: A Thinking-in-Action Approach.*[18]

Major Concepts & Definitions

NOVICE

In the novice stage of skill acquisition in the Dreyfus model, the person has no background experience of the situation in which he or she is involved. Context-free rules and objective attributes must be given to guide performance. There is difficulty discerning between relevant and irrelevant aspects of a situation. Generally, this level applies to students of nursing, but Benner has suggested that nurses at higher levels of skill in one area of practice could be classified at the novice level if placed in an unfamiliar area or situation.[7]

ADVANCED BEGINNER

The advanced beginner stage in the Dreyfus model develops when the person can demonstrate marginally acceptable performance having coped with enough real situations to note, or to have pointed out by a mentor, the recurring meaningful components of the situation. The advanced beginner has enough experience to grasp aspects of the situation.[7] Unlike attributes and features, aspects cannot be completely objectified because they require experience based on recognition in the context of the situation.

Nurses functioning at this level are guided by rules and are oriented by task completion. They have difficulty grasping the current patient situation in terms of the larger perspective. However, Dreyfus and Dreyfus[38:38] state,

Through practical experience in concrete situations with meaningful elements which neither the instructor nor student can define in terms of objective features, the advanced beginner starts intuitively to recognize these elements when they are present. We call these newly recognized elements 'situational' to distinguish them from the objective elements of the skill domain that the beginner can recognize prior to seeing concrete examples.

Clinical situations are viewed by nurses at the advanced beginner stage as a test of their abilities and the demands of the situation placed on them rather than in terms of the patient needs and responses.[21] Advanced beginners feel highly responsible for managing patient care, yet they still rely on the help of those more experienced.[21] Benner places most newly graduated nurses at this level.

COMPETENT

Through learning from actual practice situations and by following the actions of others, the advanced beginner moves to the competent level.[21] The competent stage of the Dreyfus model is typified by considerable conscious and deliberate planning that determines which aspects of the current and future situations are important and which can be ignored.[7]

"Consistency, predictability, and time management are important, and gaining a sense of mas-

Continued

tery through planning and predictability is the accomplishment."[21:20] There is an increased level of efficiency but "the focus is on time management and the nurse's organization of the task world rather than on timing in relation to the patient's needs."[21:20] The competent nurse may display hyperresponsibility for the patient, often more than is realistic, and may exhibit an ever-present and critical view of the self.[21]

The competent stage is most pivotal in clinical learning because the learner must begin to recognize patterns and determine which elements of the situation warrant attention and which can be ignored. The competent nurse devises new rules and reasoning procedures for a plan while applying learned rules for action on the basis of the relevant facts of that situation. To become proficient, the competent performer must allow the situation to guide responses.[38] Study points to the importance of active teaching and learning in the competent stage to coach nurses making the transition from competency to proficiency.

PROFICIENT

At the proficient stage of the Dreyfus model, the performer perceives the situation as a whole (the total picture) rather than in terms of aspects and the performance is guided by maxims. The proficient level is a qualitative leap beyond the competent. Now the performer recognizes the most salient aspects and has an intuitive grasp of the situation based on background understanding.[7]

Nurses at this level demonstrate a new ability to see changing relevance in a situation including the recognition and the implementation of skilled responses to the situation as it evolves. They no longer rely on preset goals for organization and they demonstrate an increased confidence in their knowledge and abilities.[21] At the proficient stage, there is much more involvement with the patient and family. The proficient stage is a transition into expertise.[22]

EXPERT

The fifth stage of the Dreyfus model is achieved when "the expert performer no longer relies on analytical principle (rule, guideline, maxim) to connect her or his understanding of the situation to an appropriate action."[7:31] Benner described the expert nurse as having an intuitive grasp of the situation and as being able to identify the region of the problem without wasting consideration on a range of alternative diagnoses and solutions. There is a qualitative change as the expert performer "knows the patient," meaning knowing typical patterns of responses and knowing the patient as a person. Key aspects of the expert nurse's practice are: (1) a clinical grasp and resource-based practice, (2) embodied know-how, (3) seeing the big picture, and (4) seeing the unexpected.[22]

The expert nurse has this ability of pattern recognition on the basis of deep experiential background. For the expert nurse, meeting the patient's actual concerns and needs is of utmost importance, even if it means planning and negotiating for a change in the plan of care. There is almost a transparent view of the self.[21]

ASPECTS OF A SITUATION

The recurring meaningful situational components recognized and understood in context because the nurse has previous experience.[7]

ATTRIBUTE OF A SITUATION

Measurable properties of a situation that can be explained without previous experience in the situation.[7]

COMPETENCY

Competency is "an interpretively defined area of skilled performance identified and described by its intent, functions, and meanings."[7:292] This term is unrelated to the competent stage of the Dreyfus model.

MAJOR CONCEPTS & DEFINITIONS—cont'd

DOMAIN

An area of practice having a number of competencies with similar intents, functions, and meanings.[7]

EXEMPLAR

An example of a clinical situation that conveys one or more intents, meanings, functions, or outcomes easily translated to other clinical situations.[7]

EXPERIENCE

Not a mere passage of time, but an active process of refining and changing preconceived theories, notions, and ideas when confronted with actual situations; implies there is a dialogue between what is found in practice and what is expected.[23]

MAXIM

A cryptic description of skilled performance that requires a certain level of experience to recognize the implications of the instructions.[7]

PARADIGM CASE

A clinical experience that stands out and alters the way the nurse perceives and understands future clinical situations.[7] Paradigm cases create new clinical understanding and open new clinical perspectives and alternatives.

SALIENCE

A perceptual stance or embodied knowledge whereby aspects of a situation stand out as more or less important.[7]

MAJOR ASSUMPTIONS

Benner[7:38] incorporated assumptions from the Dreyfus model, "that with experience and mastery the skill is transformed." She stated, "This model assumes that all practical situations are far more complex than can be described by formal models, theories and textbook descriptions."[7:178]

In her subsequent writing, Benner and her collaborators explicated the themes of nursing, person, situation, and health.

Nursing

Nursing is described as a caring relationship, an "enabling condition of connection and concern."[24:4] "Caring is primary because caring sets up the possibility of giving help and receiving help."[24:4] "Nursing is viewed as a caring practice whose science is guided by the moral art and ethics of care and responsibility."[24:xi] Benner and Wrubel[24] understand nursing practice as the care and study of the lived experience of health, illness, and disease and the relationships among these three elements.

Person

Benner and Wrubel use Heidegger's phenomenological description of person, which they describe as "A person is a self-interpreting being, that is, the person does not come into the world predefined but gets defined in the course of living a life. A person also has . . . an effortless and nonreflective understanding of the self in the world."[24:41] "The person is viewed as a participant in common meanings."[24:23]

Finally, the person is embodied. Benner and Wrubel[24] have conceptualized the major aspects of understanding that the person must deal with as: the role of the situation, the role of the body, the role of personal concerns, and the role of temporality. Together, these aspects of the person make up the person in the world. This view of the person is based on the works of Heidegger,[49] Merleau-

Ponty,[60] and Dreyfus.[34,35] Their goal is to overcome Cartesian dualism, namely, the view that the mind and body are distinct, separate entities.[70] Benner and Wrubel[24] give a central place to embodiment in their theory and define embodiment as the capacity of the body to respond to meaningful situations. On the basis of the work of Merleau-Ponty[60] and Dreyfus,[34,35,37] they outline five dimensions of the body: (1) the unborn complex, the unacculturated body of the fetus and newborn baby; (2) the habitual skilled body, the social learned postures, gestures, customs, and skills evident in bodily skills such as seeing and "body language" that are "learned over time through identification, imitation, and trial and error";[24:71] (3) the projective body, the way the body is set (predisposed) to act in specific situations (for example, opening a door or walking); (4) the actual projected body, an individual's current bodily orientation or projection in a situation that is flexible and varied to fit the situation, such as when an individual is skillful in using a keyboard; and (5) the phenomenal body, the body aware of itself, that ability to imagine and describe kinesthetic sensations.[24] Benner and Wrubel point out that nurses attend to the body and the role of embodiment in health, illness, and recovery.

Health

On the basis of the work of Heidegger[49] and Merleau-Ponty,[60] Benner and Wrubel focus "on the lived experience of being healthy and being ill."[24:7] Health is defined as what can be assessed, whereas well being is the human experience of health or wholeness. Well being and being ill are understood as distinct ways of being in the world. Health is described as not just the absence of disease and illness. Also, a person may have a disease and not experience illness because illness is the human experience of loss or dysfunction, whereas disease is what can be assessed at the physical level.[24]

Situation

Benner and Wrubel use the term *situation* rather than *environment* because situation conveys a social

environment with social definition and meaningfulness.[24] They use the phenomenological terms of *being situated* and *situated meaning*, which are defined by the person's engaged interaction, interpretation, and understanding of the situation. Benner and Wrubel stated, "To be situated implies that one has a past, present, and future and that all of these aspects . . . influence the current situation."[24:80] Persons "enter into situations with their own sets of meanings, habits, and perspectives."[24:23] "Personal interpretation of the situation is bounded by the way the individual is in it."[24:84]

THEORETICAL ASSERTIONS

Benner stated that theory is crucial to form the right questions to ask in a clinical situation; theory directs the practitioner in looking for problems and anticipating care needs. There is always more to any situation than theory predicts.[7] The skilled practice of nursing exceeds the bounds of formal theory. Concrete experience provides learning about the exceptions and shades of meaning in a situation. The knowledge embedded in practice discovers and interprets theory, precedes and extends theory, and synthesizes and adapts theory in caring nursing practice. Some of the relationship statements included in Benner's work follow:

- "Discovering assumptions, expectations, and sets can uncover an unexamined area of practical knowledge that can then be systematically studied and extended or refuted."[7:8]
- "The clinician's knowledge is embedded in perceptions rather than precepts."[7:43]
- "Perceptual awareness is central to good nursing judgment and . . . [for the expert] begins with vague hunches and global assessments that initially bypass critical analysis; conceptual clarity follows more often than it precedes."[7:xviii]
- Formal rules are limited and discretionary judgment is used in actual clinical situations.[7]
- "Knowledge . . . accrues over time in the practice of an applied discipline."[7:1]
- "Expertise develops when the clinician tests and refines propositions, hypotheses, and principle-based expectations in actual practice situations."[7:3]

LOGICAL FORM

Through qualitative descriptive research, Benner applied the Dreyfus model of Skill Acquisition to clinical nursing practice. By following Dreyfus' logical sequence, Benner was able to identify the performance characteristics and teaching-learning needs inherent at each level of skill. From her research, Benner identified 31 competencies of expert practice, which she classified inductively into seven domains of nursing practice. In reporting her research, Benner used exemplars taken directly from interviews and observation of expert practice to help the reader form a clear picture of such practice. Benner[7:218] accomplished the goal of her research, which she stated as "to uncover meanings and knowledge embedded in skilled practice . . . by bringing these meanings, skills, and knowledge into public discourse, new knowledge and understanding are constituted."

ACCEPTANCE BY THE NURSING COMMUNITY

Practice

Benner has described clinical nursing practice by using an interpretive approach. *From Novice to Expert*[7] includes several examples of the application of her work in practice settings.[33,51,69] The model has been used to aid in the development of clinical ladders of promotion, new graduate orientation programs, and clinical knowledge development seminars. Symposia focusing on excellence in nursing practice have been held for staff development, recognition, and reward and as a way to demonstrate clinical knowledge development in practice.[33]

Fenton[42] reported the use of Benner's approach in an ethnographic study of the performance of clinical nurse-specialists. She found that the nurses were functioning at an advanced level of preparation, but that "We [in nursing] have not yet developed accurate written and verbal descriptions of that advanced practice."[41:37] Balasco and Black[2] and Silver[67,68] used Benner's model as a basis for differentiating clinical knowledge development and career progression in nursing.

Neverveld[61] used Benner's rationale and format in her development of basic and advanced preceptor workshops.

Crissman and Jelsma[31] applied Benner's findings in developing a cross-training program to aid in staffing imbalances. They state, "Cross-training delineates specific performance objectives for the nurse in her novice role and provides a preceptor in the setting for the clinical area unfamiliar to her. There, as a novice, she aims to become an advanced beginner able to function independently with an experienced nurse available as a resource."[31:64D]

Benner has been cited extensively in nursing literature regarding nursing practice concerns and the role of caring in such practice. She continues to publish applications of the model to clinical situations.[8-10,20,21]

Education

Benner[5] has critiqued the concept of competency-based testing by contrasting it with the complexity of the proficiency and expert stages described in the Dreyfus Model of Skill Acquisition and the 31 competencies. In summary, she stated, "Competency-based testing seems limited to the less situational, less interactional areas of patient care where the behavior can be well defined and patient and nurse variations do not alter the performance criteria."[5:309]

Fenton[41,42] described the application of the domains of expert practice as the basis for studying the skilled performance of master's-prepared nurses. The analysis verified the performance skills of expert nurses reported in the AMICAE Project and identified new areas of skilled performance and five preliminary categories relevant for curriculum evaluation in the graduate program.

According to Barnum,[3:170] it is not Benner's development of the seven domains of nursing practice that has had the greatest impact on nursing education, but the "appreciation of the utility of the Dreyfus model in describing learning and thinking in our discipline." Nursing educators have realized that learning needs at the early stages of clinical knowledge development are different from those required at later stages. These differences must be acknowledged and valued when educators develop teaching curricula.

In *Expertise in Nursing Practice: Caring, Clinical Judgment, and Ethics*,[22] Benner, Tanner, and Chesla emphasize the importance of learning the skill of involvement and caring through practical experience, the articulation of knowledge with practice, and the use of narratives in undergraduate education.

In *Clinical Wisdom in Critical Care: A Thinking-in-Action Approach*,[18] Benner, Hooper-Kyriakidis, and Stannard urge greater attention to experiential learning and present this work as a guide to teaching. They designed a highly interactive CD-ROM to accompany this book.

Research

The preceding example by Fenton[41,42] presented an application of educational research. Lock and Gordon,[57] medical anthropologists who had been research assistants on the AMICAE Project, extended the inquiry to study the formal models used in nursing practice and medicine. They concluded that formal models may serve as maps that direct care and they can substitute knowledge and result in conformity. Gordon[46] cautions that a misuse of formal models occurs when nurses apply models without using judgment, when they use models to exert control, when they use language from models that may cover up meanings, or when they do not understand the meaning of the models. Finally, "formal models should be used with discretion" as tools and should not eclipse the relational, holistic, intuitive aspects of nursing.[7:242]

FURTHER DEVELOPMENT

Benner and Wrubel have extended the basis and interpretation of the study of clinical nursing practice in *The Primacy of Caring: Stress and Coping in Health and Illness*.[24] This work explores the philosophies affecting nurses' thinking and practice. Benner and Wrubel suggest that the adoption of a phenomenological view of a person with shared meanings in the situation gives the potential for an understanding of caring, expert nursing practice

and stress and coping. They state, "Theory must be informed by real-world experience and experiments, which are in turn subject to theoretical interpretation . . . A theory is needed that describes, interprets, and explains not an imagined ideal of nursing, but actual expert nursing as it is practiced day by day."[24:5]

Benner's application of the Dreyfus model in clinical nursing practice has provided rich descriptions of nursing as it is practiced. In the interpretation of the five levels of practice, Benner provided suggestions for matching skill level to nursing practice demands and for the development of each stage on the basis of experience. It is better to place a new graduate with a competent nurse preceptor who can explain nursing practice in ways that the beginner comprehends. The intuitive knowledge of the expert will elude beginners who do not have the experienced know-how to grasp the situation.

To date, the model provides concept definitions and in-depth descriptions of each from nursing practice. From these situated descriptions, competencies in seven domains have been derived from actual nursing practice.[31] Additionally, nine domains have been described for critical care nursing practice and the domains and competencies have been modified to reflect advanced practice nurses.[18,27,42,43] By maintaining the context of these situated performances, the descriptions are holistic or synthetic, not procedural and elemental.[7] "The competencies within each domain [are] in no way intended as an exhaustive list . . . A situation-based interpretive approach to describing nursing practice overcomes some of the problems of reductionism . . . and overcomes the problem of global and overly general descriptions based on nursing process categories."[7:45-46]

In recent research, Benner examined the role of narrative accounts in understanding the notion of good or ethical caring in expert clinical nursing practice. "The narrative memory of the actual concrete event is taken up in embodied know-how and comportment, complete with emotional responses to situations. The narrative memory can evoke perceptual or sensory memories that enhance pattern recognition."[12:16]

Dunlop[39] explored the nursing literature related to the science of caring. She draws a distinction between a science for caring and a science of caring. She states, "A science of caring implies that caring can be operationalized in some way as a set of behaviors, which can be observed, counted or measured."[39:666] Benner has taken a hermeneutical form to uncover the knowledge embedded in clinical nursing practice. Dunlop[39:668] states, "As she does this, she is also uncovering the nursing-caring with which it is deeply intertwined." Dunlop[39:668] noted that, although useful, "it does not provide us with any universal truths about caring in general or about nursing-caring in particular—indeed it does not make any such pretension."

CRITIQUE
Simplicity

Benner has developed an interpretive descriptive account of clinical nursing practice. The concepts are the levels of skilled practice from the Dreyfus model, including novice, advanced beginner, competent, proficient, and expert. She uses the five concepts to describe nursing practice from interviews, observations, and the analysis of transcripts of exemplars that nurses provide. From these descriptions,[31] competencies were identified and these were grouped into seven domains of nursing practice on the basis of common intentions and meanings. Benner's ongoing articulation research project has also produced nine domains of critical care nursing practice. The model is relatively simple in regard to the five stages of skill acquisition and it provides a comparative guide for identifying levels of nursing practice from individual nurse descriptions and observations of actual nursing practice. The interpretations are validated by consensus.

A degree of complexity is encountered in the subconcepts for differentiation among the levels of competency and the need to identify meanings and intentions. This interpretive approach is designed to overcome the constraints of the rational-technical approach to the study and description of practice. Although providing a decontextualized (object) description of the novice level of performance is possi-

ble, the limits of objectification are encountered as an understanding of the situation is required for expert performance. Clinical knowledge is relational and contextual and often deals with local, specific, historical issues. To capture the contextual and relational aspects of practice, Benner uses narrative accounts of actual clinical situations and maintains that the exemplar enables the reader to recognize similar intents and meanings, although the objective circumstances may be quite different.

Generality

The descriptive model of nursing practice has the potential for universal application as a framework, but the descriptions are limited by dependence on the actual clinical nursing situations from which they must be derived. Its use depends on the understanding of the five levels of competency and the ability to identify the characteristic intentions and meanings inherent at each level of practice. The model has universal characteristics; that is, it is not restricted by age, illness, health, or location of nursing practice. However, the characteristics of theoretical universality imply properties of operationalization for prediction that are not a part of this perspective. Indeed, this phenomenological perspective critiques the limits of "universality" in studies of human practices.

Empirical Precision

The model was empirically tested using qualitative methodologies; 31 competencies, seven domains of nursing practice, and nine domains of critical care nursing practice were derived inductively. Subsequent research suggests that the framework is applicable and useful in providing knowledge of the description of nursing practice. Benner[11] stated that "if we choose only scientific, technical and organizational strategies for legitimizing expert nursing care, we will miss the primacy of caring and the central ethic of care and responsibility embedded in expert nursing practice." It is precisely the use of alternative models of discovering nursing knowledge that makes it difficult to address the body of Benner's work within a rational-empirical framework for critique. Using the scientific approach, the nurse would look for law-like relational statements to predict practice. Instead, using the qualitative methods in an interpretive approach, Benner describes expert nursing practice in many exemplars. Positivistic science takes an alternative approach by seeking formulas and models to apply. Her work seems to be hypothesis generating rather than hypothesis testing. Benner provides no universal "how to" for nursing practice, but provides a methodology for uncovering and entering into the situated meaning of expert nursing care.

Benner's perspective is phenomenological, not cognitive. She states, "Clinical judgment and caring practices require attendance to the particular patient across time, taking into account changes and what has been learned. In this vision of clinical judgment, skilled know-how and action are linked."[15:316] Benner's interpretation of the meaning and level of nursing practice creates doubt among objective researchers who seek precision and control. The strength of the Benner model is that data-based research contributes to the science of nursing.

Although clinical nurses around the world enthusiastically received *From Novice to Expert*,[7] some academicians and administrators initially interpreted it as promoting traditionalism and devaluing education and theory for nursing practice.[29] An ongoing debate has developed over cognitive interpretations of Benner's concepts of expertise and intuition.[14,28,32,40,63]

Derivable Consequences

Benner's *From Novice to Expert*[7] model provides a general framework for identifying, defining, and describing clinical nursing practice. Benner uses a phenomenological approach to describe persons and derives meaning and abilities from interactions in life situations. The significance of Benner's research findings[23:11] lies in her conclusion that "a nurse's clinical knowledge is relevant to the extent to which its manifestation in nursing skills makes a difference in patient care and patient outcomes."

Nursing is the involved interaction with persons in a caring mode. *The Primacy of Caring*[24] further develops these themes. Benner described her work as a description of the knowledge embedded in actual nursing practice. The five levels of competencies are descriptions of the practical nursing knowledge of each level in the context of the situations described. The approach to generalization is through common meanings, skills, practices, and embodied capacities rather than through general ahistorical laws. Such common meanings, skills, and practices are socially embedded in nurse schooling, the practice and tradition of nursing. The knowledge embedded in clinical nursing practice should be brought forth as public knowledge to further a greater understanding of nursing practice. Benner[7] believes the scope and complexity of nursing practice are too extensive to rely on idealized, decontextualized views of practice or experiments. Benner[12:19] states, "The platonic quest to get to the general so that we can get beyond the vagaries of experience was a misguided turn . . . We can redeem the turn if we subject our theories to our unedited, concrete, moral experience and acknowledge that skillful ethical comportment calls us not to be beyond experience but tempered and taught by it."

The generalizations are depicted through exemplars that demonstrate relational and contextually relevant intents and aspects of clinical knowledge. This approach takes issue with the common approaches used for universality or generalization in physics and the natural sciences and claims that the basis for generalization in clinical knowledge cannot be structural or mechanistic, but must be based on common meanings and practices. The strategies for generalization are not based on abstraction through removing the situation or context (objectification), but by showing how the skilled knowledge, intent, content, and notion of good in clinical knowledge must be depicted by exemplars that illustrate the role of the situation. Benner claims that this is not a privativistic or subjectivistic approach, but an attempt to overcome the limits of subject-object descriptions. Her call is to "increase public storytelling" to validate nursing as an ethical caring practice and "to extend, alter, and preserve ethical distinctions and concerns."[12:19-20] Benner[13:35-36] states, "We have overlooked practitioner stories that demonstrate that compassion can be wise and, in the long run, less costly than 'defensive' adversarial commodified technocures." Benner's work is useful in that it has framed nursing practice from the context of what nursing actually is and does rather than from idealized theoretical descriptors that are context free.

CRITICAL THINKING *Activities*

The three patients described below are admitted to a nursing unit at the same time. Explain, describe, and provide a rationale for how a nurse at each of the stages of skill acquisition (novice, advanced beginner, competent, proficient, and expert) would do the following:

- Prioritize or categorize each patient.
- Assess each patient.
- Intervene with each patient.

1. A 69-year-old male with a history of chronic obstructive pulmonary disease has an acute exacerbation of respiratory distress. His respirations are 38 per minute, shallow, and labored and he is using the accessory muscles to assist in breathing. He is diaphoretic and pale and has decreased breath sounds bilaterally. His arterial blood gas values are pH 7.27, PO_2 59, PCO_2 57, HCO_3 21.

2. A two-year-old female is diagnosed with bilateral otitis media and she has a rectal temperature of 105.2° F. Her skin color is flushed and she has a dry cough and rhinorrhea and a pulse oximetry of 89% on room air.

3. A 35-year-old woman complains of acute onset of right lower quadrant abdominal pain and nausea and she has vomited three times. Her color is ashen, her oral temperature is 99.2° F, her pulse is 118 beats per minute, her respiration is 24 per minute, and

her blood pressure is 90/50 mm Hg. She is diagnosed with a ruptured right ovarian cyst.

REFERENCES

1. Alberti, A.M. (1991). Advancing the scope of primary nurses in the NICU. *Journal of Perinatal and Neonatal Nursing,* 5(3), 44-50.
2. Balasco, E.M. & Black, A.S. (1988). Advancing nursing practice: Description, recognition, and reward. *Nursing Administration Quarterly,* 12(2), 52-62.
3. Barnum, B.J. (1990). *Nursing theory: Analysis, application, evaluation.* Glenview, IL: Scott, Foresman.
4. Barnum, B. (1996). Foreword. In P. Benner, C. Tanner, & C. Chelsa (Eds.), *Expertise in nursing practice: Caring, clinical judgment, and ethics.* New York: Springer.
5. Benner, P. (1982, May). Issues in competency-based training. *Nursing Outlook,* 20(5), 303-309.
6. Benner, P. (1983). Uncovering the knowledge embedded in clinical practice. *Image: The Journal of Nursing Scholarship,* 15(2), 36-41.
7. Benner, P. (1984). *From novice to expert: Excellence and power in clinical nursing practice.* Menlo Park, CA: Addison-Wesley.
8. Benner, P. (1985, Feb.). The oncology clinical nurse specialist: An expert coach. *Oncology Nursing Forum,* 12(2), 40-44.
9. Benner, P. (1985, Oct.). Quality of life: A phenomenological perspective on explanation, prediction, and understanding in nursing science. *Advances in Nursing Science,* 8(1), 1-14.
10. Benner, P. (1987, Sept.). A dialogue with excellence. *American Journal of Nursing,* 87(9), 1170-1172.
11. Benner, P. (1988). Personal correspondence.
12. Benner, P. (1992). The role of narrative experience and community in ethical comportment. *Advances in Nursing Science,* 14(2), 1-21.
13. Benner, P. (1996). Embodiment, caring and ethics: A nursing perspective: The 1995 Helen Nahm lecture. *The Science of Caring,* 8(2), 30-36.
14. Benner, P. (1996). A response by P. Benner to K. Cash, Benner and expertise in nursing: A critique. *International Journal of Nursing Studies,* 33(6), 669-674.
15. Benner, P. (1999). Claiming the wisdom and worth of clinical practice. *Nursing and Health Care Perspectives,* 20(6), 312-319.
16. Benner, P. & Benner, R.V. (1979). *The new nurses' work entry: A troubled sponsorship.* New York: Tiresias.
17. Benner, P. & Benner, R.V. (1999). The clinical practice development model: Making the clinical judgment, caring and collaborative work of nurses visible. In B. Haag-Heitman (Ed.), *Clinical practice development: Using novice to expert theory* (pp. 17-42). Gaithersburg, MD: Aspen.

18. Benner, P., Hooper-Kyriakidis, P., & Stannard, D. (1999). *Clinical wisdom in critical care: A thinking-in-action approach.* Philadelphia: W.B. Saunders.

19. Benner, P. & Kramer, M. (1972, Jan.). Role conceptions and integrative role behavior of nurses in special care and regular hospital nursing units. *Nursing Research,* 21(1), 20-29.

20. Benner, P. & Tanner, C. (1987, Jan.). Clinical judgment: How expert nurses use intuition. *American Journal of Nursing,* 87(1), 23-31.

21. Benner, P., Tanner, C., & Chesla, C. (1992). From beginner to expert: Gaining a differentiated clinical world in critical care nursing. *Advances in Nursing Science,* 14(3), 13-28.

22. Benner, P., Tanner, C., & Chesla, C. (1996). *Expertise in nursing practice: Caring, clinical judgment, and ethics.* New York: Springer.

23. Benner, P. & Wrubel, J. (1982). Skilled clinical knowledge: The value of perceptual awareness. *Nurse Educator,* 7(3), 11-17.

24. Benner, P. & Wrubel, J. (1989). *The primacy of caring: Stress and coping in health and illness.* Menlo Park, CA: Addison-Wesley.

25. Benner, P. (1984). *Stress and satisfaction on the job: Work meanings and coping of mid-career men.* New York: Praeger.

26. Brykczynski, K.A. (1998). Clinical exemplars describing expert staff nursing practice. *Journal of Nursing Management,* 6, 351-359.

27. Brykczynski, K.A. (1999). An interpretive study describing the clinical judgment of nurse practitioners. *Scholarly Inquiry for Nursing Practice: An International Journal,* 13(2), 141-166.

28. Cash, K. (1995). Benner and expertise in nursing: A critique. *International Journal of Nursing Studies,* 32(6), 527-534.

29. Christman, L. (1985). Review of "From Novice to Expert" (1984) by Patricia Benner. *Nursing Administration Quarterly,* 9(4), 87-89.

30. Clifford, J. (1999). Foreword. In P. Benner, P. Hooper-Kyriakidis, & D. Stannard (Eds.), *Clinical wisdom in critical care: A thinking-in-action approach.* Philadelphia: W.B. Saunders.

31. Crissman, S. & Jelsma, N. (1990). Cross-training: Practicing effectively on two levels. *Nursing Management,* 21(3), 64a-64h.

32. Darbyshire, P. (1994). Skilled expert practice: Is it 'all in the mind'? A response to English's critique of Benner's novice to expert model. *Journal of Advanced Nursing,* 19, 755-761.

33. Dolan, K. (1984). Building bridges between education and practice. In P. Benner (Ed.), *From novice to expert: Excellence and power in clinical nursing practice* (pp. 275-284). Menlo Park, CA: Addison-Wesley.

34. Dreyfus, H.L. (1979). *What computers can't do.* New York: Harper & Row.

35. Dreyfus, H.L. (1991). *Being-in-the-world: A commentary on being and time dimension. I.* Cambridge, MA: M.I.T. Press.

36. Dreyfus, S.E. & Dreyfus, H.L. (1980, Feb.). A five-stage model of the mental activities involved in directed skill acquisition. Unpublished report supported by the Air Force Office of Scientific Research (AFSC), USAF (Contract F49620-79-c-0063), University of California at Berkeley.

37. Dreyfus, H.L. & Dreyfus, S.E. (1986). *Mind over machine.* New York: The Free Press.

38. Dreyfus, H.L. & Dreyfus, S.E. (1996). The relationship of theory and practice in the acquisition of skill. In P. Benner, C. Tanner, & C. Chesla (Eds.), *Expertise in nursing practice: Caring, clinical judgment, and ethics* (pp. 29-47). New York: Springer.

39. Dunlop, M.J. (1986). Is a science of caring possible? *Journal of Advanced Nursing,* 11, 661-670.

40. English, I. (1993). Intuition as a function of the expert nurse: A critique of Benner's novice to expert model. *Journal of Advanced Nursing,* 18, 387-393.

41. Fenton, M.V. (1984). Identification of the skilled performance of master's prepared nurses as a method of curriculum planning and evaluation. In P. Benner (Ed.), *From novice to expert: Excellence and power in clinical nursing practice* (pp. 262-274). Menlo Park, CA: Addison-Wesley.

42. Fenton, M.V. (1985). Identifying competencies of clinical nurse specialists. *Journal of Nursing Administration,* 15(12), 31-37.

43. Fenton, M.V. & Brykczynski, K.A. (1993). Qualitative distinctions and similarities in the practice of clinical nurse specialists and nurse practitioners. *Journal of Professional Nursing,* 9(6), 313-326.

44. Gadamer, G. (1970). *Truth and method.* London: Sheer & Ward.

45. Gaston, C. (1989). Inservice education: Career development for South Australian nurses. *Australian Journal of Advanced Nursing,* 6(4), 5-9.

46. Gordon, D.R. (1984). Research application: Identifying the use and misuse of formal nursing models in nursing practice. In P. Benner (Ed.), *From novice to expert: Excellence and power in clinical nursing practice* (pp. 225-243). Menlo Park, CA: Addison-Wesley.

47. Gordon, D.R. (1986). Models of clinical expertise in American nursing practice. *Social Science and Medicine,* 22(9), 953-961.

48. Hamric, A.B., Whitworth, T.R., & Greenfield, A.S. (1993). Implementing a clinically focused advancement system. *Journal of Nursing Administration,* 23(9), 20-28.

49. Heidegger, M. (1962). *Being and time.* (J. MacQuarrie, & E. Robinson, Trans.). New York: Harper & Row.

50. Henderson, V. (1989). Foreword. In P. Benner & J. Wrubel (Eds.), *The primacy of caring: Stress and coping in health and illness.* Menlo Park, CA: Addison-Wesley.

51. Huntsman, A., Lederer, J.R., & Peterman, E.M. (1984). Implementation of staff nurse III at El Camino Hospital. In P. Benner (Ed.), *From novice to expert: Excellence and power in clinical nursing practice* (pp. 244-257). Menlo Park, CA: Addison-Wesley.

52. Kierkegaard, S. (1848, 1962). *The present age.* (A. Dur, Trans.). New York: Harper & Row.

53. Kuhn, T.S. (1970). *The structure of scientific revolutions* (2nd ed.). Chicago: University of Chicago Press.

54. Lazarus, R.S. (1985). The trivialization of distress. In J.C. Rosen & L.J. Solomon (Eds.), *Preventing health risk behaviors and promoting coping with illness* (Vol. 8, pp. 279-298). Hanover, NH: University Press of New England.

55. Lazarus, R.S. & Folkman, S. (1984). *Stress appraisals and coping.* New York: Springer.

56. Lindeke, L.L., Canedy, B.H., & Kay, M.M. (1997). A comparison of practice domains of clinical nurse specialists and nurse practitioners. *Journal of Professional Nursing, 13*(5), 281-287.

57. Lock, M. & Gordon, D.R. (Eds.). (1989). *Biomedicine examined.* Boston, MA: Kluwer Academic.

58. Lynaugh, J. (1999). Foreword. In P. Benner, P. Hooper-Kyriakidis, & D. Stannard (Eds.), *Clinical wisdom in critical care: A thinking-in-action approach.* Philadelphia: W.B. Saunders.

59. Martin, L.L. (1996). Factors affecting performance of advanced nursing practice (Doctoral dissertation, Virginia Commonwealth University, School of Nursing). *Dissertation Abstracts International,* University Microfilms No. 9627443.

60. Merleau-Ponty, M. (1962). *Phenomenology of perception.* (C. Smith, Trans.). London: Routledge and Kegan Paul.

61. Neverveld, M.E. (1990, July/Aug.). Preceptorship: One step beyond. *Journal of Nursing Staff Development,* 186-189.

62. Nuccio, S.A., Lingen, D., Burke, L.J., Kramer, A., Ladewig, N., Raum, J., & Shearer, B. (1996). The clinical practice developmental model: The transition process. *Journal of Nursing Administration, 26,* 29-37.

63. Paley, J. (1996). Intuition and expertise: Comments on the Benner debate. *Journal of Advanced Nursing, 23*(4), 665-671.

64. Phillips, S. & Benner, P. (Eds.). (1994). *The crisis of care: Affirming and restoring caring practices in the helping professions.* Washington, DC: Georgetown University Press.

65. Polanyi, M. (1958). *Personal knowledge.* Chicago: University of Chicago Press.

66. Rubin, J. (1984). *Too much of nothing: Modern culture, the self and salvation in Kierkegaard's thought.* Unpublished doctoral dissertation, University of California, Berkeley.

67. Silver, M. (1986). A program for career structure: A vision becomes a reality. *The Australian Nurse, 16*(2), 44-47.

68. Silver, M. (1986). A program for career structure: From neophyte to expert. *The Australian Nurse, 16*(2), 38-41.

69. Ullery, J. (1984). Focus on excellence. In P. Benner (Ed.), *From novice to expert: Excellence and power in clinical nursing practice* (pp. 258-261). Menlo Park, CA: Addison-Wesley.

70. Visintainer, M. (1988). Review of the book "The primacy of caring: Stress and coping in health and illness." *Image: Journal of Nursing Scholarship, 20*(2), 113-114.

BIBLIOGRAPHY
Primary Sources
Books

Benner, P. (1984). *From novice to expert: Excellence and power in clinical nursing practice.* Menlo Park, CA: Addison-Wesley.

Benner, P. (1984). *Stress and job satisfaction on the job: Work meanings and coping of mid-career men.* New York: Praeger.

Benner, P. (1987). *Practica progresiva en enfermeria: Manual de comportamiento profesiona* (Spanish translation). Barcelona: Ediciones Grijalbo.

Benner, P. (1994). *Interpretive phenomenology: Embodiment, caring and ethics in health and illness.* Thousand Oaks, CA: Sage.

Benner, P. & Benner, R.V. (1979). *The new nurses' work entry: A troubled sponsorship.* New York: Tiresias Press.

Benner, P., Hooper-Kyriakidis, P., & Stannard, D. (1999). *Clinical wisdom in critical care: A thinking-in-action approach.* Philadelphia: W.B. Saunders.

Benner, P., Tanner, C., & Chesla, C. (1996). *Expertise in nursing practice: Caring, clinical judgment, and ethics.* New York: Springer.

Benner, P. & Wrubel, J. (1989). *The primacy of caring: Stress and coping in health and illness.* Menlo Park, CA: Addison-Wesley.

Gordon, S., Benner, P., & Noddings, N. (Eds.). (1996). *Caregiving readings in knowledge, practice, ethics, and politics.* Philadelphia, PA: University of Pennsylvania Press.

Phillips, S. & Benner, P. (Eds.). (1994). *The crisis of care: Affirming and restoring caring practices in the helping professions.* Washington, DC: Georgetown University Press.

Book Chapters

Allen, D., Benner, P., & Diekelmann, N. (1986). Three paradigms for nursing research-methodology implications. In P.L. Chinn (Ed.), *Nursing research methodology*. Rockville, MD: Aspen.

Benner, P. (1974). Reality testing a "reality shock" program. In M. Kramer (Ed.), *Reality shock: Why nurses leave nursing* (pp. 191-215). St. Louis: Mosby.

Benner, P. (1975). Nurses in the intensive care unit. In M. Davis, M. Kramer, & A. Straus (Eds.), *Nurses in practice: A perspective on work environment* (pp. 106-128). St. Louis: Mosby.

Benner, P. (1975). Process and persistence of value transmission. In M. Davis, M. Kramer, & A. Straus (Eds.), *Nurses in practice: A perspective on work environment* (pp. 166-176). St. Louis: Mosby.

Benner, P. (1990). The moral dimensions of caring. In J.S. Stevenson & T. Tripp-Reimer (Eds.), *Knowledge about care and caring: State of the art and future developments*. Kansas City, MO: American Academy of Nursing.

Benner, P. (1990). Performance expectations of new graduates. In J. Boller & B.J. Daly (Eds.), *Critical care in the nursing curriculum: Linking education and practice*. Laguna Niguel, CA: American Association of Critical Care Nurses.

Benner, P. (1991). Coping with cancer. In S. Baird, R. McCorkle, & M. Grant (Eds.), *Cancer nursing: A comprehensive textbook*. Philadelphia: W.B. Saunders.

Benner, P. (1991). Response to hermeneutical inquiry by Janice Thompson. In L.E. Moody (Ed.). *Advancing theory for nursing science through research* (Vol. 2). Newbury Park, CA: Sage.

Benner, P. (1994). Caring as a way of knowing and not knowing. In S. Phillips & P. Benner (Eds.), *The crisis of care: Affirming and restoring caring practices in the helping professions* (pp. 42-62). Washington, DC: Georgetown University Press.

Benner, P. (1994). Discovering challenges to ethical theory in experience-based narratives of nurses' everyday ethical comportment. In J.F. Monagle & D.C. Thomasina (Eds.), *Health care ethics: Critical issues* (pp. 401-411). Gaithersburg, MD: Aspen.

Benner, P. (1994). The role of articulation in understanding practice and experience as sources of knowledge. In J. Tully & D.M. Weinstock (Eds.), *Philosophy in a time of pluralism: Perspectives on the philosophy of Charles Taylor* (pp. 136-155). Cambridge: Cambridge University Press.

Benner, P. (1997). A dialogue between virtue ethics and care ethics. In D. Thomasma (Ed.), *The moral philosophy of Edmund Pellegrino*. Dordrecht: Kluwer.

Benner, P. (2000). The quest for control and the possibilities of care. In J. Malpas & M.A. Wrathall (Eds.), *Heidegger, coping and cognitive science: Essays in honor of Hubert L. Dreyfus* (Vol. 2). Cambridge, MA: M.I.T. Press.

Benner, P. & Benner, R.V. (1999). The clinical practice development model: Making the clinical judgment, caring and collaborative work of nurses visible. In B. Haag-Heitman (Ed.), *Clinical practice development, using novice to expert theory* (pp. 17-42). Gaithersburg, MD: Aspen.

Benner, P. & Kramer, M. (1977). Work shoes speak. In M. Kramer & C. Schmallenberg (Eds.), *Path to biculturalism* (pp. 204-232). Wakefield, MA: Contemporary Publishers.

Benner, P., Roskies, E., & Lazarus, R. (1980). Stress and coping under extreme conditions. In J.E. Dimsdale (Ed.), *Survivors, victims and perpetrators: Essays on the Nazi holocaust* (pp. 219-258). New York: Hemisphere.

Wrubel, J., Benner, P., & Lazarus, R.S. (1981). Social competence from the perspective of stress and coping. In J.D. Wine & M.D. Smye (Eds.), *Social competence* (pp. 61-99). New York: Guilford Press.

Journal Articles

Benner, P. (1981, Aug.). Retaining experienced nursing is key to quality care. *The American Nurse,* 13(8), 4, 15.

Benner, P. (1982, March). From novice to expert. *American Journal of Nursing,* 82(3), 402-407.

Benner, P. (1982, May). Issues in competency-based testing. *Nursing Outlook,* 30(5), 303-309.

Benner, P. (1983, Spring). Uncovering the knowledge embedded in clinical practice. *Image, Journal of Nursing Scholarship,* 15(2), 36-41.

Benner, P. (1985). General systems theory and nursing. *Japanese Journal of Nursing Research,* 18(1), 61-71.

Benner, P. (1985). Why does nursing need a theory? *Japanese Journal of Nursing Research,* 18(1), 3-30.

Benner, P. (1985, March/April). The oncology clinical nurse specialist: An expert coach. *Oncology Nursing Forum,* 12(2), 40-44.

Benner, P. (1985, Aug.). Preserving caring in an era of cost-containment and high technology. *Yale Nurse,* 12-20.

Benner, P. (1985, Oct.). Quality of life: A phenomenological perspective on explanation, prediction, and understanding in nursing science. *Advances in Nursing Science,* 8(1), 1-14.

Benner, P. (1986, Oct.). Advice for new graduate nurses on their first job. *The American Nurse,* 18(9), 5-9.

Benner, P. (1987, Sept.). A dialogue with excellence. *American Journal of Nursing,* 87(9), 1170-1172.

Benner, P. (1989, Dec.). *Nursing as a caring profession.* Working paper presented at the meeting of the American Academy of Nursing, Kansas City, MO.

Benner, P. (1990, Spring). Phenomenology as theory and method. *Japanese Journal of Nursing Research,* 25-34.

Benner, P. (1992). Patricia Benner: Uncovering the wonders of skilled practice by listening to nurses' stories (interview by Michael Villaire). *Critical Care Nurse,* 12(6), 82-89.

Benner, P. (1992). The role of narrative experience and community in ethical comportment. *Advances in Nursing Science,* 14(2), 1-21.

Benner, P. (1992, March). The power of our practice: A source for a national care agenda [Editorial]. *Nursing Health Care,* 13(3), 115-116.

Benner, P. (1993). The phenomenology of knowing the patient. *Image: The Journal of Nursing Scholarship,* 25(4), 273-280.

Benner, P. (1996). A response by P. Benner to K. Cash, Benner expertise in nursing: A critique. *International Journal of Nursing Studies,* 33(6), 669-674.

Benner, P. (1996). Embodiment, caring and ethics: A nursing perspective. The 1995 Helen Nahm Lecture. *Science of Caring,* 8(2), 30-36.

Benner, P. (1999). Claiming the wisdom and worth of clinical practice. *Nursing and Health Care Perspectives,* 20(6), 312-319.

Benner, P., Brennan, Sr. M.R., Kessenich, C.R., & Letvak, S.A. (1996). Critique of Silva's philosophy, science and theory: Interrelationships and implications for nursing research. *Image: The Journal of Nursing Scholarship,* 29(3), 214-215.

Benner, P., Ekegren, K., Nelson, G., Tsolinas, T., & Ferguson-Dietz, L. (1997). The nurse as a wise, skillful and compassionate stranger. *American Journal of Nursing,* 97(11), 27-34.

Benner, P. & Kramer, M. (1972, Jan./Feb.). Role conceptions and integrative role behavior of nurses in special care and regular hospital nursing units. *Nursing Research,* 21(1), 20-29.

Benner, P. & Tanner, C. (1987, Jan.). Clinical judgment: How expert nurses use intuition. *American Journal of Nursing,* 87(1), 23-31.

Benner, P., Tanner, C., & Chesla, C. (1990). The nature of clinical expertise in intensive care units. *Anthropology of Work Review,* 11(3), 16-19.

Benner, P., Tanner, C., & Chesla, C. (1992). From beginner to expert: Gaining a differentiated clinical world in critical care nursing. *Advances in Nursing Science,* 14(3), 13-28.

Benner, P. & Wrubel, J. (1982, May). Skilled clinical knowledge: The value of perceptual awareness, Part 1. *Journal of Nursing Administration,* 12(5), 11-14.

Benner, P. & Wrubel, J. (1982, May/June). Skilled clinical knowledge: The value of perceptual awareness. *Nurse Educator,* 7(3), 11-17.

Benner, P. & Wrubel, J. (1982, June). Skilled clinical knowledge: The value of perceptual awareness, Part 2. *Journal of Nursing Administration,* 12(6), 28-33.

Benner, P. & Wrubel, J. (1988). Caring comes first. *American Journal of Nursing,* 88(8), 1072-1075.

Benner, R. & Benner, P. (1991, July/Aug.). Stories from the front line. *Health Care Forum Journal,* 34, 69-74.

Benner, R.V. & Benner, P. (1979, Sept./Oct.). Follow-through evaluation: A resource for curriculum planning and development. *Nurse Educator,* 4(5), 16-21.

Brandt, S. & Benner, P. (1980, March). Infection control in hospitals: What are the challenges? *American Journal of Nursing,* 80(3), 432-434.

Diekelmann, N. & Benner, P. (1985). Three paradigms for research in nursing education. *Progressions Education Research Notes,* A Publication of Division 1: Education in the Progressions of American Educational Research Association, 7(1), 6-10.

Eaton, S. & Benner, P. (1977). Discussion stoppers in teaching. *Nursing Outlook,* 25(9), 578-583.

Malone, R.E. (1998). Whither the Almshouse? Overutilization and the role of the emergency department. *Journal of Health Politics, Policy, and Law,* 23(5), 795-822.

Marculescu, G.L. & Benner, P. (1987, Dec.). A dialogue with excellence: Early warning [Commentary]. *American Journal of Nursing,* 87(12), 1556-1558.

Meleis, A.L. & Benner, P. (1975, May). Process vs. product evaluation? *Nursing Outlook,* 23(5), 303-307.

Videotape

Moccia, P. (1987). *Nursing theory: A circle of knowledge* [Videotape]. New York: National League for Nursing.

CD-ROM

Benner, P., Stannard, D., & Hooper-Kyriakidis, P. (2000). *Clinical wisdom and interventions in critical care: A thinking-in-action approach* [CD-ROM]. Philadelphia: W.B. Saunders.

Other Sources

Dreyfus, H.L. & Rabinow, P. (1982). *Michel Foucault.* Chicago: University of Chicago Press.

Geertz, C. (1973). *The interpretation of cultures.* New York: Harper & Row.

Good, B.J. & Good, M.J.D. (1982). The meaning of symptoms: A cultural hermeneutic model for clinical practice. In L. Eisenberg & A. Kleinman (Eds.), *The relevance of social sciences for medicine.* Boston: D. Reidel.

Palmer, R.E. (1969). *Hermeneutics.* Evanston, IL: Northwestern University Press.

Taylor, C. (1971, Sept.). Interpretation and the sciences of man. *Review of Metaphysics,* 25(1), 3-34, 45-51.

Publications in Press

Benner, P. (In press). Finding the good behind the right: A dialogue between nursing and bioethics. In J.C. Fletcher & E.G. Miller (Eds.). *The nature and prospects of bioethics.* Totowa, NJ: Humana Press.

Benner, P. (In press). Learning through experience and expression: Skillful ethical comportment in nursing practice. In D. Thomasma & J.L. Kissel (Eds.). *The healthcare professional as a friend and healer.* Washington, DC: Georgetown University Press.

Benner, P. (In press). The relevance of post-Cartesian understandings of embodiment, emotion and lifeworld for rationality and agency in nursing practice. *Philosophy of Nursing.*

Benner, P. (In press). The use of narratives for reflecting on practice. *Journal of Japanese Nursing Association.*

Unpublished Manuscripts

Benner, P., Hooper, P., & Stannard, D. (1995). *Nursing therapeutics in critical care: Caring practices linked to treatment.* Unpublished manuscript, University of California, San Francisco.

Benner, P., Wrubel, J., Phillips, S., Chesla, C., & Tanner, C. (1995). *Critical caring: The knowledge and skill embedded in helping.* Unpublished manuscript, University of California, San Francisco.

Doctoral Dissertations

Brykczynski, K.A. (1985). Exploring the clinical practice of nurse practitioners (Doctoral dissertation, University of California, San Francisco). *Dissertation Abstracts International, 46,* 3789B. (University Microfilms No. DA8600592)

Chesla, C.A. (1988). Parents' caring practices and coping with Schizophrenic offspring, an interpretive study (Doctoral dissertation, University of California, San Francisco). *Dissertation Abstracts International, 49-B,* 2563. (University Microfilms No. AAD88-13331)

Day, L.J. (1999). Nursing care of potential organ donors. An articulation of ethics, etiquette and practice (Doctoral dissertation, University of California, San Francisco). *Dissertation Abstracts International, 60-B,* 5431. (University Microfilms No. AADAA-19951464)

Doolittle, N. (1990). Life after stroke (Doctoral dissertation, University of California, San Francisco). *Dissertation Abstracts International, 51-B,* 1742. (University Microfilms No. AAD90-24963)

Dunlop, M. (1990). Shaping nursing knowledge: An interpretive analysis of curriculum documents from NSW Australia (Doctoral dissertation, University of California, San Francisco). *Dissertation Abstracts International, 51-B,* 659. (University Microfilms No. AAD90-16380)

Gordon, D. (1984). Expertise, formalism, and change in American nursing practice: A case study. Medical anthropology program (Doctoral dissertation, University of California, San Francisco). *Dissertation Abstracts International, 46-A,* 738. (University Microfilms No. AAD85-09101)

Hartfield, M. (1985). Appraisal of anger situations and subsequent coping responses in hypertensive and normotensive adults: A comparison (Doctoral dissertation, University of California, San Francisco). *Dissertation Abstracts International, 46-B,* 4452. (University Microfilms No. AAD85-24005)

Hooper, P.L. (1995). Expert titration of multiple vasoactive drugs in post-cardiac surgical patients: An interpretive study of clinical judgment and perceptual acuity (Doctoral dissertation, University of California, San Francisco). *Dissertation Abstracts International, 57-B,* 238. (University Microfilms No. AAD85-19614338)

Kesselring, A. (1990). The experienced body, when taken-for-grantedness falters: A phenomenological study of living with breast cancer (Doctoral dissertation, University of California, San Francisco). *Dissertation Abstracts International, 52-B,* 1955. (University Microfilms No. AAD91-19579)

Leonard, V.W. (1993). Stress and coping in the transition to parenthood of first time mothers with career commitments: An interpretive study (Doctoral dissertation, University of California, San Francisco). *Dissertation Abstracts International, 54-A,* 3221. (University Microfilms No. AAD94-02354)

Lionberger, H. (1986). Phenomenological study of therapeutic touch in nursing practice: An interpretive study of nurses' practice of therapeutic touch (Doctoral dissertation, University of California, San Francisco). *Dissertation Abstracts International, 46-B,* 2624. (University Microfilms No. AAD85-24008)

MacIntyre, R. (1993). Sex drugs and t-cell counts in the gay community: Symbolic meanings among gay men with asymptomatic HIV infections (immune deficiency) (Doctoral dissertation, University of California, San Francisco). *Dissertation Abstracts International, 54-B,* 4601. (University Microfilms No. AAD94-06617)

Malone, R. (1995). The Almshouse revisited: Heavy users of emergency services (Doctoral dissertation, University of California, San Francisco). *Dissertation Abstracts International, 56-B,* 6036. (University Microfilms No. AADAA-19606591)

McKeever, L.C. (1988). Menopause: An uncertain passage. An interpretive study (Doctoral Dissertation, University of California, San Francisco). *Dissertation Abstracts International, 49-B,* 3677. (University Microfilms No. AAD88-24678)

Plager, K.A. (1995). Practical well-being in families with school-age children: An interpretive study (Doctoral dissertation, University of California, San Francisco). *Dissertation Abstracts International, 56-B,* 6039. (University Microfilms No. AADAA-16906593)

Popell, C.L. (1983). An interpretive study of stress and coping among parents of school-age developmentally disabled children (Doctoral dissertation, Wright Institute of Graduate Psychology). *Dissertation Abstracts International,* 44-B, 1604. (University Microfilms No. AAD83-20854)

Raingruber, B.J. (1998). Moving in a climate of care: Styles and patterns of interaction between nurse-therapists and clients: An interpretive study (Doctoral dissertation, University of California, San Francisco). *Dissertation Abstracts International,* 58-B, 6482. (University Microfilms No. AAD98-18661)

Schilder, E. (1986). The use of physical restraints in an acute care medical ward (immobilization) (Doctoral dissertation, University of California, San Francisco). *Dissertation Abstracts International,* 47-B, 4826. (University Microfilms No. AAD87-08453)

SmithBattle, L. (1992). Caring for teenage mothers and their children: Narratives of self and ethics of intergenerational caregiving (Doctoral dissertation, University of California, San Francisco). *Dissertation Abstracts International,* 53-B, 4594. (University Microfilms No. AAD93-03555)

Stainton, M.C. (1985). Origins of attachment: Culture and cue sensitivity (Doctoral dissertation, University of California, San Francisco). *Dissertation Abstracts International,* 46-B, 3786. (University Microfilms No. AAD86-00606)

Stannard, P. (1997). Reclaiming the house: An interpretive study of nurse-family interactions and activities in critical care (Doctoral dissertation, University of California, San Francisco). *Dissertation Abstracts International,* 58-B, 4147. (University Microfilms No. AAD98-06902)

Stevens, M. (1984). Adolescents coping with hospitalization for surgery (Doctoral dissertation, University of California, San Francisco). *Dissertation Abstracts International,* 45-B, 3977. (University Microfilms No. AAD85-03742)

Stuhlmiller, C. (1991). An interpretive study of appraisal and coping of rescue workers in an earthquake disaster: The Cypress collapse (Doctoral dissertation, University of California, San Francisco). *Dissertation Abstracts International,* 52-B, 4671. (University Microfilms No. AAD92-05240)

Warnian, L. (1987). *A hermeneutical study of group psychotherapy.* Unpublished doctoral dissertation, University of California, Berkeley.

Weiss, S.M. (1996). Possibility or despair: Biographies of aging (Doctoral dissertation, University of California, San Francisco). *Dissertation Abstracts International,* 57-B, 3662. (University Microfilms No. AAD96-34295)

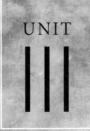

UNIT

III

Conceptual Models and Grand Theories

- *Nursing conceptual models are concepts, definitions, and propositions that specify their interrelationship to form an organized perspective for viewing phenomena specific to the discipline.*

- *Grand theories are conceptual structures that are nearly as abstract as the nursing models from which they are derived, but propose outcomes based on use and application of the model in nursing practice.*

- *Conceptual models provide different ways of thinking about nursing and address the broad metaparadigm concepts that are central to its meaning.*

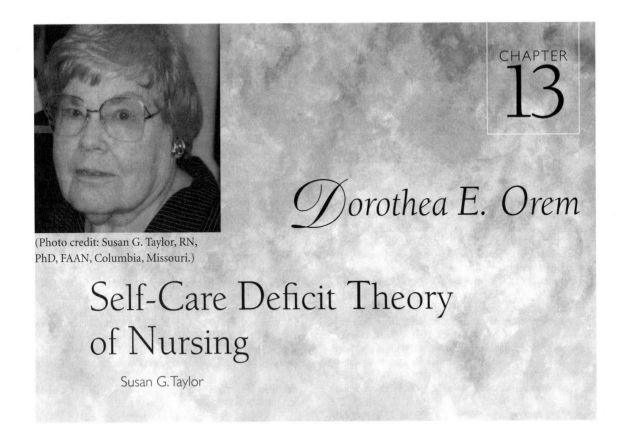

(Photo credit: Susan G. Taylor, RN, PhD, FAAN, Columbia, Missouri.)

*D*orothea E. Orem

Self-Care Deficit Theory of Nursing

Susan G. Taylor

CREDENTIALS AND BACKGROUND OF THE THEORIST

Dorothea Elizabeth Orem, one of America's foremost nursing theorists, was born in Baltimore, Maryland. Her father was a construction worker who liked fishing and her mother was a homemaker who liked reading. The younger of two daughters, Orem began her nursing career at Providence Hospital School of Nursing in Washington, DC, where she received a diploma of nursing in the early 1930s. Orem later received a B.S.N.E. from The Catholic University of America (CUA) in 1939 and, in 1946, she received an M.S.N.E. from the same university.

Her early nursing experiences included operating room nursing, private duty nursing (home and hospital), hospital staff nursing on pediatric and adult medical and surgical units, evening supervisor in the emergency room, and biological science teaching. Orem held the directorship of both the nursing school and the department of nursing at Providence Hospital, Detroit, from 1940 to 1949. After leaving Detroit, Orem spent seven years (1949 to 1957) in Indiana working in the Division of Hospital and Institutional Services of the Indiana State Board of Health. Her goal was to upgrade the quality of nursing in general hospitals throughout the state. During this time, Orem developed her definition of nursing practice.[77]

Previous authors: Susan G. Taylor, Angela Compton, Jeanne Donohue Eben, Sarah Emerson, Nergess N. Gashti, Ann Marriner Tomey, Margaret J. Nation, and Sherry B. Nordmeyer. The author acknowledges the research and editorial assistance of Sang-arun Isaramalai, MS(N), RN, doctoral student, School of Nursing, University of Missouri-Columbia.

189

In 1957, Orem moved to Washington, DC; the Office of Education, U.S. Department of Health, Education, and Welfare (DHEW) employed her as a curriculum consultant from 1958 to 1960. At DHEW, she worked on a project to upgrade practical nurse training that stimulated a need to address the question: What is the subject matter of nursing? As a result, "Guidelines for Developing Curricula for the Education of Practical Nurses" was published in 1959.[78] In 1959, Orem became an assistant professor of nursing education at CUA. She subsequently served as acting dean of the School of Nursing and as associate professor of nursing education. She continued to develop her concept of nursing and self-care at CUA. The formalization of the concepts was sometimes performed alone and sometimes with others. Members of the Nursing Models Committee at CUA and the Improvement in Nursing group, which later became the Nursing Development Conference Group (NDCG), all contributed to the development of the theory. Orem provided the intellectual leadership throughout these collaborative endeavors. In 1970, Orem left CUA and began her own consulting firm. Orem's first published book in 1971 was *Nursing: Concepts of Practice*.[80] She was editor for the NDCG as they prepared and later revised *Concept Formalization in Nursing: Process and Product*.[72-73] Georgetown University conferred Orem with the honorary degree of Doctor of Science in 1976. She received the CUA Alumni Association Award for Nursing Theory in 1980. Other honors received include Honorary Doctor of Science, Incarnate Word College, 1980; Doctor of Humane Letters, Illinois Wesleyan University (IWU), 1988; Linda Richards Award, National League for Nursing, 1991; and Honorary Fellow of the American Academy of Nursing, 1992. She was awarded the Doctor of Nursing *Honoris Causae* from the University of Missouri in 1998.

Subsequent editions of *Nursing: Concepts of Practice*[80] were published in 1980,[81] 1985,[82] 1991,[84] 1995,[85] and 2001.[87] Orem retired in 1984 and resides in Savannah, Georgia. Orem continues working, alone and with colleagues, on the development of Self-Care Deficit Nursing Theory (SCDNT).

THEORETICAL SOURCES

Although Orem cites Eugenia K. Spaulding as a great friend and teacher, she indicates that no particular nursing leader was a direct influence on her work. She believes her association with many nurses over the years provided many learning experiences and she views her work with graduate students and her collaborative work with colleagues as valuable endeavors. Although she does not credit a major influence, she does cite many other nurses' works in terms of their contributions to nursing including, but not limited to, Abdellah, Henderson, Johnson, King, Levine, Nightingale, Orlando, Peplau, Riehl, Rogers, Roy, Travelbee, and Wiedenbach. She also cites numerous authors in other disciplines including, but not limited to, Gordon Allport, Chester Barnard, René Dubos, Erich Fromm, Gartly Jaco, Robert Katz, Kurt Lewin, Ernest Nagel, Talcott Parsons, Hans Selye, Magda Arnold, William Wallace, Bernard Lonergan, and Ludwig von Bertalanffy.[85] Familiarity with these sources is necessary to gain a full understanding of Orem's work.

Orem has identified her philosophical view as that of moderate realism, as described by Wallace.[120,121] Banfield[4] presented an analysis of the metaphysical and epistemological foundations of Orem's work. Banfield[4:204] concluded that "the view of human beings as dynamic, unitary beings who exist in their environments, who are in the process of becoming, and who possess free-will as well as other essential human qualities" are foundational to SCDNT. Taylor, Geden, Isaramalai, and Wongvatunyu[109] also explored the philosophical foundations of the theory. Orem[86] detailed her views of person in a recent work. Action theory, with the perspective of the person as a deliberate actor or agent, forms the basis for the theory. Concepts of speculative and practical science are also foundational.[83] Gullifer[35:155] suggests that Orem's "insights into the patient-nurse nexus...may be viewed as being partly built upon Kantian philosophy," including the categorical imperative and the fusion of mind and body.

USE OF EMPIRICAL EVIDENCE

Orem formulated her concept of nursing in relation to self-care as part of a study on the organization and administration of hospitals, which she performed at the Indiana State Department of Health.[76] This work enabled her to formulate and express her concept of nursing. Her knowledge of the features of nursing practice situations was acquired over many years. Since the SCDNT was first published, there has been extensive empirical evidence that contributes to the development of theoretical knowledge. Much of this is incorporated into the continuing development of the theory; however, the basics of the theory remain unchanged.

Orem's views[83,87] on nursing science as practical science are basic to understanding how empirical evidence is gathered and interpreted. Practical sciences include the speculatively practical, practically practical, and applied sciences. In the most recent edition, Orem identified two sets of speculative nursing sciences: (1) nursing practice sciences and (2) foundational sciences. Nursing practice sciences include sciences of wholly compensatory nursing, partly compensatory nursing, and supportive-educative or developmental nursing. Foundational nursing sciences include the sciences of self-care, self-care agency, and human assistance. She further suggests the development of applied nursing science and basic, nonnursing sciences as a part of the empirical evidence associated with nursing practice.

MAJOR CONCEPTS & DEFINITIONS

Orem labels her self-care deficit theory of nursing as a general theory composed of three related theories: (1) the theory of self-care, which describes why and how people care for themselves; (2) the theory of self-care deficit, which describes and explains why people can be helped through nursing; and (3) the theory of nursing systems, which describes and explains relationships that must be brought about and maintained for nursing to be produced. The major concepts of these theories are identified here and discussed more fully in Orem's book, *Nursing: Concepts of Practice*[85] (Figure 13-1).

SELF-CARE

The practice of activities that maturing and mature persons initiate and perform within time frames, on their own behalf, and in the interest of maintaining life and healthful functioning and continuing personal development and well being.[85]

SELF-CARE REQUISITES

A formulated and expressed insight about actions to be performed that are known or hypothe-sized to be necessary in the regulation of an aspect(s) of human functioning and development, either continuously or under specified conditions and circumstances. A formulated self-care requisite names: (1) the factor to be controlled or managed to keep an aspect(s) of human functioning and development within the norms compatible with life and health and personal well being and (2) the nature of the required action. Formulated and expressed self-care requisite constitutes the formalized purposes of self-care. They are the reasons for which self-care is undertaken; they express the intended or desired results (the goals of self-care).[85]

UNIVERSAL SELF-CARE REQUISITES

Universally required goals to be met through self-care or dependent care have their origins in what is known and what is validated or what is in the process of being validated about human structural and functional integrity at various stages of the life cycle. Six self-care requisites common to men, women, and children are suggested:
1. The maintenance of a sufficient intake of air, water, and food.

Continued

MAJOR CONCEPTS & DEFINITIONS—cont'd

2. The provision of care associated with elimination processes and excrements.
3. The maintenance of balance between activity and rest.
4. The maintenance of balance between solitude and social interaction.
5. The prevention of hazards to human life, human functioning, and human well being.
6. The promotion of human functioning and development within social groups in accordance with human potential, known human limitations, and the human desire to be normal. Normalcy is defined as that which is essentially human and that which is in accordance with the genetic and constitutional characteristics and talents of individuals.[85]

DEVELOPMENTAL SELF-CARE REQUISITES

Developmental self-care requisites were separated from universal self-care requisites in the second edition of *Nursing: Concepts of Practice*.[81] They promote processes for life and maturation and prevent conditions deleterious to maturation or those that mitigate those effects.[85]

HEALTH DEVIATION SELF-CARE REQUISITES

These self-care requisites exist for persons who are ill or injured, who have specific forms of pathological conditions or disorders, including defects and disabilities, and who are undergoing medical diagnosis and treatment. The characteris-

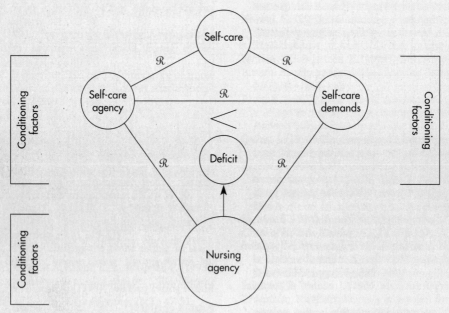

Figure 13-1 A conceptual framework for nursing. *R*, relationship; <, deficit relationship, current or projected. (From Orem, D.E. [1995]. *Nursing: Concepts of practice* (5th ed.). St. Louis: Mosby.)

tics of health deviation as conditions extending over time determine the kinds of care demands that individuals experience as they live with the effects of pathological conditions and live through their duration.

Disease or injury affects not only specific structures and physiological or psychological mechanisms, but also integrated human functioning. When integrated functioning is seriously affected (severe mental retardation, comatose states, or autism), the individual's developing or developed powers of agency are seriously impaired either permanently or temporarily. In abnormal states of health, self-care requisites arise from both the disease state and the measures used in its diagnosis or treatment.

Care measures to meet existent health-deviation self-care requisites must be made action components of individuals' systems of self-care or dependent care. The complexity of self-care or dependent-care systems is increased by the number of health-deviation requisites that must be met in specific time frames.[85]

THERAPEUTIC SELF-CARE DEMAND

The summation of care measures necessary at specific times or over a duration of time for meeting all of an individual's known self-care requisites particularized for existent conditions and for circumstances using methods appropriate for: (1) controlling or managing factors identified in the requisites, the values of which are regulatory of human functioning (sufficiency of air, water, and food); and (2) fulfilling the activity element of the requisite (maintenance, promotion, prevention, and provision).

Therapeutic self-care demand at any time: (1) describes factors in the patient or the environment that must be held steady within a range of values or brought within and held within such a range for the sake of the patient's life, health, or well being; and (2) has a known degree of instrumental

effectiveness derived from the choice of technologies and specific techniques for using changing, or in some way controlling, patient or environmental factors.[85]

SELF-CARE AGENCY

The complex acquired ability of mature and maturing persons to know and meet their continuing requirements for deliberate, purposive action to regulate their own human functioning and development.[85]

AGENT

The person who engages in a course of action or has the power to engage in a course of action.[85]

DEPENDENT-CARE AGENT

Maturing adolescents or adults who accept and fulfill the responsibility to know and meet the therapeutic self-care demand of relevant others who are socially dependent on them or to regulate the development or exercise of these persons' self-care agency.[85]

SELF-CARE DEFICIT

A relationship between the human properties of therapeutic self-care demand and self-care agency in which constituent developed self-care capabilities within self-care agency are not operable or not adequate for knowing and meeting some or all components of the existent or projected therapeutic self-care demand.[85]

NURSING AGENCY

The developed capabilities of persons educated as nurses that empower them to represent themselves as nurses and within the frame of a legitimate interpersonal relationship to act, know, and help persons in such relationships to meet their therapeutic self-care demands and to regulate the development or exercise of their self-care agency.[85]

Continued

MAJOR CONCEPTS & DEFINITIONS—cont'd

NURSING DESIGN

A professional function performed both before and after nursing diagnosis and prescription through which nurses, on the basis of reflective practical judgments about existent conditions, synthesize concrete situational elements into orderly relations to structure operational units. The purpose of nursing design is to provide guides for achieving needed and foreseen results in the production of nursing toward the achievement of nursing goals; the units taken together constitute the pattern to guide the production of nursing.[85]

NURSING SYSTEMS

Series and sequences of deliberate practical actions of nurses performed at times in coordination with actions of their patients to know and meet components of their patients' therapeutic self-care demands and to protect and regulate the exercise or development of patients' self-care agency.[85]

HELPING METHODS

A helping method from a nursing perspective is a sequential series of actions, which, if performed, will overcome or compensate for the health-associated limitations of persons to engage in actions to regulate their own functioning and development or that of their dependents. Nurses use all the methods, selecting and combining them in relation to the action demands on persons under nursing care and their health-associated action limitations:
1. Acting for or doing for another
2. Guiding and directing
3. Providing physical or psychological support
4. Providing and maintaining an environment that supports personal development
5. Teaching[85]

MAJOR ASSUMPTIONS

Assumptions basic to the general theory were formalized in the early 1970s and were first presented at Marquette University School of Nursing in 1973. Orem[85] identifies the five premises underlying the general theory of nursing:
1. Human beings require continuous, deliberate inputs to themselves and their environments to remain alive and function in accordance with natural human endowments.
2. Human agency, the power to act deliberately, is exercised in the form of care for self and others in identifying needs and making needed inputs.
3. Mature human beings experience privations in the form of limitations for action in care for self and others involving and making of life-sustaining and function-regulating inputs.
4. Human agency is exercised in discovering, developing, and transmitting ways and means to identify needs and make inputs to self and others.

5. Groups of human beings with structured relationships cluster tasks and allocate responsibilities for providing care to group members who experience privations for making required, deliberate input to self and others.

Orem lists presuppositions and propositions for the theory of self-care, the theory of self-care deficit, and the theory of nursing systems. These constitute the expression of the theories and are summarized below.[85]

THEORETICAL ASSERTIONS

Presented as a general theory of nursing, the SCDNT is expressed in three theories: (1) theory of nursing systems, (2) theory of self-care deficit, and (3) theory of self-care. The three constituent theories, taken together in relationship, constitute the SCDNT. The theory of nursing systems is the unifying theory and includes all the essential elements. It subsumes the theory of self-care deficit and the theory of self-care. The theory of self-care deficit develops the reason why a person may benefit from nursing. The theory of self-care, foundational to the others, expresses the purpose, methods, and outcome of taking care of self.

Theory of Nursing Systems

The theory of nursing systems proposes that nursing is human action; nursing systems are action systems formed (designed and produced) by nurses through the exercise of their nursing agency for persons with health-derived or health-associated limitations in self-care or dependent care. Nursing agency includes concepts of deliberate action, including intentionality and operations of diagnosis, prescription, and regulation. Figure 13-2 shows the basic nursing systems categorized according to the relationship between patient action and nurse action. Nursing systems may be produced for individuals, for persons who constitute a dependent-care unit, for groups whose members have therapeutic self-care demands with similar components or who have similar limitations for engagement in self-care or dependent care, or for families or other multiperson units.

Theory of Self-Care Deficit

The central idea of the theory of self-care deficit is that the requirements of persons for nursing are associated with the subjectivity of mature and maturing persons to health-related or healthcare-related action limitations. These limitations render them completely or partially unable to know existent and emerging requisites for regulatory care for themselves or their dependents. They also limit the ability to engage in the continuing performance of care measures to control or in some way manage factors that are regulatory of their own or their dependents' functioning and development.

Self-care deficit is a term that expresses the relationship between the action capabilities of individuals and their demands for care. Self-care deficit is an abstract concept that, when expressed in terms of

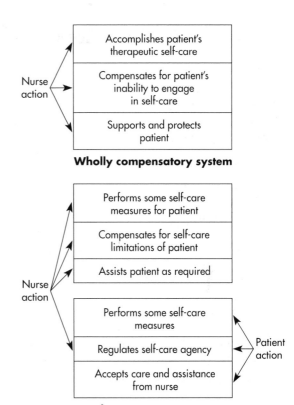

Wholly compensatory system

Partly compensatory system

Supportive-educative system

Figure **13-2** Basic nursing systems. (From Orem, D.E. [1995]. *Nursing: Concepts of practice* (5th ed.). St. Louis: Mosby.)

action limitations, provides guides for the selection of methods for helping and understanding patient roles in self-care.

Theory of Self-Care

Self-care is a human regulatory function that individuals must, with deliberation, perform themselves or have performed for them to maintain life, health, development, and well being. Self-care is an action system. The elaboration of the concepts of self-care, self-care demand, and self-care agency provide the foundation for understanding the action requirements and action limitations of persons who may benefit from nursing. Self-care, as a human regulatory function, is distinct from other types of regulation of human functioning and development, such as neuroendocrine regulation. Self-care must be learned and it must be performed deliberately and continuously in time and in conformity with the regulatory requirements of the individuals. These requirements are associated with their stages of growth and development, states of health, specific features of health or developmental states, levels of energy expenditure, and environmental factors. The theory of self-care is also extended to a theory of dependent care wherein the purpose, methods, and outcomes of care of others is expressed.[112]

LOGICAL FORM

Orem's insight led to her initial formalization and subsequent expression of a general concept of nursing. That generalization then made possible inductive and deductive thinking about nursing. The form of the theory is shown in the many models that Orem and others developed, such as those shown in Figures 13-1 and 13-2. Orem described the models and their importance to the development and understanding of the reality of the entities. The models are "directed toward knowing the structure of the processes that are operational or become operational in the production of nursing systems, systems of care for individuals or for dependent-care units or multiperson units served by nurses."[86:31] The overall theory is logically congruent.

ACCEPTANCE BY THE NURSING COMMUNITY

Orem's SCDNT has achieved a significant level of acceptance by the nursing community as evidenced by the magnitude of published material. Over 600 references can be found through a computerized

search dealing with a wide variety of subjects; therefore the following is only a sample of this literature. In a review of research performed using SCDNT or components, the number of studies and the quality of work has improved over time.[109] In reviewing articles referenced as self-care, the searcher is cautioned that not all references to self-care are references to Orem's Theory of Nursing. However, much research on self-care, not directly citing Orem's theory, is pertinent and contributes to the body of knowledge. The reader is also cautioned that not all uses of Orem's theory accurately reflect the most current state of theory development as expressed in the latest editions of *Nursing: Concepts of Practice*.[85,87] The SCDNT has great appeal to practicing nurses, as evidenced by the phone calls and e-mail messages and questions received through the SCDNT webpage. Orem's theory has been translated into Italian, French, Spanish, Dutch, and Japanese; currently, there are translations of some or all of her recent work in Germany, Thailand, and Norway, among others. Her work is used throughout the world. Practitioners of nursing in Great Britain, Taiwan, Thailand, Japan, Korea, Canada, Australia, New Zealand, South Africa, Israel, Germany, Spain, Italy, France, Belgium, the Netherlands, Bolivia, Colombia, Uruguay, and Mexico report use of Orem's theory.*

Practice

Nursing is a practice discipline; therefore the majority of research relates to questions of practice. There are some case studies in the literature, but many more are needed.[28,47] The first documented use of Orem's theory as the basis for structuring practice is found in descriptions of nurse-managed clinics at Johns Hopkins Hospital in 1973.[1,3] Since that time, there have been descriptions of the use of Orem's theory in a variety of clinical populations and age groups, from neonates to the elderly, for health promotion and care of the sick. The literature also includes the use of SCDNT in a number of ethnically and culturally diverse populations.[10,59,119,122] The

*References 12, 16, 43, 45, 56, 97, 98, 99, 124.

nursing management of pertussis was described from the SCDNT perspective.[60]

Research articles on the use of SCDNT or components in clinical practice include teaching self-care to individuals with diabetes mellitus and end-stage renal failure, hemodialysis and peritoneal dialysis, and renal transplant.* Pain assessment and control is another area that makes use of Orem's theory.[15,117,118] This research focuses on pain assessment and the prevention, control, and alleviation of pain. SCDNT is used frequently in cardiac research.[51,114,115] Cardiology nurses researched everything from self-care after a stroke to body image resulting from cardiac-related illnesses.[25] Oncology has used SCDNT with a focus on cancer prevention or on how to maintain self-care after being diagnosed with malignancies.† Dodd[17,18,19,20] has done extensive work on self-care and patients with cancer. Psychiatry and mental health research is primarily focused on the assessment and intervention of psychiatric disorders.[123] The development of positive mental health is described.[89] The self-care requisite of normalcy was explored with a mentally ill population.[92]

The elderly population is another area using Orem's theory. The elderly have many chronic illnesses and provide a variety of research topics, including health promotion, self-care for the independent elderly, and family caregiver stress.‡

In addition to the use of the theory for these clinical populations, it has been used in a variety of settings.[1,110,111] The Vancouver Health Department has done major work in designing community population-based care using Orem's conceptualizations.[21] Newark Beth Israel was one of the first acute-care hospitals to structure the nursing delivery and the documentation system from Orem's theory.[71] Some in occupational health nursing are basing their practice on SCDNT. There are many health hazards and job-related risk factors of which nurses must be aware. The ability to identify health problems, interpret findings, and draw correct conclusions is critical in occupational nursing.[57] Bingham-

ton General Hospital is using Orem's theory as part of the orientation process for their new graduate nurses. For new graduates, the first work experience is often the most difficult. There is some conflict with school teachings and work values. SCDNT helps assist these nurses in combining their school teachings with the nursing work that occurs after graduation.[24] Other future uses of the SCDNT will be on user-friendly, intuitive, computerized information systems that support nursing practices in a variety of settings.[8,66]

Orem's theory has been used to define and describe various roles for nurses within multiple settings. The clinical nurse-specialist role, the case-management role, the advanced-practice role and the primary-care role are documented as having gained meaning through the application of the theory.§ The administrative role and importance of SCDNT in designing systems of care are also described.[2,11,65] There are several reports of the use of Orem's SCDNT in the development of clinical measurement approaches. Horn and Swain's study[49] was the first major work done in this area. They developed criteria measures of nursing care focused around the universal self-care requisites and health-deviation self-care requisites. Since then, a number of other clinical instruments have been developed. In 1989, Moore and Gaffney[69] developed the Dependent Care Agent (DCA) questionnaire to measure mothers' performance of self-care activities for their children. Individual requisites for self-care are evidenced in the DCA. Hayward, Kish, Frey, Kirchner, Carr, and Wolfe[46] used Orem's theory when creating the Kidney Transplant Recipient Stress Scale, which was developed to identify stressors in renal transplant recipients. Graff, Thomas, Hollingsworth, Cohen, and Rubin[32] developed a postoperative self-assessment form with Orem's concept of the nurse assisting the patient in self-care. Riley[96] developed a COPD self-care action scale. The Denyes' Self-Care Agency Instrument (DSCAI) and the Denyes' Self-Care Practice Instrument (DSCPI) are also useful in clinical practice.[13] Much of the published literature is limited to Orem's Theory of

---

*References 3, 9, 27, 55, 58, 122.
†References 33, 34, 36, 37, 47, 75, 91, 93, 94, 95, 100.
‡References 23, 41, 53, 64, 90, 101, 116.

§References 29, 48, 50, 67, 73, 113.

Self-Care and Self-Care Deficit or other components of the theory as a way to explain practice. Orem cautions that the appropriate use of the SCDNT entails the use of all three theories: (1) self-care, (2) self-care deficit, and (3) nursing systems. Supportive-educative nursing systems have been documented as effective with pregnant women, persons with advanced heart failure, and children with cancer.[39,52,70] Winters[126] examined the use meaning of one of Orem's methods of assisting; that is, maintaining a developmental environment for persons with age-related sensory losses.

Education

This theory was first articulated in the 1950s; it was formalized and first published in 1972 for the purpose of "laying out the structure of nursing knowledge and explicating the domains of nursing knowledge."[108:8] Orem began thinking about the need for a nursing-specific knowledge structure when she was director of the school at Providence Hospital in Detroit. She wrote the chapter on nursing for a report on nursing services for the Division of Hospital and Institutional Services of the Indiana State Board of Health.[77] Orem returned to Washington, DC and took a position with the Office of Education, Vocational Section of the Technical Division, which had an ongoing project to upgrade practical nurse training. At this time, she began the more formal work of structuring her theory. She concluded that the following question needed to be answered: Why do people need nursing? Some of the elements of SCDNT emerged and were recorded in *Guides for Developing Curriculum for the Education of Practical Nurses.*[78]

After the publication of the *Guides for Developing Curriculum for the Education of Practical Nurses,*[78] Orem began working on a book, *Foundations of Nursing and Its practice,*[79] which was published privately and used at Morris Harvey College (now the University of Charleston). There are sections on education in each of Orem's subsequent book publications.

There are a number of reports in the literature describing the use of SCDNT as the basis for the curriculum.[5,6,40,42,44] At least 45 schools of nursing use SCDNT as the basis for their curriculums (data from the International Orem Society). Taylor[102,103] described the use of the theory in preservice nursing education and in teaching. The Sinclair School of Nursing, University of Missouri at Columbia has used SCDNT as the framework for curriculum and teaching since 1978. The theory is used at all levels of the curriculum and in continuing education. Oakland University, College of St. Benedict, and Anderson College are three schools with curricula designed within SCDNT. Samples of their courses may be accessed through the Internet by searching for SCDNT. An elective undergraduate course, developed to introduce students to Orem's theory as described by Berbiglia and Saenz,[6] and Hartweg,[44] describes the twenty-year experience with the theory at IWU, including the basic curriculum and the changes that have been made. IWU continues to find the SCDNT a strong and effective framework for curricular design.

Research

The research related to or derived from Orem's theory can be classified as relating to: (1) the development of research instruments for measuring the conceptual elements of the theory and (2) studies that test elements of the theory in specific populations. Research that is specific to the use of the theory in clinical situations is reviewed in the previous section on practice. This chapter does not review the research literature in which the use of SCDNT or components is merely tangential.

A number of instruments for research have been developed. The first instrument to measure the exercise of self-care agency (ESCA) was published in 1979. Since then, others have been developed and critiqued.[9] The SCDNT was the conceptual groundwork for Kearney and Fleisher's ESCA[54] in 1979, DSCAI[14] in 1980, and Hanson and Bickel's Perception of Self-Care Agency[62,63] in 1981. The SCDNT was a pivotal construct in the design of the Self-As-Carer Inventory (SCI).[30] This inventory permits individuals to express their perceived capacity to care for their self. McBride[63] did a comparative analysis of three instruments designed to measure self-care agency: (1) DSCAI, (2) Kearney and Fleisher's ESCA, and (3) Hanson and Bickel's Perception of Self-Care Agency. To identify latent traits and their relationships, a common factor analysis and canonical correlation was performed. The results supported the multidimensionality of Orem's concept of self-care agency. McBride[62] also points out that the use of only one instrument does not adequately reflect this multidimensionality. Geden and Taylor[29,31] tested the construct and the empirical validity of the SCI and found that the SCI seemed to possess strong theoretical validity, but recommended further validity testing. The Appraisal of Self-Care Agency (ASA) scale was developed to measure the core concept of Orem's SCDNT.[22] There is an extensive body of literature supporting the use of ASA with well and ill populations. The research instruments used most frequently include the DSCAI,[26,27] DSCPI,[26,27] ASA,[22] and SCI.[30] Others include Maieutic Dimensions of Self-Care Agency Scale (MDSCAS)[74] and Moore and Gaffney's DCA questionnaire.[69]

Some examples of the use of these tools follow. Moore[68] used the Child and Adolescent Self-Care Practice Questionnaire, the DSCAI, and the ESCA when she measured the self-care practices of children and adolescents. McCaleb and Edgil[64] used the DCSPI to measure self-concept and self-care practices of healthy adolescents. To assess and teach self-care to youths with diabetes mellitus, Frey and Fox[27] used the DSCPI and Denyes' Health Status Instrument with the Diabetes Self-Care Practice Instrument. For evaluation of a hemodialysis patient program and support program, the ESCA was used.[58] Whetstone and Reid[125] also used the ESCA to measure health promotion in older adults and the perceived barriers. The ESCA and the ASA were used to assess basic conditioning factors and self-care abilities related to the health of pregnant women and their infants.[38,61]

FURTHER DEVELOPMENT

Since the publication of the first edition of *Nursing: Concepts of Practice*[80] in 1971, Orem has been en-

gaged in the continual development of her conceptualizations. She has performed this work by herself and with colleagues. The sixth edition was completed and published in 2001.[87] Orem is presently working with a group of scholars, known as the Orem Study Group, to further develop the various conceptualizations and to structure nursing knowledge using the elements of the theory. This work led to the expression of a theory of dependent care and the foundational science of self-care.[88,112] A number of researchers and scholars have developed SCDNT throughout the years.[16,105-107]

Like the fifth edition, the sixth edition is organized in two focuses: (1) nursing as a unique field of knowledge and (2) nursing as practical science. It includes an expansion of content on nursing science and the theory of nursing systems. There is new work on the nature of person and interpersonal features of nursing. Orem identified many areas for further development in her descriptions of the stages of theory development.[87] She also identified the development of the science of self-care, which could include concepts such as elaboration of operational functions of self-care agency with the elements of sensation and perception, appraisal, and motivation, and determining the relevance of the foundational capabilities and dispositions to discreet acts. There is a need to focus on *person-in-the-situation* and on capabilities for *action* and *self-management*.

Allison and Renpenning[2] further developed Orem's conceptualization of nursing administration. Based on their experiences, they presented a comprehensive approach to the use of the SCDNT within a healthcare organization, including all levels of the nursing service and care delivery. Ongoing research by many nursing scholars will clarify certain conceptualizations and will demonstrate the relationship of theory and practice. Work in progress includes further development of the theory of dependent care, the use of the theory in primary care, and the development of variations in types of care systems such as the concept of collaborative care systems.[29,31] The International Orem Society for Nursing Science and Nursing Scholarship (IOS) was established in 1993. Incorporated as a not-for-profit organization, the purpose of the IOS is to advance nursing science and scholarship through the use of Dorothea E. Orem's nursing conceptualizations in nursing education, practice, and research. The IOS semiannually publishes a newsletter. Some issues can be accessed through the Internet on the Self-Care Deficit Theory home page (www.muhealth.org/nursing/scdnt/scdnt.html), which is maintained by the University of Missouri at Columbia, Sinclair School of Nursing. The Sixth International Self-Care Deficit Theory Conference, which was held in Bangkok, Thailand in February 2000, had over 300 participants from many countries. There were over 70 research presentations that demonstrated the international use of Orem's theory.

CRITIQUE
Clarity

The terms Orem uses are precisely defined. The language of the theory is consistent with the language used in action theory and philosophy. The terminology of the theory is congruent throughout. The term *self-care* has multiple meanings across disciplines; Orem has defined the term and elaborated the substantive structure of the concept in a way that is unique, but also congruent with other interpretations. There have been references to the difficulty of Orem's language; the limitation generally resides in the reader's lack of familiarity with practical science and the field of action science.

Banfield[4] and Taylor, Geden, Isaramalai, and Wongvatunyu[109] examined the philosophical basis of Orem's work. They affirmed that moderate realism is foundational to Orem's work and compatible research methods need to be used.

Simplicity

Orem's theory is expressed in a limited number of terms. These terms are defined and used consistently in the expression of the theory. Orem's general theory, SCDNT, comprises three constituent theories: (1) self-care, (2) self-care deficit, and (3) nursing systems. The self-care deficit theory of nursing is a "synthesis of knowledge about the theoretical entities self-care (and dependent-care), self-care agency

(and dependent-care agency), therapeutic self-care demand, the relational entity self-care deficit and nursing agency."[85:170]

The entity nursing system is also included. The development of the theory using these six entities is parsimonious. The relationship between and among these entities can be presented in a simple diagram. The substantive structure of the theory is found in the development of these entities. It is the depth of the concepts' development that gives the theory the complexity necessary to a practice discipline.

Generality

Orem has commented on the generality or universality of the theory:

> The self-care deficit theory of nursing is not an explanation of the individuality of a particular concrete nursing practice situation, but rather the expression of a singular combination of conceptualized properties or features common to all instances of nursing. As a general theory, it serves nurses engaged in nursing practice, in development and validation of nursing knowledge, and in teaching and learning nursing.[85:166-167]

A review of the research and other literature attests to the generality of the theory.

Empirical Precision

Orem's theory has been used for research using both qualitative and quantitative methodologies. The theoretical entities are well defined and lend themselves to measurement; however, instruments have not been developed for all entities. For example, the instrument to measure nursing agency is yet to be developed.

Furthermore, the values of the theoretical entities are not constant across populations. For example, the Theory of Self-Care Deficit is a function of the self-care requisites and basic conditioning factors. This necessitates the development of multiple instruments to measure the Theory of Self-Care Deficit. The most appropriate methods of inquiry for this theory and all nursing theories are yet to be determined. The beauty of Orem's theory is in its scope, complexity, and clinical usefulness; it is useful for generating hypotheses and adding to the body of knowledge that is nursing.

Derivable Consequences

The SCDNT differentiates the focus of nursing from other disciplines. Although other disciplines find the theory of self-care helpful and contribute to its development, the theory of nursing systems provides the unique focus for nursing. There is ample evidence in the literature that the theory is useful in developing and guiding practice and research.[104,105] It gives direction to nursing-specific outcomes related to knowing and meeting the therapeutic self-care demands, regulating the development and ESCA, and establishing self-care and self-management systems.

The theory is also useful in designing curricula for preservice, graduate, and continuing nursing education.[5,43,102,103] The theory also gives direction to nursing administration. The development of theory-based computer systems, assessment forms, and the overall structuring of the delivery of care further attests to the usefulness of the theory.[7,66,71]

The significance of Orem's work extends far beyond the development of the SCDNT. In her works, she has provided the expression of the form of nursing science as practical science with a structure for ongoing development of nursing knowledge in the stages of theory development. She has presented a visionary view of contemporary nursing practice, education, and knowledge development expressed through the general theory.

CRITICAL THINKING *Activities*

1. Orem's writings are not all expositions of the SCDNT. Review some of her writings and identify works of theory and works of application or related ideas about nursing.

2. Review the definitions provided in the glossary of the sixth edition of *Nursing: Concepts of Practice.*[87] Classify them as conceptual or operational, denotative or connotative. Explain.

3. Select a research article that purports to use SCDNT as the conceptual framework. Is the research question derived from the theory? What contribution does it make to further understanding of the theory?

4. Make a list of the definitions of nursing the theorists use. Which ones are specific to nursing? Evaluate Orem's description of the proper object of nursing. How does that relate to others?

REFERENCES

1. Allison, S.E. (1973). A framework for nursing action in a nurse conducted diabetic managed clinic. *Journal of Nursing Administration, 3*(4), 53-60.
2. Allison, S.E. & Renpenning, K. (1999). *Nursing administration in the 21st century.* Thousand Oaks, CA: Sage.
3. Backsheider, J. (1974). Self-care requirements, self-care capabilities and nursing systems in the diabetic nurse managed clinic. *American Journal of Public Health, 64*(12), 1138-1146.
4. Banfield, B. (1997). *A philosophical inquiry of Orem's self-care deficit nursing theory.* Dissertation, Wayne State University, Detroit, Michigan.
5. Berbiglia, V.A. (1991). A case study: Perspectives on a self-care deficit nursing theory-based curriculum. *Journal of Advanced Nursing, 16*(10), 1158-63.
6. Berbiglia, V.A & Saenz, J. (2000). Design, implementation, and evaluation of a self-care undergraduate elective. *The International Orem Society Newsletter, 8*(1), 2-5.
7. Bliss-Holtz, J., McLaughlin, K., & Taylor, S.G. (1990). Validating nursing theory for use within a computerized nursing information system. *Advances in Nursing Science, 13*(2), 46-52.
8. Bliss-Holtz, J., Taylor, S.G., & McLaughlin, K. (1992). Nursing theory as a base for a computerized nursing information system. *Nursing Science Quarterly, 5*(3), 124-128.
9. Bottorff, J.L. (1988). Assessing an instrument in a pilot project: The self-care agency questionnaire. *Canadian Journal of Nursing Research, 20*(1), 7-16.
10. Dashiff, C.J. (1992). Self-care capabilities in black girls in anticipation of menarche. *Health Care for Women International, 13*, 67-76.

11. Davidhizar, R. (1993). Self-care and mentors to reduce stress and enhance administrative ability. *Geriatric Nursing,* 14, 146-149.

12. Dennis, L.I. (1989). Soviet hospital nursing: A model for self-care. *Journal of Nursing Education,* 28(2), 76-77.

13. Denyes, M.J. (1980). Development of an instrument to measure self-care agency in adolescents. *Dissertation Abstracts International,* 41, 1716B.

14. Denyes, M.J. (1988). Orem's model used for health promotion: Directions from research. *Advances in Nursing,* 11(1), 13-21.

15. Denyes, M.J., Neuman, B.M., & Villarruel, A.M. (1991). Nursing actions to prevent and alleviate pain in hospitalized children. *Issues in Comprehensive Pediatric Nursing,* 14, 31-48.

16. Denyes, M.J., O'Connor, N.A., Oakley, D., & Ferguson, S. (1989). Integrating nursing theory, practice, and research through collaborative research. *Journal of Advanced Nursing,* 14(2), 141-145.

17. Dodd, M.J. (1983). Self-care for side effects of cancer chemotherapy: An assessment of nursing interventions. *Cancer Nursing,* 6(1), 63-67.

18. Dodd, M.J. (1988). Patterns of self-care in patients with breast cancer. *Western Journal of Nursing Research,* 10(1), 7-14.

19. Dodd, M.J. (1991). *Managing side effects of chemotherapy and radiation therapy for cancer: A guide for patients and families* (2nd ed.). Englewood Cliffs, NJ: Prentice Hall.

20. Dodd, M.J., Thomas, M.L., & Dibble, S.L. (1991). Self-care for patients experiencing cancer chemotherapy side effects: A concern for home care nurses. *Home Healthcare,* 9(6), 21-26.

21. Duncan, S. & Murphy, F. (1988). Embracing a conceptual model. *Canadian Nurse,* 84(4), 24-26.

22. Evers, G.C.M., Isenberg, M.A., Philipsen, H., Senten, M., & Brouns, G. (1993). Validity testing of the Dutch translation of the appraisal of the self-care agency A.S.A. scale. *International Journal of Nursing Studies,* 30(4), 331-342.

23. Fawcett, J., Ellis, V., Underwood, P., Naqvi, A., & Wilson, D. (1990). The effect of Orem's self-care model on nursing care in a nursing home setting. *Journal of Advanced Nursing,* 15, 659-666.

24. Feldsine, F.T. (1982). Options for transition into practice: Nursing process orientation program . . . bicultural approach and Orem's conceptual framework of self-care. *Journal, New York State Nurses Association,* 13(1), 11-16.

25. Folden, S.L. (1993). Effect of a supportive-educative nursing intervention on older adults' perceptions of self-care after a stroke. *Rehabilitation Nursing,* 18(3), 162-167.

26. Frey, M.A. & Denyes, M.J. (1989). Health and illness self-care in adolescents with IDDM: A test of Orem's theory. *Advanced Nursing Science,* 12(1), 67-75.

27. Frey, M.A. & Fox, M.A. (1990). Assessing and teaching self-care to youths with diabetes mellitus. *Pediatric Nursing,* 16(6), 597-599.

28. Fujita, L.Y. & Dungan, J. (1994). High risk for ineffective management of therapeutic regimen: A protocol study. *Rehabilitation Nursing,* 19(2), 75-79, 126.

29. Geden, E., Isaramalai, S., & Taylor, S.G. (2000). The value of self-care deficit nursing theory in informing the nurse practitioner's practice in primary care settings. *Nursing Science Quarterly,* 14(1): 29-33.

30. Geden, E. & Taylor, S. (1991). Construct and empirical validity of the self-as-carer inventory. *Nursing Research,* 40(1), 47-50.

31. Geden, E. & Taylor, S.G. (1999). Theoretical and empirical description of adult couples' collaborative care systems. *Nursing Science Quarterly,* 12(4), 329-334.

32. Graff, B.M., Thomas, J.S., Hollingsworth, A.O., Cohen, S.M., & Rubin, M.M. (1992). Development of a postoperative self-assessment form. *Clinical Nurse Specialist,* 6(1), 47-50.

33. Graling, P.R. & Grant, J.M. (1995). Demographics and patient treatment choice in stage I breast cancer. *AORN Journal,* 62(3), 376-384.

34. Grant, M. (1990). The effect of nursing consultation on anxiety, side effects, and self-care of patients receiving radiation therapy. *Oncology Nursing Forum,* 17(3), 31-36.

35. Gullifer, J. (1997). The acceptance of a philosophically based research culture? *International Journal of Nursing Practice,* 3, 153-158.

36. Hagoplan, G.A. (1991). The effects of a weekly radiation therapy newsletter on patients. *Oncology Nursing Forum,* 18(7), 1199-1203.

37. Hanucharurnkul, S. (1988). Predictors of self-care in cancer patients receiving radiotherapy. *Cancer Nursing,* 12(1), 21-27.

38. Hart, M.A. (1995). Orem's self-care deficit theory: Research with pregnant women. *Nursing Science Quarterly,* 8(3), 120-126.

39. Hart, M.A. & Foster, S.N. (1998). Self-care agency in two groups of pregnant women. *Nursing Science Quarterly,* 11(4), 167-171.

40. Hartweg, D.L. (1986). Self-care attitude changes of nursing students enrolled in self-care curriculum—A longitudinal study. *Research in Nursing and Health,* 9(4), 347-353.

41. Hartweg, D.L. (1990). Health promotion self-care within Orem's general theory of nursing. *Journal of Advance Nursing,* 15(1), 35-41.

42. Hartweg, D.L. (1995). Curricular decisions: Using Orem's conceptualizations to guide curriculum and student clinical practice. *International Orem Society Newsletter,* 3(1), 8-9.

43. Hartweg, D.L. (1996). Determining the adequacy of a health promotion self-care interview guide with healthy, middle-aged, Mexican-American women: A pilot study. *Health Care for Women International,* 17(1), 57-68.

44. Hartweg, D.L. (2000). Use of Orem's conceptualizations in a baccalaureate nursing program: 1980-2000. *International Orem Society Newsletter,* 8(1), 5-7.

45. Hautman, M.A. (1987). Self-care responses to respiratory illnesses among Vietnamese. *Western Journal of Nursing Research,* 9(2), 223-243.

46. Hayward, M.B., Kish, J.P., Frey, G.M., Kirchner, J.M., Carr, L.S., & Wolfe, C.M. (1989). An instrument to identify stressors in renal transplant recipients. *American Nephrology Nurses Association Journal,* 16(2), 81-84.

47. Hiromoto, B.M. & Dungan, J. (1991). Contract learning for self-care activities: A protocol study among chemotherapy outpatients. *Cancer Nursing,* 14(3), 148-154.

48. Holzemer, W.L. (1992). Linking primary health care and self-care through case management. *International Nursing Review,* 39(3), 83-89.

49. Horn, B.J. & Swain, M.A. (1977). *Development of criterion measures of nursing care* (Vols. 1 and 2). Washington, DC: National Center for Health Services Research. U.S. Department of Commerce (NTIS Publication No. 267-004 and 267-005).

50. Issel, M. (1995). Evaluating case management programs. *Maternal-Child Nursing,* 20, 67-74.

51. Jaarsma, T., Kastermans, M., Dassen, T., & Philipsen, H. (1995). Problems of cardiac patients in early recovery. *Journal of Advanced Nursing,* 21, 21-27.

52. Jaarsma, T., Halfens, R., Senten, M., Saad, H.H.A., & Dracup, K. (1998). Developing a supportive-educative program for patients with advanced heart failure within Orem's general theory of nursing. *Nursing Science Quarterly,* 11(2), 79-85.

53. Jirovec, M.M. & Kasno, J. (1993). Predictors of self-care abilities among the institutionalized elderly. *Western Journal of Nursing Research,* 15, 314-326.

54. Kearney, B. & Fleischer, B.J. (1972). Development of an instrument to measure exercise of self-care agency. *Research in Nursing Health,* 2, 25-34.

55. Keohane, N.S. & Lacey, L.A. (1991). Preparing the woman with gestational diabetes for self-care: Use of a structured teaching plan by nursing staff. *Journal of Obstetric, Gynecologic, and Neonatal Nursing,* 20(3), 189-193.

56. Kerkstra, A., Castelein, E., & Philipsen, H. (1991). Preventive home visits to elderly people by community nurses in the Netherlands. *Journal of Advanced Nursing,* 16, 631-637.

57. Komulainen, P. (1991). Occupational health nursing based on self-care theory. *AAOHN Journal,* 39(7), 333-335.

58. Korniewicz, D.M. & O'Brien, M.E. (1994). Evaluation of a hemodialysis patient education and support program. *American Nephrology Nurses Association Journal,* 21(1), 33-38.

59. Lile, J.L. & Hoffman, R. (1991). Medication-taking by the frail elderly in two ethnic groups. *Nursing Forum,* 26(4), 19-24.

60. Logue, G.A. (1997). An application of Orem's theory to the nursing management of pertussis. *Journal of School Nursing,* 13(4), 20-25.

61. Mapanga, K.G. & Andrews, C.M. (1995). The influence of family and friends' basic conditioning factors and self-care agency on unmarried teenage primiparas' engagement in contraceptive practice. *Journal of Community Health,* 12(2), 89-100.

62. McBride, S. (1987). Validation of an instrument to measure exercise of self-care agency. *Research in Nursing and Health,* 10, 311-316.

63. McBride, S. (1991). Comparative analysis of three instruments designed to measure self-care agency. *Nursing Research,* 40(1), 12-16.

64. McCaleb, A.M. & Edgil, A. (1994). Self-concept and self-care practices of healthy adolescents. *Journal of Pediatric Nursing,* 9(4), 233-238.

65. McCoy, S. (1989). Teaching self-care in a market-oriented world. *Nursing Management,* 20(5), 22-26.

66. McLaughlin, K., Taylor, S., Bliss-Holtz, J., Sayers, P., & Nickle, L. (1990). Shaping the future: The marriage of nursing theory and informatics. *Computers in Nursing,* 8(4), 174-179.

67. Mezinskis, P.M. (1998). Orem's self-care deficit theory. In A.S. Luggen (Ed.), *NGNA core curriculum for gerontological advanced practice nurses* (pp. 16-19). Thousand Oaks, CA: Sage.

68. Moore, J.B. (1995). Measuring the self-care practice of children and adolescents: Instrument development. *Maternal-Child Nursing Journal,* 23(3), 101-108.

69. Moore, J.B. & Gaffney, K.F. (1989). Development of an instrument to measure mothers' performance of self-care activities for children. *Advanced Nursing Science,* 12(1), 76-84.

70. Mosher, R.B. & Moore, J.B. (1998). The relationship of self-concept and self-care in children with cancer. *Nursing Science Quarterly,* 11(3), 116-122.

71. National League for Nursing Editorial Review Board News. (1987, Dec.). Newark Beth Israel Medical Center adopts Orem's self-care model. *Nursing and Health Care,* 8(10), 593-594.

72. Nursing Development Conference Group, Orem, D.E. (Ed.). (1972). *Concept formalization in nursing: Process and product.* Boston: Little, Brown & Co.

73. Nursing Development Conference Group, Orem, D.E. (Ed.). (1979). *Concept formalization in nursing: Process and Product* (2nd ed.). Boston: Little, Brown, & Co.

74. Norris, M.K.G. & Hill, C. (1991). The clinical nurse specialist: Developing the case manager role. *Dimensions of Critical Care Nursing,* 10(6), 346-353.

75. O'Connor, N.A. (1995). Maieutic dimensions of self-care agency: Instrument development. *Dissertation Abstracts International,* 56-05, 2563.

76. Oberst, M.T., Chang, A.S., & McCubbin, M.A. (1991). Self-care burden, stress appraisal, and mood among persons receiving radiotherapy. *Cancer Nursing,* 14(2)71-78.

77. Orem, D.E. (1956). *Hospital nursing service: An analysis.* Report to the Division of Hospital and Institutional Services of the Indiana State Board of Health. Indianapolis, IN: Division of Hospital and Institutional Services.

78. Orem, D.E. (1959). *Guides for developing curriculum for the education of practical nurses.* Washington, DC: U.S. Department of Health, Education and Welfare.

79. Orem, D.E. (1967). *Foundations of nursing and its practice.* Private Publication.

80. Orem, D.E. (1971). *Nursing: Concepts of practice.* New York: McGraw-Hill.

81. Orem, D.E. (1980). *Nursing: Concepts of practice* (2nd ed.). New York: McGraw Hill.

82. Orem, D.E. (1985). *Nursing: Concepts of practice* (3rd ed.). New York: McGraw Hill.

83. Orem, D.E. (1988, May). The form of nursing science. *Nursing Science Quarterly,* 1(2), 75-79.

84. Orem, D.E. (1991). *Nursing: Concepts of practice* (4th ed.). St. Louis, Mosby.

85. Orem, D.E. (1995). *Nursing: Concepts of practice* (5th ed.). St. Louis: Mosby.

86. Orem, D.E. (1997). Views of human beings specific to nursing. *Nursing Science Quarterly,* 10(1), 26-31.

87. Orem, D.E. (2001). *Nursing: Concepts of practice* (6th ed.). St. Louis: Mosby.

88. Orem, D.E., Denyes, M.J., & Bekel, G. (2001). Self-care: A foundational nursing science. *Nursing Science Quarterly,* 14(1), 48-54.

89. Orem, D.E. & Vardiman, E.M. (1995). Orem's nursing theory and positive mental health: Practical considerations. *Nursing Science Quarterly,* 8(4), 165-173.

90. Padula, C.A. (1992). Self-care and the elderly: Review and implications. *Public Health Nursing,* 9(1), 22-28.

91. Palmer, P. & Meyers, F.J. (1990). An outpatient approach to the delivery of intensive consolidation chemotherapy to adults with acute lymphoblastic leukemia. *Oncology Nursing Forum,* 17(4), 553-558.

92. Pickens, J. (1999). Living with serious mental illness: The desire for normalcy. *Nursing Science Quarterly,* 12(3), 233-239.

93. Rhodes, V. (1990). Nausea, vomiting, and retching. *Nursing Clinics of North America,* 25(4), 855-900.

94. Rhodes, V.A., Watson, P.M., & Hanson, B.M. (1988). Patients' descriptions of the influence of tiredness and weakness on self-care abilities. *Cancer Nursing,* 11(3), 186-194.

95. Richardson, A. (1992). Studies exploring self-care for the person coping with cancer treatment: A review. *International Journal of Nursing Studies,* 29(2), 191-204.

96. Riley, P. (1996). Development of a COPD self-care action scale. *Rehabilitation Nursing Research,* 5(1), 3-8.

97. Rodriques de la Parra, S. & Baquero, B.C. (1999). Autocuidado en el adolescente. *Revista Rol de Enfermia,* 22(4), 497-505.

98. Roy, O. & Collin, M.E.F. (1994). La personne agee atteinte de demence. *L'Infirmiere Canadienne,* 90(1), 39-43.

99. Rueda, G. (1999). Dorothea E. Orem: Aproximación a su teoría. *Revista Rol de Enfermia,* 22(4), 309-311.

100. Smith, M.C., Holcombe, J.K., & Stullenbarger, E. (1994). A meta-analysis of intervention effectiveness for symptom management in oncology nursing research. *Oncology Nursing Forum,* 21(7), 1201-1209.

101. Smits, M.W. (1992). Correlates of self-care among the independent elderly: Self-concept affects well-being. *Journal of Gerontological Nursing,* 18(9), 13-18.

102. Taylor, S.G. (1985). Curriculum development for preservice programs using Orem's theory of nursing. In J. Riehl-Sisca (Ed.), *The science and art of self-care* (pp. 25-32). Norwalk, CT: Appleton-Century-Crofts.

103. Taylor, S.G. (1985). Teaching self-care deficit theory to generic students. In J. Riehl-Sisca (Ed.), *The art and science of self-care.* New York: Appleton-Century-Crofts.

104. Taylor, S.G. (1987). Clinical decision-making from the perspective of self-care deficit theory (SCDT) (pp.78-90). In S.G. Taylor (Ed.), *Papers presented at the Sixth Annual Self-Care Deficit Nursing Theory Conference,* School of Nursing, University of Missouri-Columbia, St. Louis.

105. Taylor, S.G. (1988). Nursing theory and nursing process. *Nursing Science Quarterly,* 1(3), 111-119.

106. Taylor, S.G. (1989). The interpretation of family from the perspective of self-care deficit nursing theory. *Nursing Science Quarterly,* 2(3), 131-137.
107. Taylor, S.G. (1991). The structure of nursing diagnosis from Orem's theory. *Nursing Science Quarterly,* 4(1), 24-32.
108. Taylor, S.G. (1998). The development of self-care deficit nursing theory: An historical analysis. *International Orem Society Newsletter,* 6(2), 7-10.
109. Taylor, S., Geden, E., Isaramalai, S., & Wongvatunyu, S. (1999). Orem's self-care deficit nursing theory: Its philosophical foundation and the state of the science. *Nursing Science Quarterly,* 13(2), 104-109.
110. Taylor, S.G. & McLaughlin, K. (1991, Winter). Orem's theory and community. *Nursing Science Quarterly,* 4(4), 153-160.
111. Taylor, S.G. & Renpenning, K. (1995). The practice of nursing in multiperson situations: Family and community. In D.E. Orem (Ed.), *Nursing: Concepts of practice* (5th ed., pp. 348-380). St. Louis: Mosby.
112. Taylor, S.G., Renpenning, K., Geden, E., Neuman, B., & Hart, M. (2001). A theory of dependent care. *Nursing Science Quarterly,* 14(1), 39-47.
113. Togno-Armanasco, V.T., Olivas, G.S., & Harter, S. (1989). Developing an integrated nursing case management model. *Nursing Management,* 29(10), 26-29.
114. Utz, S.W., Hammer, J., Whitmire, V.M., & Grass, S. (1990). Perceptions of body image and health status in persons with mitral valve prolapse. *Image: Journal of Nursing Scholarship,* 22(1), 18-22.
115. Utz, S.W. & Ramos, M.C. (1993). Mitral valve prolapse and its effects: A programme of inquiry within Orem's self-care deficit theory of nursing. *Journal of Advanced Nursing,* 18, 742-751.
116. Utz, S.W., Shuster, G.F., Merwin, E., & Williams, B. (1994). A community-based smoking cessation program: Self-care behaviors and success. *Public Health Nursing,* 11(5), 291-299.
117. Vesely, C. (1995). Pediatric patient-controlled analgesia: Enhancing the self-care construct. *Pediatric Nursing,* 21(2), 124-128.
118. Villarruel, A.M. & Denyes, M.J. (1991). Pain assessment in children: Theoretical and empirical validity. *Advanced Nursing Science,* 14(2), 32-41.
119. Villarruel, A.M. & Denyes, M.J. (1997). Testing Orem's theory with Mexican Americans. *Image: Journal of Nursing Scholarship,* 29(3), 283-288.
120. Wallace, W.A. (1979). *From a realist point of view: Essays on the philosophy of science.* Washington, DC: Universal Press of America.
121. Wallace, W.A. (1996). *The modeling of nature: Philosophy of science and philosophy of nature in synthesis.* Washington, DC: The Catholic University of America Press.
122. Wang, C. (1997). The cross-cultural applicability of Orem's conceptual framework. *Journal of Cultural Diversity,* 4(2), 44-48.
123. Whall, A.L. (1994). What is the nursing treatment for depression? *Journal of Gerontological Nursing,* 42, 45.
124. Whetstone, W.R. & Hansson, A.O. (1989). Perceptions of self-care in Sweden: A cross-cultural replication. *Journal of Advanced Nursing,* 14, 962-969.
125. Whetstone, W.R. & Reid, J. (1991). Health promotion of older adults: Perceived barriers. *Journal of Advanced Nursing,* 16, 1343-1349.
126. Winters, R. (1989). Adapting the environment to age-related sensory losses. *Journal of the American Academy of Nurse Practitioners,* 1(4), 106-111.

BIBLIOGRAPHY
Primary Sources
Books

Nursing Development Conference Group, Orem, D.E. (Ed.). (1973). *Concepts formalization in nursing: Process and product.* Boston: Little, Brown, & Co.

Nursing Development Conference Group, Orem, D.E. (Ed.). (1979). *Concept formalization in nursing: Process and product* (2nd ed.). Boston: Little, Brown, & Co.

Orem, D.E. (Ed.). (1959). *Guides for developing curriculum for the education of practical nurses.* Vocational Division #274. Trade and Industrial Education #68. Washington, DC: U.S. Department of Health, Education, and Welfare.

Orem, D.E. (1971). *Nursing: Concepts of practice.* New York: McGraw-Hill.

Orem, D.E. (1980). *Nursing: Concepts of practice* (2nd ed.). New York: McGraw-Hill.

Orem, D.E. (1985). *Nursing: Concepts of practice* (3rd ed.). New York: McGraw-Hill.

Orem, D.E. (1991). *Nursing: Concepts of practice* (4th ed.). St. Louis: Mosby.

Orem, D.E. (1995). *Nursing: Concepts of practice* (5th ed.). St. Louis: Mosby.

Orem, D.E. (2001). *Nursing: Concepts of practice* (6th ed.). St. Louis: Mosby.

Orem, D.E. & Parker K.S. (Eds.). (1963). *Nurse practice education workshop proceedings.* Washington, DC: The Catholic University of America.

Orem, D.E. & Parker, K.S. (Eds.). (1964). *Nursing content in preservice nursing curriculum.* Washington, DC: The Catholic University of America Press.

Book Chapters

Orem, D.E. (1966). Discussion of paper—Another view of nursing care and quality. In K.M. Straub & K.S. Parker (Eds.), *Continuity of patient care: The role of nursing.* Washington, DC: The Catholic University of America Press.

Orem, D.E. (1969). Inservice education and nursing practice forces effecting nursing practice. In D.K. Petrowski & K.M. Staub (Eds.), *School of nursing education*. Washington, DC: The Catholic University of America Press.

Orem, D.E. (1981). Nursing: A triad of action systems. In G.E. Lasker (Ed.), *Applied systems and cybernetics. Systems research in health care, biocybernetics, and ecology* (Vol. IV). New York: Pergamon Press.

Orem, D.E. (1982). Nursing: A dilemma for higher education. In Sister A. Power (Ed.), *Words commemorated: Essays celebrating the centennial of Incarnate Word College*. San Antonio, TX: Incarnate Word College.

Orem, D.E. (1983). The self-care deficit theory of nursing: A general theory. In I. Clements & F. Roberts (Eds), *Family health: A theoretical approach to nursing care*. New York: Wiley Medical Publications.

Orem, D.E. (1984). Orem's conceptual model and community health nursing. In M.K. Asay & C.C. Ossler (Eds.), *Proceedings of the Eighth Annual Community Health Nursing Conference: Conceptual models of nursing applications in community health nursing*. Chapel Hill, NC: University of North Carolina, Department of Public Health Nursing, School of Public Health.

Orem, D.E. & Taylor, S. (1986). Orem's general theory of nursing. In P. Winstead-Fry (Ed.), *Case studies in nursing theory* (pp. 37-71). Pub. No. 15-2152. New York: National League for Nursing.

Orem, D.E. (1988). Nursing administration: A theoretical approach. In B. Henry, C. Arndt, M. DiVincenti, & A. Marriner Tomey (Eds.), *Dimensions of nursing administration*. Boston: Blackwell Scientific.

Orem, D.E. (1990). A nursing practice theory in three parts, 1956-1989. In M.E. Parker (Ed.), *Nursing theories in practice*. New York: National League for Nursing.

Journal Articles

Orem, D.E. (1962, Jan.). The hope of nursing. *Journal of Nursing Education*, 1, 5.

Orem, D.E. (1979, March). Levels of nursing education and practice. *Alumnae Magazine*, 68, 2-6.

Orem, D.E. (1985, May/June). Concepts of self-care for the rehabilitation client. *Rehabilitation Nursing*, 10(3), 33-36.

Orem, D.E. (1988, May). The form of nursing science. *Nursing Science Quarterly*, 1(2), 75-79.

Orem, D.E. (1997). Views of human beings specific to nursing. *Nursing Science Quarterly*, 10(1), 26-31.

Orem, D.E., Denyes, M.J., & Bekel, G. (2001). Self-care: A foundational nursing science.*Nursing Science Quarterly*, 14(1), 48-54.

Orem, D.E. & O'Malley, M. (1952, Aug.). Diagnosis of hospital nursing problems. *Hospitals*, 26, 63.

Orem, D.E. & Vardiman, E. (1995, Winter). Orem's nursing theory and positive mental health: Practical considerations. *Nursing Science Quarterly*, 8(4), 165-173.

Reports

Orem, D.E. (1955). *Indiana hospitals: A report. Author of three sections of 10-year report of status and problems of Indiana hospitals*. Indianapolis, IN: Indiana State Board of Health.

Orem, D.E. (1956). *Hospital nursing service: An analysis and report of a study of administrative positions in one hospital nursing service*. Indianapolis, IN: Indiana State Board of Health.

Orem, D.E., Dear, M., & Greenbaum, J. (1976). *Organization of nursing faculty responsibilities* (Project Report, Public Health Service Grant No. 03D-005-3666). Washington, DC: Georgetown University School of Nursing.

Audiotape

Orem, D.E. (1978, Dec.). *Paper presented at the Second Annual Nurse Educator Conference, New York* [Audiotape]. Available: Teach 'em, Inc., 160 E. Illinois Street, Chicago, IL 60611.

Videocassettes/Laser Disk

Fawcett, J. (1988). *The nurse theorists. Portraits of excellence: Dorothea Orem* [Videotape]. Available: Fuld Video Project, Studio III, 370 Hawthorne Avenue, Oakland, CA 94609.

Fawcett, J. (1992). *Excellence in action: Dorothea Orem* [Videotape]. Oakland, CA: Studio III. Available: Fuld Video Project, Studio III, 370 Hawthorne Avenue, Oakland, CA 94609.

Fawcett, J. (1997). *Dorothea Orem: Self-care framework* [Videotape]. Athens, OH: FITNE, Inc.

National League for Nursing. (1987). *Nursing theory: A circle of knowledge* [Videotape]. Available: The author, 10 Columbus Circle, New York, NY 10019.

Secondary Sources
Book Reviews

[Review of the book *Nursing: Concepts of practice*]. (1971, Dec.). *Canadian Nurse*, 67, 47.

[Review of the book *Nursing: Concepts of practice*]. (1972, Jan.). *Supervisor Nurse*, 3, 45-46.

[Review of the book *Nursing: Concepts of practice*]. (1972, July). *American Journal of Nursing*, 72, 1330.

[Review of the book *Nursing: Concepts of practice* (2nd ed.)]. (1980, Nov.). *Registered Nurse Association of British Columbia*, 12, 25.

[Review of the book *Nursing: Concepts of practice* (2nd ed.)]. (1981, Oct.). *AORN Journal*, 24, 776.

[Review of the book *Nursing: Concepts of practice* (2nd ed.)]. (1982, Oct.). *Nursing Times*, 78, 1671.

[Review of the book *Nursing: Concepts of practice* (2nd ed.)]. (1983, Jan.). *Journal of Advanced Nursing*, 8(1), 89.

Dissertations (since 1990)

Aish, A.E. (1993). An investigation of a nursing system to support nutritional self-care in post myocardial infarction patients. *Dissertation Abstracts International,* 53, 362B.

Alfred, N. (1990). Effect of a health promotion program on self-care agency of children. *Dissertation Abstracts International,* 51, 3777B.

Anderson, J.A.M. (1996). Basic conditioning factors, self-care agency, self-care, and well-being in homeless adults. *Dissertation Abstracts International,* 57, 2473B.

Baiardi, J.M. (1997).The influence of health status, burden, and degree of cognitive impairment on the self-care agency and dependent-care agency of caregivers of elders. *Dissertation Abstracts International,* 58, 5885B.

Baker, L.K. (1991). Predictors of self-care in adolescents with cystic fibrosis: A test and explication of Orem's theories of self-care and self-care deficit. *Dissertation Abstracts International,* 53, 1290B.

Baker, S.P. (1993). The relationship of self-care agency and self-care actions to caregivers' strain as perceived by female family caregivers of elderly parents. *Dissertation Abstracts International,* 54, 1884B.

Banfield, B.E. (1997). A philosophical inquiry of Orem's Self-Care Deficit Nursing Theory. *Dissertation Abstracts International,* 58, 5885B.

Beatty, E.R. (1991). Locus-of-control, self-actualization and self-care agency among registered nurses. *Dissertation Abstracts International,* 52, 3523B.

Beecroft, P.C. (1990). The effects of cognitive restructuring and assertion skills training on the self-efficacy and self-care agency of adolescents undergoing hemodialysis. *Dissertation Abstracts International,* 51, 5243B.

Bennett, J.A. (1994). The effects of empathy, knowledge, and attitudes about AIDS care: An exploration of Orem's concept of nursing agency using propositions from Travelbee's theory of interpersonal relations in nursing. *Dissertation Abstracts International,* 54, 4598B.

Bess, C.J. (1995). Abilities and limitation of adult type II diabetic patients with integrating of self-care practices into their daily lives. *Dissertation Abstracts International,* 56, 3688B.

Brown, K.L.G. (1996). Grief as a basic conditioning factor affecting the self-care agency and self-care of family caregivers of persons with neurotrauma. *Dissertation Abstracts International,* 57, 7447B.

Budd, S.P. (1992). Women's health study: Self-efficacy and the rehabilitation experiences. *Dissertation Abstracts International,* 53, 12913B.

Burkett, M.T.E. (1991). Relationships among reminiscence, self-esteem, and physical functioning in older African-American women. *Dissertation Abstracts International,* 51, 3318B.

Canty, J.L. (1993). An investigation of life change events, hope, and self-care agency in inner city adolescents. *Dissertation Abstracts International,* 54, 2992B.

Carroll, D.L. (1993). Recovery in the elderly after coronary artery bypass surgery. *Dissertation Abstracts International,* 54, 2992B.

Chen, Y.M. (1996). Relationships among health control orientation, self-efficacy, self-care, and subjective well-being in the elderly with hypertension. *Dissertation Abstracts International,* 57, 3652B.

Cofield, N.A. (1991). Effect of a health promotion program on self-care agency of children. *Dissertation Abstracts International,* 51, 3777B.

Cull, V.V. (1995). Exposure to violence and self-care practices of adolescents. *Dissertation Abstracts International,* 56, 3690B.

Cunningham, G.D. (1990). Health promoting self-care behaviors in the community older adult. *Dissertation Abstracts International,* 50, 4968B.

Cutler, C.G. (1998). The relationship of self-care agency, self-efficacy, and social support to post-hospitalization adjustment of patients with a mood disorder. *Dissertation Abstracts International,* 59, 0600B.

Demasters, J.J. (1999). Women and the hormone replacement therapy decision: A study of concerns, values, and behaviors using a multiattribute utility model. *Dissertation Abstracts International,* 59, 5784B.

Dennis, C. (1998). Self-care agency, learned helplessness, and health status in elderly adults. *Dissertation Abstracts International,* 59, 1582B.

Dowd, T.T. (1994). Relationship among health state factors, foundational capabilities, and urinary incontinence self-care in women. *Dissertation Abstracts International,* 55, 1376B.

Emerson, E.A. (1992). Playing for health: The process of play and self-expression in children who have experienced a sexual trauma. *Dissertation Abstracts International,* 53, 2784B.

Folden, S.L. (1990). The effect of supportive-educative nursing interventions on poststroke older adults' self-care perceptions. *Dissertation Abstracts International,* 52, 159B.

Fordham, P.N. (1990). A Q analysis of nursing behaviors which facilitate the grief work of parents with a premature infant in a neonatal intensive care unit. *Dissertation Abstracts International,* 51, 661B.

Freeman, E.M. (1992). Self-care agency in gay men with HIV infection. *Dissertation Abstracts International,* 53, 3400.

Fuller, F.J. (1992). Health of elderly male dependent-care agents for a spouse with Alzheimer's disease. *Dissertation Abstracts International,* 53, 4589B.

Gallegos, E.C. (1997). The effect of social, family and individual conditioning factors on self-care agency and self-care of adult Mexican women. *Dissertation Abstracts International,* 58, 5889B.

Good, M.P.L. (1992). Comparison of the effects of relaxation and music on post-operative pain. *Dissertation Abstracts International,* 53, 1783B.

Greenfield, P.H. (1990). A comparison of the self-care ability of employed women who have and have not maintained weight loss. *Dissertation Abstracts International,* 50, 3398B.

Haas, D.L. (1991). The relationship between coping dispositions and power components of dependent-care agency in parents of children with special health care needs. *Dissertation Abstracts International,* 52, 1351B.

Harris, J.L. (1990). Self-care actions of chronic schizophrenics associated with meeting solitude and social interaction self-care requisites. *Dissertation Abstracts International,* 50, 3920B.

Hart, M.A. (1993). Self-care agency and prenatal care actions: Relationships to pregnancy outcomes. *Dissertation Abstracts International,* 55, 364B.

Hartweg, D.L. (1991). Health promotion self-care actions of healthy, middle-aged women. *Dissertation Abstracts International,* 52, 6316B.

Horsburgh, M.E. (1994). The contribution of personality to adult well-being: A test and explication of Orem's theory of self-care. *Dissertation Abstracts International,* 56, 1346B.

Huddleston, D.S.T. (1991). *Determinants of self-care response patterns of perimenopausal women.* Unpublished doctoral dissertation, University of Illinois at Chicago, Health Sciences Center.

Humphrey, J.C. (1990). Dependent-care directed toward the prevention of hazards to life, health, and well-being in mothers and children who experience family violence. *Dissertation Abstracts International,* 51, 1744B.

Hurst, J.D. (1991). The relationship among self-care agency, risk-taking, and health risks in adolescents. *Dissertation Abstracts International,* 52, 1352B.

Jackson, E.M. (1991). Dimensions of nursing home care. *Dissertation Abstracts International,* 53, 865A.

James, K.S. (1991). Factors related to self-care agency and self-care practices of obese adolescents. *Dissertation Abstracts International,* 52, 1955B.

Jesek-Hale, S.R. (1994). Self-care agency and self-care pregnant adolescents: A test of Orem's theory. *Dissertation Abstracts International,* 56, 173B.

Keatley, V.M. (1998). Critical incident stress in generic baccalaureate students. *Dissertation Abstracts International,* 59, 2124B.

Kennedy, L.M. (1991). The effectiveness of a self-care medication education protocol on the home medication behaviors of recently hospitalized elderly. *Dissertation Abstracts International,* 51, 3779B.

Kerschbaumer, R.M. (1994). An educational model for nursing and midwifery education in Malawi, Central Africa. *Dissertation Abstracts International,* 54, 6134B.

Kleinbeck, S.V.M. (1996). Postdischarge surgical recovery of adult laparoscope outpatients. *Dissertation Abstracts International,* 57, 989B.

Koster, M.K. (1995). A comparison of the relationship among self-care agency, self-determinism, and absenteeism in two groups of school-age children. *Dissertation Abstracts International,* 56, 541B.

Lee, M.B. (1996). Power, self-care, and health in women living in urban squatter settlements in Karachi, Pakistan: A test of Orem's theory. *Dissertation Abstracts International,* 57, 7451B.

Mapanga, K.G. (1994). The influence of family and friends' basic conditioning factors, and self-care agency on unmarried teenage primiparas' engagement in contraceptive practice. *Dissertation Abstracts International,* 55, 5285B.

McCaleb, K.A. (1991). Self-concept and self-care practices of health adolescents. *Dissertation Abstracts International,* 52, 3529B.

McDermott, M.A.N. (1990). The relationship between learned helplessness and self-care agency in adults as a function of gender and age. *Dissertation Abstracts International,* 50, 3403B.

McQuiston, C.M. (1993). Basic conditioning factors and self-care agency of unmarried women at risk for sexually transmitted disease. *Dissertation Abstracts International,* 53, 368B.

Metcalfe, S.A. (1997). Self-care actions as a function of the therapeutic self-care demand and self-care agency in individuals with chronic obstructive pulmonary disease. *Dissertation Abstracts International,* 57, 7453B.

Morgan, M.J. (1998). Self-care agency in people with end-stage renal disease. *Dissertation Abstracts International,* 59, 1048B.

Neuman, B. (1996). Relationship between children's descriptions of pain, self-care, and dependent-care and basic conditioning factors of development, gender, and ethnicity: "Bears in my throat." *Dissertation Abstracts International,* 57, 2482B.

Nicolas, P.K. (1991). Hardiness, self-care practices, and perceived health status in the elderly. *Dissertation Abstracts International,* 52, 1957B.

O'Connor, N.A. (1995). Maieutic dimensions of self-care agency: Instrument development. *Dissertation Abstracts International,* 56, 2563B.

Ortiz-Martinez, M.A. (1994). The self-care model for nursing in Puerto Rico: A cross-cultural study of the implementation of change. *Dissertation Abstracts International,* 56, 3696B.

Patterson, D.L.F. (1992). Self-care of menstrual health in collegiate athletes. *Dissertation Abstracts International,* 53, 5647B.

Pavlides, C.C. (1993). The relationship among complexity of medication, functional ability, and adherences to prescribed medication regimen in the homebound older adult. *Dissertation Abstracts International,* 54, 1336B.

Pettine, A. (1995). Development of self-care: A problem for elementary-age children? *Dissertation Abstracts International*, 56, 3479B.

Pressly, K.B. (1994). Relationship of psychosocial characteristics and the occurrence of infectious complications in continuous ambulatory peritoneal dialysis patients. *Dissertation Abstracts International*, 54, 50095B.

Ransom, J.E. (1988). Factors related to safer sex behaviors in young college students. *Dissertation Abstracts International*, 59, 2126B.

Renker, P.R. (1998). Physical abuse, social support, self-care agency, self-care practices, and late adolescent pregnancy outcomes. *Dissertation Abstracts International*, 58, 5891B.

Robinson, M.K. (1996). Determinants of functional status in chronically ill adults. *Dissertation Abstracts International*, 56, 5424B.

Rowles, C.J. (1993). The relationship of selected personal and organizational variables and the tenure of directors of nursing in nursing homes. *Dissertation Abstracts International*, 53, 4593B.

Rozmus, C.L. (1991). A description of the maternal decision-making process regarding circumcision. *Dissertation Abstracts International*, 51, 3787B.

Schlatter, B.L. (1991). Control and satisfaction with the birth experience. *Dissertation Abstracts International*, 52, 164B.

Schmidt, C.A. (1997). Mothers' views concerning the development of self-care agency in school-age children with diabetes. *Dissertation Abstracts International*, 59, 0162B.

Schott-Baer, D. (1991). Family culture, family resources, dependent care, care-giver burden and self-care agency of spouses of cancer patients. *Dissertation Abstracts International*, 51, 3327B.

Simmons, S.J. (1990). Self-care agency and health-promoting behavior of a military population. *Dissertation Abstracts International*, 51, 22900B.

Slusher, I.L. (1994). Self-care agency and self-care practice of adolescent primiparas during the in-hospital post-partum period. *Dissertation Abstracts International*, 55, 3240B.

Sonninen, A. L. (1997). Testing reliability and validity of the Finnish version of the appraisal of self-care agency (ASA) scale with elderly Finns. *Dissertation Abstracts International*, 60, 0604C.

Spezia, M.A. (1991). Family responses and self-care activities in school-age children with diabetes. *Dissertation Abstracts International*, 52, 2997B.

Stonebraker, D.H. (1991). The relationship between self-care agency, self-care, and health in the pregnant adolescent. *Dissertation Abstracts International*, 53, 2789B.

St. Onge, J.L. (1990). The relationship of self-care agency to health-seeking behaviors in Caucasian and Black U.S. veterans. *Dissertation Abstracts International*, 50, 3926B.

Tiansawad, S. (1995). Self-care abilities and practices for prevention of HIV infection among rural Thai women who attended mobile family planning clinic. *Dissertation Abstracts International*, 55, 3241B.

Urbancic, J.C. (1992). The relationship between empowerment support, motivation, for self-care, mental health self-care, well-being, and incest trauma resolution in adult female survivors. *Dissertation Abstracts International*, 54, 1896B.

Vannoy, B.E. (1990). Relationships among basic conditioning factors, motivational dispositions, and the power elements of self-care agency in people beginning a weight loss program. *Dissertation Abstracts International*, 51, 1197B.

Villarruel, A.M. (1993). Mexican-American cultural meanings, expressions, self-care and dependent-care actions associated with experiences of pain. *Dissertation Abstracts International*, 55, 372B.

Vogt, C.A. (1995). A comparison of educational models in determining patients' knowledge and behaviors concerning advance directives. *Dissertation Abstracts International*, 55, 3843B.

Wang, H.H. (1998). A model of self-care and well-being of rural elderly women in Taiwan. *Dissertation Abstracts International*, 59, 2689B.

West, P.P. (1993). The relationship between depression and self-care agency in young adult women. *Dissertation Abstracts International*, 55, 372B.

Zehnder, N.R. (1996). The influence of basic conditioning factors on menopausal self-care agency and menopausal self-care in midlife women. *Dissertation Abstracts International*, 57, 7460B.

Books

Chinn, P.L. & Jacobs, M.K. (1987). *Theory and nursing: A systematic approach.* St. Louis: Mosby.

Dennis, C.M. (1997). *Self-care deficit nursing theory: Concepts and applications.* St. Louis: Mosby.

Fawcett, J. (2000). *Analysis and evaluation of contemporary nursing knowledge: Nursing models and theories.* Philadelphia: F.A. Davis.

Fitzpatrick, J. & Whall, A. (1983). *Conceptual models of nursing: Analysis and application.* Bowie, MD: Robert J. Brady.

Fitzpatrick, J.J., Whall, A.L., Johnston, R.L., & Floyd, J.A. (1982). *Nursing models and their psychiatric mental health applications.* Bowie, MD: Robert J. Brady.

Hartweg, D.L. (1991). *Dorothea Orem: Self-care deficit theory.* Thousand Oaks, CA: Sage Publications.

Horn, B.J. & Swain, M.A. (1977). *Development of criterion measures of nursing care* (Vols. 1 and 2, NTIS Publication No. 267-004 and 267-005). Washington, DC: National Center for Health Services Research, U.S. Department of Commerce.

Kin, H.S. (1983). *The nature of theoretical thinking in nursing.* Norwalk, CT: Appleton-Century-Crofts.

Leddy, S. & Pepper, J.M. (1985). *Conceptual bases of professional nursing*. Philadelphia: J.B. Lippincott.

Meleis, A.J. (1997). *Theoretical nursing: Development and progress* (3rd ed.). Philadelphia: J.B. Lippincott.

National League for Nursing. (1978). *Theory development: What, why, how?* (Publication No. 15-1708, pp. 73-74). New York: National League for Nursing.

Nursing Theories Conference Group, J.B. George (Chairperson). (1980). *Nursing theories: The base for professional practice*. Englewood Cliffs, NJ: Prentice Hall.

Parker, M.E. (1990). *Nursing theories in practice*. New York: National League for Nursing.

Parse, R.R. (1987). *Nursing science*. Philadelphia: W.B. Saunders.

Polit, D.F. & Hungler, B.P. (1987). *Nursing research principles and methods* (3rd ed.). Philadelphia: J.B. Lippincott.

Torres, G. (1986). *Theoretical foundations of nursing*. Norwalk, CT: Appleton-Century-Crofts.

Winstead-Fry, P. (1986). *Case studies in nursing theory*. New York: National League for Nursing.

Book Chapters

Berbiglia, V.A. (1997). Orem's self-care deficit theory in nursing practice. In M.R. Alligood & A. Marriner Tomey (Eds.), *Nursing theory: Utilization and application* (pp. 129-152). St. Louis: Mosby.

Calley, J.M., Dirksen, M., Engalla, M., & Hennrich, M.L. (1980). The Orem self-care nursing model. In J.P. Riehl & C. Roy (Eds.), *Conceptual models for nursing practice* (pp. 302-314). New York: Appleton-Century-Crofts.

Coleman, L.J. (1980). Orem's self-care nursing model. In J.P. Riehl & C. Roy (Eds.), *Conceptual models for nursing practice* (pp. 315-328). New York: Appleton-Century-Crofts.

Fawcett, J. (1984). Orem's self-care model. In J. Fawcett (Ed.), *Analysis and evaluation of conceptual models in nursing* (pp. 175-210). Philadelphia: F.A. Davis.

Fawcett, J. (2000). Orem's self-care framework. In J. Fawcett (Ed.), Analysis and evaluation of contemporary nursing knowledge (pp. 259-360). Philadelphia: F.A. Davis.

Foster, P.C. & Janssens, N.P. (1980). Dorothea E. Orem. In Nursing Theories Conference Group, J.B. George (Chairperson), *Nursing theories: The base for professional practice* (pp. 91-106). Englewood Cliffs, NJ: Prentice-Hall.

Goldstein, N., Zink, M., Stevenson, L., Anderson, M., Woolery, L., & DePompdo, T. (1983). Self-care: A framework for the future. In P.L. Chinn (Ed.), *Advances in nursing theory development* (pp. 107-121). Rockville, MD: Aspen Systems.

Horn, B.J. (1978). Development of criterion measures of nursing care (abstract). In *Communicating nursing research: New approaches to communicating nursing research* (Vol. 11). Boulder, CO: Western Interstate Commission for Higher Education.

Horn, B.J. & Swain, M.A. (1976). An approach to development of criterion measures for quality patient care. In *Issues in evaluation research*. Kansas City, MO: American Nurses Association.

Johnston, R.L. (1982). Individual psychotherapy: Relationships of theoretical approaches to nursing conceptual models. In J. Fitzpatrick, A. Whall, R. Johnston, & J. Floyd, (Eds.), *Nursing models and their psychiatric mental health applications* (pp. 56-60). Bowie, MD: Robert J. Brady.

Johnston, R.L. (1983). Orem self-care model of nursing. In J. Fitzpatrick & A. Whall (Eds.), *Conceptual models of nursing, analysis and application* (pp. 137-156). Bowie, MD: Robert J. Brady.

Kinlein, M.L. (1977). *Independent nursing practice with clients* (pp. 15-24). Philadelphia: J.B. Lippincott.

Meleis, A.I. (1985). Dorothea Orem. In A.I. Meleis (Ed.), *Dorothea Orem* (pp. 284-296). Philadelphia: J.B. Lippincott.

Mezinskis, P.M. (1998). Orem's self-care deficit theory. In A.S. Luggen, (Ed.), *NGNA core curriculum for gerontological advance practice nurses* (pp. 16-19). Thousand Oaks, CA: Sage.

Roy, C. (1980). A case study viewed according to different models. In J.P. Riehl & C. Roy (Eds.), *Conceptual models for nursing practice* (pp. 385-386). New York: Appleton-Century-Crofts.

Spangler, Z.S. & Spangler, W.O. (1983). Self-care: A testable model. In P.L. Chinn (Ed.), *Advances in nursing theory development* (pp. 89-105). Rockville, MD: Aspen Systems.

Stanton, M. (1980). Nursing theories and the nursing process. In Nursing Theories Conference Group, J.B. George (Chairperson), *Nursing theories: The base for professional practice* (pp. 213-217). Englewood Cliffs, NJ: Prentice Hall.

Sullivan, T.J. (1980). Self-care model for nursing. In *Directions for nursing in the 80's*. Kansas City, MO: American Nurses Association.

Taylor, S.G. (1990). Nursing practice applications of self-care deficit nursing theory. In M. Parker (Ed.), *Nursing theories in practice* (pp. 61-70). New York: National League for Nursing.

Taylor, S.G. & Renpenning, K. (1995). Nursing in multiperson situations: Family and community. In D.E. Orem (Ed.), *Nursing: Concepts of practice* (5th ed., pp. 348-380). St. Louis: Mosby.

Thibodeau, J.A. (1983). An eclectic model: The Orem model. In J.A. Thibodeau (Ed.), *Nursing models: Analysis and evaluation* (pp. 125-140). Monterey, CA: Wadsworth Health Sciences Division.

Underwood, P.R. (1980). Facilitating self-care. In P. Potheir (Ed.), *Psychiatric nursing: A basis text*. Boston: Little, Brown.

Other Resources

Copies of papers presented at the Fifth, Sixth, and Seventh Annual Self-Care Deficit Nursing Theory Conferences and the First, Second, Third, and Fourth International Self-Care Deficit Nursing Theory Conferences are available. These include papers by Orem and others.

Also available are introductory videotapes. Order from the University of Missouri-Columbia, Sinclair School of Nursing, Nursing Outreach and Distance Education, S266 School of Nursing Building, Columbia, MO 65211, (573) 882-0216.

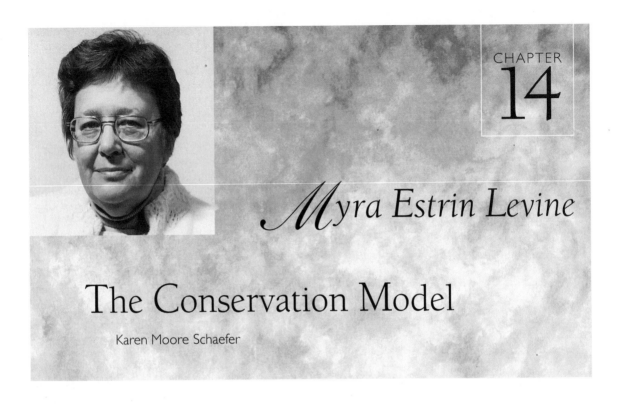

Myra Estrin Levine

The Conservation Model

Karen Moore Schaefer

CREDENTIALS AND BACKGROUND OF THE THEORIST

Myra Estrin Levine[32] obtained a diploma from Cook County School of Nursing in 1944, an S.B. from the University of Chicago in 1949, an M.S.N. from Wayne State University in 1962, and she has taken postgraduate courses at the University of Chicago. Hutchins' curriculum was being taught to undergraduate students at the University of Chicago. All students took a year-long survey in the biological, physical, and social sciences and the humanities. The students read and analyzed primary work under the guidance of distinguished professors. Irene Beland became Levine's mentor during her graduate studies at Wayne State and she directed Levine's attention to many of the authors who greatly influenced Levine's thinking.[34,36,50]

Previous authors: Karen Moore Schaefer, Gloria S. Artigue, Karen J. Foli, Tamara Johnson, Ann Marriner Tomey, Mary Carolyn Poat, LaDema Poppa, Roberta Woeste, and Susan T. Zoretich.

Levine has enjoyed a varied career. She has been a private duty nurse (1944), a civilian nurse in the U.S. Army (1945), a preclinical instructor in the physical sciences at Cook County (1947 to 1950), the director of nursing at Drexel Home in Chicago (1950 to 1951), and a surgical supervisor at both the University of Chicago Clinics (1951 to 1952) and Henry Ford Hospital in Detroit (1956 to 1962). Levine worked her way up the academic ranks at Bryan Memorial Hospital in Lincoln, Nebraska (1951), Cook County School of Nursing (1963 to 1967), Loyola University (1967 to 1973), Rush University (1974 to 1977), and the University of Illinois (1962 to 1963, 1977 to 1987). She chaired the Department of Clinical Nursing at Cook County School of Nursing (1963 to 1967) and coordinated the graduate nursing program in oncology at Rush University (1974 to 1977). Levine[33] was the director of the Department of Continuing Education at Evanston Hospital (March to June 1974) and a consultant to the department (July 1974 to 1976). She was an adjunct associate professor of Humanistic Studies at the University of Illinois (1981 to 1987). In 1987, she became a Professor Emerita, Medical Surgical Nursing, at the University of Illinois at Chicago. In 1974, Levine went to Tel-Aviv University, Israel, as a visiting associate professor and returned as a visiting professor in 1982. She was also a visiting professor at Recanati School of Nursing, Ben Gurion University of the Negev, at Beer Sheva, Israel (March to April, 1982).[39]

Levine has received numerous honors, including charter fellow of the American Academy of Nursing (1973), honorary member of the American Mental Health Aid to Israel (1976), and honorary recognition from the Illinois Nurses' Association (1977). She was the first recipient of the Elizabeth Russell Belford Award for excellence in teaching from Sigma Theta Tau (1977). Both the first and second editions of her book *Introduction to Clinical Nursing*[28,29] received *American Journal of Nursing* Book of the Year awards and her 1971 book, *Renewal for Nursing,*[27] was translated into Hebrew.[27,32] Levine[32,37] was listed in *Who's Who in American Women* (1977 to 1988) and in *Who's Who in American Nursing* (1987). She was elected fellow of the Institute of Medicine of Chicago (1987 to 1991). The Alpha Lambda Chapter of Sigma Theta Tau recognized Levine for her outstanding contributions to nursing in 1990. In January 1992, she was awarded an honorary doctorate of humane letters from Loyola University, Chicago.[43,46] Levine was an active leader in the American Nurses Association and the Illinois Nurses' Association. After her retirement in 1987, she remained active in theory development and encouraged questions and research about her theory.[49,51]

A dynamic speaker, she was a frequent presenter on programs, workshops, seminars, and panels and a prolific writer regarding nursing and education. Levine[44,47] has also served as a consultant to hospitals and schools of nursing. Although she never intended to develop theory, she provided an organizational structure for teaching medical-surgical nursing and a stimulus for theory development. "The Four Conservation Principles of Nursing"[23] was the first statement of the conservation principles. Other preliminary work included "Adaptation and Assessment: A Rationale for Nursing Intervention,"[22] "For Lack of Love Alone,"[24] and "The Pursuit of Wholeness."[25] The first edition of her book using the conservation principles, *Introduction to Clinical Nursing,*[28] was published in 1969. She addressed the consequences of the four conservation principles in "Holistic Nursing."[26] The second edition of *Introduction to Clinical Nursing*[29] was published in 1973. Since then, Levine[30,31] has presented the conservation principles at nurse theory conferences, some of which have been audiotaped, and at the Allentown College of St. Francis de Sales Conferences in April 1984.

In 1989, substantial change and clarification about her theory was published in her chapter "Four Conservation Principles: Twenty Years Later" in Riehl's book *Conceptual Models for Nursing Practice.*[40] Levine elaborates on how redundancy characterizes availability of adaptive responses when stability is threatened. Adaptation processes establish a body economy to safeguard the individual's stability. The outcome of adaptation is conservation.

In 1991, she explicitly linked health to the process of conservation to clarify that the Conservation Model views health as one of its essential components.[42] Conservation, through treatment, focuses on integrity and the reclamation of oneness of the whole person.

Levine died on March 20, 1996 at the age of 75. She leaves a legacy as an educator, scholar, administrator, student, wife, mother, friend, and nurse.[53] Just before her untimely death, she had the opportunity to assure her colleagues that spirituality was an implicit part of personhood and essential to the maintenance of personal integrity.[47]

THEORETICAL SOURCES

From Beland's presentation of the theory of specific causation and multiple factors, Levine learned historical viewpoints of diseases and learned that the way people think about disease changes over time.[2] Beland directed Levine's attention to numerous authors who became influential in Levine's thinking, including Kurt Goldstein, Edward T. Hall, Sir Arthur Sherrington, and Rene Dubos.[7,8,14,15,62] Levine uses

James E. Gibson's definition of perceptual systems, Erik Erikson's differentiation between total and whole, Hans Selye's stress theory, and M. Bates' models of external environment.[1,9,10,13,61] Levine was proud that Martha Rogers was her first editor.[34,36,57] She acknowledged Nightingale's contribution to her thinking about the "guardian activity" of observation used by nurses to "save lives and increase health and comfort."[45:42]

USE OF EMPIRICAL EVIDENCE

Levine believed that specific nursing activities could be deducted from scientific principles. The scientific theoretical sources have been well researched. She based much of her work on accepted science principles.[35,38]

MAJOR CONCEPTS & DEFINITIONS

The three major concepts of the Conservation Model are wholeness, adaptation, and conservation.

WHOLENESS (HOLISM)

"Whole, health, hale are all derivations of the Anglo-Saxon word *hal*."[30] Levine based her use of wholeness on Erikson's description of wholeness as an open system. Levine[9:92,25:94,31] quotes Erikson, who states, "Wholeness emphasizes a sound, organic, progressive, mutuality between diversified functions and parts within an entirety, the boundaries of which are open and fluent." Levine[49] believed that Erikson's definition set up the option of exploring the parts of the whole to understand the whole. Integrity means the oneness of the individuals, emphasizing that they respond in an integrated, singular fashion to environmental challenges.

ADAPTATION

"Adaptation is a process of change whereby the individual retains his integrity within the realities of his internal and external environment."[29:11,36] Conservation is the outcome. Some adaptations are successful and some are not. Adaptation is a matter of degree, not an all-or-nothing process.[29,36] There is no such thing as maladaptation.

Levine[43] speaks of three characteristics of adaptation: (1) historicity, (2) specificity, and (3) redundancy. Levine[43:5] states, " . . . every species has fixed patterns of responses uniquely designed to ensure success in essential life activities, demonstrating that adaptation is both historical and specific." In addition, adaptive patterns may be hidden in the individual's genetic code. Redundancy represents the fail-safe options available to individuals to ensure adaptation. Loss of redundant choices either through trauma, age, disease, or environmental conditions makes it difficult for the individual to maintain life. Levine[43:6] suggests "the possibility exists that aging itself is a consequence of failed redundancy of physiological and psychological processes."

Environment

Environment is "where we are constantly and actively involved."[39] The person and his or her relationship to the environment is what counts.[32]

Levine also views each individual as having his or her own environment, both internally and externally. Nurses can relate the internal environment as the physiological and pathophysiological aspects of the patient. Levine uses Bates' definition of the external environment[1] and suggests three levels: (1) perceptual, (2) operational, and (3) conceptual. These levels give dimension to the interactions between individuals and their environments. The perceptual level includes the aspects of the world that individuals are able to intercept and interpret with their sense organs. The operational level contains things that affect individuals physically although they cannot directly perceive them, such as microorganisms. At the conceptual level,

MAJOR CONCEPTS & DEFINITIONS—cont'd

the environment is constructed from cultural patterns, characterized by a spiritual existence, and mediated by the symbols of language, thought, and history.[29]

Organismic Response

The capacity of the individual to adapt to his or her environmental condition is called the organismic response. It can be divided into four levels of integration: (1) fight or flight, (2) inflammatory response, (3) response to stress, and (4) perceptual awareness. Treatment focuses on the management of these responses to illness and disease.[29]

Fight or Flight The most primitive response is the fight or flight syndrome. The individual perceives that he or she is threatened, whether or not a threat actually exists. Hospitalization, illness, and new experiences elicit a response. The individual responds by being on the alert to find more information and to ensure his or her safety and well being.[29]

Inflammatory Response This defense mechanism protects the self from insult in a hostile environment. It is a way of healing. The response uses available energy to remove or keep out unwanted irritants or pathogens. It is limited in time because it drains the individual's energy reserves. Environmental control is important.[29]

Response to Stress Selye[61] described the stress response syndrome to predictable, nonspecifically induced organismic changes. The wear and tear of life is recorded on the tissues and reflects long-term hormonal responses to life experiences that cause structural changes. It is characterized by irreversibility and influences the way patients respond to nursing care.

Perceptual Awareness This response is based on the individual's perceptual awareness. It occurs only as the individual experiences the world around him or her. The individual uses this response to seek and maintain safety. It is information seeking.[23,24]

Trophicognosis

Levine recommended trophicognosis as an alternative to nursing diagnosis. It is a scientific method to reach a nursing care judgment.[21]

CONSERVATION

Conservation is from the Latin word *conservatio*, meaning to keep together.[17,29,30] "Conservation describes the way complex systems are able to continue to function even when severely challenged."[41:192] Through conservation, individuals are able to confront obstacles, adapt accordingly, and maintain their uniqueness. "The goal of conservation is health and the strength to confront disability" as " . . . the rules of conservation and integrity hold" in all situations where nursing is required.[22,42:193-195,49] The primary focus of conservation is keeping together of the wholeness of the individual. Although nursing interventions may deal with one particular conservation principle, nurses must also recognize the influence of the other conservation principles.[41,42]

Levine's model[29] stresses nursing interactions and interventions that are intended "to keep together the unique and individual resources that each individual brings to his predicament." Those interactions are based on the scientific background of the conservation principles. Conservation focuses on achieving a balance of energy supply and demand within the biological realities unique to the individual. Nursing care is based on scientific knowledge and nursing skills. There are four conservation principles.

Conservation Principles

The goals of the Conservation Model are achieved through interventions that attend to the conservation principles.

Conservation of Energy The individual requires a balance of energy and a constant renewal of energy to maintain life activities. Processes such as healing and aging challenge that energy. This sec-

Continued

MAJOR CONCEPTS & DEFINITIONS—cont'd

ond law of thermodynamics applies to everything in the universe, including people.

Conservation of energy has long been used in nursing practice even with the most basic procedures. Nursing interventions "scaled to the individual's ability are dependent upon providing care that makes the least additional demand possible."[42:197,198]

Conservation of Structural Integrity Healing is a process of restoring structural and functional integrity in defense of wholeness.[41] The disabled are guided to a new level of adaptation.[49] Nurses can limit the amount of tissue involved in disease by early recognition of functional changes and by nursing interventions.

Conservation of Personal Integrity Self-worth and a sense of identity are important. The most vulnerable become patients. This begins with the

erosion of privacy and the creation of anxiety. Nurses can show patients respect by calling them by name, respecting their wishes, valuing personal possessions, providing privacy during procedures, supporting their defenses, and teaching them. "The nurse's goal is always to impart knowledge and strength so that the individual can resume a private life—no longer a patient, no longer dependent."[41:199] The sanctity of life is manifested in all people. "The conservation of personal integrity includes recognition of the holiness of each person."[48:40]

Conservation of Social Integrity Life gains meaning through social communities and health is socially determined. Nurses fulfill professional roles, provide for family members, assist with religious needs, and use interpersonal relationships to conserve social integrity.[24,25,36]

MAJOR ASSUMPTIONS

Introduction to Clinical Nursing[29] is a text for beginning nursing students that uses the conservation principles as an organizing framework. Although not specifically stated as assumptions, Levine[29:151] values "a holistic approach to care of all people, well or sick." Her respect for the individuality of each person is noted in the following statements: "Ultimately, decisions for nursing interventions must be based on the unique behavior of the individual patient" and "Patient centered nursing care means individualized nursing care . . . and as such he requires a unique constellation of skills, techniques, and ideas designed specifically for him."[29:6]

Schaefer[60] identified the following statements as assumptions about the model:

1. The person can only be understood in the context of his or her environment.[29]
2. "Every self-sustaining system monitors its own behavior by conserving the use of the resources required to define its unique identity."[43:4]
3. Human beings respond in a singular, yet integrated, fashion.[26]

Nursing

Levine stated the following about nursing: "Nursing is a human interaction."[29:1] "Professional nursing should be reserved for those few who can complete a graduate program as demanding as that expected of professionals in any other discipline. . . . There will be very few professional nurses."[20:214] "Nursing practice—and this includes the teaching of nurses—has always mirrored prevailing theories of health and disease."[19,23:240,44] "It is the nurse's task to bring a body of scientific principles, on which decisions depend, into the precise situation which she shares with the patient. Sensitive observation and the selection of relevant data form the basis for her assessment of his nursing requirements."[22:2452] "The nurse participates actively in every patient's enironment and much of what she does supports his adjustments as he struggles in the predicament of illness."[22:2452] The essence of Levine's theory[22:2453,29:13,36] is that "when nursing intervention influences adaptation favorably, or toward renewed social well-being, then the nurse is acting in a therapeutic sense; when the response is unfavorable, the nurse provides supportive care." "The goal of nursing is to promote adaptation and maintain wholeness."[26:258]

Person

Person is described as a holistic being; wholeness is integrity.[43] Integrity means that the person has freedom of choice and movement. The person has a sense of identity and self-worth. Levine[43:8-9] also described person as a "system of systems, and in its wholeness expresses the organization of all the contributing parts." Persons experience life as change through adaptation with the goal of conservation. According to Levine,[40:326] "The life process is the process of changes."

Health

Health is socially determined by the ability to function in a reasonably normal manner.[25] Health is predetermined by social groups and it is not just an absence of pathological conditions. Health is the return to self; individuals are free and able to pursue their own interests within the context of their own resources. Levine[48] stressed, "It is important to keep in mind that health is also culturally determined—it is not an entity on its own, but rather a definition imparted by the ethos and beliefs of the groups to which individuals belong." Even for a single individual, the definition of health will change over time.

Environment

Environment is the "context in which we live our lives."[34] It is not a passive backdrop. "We are active participants in it."[34]

THEORETICAL ASSERTIONS

Levine's work was intended to provide an organizational structure for teaching medical-surgical nursing rather than to develop theory; therefore she did not explicitly identify theoretical assertions. Although many theoretical assertions can be generated from her work, the four major assertions follow:

1. "Nursing intervention is based on the conservation of the individual patient's energy"[23:49,29:13]

2. "Nursing intervention is based on the conservation of the individual patient's structural integrity."[23:56,29:13]

3. Nursing intervention is based on the conservation of the individual patient's personal integrity."[23:56,29:13]

4. "Nursing intervention is based on the conservation of the individual patient's social integrity."[24:57,29:14]

LOGICAL FORM

Levine primarily uses deductive logic. In developing her model, Levine integrates theories and concepts from the humanities and the sciences of nursing, physiology, psychology, and sociology. She uses the information to analyze nursing practice situations and describe nursing skills and activities. With the assistance of many of her students and colleagues and through her own personal health encounters, she has experienced the Conservation Model and its principles operating in practice.

ACCEPTANCE BY THE NURSING COMMUNITY

Practice

Levine helps define what nursing is by identifying the activities it encompasses and giving the scientific principles behind them. Conservation principles as a framework are not limited to nursing care in the hospital, but can be generalized and used in every environment, hospital, or community.[42,43] Conservation principles, levels of integration, and other concepts can be used in numerous contexts.[41] Hirschfeld[17] has used the principles of conservation in the care of the older adult. Savage and Culbert[58] used the Conservation Model to establish a plan of care for infants. Dever[6] based her care of children on the Conservation Model. Roberts, Fleming, and Yeates-Giese[56] designed interventions for women in labor on the basis of the Conservation Model. Mefford[52] tested a Theory of Health Promotion for Preterm Infants derived from Levine's Conservation Model of Nursing and found a significant inverse relationship between the consistency of caregiver and the age at which the infant achieved health and an inverse relationship between the use of resources by preterm infants during the initial hospital stay and the consistency of caregivers. Cooper[5] developed a framework for wound care focusing on structural integrity while integrating all the integrities. Webb[65] used the Conservation Model to provide care for patients undergoing cancer treatment. Roberts, Brittin, Cook, and deClifford[54,55] used the Conservation Model to study the boomerang pillow technique effect on respiratory capacity. Taylor[63] used them to measure the outcomes of nursing care and used them again in her textbook, *Neurological Dysfunction and Nursing Interventions.*[64] Jost[18] used the model to develop an assessment of the needs of staff during the experience of change.

Conservation principles have been used as frameworks for numerous practice settings in cardiology, obstetrics, gerontology, acute care (neurology), pediatrics, long-term care, emergency care, primary care, neonatology, critical care areas, and in the homeless community.[58,59]

Education

Levine wrote *Introduction to Clinical Nursing,*[29] a textbook for beginning students that introduced new material into the curricula. She presented an early discussion of death and dying and believed that women should be awakened after a breast biopsy and consulted about the next step.[29,34,36]

Introduction to Clinical Nursing[29] provides an organizational structure for teaching medical-surgical nursing to beginning students. In both the 1969 and 1973 editions, Levine presents a model at the end of each of the first nine chapters.[28,29] Each model contains objectives, essential science concepts, and nursing process to give nurses a foundation for nursing activities. These models are not part of the Conservation Model. The Conservation Model is addressed in the Introduction and in Chapter 10 of the introductory text. The teachers' manual that accompanies the text remains a timely source of educational principles that may be helpful to both beginning teachers and seasoned teachers who may benefit from a review of educational roots.[34]

Critics argue that, although the text is labeled introductory, a beginning student would need a fairly extensive background in physical and social science to use it.[3] A critic of the second edition suggests that the emphasis of scientific principles is a definite strength, but the text's weakness is that it does not present adequate examples of pathological profiles when disturbances are discussed.[4] For this reason, this one reviewer recommends that the text be used as a supplementary or complementary text, not a primary text.[4]

Hall[16] indicates that Levine's model is used as a curriculum model. More recently, the model has been successfully integrated into undergraduate and graduate curricula. Several graduate students have used Levine's model for theses and dissertations.[34,46,47,52,59]

Research

Fitzpatrick and Whall[12:115] state, "All in all, Levine's model served as an excellent beginning. Its contribution has added a great deal to the overall development of nursing knowledge." However, Fawcett[11:208] states that to establish credibility, "more systematic evaluations of the use of the model in various clinical situations are needed, as are studies that test conceptual-theoretical-empirical structures directly derived from or linked with the conservation principles." Many research questions can be generated from Levine's model. Several graduate students have used the conservation principles as a framework for their research.[36,47]

FURTHER DEVELOPMENT

Levine and others have worked on using the conservation principles as the basis of a taxonomy of nursing diagnosis. However, further development of this concept has been deferred since the American Nurses Association took over nursing diagnosis in 1992.[46] Additional work has been done on use of Levine's Model in administration and with the frail elderly. Most recently, the model was used to develop a Theory of Health Promotion in Preterm Infants.[52] It has great potential for studies of sleep disorders and in the development of collaborative and primary care practices.

CRITIQUE
Clarity

Levine's model possesses clarity. Fitzpatrick and Whall[12] believe that Levine's work is both internally and externally consistent. Fawcett[11:208] states that "Levine's Conservation Model provides nursing with a logically congruent, holistic view of the person." The model has numerous terms; however, Levine adequately defines them for clarity.

Simplicity

Although the four conservation principles appear simple initially, they contain subconcepts and multiple variables. Nevertheless, this model is still one of the simpler ones that have emerged.

Generality

The four conservation principles can be used in all nursing contexts.

Empirical Precision

Levine used deductive logic to develop her model, which can be used to generate research questions. As she lived her conservation model, she verified the use of inductive reasoning to further develop and inform her model.[41]

Derivable Consequences

Although some authors question the level of contribution Levine's model provides, the four conservation principles are recognized as one of the earliest nursing models. Furthermore, it has continued to have utility for nursing practice and research and is receiving increased recognition in this twenty-first century.

CRITICAL THINKING *Activities*

1. Keep a reflective journal about a personal health or illness experience or that of someone very close. Reflect on the experience and its consistency with the Conservation Model. Consider how to modify, expand, or delimit the model to better provide a context in which to explain the experience.

2. Levine[47:41] stated, "Every ethnic group defines health and illness in context of its cherished beliefs." Visit a nearby museum and evaluate how artistic expression captures the beliefs of different ethnic groups. Explore how these beliefs may shape the definitions of health and compare it with Levine's approach to health and illness. On the basis of the ethnically derived definition of health, propose ethnically appropriate interventions using Levine's conservation principles.

3. Watch the movie *City of Joy*. Use examples from the movie to support or refute the propositional statements that Levine made about the environment and the relationships with person, nursing, and health and illness.

REFERENCES

1. Bates, M. (1967). A naturalist at large. *Natural History,* 76(6), 8-16.
2. Beland, I. (1971). *Clinical nursing: Pathophysiological and psychosocial implications* (2nd ed.). New York: Macmillan.
3. [Review of the book *Introduction to clinical nursing*]. (1970, Jan.). *Canadian Nurse,* 66, 42.
4. [Review of the book *Introduction to clinical nursing* (2nd ed.)]. (1974, May). *Canadian Nurse,* 70, 39.
5. Cooper, D.H. (1990). Optimizing wound healing: A practice within nursing domains. *Nursing Clinics of North America,* 25(1), 165-180.
6. Dever, M. (1991). Care of children. In K.M. Schaefer & J.B. Pond (Eds.), *The conservation model: A framework for nursing practice* (pp. 71-82). Philadelphia: F.A. Davis.
7. Dubos, R. (1961). *Mirage of health.* Garden City, NY: Doubleday.
8. Dubos, R. (1965). *Man adapting.* New Haven, CT: Yale University Press.
9. Erikson, E.H. (1964). *Insight and responsibility.* New York: W.W. Norton.
10. Erikson, E.H. (1968). *Identity: Youth and crisis.* New York: W.W. Norton.

11. Fawcett J. (1995). Levine's conservation model. In J. Fawcett (Ed.), *Analysis and evaluation of conceptual models of nursing* (pp. 165-215). Philadelphia: F.A. Davis.

12. Fitzpatrick, J.J. & Whall, A.L. (1983). *Conceptual models of nursing: Analysis and application.* Bowie, MD: Robert J. Brady.

13. Gibson, J.E. (1966). *The senses considered as perceptual systems.* Boston: Houghton Mifflin.

14. Goldstein, K. (1963). *The organism.* Boston: Beacon Press.

15. Hall, E.T. (1966). *The hidden dimension.* Garden City, NY: Doubleday.

16. Hall, K.V. (1979). Current trends in the use of conceptual frameworks in nursing education. *Journal of Nursing Education,* 18(4), 26-29.

17. Hirschfeld, M.J. (1976). The cognitively impaired older adult. *American Journal of Nursing,* 76, 1981-1984.

18. Jost, S.G. (2000). An assessment and intervention strategy for managing. *Journal of Nursing Administration,* 30(1), 34-40.

19. Levine, M.E. (1963). Florence Nightingale: The legend that lives. *Nursing Forum,* 2(4), 24-35.

20. Levine, M.E. (1965, June). The professional nurse and graduate education. *Nursing Science,* 3, 206.

21. Levine, M.E. (1966). Trophicognosis: An alternative to nursing diagnosis. *American Nurses Association Regional Clinical Conferences,* 2, 55-70.

22. Levine, M.E. (1966, Nov.). Adaptation and assessment: A rationale for nursing intervention. *American Journal of Nursing,* 66, 2450.

23. Levine, M.E. (1967). The four conservation principles of nursing. *Nursing Forum,* 6, 45.

24. Levine, M.E. (1967, Dec.). For lack of love alone. *Minnesota Nursing Accent,* 39, 179.

25. Levine, M.E. (1969, Jan.). The pursuit of wholeness, *American Journal of Nursing,* 69, 93.

26. Levine, M.E. (1971, June). Holistic nursing. *Nursing Clinics of North America,* 6, 253.

27. Levine, M.E. (1971). *Renewal for nursing.* Philadelphia: F.A. Davis.

28. Levine, M.E. (1969). *Introduction to clinical nursing.* Philadelphia: F.A. Davis.

29. Levine, M.E. (1973). *Introduction to clinical nursing* (2nd ed.). Philadelphia: F.A. Davis.

30. Levine, M.E. (1978). *Nursing theory.* [Audiotape]. Paper presented at the Second Annual Nurse Educators' Conference, New York.

31. Levine, M.E. (1984, April). *A conceptual model for nursing: The four conservation principles.* Proceedings from Allentown College of St. Francis Conference.

32. Levine, M.E. (1984). Curriculum vitae.

33. Levine, M.E. (1984). Personal correspondence.

34. Levine, M.E. (1984). Telephone interviews.

35. Levine, M.E. (1985). Personal correspondence.

36. Levine, M.E. (1985). Telephone interviews.

37. Levine, M.E. (1988). Curriculum vitae.

38. Levine, M.E. (1988). Personal correspondence.

39. Levine, M.E. (1988). Telephone interviews.

40. Levine, M.E. (1989). The four conservation principles: Twenty years later. In J. Riehl (Ed.), *Conceptual models for nursing practice* (3rd ed., pp. 325-337). New York: Appleton-Century-Crofts.

41. Levine, M.E. (1989). Personal communication via letter.

42. Levine, M.E. (1990). Conservation and integrity. In M. Parker (Ed.), *Nursing theories in practice* (pp. 189-201). New York: National League for Nursing.

43. Levine, M.E. (1991). The conservation principles: A model for health. In K. Schaefer & J. Pond (Eds.), *Levine's conservation model: A framework for nursing practice* (pp. 1-11). Philadelphia: F.A. Davis.

44. Levine, M.E. (1992). Curriculum vitae.

45. Levine, M.E. (1992). Nightingale redux. In B.S. Barnum (Ed.), *Nightingale's notes on nursing* (pp. 39-43). Philadelphia: J.B. Lippincott.

46. Levine, M.E. (1992). Personal correspondence.

47. Levine, M.E. (1992). Telephone interviews.

48. Levine, M.E. (1995). Personal correspondence.

49. Levine, M.E. (1996). The conservation principles: A retrospective. *Nursing Science Quarterly,* 9(1), 38-41.

50. Levine, M.E. & Levine, E.B. (1965, Dec.). Hippocrates: Father of nursing too. *American Journal of Nursing,* 65, 86.

51. *The nursing theorist: Portraits of excellence: Myra Levine* [Videotape]. (1988). Oakland, CA: Studio III.

52. Mefford, L.C. (2000). *The relationships of nursing care to health outcomes of preterm infants: Testing a theory of health promotion for preterm infants based on Levine's Conservation Model.* Unpublished doctoral dissertation, University of Tennessee, Knoxville.

53. Pond, J.B. (1996). Myra Levine, nurse educator and scholar dies. *Nursing Spectrum,* 5(8), 8.

54. Roberts, K.L., Brittin, M., Cook, M., & deClifford, J. (1994). Boomerang pillows and respiratory capacity. *Clinical Nursing Research,* 3(2), 157-165.

55. Roberts, K.L., Britton, M., & deClifford, J. (1995). Boomerang pillows and respiratory capacity in frail elderly women. *Clinical Nursing Research,* 4(4), 465-471.

56. Roberts, J.E., Fleming, N., & Yeates-Giese, D. (1991). Perineal integrity. In K.M. Schaefer & J.B. Pond (Eds.), *The conservation model: A framework for nursing practice* (pp. 61-70). Philadelphia: F.A. Davis.

57. Rogers, M.E. (1970). *An introduction to the theoretical basis of nursing.* Philadelphia: F.A. Davis.

58. Savage, T.A. & Culbert C. (1989). Early intervention: The unique role of nursing. *Journal of Pediatric Nursing,* 4(5), 339-345.
59. Schaefer, K.M. & Pond, J.B. (Eds.) (1991). *Levine's conservation model: A framework for nursing practice.* Philadelphia: F.A. Davis.
60. Schaefer, K.M. (1996). Levine's Conservation Model: Caring for women with chronic illness. In P.H. Walker & B. Neuman (Eds.), *Blueprint for use of nursing models: Education, research, practice and administration.* New York: National League for Nursing.
61. Selye, H. (1956). *The stress of life.* New York: McGraw-Hill.
62. Sherrington, A. (1906). Integrative function of the nervous system. New York: Charles Scribner's Sons.
63. Taylor, J.W. (1974). Measuring the outcomes of nursing care. *Nursing Clinics of North America,* 9, 337-348.
64. Taylor, J. & Ballenger, S. (1980). *Neurological dysfunction and nursing interventions.* New York: McGraw-Hill.
65. Webb, H. (1993). Holistic care following a palliative Hartmann's procedure. *British Journal of Nursing,* 2(2), 128-132.

BIBLIOGRAPHY
Primary Sources
Books

Levine, M.E. (1969). *Introduction to clinical nursing.* Philadelphia: F.A. Davis.
Levine, M.E. (1971). *Renewal for nursing.* Philadelphia: F.A. Davis. (Translated into Hebrew, Am Oved, Jerusalem, 1978.)
Levine, M.E. (1973). *Introduction to clinical nursing* (2nd ed.). Philadelphia: F.A. Davis.

Book Chapters

Levine, M.E. (1964). Nursing service. In M. Leeds & H. Shore (Eds.), *Geriatric institutional management.* New York: G.J.P. Putnam & Sons.
Levine, M.E. (1972). Benoni. *American Journal of Nursing,* 72(3), 466-468.
Levine, M.E. (1973). Adaptation and assessment: A rationale for nursing intervention. In M.E. Hardy (Ed.), *Theoretical foundations for nursing.* New York: Irvington.
Levine, M.E. (1988). Myra Levine. In T.M. Schorr & A. Zimmerman (Eds.), *Making choices, taking chances: Nursing leaders tell their stories.* St. Louis: Mosby.
Levine, M.E. (1989). The four conservation principles: Twenty years later. In J. Riehl (Ed.), *Conceptual models for nursing practice* (3rd ed.). New York: Appleton-Century-Crofts.
Levine, M.E. (1990). Conservation and integrity. In M. Parker (Ed.), *Nursing theories in practice* (pp. 189-201). New York: National League for Nursing.
Levine, M.E. (1991). The conservation principles: A model for health. In K. Schaefer & J. Pond (Eds.), *Levine's conservation model: A framework for nursing practice* (pp. 1-11). Philadelphia: F.A. Davis.
Levine, M.E. (1992). Nightingale redux. In B.S. Barnum (Ed.), *Nightingale's notes on nursing: Commemorative edition with commentaries by nursing theorists.* Philadelphia: J.B. Lippincott.
Levine, M.E. (1994). Some further thoughts on nursing rhetoric. In J.F. Kikuchi & H. Simmons (Eds.), *Developing a philosophy of nursing* (pp. 104-109). Thousand Oaks, CA: Sage.

Journal Articles

Levine, M.E. (1963). Florence Nightingale: The legend that lives. *Nursing Forum,* 2(4), 24-35.
Levine, M.E. (1964, Feb.). Not to startle, though the way were steep. *Nursing Science,* 2, 58-67.
Levine, M.E. (1964, Dec.). There need be no anonymity. *First,* 18(9), 4.
Levine, M.E. (1965). Trophicognosis: An alternative to nursing diagnosis. *ANA Regional Clinical Conferences,* 2, 55-70.
Levine, M.E. (1965, June). The professional nurse and graduate education. *Nursing Science,* 3, 206-214.
Levine, M.E. (1966, Nov.). Adaptation and assessment: A rationale for nursing intervention. *American Journal of Nursing,* 66(11), 2450-2453.
Levine, M.E. (1967). The four conservation principles of nursing. *Nursing Forum,* 6, 45-59.
Levine, M.E. (1967, May). Medicine-nursing dialogue belongs at patient's bedside. *Chart,* 64(5), 136-137.
Levine, M.E. (1967, July). This I believe: About patient-centered care. *Nursing Outlook,* 15, 53-55.
Levine, M.E. (1967, Dec.). For lack of love alone. *Accent,* 39(7), 179-202.
Levine, M.E. (1968, Feb.). Knock before entering personal space bubbles (part 1). *Chart,* 65(2), 58-62.
Levine, M.E. (1968, March). Knock before entering personal space bubbles (part 2). *Chart,* 65(3), 82-84.
Levine, M.E. (1968, April). The pharmacist in the clinical setting: A nurse's viewpoint. *American Journal of Hospital Pharmacy,* 25(4), 168-171. (Also translated into Japanese and published in Kyushu National Hospital Magazine for Western Japan.)
Levine, M.E. (1969). Nursing for the 21st century. *National Student Association.*
Levine, M.E. (1969, Jan.). The pursuit of wholeness. *American Journal of Nursing,* 69, 93-98.
Levine, M.E. (1969, Feb.). Constructive student power. *Chart,* 66(2), 42FF.
Levine, M.E. (1969, Oct.). Small hospital—Big nursing. *Chart,* 66, 265-269.
Levine, M.E. (1969, Nov.). Small hospital—Big nursing. *Chart,* 66, 310-315.

Levine, M.E. (1970). Dilemma. *ANA Clinical Conferences*, 338-342.

Levine, M.E. (1970, April). Breaking through the medications mystique. *American Journal of Hospital Pharmacy*, 27(4), 294-299; *American Journal of Nursing*, 70(4), 799-803.

Levine, M.E. (1970, July/Dec.). Symposium on a drug compendium: View of a nursing educator. *Drug Information Bulletin*, 133-135.

Levine, M.E. (1970, Oct.). The intransigent patient. *American Journal of Nursing*, 70, 2106-2111.

Levine, M.E. (1971, May). Consider implications for nursing in the use of physician's assistant. *Hospital Topics*, 49, 60-63.

Levine, M.E. (1971, June). Holistic nursing. *Nursing Clinics of North America*, 6, 253-264.

Levine, M.E. (1971, June). The time has come to speak of health care. *AORN Journal*, 13, 37-43.

Levine, M.E. (1972). Benoni. *American Journal of Nursing*, 72(3), 466-468.

Levine, M.E. (1972). Nursing educators—An alienating elite? *Chart*, 69(2), 56-61.

Levine, M.E., Moschel, P., Taylor, J., & Ferguson, G. (1972, March). Nursing grand rounds: Complicated case of CVA. *Nursing '72*, 2(3), 3-34.

Levine, M.E., Line, L., Boyle, A., & Kopacewski, E. (1972, May). Nursing grand rounds: Insulin reactions in a brittle diabetic, *Nursing '72*, 2(5), 6-11.

Levine, M.E., Scanlon, M., Gregor, P., King, R., & Martin, N. (1972, June). Issues in rehabilitation: The quadriplegic adolescent. *Nursing '72*, 2, 6.

Levine, M.E., Zoellner, J., Ozmon, B., & Simunek, E. (1972, Sept.). Nursing grand rounds: Severe trauma, *Nursing '72*, 2(9), 33-38.

Levine, M.E., Hallberg, C., Kathrein, M., & Cox, R. (1972, Oct.). Nursing grand rounds: Congestive failure. *Nursing '72*, 2(10), 18-23.

Levine, M.E. (1973). On creativity in nursing. *Image*, 3(3), 15-19.

Levine, M.E. (1973, Nov.). A letter from Myra, *Chart*, 70(9).

Levine, M.E. (1974, Oct.). The pharmacist's clinical role in interdisciplinary care: A nurse's viewpoint. *Hospital Formulary Management*, 9, 47.

Levine, M.E. (1975, Jan./Feb.). On creativity in nursing. *Nursing Digest*, 3, 38-40.

Levine, M.E. (1977, May). Nursing ethics and the ethical nurse. *American Journal of Nursing*, 77, 845-849.

Levine, M.E. (1978, June). Cancer chemotherapy: A nursing model. *Nursing Clinics of North America*, 13(2), 271-280.

Levine, M.E. (1978, July). Kapklavoo and nursing, too [Editorial]. *Research in Nursing and Health*, 1(2), 51.

Levine, M.E. (1978, Nov.). Does continuing education improve nursing practice? *Hospitals*, 52(21), 138-140.

Levine, M.E. (1979). Knowledge base required by generalized and specialized nursing practice. *ANA Publications*, (G-127), 57-69.

Levine, M.E. (1980). The ethics of computer technology in health care. *Nursing Forum*, 19(2), 193-198.

Levine, M.E. (1982, March/April). Bioethics of cancer nursing. *Rehabilitation Nursing*, 7, 27-31, 41.

Levine, M.E. (1982, March/April). The bioethics of cancer nursing. *Journal of Enterostomal Therapy*, 9, 11-13.

Levine, M.E. (1988, Feb.). Antecedents from adjunctive disciplines: Creation of nursing theory. *Nursing Science Quarterly*, 1(1), 16-21.

Levine, M.E. (1988, June). What does the future hold for nursing? 25th Anniversary Address, 18th District. *Illinois Nurses Association Newsletter*, XXIV(6), 1-4.

Levine, M.E. (1989). Beyond dilemma. *Seminars in Oncology Nursing*, 5, 124-128.

Levine, M.E. (1989). The ethics of nursing rhetoric. *Image: The Journal of Nursing Scholarship*, 21(1), 4-5.

Levine, M.E. (1989). Ration or rescue: The elderly in critical care. *Critical Care Nursing*, 12(1), 82-89.

Levine, M.E. (1995). The rhetoric of nursing theory. *Image: The Journal of Nursing Scholarship*, 27(1), 11-14.

Levine, M.E. (1996). On the humanities in nursing. *Canadian Journal of Nursing Research*, 27(2), 19-23.

Levine, M.E. (1996). The conservation principles: A retrospective. *Nursing Science Quarterly*, 9(1), 38-41.

Audiotapes

Levine, M.E. (1978, Dec.). *Nursing theory* [Audiotape]. Paper presented at the Second Annual Nurse Educator Conference, New York. Available: Teach 'em Inc., 160 E. Illinois Street, Chicago, IL 60611.

Levine, M.E. (1984, May). *Application-practice/research/education* [Audiotape]. Paper presented at Nursing Theory Conference, Boyle, Letoueneau Conference, Edmonton, Canada. Available: Ed Kennedy, Kennedy Recording, R.R.5, Edmonton, Alberta, Canada TSP4B7 (403-470-0013).

Videotape

Fawcett, J. (1988). *The nursing theorist: Portraits of excellence: Myra Levine* [Videotape]. Oakland: Studio III. Available: Fuld Video Project, 370 Hawthorne Avenue, Oakland, CA 94609.

Proceedings

Levine, M.E. (1976, Jan.). *On the nursing ethnic and the negative command*. Proceedings of the Intensive Conference, Faculty of the University of Illinois Medical Center. Philadelphia: Society for Health and Human Values.

Levine, M.E. (1977). *History of nursing in Illinois.* Proceedings of the Bicentennial Workshop of the University of Illinois College of Nursing. Chicago: University of Illinois Press.

Levine, M.E. (1977). *Primary nursing: Generalist and specialist education.* Proceedings of the American Academy of Nursing. Kansas City, MO: American Academy of Nursing.

Levine, M.E. (1984, April). *A conceptual model for nursing: The four conservation principles.* Proceedings for a Conference on Nursing Education, Allentown College of St. Francis de Sales, PA.

Levine, M.E. (1985). What's wrong about rights? In A. Carmi & S. Schneider (Eds.), *Proceedings of the 1st International Congress of Nursing Law and Ethics.* Berlin: Springer-Verlag.

Interviews

Levine, M.E. (1984). Telephone interviews.
Levine, M.E. (1985). Telephone interviews.
Levine, M.E. (1988). Telephone interviews.
Levine, M.E. (1992). Telephone interviews.

Correspondence

Levine, M.E. (1984). Curriculum vitae.
Levine, M.E. (1984). Personal correspondence.
Levine, M.E. (1985). Personal correspondence.
Levine, M.E. (1988). Personal correspondence.
Levine, M.E. (1992). Personal correspondence.

Secondary Sources

Book Reviews

[Review of the book *Introduction to clinical nursing*]. (1969, Sept./Oct.). *Bedside Nurse, 2,* 4.

[Review of the book *Introduction to clinical nursing*]. (1970, Jan.). *American Journal of Nursing, 70,* 99.

[Review of the book *Introduction to clinical nursing*]. (1970, Jan.). *Canadian Nurse, 66,* 42.

[Review of the book *Introduction to clinical nursing*]. (1970, Feb.). *Nursing Outlook, 18,* 20.

[Review of the book *Introduction to clinical nursing*]. (1970, Oct.). *American Journal of Nursing, 70,* 2220.

[Review of the book *Introduction to clinical nursing*]. (1971, April). *Nursing Mirror, 132,* 43.

[Review of the book *Introduction to clinical nursing*]. (1971, Nov.). *Bedside Nurse, 4,* 2.

[Review of the book *Introduction to clinical nursing*]. (1971, Dec.). *Canadian Nurse, 76,* 47.

[Review of the book *Introduction to clinical nursing*]. (1971, Dec.). *Nursing Mirror, 133,* 16.

[Review of the book *Introduction to clinical nursing*]. (1974, Feb.). *American Journal of Nursing, 74,* 347.

[Review of the book *Introduction to clinical nursing*]. (1974, May). *Canadian Nurse, 70,* 39.

[Review of the book *Introduction to clinical nursing*]. (1974, May). *Nursing Outlook, 22,* 301.

[Review of the book *Renewal for nursing*]. (1971, Aug.). *Supervisor Nurse, 2,* 68.

[Review of the book *Renewal for nursing*]. (1971, Dec.). *AANA Journal, 49,* 495.

[Review of the book *Renewal for nursing*]. (1971, Dec.). *Canadian Nurse, 67,* 47.

[Review of the book *Renewal for nursing*]. (1971, Dec.). *Nursing Mirror, 133,* 16.

Book Chapters

Fawcett, J. (1995). Levine's conservation model. In J. Fawcett (Ed.), *Analysis and evaluating of conceptual models of nursing* (pp. 165-215). Philadelphia: F.A. Davis.

Leonard, M.K. (1990). Myra Estrin Levine. In J.B. George (Ed.), *Nursing theories: The base for professional nursing practice* (pp. 181-192). Englewood Cliffs, NJ: Prentice Hall.

MacLean, S.L. (1989). Activity intolerance: Cues for diagnosis. In R.M. Carroll-Johnson (Ed.), *Classification proceedings of the eighth annual conference of North American Nursing Diagnosis Association* (pp. 320-327). Philadelphia: J.B. Lippincott.

McLane, A. (1987). Taxonomy and nursing diagnosis, a critical view. In A. McLane (Ed.). *Classification proceedings of the seventh annual conference of Nursing of North America.* St. Louis: Mosby.

Meleis, A.I. (1985). Myra Levine. In A.I. Meleis (Ed.), *Theoretical nursing: Development and progress* (pp. 275-283). Philadelphia: J.B. Lippincott.

Peiper, B.A. (1983). Levine's nursing model. In J.J. Fitzpatrick & A.L. Whall (Eds.), *Conceptual models of nursing: Analysis and application* (pp. 101-115). Bowie, MD: Robert J. Brady.

Pond, J.B. (1990). Application of Levine's conservation model to nursing the homeless community. In M.E. Parker (Ed.), *Nursing theories in practice* (pp. 203-215). New York: National League for Nursing.

Schaefer, K.M. (1990). A description of fatigue associated with congestive heart failure: Use of Levine's conservation model. In M.E. Parker (Ed.), *Nursing theories in practice* (pp. 217-237). New York: National League for Nursing.

Schaefer, K.M. (1996). Levine's conservation model: Caring for women with chronic illness. In P.H. Walker & B. Neuman (Eds.), *Blueprint for use of nursing models: Education, research, practice and administration* (pp. 187-228). New York: National League for Nursing Press.

Schaefer, K.M. (2000). Levine's Conservation Model: A model for the future of nursing. In Parker, M.E. (Ed.), *Nursing theories and nursing practice* (pp. 103-124). Philadelphia: F.A. Davis.

Books

Barnum, B.J.S. (1994). *Nursing theory: Analysis application evaluation* (4th ed.). Philadelphia: J.B. Lippincott.

Chinn, P.L. & Kramer, M.K. (1995). *Theory and nursing: A systematic approach* (4th ed.). St. Louis: Mosby.

Clark, M.J. (1992). *Nursing in the community.* Norwalk, CN: Appleton & Lange.

Dubos, R. (1961). *Miracle of health.* Garden City, NY: Doubleday.

Dubos, R. (1965). *Man adapting.* New Haven, CT: Yale University Press.

Erikson, E.H. (1964). *Insight and responsibility.* New York: W.W. Norton.

Erikson, E.H. (1968). *Identity: Youth and crisis.* New York: W.W. Norton.

Gibson, J.E. (1966). *The senses considered as perceptual systems.* Boston: Houghton Mifflin.

Goldstein, K. (1963). *The organism.* Boston: Beacon Press.

Griffith-Kenney, J.W. & Christensen, P. (1986). *Nursing process: Application of theories, frameworks, and models* (pp. 6, 24-25), St. Louis: Mosby.

Hall, E. (1966). *The hidden dimension.* Garden City, NY: Doubleday.

Rogers, M.E. (1970). *An introduction to the theoretical basis of nursing.* Philadelphia: F.A. Davis.

Selye, H. (1956). *The stress of life.* New York: McGraw-Hill.

Sherrington, A. (1906). *Integrative function of the nervous system.* New York: Charles Scribner & Sons.

Taylor, J. & Ballenger, S. (1980). *Neurological dysfunction and nursing interventions.* New York: McGraw-Hill.

Journal Articles

Bates, M. (1967). A naturalist at large. *Natural History,* 76(6), 8-16.

Brunner, M. (1985). A conceptual approach to critical care nursing using Levine's model. *Focus on Critical Care,* 12(2), 39-40.

Bunting, S.M. (1988, Nov.). The concept of perception in selected nursing theories. *Nursing Science Quarterly,* 1(4), 168-174.

Cooper, D.M. (1990, March). Optimizing wound healing: A practice within nursing's domain. *Nursing Clinics of North America,* 25(1), 165-180.

Crawford-Gamble, P.E. (1986). An application of Levine's conceptual model. *Perioperative Nursing Quarterly,* 2(1), 64-70.

Fawcett, J., Tulman, L., & Samarel, N. (1995). Enhancing function in life transitions and serious illness. *Advance Practice Nursing Quarterly,* 1, 50-57.

Flaskerud, J.H. & Halloran, E.J. (1980). Areas of agreement in nursing theory development. *Advances in Nursing Science,* 3(1), 1-7.

Foreman, M.D. (1989, Feb.). Confusion in the hospitalized elderly: Incidence, onset, and associated factors. *Research in Nursing and Health,* 12(1), 21-29.

Hall, K.V. (1979). Current trends in the use of conceptual frameworks in nursing education. *Journal of Nursing Education,* 18(4), 26-29.

Happ, M.B., Williams, C.C., Strumpf, N.E., & Burger, S.G. (1996). Individualized care for frail elderly: Theory and practice. *Journal of Gerontological Nursing,* 22(3), 6-14.

Hirschfeld, M.J. (1976). The cognitively impaired older adult. *American Journal of Nursing,* 76, 1981-1984.

Jost, S.G. (2000). An assessment and intervention strategy for managing staff needs during change. *Journal of Nursing Administration,* 30(1), 34-40.

Langer, V.S. (1990, Oct.). Minimal handling protocol for the intensive care nursery. *Neonatal Network-Journal of Neonatal Nursing,* 9(3), 23-27.

Lynn-McHale, D.J. & Smith, A. (1991, May). Comprehensive assessment of families of the critically ill. *AACN Clinical Issues in Critical Care Nursing,* 2(2), 195-209.

Molchany, C.B. (1992). Ventricular septal and free wall rupture complicating acute MI. *Journal of Cardiovascular Nursing,* 6(4), 38-45.

Newport, M.A. (1984). Conserving thermal energy and social integrity in the newborn. *Western Journal of Nursing Research,* 6(2), 175-197.

O'Laughlin, K.M. (1986). Change in bladder function in the woman undergoing radical hysterectomy for cervical cancer. *Journal of Obstetrical, Gynecological and Neonatal Nursing,* 15(5), 380-385.

Roberts, K.L., Britton, M., Cook, M., & deClifford, J. (1994). Boomerang pillows and respiratory capacity. *Clinical Nursing Research,* 3(2), 157-165.

Roberts, K.L., Britton, M., & deClifford, J. (1995). Boomerang pillows and respiratory capacity in frail elderly women. *Clinical Nursing Research,* 4(4), 465-471.

Savage, T.V. & Culbert, C. (1989). Early intervention: The unique role of nursing. *Journal of Pediatric Nursing,* 4(5), 339-345.

Schaefer, K.M. (1997). Levine's conservation model in nursing practice. In M.R. Alligood and A. Marriner-Tomey (Eds.), *Nursing theory: Utilization and application* (pp. 89-107). St. Louis: Mosby.

Schaefer, K.M. & Shober-Potylycki, M.J. (1993). Fatigue in congestive heart failure: Use of Levine's conservation model. *Journal of Advanced Nursing,* 18, 260-268.

Schaefer, K.M. & Pond, J. (1994). Levine's conservation model as a guide to nursing practice. *Nursing Science Quarterly,* 7(2), 53-54.

Schaefer, K.M., Swavely, D., Rothenberger, C., Hess, S., & Willistin, D. (1996). Sleep disturbances post coronary artery bypass surgery. *Progress in Cardiovascular Nursing,* 11(1), 5-14.

Taylor, J.W. (1989). Levine's conservation principles: Using the model for nursing diagnosis in a neurological setting. In J.P. Riehl-Sisca (Ed.), *Conceptual models for nursing practice* (3rd ed., pp. 349-358). Norwalk, CT: Appleton & Lange.

Tillich, P. (1961). The meaning of health. *Perspectives in Biology and Medicine, 5,* 92-100.

Tompkins, E.S. (1980). Effect of restricted mobility and dominance on perceived duration. *Nursing Research, 29*(6), 333-338.

Tribotti, S. (1990). Admission to the neonatal intensive care unit: Reducing the risks. *Neonatal Network, 8*(4), 17-22.

Webb, H. (1993). Holistic care following a palliative Hartmann's procedure. *British Journal of Nursing, 2*(2), 128-132.

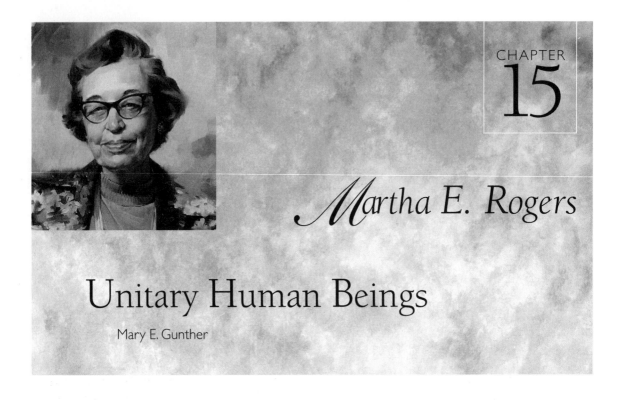

*M*artha E. Rogers

Unitary Human Beings

Mary E. Gunther

CREDENTIALS AND BACKGROUND OF THE THEORIST

Martha Elizabeth Rogers, the eldest of four children of Bruce Taylor Rogers and Lucy Mulholland Keener Rogers, was born May 12, 1914, in Dallas, Texas. Soon after her birth, her family returned to Knoxville, Tennessee. She began her college education studying science at the University of Tennessee (1931 to 1933). Receiving her nursing diploma from Knoxville General Hospital School of Nursing (1936), she quickly obtained a B.S. from George Peabody College in Nashville, Tennessee (1937). Her other degrees include an M.A. in public health nursing supervision from Teachers College, Columbia University, New York (1945) and an M.P.H. (1952) and an Sc.D. (1954) from Johns Hopkins University in Baltimore.

Previous authors: Kaye Bultemeier, Mary Gunther, Joann Sebastian Daily, Judy Sporleder Maupin, Cathy A. Murray, Martha Carole Satterly, Denise L. Schnell, and Therese L. Wallace. Earlier editions of this chapter were critiqued by Dr. Lois Meier and Dr. Martha Rogers.

Rogers' early nursing practice was in rural public health nursing in Michigan and in visiting nurse supervision, education, and practice in Connecticut. Rogers subsequently established the Visiting Nurse Service of Phoenix, Arizona. For 21 years (1954 to 1975), she was professor and head of the Division of Nursing at New York University. After 1975, she continued her duties as professor until she became professor emerita in 1979. She held this title until her death on March 13, 1994 at the age of 79.

Rogers' publications include three books and more than 200 articles. She lectured in 46 states, the District of Columbia, Puerto Rico, Mexico, the Netherlands, China, Newfoundland, Columbia, Brazil, and other countries.[48] Rogers received honorary doctorates from such renowned institutions as Duquesne University, University of San Diego, Iona College, Fairfield University, Emory University, Adelphi University, Mercy College, and Washburn University of Topeka. The numerous awards for her contributions and leadership in nursing include citations for "Inspiring Leadership in the Field of Intergroup Relations" by Chi Eta Phi Sorority, "In Recognition of Your Outstanding Contribution to Nursing" by New York University, and "For Distinguished Service to Nursing" by Teachers College. In addition, New York University houses the Martha E. Rogers Center for the Study of Nursing Science. In 1996, Rogers was posthumously inducted into the American Nurses Association Hall of Fame.

In 1988, colleagues and students joined her in forming the Society of Rogerian Scholars (SRS) and immediately began publishing *Rogerian Nursing Science News,* a members' newsletter, to disseminate theory developments and research studies.[37] In 1993, SRS began publishing an annual refereed journal, *Visions: The Journal of Rogerian Nursing Science.*[37] The society maintains and administers the Martha E. Rogers Fund. Keeping pace with the newest information technology, Rogers has a website based in Wales called "Nurse-Rogers" (http://www.uwcm.ac.uk/uwcm/ns/martha/homepage.html) and New York University's "Martha E. Rogers Listserv" (http://www.nyu.edu/pages/nursing/rogers.html).

A verbal portrait of Rogers includes such descriptive terms as stimulating, challenging, controversial, idealistic, visionary, prophetic, philosophical, academic, outspoken, humorous, blunt, and ethical. Rogers remains a widely recognized scholar honored for her contributions and leadership in nursing. Butcher[12:114] noted, "Rogers, like Nightingale, was extremely independent, a determined, perfectionist individual who trusted her vision despite skepticism." Colleagues consider her one of the most original thinkers in nursing as she synthesized and resynthesized knowledge into "an entirely new system of thought."[12:111]

THEORETICAL SOURCES

Rogers' grounding in the liberal arts and sciences is apparent in both the origin and development of her conceptual model published in 1970 as *An Introduction to the Theoretical Basis of Nursing.*[44] Aware of the interrelatedness of knowledge, Rogers credited scientists from multiple disciplines with influencing the development of the Science of Unitary Human Beings. Rogerian science emerged from the knowledge bases of anthropology, psychology, sociology, astronomy, religion, philosophy, history, biology, physics, mathematics, and literature to create a model of unitary human beings and the environment as energy fields integral to the life process.[21] Within nursing, the origins of Rogerian science can be traced to Nightingale's proposals and statistical data placing the human being within the framework of the natural world. This "foundation for the scope of modern nursing" began nursing's investigation of the relationship between human beings and the environment.[44:30] Newman[40:9] describes the Science of Unitary Human Beings as "the study of the moving, intuitive experience of nurses in mutual process with those they serve."

USE OF EMPIRICAL EVIDENCE

Being an abstract conceptual system, the Science of Unitary Human Beings does not directly identify testable empirical indicators. Rather, it specifies a world view and philosophy used to identify the phenomena of concern to the discipline of nursing. As mentioned previously, Rogers' model emerged from multiple knowledge sources; the most readily apparent of these are the nonlinear dynamics of quantum physics and general system theory.

Evident in her model is the influence of Einstein's theory of relativity[20] in relation to space time and Burr and Northrop's electrodynamic theory[11] relating to electrical fields. By the time von Bertalanffy[54] introduced general system theory, theories regarding a universe of open systems were beginning to affect the development of knowledge within all disciplines. With general system theory, the term *negentrophy* was brought into use to signify increasing order, complexity, and heterogeneity in direct contrast to the previously held belief that the universe was winding down. Rogers, however, refined and purified general system theory by denying hierarchical subsystems, the concept of single causation, and predictability of a system's behavior through investigations of its parts.

The introduction of the theory of relativity, of quantum theory, and of probability fundamentally challenged the prevailing absolutism. As new knowledge escalated, the traditional meanings of homeostasis, steady state, adaptation, and equilibrium were seriously questioned. The closed system, entropic model of the universe was no longer adequate to explain phenomena and evidence continued to accumulate in support of a universe of open systems.[52] Today, Rogers' model is validated by the continuing development within other disciplines of the acausal, nonlinear dynamics of life. Most notable of this development is that of chaos theory, quantum physics' contribution to the science of complexity (or wholeness), that is blurring the boundaries between the disciplines, allowing an exploration and deepening of the understanding of the totality of human experience.

MAJOR CONCEPTS & DEFINITIONS

In 1970, Rogers' conceptual model of nursing rested on a set of basic assumptions that described the life process in human beings. Wholeness, openness, unidirectionality, pattern and organization, sentience, and thought characterized the life process.[44]

Rogers postulates that human beings are dynamic energy fields integral with environmental fields. Both human and environmental fields are identified by pattern and characterized by a universe of open systems. In her 1983 paradigm, Rogers postulated four building blocks for her model: (1) energy field, (2) a universe of open systems, (3) pattern, and (4) four dimensionality.[45]

Rogers consistently updated the conceptual model through revision of the homeodynamic principles. Such changes corresponded with scientific and technological advances. In 1983, Rogers[45] changed her wording from that of unitary man to unitary human being to remove the concept of gender. Additional clarification of unitary human beings as separate and different from the term *holistic* stressed the unique contribution of nursing to healthcare. In 1992, four dimensionality evolved into pandimensionality. Rogers' fundamental postulates have remained consistent since their introduction; her subsequent writings served to clarify the articulation of her original ideas.

ENERGY FIELD

An energy field constitutes the fundamental unit of both the living and the nonliving. Field is a unifying concept and energy signifies the dynamic nature of the field. Energy fields are infinite and pandimensional. Two fields are identified: (1) the human field and (2) the environmental field.[45] "Specifically human beings and environment are energy fields."[47:2] The unitary human being (human field) is defined as an irreducible, indivisible, pandimensional energy field identified by pattern and manifesting characteristics that are specific to the whole and that cannot be predicted from knowledge of the parts. The environmental field is defined as an irreducible, pandimensional energy field identified by pattern and integral with the human field. Each environmental field is specific to its given human field. Both change continuously, creatively, and integrally.[51]

UNIVERSE OF OPEN SYSTEMS

The concept of the universe of open systems holds that energy fields are infinite, open, and integral with one another.[45] The human and the environmental field are in continuous process and are open systems.

PATTERN

Pattern identifies energy fields. It is the distinguishing characteristic of an energy field and is perceived as a single wave. The nature of the pattern changes continuously, innovatively, and these changes give identity to the energy field. Each human field pattern is unique and is integral with the environmental field.[45] Manifestations emerge as a human-environmental mutual process. Pattern is an abstraction; it reveals itself through manifestation. "Manifestations of pattern have been described as unique and refer to behaviors, qualities, and characteristics of the field"[15:30] A sense of self is a field manifestation, the nature of which is unique to each individual. Some variations in pattern manifestations have been described in phrases such as longer versus shorter rhythms, pragmatic versus imaginative, and time experienced as fast or slow. Pattern is continually changing and may manifest disease, illness, feelings, or pain.[57] Pattern change is continuous, innovative, and relative.

PANDIMENSIONALITY

Rogers defines pandimensionality as a nonlinear domain without spatial or temporal attributes. The term pandimensional provides for an infinite domain without limit. It best expresses the idea of a unitary whole.[51]

MAJOR ASSUMPTIONS

Nursing

Nursing is a learned profession, both a science and an art. It is an empirical science and, like that of other sciences, it lies in the phenomenon central to its focus. Rogerian nursing focuses on concern with people and the world in which they live, a natural fit for nursing care, as it encompasses people and their environments. The integrality of people and their environments, operating from a pandimensional universe of open systems, points to a new paradigm and initiates the identity of nursing as a science. The purpose of nursing is to promote health and well being for all persons. The art of nursing is the creative use of the science of nursing for human betterment.[52] "Professional practice in nursing seeks to promote symphonic interaction between human and environmental fields, to strengthen the integrity of the human field, and to direct and redirect patterning of the human and environmental fields for realization of maximum health potential."[44:122] Nursing exists for the care of people and the life process of humans.

Person

Rogers defines person as an open system in continuous process with the open system that is the environment (integrality). She defines unitary human being as an "irreducible, indivisible, pandimensional energy field identified by pattern and manifesting characteristics that are specific to the whole."[51:29] Human beings "are not disembodied entities, nor are they mechanical aggregates. . . . Man is a unified whole possessing his own integrity and manifesting characteristics that are more than and different from the sum of his parts."[44:46-47] Within a conceptual model specific to nursing's concern, people and their environment are perceived as irreducible energy fields integral with one another and continuously creative in their evolution.

Health

Rogers uses health in many of her earlier writings without clearly defining the term. She uses the term *passive health* to symbolize wellness and the absence of disease and major illness.[44] Her promotion of positive health connotes direction in helping people with opportunities for rhythmic consistency.[44]

Rogers uses health as a value term defined by the culture or individual. Health and illness are manifestations of pattern and are considered "to denote behaviors that are of high value and low value."[25:248] Events manifested in the life process indicate the extent to which man achieves maximum health according to some value systems. In Rogerian science, the phenomena central to nursing's conceptual system is the human life process. The life process has its own dynamic and creative unity, inseparable from the environment, and is characterized by the whole.[44]

In *Dimensions of Health: A View from Space,* [47] Rogers reaffirms the original theoretical assertions, adding philosophical challenges to the prevailing perception of health. Stressing a new worldview that focuses on people and their environment, she lists iatrogenesis, nosocomial conditions, and hypochrondriasis as the major health problems in the United States. Rogers[47:2] writes, "A new world view compatible with the most progressive knowledge available is a necessary prelude to studying human health and to determining modalities for its promotion whether on this planet or in the outer reaches of space."

Environment

Rogers[51:29] defines environment as "an irreducible, pandimensional energy field identified by pattern and manifesting characteristics different from those of the parts. Each environmental field is specific to its given human field. Both change continuously and creatively."

Environmental fields are infinite and change is continuously innovative, unpredictable, and characterized by increasing diversity. Environmental and human fields are identified by wave patterns manifesting continuous change. Environmental and human fields are in continuous and mutual process.[5]

THEORETICAL ASSERTIONS

The principles of homeodynamics postulate a way of perceiving unitary human beings. The evolution of these principles from 1970 to 1994 is depicted in Table 15-1. Rogers[44:96] writes, "The life process is homeodynamic. . . . These principles postulate the way the life process is and predict the nature of its evolving." Rogers identified the principles of helicy, resonancy, and integrality. The helicy principle describes spiral development in continuous, nonrepeating, and innovative patterning. Rogers' articulation of the principle of helicy describing the nature of change evolved from probabilistic to unpredictable while remaining continuous and innovative. According to the principle of resonancy, patterning changes with development from lower to higher frequency; that is, with varying degrees of intensity. Resonancy embodies wave frequency and energy field pattern evolution. Integrality, the third principle of homeodynamics, stresses the continuous mutual process of person and environment. The principles of homeodynamics evolved into a concise and clear description of the nature of change within human and environmental energy fields.

In 1970, Rogers identified five assumptions that are also theoretical assertions supporting her model derived from literature on human beings, physics, mathematics, and behavioral science:

1. "Man is a unified whole possessing his own integrity and manifesting characteristics more than and different from the sum of his parts" (energy field).[44:47]
2. "Man and environment are continuously exchanging matter and energy with one another" (openness).[44:54]
3. "The life process evolves irreversibly and unidirectionally along the space-time continuum" (helicy).[44:59]
4. "Pattern and organization identify man and reflect his innovative wholeness" (pattern and organization).[44:65]
5. "Man is characterized by the capacity for abstraction and imagery, language and thought, sensation, and emotion" (sentient, thinking being).[44:73]

LOGICAL FORM

Rogers uses a dialectic method as opposed to a logistical, problematic, or operational method; that is, Rogers explains nursing by referring to broader principles that explain human beings. She then explains human beings through principles that characterize the universe. The method is based on the perspective of a whole that organizes the parts.[39]

Rogers' model of unitary human beings is deductive and logical. The theory of relativity, general system theory, electrodynamic theory of life, and many other theories contributed ideas for Rogers' model. Unitary human beings and environment, the central components of the model, are integral with one another. The basic building blocks of her model are energy field, openness, pattern, and pandimensionality providing a new worldview. These concepts form the

Table **15-1**

Evolution of Principles of Homeodynamics: 1970, 1980, 1983, 1986, and 1992				
AN INTRODUCTION TO THE THEORETICAL BASIS OF NURSING, 1970	**NURSING: A SCIENCE OF UNITARY MAN, 1980**	**SCIENCE OF UNITARY HUMAN BEINGS: A PARADIGM FOR NURSING, 1983**	**DIMENSIONS OF HEALTH: A VIEW FROM SPACE, 1986**	**NURSING SCIENCE AND THE SPACE AGE, 1992**
RESONANCY Continuously propagating series of waves between man and environment	RESONANCY The continuous change from lower to higher frequency wave patterns in the human and environmental fields	RESONANCY The continuous change from lower to higher frequency wave patterns in human and environmental fields	RESONANCY The continuous change from lower to higher frequency wave patterns in human and environmental fields	RESONANCY The continuous change from lower to higher frequency wave patterns in human and environmental fields
HELICY Continuous, innovative change growing out of mutual interaction of man and environment along a spiraling, longitudinal axis bound in space time	HELICY Nature of change between human and environmental fields is continuously innovative, probabilistic, and increasingly diverse, manifesting nonrepeating rhythmicities	HELICY The continuous, innovative, probabilistic, increasing diversity of human and environmental field patterns, characterized by nonrepeating rhythmicities	HELICY The continuous, innovative, probabilistic, increasing diversity of human and environmental characterized by nonrepeating rhythmicities	HELICY The continuous, innovative, unpredictable, increasing diversity of human and environmental field patterns
RECIPROCY Continuous mutual interaction between the human field and environmental field				

Continued

Table 15-1

Evolution of Principles of Homeodynamics: 1970, 1980, 1983, 1986, and 1992—cont'd				
AN INTRODUCTION TO THE THEORETICAL BASIS OF NURSING, 1970	NURSING: A SCIENCE OF UNITARY MAN, 1980	SCIENCE OF UNITARY HUMAN BEINGS: A PARADIGM FOR NURSING, 1983	DIMENSIONS OF HEALTH: A VIEW FROM SPACE, 1986	NURSING SCIENCE AND THE SPACE AGE, 1992
SYNCHRONY	COMPLE-MENTARITY	INTEGRALITY	INTEGRALITY	INTEGRALITY
Change in the human field and simulta-neous state of environmental field at any given point in space time	The continuous, mutual, simultaneous interaction between human and environ-mental fields	The continuous, mutual human field and environ-mental field process	The continuous, mutual human field and environ-mental field process	The continuous, mutual human field and environ-mental field process

Conceptualized by Joann Daily from the following sources: Riehl, J.P. & Roy, C. (Eds.). (1980). *Conceptual models for nursing practice* (2nd ed.). New York: Appleton-Century-Crofts; Rogers, M.E. (1970). *An introduction to the theoretical basis of nursing.* Philadelphia: F.A. Davis; Rogers, M.E. (1983). Science of unitary human beings: A paradigm for nursing. In I.W. Clements & F.B. Roberts (Eds.), *Family health: A theoretical approach to nursing care.* New York: John Wiley & Sons.

Revised by Denise Schnell and Therese Wallace in 1988 to include: Rogers, M.E. (1986). *Dimensions of health: A view from space,* obtained through correspondence with Martha Rogers, March 1988.

Updated by Cathy Murray from the following source: Rogers, M.E. (1992). Nursing science and the space age. *Nursing Science Quarterly,* 5(1), 27-34.

basis of an abstract conceptual system defining nursing and health. From the abstract conceptual system, Rogers derives the principles of homeodynamics, which postulate the nature and direction of human beings' evolution. Although Rogers invents the words homeodynamics (similar state of change and growth), helicy (evolution), resonancy (intensity of change), and integrality (wholeness), all definitions are etymologically consistent and logical.

ACCEPTANCE BY THE NURSING COMMUNITY

Practice

The Rogerian model is an abstract system of ideas from which to approach the practice of nursing.

Rogers' model, stressing the totality of experience and existence, is relevant in today's healthcare system where continuum of care is more important than episodic illness and hospitalization. The model provides the abstract philosophical framework from which to view the unitary human-environmental field phenomenon. Within the Rogerian framework, nursing is based on theoretical knowledge that guides nursing practice. The professional practice of nursing is creative and imaginative and exists to serve people. It is rooted in intellectual judgment, abstract knowledge, and human compassion.

Historically, nursing has equated practice with the practical and theory with the impractical. More appropriately, theory and practice are two related components in a unified nursing practice. Alligood[2] articulates how theory and practice direct and guide each other as they expand and increase nursing knowledge. Nursing knowledge provides the framework for the emergent artistic application of nursing care.[44]

Within Rogers' model, the critical thinking process directing practice can be divided into three components: (1) pattern appraisal, (2) mutual patterning, and (3) evaluation. Cowling[16] introduced a template for pattern-based nursing practice. The template emerged from Rogerian science and is widely accepted by nurses functioning within the Rogerian model. Bultemeier,[9] who expanded on the ideas of Cowling and articulated Rogerian nursing from a theoretical and practice stance, outlined further clarification of practice from the unitary perspective.

Cowling[17,19] states that pattern appraisal is meant to avoid, if not transcend, reductionistic categories of physical, mental, spiritual, emotional, cultural, and social assessment frameworks. Through observation and participation, the nurse focuses on human expressions of reflection, experience, and perception to form a profile of the patient. Mutual exploration of emergent patterns allows identification of unitary themes predominant in pandimensional human-environmental field process. Mutual understanding implies knowing participation, but does not lead to the nurse prescribing change or predicting outcomes. As Cowling[19:31] explains, "A critical feature of the unitary pattern appreciation process, and also of healing through appreciating wholeness, is a willingness on the part of the scientist/practitioner to let go of expectations about change." Evaluation centers on the perceptions emerging during mutual patterning.

Noninvasive patterning modalities used within Rogerian practice include, but are not limited to, therapeutic touch, guided imagery, meditation, self-reflection, guided reminiscence, journal keeping, humor, hypnosis, sleep hygiene, dietary manipulation, and physical exercise.[1,8,15,35,42] Barrett[6:138] notes that integral to these modalities are "meaningful dialogue, centering, and pandimensional authenticity (genuineness, trustworthiness, accep-

tance, and knowledgeable caring)." Nurses participate in the lived experience of health in a multitude of roles, including "facilitators and educators, advocates, assessors, planners, coordinators, and collaborators" by accepting diversity, recognizing patterns, viewing change as positive, and accepting the connectedness of life.[35:27] These roles may require the nurse to "let go of traditional ideas of time, space, and outcome."[36:115]

The Rogerian model provides a challenging and innovative framework from which to plan and implement nursing practice, which Barrett[6:136] defines as the "continuous process (of voluntary mutual patterning) whereby the nurse assists clients to freely choose with awareness ways to participate in their well-being."

Education

Rogers clearly articulated guidelines for the education of nurses within the Science of Unitary Human Beings. Rogers discusses structuring the nursing education programs to teach nursing as a science and as a learned profession. Barrett[5:306] calls Rogers a "consistent voice crying out against antieducationalism and dependency." Rogers' model clearly articulates values and beliefs about human beings, health, nursing, and the educational process. As such, it has been used to guide curriculum development in all levels of nursing education.[5,29,38] Rogers[50:11] stated that nurses must commit to lifelong learning and noted that "the nature of the practice of nursing (the use of knowledge for human betterment) is rooted in what one knows and in the imagination, creativity, compassion, and skill one uses."

Rogers advocated separate licensure for nurses prepared with an associate degree and those with a baccalaureate degree, recognizing that there is a difference between the technically oriented and the professional nurse. In her view, the professional nurse needs to be well rounded and educated in the humanities, sciences, and nursing. Such a program would include a basic education in language, mathematics, logic, philosophy, psychology, sociology, music, art, biology, microbiology, physics, and chemistry; elective courses could include economics, ethics, political science, anthropology, and computer science.[5] In regard to the research component of the curriculum, Rogers[52:34] stated:

> Undergraduate students need to be able to identify problems, to have tools of investigation and to do studies that will allow them to use knowledge for the improvement of practice, and they should be able to read the literature intelligently. People with master's degrees ought to be able to do applied research. . . . The theoretical research, the fundamental basic research is going to come out of doctoral programs of stature that focus on nursing as a learned field of endeavor.

Barrett[5] notes that with increasing use of technology and severity of illness of hospitalized patients, students may be limited to observational experiences in these institutions. Therefore the acquisition of manipulative technical skills must be accomplished in practice laboratories and alternative sites, such as clinics and home health agencies. Other sites for education include health-promotion programs, managed-care programs, homeless shelters, and senior centers.[5]

Research

Rogers' conceptual model provides a stimulus and direction for research and theory development in nursing science. Fawcett,[22] who insists that the level of abstraction affects direct applicability, endorses the designation of the Science of Unitary Human Beings as a conceptual model rather than a grand theory. She states clearly that the purpose of the work determines its category. If, as in the case of the Science of Unitary Human Beings, the purpose of the work is to "articulate a body of distinctive knowledge," the work is a conceptual model.[22:27]

Emerging from Rogers' model are theories that explain human phenomena and direct nursing practice. The Rogerian model, with its implicit assumptions, provides broad principles that conceptually direct theory development. The conceptual model provides a stimulus and direction for scientific activity. Relationships among identified phenomena generate both grand theories (further development of one aspect of the model) and middle-range theories (description, explanation, or prediction of concrete aspects).[22]

Two prominent grand nursing theories grounded in Rogers' model are Newman's Health as Expanding Consciousness and Parse's Human Becoming.[22] Numerous middle-range theories have emerged out of Rogers' three homeodynamic principles: (1) helicy, (2) resonancy, and (3) integrality. Exemplars of middle-range theories derived from the principles of Rogers' model include Power-As-Knowing-Participation-in-Change (helicy), the Theory of Perceived Dissonance (resonancy), and the Theory of Interactive Rhythms (integrality) (Figure 15-1).[4,8,26]

Rogers[46] maintains that research in nursing must examine unitary human beings as integral with their environment. Therefore the intent of nursing research is to examine and understand a phenomenon and, from this understanding, design patterning activities that promote healing. To obtain a clearer understanding of lived experiences, the person's perception and sentient awareness of what is occurring are imperative. The variety of events associated with human phenomena provides the experiential data for research that is directed toward capturing the dynamic, ever-changing life experiences of human beings. Selecting the correct methodology for examining the person and the environment as health-related phenomena is the challenge of the Rogerian researcher. Both quantitative and qualitative approaches have been used in the Science of Unitary Human Beings research although not all researchers agree that both are appropriate. Researchers do agree that ontological and epistemological congruence between the model and the approach must be considered and reflected by the research question.[7] Quantitative experimental and quasiexperimental designs are not appropriate as their purpose is to reveal causal relationships. Descriptive, explanatory, and correlational designs are more appropriate as they recognize "the unitary nature of the phenomenon of interest" and may "propose evidence of patterned mutual change among variables."[53:132]

Principles of Homodynamics

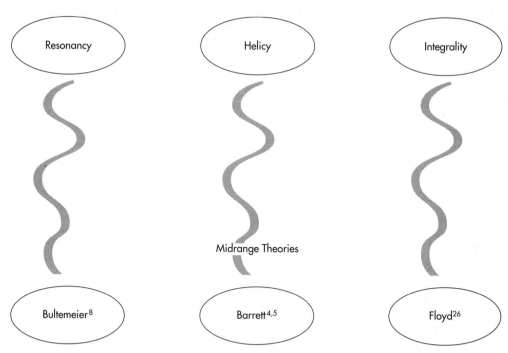

Figure **15-1** Theory development within the Science of Unitary Human Beings.

Specific research methodologies emerging from midrange theories based on the Rogerian model capture the human-environment phenomena. As a means of capturing the unitary human being, Cowling describes the process of pattern appreciation using the combined research and practice case study method. Case study attends to the whole person (irreducibility), aims at comprehending the essence (pattern), and respects the inherent interconnectedness of phenomena.[18] A pattern profile is composed through a synopsis and synthesis of the data.[7] Other innovative methods of recording and entering the human-environmental field phenomenon include photodisclosure, hermeneutic text interpretation, and the measurement of the effect of dialogue combined with noninvasive modalities.[3,10,33]

Rogerian instrument development is extensive and ever evolving. A wide range of instruments for measuring human-environment field phenomena has emerged (Table 15-2). The continual emergence of midrange theories, methodologies, and instruments demonstrate recognition of the importance of Rogerian science to nursing.

FURTHER DEVELOPMENT

Rogers[46:4] believed that knowledge development within her model was a "never-ending process" using "a multiplicity of knowledge from many sources . . . to create a kaleidoscope of possibilities." Recent explorations by Rogerian scholars into Buddhist, Hindu, and Aborigine philosophies exemplify this belief in an essential unity.[34]

Fawcett[22] identified three rudimentary theories developed by Rogers from the science of unitary human beings: (1) theory of accelerating evolution, (2) theory of rhythmical correlates of change, and (3) theory of paranormal phenomena. Further explication and testing of these theories and the homeodynamic principles will contribute to nursing science knowledge.

Table **15-2**

Instruments Developed within Rogers' Science of Unitary Human Beings

INSTRUMENT	CONSTRUCT	AUTHOR
Power-As-Knowing-Participation-in-Change (PKPCT)	Power	E.A.M. Barrett[4]
Mutual Exploration of the Healing Human-Environment Field Relationship	Healing human-environmental mutual process	J.T. Carboni[14]
Human Field Motion Test (HFMT)	Human field motion	H.M. Ference[23,24]
Index of Field Energy (IFE)	Human field dynamics	S.H. Gueldner[27]
Diversity of Human Field Pattern Scale (DHFPS)	Human field pattern diversity	M. Hastings-Tolsma[28]
Human Field Image Metaphor Scale	Individual awareness of the infinite wholeness of the human field	L. Johnston[30]
Person-Environment Participation Scale (PEPS)	Experience of continuous human-environment mutual process	S. Leddy[31]
Leddy Healthiness Scale	Healthiness	S. Leddy[32]
Temporal Experience Scale (TES)	Subjective experience of temporal awareness	J. Paletta[41]
Assessment of Dream Experience	Dreaming as a beyond waking experience	J. Watson[55]
Perceived Field Motion Scale (PFM)	Human field motion	A. Yarcheski & N. Mahon[58]
Human Field Rhythms	Experience of rhythms in human-environmental field mutual process	A. Yarcheski & N. Mahon[58]

Modified from Instruments developed within Rogers' science of unitary human beings. (1996). *Rogerian Nursing Science News,* 8(4), 9-12.

CRITIQUE

Simplicity

Ongoing studies and work within the model have served to simplify and clarify some of the concepts and relationships. However, when the model is examined in total perspective, some still classify it as complex. With its continued use in practice, research, and education, nurses will come to appreci-ate the model's elegant simplicity. As Whall[56:154] notes, "With only three principles, a few major concepts, and five assumptions, Rogers has explained the nature of man and the life process."

Generality

Rogers' conceptual model is abstract and therefore generalizable and powerful. It is broad in scope, providing a framework for the development of nursing knowledge through the generation of grand and middle-range theories.

Empirical Precision

Early criticisms of the model identified its major limitations as difficulty in understanding the principles, lack of operational definitions, and inadequate tools for measurement.[13] Drawing on knowledge from a multitude of scientific fields, Rogers' conceptual model is deductive in logic with the inherent lack of immediate empirical support.[5] As Fawcett[22:29] points out, failure to properly categorize the work as a conceptual model rather than a theory leads to "considerable misunderstandings and inappropriate expectations," which can result in the work being labeled inadequate.

As noted earlier, the development of the model by Rogerian scientists has resulted in the generation of testable theories accompanied by tools of measurement.

Derivable Consequences

Rogers' science has the fundamental intent of understanding human evolution and its potential. It "coordinates a universe of open systems to identify the focus of a new paradigm and initiate nursing's identity as a science."[49:182]

Although all the metaparadigm concepts are explored, the emphasis is on the integrality of human-environment field phenomena. Rogers[24] suggested many ideas for future studies; on the basis of this and the research of others, it can be said that the conceptual model is useful. Such utility has been proven in the arenas of practice, education, and research.

CONCLUSION

The Rogerian model emerged from a broad historical base and has moved to the forefront as scientific knowledge has evolved. Understanding the concepts and principles of the Science of Unitary Human Beings requires a foundation in general education, a willingness to let go of the traditional, and an ability to perceive the world in a new and creative way. Emerging from a strong educational base, the model provides a challenging framework from which to provide nursing care. The abstract ideas expounded in the Rogerian model and their congruence with modern scientific knowledge spur new and challenging theories that further the understanding of the unitary human being. Nursing scholars and practitioners are carrying Rogers' ideas into the next century.

CRITICAL THINKING *Activities*

1. Identify philosophical tenets from Nightingale that contributed to the basis for the development of the Rogerian model.

2. Discuss three main areas in which Rogerian science has had an impact on current nursing education.

3. Analyze your clinical practice and identify areas where practice based on Rogerian science would improve nursing care. Enumerate what the changes would be and identify anticipated positive outcomes.

4. Review two research articles grounded in Rogerian science. If possible, identify the midrange theory that guided the research process. From what principle of homeodynamics was the midrange theory derived?

REFERENCES

1. Alligood, M.R. (1991). Guided reminiscence: A Rogerian based intervention. *Rogerian Nursing Science News, 3*(3), 1-3.
2. Alligood, M.R. (1994). Toward a unitary view of nursing practice. In M. Madrid & E.A.M. Barrett (Eds.), *Rogers' scientific art of nursing practice* (pp. 223-240). New York: National League for Nursing.
3. Alligood, M.R. & Fawcett, J. (1999). Acceptance of an invitation to dialogue: Examination of an interpretive approach for the science of unitary human beings. *Visions: Journal of Rogerian Nursing Science, 7*(1), 5-13.

4. Barrett, E.A.M. (1990). An instrument to measure power-as-knowing-participation-in-change. In O. Strickland & C. Waltz (Eds.), *The measurement of nursing outcomes: Measuring clients self-care and coping skills* (Vol. 4, pp. 159-180). New York: Springer.

5. Barrett, E.A.M. (1990). *Visions of Rogers' science-based nursing*. New York: National League for Nursing.

6. Barrett, E.A.M. (1998). A Rogerian practice methodology for health patterning. *Nursing Science Quarterly*, 11(4), 136-138.

7. Barrett, E.A.M., Cowling, W.R., Carboni, J.T., & Butcher, H.K. (1997). Unitary perspectives on methodological practices. In M. Madrid (Ed.), *Patterns of Rogerian knowing* (pp. 47-62). New York: National League for Nursing.

8. Bultemeier, K. (1993). *Photographic inquiry of the phenomenon premenstrual syndrome within the Rogerian derived theory of perceived dissonance*. Doctoral dissertation, University of Tennessee, Knoxville.

9. Bultemeier, K. (1996). Rogers' science of unitary human beings in nursing practice. In M.R. Alligood & A. Marriner Tomey (Eds.), *Nursing theory: Utilization and application* (pp. 153-174). St. Louis: Mosby.

10. Bultemeier, K. (1997). Photo-disclosure: A research methodology for investigating the unitary human being. In M. Madrid (Ed.), *Patterns of Rogerian knowing*. New York: National League for Nursing Press.

11. Burr, H.S. & Northup, F.S.C. (1935). The electrodynamic theory of life. *Quarterly Review of Biology*, 10, 322-323.

12. Butcher, H.K. (1999). Rogerian ethics: An ethical inquiry into Rogers' life and science. *Nursing Science Quarterly*, 5, 111-118.

13. Butterfield, S.E. (1983). In search of commonalties: Analysis of two theoretical frameworks. *International Journal of Nursing Studies*, 20(1), 15-22.

14. Carboni, J.T. (1992). Instrument development and the measurement of unitary constructs. *Nursing Science Quarterly*, 5, 134-142.

15. Clarke, P.N. (1986). Theoretical and measurement issues in the study of field phenomena. *Advances in Nursing Science*, 9(1), 29-39.

16. Cowling, W.R. (1990). A template for nursing practice. In E.A.M. Barrett (Ed.), *Visions of Rogers' science-based nursing* (pp. 45-65). New York: National League for Nursing.

17. Cowling, W.R. (1993). Unitary knowing in nursing practice. *Nursing Science Quarterly*, 6(4), 201-207.

18. Cowling, W.R. (1998). Unitary case inquiry. *Nursing Science Quarterly*, 11(4), 139-141.

19. Cowling, W.R. (2000). Healing as appreciating wholeness. *Advances in Nursing Science*, 22(3), 16-32.

20. Einstein, A. (1961). *Relativity*. New York: Crown.

21. Falco, S.M. & Lobo, M.L. (1980). Martha E. Rogers. In Nursing Theories Conference Group, *Nursing theories: The base for professional practice* (pp. 164-183). Englewood Cliffs, NJ: Prentice Hall.

22. Fawcett, J. (1995). *Analysis and evaluation of conceptual models of nursing* (3rd ed.). Philadelphia: F.A. Davis.

23. Ference, H.M. (1986). Foundations of a nursing science and its evolution: A perspective. In V.M. Malinski (Ed.), *Explorations in Martha Rogers' science of unitary human beings* (pp. 35-44). Norwalk, CT: Appleton-Century-Crofts.

24. Ference, H.M. (1986). The relationship of time experience, creativity traits, differentiation, and human field motion. In V.M. Malinski (Ed.), *Explorations in Martha Rogers' science of unitary human beings* (pp. 95-106). Norwalk, CT: Appleton-Century-Crofts.

25. Fitzpatrick, J.J. & Whall, A.L. (1983). *Conceptual models of nursing: Analysis and application*. Bowie, MD: Robert J. Brady.

26. Floyd, J.A. (1983). Research using Rogers' conceptual system: Development of a testable theorem. *Advances in Nursing Science*, 5(2), 37-48.

27. Gueldner, S.H. (1993). *Index of field energy: A psychometric analysis*. Unpublished manuscript.

28. Hastings-Tolsma, M.T. (1992). The relationship of diversity of human field pattern to risk-taking and time experience: An investigation of Rogers' principles of homeodynamics. *Dissertation Abstracts International*, 53, 4029B.

29. Hellvig, S.D. & Ferrante, S. (1993). Martha Rogers' model in associate degree education. *Nurse Educator*, 18(5), 25-27.

30. Johnston, L.W. (1994). Psychometric analysis of Johnston's human field image metaphor scale. *Visions: The Journal of Rogerian Nursing Science*, 2(1), 7-11.

31. Leddy, S.K. (1995). Measuring mutual process: Development and psychometric testing of the person-environment participation scale. *Visions: The Journal of Rogerian Nursing Science*, 3(1), 20-31.

32. Leddy, S.K. (1996). Development and psychometric testing of the Leddy healthiness scale. *Research in Nursing and Health*, 19(5), 431-440.

33. Leddy, S. K. & Fawcett, J. (1997). Testing the theory of healthiness: Conceptual and methodological issues. In M. Madrid (Ed.), *Patterns of Rogerian knowing* (pp. 75-86). New York: National League for Nursing.

34. Madrid, M. (Ed.). (1997). *Patterns of Rogerian knowing*. New York: National League for Nursing.

35. Malinksi, V.M. (1986). *Explorations on Martha Rogers' science of unitary human beings*. New York: Appleton-Century-Crofts.

36. Malinski, V.M. (1997). Rogerian health patterning: Evolving into the 21st century. *Nursing Science Quarterly*, 10(3), 115-116.

37. Malinski, V.M. & Barrett, E.A.M. (1994). *Martha E. Rogers: Her life and her work.* Philadelphia: F.A. Davis.
38. Mathwig, G.M., Young, A.A., & Pepper, J.M. (1990). Using Rogerian science in undergraduate and graduate nursing education. In E.A.M. Barrett (Ed.), *Visions of Rogers' science-based nursing* (pp. 319-334). New York: National League for Nursing.
39. McHugh, M. (1986). Nursing process: Musings on the method. *Holistic Nursing Practice,* 1(1), 21-28.
40. Newman, M.A. (1997). A dialogue with Martha Rogers and David Bohm about the science of unitary human beings. In M. Madrid (Ed.), *Patterns of Rogerian knowing* (pp. 3-10). New York: National League for Nursing.
41. Paletta, J.L. (1990). The relationship of temporal experience to human time. In E.A.M. Barrett (Ed.), *Visions of Rogers' science-based nursing* (pp. 239-254). New York: National League for Nursing.
42. Parker, K.P. (1989). The theory of sentience evolution: A practice-level theory of sleeping, waking, and beyond waking patterns based on the science of unitary human beings. *Rogerian Nursing Science News,* 2(1), 4-6.
43. Phillips, J. (1997). Evolution of the science of unitary human beings. In M. Madrid (Ed.), *Patterns of Rogerian knowing* (pp. 11-27). New York: National League for Nursing.
44. Rogers, M.E. (1970). *An introduction to the theoretical basis of nursing.* Philadelphia: F.A. Davis.
45. Rogers, M.E. (1983). Science of unitary human beings: A paradigm for nursing. In I.W. Clements & F.B. Roberts (Eds.), *Family health: A theoretical approach to nursing care* (pp. 219-227). New York: John Wiley & Sons.
46. Rogers, M.E. (1986). Science of unitary human beings. In V.M. Malinski (Ed.), *Explorations in Martha Rogers' science of unitary human beings* (pp. 3-8). Norwalk, CT: Appleton-Century-Crofts.
47. Rogers, M.E. (1986, Sept.). *Dimensions of health: A view from space.* Paper presented at the conference on "Law and Life in Space," September 12, 1986. Center for Aerospace Sciences, University of North Dakota.
48. Rogers, M.E. (1988, March). Personal correspondence.
49. Rogers, M.E. (1989). Nursing: A science of unitary human beings. In J.P. Riehl-Sisca (Ed.), *Conceptual models for nursing practice* (3rd ed., pp. 181-188). Norwalk, CT: Appleton-Century-Crofts.
50. Rogers, M.E. (1990). Space-age paradigm for new frontiers in nursing. In M.E. Parker (Ed.), *Nursing theories in practice* (pp.105-114). New York: National League for Nursing.
51. Rogers, M.E. (1994). Nursing science evolves. In M. Madrid & E.A.M. Barrett (Eds.), *Rogers' scientific art of nursing practice* (pp. 3-9). New York: National League for Nursing.
52. Rogers, M.E. (1994). The science of unitary human beings: Current perspectives. *Nursing Science Quarterly,* 7(1), 33-35.
53. Sherman, D.W. (1997). Rogerian science: Opening new frontiers of nursing knowledge through its application in quantitative research. *Nursing Science Quarterly,* 10(3), 131-135.
54. von Bertalanffy, L. (1960). *General system theory: Foundations, developments, application.* New York: George Braziller.
55. Watson, J. (1993). Relationship of sleep-wake rhythm, dream experience, human field motion, and time experience in older women. *Dissertation Abstracts International,* 54(12), 6137B.
56. Whall, A.L. (1987). A critique of Rogers' framework. In R.R. Parse (Ed.), *Nursing science: Major paradigms, theories, and critiques* (pp. 147-158). Philadelphia: W.B. Saunders.
57. Wright, S.M. (1987, Sept.). The use of therapeutic touch in the management of pain. *Nursing Clinics of North America,* 22(3), 705-713.
58. Yarcheski, A. & Mahon, N.E. (1991). An empirical test of Rogers' original and revised theory of correlates in adolescents. *Research in Nursing and Health,* 14, 447-455.

BIBLIOGRAPHY
Primary Sources
Books

Rogers, M.E. (1961). *Educational revolution in nursing.* New York: Macmillan.
Rogers, M.E. (1964). *Reveille in nursing.* Philadelphia: F.A. Davis.
Rogers, M.E. (1970). *An introduction to the theoretical basis of nursing.* Philadelphia: F.A. Davis.

Book Chapters

Rogers, M.E. (1969). Nursing research: Relevant to practice? *Proceedings of the fifth nursing research conference.* New York: American Nurses Association.
Rogers, M.E. (1977). Nursing: To be or not to be. In B. Bullough & V.Bullough (Eds.), *Expanding horizons for nursing.* New York: Springer.
Rogers, M.E. (1978). Emerging patterns in nursing education. In *Current perspectives in nursing education* (Vol. II, p. 1-8). St. Louis: Mosby.
Rogers, M.E. (1980). Nursing: A science of unitary man. In J.P. Reihl & C. Roy (Eds.), *Conceptual models for nursing practice* (2nd ed., pp. 329-337). New York: Appleton-Century-Crofts.
Rogers, M.E. (1981). Science of unitary man: A paradigm for nursing. In G.E. Laskar (Ed.), *Applied systems and cybernetics* (Vol. IV, pp. 1719-1722). New York: Pergamon.

Rogers, M.E. (1983). Beyond the horizon. In N.L. Chaska (Ed.), *The nursing profession: A time to speak.* New York: McGraw-Hill.

Rogers, M.E. (1983). The family coping with a surgical crisis: Analysis and application of Rogers' theory to nursing care (Rogers' response). In I.W. Clements & F.B. Roberts (Eds.), *Family health: A theoretical approach to nursing care.* New York: John Wiley & Sons.

Rogers, M.E. (1985). High touch in a high-tech future. In National League for Nursing, *Perspectives in nursing— 1985-1987* (pp. 25-31). New York: National League for Nursing.

Rogers, M.E. (1985). Nursing education: Preparing for the future. In National League for Nursing, *Patterns of education: The unfolding of nursing* (pp. 11-14). New York: National League for Nursing.

Rogers, M.E. (1985). Science of unitary human beings: A paradigm for nursing. In R. Wood & J. Kekhababh (Eds.), *Examining the cultural implications of Martha E. Rogers' science of unitary human beings* (pp. 13-23). Lecompton, KS: Wood-Kekhababh Associates.

Rogers, M.E. (1986). Science of unitary human beings. In V.M. Malinski (Ed.), *Explorations on Martha Rogers: Science of unitary human beings* (pp. 3-8). Norwalk, CT: Appleton-Century-Crofts.

Rogers, M.E. (1987). Nursing research in the future. In J. Roode (Ed.), *Changing patterns in nursing education* (pp. 121-123). New York: National League for Nursing.

Rogers, M.E. (1987). Rogers' science of unitary human beings. In R.R. Parse (Ed.), *Nursing science: Major paradigms, theories, and critiques* (pp. 139-146). Philadelphia: W.B. Saunders.

Rogers, M.E. (1989). Nursing: A science of unitary human beings. In J.P. Riehl-Sisca (Ed.), *Conceptual models for nursing practice* (3rd ed., pp. 181-188). Norwalk, CT: Appleton & Lange.

Rogers, M.E. (1990). Nursing: Science of unitary, irreducible, human beings: Update 1990. In E.A.M. Barrett (Ed.), *Visions of Rogers' science-based nursing.* New York: National League for Nursing.

Rogers, M.E. (1992). Nightingale's notes on nursing: Prelude to the 21st century. In F. Nightingale, *Notes on nursing: What it is and what it is not* (Commemorative edition, pp. 58-62). Philadelphia: J.B. Lippincott.

Rogers, M.E., Doyle, M.B., Racolin, A., & Walsh, P.C. (1990). A conversation with Martha Rogers on nursing in space. In E.A.M. Barrett (Ed.), *Visions of Rogers' science-based nursing* (pp. 375-386). New York: National League for Nursing.

Journal Articles

Rogers, M.E. (1963). Building a strong educational foundation. *American Journal of Nursing, 63,* 94-95.

Rogers, M.E. (1963). Some comments on the theoretical basis of nursing practice. *Nursing Science, 1,* 11-13, 60-61.

Rogers, M.E. (1963). The clarion call. *Nursing Science, 1,* 134-135.

Rogers, M.E. (1964). Professional standards: Whose responsibility? *Nursing Science, 2,* 71-73.

Rogers, M.E. (1965). Collegiate education in nursing [Editorial]. *Nursing Science, 3*(5), 362-365.

Rogers, M.E. (1965). Higher education in nursing [Editorial]. *Nursing Science, 3*(6), 443-445.

Rogers, M.E. (1965). Legislative and licensing problems in health care. *Nursing Administration Quarterly, 2,* 71-78.

Rogers, M.E. (1965). What the public demands of nursing today. *Registered Nursing, 28,* 80.

Rogers, M.E. (1966). Doctoral education in nursing. *Nursing Forum, 5*(2), 75-82.

Rogers, M.E. (1968). Nursing science: Research and researchers, *Teachers College Record, 69,* 469.

Rogers, M.E. (1969). Nursing education for professional practice. *Catholic Nurse, 18*(1), 28-37, 63-64.

Rogers, M.E. (1969). Preparation of the baccalaureate degree graduate. *New Jersey State Nurses Association Newsletter, 25*(5), 32-37.

Rogers, M.E. (1970). Yesterday a nurse, tomorrow a manager: What now? *Journal of New York State Nurses Association, 1*(1), 15-21.

Rogers, M.E. (1972). Nursing: To be or not to be? *Nursing Outlook, 20*(1), 42-46.

Rogers, M.E. (1972). Nursing's expanded role . . . and other euphemisms. *Journal of New York State Nurses Association, 3*(4), 5-10.

Rogers, M.E. (1975). Euphemisms and nursing's future. *Image, 7,* 3-9.

Rogers, M.E. (1975). Forum: Professional commitment in nursing. *Image, 2,* 12-13.

Rogers, M.E. (1975). Nursing is coming of age. *American Journal of Nursing, 75*(10), 1834-1843,1859.

Rogers, M.E. (1975). Reactions to the two foregoing presentations. NLN Pub. No. 15-1456. *Nursing Outlook, 20,* 436.

Rogers, M.E. (1975). Research is a growing word. *Nursing Science, 31,* 283-294.

Rogers, M.E. (1975). Yesterday a nurse, today a manager: What now? *Image, 2,* 12-13.

Rogers, M.E. (1977). Legislative and licensing problems in health care. *Nursing Administration Quarterly, 2*(3), 71-78.

Rogers, M.E. (1978). A 1985 dissent [Peer review]. *Health/PAC Bulletin, 80,* 32-35.

Rogers, M.E. (1979). Contemporary American leaders in nursing: An oral history. An interview with Martha E. Rogers. *Kango Tenbo, 4*(12), 1126-1138.

Rogers, M.E. (1985). The nature and characteristics of professional education for nursing. *Journal of Professional Nursing,* 1(6), 381-383.

Rogers, M.E. (1985). The need for legislation for licensure to practice professional nursing. *Journal of Professional Nursing,* 1(6), 384.

Rogers, M.E. (1988). Nursing science and art: A prospective. *Nursing Science Quarterly,* 1(3), 99-102.

Rogers, M.E. (1989). Creating a climate for the implementation of a nursing conceptual framework. *Journal of Continuing Education in Nursing,* 20(3), 112-116.

Rogers, M.E. (1990). AIDS: Reason for optimism. *Philippine Journal of Nursing,* 60(2), 2-3.

Rogers, M.E. (1992). Nursing science and the space age. *Nursing Science Quarterly,* 5(1), 27-34.

Rogers, M.E. (1994). The science of unitary human beings: Current perspectives. *Nursing Science Quarterly,* 7(1), 33-35.

Rogers, M.E. & Malinski, V. (1989). Vital signs in the science of unitary human beings. *Rogerian Nursing Science News,* 1(3), 6.

Audiotapes

Rogers, M.E. (1978). *Application of theory in education and service* [Audiotape]. Available: Teach 'em Inc., 160 E. Illinois Street, Chicago, IL 60611.

Rogers, M.E. (1978). *Nursing science: A science of unitary mass* [Audiotape]. Distinguished Lecture Series, Wright State University, Dayton, OH.

Rogers, M.E. (1980). *The science of unitary man. Tape I: Unitary man and his world: A paradigm for nursing* [Audiotape]. New York: Media for Nursing.

Rogers, M.E. (1980). *The science of unitary man. Tape II: Developing an organized abstract system* [Audiotape]. New York: Media for Nursing.

Rogers, M.E. (1980). *The science of unitary man. Tape III: Principles and theories* [Audiotape]. New York: Media for Nursing.

Rogers, M.E. (1980). *The science of unitary man. Tape IV: Theories of accelerating change, paranormal phenomenon, and other events* [Audiotape]. New York: Media for Nursing.

Rogers, M.E. (1980). *The science of unitary man. Tape V: Health and illness* [Audiotape]. New York: Media for Nursing.

Rogers, M.E. (1980). *The science of unitary man. Tape VI: Interventive modalities: Translating theories into practice* [Audiotape]. New York: Media for Nursing.

Rogers, M.E. (1984). *Paper presented at Nurses Theorist Conference, Edmonton, Alberta, Canada* [Audiotape]. Available: Kennedy Recordings, R.R. 5, Edmonton, Alberta, Canada TSP 4B7 (403-470-0013).

Rogers, M.E. (1987). *Rogers' framework* [Audiotape]. Nurse Theorist Conference held in Pittsburgh, PA. Available: Meetings International, 1200 Delor Avenue, Louisville, KY 40217.

Videotapes

Distinguished leaders in nursing—Martha Rogers [Videotape]. (1982). Available: National Institutes of Health, National Library of Medicine, Bethesda, MD 20894 and from Sigma Theta Tau International, 550 West North Street, Indianapolis, IN 46202. Capitol Heights, MD: The National Audiovisual Center.

National League for Nursing. (1987). *Nursing theory: A circle of knowledge* [Videotape]. Available: National League for Nursing, 10 Columbus Circle, New York, NY 10019. New York: The author.

Rogers, M.E. (1984). *The science of unitary man. An interview with Martha Rogers with E. Donnelly* [Videotape]. Bloomington, IN: Indiana University School of Nursing.

Rogers, M.E. (1987). *Rogers' framework* [Videotape]. Nurse Theorist Conference held in Pittsburgh, PA. Available: Meetings International, 1200 Delor Avenue, Louisville, KY 40217.

The nurse theorist: Portraits of Excellence—Martha Rogers [Videotape]. (1988). Available: Fuld Video Project, Studio III, 370 Hawthorne Avenue, Oakland, CA 94609. Oakland, CA: Studio III.

Lectures

Rogers M.E. (1962). *Viewpoints—critical areas for nursing education in baccalaureate and higher degree programs.* An address given at the meeting of the Council of Member Agencies of the Department of Baccalaureate and Higher Degree Programs, Williamsburg, VA, March 26, 1962. New York: National League for Nursing, Department of Baccalaureate and Higher Degree Programs.

Rogers, M.E. (1984). *Current issues for nursing in the next decade.* Indiana Central University, Indianapolis.

Rogers, M.E. (1992). *Science and philosophy merge for a new reality.* Keynote speaker at the Fourth Annual Rosemary Ellis Scholars' Retreat, Case Western Reserve University, Cleveland, OH.

Dissertation

Rogers, M.E. (1954). *The association of maternal and fetal factors with the development of behavior problems among elementary school children.* Doctor of Science dissertation. Baltimore: Johns Hopkins University.

Secondary Sources
Books

Alligood, M.R. & Marriner Tomey, A. (1997). *Nursing theory: Utilization and application.* St. Louis: Mosby.

Argyris, C. & Schon, D. (1974). *Theory in practice.* San Francisco: Jossey-Bass.

Barnum, B.J. (1994). *Nursing theory: Analysis, application, evaluation.* Philadelphia: J.B. Lippincott.

Barrett, E.A.M. (1990). *Visions of Rogers' science-based nursing.* New York: National League for Nursing.

Chinn, P.L. & Kramer, M.K. (1991). *Theory and nursing: A systematic approach.* (3rd ed.). St. Louis: Mosby.

Fitzpatrick, J.J. & Whall, A.L. (1983). *Conceptual models of nursing: Analysis and application.* Bowie, MD: Robert J. Brady.

George, J.B. (1985). *Nursing theories: The base for professional nursing practice* (2nd ed.). Englewood Cliffs, NJ: Prentice-Hall.

Hanchett, E.S. (1979). *Community health assessment: A conceptual tool kit.* New York: John Wiley & Sons.

Lutjens, L.J.R. (1991). *Martha Rogers: The science of unitary human beings.* Newbury Park, CA: Sage Publications.

Madrid, M. & Barrett, E.A.M. (1994). *Rogers' scientific art of nursing practice.* New York: National League for Nursing.

Malinski, V.M. (Ed.). (1986). *Explorations on Martha Rogers' science of unitary human beings.* Norwalk, CT: Appleton-Century-Crofts.

Meleis, A.J. (1991). *Theoretical nursing: Development and progress* (2nd ed.). Philadelphia: J.B. Lippincott.

Newman, M.A. (1979). *Theory development in nursing.* Philadelphia: F.A. Davis.

Parse, R.R. (1981). *Man-living-health: A theory of nursing.* New York: John Wiley & Sons.

Riehl-Sisca, J.P. & Roy, C. (Eds.). (1989). *Conceptual models for nursing practice* (3rd ed.). Norwalk, CT: Appleton & Lange.

Sarter, B. (1988). *The stream of becoming: A study of Martha Rogers' theory.* New York: National League for Nursing.

Book Chapters

Alligood, M.R. (1986). The relationship of creativity, actualization, and empathy in unitary human development. In V.M. Malinski (Ed.), *Explorations on Martha Rogers' science of unitary human beings* (pp. 145-153). Norwalk, CT: Appleton-Century-Crofts.

Alligood, M.R. (1989). Rogers' theory and nursing administration: A perspective on health and environment. In B. Henry, C. Arndt, M. DeVincenti, & A. Marriner Tomey (Eds.), *Dimensions of nursing administration: Theory, research, education, practice* (pp. 105-111). Boston: Blackwell Scientific.

Andersen, M. & Hockman, E.M. (1997). Well-being and high-risk drug use among active drug users. In M. Madrid (Ed.), *Patterns of Rogerian knowing* (pp. 152-166). New York: National League for Nursing.

Barrett, E.A.M. (1986). Investigation of the principle of helicy: The relationship of human field motion and power. In V.M. Malinski (Ed.), *Explorations on Martha Rogers' science of unitary human beings* (pp. 173-184). Norwalk, CT: Appleton-Century-Crofts.

Barrett, E.A.M., Caroselli, C., Smith, A.S., & Smith, D.W. (1997). Power as knowing participation in change: Theoretical, practice, and methodological, issues, insights, and ideas. In M. Madrid (Ed.), *Patterns of Rogerian knowing* (pp. 31-46). New York: National League for Nursing.

Bultemeier, K., Gunther, M., Daily, J.S., Maupin, J.S., Murray, C.A., Satterly, M.C., Schnell, D.L., & Wallace, T.L. (1998). Martha E. Rogers: Unitary human beings. In A. Marriner Tomey & M.R. Alligood (Eds.), *Nursing theorists and their work* (4th ed., pp. 207-226). St. Louis: Mosby.

Butcher, H.K. (1993). Kaleidoscoping in life's turbulence: From Seurat's art to Rogers' nursing science. In M.E. Parker (Ed.), *Patterns of nursing theories in practice* (pp. 183-198). New York: National League for Nursing.

Cowling, W.R. (1986). The relationship of mystical experience, differentiation, and creativity in college students. In V.M. Malinski (Ed.), *Explorations on Martha Rogers' science of unitary human beings* (pp. 131-140). Norwalk, CT: Appleton-Century-Crofts.

Cowling, W.R. (1986). The science of unitary human beings: Theoretical issues, methodological challenges, and research realities. In V.M. Malinski (Ed.), *Explorations on Martha Rogers' science of unitary human beings* (pp. 35-44). Norwalk, CT: Appleton-Century-Crofts.

Cowling, W.R. (1997). Pattern appreciation: The unitary science/practice for essence. In M. Madrid (Ed.), *Patterns of Rogerian knowing* (pp. 129-142). New York: National League for Nursing.

Field, I. & Newman, M. (1982). Clinical application of the unitary man framework: Case study analysis (1980). In M.J. Kim & D.A. Moritz (Eds.), *Classification of nursing diagnosis: Proceedings of the third and fourth national conference.* New York: McGraw-Hill.

Field, S. (1997). The scientific art of medical practice. In M. Madrid (Ed.), *Patterns of Rogerian knowing* (pp. 267-284). New York: National League for Nursing.

Gold, J. (1997). Practicing medicine in the nineties with an emphasis on the unitary perspective of patient care. In M. Madrid (Ed.), *Patterns of Rogerian knowing* (pp. 257-266). New York: National League for Nursing.

Gold, J. (1997). The practice of nursing from a unitary perspective. In M. Madrid (Ed.), *Patterns of Rogerian knowing* (pp. 249-256). New York: National League for Nursing.

Gueldner, S.H. (1986). The relationship between imposed motion and human field motion in elderly individuals living in nursing homes. In V.M. Malinski (Ed.), *Explorations on Martha Rogers' science of unitary human beings* (pp. 161-170). Norwalk, CT: Appleton-Century-Crofts.

Hanchett, E.S. (1997). Traditions of mysticism and Rogerian science. In M. Madrid (Ed.), *Patterns of Rogerian knowing* (pp. 103-111). New York: National League for Nursing.

Horvath, B. (1997). The pandimensional nurse manager. In M. Madrid (Ed.), *Patterns of Rogerian knowing* (pp. 211-217). New York: National League for Nursing.

Ireland, M. (1997). Pediatric acquired immunodeficiency syndrome (AIDS) studied from a Rogerian perspective: A sense of hope. In M. Madrid (Ed.), *Patterns of Rogerian knowing* (pp. 143-151). New York: National League for Nursing.

Joseph, L. (1990). Practical application of Rogers' theoretical framework for nursing. In M.E. Parker (Ed.), *Nursing theories in practice* (pp. 115-125). New York: National League for Nursing.

Madrid, M. & Winstead-Fry, P. (1986). Rogers' conceptual model. In P. Winstead-Fry (Ed.), *Case studies in nursing theory.* New York: National League for Nursing.

Malinski, V.M. (1986). Contemporary science and nursing: Parallels with Rogers. In V.M. Malinski (Ed.), *Explorations of Martha Rogers' science of unitary human beings* (pp. 15-24). Norwalk, CT: Appleton-Century-Crofts.

Malinski, V.M. (1986). Further ideas from Martha Rogers. In V.M. Malinski (Ed.), *Explorations of Martha Rogers' science of unitary human beings* (pp. 9-14). Norwalk, CT: Appleton-Century-Crofts.

Malinski, V.M. (1986). Nursing practice within the science of unitary human beings. In V.M. Malinski (Ed.), *Explorations of Martha Rogers' science of unitary human beings* (pp. 25-32). Norwalk, CT: Appleton-Century-Crofts.

Malinski, V.M. (1986). The relationship between hyperactivity in children and perception of short wavelength light. In V.M. Malinski (Ed.), *Explorations of Martha Rogers' science of unitary human beings* (pp. 107-116). Norwalk, CT: Appleton-Century-Crofts.

Malinski, V.M. (1997). The relationship of temporal experience and power as knowing participation in change in depressed and nondepressed women. In M. Madrid (Ed.), *Patterns of Rogerian knowing* (pp. 197-208). New York: National League for Nursing.

Mandl, A. (1997). A plea to educate the public about Martha Rogers' science of unitary human beings. In M. Madrid (Ed.), *Patterns of Rogerian knowing* (pp. 236-238). New York: National League for Nursing.

Matas, K.E. (1997). Therapeutic touch: A model for community-based health promotion. In M. Madrid (Ed.), *Patterns of Rogerian knowing* (pp. 218-229). New York: National League for Nursing.

McDonald, S.F. (1986). The relationship between visible lightwaves and the experience of pain. In V.M. Malinski (Ed.), *Explorations of Martha Rogers' science of unitary human beings* (pp. 119-126). Norwalk, CT: Appleton-Century-Crofts.

McNiff, M.A. (1997). Power, perceived health, and life satisfaction in adults with long-term care needs. In M. Madrid (Ed.), *Patterns of Rogerian knowing* (pp. 177-186). New York: National League for Nursing.

Meleis, A.I. (1985). Martha Rogers. In A.I. Meleis (Ed.), *Theoretical nursing: Development and progress.* Philadelphia: J.B. Lippincott.

Rawnsley, M.M. (1986). The relationship between the perception of the speed of time and the process of dying. In V.M. Malinski (Ed.), *Explorations of Martha Rogers' science of unitary human beings* (pp. 79-90). Norwalk, CT: Appleton-Century-Crofts.

Reed, P.G. (1997). The place of transcendence in nursing's science of unitary human beings: Theory and practice. In M. Madrid (Ed.), *Patterns of Rogerian knowing* (pp. 187-196). New York: National League for Nursing.

Reeder, F. (1986). Basic theoretical research in the conceptual system of unitary human beings. In V.M. Malinski (Ed.), *Explorations of Martha Rogers' science of unitary human beings* (pp. 45-64). Norwalk, CT: Appleton-Century-Crofts.

Reeder, F. (1997). Mysticism/spirituality of Aborigine people and Rogerian science. In M. Madrid (Ed.), *Patterns of Rogerian knowing* (pp. 120-126). New York: National League for Nursing.

Sarter, B. (1997). Hindu mysticism: The realization of integrality. In M. Madrid (Ed.), *Patterns of Rogerian knowing* (pp. 112-119). New York: National League for Nursing.

Watson, J. (1997). Using Rogers' model to study sleep-wake pattern changes in older women. In M. Madrid (Ed.), *Patterns of Rogerian knowing* (pp. 167-176). New York: National League for Nursing.

Watson, J., Barrett, E.A.M., Hastings-Tolsma, M., Johnston, L., & Gueldner, S. (1997). Measurement in Rogerian science: A review of selected instruments. In M. Madrid (Ed.), *Patterns of Rogerian knowing* (pp. 87-99). New York: National League for Nursing.

Woodward, T.A. & Heggie, J. (1997). Rogers in reality: Staff nurse application of the science of unitary human beings in the clinical setting following changes in an orientation program. In M. Madrid (Ed.), *Patterns of Rogerian knowing* (pp. 239-248). New York: National League for Nursing.

Journal Articles

Aggleton, P. & Chalmers, H. (1984). Models and theories: Rogers' unitary field model. Within the bounds of the nursing process—Part 4. *Nursing Times,* 80(50), 35-39.

Allanach, E.J. (1988). Perceived supportive behaviors and nursing occupational stress: An evolution of consciousness. *Advances in Nursing Science,* 10(2), 73-82.

Alligood, M.R. (1990). Rogers' theory: Research to practice. *Rogerian Nursing Science News,* 2(3), 2-4.

Alligood, M.R. (1991). Testing Rogers' theory of accelerating change: The relationships among creativity, actualization, and empathy in persons 18 to 92 years of age. *Western Journal of Nursing Research,* 13(1), 84-96.

Anderson, M. (1980). A psychosocial screening tool for ambulatory health-care clients: A pilot study of validity. *Nursing Research,* 29(6), 347-351.

Anderson, M.D. & Smereck, G.A.D. (1992). The consciousness rainbow: An explication of Rogerian field pattern manifestations. *Nursing Science Quarterly,* 5(2), 72-79.

Anonymous. (1990). Mission statement of the Society of Rogerian Scholars. *Rogerian Nursing Science News,* 3(1), 6-7.

Armstrong, M.A. & Kelly, A.E. (1995). More than the sum of their parts: Martha Rogers and Hildegard Peplau. *Archives of Psychiatric Nursing,* 9(1), 40-44.

Atwood, J.R. & Gill-Rogers, B.P. (1984). Metatheory, methodology, and practicality: Issues in research uses of Rogers' science of unitary man. *Nursing Research,* 33(2), 88-91.

Barrett, E.A.M. (1988). Using Rogers' science of unitary human beings in nursing practice. *Nursing Science Quarterly,* 1(2), 50-51.

Barrett, E.A.M. (1993). Virtual reality: A health patterning modality for nursing in space. *Visions: The Journal of Rogerian Nursing Science,* 1(1), 10-21.

Barrett, E.A.M. (1996). Canonical correlation analysis and its use in Rogerian research. *Nursing Science Quarterly,* 9(2), 50-52.

Bateau, J. (1985, May/June). Case study in family therapy: A Rogers/Minuchin reformation. *Michigan Nurse,* 58(3), 7-9.

Batra, C. (1995). Theory based curricula and utilization of Martha Rogers' framework in undergraduate and graduate programs. *Rogerian Nursing Science News,* 8(2), 8-9.

Benedict, S.C. & Burge, J.M. (1990). The relationship between human field motion and preferred visible wavelengths. *Nursing Science Quarterly,* 3(2), 73-80.

Bernado, M.L. (1996). Parent-reported injury-associated behaviors and life events among injured, ill, and well preschool children. *Journal of Pediatric Nursing,* 11(2), 100-110.

Biley, F. (1990). Rogers' model: An analysis. *Nursing-Oxford,* 4(15), 31-33.

Biley, F.C. (1992). The perception of time as a factor in Rogers' science of unitary human beings: A literature review. *Journal of Advanced Nursing,* 17(9), 1141-1145.

Biley, F.C. (1993). Energy fields nursing: A brief encounter of a unitary kind. *International Journal of Nursing Studies,* 30(6), 519-525.

Biley, F.C. (1996). Rogerian science, phantoms, and therapeutic touch: Exploring potentials. *Nursing Science Quarterly,* 9(4), 165-169.

Biley, F.C. (1998). The beat generation and beyond: Popular culture and the development of the science of unitary human beings. *Visions: The Journal of Rogerian Nursing Science,* 6(1), 5-12.

Blair, C. (1979). Hyperactivity in children: Viewed within the framework of synergistic man. *Nursing Forum,* 18, 293-303.

Bramlett, N.H., Gueldner, S.H., & Sowell, R.L. (1990). Consumer-centric advocacy: Its connection to nursing frameworks. *Nursing Science Quarterly,* 3(4), 156-61.

Bramlett, N.H., Gueldner, S.H., & Boettcher, J.H. (1993). Reflections on the science of unitary human beings in terms of Kuhn's requirement for explanatory power. *Visions: The Journal of Rogerian Nursing Science,* 1(1), 22-35.

Braunstein, M.S. (1998). Evaluation of nursing practice: Process and critique. *Nursing Science Quarterly,* 11(2), 64-68.

Brouse, S.H. (1985). Effect of gender role identity on patterns of feminine and self-concept scores from late pregnancy to early postpartum. *Advances in Nursing Science,* 7(3), 32-48.

Buczny, B. (1990). Nursing care of the terminally ill client. Applying Martha Rogers' conceptual framework. *Home Health Nurse,* 7(4), 13-18.

Bush, M.R. (1997). Influence of health locus of control and parental health perceptions as follow-through with school health nurse referral. *Issues in Comprehensive Pediatric Nursing,* 20(3), 175-182.

Butcher, H.K. (1996). A unitary field pattern portrait of dispiritedness in later life. *Visions,* 4(1), 41-58.

Butcher, H.K. (1998). Crystallizing the processes of the unitary field pattern portrait research method. *Visions: The Journal of Rogerian Nursing Science,* 6(1), 13-26.

Butcher, H.K. (1999). The artistry of Rogerian practice. *Visions: The Journal of Rogerian Nursing Science,* 7(1), 49-54.

Butcher, H.K. (1999). Weaving a theoretical tapestry supporting pandimensionality: Deep connectedness in the multiverse. *Visions: The Journal of Rogerian Nursing Science,* 6(1), 51-55.

Butcher, H.K. & Parker, N.I. (1988). Guided imagery within Rogers' science of unitary human beings: An experimental study. *Nursing Science Quarterly,* 1(3), 103-110.

Carboni, J.T. (1991). A Rogerian theoretical tapestry. *Nursing Science Quarterly, 4*(3), 130-136.

Carboni, J.T. (1995). A Rogerian process of inquiry. *Nursing Science Quarterly, 5*(1), 22-34.

Carboni, J.T. (1995). Enfolding health-as-wholeness-and-harmony: A theory of Rogerian nursing practice. *Nursing Science Quarterly, 8*(2), 71-78.

Change through environmental interaction makes aging exciting: An interview with Martha Rogers. (1985). *Journal of Gerontological Nursing, 11*(2), 35-36.

Christensen, P., Sowell, R., & Gueldner, S.H. (1993). Nursing in space: Theoretical foundations and potential practice applications within Rogerian science. *Visions: The Journal of Rogerian Nursing Science, 1*(1), 36-44.

Compton, M.A. (1989). A Rogerian view of drug abuse: Implications for nursing. *Nursing Science Quarterly, 2*(2), 98-105.

Davidson, A.W. (1992). Choice patterns: A theory of the human-environment relationship. *Rogerian Nursing Science News, 5*(1), 4-5.

Denham, G. (1992). Toward the development of a theory of unitary perception. *Rogerian Nursing Science News, 5*(1), 7.

Donahue, L. & Alligood, M.R. (1995). A description of the elderly from self-selected attributes. *Visions: The Journal of Rogerian Nursing Science, 3*(1), 12-19.

Dykeman, M.C. & Loukissa, D. (1993). The science of unitary human beings: An integrative review. *Nursing Science Quarterly, 6*(4), 179-188.

Fawcett, J. (1975). Family as a living open system: Emerging conceptual framework for nursing. *International Nursing Review, 22*(4), 113-116.

Fawcett, J. (1977). Relationship between identification and patterns of change in spouses' body images during and after pregnancy. *International Journal of Nursing Studies, 14*(4), 199-213.

Fawcett, J. (1996). Issues of (in)compatibility between the worldview and research rules of the science of unitary human beings: An invitation to dialogue. *Visions: The Journal of Rogerian Nursing Science, 4*(1), 5-11.

Floyd, J.A. (1984). Interaction between personal sleep-wake rhythms and psychiatric hospital rest-activity schedule. *Nursing Research, 33*(5), 255-259.

Garon, M. (1991). Assessment and management of pain in the home care setting: Application of Rogers' science of unitary human beings. *Holistic Nursing Practice, 6*(1), 47-57.

Garon, M. (1992). Contributions of Martha Rogers to the development of nursing theory. *Nursing Outlook, 40*(2), 67-72.

Gibson, A. (1996). Personal experiences of individuals using meditations from a metaphysical source. *Visions: The Journal of Rogerian Nursing Science, 4*(1), 12-23.

Gill, B.P. & Atwood, J.R. (1981). Reciprocy and helicy used to relate MEGF and wound healing. *Nursing Research, 30*(2), 68-72.

Goldberg, W.G. & Fitzpatrick, J.J. (1980). Movement therapy with the aged. *Nursing Research, 29*(6), 339-346.

Greiner, D.S. (1991). Rhythmicities. *Nursing Science Quarterly, 4*(1), 21-23.

Griffin, W.M., Moore, P., Ruge, C., & Weiler-Crespo, W. (1996). Martha E. Rogers' nursing science: Application to therapeutic touch. *Rogerian Nursing Science News, 8*(3), 9-12.

Halkitis, P.N. & Kirton, C. (1999). Self-strategies as means of enhancing adherence to HIV antiretroviral therapies: A Rogerian approach. *Journal of the New York State Nurses Association, 30*(2), 22-27.

Hanchett, E.S. (1990). Nursing models and community as client(public health/community health nursing. *Nursing Science Quarterly, 3*(2), 67-72.

Hanchett, E.S. (1992). Concepts from Eastern philosophy and Rogers' science of unitary human beings. *Nursing Science Quarterly, 5*(4), 164-170.

Hanchett, E.S. (1999). Field phenomena and outcomes research on the brink of a quantum leap? *Visions: The Journal of Rogerian Nursing Science, 7*(1), 44-48.

Hardin, S.R. (1997). Culture: A manifestation of pattern. *Journal of Multicultural Nursing and Health, 3*(3), 21-23.

Heggie, J.R., Schoenmehl, P.A., Chang, M.K., & Grieco, C. (1989). Selection and implementation of Dr. Martha Rogers' nursing conceptual model in an acute care setting. *Clinical Nurse Specialist, 3*(3), 143-147.

Heidt, P. (1981). Effect of therapeutic touch on anxiety level of hospitalized patients. *Nursing Research, 30*(1), 32-37.

Instruments developed within Rogers' science of unitary human beings. (1996). *Visions: The Journal of Rogerian Nursing Science, 8*(4), 9-12.

Iveson, J. (1982). The four dimensional nurse. The Rogers' model of nursing. *Nursing Mirror, 155*(22), 52.

Johnson, M.O. (1996). A mutual field manifestation: Substance abuse and nursing. *Visions: The Journal of Rogerian Nursing Science, 4*(1), 24-30.

Keller, E. & Bzdek, V.M. (1986). Effects of therapeutic touch on tension headache pain. *Nursing Research, 35*(2), 101-106.

Kim, H.S. (1983). Use of Rogers' conceptual system in research: Comments. *Nursing Research, 32*(2), 89-91.

Klemm, P.R. & Stashinko, E.E. (1997). Martha Rogers' science of unitary human beings: A participative teaching-learning approach. *Journal of Nursing Education, 36*(7), 341-343.

Kodiath, M.F. (1991). A new view of the chronic pain client. *Holistic Nursing Practice, 6*(1), 41-46.

Kreiger, D. (1990). Compassion as power: Clinical implications of therapeutic touch. *Rogerian Nursing Science News, 3*(1), 1-5.

Levine, N.H. (1976). A conceptual model for obstetric nursing. *Journal of Obstetric, Gynecologic, and Neonatal Nursing,* 5(2), 9-15.

Malinski, V.M. (1991). The experience of laughing at oneself in older couples. *Nursing Science Quarterly,* 4(2), 69-75.

Malinski, V.M. (1993). Therapeutic touch: The view from Rogerian science. *Visions: The Journal of Rogerian Nursing Science,* 1(1), 45-54.

Malinski, V.M. (1994). Spirituality: A pattern manifestation of the human/environment mutual process. *Visions: The Journal of Rogerian Nursing Science,* 2(1), 12-18.

Malinski, V.M. (1999). Participating, transforming, celebrating: The dance of unitary becoming. *Visions: The Journal of Rogerian Nursing Science,* 7(1), 14-23.

Mason, T. & Patterson, R. (1990). A critical review of the use of Rogers' model within a special hospital: A single case study. *Journal of Advanced Nursing,* 15(2), 130-141.

Matas, K.E. (1997). Human patterning and chronic pain. *Nursing Science Quarterly,* 10(2), 88-96.

McFarlane, E.A. (1980). Nursing theory: Comparison of four theoretical proposals. *Journal of Advanced Nursing,* 5(1), 3-19.

Meehan, T.C. (1988). Theory development. *Rogerian Nursing Science News,* 1(2), 4-8.

Miller, L.A. (1979). An explanation of therapeutic touch using the science of unitary man. *Nursing Forum,* 18, 278-287.

Moccia, P. (1985). A further investigation of "dialectical thinking as a means to understanding systems-in-development: Relevance to Rogers' principles." *Advances in Nursing Science,* 7(4), 33-38.

Nicoll, L.H., Meyer, P.A., & Abraham, I.L. (1985). Critique: External comparison of conceptual nursing models. *Advances in Nursing Science,* 7(4), 1-9.

Novak, D.M. (1999). Perception of menopause and its application to Rogers' science of unitary human beings. *Visions: The Journal of Rogerian Nursing Science,* 7(1), 24-29.

Papowitz, L. (1986). During resuscitation, some patients face a life-or-death choice that no one else will know about—Unless they ask. *American Journal of Nursing,* 86, 416-418.

Patty, C.M. (1999). Teaching affective competencies to surgical technologists. *AORN Journal,* 70(5), 778-781.

Peterson, M. (1987). Time and nursing process. *Holistic Nursing Practice,* 1(3), 72-80.

Phillips, B.B. & Bramlett, M.H. (1994). Integrated awareness: A key to the pattern of mutual process. *Visions: The Journal of Rogerian Nursing Science,* 2(1), 19-34.

Phillips, J.R. (1989). Science of unitary human beings: Changing research perspectives. *Nursing Science Quarterly,* 2(2), 57-60.

Phillips, J.R. (1991). Human field research. *Nursing Science Quarterly,* 4(4), 142-143.

Phillips, J.R. (2000). Rogerian nursing science and research: A healing process for nursing. *Nursing Science Quarterly,* 13(3), 196-201.

Porter, L.S. (1998). Reducing teenage and unintended pregnancies through client-centered and family-focused school-based family planning. *Journal of Pediatric Nursing,* 13(3), 158-163.

Reed, P.G. (1986). Developmental resources and depression in the elderly. *Nursing Research,* 35(6), 368-374.

Reed, P.G. (1987). Constructing a conceptual framework for psychosocial nursing. *Journal of Psychosocial Nursing and Mental Health Services,* 25(2), 24-28.

Reed, P.G. (1991). Toward a nursing theory of self-transcendence: Deductive reformulation using developmental theories. *Advances in Nursing Science,* 13(4), 64-77.

Reed, P.G., Fitzpatrick, J.J., Donovan, M.J., & Johnston, R.L. (1982). Suicidal crises: Relationship to the experience of time [Abstract]. *Nursing Research,* 31, 122.

Reeder, F. (1993). The science of unitary human beings and interpretive human science. *Nursing Science Quarterly,* 6(1), 13-24.

Reeder, F.M. (1999). Energy: Its distinctive meanings. *Nursing Science Quarterly,* 12(1), 6-8.

Roberts, K.L. (1985). Theory of nursing as curriculum content. *Journal of Advanced Nursing,* 10, 209-215.

Rush, M.N. (1997). A study of the relations among perceived social support, spirituality, and power as knowing participation in change among sober female alcoholics within the science of unitary human beings. *Journal of Addiction Nursing,* 9(4), 146-155.

Samarel, N. (1992). The experience of receiving therapeutic touch. *Journal of Advanced Nursing,* 17(6), 651-657.

Samarel, N. (1997). Therapeutic touch, dialogue, and women's experiences in breast cancer surgery. *Holistic Nursing Practice,* 12(1), 62-70.

Samarel, N., Fawcett, J., Davis, N.M., & Ryan, F.M. (1998). Effects of dialogue and therapeutic touch on preoperative and postoperative experiences of breast cancer surgery: An exploratory study. *Oncology Nursing Forum,* 25(8), 1369-1376.

Sarter, B. (1989). Some critical philosophical issues in the science of unitary human beings. *Nursing Science Quarterly,* 2(2), 74-78.

Schneider, P.E. (1995). Focusing awareness: The process of extraordinary healing from a Rogerian perspective. *Visions: The Journal of Rogerian Nursing Science,* 3(1), 32-43.

Schodt, C.M. (1989). Parental-fetal attachment and couvade: A study of patterns of human-environment integrality. *Nursing Science Quarterly,* 2(2), 88-97.

Schroeder, C. (1991). Disembodiment or "where's the body in field theory?" *Nursing Science Quarterly,* 4(4), 146-148.

Sherman, D.W. (1996). Nurses' willingness to care for AIDS patients and spirituality, social support, and death anxiety. *Image,* 28(3), 205-213.

Skillman, L. (1991). A challenge to our current methods for studying and understanding human mutual processing. *Rogerian Nursing Science News,* 3(3), 4-7.

Smith, C.S. (1988). Testing propositions derived from Rogers' conceptual system. *Nursing Science Quarterly,* 1(2), 60-67.

Smith, D.W. (1994). Toward developing a theory of spirituality. *Visions: The Journal of Rogerian Nursing Science,* 2(1), 35-43.

Smith, D.W. (1995). Power and spirituality in polio survivors: A study based on Rogers' science. *Nursing Science Quarterly,* , 8(3), 133-139.

Smith, M.C. (1991). Affirming the unitary perspective. *Nursing Science Quarterly,* 4(4), 148-152.

Smith, M.C. (1999). Caring and the science of unitary human beings. *Advances in Nursing Science,* 21(4), 14-28.

Smith, M.C. & Reeder, F. (1998). Clinical outcomes research and Rogerian science: Strange or emergent bedfellows? *Visions: The Journal of Rogerian Nursing Science,* 6(1), 27-38.

Smith, M.J. (1986). Human-environment process: A test of Rogers' principle of integrality. *Advances in Nursing Science,* 9(1), 21-28.

Smith, M.J. (1989). Four-dimensionality: Where to go with it. *Nursing Science Quarterly,* 2(2), 56.

Thompson, J.E. (1990). Finding the borderline's border: Can Martha Rogers help? *Perspectives in Psychiatric Care,* 26(4), 7-10.

Todaro-Franceschi, V. (1999). The idea of energy as phenomenon and Rogerian science: Are they congruent? *Visions: The Journal of Rogerian Nursing Science,* 7(1), 30-41.

Ulys, L.R. (1987). Foundational studies in nursing: Orem, King, and Rogers. *Journal of Advanced Nursing,* 12(3), 275-280.

Watson, J. (1996). Issues with measuring time experience in Rogers' conceptual model. *Visions: The Journal of Rogerian Nursing Science,* 4(1), 31-40.

Watson, J. (1999). Exploring the concept of beyond waking experience. *Visions: The Journal of Rogerian Nursing Science,* 6(1), 39-46.

Whall, L. M. (1999). Exercise: A unitary concept. *Nursing Science Quarterly,* 12(1), 68-72.

Whelton, B.J. (1979). An operationalization of Martha Rogers' theory throughout the nursing process. *International Journal of Nursing Studies,* 16(1), 7-20.

Wilson, L.M. & Fitzpatrick, J.J. (1984). Dialectic thinking as a means of understanding systems-in-development: Relevance to Rogers' principles. *Advances in Nursing Science,* 6(2), 24-41.

Yarcheski, A. & Mahon, N.E. (1995). Rogers' pattern manifestations and health in adolescents. *Western Journal of Nursing Research,* 17(4), 383-397.

Young, A.A. & Keil, C. (1981, April). The Washburn nursing curriculum: Interpreting Martha Rogers in the Land of Oz. *Kansas Nurse,* 56(4), 7-8.

Doctoral Dissertations

Allen, V.L.R. (1988). *The relationships of time experience, human field motion, and clairvoyance: An investigation in the Rogerian conceptual framework.* Unpublished doctoral dissertation, New York University.

Barrett, E.A. (1983). *An empirical investigation of Rogers' principle of helicy: The relationship of human field complexity, human field motion, and power.* Unpublished doctoral dissertation, New York University.

Bays, C. (1995). *Older adults descriptions of hope after a stroke.* Unpublished doctoral dissertation, University of Cincinnati.

Bernardo, L.M. (1993). *Parent-reported injury-associated behaviors and life events among injured, ill, and well preschool children.* Unpublished doctoral dissertation, New York University.

Bowles, D.J.N. (1999). *Exploring pattern manifestation through critical incident analysis of nurse educators and clinicians.* Unpublished doctoral dissertation, Spalding University.

Bramlett, M.H. (1990). *Power, creativity and reminiscence in the elderly.* Unpublished doctoral dissertation, Medical College of Georgia.

Bray, J.D. (1989). *The relationships of creativity, time experience and mystical experience.* Unpublished doctoral dissertation, New York University.

Brown, P.W. (1992). *Sibling relationship qualities following the crisis of divorce.* Unpublished doctoral dissertation, University of Miami.

Bultemeier, K. (1993). *Photographic inquiry of the phenomenon premenstrual syndrome within the Rogerian derived theory of perceived dissonance.* Unpublished doctoral dissertation, University of Tennessee, Knoxville.

Butcher, H.K. (1994). *A unitary field pattern portrait of dispiritedness in later life.* Unpublished doctoral dissertation, University of South Carolina.

Carboni, J.T. (1997). *Coming home: An investigation of the enfolding-unfolding movement of human environmental energy field patterns within the nursing home setting and the enfoldment of health-as-wholeness-and-harmony by the nurse and client.* Unpublished doctoral dissertation, University of Rhode Island.

Caroselli-Dervan, C. (1991). *The relationship of power and feminism in female nurse executives in acute care hospitals.* Unpublished doctoral dissertation, New York University.

Conner, G.K. (1986). *The manifestations of human field motion, creativity, and time experience patterns of female and male parents.* Unpublished doctoral dissertation, University of Alabama, Birmingham.

Cowling, W.R. (1982). *The relationship of mystical experience, differentiation, and creativity in college students: An empirical investigation of the principle of helicy in Rogers' science of unitary man.* Unpublished doctoral dissertation, New York University.

Daffron, J.M. (1988). *Patterns of human field motion and human health.* Unpublished doctoral dissertation, Texas Women's University.

De Sevo, M. (1991). *Temporal experience and the preference for musical sequence complexity: A study based on Martha Rogers' conceptual system.* Unpublished doctoral dissertation, New York University.

Dixon, D.S. (1994). *An exploration of the sleep patterns of individuals when their environment changes from home to hospital.* Unpublished doctoral dissertation, University of Cincinnati.

Dominguez, L.M. (1996). *The lived experience of women with Mexican heritage with HIV/AIDS.* Unpublished doctoral dissertation, University of Arizona.

Doyle, M.B. (1995). *Mental health nurses' imagination, power, and empathy: A descriptive study using Rogerian nursing science.* Unpublished doctoral dissertation, New York University.

Evans, B.A. (1990). *The relationship among a pattern of influence in the organizational environment, power of the nurse, and the nurse's empathic attributes: A manifestation of integrality.* Unpublished doctoral dissertation, Case Western University.

Ference, H. (1979). *The relationship of time experience, creativity traits, differentiation, and human field motion.* Unpublished doctoral dissertation, New York University.

Gabor, L.M. (1994). *Understanding the impact of chronically ill and/or developmentally disabled children on low-income, single parent families.* Unpublished doctoral dissertation, University of Nevada.

Garrard, C.T. (1995). *The effect of therapeutic touch on stress reduction and immune function in person with AIDS.* Unpublished doctoral dissertation, University of Alabama, Birmingham.

Girardin, B.W. (1990). *The relationship of lightwave frequency to sleepwakefulness frequency in well, full-term, Hispanic neonates.* Unpublished doctoral dissertation, Wayne State University.

Gueldner, S.H. (1983). *A study of the relationship between imposed motion and human field motion in elderly individuals living in nursing homes.* Unpublished doctoral dissertation, University of Alabama, Birmingham.

Guthrie, B.J. (1987). *The relationships of tolerance of ambiguity, preference for processing information in the mixed mode to differentiation in female college students: An empirical investigation of the homeodynamic principle of helicy.* Unpublished doctoral dissertation, New York University.

Hastings-Tolsma, M.T. (1992). *The relationship of diversity of human field pattern to risk-taking and time experience: An investigation of Rogers' principles of homeodynamics.* Unpublished doctoral dissertation, New York University.

Headley, J.A. (1997). *Chemotherapy-induced ovarian failure in women with breast cancer.* Unpublished doctoral dissertation, Texas Women's University.

Hills, R.G.S. (1998). *Maternal field patterning of awareness, wakefulness, human field motion, and well-being in mothers with six month old infants: A Rogerian perspective.* Unpublished doctoral dissertation, Wayne State University.

Hindman, M.L. (1993). *Humor and field energy in older adults.* Unpublished doctoral dissertation, Medical College of Georgia.

Horvath, B. (1998). *The relation of the clinical application of music and mood in persons receiving treatment for alcoholism.* Unpublished doctoral dissertation, New York University.

Johnson, E.E. (1996). *Health choice-making: The experience, perception, expression of older women.* Unpublished doctoral dissertation, University of South Carolina.

Johnston, L.W. (1993). *The development of the human field image metaphor scale.* Unpublished doctoral dissertation, Medical College of Georgia.

Kells, K.J. (1995). *Sensing presence as open or closed space: A phenomenological inquiry on blind individuals' experiences of obstacle detection.* Unpublished doctoral dissertation, University of Colorado Health Sciences Center.

Kilker, M.J. (1994). *Transformational and transactional leadership styles: An empirical investigation of Rogers' principle of integrality.* Unpublished doctoral dissertation, Columbia University.

Kim, H. (1990). *Patterning of parent-fetal attachment during the experience of guided imagery: An experimental investigation of Martha Rogers' human-environment integrality.* Unpublished doctoral dissertation, Columbia University.

Krause, D.A. (1991). *The impact of an individually tailored nursing intervention on human field patterning in clients who experience dyspnea.* Unpublished doctoral dissertation, University of Miami.

Lothian, J.A. (1989). *Continuing to breastfeed.* Unpublished doctoral dissertation, New York University.

Mahoney, J. (1998). *The relationship of power and actualization to job satisfaction in female home health care nurses.* Unpublished doctoral dissertation, New York University.

Malinski, V. (1980). *The relationship between hyperactivity in children and perception of short wave length light: An investigation into the conceptual system proposed by Martha E. Rogers.* Unpublished doctoral dissertation, New York University.

McEvoy, M.D. (1987). *The relationships among the experience of dying, the experience of paranormal events, and creativity in adults.* Unpublished doctoral dissertation, New York University.

McNiff, M.A. (1995). *A study of the relationship of power, perceived health, and life satisfaction in adults with long-term care needs based on Martha E. Rogers' science of unitary human beings.* Unpublished doctoral dissertation, New York University.

Mellow, J.I. (1993). *The relationship of back massage to a person's patterning, using Martha Rogers' nursing theory.* Unpublished doctoral dissertation, University of Nevada.

Mersmann, C.A. (1993). *Therapeutic touch and milk letdown in mothers of non-nursing preterm infants.* Unpublished doctoral dissertation, New York University.

Morris, D.L.Y. (1991). *An exploration of elders' perceptions of power and well-being.* Unpublished doctoral dissertation, Case Western Reserve University.

Moulton, P.J. (1994). *An investigation of the relationship of power and empathy in nurse executives.* Unpublished doctoral dissertation, New York University.

Muscari, M.E. (1992). *Binge/purge behaviors and attitudes as manifestation of relational patternings in a woman with bulimia nervosa.* Unpublished doctoral dissertation, Adelphi University.

Nellett, G.H. (1998). *The caregiver's experience of deliberative mutual pattern with pain-ridden substance abusers.* Unpublished doctoral dissertation, Loyola University of Chicago.

Quinn, A.A. (1989). *Integrating a changing me: A grounded theory of the process of menopause for perimenopausal women.* Unpublished doctoral dissertation, University of Colorado.

Raile, M.M. (1982). *The relationship of creativity, actualization, and empathy in unitary human development: A descriptive study of Rogers' principle of helicy.* Unpublished doctoral dissertation, New York University.

Rankin, M.K. (1984). *Effect of sound wave repatterning on symptoms of menopausal women.* Unpublished doctoral dissertation, Texas Women's University.

Rapacz, K.E. (1991). *Human patterning and chronic pain.* Unpublished doctoral dissertation, Case Western Reserve University.

Rawnsley, M. (1977). *Relationships between the perception of the speed of time and the process of dying: An empirical investigation of the holistic theory of nursing proposed by Martha Rogers.* Unpublished doctoral dissertation, Boston University.

Reeder, F. (1984). *Nursing research, holism, and philosophies of science: Points of congruence between Edmund Husseerl and Martha E. Rogers.* Unpublished doctoral dissertation, New York University.

Rizzo, J.A. (1990). *An investigation of the relationships of life satisfaction, purpose in life, and power in individuals sixty-five years and older.* Unpublished doctoral dissertation, New York University.

Rush, M.M. (1995). *A study of the relations among perceived social support, spirituality, and power as knowing participation in change among sober female alcoholics in Alcoholics Anonymous within the science of unitary human beings.* Unpublished doctoral dissertation, New York University.

Sarter, B.V. (1984). *The stream of becoming: A metaphysical analysis of Rogers' model of unitary man.* Unpublished doctoral dissertation, New York University.

Schodt, C.M. (1989). *Patterns of parent-fetus attachment and the couvade syndrome: An application of human-environment integrality as postulated in the science of unitary human beings.* Unpublished doctoral dissertation, New York University.

Sherman, D.W. (1993). *An investigation of the relationships among spirituality, perceived social support, death anxiety, and nurses' willingness to care for AIDS patients.* Unpublished doctoral dissertation, New York University.

Smith, M.C. (1986). *An investigation of the effects of different sound frequencies on vividness and creativity of imagery.* Unpublished doctoral dissertation, New York University.

Smyth, P.E. (1999). *Reducing immunization pain perception in preschoolers with therapeutic touch.* Unpublished doctoral dissertation, University of Alabama, Birmingham.

Straneva, J.A. (1992). *Therapeutic touch and in vitro erythropoiesis.* Unpublished doctoral dissertation, Indiana University School of Nursing.

Wall, J.M. (1999). *An exploration of hope and power among lung cancer patients who have and have not participated in a preoperative exercise program.* Unpublished doctoral dissertation, New York University.

Watson, J. (1993). *The relationships of sleep-wake rhythm, dream experience, human field motion, and time experience in older women.* Unpublished doctoral dissertation, New York University.

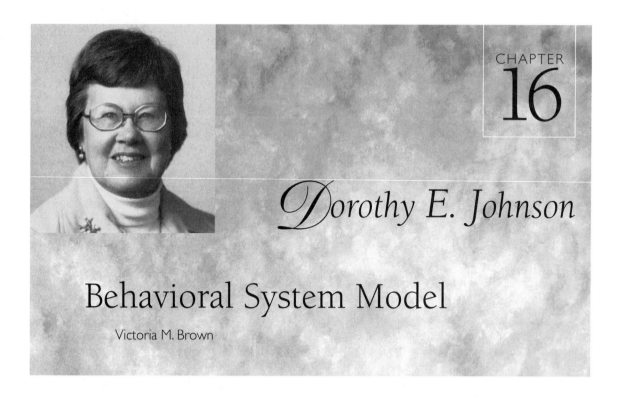

Dorothy E. Johnson

Behavioral System Model

Victoria M. Brown

CREDENTIALS AND BACKGROUND OF THE THEORIST

Dorothy E. Johnson was born on August 21, 1919 in Savannah, Georgia. She received her A.A. from Armstrong Junior College in Savannah, Georgia (1938); her B.S.N. from Vanderbilt University in Nashville, Tennessee (1942); and her M.P.H. from Harvard University in Boston (1948).

Johnson's professional experiences involved mostly teaching, although she was a staff nurse at the Chatham-Savannah Health Council from 1943 to 1944. She had been an instructor and an assistant professor in pediatric nursing at Vanderbilt University School of Nursing. From 1949 until her retirement in 1978 and her subsequent move to Florida, Johnson was an assistant professor of pediatric nursing, an associate professor of nursing, and a

Previous authors: Victoria M. Brown, Sharon S. Conner, Linda S. Harbour, Jude A. Magers, and Judith K. Watt.
The author wishes to express appreciation to Dr. Bonnie Holaday for her assistance.

professor of nursing at the University of California in Los Angeles.

In 1955 and 1956, Johnson was a pediatric nursing advisor assigned to the Christian Medical College School of Nursing in Vellore, South India. In addition, from 1965 to 1967, she chaired the committee of the California Nurses' Association that developed a position statement on specifications for the clinical specialist. Johnson's publications[25] include four books; more than 30 articles in periodicals; and many papers, reports, proceedings, and monographs.

Of the many honors she received, Johnson[27] was proudest of the 1975 Faculty Award from graduate students, the 1977 Lulu Hassenplug Distinguished Achievement Award from the California Nurses' Association, and the 1981 Vanderbilt University School of Nursing Award for Excellence in Nursing. She died in February, 1999 at the age of 80.[15] She was pleased that her Behavioral System Model had been found useful in furthering the development of a theoretical basis for nursing and was being used as a model for nursing practice on an institution-wide basis, but she reported that her greatest source of satisfaction came from following the productive careers of her students.[29]

THEORETICAL SOURCES

Johnson's Behavioral System Theory springs from Nightingale's belief that nursing's goal is to help individuals prevent or recover from disease or injury.[34] The science and art of nursing should focus on the patient as an individual and not on the specific disease entity.[28] Johnson reports that the Behavioral System Model is based on a preexistent body of knowledge developed over years by a number of different disciplines.

She used the work of behavioral scientists in psychology, sociology, and ethnology to develop her theory. Talcott Parsons is acknowledged specifically in early developmental writings presenting concepts of the behavioral system model.[18] She relies heavily on the systems theory and uses concepts and definitions from Rapoport, Chinn, and Buckley.[25] The structure of the Behavioral System Theory is patterned after a systems model; a system is defined as consisting of interrelated parts functioning together to form a whole. In her writings, Johnson conceptualizes a person as a behavioral system in which the functioning outcome is the observed behavior. An analogy to the Behavioral System Theory is the Biological System Theory in which a person is viewed as a biological system consisting of biological parts and disease is an outcome of biological system disorder.

Johnson notes that, although the literature indicates others support the idea that a person is a behavioral system and that a person's specific response patterns form an organized and integrated whole, as far as she knows, the idea is original with her. Just as the development of knowledge of the whole biological system was preceded by knowledge of the parts, the development of knowledge of behavioral systems is focused on specific behavioral responses. Empirical literature supporting the notion of the behavioral system as a whole and its usefulness as a framework for nursing decisions in research, educa-

tion, and nursing practice has accumulated consistently since it was first introduced.*

Developing the Behavioral System Theory from a philosophical perspective, Johnson[25] writes that nursing contributes by facilitating effective behavioral functioning in the patient before, during, and after illness. She uses concepts from other disciplines, such as social learning, motivation, sensory stimulation, adaptation, behavioral modification, change process, tension, and stress to expand her theory for the practice of nursing.

USE OF EMPIRICAL EVIDENCE

Some of the concepts Johnson has identified and defined in her theory are supported in the literature. Leitch and Escolona point out that tension produces behavioral changes and that the manifestation of tension by an individual depends on both internal and external factors.[20] Johnson[17] uses the work of Selye, Grinker, Simmons, and Wolff to support the idea that specific patterns of behavior are reactions to stressors from biological, psychological, and sociological sources, respectively. Johnson[18] suggested a difference in her model from Selye's conception of stress. Johnson's concept of stress[18:7-8] "follows rather closely Caudill's conceptualization; that is, that stress is a process in which there is interplay between various stimuli and the defenses erected against them. Stimuli may be positive in that they are present, or negative in that something desired or required is absent." Selye[18:8] "conceives stress as 'a state manifested by the specific syndrome which consists of all the nonspecifically induced changes within a biologic system.'"

In *Conceptual Models for Nursing Practice*,[25] Johnson describes seven subsystems that comprise her behavioral system. To support the attachment-affiliative subsystem, she cites the work of Ainsworth and Robson.[25] Heathers, Gerwitz, and Rosenthal have described and explained dependency behavior, another subsystem defined by Johnson.[25] The response systems of ingestion and elimination, as de-

*References 1, 6, 7, 10, 11, 12, 13, 14, 29, 30, 31, 33, 37, 40, 41, 42, 43, 44, 47.

scribed by Walike, Mead, and Sears, are also parts of Johnson's behavior system.[25] The work of Kagan and Resnik is used to support the sexual subsystem.[25] The aggressive/protective subsystem, which functions to protect and preserve, is supported by Lorenz and Feshbach.[9,25,32] According to Atkinson, Feather, and Crandell, physical, creative, mechanical, and social skills are manifested by achievement behavior, another subsystem identified by Johnson.[25]

Another subsystem, restorative, has been suggested by faculty and clinicians to include behaviors such as sleep, play, and relaxation.[12] Although John-

son[29] agrees that "there may be more or fewer subsystems" than originally identified, she does not accept restorative as a subsystem of the behavioral system model. She believes that sleep is primarily a biological force, not a motivational behavior. She suggests that many of the behaviors identified in infants during their first years of life, such as play, are actually achievement behaviors. Johnson[29] states that there may be a need to examine the possibility of an eighth subsystem that addresses explorative behaviors; further investigation may delineate it as a subsystem separate from the achievement subsystem.

MAJOR CONCEPTS & DEFINITIONS

BEHAVIOR

Johnson accepts the definition of behavior as expressed by the behavioral and biological scientists; that is, the output of intraorganismic structures and processes as they are coordinated and articulated by and responsive to changes in sensory stimulation. Johnson[25] focuses on behavior affected by the actual or implied presence of other social beings that has been shown to have major adaptive significance.

SYSTEM

Using Rapoport's 1968 definition of system, Johnson[25:208] states, "A system is a whole that functions as a whole by virtue of the interdependence of its parts." She accepts Chinn's statement that there is "organization, interaction, interdependency, and integration of the parts and elements."[25:208] In addition, a person strives to maintain a balance in these parts through adjustments and adaptations to the impinging forces.

BEHAVIORAL SYSTEM

A behavioral system encompasses the patterned, repetitive, and purposeful ways of behaving. These ways of behaving form an organized and integrated functional unit that determines and limits the interaction between the person and his or her environment and establishes the relation-

ship of the person to the objects, events, and situations within his or her environment. Usually the behavior can be described and explained. A person as a behavioral system tries to achieve stability and balance by adjustments and adaptations that are successful to some degree for efficient and effective functioning. The system is usually flexible enough to accommodate the influences affecting it.[25]

SUBSYSTEMS

The behavioral system has many tasks to perform; therefore parts of the system evolve into subsystems with specialized tasks. A subsystem is "a minisystem with its own particular goal and function that can be maintained as long as its relationship to the other subsystems or the environment is not disturbed."[25:221] The seven subsystems identified by Johnson are open, linked, and interrelated. Input and output are components of all seven subsystems.[12]

Motivational drives direct the activities of these subsystems, which are continually changing through maturation, experience, and learning. The systems described appear to exist cross culturally and are controlled by biological, psychological, and sociological factors. The seven identified subsystems are attachment/affiliative, dependency, ingestive, eliminative, sexual, achievement, and aggressive/protective.[25]

Attachment/Affiliative Subsystem

The attachment/affiliative subsystem is probably the most critical because it forms the basis for all social organization. On a general level, it provides survival and security. Its consequences are social inclusion, intimacy, and formation and maintenance of a strong social bond.[25]

Dependency Subsystem

In the broadest sense, the dependency subsystem promotes helping behavior that calls for a nurturing response. Its consequences are approval, attention or recognition, and physical assistance. Developmentally, dependency behavior evolves from almost total dependence on others to a greater degree of dependence on self. A certain amount of interdependence is essential for the survival of social groups.[25]

Ingestive Subsystem

The ingestive and eliminative subsystems should not be seen as the input and output mechanisms of the system. All subsystems are distinct subsystems with their own input and output mechanisms. The ingestive subsystem "has to do with when, how, what, how much, and under what conditions we eat."[25:213] "It serves the broad function of appetitive satisfaction."[25:213] This behavior is associated with social, psychological, and biological considerations.[25]

Eliminative Subsystem

The eliminative subsystem addresses "when, how, and under what conditions we eliminate."[25:213] As with the ingestive subsystem, the social and psychological factors are viewed as influencing the biological aspects of this subsystem and may be, at times, in conflict with the eliminative subsystem.[34]

Sexual Subsystem

The sexual subsystem has the dual functions of procreation and gratification. Including, but not limited to, courting and mating, this response system begins with the development of gender role identity and includes the broad range of sex-role behaviors.[25]

Achievement Subsystem

The achievement subsystem attempts to manipulate the environment. Its function is control or mastery of an aspect of self or environment to some standard of excellence. Areas of achievement behavior include intellectual, physical, creative, mechanical, and social skills.[25]

Aggressive/Protective Subsystem

The aggressive/protective subsystem's function is protection and preservation. This follows the line of thinking of ethologists such as Lorenz[32] and Feshbach[9] rather than the behavioral reinforcement school of thought, which contends that aggressive behavior is not only learned, but has a primary intent to harm others. Society demands that limits be placed on modes of self-protection and that people and their property be respected and protected.[25]

EQUILIBRIUM

Johnson[20] states that equilibrium is a key concept in nursing's specific goal. It is defined "as a stabilized but more or less transitory, resting state in which the individual is in harmony with himself and with his environment."[20:65] "It implies that biological and psychological forces are in balance with each other and with impinging social forces."[19:11] It is "not synonymous with a state of health, since it may be found either in health or illness."[19:11]

Continued

TENSION

"The concept of tension is defined as a state of being stretched or strained and can be viewed as an end-product of a disturbance in equilibrium."[18:10] Tension can be constructive in adaptive change or destructive in inefficient use of energy, hindering adaptation and causing potential structural damage.[18] Tension is the cue to disturbance in equilibrium.[19]

STRESSOR

Internal or external stimuli that produce tension and result in a degree of instability are called stressors. "Stimuli may be positive in that they are present; or negative in that something desired or required is absent. [Stimuli] . . . may be either endogenous or exogenous in origin [and] may play upon one or more of our linked open systems."[19:13] The open-linked systems are in constant interchange. The open-linked systems include the physiological, personality, and meaningful small group (the family) systems and the larger social system.[19]

MAJOR ASSUMPTIONS

Nursing

Nursing, as perceived by Johnson, is an external force acting to preserve the organization of the patient's behavior by means of imposing regulatory mechanisms or by providing resources while the patient is under stress.[34] An art and a science, it supplies external assistance both before and during system balance disturbance and therefore requires knowledge of order, disorder, and control.[13,25] Nursing activities do not depend on medical authority, but they are complementary to medicine.

Person

Johnson[25] views the person as a behavioral system with patterned, repetitive, and purposeful ways of behaving that link the person to the environment. An individual's specific response patterns form an organized and integrated whole.[23] A person is a system of interdependent parts that requires some regularity and adjustment to maintain a balance.[25]

Johnson[25] further assumes that a behavioral system is essential to the individual. When strong forces or lower resistance disturb behavioral system balance, the individual's integrity is threatened.[34] A person's attempt to reestablish balance may require an extraordinary expenditure of energy, which leaves a shortage of energy to assist biological processes and recovery.[34]

Health

Johnson perceives health as an elusive, dynamic state influenced by biological, psychological, and social factors. Health is a desired value by health professionals and focuses on the person rather than the illness.[34]

Health is reflected by the organization, interaction, interdependence, and integration of the subsystems of the behavioral system.[25] An individual attempts to achieve a balance in this system, which will lead to functional behavior. A lack of balance in the structural or functional requirements of the subsystems leads to poor health. When the system requires a minimal amount of energy for maintenance, a larger supply of energy is available to affect biological processes and recovery.[34]

Environment

In Johnson's theory, the environment consists of all the factors that are not part of the individual's behavioral system, but influence the system, some of which can be manipulated by the nurse to achieve the health goal for the patient.[34] The individual links to and interacts with the environment.[16] The behavioral system attempts to maintain equilibrium in response to environmental factors by adjusting and adapting to the forces that impinge on it. Excessively strong environmental forces disturb the behavioral system balance and threaten the person's stability. An unusual amount of energy is required for the system to reestablish equilibrium in the face of continuing forces.[34] When the environment is stable, the individual is able to continue with successful behaviors.

THEORETICAL ASSERTIONS

Johnson's Behavioral System Theory addresses two major components: (1) the patient and (2) nursing. The patient is a behavioral system with seven interrelated subsystems (Figure 16-1).

Each subsystem can be described and analyzed in terms of structure and functional requirements. The four structural elements that have been identified include: (1) drive, or goal; (2) set, predisposition to act; (3) choice, alternatives for action; and (4) behavior.[25]

Each of the subsystems has the same three functional requirements: (1) protection, (2) nurturance, and (3) stimulation.[34] The system and subsystems tend to be self-maintaining and self-perpetuating as long as internal and external conditions remain orderly and predictable. If the conditions and resources necessary to their functional requirements are not met, or the interrelationships among the subsystems are not harmonious, dysfunctional behavior results.[25]

The responses by the subsystems are developed through motivation, experience, and learning and are influenced by biological, psychological, and social factors.[25] The behavioral system attempts to achieve balance by adapting to internal and environmental stimuli. The behavioral system is made up of "all the patterned, repetitive, and purposeful ways of behaving that characterize each man's life."[25:209] This functional unit of behavior "determines and limits the interaction of the person and his environment and establishes the relationship of the person

with the objects, events, and situations in his environment."[25:209] "The behavioral system manages its relationship with its environment."[25:209] The behavioral system appears to be active and not passive. The nurse is external to and interactive with the behavioral system.

A state of instability in the behavioral system results in a need for nursing intervention. Identification of the source of the problem in the system leads to appropriate nursing action that results in the maintenance or restoration of behavioral system balance.[34] Nursing is seen as an external regulatory force that acts to restore the balance in the behavioral system.[25]

LOGICAL FORM

By studying the literature of other disciplines and observing specifics in her practice, nursing literature, and research, Johnson used the logical forms of deductive and inductive reasoning to develop her theory. She states that a common core exists in nursing, a core that practitioners use in many settings and with varying populations.[16] Johnson[24] used her observations of behavior over many years to formulate a general theory of the person as a behavioral system.

ACCEPTANCE BY THE NURSING COMMUNITY
Practice

According to Johnson,[25] the Behavioral System Theory provides direction for practice, education, and research. The goal of the theory is to use protection, nurturing, and stimulation to maintain and restore balance in the patient and a more optimal level of functioning. This is congruent with the goals of nursing.

Johnson does not use the term *nursing process*. Assessment, disorders, treatment, and evaluation are concepts referred to in a variety of Johnson's works. "For the practitioner, conceptual models provide a diagnostic and treatment orientation, and thus are of considerable practical import."[22:2] The nursing process becomes applicable in the behavioral system

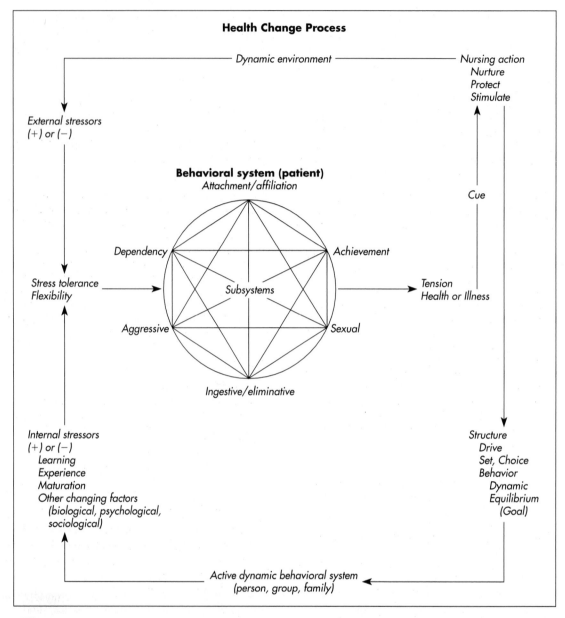

Figure 16-1 Johnson's Behavioral System Model. (Conceptualized by Jude A. Magers.)

model when behavioral malfunction occurs "that is in part disorganized, erratic, and dysfunctional. Illness or other sudden internal or external environmental change is most frequently responsible for such malfunctions."[25:212] "Assistance is appropriate

at those times the individual is experiencing stress of a health-illness nature which disturbs equilibrium, producing tension."[18:6]

Johnson[16] implies that the initial nursing assessment begins when the cue tension is observed and signals disequilibrium. Sources for assessment data can be through history taking, testing, and structural observations.[25] "The behavioral system is thought to determine and limit the interaction between the person and his environment."[22:3] This suggests that the accuracy and quantity of the data obtained during nursing assessment are not controlled by the nurse, but by the patient (system). The only observed part of the subsystems structure is behavior. Six internal and external regulators have been identified that "simultaneously influence and are influenced by behavior" including biophysical, psychological, developmental, sociocultural, family, and physical environmental regulators.[38:157]

The nurse must be able to access information related to goals, sets, and choices that make up the structural subsystems. "One or more of [these] subsystems is likely to be involved in any episode of illness, whether in an antecedent or a consequential way or simply in association, directly or indirectly with the disorder or its treatment."[22:3] Accessing the data is critical to accurate statement of the disorder.

Johnson does not define specific disorders, but she does state two general categories of disorders on the basis of the relationship to the biological system.[22] Disorders are

> those which are related tangentially or peripherally to disorder in the biological system; that is, they are precipitated simply by the fact of illness or the situational context of treatment; and . . . those [disorders] which are an integral part of a biological system disorder in that they are either directly associated with or a direct consequence of a particular kind of biological system disorder or its treatment.[22:7]

The "means of management" or interventions do consist in part of the provision of nurturance, protection, and stimulation.[22:7,25] The nurse may provide "temporary imposition of external regulatory and control mechanisms, such as inhibiting ineffective behavioral responses, and assisting the patient to acquire new responses."[22:6] Johnson[25:211] suggests that techniques may include "teaching, role modeling, and counseling." If a problem or disorder is an-

ticipated, preventive nursing action is appropriate with adequate methodologies.[25] Nurturance, protection, and stimulation are as important for preventive nursing care or health promotion as they are for managing illness.

The outcome of nursing intervention is behavioral system equilibrium. "More specifically, equilibrium can be said to have been achieved at that point at which the individual demonstrates a degree of constancy in his pattern of functioning, both internally and interpersonally."[18:9] The evaluation of the nursing intervention is based on whether it made "a significant difference in the lives of the persons involved."[25:215]

The Behavioral System Model has been operationalized through the development of several assessment instruments. In 1974, Grubbs[12] used the theory to develop an assessment tool and a nursing process sheet based on Johnson's seven subsystems. Questions and observations related to each subsystem provided tools with which to collect important data that assist in discovering other choices of behavior that will enable the patient to accomplish his or her goal of health.

That same year, Holaday[14] used the theory as a model to develop an assessment tool when caring for children. This tool allowed the nurse to objectively describe the child's behavior and to guide nursing action.

Derdiarian investigated the effects of using two systematic assessment instruments on patient and nurse satisfaction. The Johnson Behavioral System Model was used to develop a self-report and observational instrument to be implemented with the nursing process. The Derdiarian Behavioral System Model (DBSM) instrument included assessment of the restorative subsystem and the seven subsystems advocated by Johnson. The results indicated that implementation of the instruments provided a more comprehensive and systematic approach to assessment and intervention, thereby increasing patient and nurse satisfaction with care.[6]

Lanouette and St-Jacques[31] used Johnson's model to compare the coping abilities and perceptions of families with premature infants with families of full-term infants. The results indicated that positive coping skills were relative to bonding with the infant, using resources, solving problems, and making decisions. Lanouette and St-Jacques suggested that improvement in nursing care practices in nursery, hospital, and community settings might have contributed to this outcome. This supported Johnson's statement[29] that "the effective use of nurturance, protection, and stimulation during maternal contact at birth could significantly reduce the behavioral system problems we see today."

Case studies have documented the use and evaluation of the Johnson Behavioral System Theory in clinical practice. In 1980, Rawls[40] used the theory to systematically assess a patient who was facing the loss of function in one arm and hand. Herbert[13] reported the outcomes of a nursing care plan developed for an elderly stroke patient. Rawls and Herbert concluded that Johnson's theory provided a theoretical base that predicted the results of nursing interventions, formulated standards for care, and administered holistic care. Fruehwirth[10] found it equally effective in assessing and intervening with a support group for the caregivers of Alzheimer's disease patients.

Recent studies of nursing practice using Johnson's model have focused on decision making and evaluation of outcomes. Grice[11] found that the nurse, patient, and situational characteristics influenced assessment and decision making for the administration of antianxiety and antipsychotic medication for psychiatric inpatients at certain hours.

Benson[1] conducted a review of research literature on the fear of crime among older adults. The Behavioral System Model was used to describe the "hazards of fear of crime" that could cause disturbances in the ingestive, dependency, achievement, affiliative, and aggressive-protective subsystems.[1:26] Patient and community-focused interventions were presented to improve quality of care and quality of life of older adults.

Lachicotte and Alexander[30] examined the use of Johnson's Behavioral System Model as a framework for nursing administrators to use when making decisions concerning the management of impaired nurses. They suggested that, by viewing all levels of the environment, the framework encouraged the nurse administrators to assess the imbalance in the nursing system when nurse impairment exists and evaluate the "system's state of balance in relationship to the method chosen to deal with nurse impairment."[30:103] The results of the study indicated that nurse administrators preferred an assistive approach when dealing with nurse impairment. It was believed that "when the impaired nurse is confronted and assisted, equilibrium begins to be restored and balance brought back to the system."[30:103]

At the University of California, Los Angeles, the Neuropsychiatric Institute and Hospital has used Johnson's Behavioral System Model as the basis of their psychiatric nursing practice for many years.[37] "Patients are assessed and behavioral data are classified by subsystem. Nursing diagnoses are formulated that reflect the nature of the ineffective behavior and its relationship to the regulators in the environment."[38:154] A study comparing the diagnostic labels generated from the Johnson Behavioral System Model to the North American Nursing Diagnosis Association list indicated that the Johnson Behavioral System Model was better at distinguishing the problems and the etiology.[38]

It has become increasingly important to document nursing care and demonstrate the effectiveness of the care on patient outcomes. Using Johnson's model, Poster, Dee, and Randell[37] found a positive relationship between nursing interventions and the achievement of patient outcomes at discharge. They state that "a nursing theoretical framework made it possible to prescribe nursing care as a distinction from medical care."[37:73]

Dee, van Servellen, and Brecht[4] examined the effects of managed healthcare on patient outcomes using Johnson's Behavioral System Model. Upon admission, nurses develop a behavioral profile by assessing the eight subsystems, determine the balance or imbalance of the subsystems, and rate the impact of the six regulators. This is used to determine the nursing diagnoses, plan of action, and evaluation of care for each patient. The results of this study indicated significant improvement in the level of functioning upon discharge for patients with shorter hospital stays.

Education

Loveland-Cherry and Wilkerson[34] analyzed Johnson's theory and concluded that it has utility in nursing education. A curriculum based on a person as a behavioral system would have definite goals and straightforward course planning. Study would center on the patient as a behavioral system and its dysfunction, which would require use of the nursing process. In addition to an understanding of systems theory, the student would need knowledge from the social and behavioral disciplines and the physical and biological sciences. The model has been used in practice and educational institutions in the United States, Canada, and Australia.[11,36]

Research

Johnson[22:7] stated that nursing research would need to "identify and explain the behavioral system disorders which arise in connection with illness, and develop the rationale for the means of management." Theory derived from the Behavioral System Model leads the researcher in one of two directions. One researcher might investigate the functioning of the system and subsystems by focusing on the basic sciences.[34] In addition to the growing body of knowledge concerning the patterning of behavior from infancy to adolescence and during aging, there is a need for more knowledge about the response systems within the behavioral systems of individuals between adolescence and aging.[39] Another researcher might concentrate on investigating methods of gathering diagnostic data or problem-solving activities as they influence the behavioral system.[39]

Small[42] used Johnson's theory as a conceptual framework to use when caring for visually impaired children. By evaluating and comparing the perceived body image and spatial awareness of normally sighted children with those of visually impaired children, Small found that the sensory deprivation of visual impairment affected the normal development of the child's body image and the awareness of his body in space. She concluded that when the human system is subjected to excessive stress, the goals of the system could not be maintained.

Wilkie, Lovejoy, Dodd, and Tesler[47] examined cancer pain control behaviors with the use of Johnson's Behavioral System Model. The results of the study demonstrated that, with high pain intensity, persons used known behaviors to protect themselves from the pain. This supported the assumption that "aggressive/protective subsystem behaviors are developed and modified over time to protect the individual from pain and these behaviors represent some of the patient's pain control choices."[47:729]

These findings were supported in a recent study that examined the "meanings associated with self-report and self-management decision making" of cancer patients with metastatic bone pain.[2:101] Pain provided an incentive to seek treatment from healthcare providers; therefore it was a protective mechanism. Yet the results indicated that most of the cancer patients did not take pain medication as often as prescribed and preferred nonpharmacological methods, such as positioning or distraction, as their pain control choices.

Believing the model had potential in preventive care, Majesky, Brester, and Nishio[35] used it to construct a tool to measure patient indicators of nursing care. Holaday,[14] Rawls,[40] and Stamler[43] have conducted research using one subsystem. Derdiarian[7] examined the relationships between the aggressive and protective subsystem and the other subsystems. Her findings supported the proposition that the subsystems are interactive, interdependent, and integrated; therefore Derdiarian supported Johnson's contention that "changes in a subsystem resulting from illness cannot be well understood without understanding their relationship to changes in the other subsystems."[7:219]

Damus[3] tested the validity of Johnson's theory by comparing serum alanine aminotransferase (ALT) values in patients exposed to hepatitis B with the number of nursing diagnoses. Damus[3] correlated the physiological disorder of elevated ALT values with behavioral disequilibrium and found that disorder in one area reflected disorder in another area.

Nurse researchers have demonstrated the usefulness of Johnson's theory in clinical practice. The majority of these studies have been conducted with individuals with long-term illnesses or chronic illnesses; for example, those with AIDS, chronic pain, cancer, and psychiatric illnesses.* Studies have documented the effectiveness of using the model with children, adolescents, and the elderly population. Based on extensive practice, instrument development, and research, Holaday[14] concluded that the user of Johnson's theory was provided with a guide for planning and giving care based on scientific knowledge.

FURTHER DEVELOPMENT

Johnson believes people are active beings constantly seeking to adjust to their environments and that they adjust their environments to achieve better functioning for themselves. Therefore she views the behavioral system as active rather than merely reactive.[18] As the model allows for this belief, it can also be studied.

Primarily, the theory has been associated with individuals. Johnson believes groups of individuals can be considered groups of interactive behavioral systems. Use of her theory with families and other groups needs more visibility.[21]

As a result of the current emphasis on health promotion and maintenance and illness and injury prevention, theory could be derived from the model recognizing behavior disorders in these areas. This could be an important area for further development.

It should be noted that preventive nursing (to prevent behavioral system disorder) is not the same as preventive medicine (to prevent biological system disorders) and disorders in both cases must be identified and explicated before approaches to prevention can be developed. At this point, not even medicine has developed very many specific preventive measures (immunizations for some infectious diseases and protection against some vitamin deficiency diseases are notable exceptions). There are a number of general approaches to better health, including adequate nutrition, safe water, and exercise, which are applicable contributing to prevention of some disorders. It is a small wonder that preventive nursing remains to be developed; this is true no matter what model or theory for nursing is used.[27]

Riegel[41:74] reviewed the literature to identify major factors that predict "cardiac crippled behaviors or dependency following a myocardial infarction." Social support, self-esteem, anxiety, depression, and perceptions of functional capacity were considered the primary factors affecting psychological adjustment to chronic coronary heart disease. This emphasized the effect of social support or nurturing on the structure and function of the dependency subsystem.

Johnson[29] states, "If care takers were aware of how their behaviors and family behaviors interact with patients to encourage dependency behaviors at the beginning of illness, they could easily prevent many dysfunctional problems."

Further development could identify nursing actions that would facilitate appropriate functioning of the system toward disease prevention and health maintenance. Rather than expending energy developing nursing interventions in response to the consequences of disequilibrium, nurses need to learn how to identify precursors of disequilibrium and respond with preventive interventions.

Assuming that a community is a geographical area, a subpopulation, or any aggregate of people and assuming that a community can benefit from nursing interventions, the behavioral system framework can be applied to community health. A community can be described as a behavioral system with interacting subsystems that have structural elements and functional requirements. For example, mothers of chronically ill children have functional requirements needed to maintain stability within the achievement subsystem. The interaction of environmental factors such as "economic, educational, and employment influence mothers' caretaking skills."[44:97]

Communities have goals, norms, choices, and actions in addition to needing protection, nurturance, and stimulation. The community reacts to internal and external stimuli, which results in functional or dysfunctional behavior. An example of an external stimulus is health policy and an example of dysfunctional behavior is a high infant-mortality rate. The behavioral system consists of yet undefined subsystems that are organized, interacting, interdependent, and integrated. Physical, biological, and psychosocial factors also affect community behavior.

*References 2, 4, 5, 8, 11, 33, 45, 46.

CRITIQUE
Simplicity

Johnson's theory is relatively simple in relation to the number of concepts. A person is described as a behavioral system composed of seven subsystems. Nursing is an external regulatory force. However, the theory is potentially complex because there is a number of possible interrelationships between and among the behavioral system, its subsystems, and the forces impinging on them. At this point, however, only a few of the potential relationships have been explored.

Generality

Johnson's theory is relatively unlimited when applied to sick individuals, but it has not been used as much with well individuals or groups. Johnson perceives a person as a behavioral system comprised of seven subsystems, aggregates of interactive behavioral systems. Initially, Johnson[26] did not clearly address nonillness situations or preventive nursing. In later publications, Johnson emphasized the role of nurses in preventive healthcare of individuals and for society. She stated, "Nursing's special responsibility for health is derived from its unique social mission. Nursing needs to concentrate on developing preventive nursing to fulfill its social obligations."[28:26]

Empirical Precision

Empirical precision is achieved by identifying empirical indicators for the theory because models contain abstract concepts. Empirical precision improves when the subconcepts and the relationships between and among the subconcepts become better defined and empirical indicators are introduced to the science. The units and the relationships between the units in Johnson's theory are consistently defined and used. So far, a moderate degree of empirical precision has been demonstrated in research using Johnson's model. However, throughout Johnson's writings, terms such as balance, stability, and equilibrium, adjustments and adaptations, disturbances, disequilibrium, and behavioral disorders are used interchangeably, which confounds their meanings. The clarity of definitions in the subsystems improves the model's empirical precision.

Derivable Consequences

Johnson's model guides nursing practice, education, and research; generates new ideas about nursing; and differentiates nursing from other health professions. By focusing on behavior rather than biology, the theory clearly differentiates nursing from medicine, although the concepts overlap with the psychosocial professions.

Johnson's Behavioral System Theory provides a conceptual framework for nursing education, practice, and research. The theory has directed questions for nursing research. It has been analyzed and judged to be appropriate as a basis for the development of a nursing curriculum. Practitioners and patients have judged the resulting nursing actions to be satisfactory.[25] The theory has potential for continued utility in nursing to achieve valued nursing goals.

CRITICAL THINKING *Activities*

1. In a practice setting, use Johnson's Behavioral System Model to guide your practice for one day. Describe how the use of this model affected your approach to assessing needs, making and prioritizing nursing decisions, and evaluating outcomes.

2. Identify the strengths and limitations of the model for preventive care in a community setting.

3. Develop a teaching plan for an Alzheimer patient and his or her family using Johnson's Behavioral System Model.

4. Design a research study to examine the evaluation outcomes of managed care in your practice setting using this model.

REFERENCES

1. Benson, S. (1997). The older adult and fear of crime. *Journal of Gerontological Nursing, 23*(10), 24-31.

2. Coward, D.D. & Wilkie, D.J. (2000). Metastatic bone pain: Meanings associated with self-report and self-management decision making. *Cancer Nursing*, 23(2), 101-108.

3. Damus, K. (1980). An application of the Johnson behavioral system model for nursing practice. In J.P. Riehl & C. Roy (Eds.), *Conceptual models for nursing practice* (2nd ed.). New York: Appleton-Century-Crofts.

4. Dee, V., van Servellen, G., & Brecht, M. (1998). Managed behavioral health care patients and their nursing care problems, level of functioning, and impairment on discharge. *Journal of American Psychiatric Nurses Association*, 4(2), 57-66.

5. Derdiarian, A.K. (1988). Sensitivity of the Derdiarian Behavioral System Model instrument to age, site, and stage of cancer: A preliminary validation study. *Scholarly Inquiry for Nursing Practice*, 2(2), 103-24.

6. Derdiarian, A.K. (1990). Effects of using systematic assessment instruments on patient and nurse satisfaction with nursing care. *Oncology Nursing Forum*, 17(1), 95-100.

7. Derdiarian, A.K. (1991). Effects of using a nursing model-based assessment instrument on quality of nursing care. *Nursing Administration Quarterly*, 15(3), 1-16.

8. Derdiarian, A.K. & Schobel, D. (1990). Comprehensive assessment of AIDS patients using the behavioral systems model for nursing practice instrument. *Journal of Advanced Nursing*, 15(4), 436-46.

9. Feshbach, S. (1970). Aggression. In P. Mussen (Ed.), *Carmichael's manual of child psychology* (3rd ed.). New York: John Wiley & Sons.

10. Fruehwirth, S.E.S. (1989). An application of Johnson's behavioral model: A case study. *Journal of Community Health Nurse*, 6(2), 61-71.

11. Grice, S.L. (1997). *Nurses' use of medication for agitation for the psychiatric inpatient*. Unpublished doctoral dissertation, Catholic University of America.

12. Grubbs, J. (1980). *An interpretation of the Johnson behavioral system model for nursing practice* (2nd ed.). New York: Appleton-Century-Crofts.

13. Herbert, J. (1989). A model for Anna . . . using the Johnson model of nursing in the care of one 75-year-old stroke patient. *The Journal of Clinical Practice, Education and Management*, 3(42), 30-4.

14. Holaday, B. (1980). Implementing the Johnson model for nursing practice. In J.P. Riehl, & C. Roy (Eds.), *Conceptual models for nursing practice* (2nd ed.). New York: Appleton Century-Crofts.

15. Holaday, B. (2000, June). Personal correspondence.

16. Johnson, D.E. (1959, April). A philosophy of nursing. *Nursing Outlook*, 7, 198-200.

17. Johnson, D.E. (1959, May). The nature of a science of nursing. *Nursing Outlook*, 7, 291-294.

18. Johnson, D.E. (1961, Jan.). *Nursing's specific goal in patient care*. Unpublished lecture, Faculty Colloquium, School of Nursing, University of California, Los Angeles.

19. Johnson, D.E. (1961, June). *A conceptual basis for nursing care*. Unpublished lecture, Third Conference, C.E. Program, University of California, Los Angeles.

20. Johnson, D.E. (1961, Nov.). The significance of nursing care. *American Journal of Nursing Studies*, 61, 63-66.

21. Johnson, D.E. (1965, April). *Is nursing meeting the challenge of family needs?* Unpublished lecture, Wisconsin League for Nursing, Madison, Wisconsin.

22. Johnson, D.E. (1968, April). *One conceptual model of nursing*. Unpublished lecture, Vanderbilt University, Nashville, Tennessee.

23. Johnson, D.E. (1968, May/June). Theory in nursing: Borrowed and unique. *Nursing Research*, 17, 206-209.

24. Johnson, D.E. (1974, Sept./Oct.). Development of theory: A requisite for nursing as a primary health profession. *Nursing Research*, 23, 372-377.

25. Johnson, D.E. (1980). The behavioral system model for nursing. In J.P. Riehl & C. Roy (Eds.), *Conceptual models for nursing practice* (2nd ed.). New York: Appleton-Century-Crofts.

26. Johnson, D.E. (1984). Curriculum vitae.

27. Johnson, D.E. (1984). Personal correspondence.

28. Johnson, D.E. (1992). Origins of behavioral system model. In F. Nightingale (Ed.), *Notes on nursing* (Commemorative Edition, pp. 23-28). Philadelphia: J.B. Lippincott.

29. Johnson, D.E. (1996). Personal communication.

30. Lachicotte, J.L. & Alexander, J.W. (1990). Management attitudes and nurse impairment. *Nursing Management*, 21(9), 102-110.

31. Lanouette, M. & St-Jacques, A. (1994). Premature infants and their families. *Canadian Nurse*, 90(9), 36-9.

32. Lorenz, K. (1966). *On aggression*. New York: Harcourt.

33. Lovejoy, N. & Moran, T. (1988). Selected AIDS beliefs, behaviors and information needs of homosexual/bisexual men with AIDS or ARC. *International Journal of Nursing Studies*, 25(3), 207-216.

34. Loveland-Cherry, C. & Wilkerson, S. (1983). Dorothy Johnson's behavioral systems model. In J. Fitzpatrick & A. Whall (Eds.), *Conceptual models of nursing: Analysis and application*. Bowie, MD: Robert J. Brady.

35. Majesky, S.J., Brester, M.H., & Nishio, K.T. (1978). Development of a research tool: Patient indicators of nursing care. *Nursing Research*, 27(6), 365-371.

36. Orb, A. & Reilly, D.E. (1991). Changing to a conceptual base curriculum. *International Nursing Review*, 38(2), 56-60.

37. Poster, E.C., Dee, V., & Randell, B.P. (1997). The Johnson Behavioral Systems Model as a framework for patient outcome evaluation. *Journal of American Psychiatric Nurses Association, 3*(3), 73-80.

38. Randell, B.P. (1991). NANDA versus the Johnson behavioral systems model: Is there a diagnostic difference? In R.M. Carroll-Johnson (Ed.), *Classification of nursing diagnosis: Proceedings of the ninth conference.* Philadelphia: J.P. Lippincott.

39. Randell, B.P. (1992). Nursing theory: The 21st century. *Nursing Science Quarterly, 5*(4), 176-184.

40. Rawls, A. (1980). Evaluation of the Johnson behavioral model in clinical practice: Report of a test and evaluation of the Johnson theory. *Image,* 12, 13-16.

41. Riegel, B. (1989). Social support and psychological adjustment to chronic coronary heart disease: Operalization of Johnson's behavioral system model. *Advances in Nursing Science, 11*(2), 74-84.

42. Small, B. (1980). Nursing visually impaired children with Johnson's model as a conceptual framework. In J.P. Riehl & C. Roy (Eds.), *Conceptual models for nursing practice* (2nd ed.). New York: Appleton-Century-Crofts.

43. Stamler, C. (1971). Dependency and repetitive visits to nurses' office in elementary school children. *Nursing Research,* 20(3), 254-255.

44. Turner-Henson, A. (1992). *Chronically ill children's mothers' perceptions of environmental variables.* Unpublished doctoral dissertation, University of Alabama at Birmingham.

45. Wheeler, K. (1989). Self-psychology's contributions to understanding stress and implications for nursing. *Journal of Advanced Medical-Surgical Nursing,* 1(4), 1-10.

46. Wilkie, D.J. (1990). Cancer pain management: State-of-the-art nursing care. *Nursing Clinics of North America,* 25(2), 331-43.

47. Wilkie, D., Lovejoy, N., Dodd, M., & Tesler, M. (1988). Cancer pain control behaviors: Description and correlation with pain intensity. *Oncology Nursing Forum,* 15(6), 723-731.

BIBLIOGRAPHY
Primary Sources
Book Chapters

Johnson, D.E. (1964, June). Is there an identifiable body of knowledge essential to the development of a generic professional nursing program? In M. Maker (Ed.), *Proceedings of the first interuniversity faculty work conference.* Stowe, VT: New England Board of Higher Education.

Johnson, D.E. (1973). Medical-surgical nursing: Cardiovascular care in the first person. In American Nurses Association, *ANA Clinical Sessions* (pp. 127-134). New York: Appleton-Century-Crofts.

Johnson, D.E. (1976). Foreword. In J.R. Auger (Ed.), *Behavioral systems and nursing.* Englewood Cliffs, NJ: Prentice-Hall.

Johnson, D.E. (1978). State of the art of theory development in nursing. In National League for Nursing, *Theory development: What, why, how?* NLN Pub. No. 15-1708. New York: National League for Nursing.

Johnson, D.E. (1980). The behavioral system model for nursing. In J.P. Riehl & C. Roy (Eds.), *Conceptual models for nursing practice* (2nd ed.). New York: Appleton-Century-Crofts.

Johnson, D.E. (1990). The Behavioral System Model for nursing. In M.E. Parker (Ed.), *Nursing theories in practice.* New York: National League for Nursing.

Johnson, D.E. (1992). Origins of behavioral system model. In F. Nightingale (Ed.), *Notes on nursing* (Commemorative Edition, pp. 23-28). Philadelphia: J.B. Lippincott.

Journal Articles

Johnson, D.E. (1943, March). Learning to know people. *American Journal of Nursing,* 43, 248-252.

Johnson, D.E. (1954). Collegiate nursing education. *College Public Relations Quarterly,* 5, 32-35.

Johnson, D.E. (1959, April). A philosophy of nursing. *Nursing Outlook,* 7, 198-200.

Johnson, D.E. (1959, May). The nature of a science of nursing. *Nursing Outlook,* 7, 291-294.

Johnson, D.E. (1961, Oct.). Patterns in professional nursing education. *Nursing Outlook,* 9, 608-611.

Johnson, D.E. (1961, Nov.). The significance of nursing care. *American Journal of Nursing,* 61, 63-66.

Johnson, D.E. (1962, July/Aug.). Professional education for pediatric nursing. *Children,* 9, 153-156.

Johnson, D.E. (1964, Dec.). Nursing and higher education. *International Journal of Nursing Studies,* 1, 219-225.

Johnson, D.E. (1965, Sept.). Today's action will determine tomorrow's nursing. *Nursing Outlook,* 13, 38-41.

Johnson, D.E. (1965, Oct.). Crying in the newborn infant. *Nursing Science,* 3, 339-355.

Johnson, D.E. (1966, Jan.). Year round programs set the pace in health careers promotion. *Hospitals,* 40, 57-60.

Johnson, D.E. (1966, Oct.). Competence in practice: Technical and professional. *Nursing Outlook,* 14, 30-33.

Johnson, D.E. (1967). Professional practice in nursing. *NLN Convention Papers,* 23, 26-33.

Johnson, D.E. (1967, April). Powerless: A significant determinant in patient behavior? *Journal of Nursing Educators,* 6, 39-44.

Johnson, D.E. (1968). Critique: Social influences on student nurses in their choice of ideal and practiced solutions to nursing problems. *Communicating Nursing Research, 1,* 150-155.

Johnson, D.E. (1968, April). Toward a science in nursing. *Southern Medical Bulletin, 56,* 13-23.

Johnson, D.E. (1968, May/June). Theory in nursing: Borrowed and unique. *Nursing Research, 17,* 206-209.

Johnson, D.E. (1974, Sept./Oct.). Development of theory: A requisite for nursing as a primary health profession. *Nursing Research, 23,* 372-377.

Johnson, D.E. (1982, Spring). Some thoughts on nursing. *Clinical Nurse Specialist, 3,* 1-4.

Johnson, D.E. (1987, July/Aug.). Evaluating conceptual models for use in critical care nursing practice. *Dimensions of Critical Care Nursing, 6,* 195-197.

Johnson, D.E., Wilcox, J.A., & Moidel, H.C. (1967). The clinical specialist as a practitioner. *American Journal of Nursing, 67,* 2298-2303.

McCaffery, M. & Johnson, D.E. (1967). Effect of parent group discussion upon epistemic responses. *Nursing Research, 16,* 352-358.

Audiotape

Johnson, D.E. (1978, Dec.). *Paper presented at the Second Annual Nurse Educator Conference, New York* [Audiotape]. Available: Teach 'em Inc., 160 E. Illinois Street, Chicago, IL 60611.

Videotape

The nurse theorists: Portraits of excellence: Dorothy Johnson [Videotape]. (1988). Oakland, CA: Studio III. Available: Fuld Video Project, 370 Hawthorne Avenue, Oakland, CA 94609.

Unpublished Lectures

Johnson, D.E. (1961). *A conceptual basis for nursing care.* Presentation given at the Third Conference, C.E. Program, University of California, Los Angeles.

Johnson, D.E. (1961). *Nursing's specific goal in patient care.* Presentation given at Faculty Colloquium, University of California, Los Angeles.

Johnson, D.E. (1965). *Is nursing meeting the challenge of family needs?* Presentation given to the Wisconsin League for Nursing at Madison, Wisconsin.

Johnson, D.E. (1968). *One conceptual model of nursing.* Lecture given at Vanderbilt University, Nashville, TN.

Johnson, D.E. (1976). *The search for truth.* Presentation to Sigma Theta Tau, University of California, Los Angeles.

Johnson, D.E. (1977). *The behavioral system model for nursing.* Sigma Theta Tau Conference, University of California, Los Angeles.

Johnson, D.E. (1978). *The behavioral system model: Then and now.* Presentation given to Vanderbilt University, Nashville, TN.

Johnson, D.E. (1982). *Conceptual frameworks or models.* Presentation at Wheeling College, West Virginia.

Johnson, D.E. (1986). *The search for truth.* Presentation to Sigma Theta Tau, University of Miami, Miami, FL.

Correspondence

Johnson, D.E. (1984, Feb.). Curriculum vitae.

Johnson, D.E. (1984, Feb.). Personal correspondence.

Johnson, D.E. (1988, March). Personal correspondence.

Johnson D.E. (1996, Aug.). Personal communication.

Secondary Sources
Books

Auger, J.R. (1976). *Behavioral systems and nursing.* Englewood Cliffs, NJ: Prentice-Hall.

Chinn, P.L. & Kramer, M.K. (1995). *Theory and nursing: A systematic approach* (4th ed.). St. Louis: Mosby.

Fawcett, J. (1995). *Analysis and evaluation of conceptual models of nursing* (3rd ed.). Philadelphia: F.A. Davis.

Feshbach, S. (1970). Aggression. In P. Mussen (Ed.), *Carmichael's manual of child psychology* (3rd ed.). New York: John Wiley & Sons.

Fitzpatrick, J.J. & Whall, A.L. (1996). *Conceptual models of nursing: Analysis and application* (3rd ed.). Norwalk, CT: Appleton & Lange.

Fitzpatrick, J.J., Whall, A., Johnston, R., & Floyd, J. (1982). *Nursing models and their psychiatric mental health applications.* Bowie, MD: Robert J. Brady.

Hoeman, S.P. (1996). Conceptual bases for rehabilitation nursing. In S.P. Hoeman (Ed.), *Rehabilitation nursing: Process and application* (2nd ed., p. 7). St. Louis: Mosby.

Infante, M.S. (1982). *Crisis theory: A framework for nursing practice.* Reston, VA: Reston Publishing.

Kim, H.S. (1983). *The nature of theoretical thinking in nursing.* Norwalk, CT: Appleton-Century-Crofts.

Parker, M.E. (1990). *Nursing theories in practice.* New York: National League for Nursing.

Riehl-Sisca, J.P. (1989). *Conceptual models for nursing practice.* New York: Appleton-Century-Crofts.

Dissertations

Dee, V. (1986). Validation of a patient classification instrument for psychiatric patients based on the Johnson model for nursing. *Dissertation Abstracts International, 47,* 4822B.

Grice, S.L. (1997). *Nurses' use of medication for agitation for the psychiatric inpatient.* Unpublished doctoral dissertation, The Catholic University of America.

Lovejoy, N.C. (1981). *An empirical verification of the Johnson behavioral system model for nursing.* Unpublished doctoral dissertation, University of Alabama, Birmingham.

Riegal, B.J. (1991). *Social support and cardiac invalidism following myocardial infarction.* Unpublished doctoral dissertation, University of California, Los Angeles.

Turner-Henson, A. (1992). *Chronically ill children's mothers' perceptions of environmental variables.* Unpublished doctoral dissertation, University of Alabama at Birmingham.

Book Chapters

Damus, K. (1974). An application of the Johnson behavioral system model for nursing practice. In J.P. Riehl & C. Roy (Eds.), *Conceptual models for nursing practice* (pp. 218-233). New York: Appleton-Century-Crofts.

Damus, K. (1980). An application of the Johnson behavioral system model for nursing practice. In J.P. Riehl & C. Roy (Eds.), *Conceptual models for nursing practice* (2nd ed., pp. 274-289). New York: Appleton-Century-Crofts.

Dee, B. (1990). Implementation of the Johnson model: One hospital's experience. In M.E. Parker (Ed.), *Nursing theories in practice* (pp. 33-44). New York: National League for Nursing.

Derdiarian, A.K. (1993). Application of the Johnson behavioral system model in nursing practice. In M.E. Parker (Ed.), *Patterns of nursing theories in practice* (pp. 285-298). Publication No. 15-2548. New York: National League for Nursing.

Derdiarian, A.K. (1993). The Johnson system model in nursing practice. In M.E. Parker (Ed.), *Patterns of nursing theories in practice* (pp. 285-298). Publication No. 15-2548. New York: National League for Nursing.

Fawcett, J. (1995). Johnson's behavioral systems model. In J. Fawcett (Ed.), *Analysis and evaluation of conceptual models of nursing* (3rd ed., pp. 67-107). Philadelphia: F.A. Davis.

Glennin, C.G. (1980). Formulation of standards of nursing practice using a nursing model. In J.P. Riehl & C. Roy (Eds.), *Conceptual models for nursing practice* (2nd ed., pp. 290-310). New York: Appleton-Century-Crofts.

Grubbs, J. (1974). An interpretation of the Johnson behavioral systems model for nursing practice. In J.P. Riehl & C. Roy (Eds.), *Conceptual models for nursing practice* (pp. 160-194). New York: Appleton-Century-Crofts.

Grubbs, J. (1980). An interpretation of the Johnson behavioral system model for nursing practice. In J.P. Riehl & C. Roy (Eds.), *Conceptual models for nursing practice* (2nd ed., pp. 217-249). New York: Appleton-Century-Crofts.

Holaday, B. (1974). Implementing the Johnson model for nursing practice. In J.P. Riehl & C. Roy (Eds.), *Conceptual models for nursing practice* (2nd ed., pp. 197-206). New York: Appleton-Century-Crofts.

Holaday, B. (1980). Implementing the Johnson model for nursing practice. In J.P. Riehl & C. Roy (Eds.), *Conceptual models for nursing practice* (2nd ed., pp. 255-263). New York: Appleton-Century-Crofts.

Holaday, B. (1997). Johnson's behavioral system model in nursing practice. In M.R. Alligood & A. Marriner Tomey (Eds.), *Nursing theory: Utilization and application* (pp. 49-70). St. Louis: Mosby.

Holaday, B., Turner-Henson, A., & Swan, J. (1996). The Johnson behavioral system model: Explaining activities of chronically ill children. In P.H. Walker & B. Neuman (Eds.), *Blueprint for use of nursing models: Education, research, practice and administration* (pp. 33-63). Publication No. 14-2696. New York: National League for Nursing.

Lewis, C. & Randell, B.P. (1991). Alteration in self-care: An instance of ineffective coping in the geriatric patient. In R.M. Carroll-Johnson (Ed.), *Classification of nursing diagnoses: Proceedings of the ninth conference.* Philadelphia: J.B. Lippincott.

Loveland-Cherry, C. & Wilkerson, S.A. (1983). Dorothy Johnson's behavioral systems model. In J.P. Fitzpatrick & A.L. Whall (Eds.), *Conceptual models of nursing: Analysis and application* (pp. 117-135). Bowie, MD: Robert J. Brady.

Meleis, A.I. (1985). Dorothy Johnson. In A.I. Meleis (Ed.), *Theoretical nursing: Development and progress* (pp. 195-205). Philadelphia: JB Lippincott.

Randell, B.P. (1991). NANDA versus the Johnson behavioral system model: Is there a diagnostic difference? In R.M. Carroll-Johnson (Ed.), *Classification of nursing diagnosis: Proceedings of the ninth conference.* Philadelphia: J.B. Lippincott.

Riehl, J.P. & Roy, C. (1980). Appendix: Nursing assessment tool using Johnson model. In J.P. Riehl & C. Roy (Eds.), *Conceptual models for nursing practice* (2nd ed., pp. 250-254). New York: Appleton-Century-Crofts.

Skolny, M.S. & Riehl, J.P. (1974). Hope: Solving patient and family problems by using a theoretical framework. In J.P. Riehl & C. Roy (Eds.), *Conceptual models for nursing practice* (pp. 206-218). New York: Appleton-Century-Crofts.

Small, B. (1980). Nursing visually impaired children with Johnson's model as a conceptual framework. In J.P. Riehl & C. Roy (Eds.), *Conceptual models for nursing practice* (2nd ed., pp. 264-273). New York: Appleton-Century-Crofts.

Steven, B.J. (1979). Criteria for evaluating theories. In B.J. Stevens (Ed.), *Nursing theory: Analysis, application, evaluation* (pp. 49-67). Boston: Little, Brown.

Wesley, R.L. (1991). Johnson's behavioral systems model. In D. Moreau & K. Zimmerman (Eds.), *Nursing theories and models* (pp. 60-63). Springhouse, PA: Springhouse.

Directional and Biographical Sources

Henderson, J. (1957-1959). *Nursing studies index* (Vol. IV). Philadelphia: J.B. Lippincott.

Journal Articles

Abdellah, F.G. (1969). Dept. HEW-Health administration center of health services research and development health services. *Nursing Research, 18*(5), 390-393.

Adam, E. (1983). Frontiers of nursing in the 21st century: Development of models and theories on the concept of nursing. *Journal of Advanced Nursing, 8,* 41-45.

Ainsworth, M. (1964). Patterns of attachment behavior shown by the infant in interaction with mother. *Merrill Palmer Quarterly, 10*(1), 51-58.

Arndt, C. (1970). Role sharing in diversified role set director of nursing service. *Nursing Research, 19*(3), 253-259.

Auger, J. & Dee, V. (1983). Patient classification system based on the behavioral system model of nursing. Part I. *Journal of Nursing Administration, 13*(4), 38-43.

Bates, B. (1970). Doctor and nurse, changing nurse, and relations. *New England Journal of Medicine, 283,* 129-130.

Benson, S. (1997). The older adult and fear of crime. *Journal of Gerontological Nursing, 23*(10), 24-31.

Botha, M.E. (1989). Theory development in perspective: The role of conceptual frameworks and models in theory development. *Journal of Advanced Nursing, 14,* 49-55.

Brandt, E.M. (1967). Comparison of on job performance of graduates with school of nursing objectives. *Nursing Research, 16*(1), 50-60.

Brester, M.H., Majesky, S.J., & Nishio, K.T. (1978, Nov./Dec.). Development of a research tool: Patient indicators of nursing care. *Nursing Research, 27,* 365-371.

Broncatello, K.F. (1980). Anger in action: Application of the model. *Advances in Nursing Science, 2*(2), 13-24.

Bullough, B. (1976). Influences in role expansion. *American Journal of Nursing, 76*(9), 1476-1481.

Chance, K.S. (1982). Nursing models: A requisite for professional accountability. *Advances in Nursing Science, 4*(2), 57-65.

Conway, B. (1971). Effects of hospitalization on adolescence. *Adolescence, 6*(21), 77-92.

Coward, D.D. & Wilkie, D.J. (2000). Metastatic bone pain: Meanings associated with self-report and self-management decision making. *Cancer Nursing, 23*(2), 101-108.

Crawford, G. (1982). The concept of pattern in nursing, conceptual development and measurement. *Advances in Nursing Science, 5*(1), 1-6.

Craig, S.L. (1980). Theory development and its relevance for nursing. *Journal of Advanced Nursing, 5*(4), 349-355.

Darnell, R.E. (1973). Promotion of interest in role of physician association as a potential career opportunity for nurses' alternative strategy. *Social Science and Medicine, 7*(7), 495.

Dee, U. & Auger, J.A. (1983, May). A patient classification system based on behavioral system model of nursing. Part II. *Journal of Nursing Administration, 13,* 18-23.

Dee, V., van Servellen, G., & Brecht, M. (1998). Managed behavioral health care patients and their nursing care problems, level of functioning, and impairment on discharge. *Journal of American Psychiatric Nurses Association, 4*(2), 57-66.

Derdiarian, A.K. (1983, July/Aug.). An instrument for theory and research development using the behavioral system model for nursing: The cancer patient. Part I. *Nursing Research, 32,* 196-201.

Derdiarian, A.K. (1988). Sensitivity of the Derdiarian Behavioral System Model instrument to age, site, and stage of cancer: A preliminary validation study. *Scholarly Inquiry for Nursing Practice, 2*(2), 103-24.

Derdiarian, A.K. (1990). Effects of using systematic assessment instruments on patient and nurse satisfaction with nursing care. *Oncology Nursing Forum, 17*(1), 95-100.

Derdiarian, A.K. (1990). The relationship among the subsystems of Johnson's behavioral system model. *Image Journal of Nursing Scholarship, 22*(4), 219-224.

Derdiarian, A.K. (1991). Effects of using a nursing model-based assessment instrument on quality of nursing care. *Nursing Administration Quarterly, 15*(3), 1-16.

Derdiarian, A.K. & Forsythe, A.B. (1983, Sept./Oct.). An instrument for theory and research development using the behavioral systems model for nursing: The cancer patient. Part II. *Nursing Research, 32,* 260-266.

Derdiarian, A.K. & Schobel, D. (1990). Comprehensive assessment of AIDS patients using the behavioral systems model for nursing practice instrument. *Journal of Advanced Nursing, 15*(4), 436-46.

Evans, R.T. (1969). Exploration of factors involved in maternal adaption to breastfeeding. *Nursing Research, 18*(1), 28-33.

Flint, R.T. (1969). Recent issues in nursing manpower review. *Nursing Research, 18*(3), 217-222.

Fritz, E. (1966). Baccalaureate nursing education: What is its job? *American Journal of Nursing, 66*(6), 1312-1316.

Fruehwirth, S.E.S. (1989). An application of Johnson's behavioral model: A case study. *Journal Community Health Nurse, 6*(2), 61-71.

Georgopo, B.S. (1970). Nursing Kardex behavior in an experimental study of patient units with and without clinical nurse specialists. *Nursing Research, 19*(3), 196-218.

Godley, S.T. (1976). Community based orientation and mobility programs. *Nursing Outlook, 70*(10), 429-432.

Gortner, S.R. (1977). Overview of nursing research in United States. *Nursing Research, 26*(1), 16-23.

Gray, S.E. (1977). Do graduates of technical and professional nursing programs differ in practice? *Nursing Research, 26*(5), 368-373.

Greaves, F. (1980). Objectively toward curriculum improvement in nursing education in England and Wales. *Journal of Advanced Nursing, 5*, 591-599.

Hadley, B.J. (1969). Evolution of a conception of nursing. *Nursing Research, 18*(5), 400-405.

Hall, B.P. (1981). The change paradigm in nursing: Growth versus persistence. *Advances in Nursing Science, 3*(4), 1-6.

Herbert, J. (1989). A model for Anna. . .using the Johnson model of nursing in the care of one 75-year-old stroke patient. *The Journal of Clinical Practice, Education and Management, 3*(42), 30-4.

Hogstel, M.O. (1977). Associate degree and baccalaureate graduates: Do they function differently? *American Journal of Nursing, 77*(10), 1598-1600.

Holaday, B. (1974). Achievement behavior in chronically ill children. *Nursing Research, 23*, 25-30.

Holaday, B. (1981). Maternal response to their chronically ill infants' attachment behavior of crying. *Nursing Research, 30*, 343-348.

Holaday, B. (1982). Maternal conceptual set development: Identifying patterns of maternal response to chronically ill infant crying. *Maternal-Child Nursing Journal, 11*(1), 47-58.

Holaday, B. (1987). Patterns of interaction between mothers and their chronically ill infants. *Maternal Child Nursing Journal, 16*, 29-36.

Iveson-Iveson, J. (1982). Standards of behavior . . . theories of nursing practice . . . the Johnson model. *Nursing Mirror, 155*(20), 38.

Ketefian, S. (1981). Critical thinking: Educational preparation and development of moral judgment among selected groups of practicing nurses. *Nursing Research, 30*(2), 98-103.

Kohnk, M.F. (1973). Do nursing educators practice what is preached? *American Journal of Nursing, 73*(9), 1571.

Lanouette, M. & St-Jacques, A. (1994). Premature infants and their families. *Canadian Nurse, 90*(9), 36-9.

Lovejoy, N. (1983). The leukemic child's perceptions of family behaviors. *Oncology Nursing Forum, 10*(4), 20-25.

Lovejoy, N. & Moran, T. (1988). Selected AIDS beliefs, behaviors and information needs of homosexual/bisexual men with AIDS or ARC. *International Journal of Nursing Studies, 25*(3), 207-16.

Ma T. & Gandet, D. (1997). Assessing the quality of our end-stage renal disease client population. *Journal of the Canadian Association of Nephrology Nurses and Technicians, 7*(2), 13-16.

Magnani, L.E. (1990). Hardiness, self-perceived health, and activity among independently functioning older adults . . . including commentary by Hadley B.J. *Scholarly Inquiry for Nursing Practice, 4*(3), 171-88.

Majesky, S.J. (1978). Development of a research tool: Patient indicators of nursing care. *Nursing Research, 27*(6), 365-371.

Mauksch, I.G. (1972). Prescription for survival. *American Journal of Nursing, 72*(12), 2189-2193.

McCain, R.F. (1965, April). Systematic investigation of medical-surgical nursing content. *Journal of Nursing Education, 4*, 23-31.

McFarlane, E.A. (1980). Nursing theory: Comparison of four theoretical proposals. *Journal of Advanced Nursing, 5*, 3-19.

McQuaid, E.A. (1979). How do graduates of different types of programs perform on state boards? *American Journal of Nursing, 79*(2), 305-308.

Newman, M.A. (1994). Theory for nursing practice. *Nursing Science Quarterly, 7*(4), 153-157.

Niemela, K., Poster, E.C., & Moreau, D. (1992). The attending nurse: A new role for the advanced clinician . . . adolescent inpatient unit. *Journal of Child and Adolescent Psychiatric and Mental Health Nursing, 5*(3), 5-12.

Orb, A. & Reilly, D.E. (1991). Changing to a conceptual base curriculum. *International Nursing Review, 38*(2), 56-60.

Poster, E.C. & Beliz, L. (1992). The use of the Johnson behavioral system model to measure changes during adolescent hospitalization. *International Journal of Adolescence and Youth, 4*, 73-84.

Poster, E.C., Dee, V., & Randell, B.P. (1997). The Johnson Behavioral Systems Model as a framework for patient outcome evaluation. *Journal of American Psychiatric Nurses Association, 3*(3), 73-80.

Randell, B.P. (1992). Nursing theory: The 21st century. *Nursing Science Quarterly, 5*(4), 176-184.

Rawls, A.C. (1980, Feb.). Evaluation of the Johnson behavioral model in clinical practice. *Image, 12*, 13-16.

Reynolds, W. & Cormack, D. (1991). An evaluation of the Johnson behavioral system model of nursing. *Journal of Advanced Nursing, 16*(9), 1122-1130.

Rickelma, B.L. (1971). Bio-psycho-social linguistics conceptual approach to nurse-patient interaction. *Nursing Research, 20*(5), 398-403.

Riegel, B. (1989). Social support and psychological adjustment to chronic coronary heart disease: Operationalization of Johnson's behavioral system model. *Advances in Nursing Science, 11*(2), 74-84.

Rogers, C.G. (1973). Conceptual models as guides to clinical nursing specialization. *Journal of Nursing Education, 12*(4), 2-6.

Rogers, J.C. (1982, Jan.). Order and disorder in medicine and occupational therapy. *American Journal of Occupational Therapy, 36*, 29-35.

Scher, M.E. (1975). Stereotyping and role conflicts between medical students and psychiatric nurses. *Hospital and Community Psychiatry, 26*(4), 219-221.

Secrest, H.P. (1968). Nurses and collaborative peritonatal research project. *Nursing Research, 17*, 292.

Smith, M.C. (1974). Perceptions of head nurses, clinical nurse specialists, nursing educators and nursing office personnel re: Performance of selected nursing activities. *Nursing Research, 23*(6), 505-510.

Smith, M.C. (1976). Patient responses to being transferred during hospitalization. *Nursing Research, 25*(3), 192-196.

Smithern, C. (1969). Vocal behavior of infants as related to nursing procedures of rocking. *Nursing Research, 18*(3), 256-258.

Sorrentino, E.A. (1991). Making theories work for you. *Nursing Administration Quarterly, 15*(3), 54-59.

Stamler, C. (1971). Dependency and repetitive visits to nurses' offices in elementary school children. *Nursing Research, 20*(3), 254-255.

Stevens, B.J. (1971). Analysis of structural forms used in nursing curricula. *Nursing Research, 20*(5), 388-397.

Taylor, S.D. (1975). Bibliography on nursing research 1950-1975. *Nursing Research, 24*(3), 207-225.

Vaillot, M.C. (1970). Hope: Restoration of being. *American Journal of Nursing, 10*(2), 268.

Waltz, C.F. (1978). Faculty influence on nursing students' preference in practice. *Nursing Research, 27*(2), 89-97.

Waters, V.H. (1972). Nursing practice: Implemental and supplemental. *Nursing Research, 21*(2), 124-131.

Wheeler, K. (1989). Self-psychology's contributions to understanding stress and implications for nursing. *Journal of Advanced Medical-Surgical Nursing, 1*(4), 1-10.

White, M.B. (1972). Importance of selected nursing activities. *Nursing Research, 21*(1), 4-14.

Wilkie, D.J. (1990). Cancer pain management: State-of-the-art nursing care. *Nursing Clinics of North America, 25*(2), 331-43.

Wilkie, D., Lovejoy, N., Dodd, M., & Tesler, M. (1988). Cancer pain control behaviors: Description and correlation with pain intensity. *Oncology Nursing Forum, 15*(6), 723-731.

Zbilut, J.P. (1978). Epistemologic constraints to development of a theory of nursing. *Nursing Research, 27*(2), 128-129.

Other Sources

Ainsworth, M. (1964). Patterns of attachment behavior shown by the infant in interaction with mother. *Merrill-Palmer Quarterly, 10*(1), 51-58.

Ainsworth, M. (1972). Attachment and dependency: A comparison. In J. Gewirtz (Ed.), *Attachment and dependency.* Englewood Cliffs, NJ: Prentice-Hall.

Aita, V.A. (1995). *Toward improved practice: Formal prescriptions and informal expressions of compassion in American nursing during the 1950s.* Unpublished doctoral dissertation, University of Nebraska Medical Center.

Atkinson, J.W. (1966). *Feather NT: A theory of achievement maturation.* New York: John Wiley & Sons.

Buckley, W. (Ed.). (1968). *Modern systems research for the behavioral scientist.* Chicago: Aldine.

Chin, R. (1961). The utility of system models and developmental models for practitioners. In K. Benne, W. Bennis, & R. Chin (Eds.), *The planning of change.* New York: Holt, Rinehart, & Winston.

Crandal, V. (1963). Achievement. In H.W. Stevenson (Ed.), *Child psychology.* Chicago: University of Chicago Press.

Dimino, E. (1988). Needed: Nursing research questions which test and expand our conceptual models of nursing. *Virginia Nurse, 56*(3), 43-6.

Feshbach, S. (1970). Aggression. In P. Mussen (Ed.), *Carmichael's manual of child psychology* (3rd ed., Vol. 2). New York: John Wiley & Sons.

Gerwitz, J. (Ed.). (1972). *Attachment and dependency.* Englewood Cliffs, NJ: Prentice-Hall.

Grinker, R.R. (Ed.). (1956). *Toward a unified theory of human behavior.* New York: Basic Books.

Heathers, G. (1955). Acquiring dependence and independence: A theoretical orientation. *Journal of General Psychology, 87,* 277-291.

Kagan, J. (1964). Acquisition and significance of sex typing and sex role identity. In M.L. Hoffman & L.W. Hoffman, (Eds.), *Review of child development research.* New York: Russell Sage Foundation.

Leitch, M. & Escalona, E. (1949). The reaction of infants to stress. In *Psychoanalytic study of the child* (Vols. 3-4). New York: International Universities Press.

Lorenz, K. (1966). *On aggression.* New York: Harcourt.

Mead, M. (Ed.). (1953). *Cultural patterns and technical change.* Paris: World Federation for Mental Health, United Nations Educational, Scientific, and Cultural Organization.

Rapoport, A. (1968). Foreword. In W. Buckley (Ed.), *Modern systems research for the behavioral scientist.* Chicago: Aldine.

Resnik, H.L.P. (1972). *Sexual behaviors.* Boston: Little, Brown.

Robson, K.S. (1967). Patterns and determinants of maternal attachment. *Journal of Pediatrics, 77,* 976-985.

Rosenthal, M. (1967). The generalization of dependency from mother to a stranger. *Journal of Child Psychology and Psychiatry, 8,* 177-183.

Sears, R., Macoby, E., & Levin, H. (1954). *Patterns of child rearing.* White Plains, NY: Row, Peterson.

Selye, H. (1956). *The stress of life.* New York: McGraw-Hill.

Simmons, L.W. & Wolff, H.G. (1954). *Social science in medicine.* New York: Russell Sage Foundation.

Walike, B., Jordan, H.A., & Stellar, E. (1969). Studies of eating behavior. *Nursing Research, 18,* 108-113.

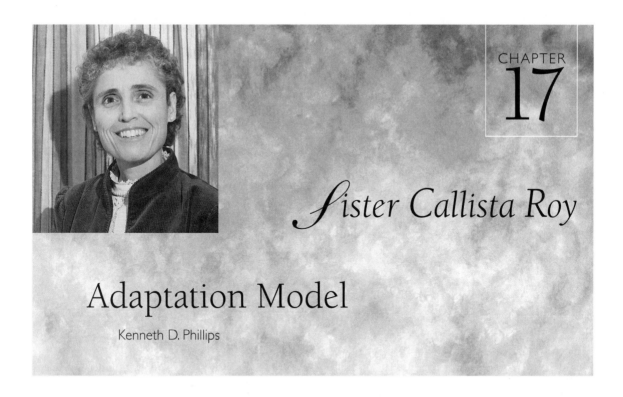

$\int$ ister Callista Roy

Adaptation Model

Kenneth D. Phillips

CREDENTIALS AND BACKGROUND OF THE THEORIST

Sister Callista Roy, a member of the Sisters of Saint Joseph of Carondelet, was born on October 14, 1939 in Los Angeles, California. She received a B.A. in nursing in 1963 from Mount Saint Mary's College in Los Angeles and an M.S.N. from the University of California, Los Angeles in 1966. After earning her nursing degrees, Roy began her education in sociology, receiving both an M.A. in sociology in 1973 and a Ph.D. in sociology in 1977 from the University of California.

While working toward her master's degree, Roy was challenged in a seminar with Dorothy E. Johnson to develop a conceptual model for nursing. While

Previous authors: Kenneth D. Phillips, Carolyn L. Blue, Karen M. Brubaker, Julia M.B. Fine, Martha J. Kirsch, Katherine R. Papazian, Cynthia M. Riester, and Mary Ann Sobiech.
The author wishes to express appreciation to Sister Callista Roy for critiquing the chapter.

working as a pediatric staff nurse, Roy had noticed the great resiliency of children and their ability to adapt in response to major physical and psychological changes. Roy was impressed by adaptation as an appropriate conceptual framework for nursing. Roy developed the basic concepts of the model while she was a graduate student at the University of California, Los Angeles from 1964 to 1966. Roy began operationalizing her model in 1968 when Mount Saint Mary's College adopted the adaptation framework as the philosophical foundation of the nursing curriculum. The Roy Adaptation Model (RAM) was first presented in the literature in an article published in *Nursing Outlook* in 1970 entitled, "Adaptation: A Conceptual Framework for Nursing."[71]

Roy was an associate professor and chairperson of the Department of Nursing at Mount Saint Mary's College until 1982. She was promoted to the rank of professor in 1983 at both Mount St. Mary's College and the University of Portland. She helped

269

initiate and taught in a summer masters program at the University of Portland. From 1983 to 1985, she was a Robert Wood Johnson Post Doctoral Fellow at the University of California, San Francisco as a clinical nurse scholar in neuroscience. During this time, she conducted research on nursing interventions for cognitive recovery in head injuries and on the influence of nursing models on clinical decision making. In 1987, Roy began the newly created position of nurse theorist at Boston College School of Nursing.[97]

Roy has published many books, chapters, and periodical articles and has presented numerous lectures and workshops focusing on her nursing adaptation theory.[85] The most recent refinement and restatement of the RAM is published in her 1999 book, *The Roy Adaptation Model*.[86]

Roy is a member of Sigma Theta Tau and she received the National Founder's Award for Excellence in Fostering Professional Nursing Standards in 1981. Her achievements include an Honorary Doctorate of Humane Letters by Alverno College (1984), Honorary Doctorates from Eastern Michigan University (1985) and St. Joseph's College in Maine (1999), and an A.J.N. Book of the Year Award for *Essentials of the Roy Adaptation Model*[2] (1986). Roy has been recognized in the World Who's Who of Women (1979), Personalities of America (1978), as a Fellow of the American Academy of Nursing (1978); recipient of a Fulbright Senior Scholar Award from the Australian-American Educational Foundation (1989); and the Martha Rogers Award for Advancing Nursing Science from the National League for Nurses (1991).

THEORETICAL SOURCES

Derivation of the RAM for nursing included a citation of Harry Helson's work in psychophysics that extended to social and behavioral sciences.[81] In Helson's Adaptation Theory, adaptive responses are a function of the incoming stimulus and the adaptive level.[81] A stimulus is any factor that provokes a response. Stimuli may arise from either the internal or the external environment.[81] The adaptation level is made up of the pooled effect of three classes of stimuli: (1) focal stimuli, which immediately confront the individual; (2) contextual stimuli, which are all other

stimuli present that contribute to the effect of the focal stimulus; and (3) residual stimuli, environmental factors whose effects are unclear in a given situation. Helson's work developed the concept of the adaptation level zone, which determines whether a stimulus will elicit a positive or a negative response. According to Helson's theory, adaptation is a process of responding positively to environmental changes.[90]

Roy[90] combined Helson's work with Rapoport's definition of system to view the person as an adaptive system. With Helson's Adaptation Theory as a foundation, Roy[71] developed and further refined the model with concepts and theory from Dohrenwend, Lazarus, Mechanic, and Selye. Roy gave special credit to coauthors Driever (for outlining subdivisions of self-integrity) and Martinez and Sato (for identifying common and primary stimuli affecting the modes). Other co-workers also elaborated the concepts: Pousch-Teddrow and Van Landingham for the interdependence mode and Randall for the role function mode.

After the development of her model, Roy presented it as a framework for nursing practice, research, and education.[111] According to Roy[72] more than 1500 faculty and students have contributed to the theoretical development of the adaptation model. By 1987, it was estimated that over 100,000 nurses in the United States and Canada had been prepared to practice using the Roy model.

In *Introduction to Nursing: An Adaptation Model*,[76] Roy discussed self-concept and group-identity mode. She and her collaborators cited the work of Coombs and Snygg regarding self-consistency and major influencing factors of self-concept.[81] Social interaction theories are cited to provide a theoretical basis. For example, Roy[81] notes that Cooley indicates that in Epstein's publication, self-perception is influenced by perceptions of other's responses. She points out that Mead expands the idea by hypothesizing that self-appraisal uses the *generalized other*. Roy builds on Sullivan's suggestion that self arises from social interaction.[81] Gardner and Erickson support Roy's developmental approaches.[81] The other modes—physiological-physical, role function, and interdependence—were drawn similarly from biological and behavioral sciences for an understanding of the person.

Additional development of the model occurred in the later 1900s and into the twenty-first century. These developments included updated scientific and philosophical assumptions; a redefinition of adaptation and adaptation levels; extension of the adaptive modes to group-level knowledge development; and analysis, critique, and synthesis of the first 25 years of research based on the RAM. Roy agrees with other theorists who believe that changes in the person-environment systems of the earth are so extensive that a major epoch is ending.[14,15] During the 67 million years of the Cenozoic era, the Age of Mammals and an era of great creativity, human life appeared on earth. During this era, humankind has had little or no influence on the universe.[84] "As the era closes, humankind has taken extensive control of the life systems of the earth. Roy claims that we are now in the position of deciding what kind of universe we will inhabit."[84:42] Roy "has made the foci of assumptions of the 21st century mutual complex person and environment self-organization and a meaningful destiny of convergence of the universe, persons, and environment in what can be considered a supreme being or God."[86:395] According to Roy,[84:42,86:395] "persons are coextensive with their physical and social environments," and they "share a destiny with the universe and are responsible for mutual transformations." Developments of the model related to the integral relationship between person and the environment have been influenced by Pierre Teilhard de Chardin's law of progressive complexity and increasing consciousness[15,16] and the work of Swimme and Berry.[98]

USE OF EMPIRICAL EVIDENCE

The use of the RAM in nursing practice led to further clarification and refinement. A 1971 pilot research study and a survey research study from 1976 to 1977 led to some tentative confirmations of the model.[79]

From this beginning, the RAM has been supported through research in practice and in education.* In 1999, a group of seven scholars working with Roy conducted an analysis, critique, and synthesis of 163 studies based on the RAM that had been published in 44 English-speaking journals on five continents and dissertations and theses from the United States. From the 163 studies, 116 met the criteria established for testing propositions from the model. Twelve generic propositions based on Roy's earlier work were derived. To synthesize the research, the findings of each study were used to state ancillary and practice propositions and support for the propositions were examined. Of the 265 propositions tested, 216 (82%) were supported.

*References 6, 24, 50, 52, 89, 110.

MAJOR CONCEPTS & DEFINITIONS

SYSTEM

A system is "a set of parts connected to function as a whole for some purpose and that does so by virtue of the interdependence of its parts."[86:32] In addition to having wholeness and related parts, "systems also have inputs, outputs, and control and feedback processes."[3:7]

ADAPTATION LEVEL

"Adaptation level represents the condition of the life processes described on three levels as integrated, compensatory, and compromised."[86:30] A person's adaptation level is "a constantly changing point, made up of focal, contextual, and residual stimuli, which represent the person's own standard of the range of stimuli to which one can respond with ordinary adaptive responses."[81:27-28]

ADAPTATION PROBLEMS

Adaptation problems are "broad areas of concern related to adaptation. These describe the difficulties related to the indicators of positive adaptation."[86:65] Roy[81:89-90] states, "It can be noted at this point that the distinction being made between adaptation problems and nursing diagnoses is

Continued

MAJOR CONCEPTS *&* DEFINITIONS—cont'd

based on the developing work in both of these fields. At this point, adaptation problems are seen not as nursing diagnoses, but as areas of concern for the nurse related to adapting person or group (within each adaptive mode)."

FOCAL STIMULUS

The focal stimulus is "the internal or external stimulus most immediately confronting the human system."[86:31]

CONTEXTUAL STIMULI

Contextual stimuli "are all other stimuli present in the situation that contribute to the effect of the focal stimulus."[86:31] That is, "contextual stimuli are all the environmental factors that present to the person from within or without but which are not the center of the person's attention and/or energy."[3:9]

RESIDUAL STIMULI

Residual stimuli "are environmental factors within or without the human system with effects in the current situation that are unclear."[86:32]

COPING PROCESSES

Coping processes "are innate or acquired ways of interacting with the changing environment."[86:31]

INNATE COPING MECHANISMS

Innate coping mechanisms "are genetically determined or common to the species and are generally viewed as automatic processes; humans do not have to think about them."[86:46]

ACQUIRED COPING MECHANISMS

Acquired coping mechanisms "are developed through strategies such as learning. The experiences encountered throughout life contribute to customary responses to particular stimuli."[86:46]

REGULATOR SUBSYSTEM

Regulator is "a major coping process involving the neural, chemical, and endocrine systems."[86:32]

COGNATOR SUBSYSTEM

Cognator is "a major coping process involving four cognitive-emotive channels: perceptual and information processing, learning, judgment, and emotion."[86:31]

ADAPTIVE RESPONSES

Adaptive responses are those "that promote integrity in terms of the goals of human systems."[86:30]

INEFFECTIVE RESPONSES

Ineffective responses are those "that do not contribute to integrity in terms of the goals of the human system."[86:31]

INTEGRATED LIFE PROCESS

Integrated life process refers to the "adaptation level at which the structures and functions of a life process are working as a whole to meet human needs."[86:31]

PHYSIOLOGICAL-PHYSICAL MODE

The physiological mode "is associated with the physical and chemical processes involved in the function and activities of living organisms."[86:102] Five needs are identified in the physiological-physical mode relative to the basic need of physiological integrity: (1) oxygenation, (2) nutrition, (3) elimination, (4) activity and rest, and (5) protection.[86] Complex processes that include the senses; fluid, electrolyte, and acid-base balance; neurological function; and endocrine function contribute to physiological adaptation. The basic need of the physiological mode is physiological integrity.[86] The physical mode is "the manner in which the collective human adaptive system manifests adaptation relative to basic operating re-

MAJOR CONCEPTS & DEFINITIONS—cont'd

sources, participants, physical facilities, and fiscal resources."[86:104] The basic need of the physical mode is operating integrity.

SELF-CONCEPT-GROUP IDENTITY MODE

The self-concept-group identity mode is one of the three psychosocial modes and "it focuses specifically on the psychological and spiritual aspects of the human system. The basic need underlying the individual self-concept mode has been identified as psychic and spiritual integrity, or the need to know who one is so that one can be or exist with a sense of unity, meaning, and purposefulness in the universe."[86:107] "Self-concept is defined as the composite of beliefs and feelings about oneself at a given time and is formed from internal perceptions and perceptions of others' reactions."[86:107] Its components include: (1) the physical self, which involves sensation and body-image and (2) the personal self, which is made up of self-consistency, self-ideal or expectancy, and the moral-ethical-spiritual self.[86] The group identity mode "reflects how people in groups perceive themselves based on environmental feedback. The group identity mode is comprised of interpersonal relationships, group self-image, social milieu, and culture"[86:108] The basic need of the group identity mode is identity integrity.[86]

ROLE FUNCTION MODE

The role function mode "is one of two social modes and focuses on the roles the person occupies in society. A role, as the functioning unit of society, is defined as a set of expectations about how a person occupying one position behaves toward a person occupying another position. The basic need underlying the role function mode has been identified as social integrity—the need to know who one is in relation to others so that one can act."[41:109-110] Persons perform primary, secondary, and tertiary roles. These roles are carried out with both instru-

mental and expressive behaviors. Instrumental behavior is "the actual physical performance of a behavior."[1:348] Expressive behaviors are "the feelings, attitudes, likes or dislikes that a person has about a role or about the performance of a role."[1:348] "The primary role determines the majority of behavior engaged in by the person during a particular period of life. It is determined by age, sex, and developmental stage."[1:349] "Secondary roles are those that a person assumes to complete the task associated with a developmental stage and primary role."[1:349] "Tertiary roles are related primarily to secondary roles and represent ways in which individuals meet their role associated obligations . . . . Tertiary roles are normally temporary in nature, freely chosen by the individual, and may include activities such as clubs or hobbies."[1:349]

> The major roles that one plays can be analyzed by imagining a tree formation. The trunk of the tree is one's primary role, that is, one's developmental level—for example, generative adult female. Secondary roles branch off from this—for example, wife, mother, teacher. Finally, tertiary roles branch off from secondary roles—for example, the mother role might involve the role of PTA president for a given period of time. Each of these roles is seen as occurring in a dyadic relationship, that is with a reciprocal role.[86:44]

INTERDEPENDENCE MODE

The interdependence mode

> focuses on close relationships of people (individually and collectively) and their purpose, structure, and development. . . . Interdependent relationships involve the willingness and ability to give to others and accept from them aspects of all that one has to offer such as love, respect, value, nurturing, knowledge, skills, commitments, material possessions, time, and talents.[86:111]

The basic need of this mode is termed relational integrity.[86] "Two specific relationships are the focus of the interdependence mode as it

Continued

applies to individuals. The first is with significant others, persons who are the most important to the individual. The second is with support systems, that is, others contributing to meeting interdependence needs."[86:112] Two major areas of interdependence behaviors have been identified, receptive behavior and contributive behavior. These behaviors apply respectively to the "receiving and

giving of love, respect and value in interdependent relationships."[86:112]

PERCEPTION

"Perception is the interpretation of a stimulus and the conscious appreciation of it."[66:169] Perception links the regulator with the cognator and connects the adaptive modes.[67]

MAJOR ASSUMPTIONS

Assumptions from systems theory and assumptions from adaptation-level theory have been combined into a single set of scientific assumptions. From systems theory, human adaptive systems are viewed as systems with interactive parts that act in unity for some purpose. Human adaptive systems are complex, multifaceted, and respond to myriad environmental stimuli to achieve adaptation. With their ability to adapt to environmental stimuli, humans have the capacity to create changes in the environment.[86] Drawing on characteristics of creation spirituality by Swimme and Berry,[98] Roy combined the assumptions of humanism and veritivity into a single set of philosophical assumptions. Humanism asserts that the person and human experiences are essential to knowing and valuing and that they share in creative power. Veritivity affirms the belief in the purpose, value, and meaning of all human life. These scientific and philosophical assumptions have been refined for use in the model in the twenty-first century (Box 17-1).

Adaptation

In her most recent book, Roy[86] has further defined adaptation for use in the twenty-first century. According to Roy,[86:30] adaptation refers to "the process and outcome whereby thinking and feeling persons as individuals or in groups, use conscious awareness and choice to create human and environmental integration." Rather than a system simply striving to

respond to environmental stimuli to maintain integrity, every human life is purposeful in a universe that is creative and persons are inseparable from their environment.

Nursing

Roy[86:4] defines nursing broadly as a "health care profession that focuses on human life processes and patterns and emphasizes promotion of health for individuals, families, groups, and society as a whole." Specifically, Roy[86] defines nursing according to her model as the science and practice that expands adaptive abilities and enhances person and environmental transformation. She identifies nursing activities as the assessment of behavior and the stimuli that influence adaptation. Nursing judgments are based on the assessment and interventions are planned to manage the stimuli. Roy[81] differentiates nursing as a science from nursing as a practice discipline. Nursing science is "a developing system of knowledge about persons that observes, classifies, and relates the processes by which persons positively affect their health status."[81:3-4] Nursing as a practice discipline is "nursing's scientific body of knowledge used for the purpose of providing an essential service to people, that is, promoting ability to affect health positively."[81:3-4] "Nursing acts to enhance the interaction of the person with the environment—to promote adaptation."[3:20]

Roy's goal of nursing[86:19] is "the promotion of adaptation for individuals and groups in each of the four adaptive modes thus contributing to health, quality of life, and dying with dignity." Nursing fills a unique role as a facilitator of adaptation by assessing behavior in each of these four adaptive modes and factors influencing adaptation and by intervening to promote adaptive abilities and to enhance environment interactions.[86]

Person

According to Roy, humans are holistic, adaptive systems. "As an adaptive system, the human system is described as a whole with parts that function as unity for some purpose. Human systems include people as individuals or in groups including families, organizations, communities, and society as a whole."[86:31] Despite their great diversity, all persons are united in a common destiny.[86] "Human systems have thinking and feeling capacities, rooted in consciousness and meaning, by which they adjust effectively to changes in the environment and, in turn, affect the environment."[86:36] Persons and the earth have common patterns and mutuality of relations and meaning.[86] Roy[86] defined the person as the main focus of nursing; the recipient of nursing care; a living, complex, adaptive system with internal processes (cognator and regulator) acting to maintain adaptation in the four adaptive modes (physiological, self-concept, role function, and interdependence).

Health

"Health is a state and a process of being and becoming integrated and a whole person. It is a reflection of adaptation, that is, the interaction of the person and the environment."[3:21] Roy[81] derived this definition from the thought that adaptation is a process of promoting physiological, psychological, and social integrity and that integrity implies an unimpaired condition leading to completeness or unity. In her earlier work, Roy viewed health along a continuum flowing from death and extreme poor health to high-level and peak wellness.[6] Roy's recent writings[86] have focused more on health as a process in which health and illness can coexist. Drawing on the writings of Illich, Roy[86:52] wrote "health is not

Box 17-1

Vision Basic to Concepts for the Twenty-First Century

SCIENTIFIC ASSUMPTIONS
- Systems of matter and energy progress to higher levels of complex self-organization.
- Consciousness and meaning are constitutive of person and environment integration.
- Awareness of self and environment is rooted in thinking and feeling.
- Humans by their decisions are accountable for the integration of creative processes.
- Thinking and feeling mediate human action.
- System relationships include acceptance, protection, and fostering of interdependence.
- Persons and the earth have common patterns and integral relationships.
- Persons and environment transformations are created in human consciousness.
- Integration of human and environment meanings results in adaptation.

PHILOSOPHICAL ASSUMPTIONS
- Persons have mutual relationships with the world and God.
- Human meaning is rooted in an omega point convergence of the universe.
- God is ultimately revealed in the diversity of creation and is the common destiny of creation.
- Persons use human creative abilities of awareness, enlightenment, and faith.
- Persons are accountable for the processes of deriving, sustaining, and transforming the universe.

From Roy, C. & Andrews, H. (1999). *The Roy adaptation model* (2nd ed., p. 35). Stamford, CT: Appleton & Lange.

freedom from the inevitability of death, disease, un-happiness, and stress, but the ability to cope with them in a competent way."

Health and illness are one inevitable, coexistent dimension of the person's total life experience.[70] Nursing is concerned with this dimension. When mechanisms for coping are ineffective, illness results. Health ensues when humans continually adapt. As people adapt to stimuli, they are free to respond to other stimuli. The freeing of energy from ineffective coping attempts can promote healing and enhance health.[81]

Environment

According to Roy,[86:31] environment is "all the conditions, circumstances, and influences surrounding and affecting the development and behavior of persons or groups, with particular consideration of the mutuality of person and earth resources that includes focal, contextual, and residual stimuli." "It is the changing environment [that] stimulates the person to make adaptive responses."[3:18] Environment is the input into the person as an adaptive system involving both internal and external factors. These factors may be slight or large, negative or positive. However, any environmental change demands increasing energy to adapt to the situation. Factors in the environment that affect the person are categorized as focal, contextual, and residual stimuli.

THEORETICAL ASSERTIONS

Roy's model focuses on the concept of adaptation of the person. Her concepts of nursing, person, health, and environment are all interrelated to this central concept. The person continually scans the environment for stimuli. Ultimately, a response is made and adaptation occurs. That adaptive response may be either an adaptive or an ineffective response. Adaptive responses are those that promote integrity and help the person to achieve the goals of adaptation; that is, survival, growth, reproduction, mastery, and person and environmental transformations. Ineffective responses are responses that fail to achieve or threaten the goals of adaptation. Nursing has a unique goal to assist the person's adaptation effort by managing the

environment. The result is attainment of an optimum level of wellness by the person.[*]

As an open living system, the person receives inputs or stimuli from both the environment and the self. The adaptation level is determined by the combined effect of the focal, contextual, and residual stimuli. Adaptation occurs when the person responds positively to environmental changes. This adaptive response promotes the integrity of the person, which leads to health. Ineffective responses to stimuli leads to the disruption of the integrity of the person.[†]

There are two interrelated subsystems in Roy's model (Figure 17-1). The primary, functional, or control processes subsystem consists of the regulator and the cognator. The secondary, effector subsystem consists of four adaptive modes: (1) physiological needs, (2) self-concept, (3) role function, and (4) interdependence.[‡]

Roy views the regulator and cognator as methods of coping. The regulator coping subsystem, by way of the physiological adaptive mode, "responds automatically through neural, chemical, and endocrine coping processes."[3:14] The cognator coping subsystem, by way of the self-concept, interdependence, and role-function adaptive modes "responds through four cognitive-emotive channels: perceptual information processing, learning, judgment, and emotion."[3:14] Perception of the person links the regulator with the cognator in that "input into the regulator is transformed into perceptions. Perception is a process of the cognator. The responses following perception are feedback into both the cognator and the regulator."[34:67]

The four adaptive modes of the two subsystems in Roy's model provide form or manifestations of cognator and regulator activity. Responses to stimuli are carried out through four adaptive modes. The physiological-physical adaptive mode is concerned with the way humans interact with the environment through physiological processes to meet the basic needs of oxygenation, nutrition, elimination, activity and rest, and protection. The self-concept-group

---

*References 2, 68, 71, 72, 79, 81, 88, 90.
†References 2, 68, 71, 72, 79, 81, 88.
‡References 2, 47, 51, 52, 70, 72, 74.

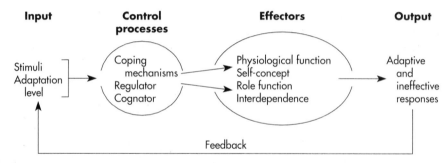

Figure **17-1** **Person as an adaptive system.** (From Roy, C. [© 1984]. *Introduction to nursing: An adaptation model* [2nd ed., p. 30]. Englewood Cliffs, NJ: Prentice Hall. Reprinted by permission of Prentice-Hall, Inc., Englewood Cliffs, NJ.)

identity adaptive mode is concerned with the need to know who one is and how to act in society. An individual's self-concept is defined by Roy as "the composite of beliefs or feelings that an individual holds about him or her self at any given time."[86:49] An individual's self-concept is comprised of the physical self (body sensation and body image) and personal self (self-consistency, self-ideal, and moral-ethical-spiritual self). The role function adaptive mode describes the primary, secondary, and tertiary roles that an individual performs in society. A role describes the expectations about how one person behaves toward another person. The interdependence adaptive mode deals with the interactions of people in society. The major task of the interdependence adaptive mode is for persons to give and receive love, respect, and value. The most important components of the interdependence adaptive mode are a person's significant other (spouse, child, friend, or God) and his or her social support system. The purpose of the four adaptive modes is to achieve physiological, psychological, and social integrity.[86] Interrelated propositions of the cognator and regulator subsystems link the systems of the adaptive modes (Figure 17-2).[24]

The person as a whole is made up of six subsystems. These subsystems (the regulator, cognator, and the four adaptive modes) are interrelated to form a complex system for the purpose of adaptation. Relationships among the four adaptive modes occur when internal and external stimuli affect more than one mode; when disruptive behavior occurs in more

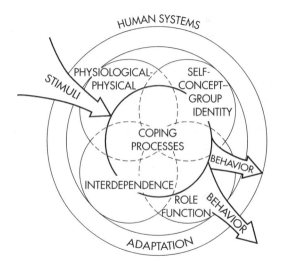

Figure **17-2** **Diagrammatic representation of human adaptive systems.** (From Roy, C. & Andrews, H. [© 1999]. *The Roy adaptation model* [2nd ed.]. Norwalk, CT: Appleton & Lange. Reprinted by permission of Pearson Education, Inc., Upper Saddle River, NJ.)

than one mode; or when one mode becomes the focal, contextual, or residual stimulus for another mode.[6,13,50]

In regard to human social systems, Roy broadly categorizes the control processes into the stabilizer and innovator subsystems. The stabilizer system is analogous to the regulator subsystem of the individual and is concerned with stability. To maintain the system, the stabilizer subsystem involves organizational structure, cultural values, and regulation of daily activities of the system. The innovator subsystem is associated with the cognator subsystem of the individual and is concerned with creativity, change, and growth.[86]

LOGICAL FORM

The RAM of nursing is both deductive and inductive. It is deductive in that much of Roy's theory is derived from Helson's psychophysics theory. Helson developed the concepts of focal, contextual, and residual stimuli, which Roy[72] redefined within nursing to form a typology of factors related to adaptation levels of persons. Roy also uses other concepts and theory outside the discipline of nursing and synthesizes these within her adaptation theory.

Roy's adaptation theory is inductive in that she developed the four adaptive modes from research and nursing practice experiences of herself, her colleagues, and her students. Roy[76,79,81] built on the conceptual framework of adaptation and developed a step-by-step model by which nurses use the nursing process to administer nursing care to promote adaptation in situations of health and illness.

ACCEPTANCE BY THE NURSING COMMUNITY

Practice

With use of Roy's six-step nursing process, the nurse: (1) assesses the behaviors manifested from the four adaptive modes; (2) assesses the stimuli for those behaviors and categorizes them as focal, contextual, or residual stimuli; (3) makes a statement or nursing diagnosis of the person's adaptive state; (4) sets goals to promote adaptation; (5) implements interventions aimed at managing the stimuli to promote adaptation; and (6) evaluates whether the adaptive goals have been met. By manipulating the stimuli and not the patient, the nurse enhances "the interaction of the person with their environment, thereby promoting health."[2:51]

Brower and Baker[6] consider Roy's model useful for nursing practice because it outlines the features of the discipline and provides direction for practice, education, and research. The model considers goals, values, the patient, and practitioner interventions. Brower and Baker view Roy's nursing process as well developed. The two-level assessment assisted in identification of nursing goals and diagnoses. They also note the need for continued work on a typology of nursing and on organizing categories of nursing interventions.

It is a valuable theory for nursing practice because it includes a goal that is specified as the aim for activity and prescription for activities to realize the goal.[18] The goal of the model is the person's adaptation in four adaptive modes in situations of health and illness. The prescriptions or interventions are the management of stimuli by removing, increasing, decreasing, or altering them. These prescriptions can be obtained by listing practice-related hypotheses generated by the model.[81]

The nursing process is well suited for use in a practice setting. The two-level assessment is unique to this model and leads to the identification of adaptation problems or nursing diagnosis. Work has been performed on developing a typology of nursing diagnoses from the perspective of the RAM.[81,90] Intervention is based specifically on the model, but there is a need to develop an organization of categories of nursing interventions.[90]

Wagner described use of the model in practice by graduate nursing students.[110] The students identified blending in the psychosocial modes of self-concept, role function, and interdependence as they decided where a given behavior belonged. They also reported that the nursing process seemed lengthy and took much time to complete. The model was useful in inpatient settings, except in intensive care units where rapid changes in the patient's condition occurred. The students found it easier to use the model in outpatient settings such as clinics and physician's offices.[110] A major strength of the model was that it provided a system that accounted for physical needs and psychosocial needs. It was particularly useful in the pediatric setting because it allowed for assessment of the covert psychological needs of children.

Mitchell and Pilkington[53] are also of the notion that the complexity of the assessment process would not be useful in a rapidly changing environment such as labor and delivery or critical care. They have also discussed the linearity of the six-step nursing process in the model and held that it is not realistic in practice settings. They questioned that the model provides direction for priority setting for interventions.

Mitchell and Pilkington[53] did find Roy's model useful for patients receiving care when they could participate in care planning and problem solving. They reported that the patients learned about healthier behaviors and ineffective behaviors. Mitchell and Pilkington[53] suggest that the patient may be viewed as passive in the nursing process when the nurse is viewed as the change agent.

In 1989, Hamner[38] discussed the Roy model and how it could be applied to nursing care in a cardiac care unit (CCU). The model is described as enhancing care in the CCU and being consistent with the nursing process. Hamner also reported that all patients' behavior was assessed using the model and that none was excluded. Hamner[38] discovered that the Roy model provides a structure in which manipulation of stimuli are not overlooked as it emphasized identifying and reinforcing positive behavior, which speeded recovery.

Frank and Lang[33] used the RAM to analyze disturbances in the sexual role performance of alcoholics. In the physiological mode, alcohol use was shown to alter sex hormone function and depress sexual response. In the role performance mode, there was an inconsistency between alcoholic men and women about the effect of alcohol on sexual performance and the depressant effects that alcohol has on sexual performance. For example, alcoholic men believe that their sexual pleasure increased with alcohol use even when their physiological response decreased, such as difficulty in maintaining an erection after increased alcohol consumption. In the self-concept role, alcoholics may use alcohol to increase their self-concept. In the interdependence mode, the decreased quality of a relationship as a result of alcohol use may prompt prolonged drinking bouts.

Giger, Davidhizar, and Miller[36] evaluated the RAM and the Nightingale theory as a means of providing care for patients in the operating room (OR).

They discovered many similarities and some differences between the models. Both described the metaparadigm of nursing in relation to the models and defined the interrelatedness among concepts. Both are deductive, both provide a systems model, and both provide an open systems model. They viewed Roy's model as a testable, practice theory and viewed Nightingale's theory as an untestable, grand theory. The main focus of Nightingale's theory is environment, whereas Roy's theory focuses on the person and the person's adaptation. Nightingale saw the person as having a passive role and the nurse an active role, whereas Roy sees the person as an active participant and the nurse more as a guide. Giger, Davidhizar, and Miller[36] concluded that the OR nurse should use various nursing theories and models to care for patients in the OR and that both works (Roy and Nightingale) could be applied quite easily.

Piazza and Foote[63] have found Roy's model useful for rehabilitation nursing practice. The rehabilitation patient frequently encounters changes in all adaptive modes. The model provides a holistic approach for the care of patients in all four modes.

Galligan[34] reported that Roy's model was useful to nurses caring for young, hospitalized children. Schmitz[91] used the model in the community setting for patients receiving home healthcare. The model reportedly enabled needs assessment, goal setting, and prioritization of goals. Interventions and evaluations were observed to be more efficient and effective as outcomes.

In May 1979, three nursing administrators initiated a pilot study using the model in an 18-bed unit in Arlington, Virginia. Evaluation and revision of the nursing assessment tools were conducted and, by April 1980, the model was in use in practice. Early research suggests that it enhanced patient satisfaction and improved health outcomes.[51] Consistent with the model, the nurses began to enhance their professionalism by writing complete care plans and phrasing patient problems in terms of nursing diagnoses. A year after initiation, the model was still supported by the staff. The group directors cautioned that the model required diligence in applying it in practice. They also suggested that further validation of the theory was needed.[51]

In September 1981, a research study was published that dealt with problems associated with nursing home applications for elderly persons.[24] The research was performed within the framework of the adaptation model. The research design was used to identify adaptation problems and hypotheses were formulated. The study concluded that, "As a broad conceptual framework, the Roy Adaptation Nursing Model served as a useful tool for systematically gathering responses regarding adaptation problems experienced by the elderly persons and their significant others."[24:364] The RAM has been applied to the care of elderly patients with Alzheimer's disease.[99]

Fitzpatrick, Whall, Johnston, and Floyd[32] also found Roy's model useful in the psychological assessment of the family. They used the model to analyze role function needs and interdependence needs, which may lead to maladaption in a troubled family system. They asserted that the nurse, as the environmental change agent, could improve a maladaptive family system.

Another research study used the model to analyze the content of 20 interviews of parents whose children had been recently diagnosed with cancer. Although operational definitions of Roy's adaptation modes were used in the study, the origins of the definitions remain unclear. Smith, Garvis, and Martinson[96] found the framework applicable as a result of its ability to treat multiple patient variables.

In 1986, Logan[48] described the practical use of the model and explored its appropriateness for palliative care nursing and its applicability in improving care of the dying patient. Logan[48] noted that basic assumptions of the Roy model seemed to correlate with the palliative care philosophy, except that terminology relating to goals differed. A utility index was used to assess the usefulness of the model on the basis of feasibility, practicality, compatibility, social benefit, and completeness. The Roy nursing process is very well illustrated by Logan's application of the model with an oncology case study. The nursing care plan is described in detail and includes analysis of diagnoses and behaviors. Logan makes suggestions for improving the model's language in the use of like words when describing like things.

In addition, the RAM has been evaluated for the care of patients with breast cancer, colorectal cancer, ulcerative colitis, colectomy, depression, quadriplegia, dermatomyositis, Alzheimer's disease, and leukemia.* The RAM has been applied to assessment and intervention for the adaptational needs of patients with chronic renal failure on hemodialyisis.[43] Samarel and colleagues[92] used the RAM as a guiding framework to create a resource kit for women with breast cancer that dealt with information needs in each of the four adaptive modes.

De Villers[17] demonstrated how clinical nurse specialists could use the RAM to help delineate their roles as expert practitioners in the obstetrical and gynecological setting. She applied Roy's steps of the nursing process and gave specific examples or expert care from each of the adaptive modes. Eaganhouse[23] has used the RAM to plan a preterm birth prevention program in a community hospital. Likewise, Phillips[62] used the RAM to demonstrate holistic nursing care for persons with cervical cancer and HIV disease. As another example, the RAM has been used as a theoretical basis and an organizing framework to provide group psychotherapy in a 15-bed acute inpatient psychiatric unit.[44] Use of the RAM facilitates advanced practice nurses to address the holistic needs of their patients, including their physiological needs.

The RAM has been analyzed for use in accident and emergency nursing, maternity nursing, neonatal intensive care units, rehabilitation nursing, community health nursing, nursing administration, and a rehabilitation program for women with breast cancer.† A number of healthcare agencies have begun implementing the RAM as a basis for nursing practice. Roy has compiled a list of experienced resource persons who can assist with this work in the United States and Canada.

Education

The adaptation model has also been useful in the educational setting and is currently in use at Mount

---

*References 7, 8, 10, 11, 37, 39, 54, 64, 95, 112, 113.
†References 19, 30, 40, 42, 45, 49, 54, 63, 93.

Saint Mary's College Department of Nursing in Los Angeles.[81] Mount Saint Mary's program demonstrates the relationship of nursing theory to nursing education. Three vertical strands run throughout the curriculum: (1) the adapting person (theory strand), (2) health-illness (theory strand), and (3) nursing management (practice strand). There are two horizontal strands in the curriculum: (1) nursing process and (2) student adaptation and leadership. The horizontal strands enhance the theory and practice of the vertical strands. All strands within the curriculum build in complexity from one level to the next.[78] In addition, the model allows for increasing knowledge in the areas of both theory and practice.[73,83]

Roy[73,78] states that the model defines the distinct purpose of nursing for students, which is to promote adaptation of person in each of the adaptive modes in situations of health and illness. The model also distinguishes nursing science from medical science by having the content of these areas taught in separate courses. She stresses collaboration, but delineates separate goals for nurses and physicians. According to Roy,[72] it is the nurse's goal to help the patient put his or her energy into getting well, whereas the medical student focuses on the patient's position on the health-illness continuum with the goal of causing movement along the continuum. She views the model as a valuable tool to analyze the distinctions between the two professions of nursing and medicine. Roy[78] believes that curricula based on this model help in theory development by the students, who also learn how to test theories and recognize new theoretical insights. Roy[72] suggests that the model is advantageous for integrated curricula and that it clarifies objectives, identifies content, and specifies patterns for teaching and learning.

In the early 1980s, the School of Nursing at the University of Ottawa experienced a major curriculum change.[58] The curriculum change included incorporating a nursing model on which to base the new curriculum. The RAM was one of the models to be included in the first year of the baccalaureate program. The professors met four challenges during the change: (1) adapting the course to be congruent with the Roy model, (2) developing teaching tools suitable for student learning, (3) sequencing content for student learning, and (4) obtaining competent role models. These challenges were met and the faculty continues to evaluate and modify the course.

In 1976, the model was used for curriculum development of a practitioner program at the University of Miami in Florida. Organization of curriculum content and selections of student learning experiences were derived from the model. Course objectives included identifying adaptive problems and distinguishing between effective and ineffective coping mechanisms. Application of the model resulted in decreased anxiety in the students and provided a framework to give direction to the education of practitioners.[6] Carveth[12] proposed the use of conceptual models as one means of improving the scientific knowledge base in nurse-midwifery. Carveth[12] asserted that the use of Roy's model would assist nurse-midwives to systematically study, communicate, define, and describe their interdependent role.

Throughout the 1970s and 1980s, the Roy model was implemented as a basis for curriculum development in associate-degree diploma, baccalaureate, and higher-degree programs in many countries. Articles and books on Roy's model have been published in several languages, including Portuguese, Japanese, and French. Roy and her colleagues have provided consultation for this work in more than 30 schools in the United States, Canada, and abroad.

Research

Development and testing of theories. If research is to affect practitioners' behavior, it must be directed at testing and retesting theories derived from conceptual models for nursing practice. Roy[81] has stated that theory development and the testing of developed theories are the highest priorities for nursing. The model is able to generate many testable hypotheses that need to be researched.

As previously stated, Roy's theory has generated a number of general propositions. From these general propositions, specific hypotheses can be developed and tested. Hill and Roberts[41] have demonstrated the development of testable hypotheses from the model, as has Roy. Data to validate or support the model is created by the testing of such hypotheses; the model is beginning to generate more of this type of research.[100] Lutjens[49] derived a theory from the RAM and has applied this theory to social organizations.

Roy[71] has identified a set of concepts forming a model from which the process of observation and classification of facts would lead to postulates. The postulates concern the occurrence of adaptation problems, coping mechanisms, and interventions based on laws derived from factors making up the response potential of the focal, contextual, and residual stimuli. Roy[73-75] has outlined a typology of adaptation problems or nursing diagnoses. Research and testing are needed in the area of typology and categories of interventions that fit into the model. General propositions that need to be tested have also been developed.[88]

Practice-based research. A group of graduate students at DePaul University tested the model in a number of practice situations.[96] The students adapted an assessment tool and tested the model in episodic settings in a variety of units in different hospitals. They also used distributive settings in physicians' offices, industrial health settings, and outpatient clinics. The students concluded that the model provided a good framework for ordering a variety of observations and was flexible enough to be used in both episodic and distributive settings.[96] The study provided empirical support for the model in the area of the process of assessment within the four adaptive modes.

Limadri[47] studied the model as a conceptual framework in her descriptive research study and in her practice with abused women in an outpatient setting. She identified patterns of help-seeking behaviors in a group of 40 abused women. From her experiences in practice, Limadri analyzed the model's construct interrelationships and expanded Roy's original model to illustrate a conceptualization of the abused women's adaptive response in help-seeking behaviors. She also reported that the modes overlap, but found that "the model proves a useful framework to identify the complex needs of the client."[47:58-59]

In 1987, Silva[95] used the Roy model to structure the perceived needs of family members of patients undergoing surgery. The four modes were reflected in responses to a questionnaire, but the patterning of relationships was somewhat different from that suggested by the model. Some needs classified in the psychosocial modes were found to be interrelated, whereas other needs theoretically related to these modes appeared independent. Silva found the physiological mode to be relatively independent of the three psychosocial modes. She suggested further refinement of the modes to clarify the interdependent and interrelated areas of each. Roy,[82] in her response to this article, commends Silva's use of factor analysis for exploring and testing the model and contributing to the basic science of adaptation nursing.

Brydolf and Segesten[7] used the RAM to assess long-term physiological adaptation in 30 young persons with ulcerative colitis who had undergone a colectomy. The model helped them track the symptoms. Twenty-four of the young persons reported significant problems related to nutrition, elimination, activity and rest, and protection, whereas six subjects reported no adaptation problems.

Pittman[65] studied wellness promotion behaviors among school-aged children using a Q-sort methodology. Four factors related to wellness promotion behaviors represented the four adaptive modes. An important finding was that the self-concept adaptive mode was represented by the most enabling wellness promotion behaviors.

Nuamah, Cooley, Fawcett, and McCorkle[60] studied quality of life in 515 cancer patients. The researchers clearly established linkages between the concepts of the RAM, the middle-range theory concepts, and the empirical indicators. Focal and contextual stimuli were identified. Variables in each of the adaptive modes were operationalized. Using structural equation modeling, the researchers found that two of the environmental stimuli (adjuvant cancer treatment and severity of the disease) explained 59% of the variance in the biopsychosocial indicators of the latent variable health-related quality of life. Their findings supported the proposition of the RAM that environmental stimuli influence biopsychosocial responses.

Samarel and colleagues[92] used the RAM to study women's perceptions of adaptation to breast cancer in a sample of 70 women who were participating in an experimental support and education group. The experimental group received coaching; the control group received no coaching. Using quantitative content analysis of structured telephone interviews, the researchers found that 51 of 70 women (72.9%) experienced a positive change toward their breast cancer over the study period, which was indicative of adaptation to the breast cancer. The researchers report qualitative indicators of adaptation for each of Roy's four adaptive modes.

Modrcin-Talbott, Pullen, Zandstra, Ehrenberger, and Muenchen[56-57] have studied self-esteem from the perspective of the RAM in 140 well adolescents and 77 adolescents in an outpatient mental health setting. The adolescents were grouped as early (12 to 14 years), middle (15 to 16 years), or late adolescence (17 to 19 years). Well adolescents were conveniently recruited from a large, Southeastern church. Self-esteem in well adolescents did not differ by age group, gender, or whether or not they smoked tobacco. Well adolescents who exercised regularly did score higher on self-esteem. Significant negative relationships were found between self-esteem and depression, state anger, trait anger, anger-in, anger-out, anger control, and anger expression. In the second study, the adolescents were sampled from participants of regularly scheduled group sessions as part of an outpatient psychiatric treatment program. Self-esteem significantly differed by age group, with older adolescents scoring lowest on self-esteem. Self-esteem did not differ by gender or whether or not they smoked tobacco. A significant negative relationship was observed between self-esteem and depression. Unlike their study in well adolescents, no statistically significant relationship was found between self-esteem and the dimensions of anger. Self-esteem was not significantly related to parental alcohol usage in either group.

Bournaki[5] studied the correlates of pain-related responses to venipunctures in 94 school-aged children. Using canonical correlation, she examined the relationship of a set of correlates that included age, gender, past painful experiences, temperament, general and medical fears, and child-rearing practices on the school-aged children's subjective, behavioral, and heart-rate responses to a venipuncture. Age and threshold (a dimension of temperament) correlated with pain quality, behavioral responses, and heart rate, accounting for 12% of the variance. Age, distractibility (temperament), and threshold (temperament) explained 5.7% of the variance. The researcher concluded that the findings support the multidimensionality of pain as conceptualized by the RAM.

Gallagher[35] conducted a pilot study to discern if a relationship exists between urogenital distress and the psychosocial impact of urinary incontinence in 17 elderly women. The researcher found significant relationships between urogenital distress and physical activity, social relationships, and travel, which are dimensions of the psychosocial impact of urinary incontinence. Although the findings are inconclusive because there was a small sample size, the study was framed well in the RAM and provided important information for future studies.

Fawcett, Sidney, Riley-Lawless, and Hanson[27] conducted an exploratory study of the relationship between alternative therapies, functional status, and symptom severity among 16 people with multiple sclerosis. They found a negative correlation between the number of alternative therapies used and functional status (r = -.42) and a positive correlation between the number of symptoms experienced and the number of alternative therapies used by the participants. All participants reported a decrease in symptom severity as a direct result of having used alternative therapies (t = 6.45, p < .0005).

Development of programs of research. A program of research has been developed around various aspects of the childbirth experience.* Fawcett and Tulman[28,101] used the model for the design of studies measuring functional status after childbirth. They used the model for retrospective and longitudinal studies of variables associated with functional status during the postpartum period. The model was also used for ongoing studies of functional status during pregnancy and after the diagnosis of breast cancer. The model facilitated the selection of study variables and clarified thinking about the classification of

*References 20, 25, 26, 31, 102, 104-106.

study variables. The model was a useful guide for the design and conduct of studies of functional status.

Fawcett[25] used the RAM as a guide to design four studies. The first was a retrospective survey of cesarean birth parents, which revealed the need for detailed information about the events surrounding the cesarean birth. The second was a field test of a nursing intervention that consisted of a pamphlet with information about cesarean births with follow-up discussion of the pamphlet content. The third was a field test of a different version of the pamphlet intervention and focused discussion about cesarean birth. The fourth study is an ongoing experiment that tests the effects of nursing intervention on responses to unplanned cesarean birth. The purpose of all the studies was to determine whether responses to unplanned cesarean birth are adaptive or ineffective. The survey and field tests provided support for the RAM "in as much as the modes of adaptation were sufficiently comprehensive to permit classification of all data."[25:1423]

Fawcett, Tulman, and Spedden[30] studied the perceptions of women who experienced a vaginal birth after cesarean birth (VBAC). The researchers compared the women's perceptions of the VBAC with their perception of the past cesarean by use of the Perception of the Birth Scale. Although women reported positive perceptions of the VBAC, their perceptions were significantly less positive than women who delivered vaginally.

A program of research related to functional status in patients with cancer is being developed.[103] An instrument has been developed to measure functional status in this population of patients.[107]

Pollock[66] has developed a program of research around the concept of adaptation to chronic illness. Over a seven-year period, 597 adults with various chronic illnesses have participated. Significant differences related to physiological adaptation have been found; however, no differences in psychosocial adaptation have been identified.

The University of Montreal Research Team in Nursing Science[21,46] is studying adaptation to a variety of environmental stimuli. Four groups of individuals were included in their studies: (1) informal family caregivers of a demented relative at home, (2) informal family caregivers of a psychiatrically ill relative at home, (3) nurses as professional caregivers in geriatric institutions, and (4) aged spouses in the community. Using linear structural relations (LISREL), perceived stress (focal stimulus), social support (contextual stimulus), and passive and avoidance coping (coping mechanism) were directly or indirectly linked to psychological distress. This finding supports Roy's proposition that coping promotes adaptation.

Development of adaptation research instruments. The RAM has provided the theoretical basis for the development of a number of research instruments. An instrument has been developed to measure functional status during pregnancy and childbirth and after childbirth.[29,104,109] An instrument has been developed to measure role function changes exhibited by new fathers.[108] Tulman, Fawcett, and McEvoy[107] developed the Inventory of Functional Status-Cancer to measure functional status in women with cancer. Zhan and Shen[114] developed an instrument to measure self-consistency in elderly people with chronic conditions. By use of Roy's self-concept adaptive mode, Phillips[61] developed the Phillips Stigma Questionnaire-AIDS to measure internalized stigma in persons with HIV infection. Modrcin-McCarthy, McCue, and Walker[55] used the RAM to develop a clinical tool that may be used to identify actual and potential stressors of fragile premature infants and to implement care for them. This tool measured the signs of stress, touch interventions, reduction of pain, environmental considerations, state, and stability (STRESS). Burgess and Fawcett[9] have developed a comprehensive sexual assault assessment tool (CSAAT) that reflects the major concepts of the RAM. The purpose of the CSAAT is to collect data about the victims and offenders in cases of rape and sexual assault. Newman[59] used the RAM to develop an instrument to measure the functional status of a caregiver of a child in a body cast (IFSCCBC).

Need for further testing. Silva[94] has pointed out that using a conceptual framework for a research study is not theory testing. Many of the early researchers who used Roy's model did not actually test propositions or hypotheses of her model, but have provided face validity for its usefulness as a framework to guide the study. Theory derived from a conceptual framework must be made explicit; therefore the need is for the development and testing of middle-range theories derived from the RAM. Some research of this nature has been conducted on the model, but more is needed for further validation and development of new areas. The model does generate many testable hypotheses related to both practice and nursing theory.

FURTHER DEVELOPMENT

The RAM is an approach to nursing that has made and continues to make a significant contribution to the body of nursing knowledge, but a few areas remain for development of the model. A more thoroughly defined typology of nursing diagnoses and an organization of categories of interventions would facilitate its use in nursing practice. Overlapping in the psychosocial categories of self-concept, role function, and interdependence continues to be noted by Roy researchers. Roy has recently redefined health, deemphasizing the concept of a health-illness continuum, and conceptualizing health as integration and wholeness of the person. This approach incorporates the adaptive mechanisms of the comatose patient in response to tactile and verbal stimuli more clearly. However, because health was not conceptualized in this manner in the earlier work, this opens up a new area for research.

There appear to be problems involved in using the model in an intensive care unit, where situations change rapidly. Roy has used the model herself in these types of settings and she notes that it is helpful to use a system for setting priorities with the model. When a priority-setting system is used in conjunction with the model, it might be better suited for use in a critical-care setting.[77] For instance, the priority of nursing care for a patient having a cardiac arrest is the physiological adaptive mode. Whether the patient lives or dies, the other adaptive modes begin to emerge as a priority and nursing care can then be focused on the other modes. A chapter regarding life closure was added to the 1984 edition of *Introduction to Nursing: An Adaptation Model.*[81] Support and encouragement of adaptation to the dying process is an integral component of nursing. According to Roy,[86:381] life closure "is the process through which a person resolves the issue of the meaning of one's life and accepts the reality of eventual death."

Of great significance is the work of Roy and Roberts[90] as they used elements of the model to construct a series of propositions for each subsystem and mode. They acknowledge that the propositions are simplistic, implying linear bivariate relationships, and they suggest further work is necessary. However, this work gives helpful starting points for theory-testing research to validate the subsystems of the model. Roy sees a possibility of combining these propositions into interrelated systems and building actual theory. Note that Roy classifies her model as a conceptualization of nursing, from which theory may be derived, and calls for more middle-range theory development in nursing.[80]

Limadri[47] reviewed that work and concluded that Roy and Roberts[90] obscured the regulator mechanism and the physiological mode by superimposing one on the other in forming propositions. She further suggested a rather sweeping modification; that is, grouping the physiological mode into a category of the biological self and grouping the other three modes into the psychosocial self. Similarly, Fitzpatrick, Whall, Johnston, and Floyd[32] reformulated the model to include the alternative nursing intervention strategy of increasing the adaptation range and manipulating stimuli. These examples illustrate the use of Roy's model as it contributes to the science and practice of nursing.

Artinian[4] had attempted to strengthen the Roy model through conceptual problem solving. She believed that strengthening the model would aid in knowledge development. She identified four areas of conceptual problems in the model: (1) health and adaptation, (2) adaptation versus coping, (3) the person as an adaptive system, and (4) goals of adaptation. Artinian suggested that the state of health was synonymous with the end state of adaptation and the process of health was synonymous with the process of adaptation. She thought that this overlap might lead to confusion within the Roy framework. Therefore she proposed that adaptation refer to the process by which health is obtained and that health refer to a state of integration and wholeness. Roy's recent updates that are included in this chapter are in line with Artinian's recommendations (see Figure 17-1).

In the Roy model, coping and adaptation *are* viewed as synonymous. Artinian[4] suggested that the two terms be used synonymously and that the definition of adaptation include the meaning portrayed by Dubos. In this way, the model would be brought up to date and have consistency between the definition of adaptation and the assumptions. Artinian proposed that the positive feedback process was congruent with Roy's assumptions, but that it has not been described in the adaptation model. She suggested that positive and negative feedback processes be incorporated into the model. Finally, she thought that the goals of adaptation could be expanded to include attaining self-actualization, carrying out role functions, and achieving affectional adequacy. These goals would incorporate Roy's holistic and humanistic view of the person.

CRITIQUE
Clarity

According to Chinn and Jacobs,[13:140] "clarity requires the semantic and structural organization of goals, assumptions, concepts, definitions, relationships, and structure into a logically coherent whole."

In an early critique of the RAM, Duldt and Giffin[22] stated that Roy's arrangement of concepts is logical, but that the development of definitions is inadequate related to her original format. Terms and concepts borrowed from other disciplines are not redefined for nursing. Roy's theory examples tend to use a biopsychosocial set as the principle for organizing rather than the adaptive modes and the internal processors. One limitation Duldt and Giffin cited is that Roy claimed to follow a holistic view, but omitted spiritual, humanistic, and existential aspects of being a person. Instead, "man is defined as a survival-oriented, behaviorist (condition-response), amoral, living system."[22:246]

In recent writings, Roy[86:35] has acknowledged the holistic nature of persons who exist in a universe that is "progressing in structure, organization, and complexity. Rather than a system acting to maintain itself, the emphasis shifts to the purposefulness of human existence in a universe that is creative." Roy[86:35] contends that persons have mutual, integral, and simultaneous relationships with the universe and God and that as humans they "use their creative abilities of awareness, enlightenment, and faith in the processes of deriving, sustaining, and transforming the universe." Using these creative abilities, persons (sick or well) are active participants in their care and are able to achieve a higher level of adaptation (health).

Mastal and Hammond[50] discussed difficulties with Roy's model in classifying certain behaviors because concept definitions overlapped. The problem dealt with theory conceptualization and the need for mutually exclusive categories to classify human behavior. Conceptualizing a person's position on the health-illness continuum is no longer a problem because Roy recently redefined health as personal integration. Other researchers have referred to difficulty in classifying behavior exclusively in one adaptive mode.[47] However, this observation supports Roy's proposition that behavior in one adaptive mode affects and is affected by the other modes.

Simplicity

The Roy model includes the concepts of nursing, person, health-illness, environment, adaptation, and nursing activities. It also includes two subconcepts (regulator and cognator) and four effector modes (physiological, self-concept, role function, and interdependence). This model has several major concepts and subconcepts; therefore it has numerous relational statements and is complex.

Generality

Roy[81] defines her model as drawn from multiple middle-range theories and advocates multiple middle-range theories for use in nursing. Middle-range theories are testable and have sufficient generality to be scientifically interesting.[111] The RAM's broad scope is an advantage because it may be used for other theory building and testing in studying smaller ranges of phenomena.[69] Roy's model[87] is generalizable to all settings in nursing practice, but is limited in scope because it primarily addresses the concept of person-environment adaptation and focuses primarily on the patient. Information on the nurse is implied.

Empirical Precision

Increasing complexity within theories often helps increase empirical precision. When subcomponents are designated within the theory, the empirical precision increases, assuming the broad concepts are based in reality.[13]

Roy's broad concepts stem from theory in physiological psychology, psychology, sociology, and nursing; therefore empirical data indicate that this general theory base has substance. Roy's model offers direction for researchers who want to incorporate physiological phenomena in their studies.

Roy[71,79] studied and analyzed 500 samples of patient behaviors collected by nursing students. From this analysis, Roy proposed her four adaptive modes in man.

Roy[88,90] identifies many propositions in relation to the regulator and cognator mechanisms and the self-concept, role function, and interdependence modes. These propositions have varying degrees of support from general theory and empirical data. Most of the propositions are relational statements and can be tested.[100] Over the years, many testable hypotheses have been derived from the model.[41]

The greatest needs to increase empirical precision of the RAM are for researchers to continue to build middle-range theory based on the RAM and to develop empirical referents specifically designed to measure concepts proposed in the derived theory. Roy has explicated a great number of propositions, theorems, and axioms that serve well in the development of middle-range theory. The holistic nature of the model serves well for nurse researchers who are interested in the complex reaction between physiological and psychosocial adaptive processes.

Derivable Consequences

Derivable consequences refer to how practically useful, important, and generally sufficient the theory is in relation to achieving valued nursing outcomes. The theory needs to guide research and practice, generate ideas, and differentiate the focus of nursing from other service professions.[13]

The RAM has a clearly defined nursing process and can be useful in guiding clinical practice. The model provides direction in providing nursing care that addresses the holistic needs of the patient. The model is also capable of generating new information through the testing of the hypotheses that have been derived from it.[87,96]

CONCLUSION

Meleis[52] asserts that there are three types of nursing theorists: (1) those who focus on needs, (2) those who focus on interaction, and (3) those who focus on outcome. The RAM is classified as an outcome theory, defined by Meleis as "a well-articulated conception of man as a nursing client and of nursing as an external regulatory mechanism."[52:180] Roy, in applying the concepts of system and adaptation to person as the patient of nursing, has presented her articulation of the person for nurses to use as a tool in practice, education, and research. Her conceptions of person and of the nursing process contribute to the science and the art of nursing. The RAM deserves further study and development by nursing educators, researchers, and practitioners.

CRITICAL THINKING *Activities*

A 23-year-old male patient is admitted with a fracture of C6 and C7 that resulted in quadriplegia. He was injured during a football game at the university where he is currently a senior. His career as quarterback had been very promising. At the time of the injury, contract negotiations were in progress with a leading professional football team.

1. Use Roy's criteria to identify focal and contextual stimuli for each of the four adaptive modes.

2. Consider what adaptations would be necessary in each of the four adaptive modes: (1) physiological, (2) self-concept, (3) interdependence, and (4) role function.

3. Create an intervention for each of the adaptive modes that will promote adaptation.

REFERENCES

1. Andrews, H. (1991). Overview of the role function mode. In C. Roy & H. Andrews (Eds.), *The Roy adaptation model: The definitive statement* (pp. 347-361). Norwalk, CT: Appleton & Lange.
2. Andrews, H. & Roy, C. (1986). *Essentials of the Roy adaptation model.* Norwalk, CT: Appleton-Century-Crofts.
3. Andrews, H. & Roy, C. (1991). Essentials of the Roy adaptation model. In C. Roy & H. Andrews (Eds.), *The Roy adaptation model: The definitive statement* (pp. 3-25). Norwalk, CT: Appleton & Lange.
4. Artinian, N.T. (1990). Strengthening the Roy adaptation model through conceptual clarification: Commentary and response. *Nursing Science Quarterly,* 3(2), 60-64.
5. Bournaki, M. (1997). Correlates of pain-related responses to venipunctures in school-age children. *Nursing Research,* 40(3), 147-154.
6. Brower, H.T.F. & Baker, B.J. (1976, Nov.). The Roy adaptation model: Using the adaptation model in a practitioner curriculum. *Nursing Outlook,* 24, 686-689.
7. Brydolf, M. & Segesten, K. (1994). Physical health in young subjects after colectomy: An application of the Roy model. *Journal of Advanced Nursing,* 20(3), 500-508.
8. Brydolf, M. & Segesten, K. (1996). Living with ulcerative colitis: Experiences of adolescents and young adults. *Journal of Advanced Nursing,* 23(1), 39-47.
9. Burgess, A.W. & Fawcett, J. (1996). The comprehensive sexual assault assessment tool. *Nurse Practitioner,* 21(4), 71-76.
10. Campbell, J.M. (1992). Treating depression in well older adults: Use of diaries in cognitive therapy. *Issues in Mental Health Nursing,* 13(1), 19-27.
11. Campbell, T. & Lunn, D. (1999). Colorectal cancer. Part 3: Patient care. *Professional Nurse,* 15(2), 117-121.
12. Carveth, J.A. (1987). Conceptual models in nurse-midwifery. *Journal of Nurse-Midwifery,* 32(1), 20-25.
13. Chinn, P. & Jacobs, M.K. (1987). *Theory and nursing: A systematic approach.* St. Louis: Mosby.
14. Davies, P. (1988). *The cosmic blueprint.* New York: Simon and Schuster.
15. De Chardin, P.T. (1966). *Man's place in nature.* New York: Harper & Row.
16. De Chardin, P.T. (1969). *Human energy.* New York: Harper & Row.
17. De Villers, M.J. (1998). The clinical nurse specialist as expert practitioner in the obstetrical/gynecological setting. *Clinical Nurse Specialist,* 12(5), 193-199.
18. Dickoff, J., James, P., & Weidenbach, E. (1968, May). Theory in practice discipline. Part I. Practice oriented theory. *Nursing Research,* 17, 413-415.
19. Dixon, E.L. (1999). Community health nursing practice and the Roy adaptation model. *Public Health Nursing,* 16(4), 290-300.
20. Drake, M.L., Verhulst, D., & Fawcett, J. (1988). Physical and psychological symptoms experienced by Canadian women and their husbands during pregnancy and the postpartum. *Journal of Advanced Nursing,* 13(4), 436-440.
21. Ducharme, F., Ricard, N., Duquette, A., Levesque, L., & Lachance, L. (1998). Testing of a longitudinal model from the Roy adaptation model. *Nursing Science Quarterly,* 11(4), 149-159.
22. Duldt, B. & Giffin, K. (1985). *Theoretical perspectives for nursing* (pp. 242-247). Boston: Little, Brown.
23. Eaganhouse, D.J. (1994). A nursing model for a community hospital preterm birth prevention program. *Journal of Obstetrical and Gynecological Nursing,* 23(9), 756-766.
24. Farkas, L. (1981, March). Adaptation problems with nursing home application for elderly persons: An application of the Roy adaptation nursing model. *Journal of Advanced Nursing,* 6, 363-368.
25. Fawcett, J. (1990). Preparation for caesarian childbirth: Derivation of a nursing intervention from the Roy adaptation model. *Journal of Advanced Nursing,* 15(2), 1418-1425.
26. Fawcett, J., Bliss-Holtz, V.J., Haas, M.B., Leventhal, M., & Rubin, M. (1986). Spouses' body image changes during and after pregnancy: A replication and extension. *Nursing Research,* 35(4), 220-223.
27. Fawcett, J., Sidney, J.S., Riley-Lawless, K., Hanson, M.J.S. (1996). An exploratory study of the relationship between alternative therapies, functional status, and symptom severity among people with multiple sclerosis. *Journal of Holistic Nursing,* 14(2), 115-129.
28. Fawcett, J. & Tulman, L. (1990). Building a program of research from the Roy adaptation model of nursing. *Journal of Advanced Nursing,* 15(6), 720-725.

29. Fawcett, J., Tulman, L., & Myers, S.T. (1988). Development of the inventory of functional status after childbirth. *Journal of Nurse Midwifery,* 33(6), 252-260.

30. Fawcett, J., Tulman, L., & Spedden, J.P. (1994). Responses to vaginal birth after cesarean section. *JOGNN: Journal of Obstetric, Gynecologic, and Neonatal Nursing,* 23(3), 253-259.

31. Fawcett, J. & York, R. (1986). Spouses' physical and psychological symptoms during pregnancy and the postpartum. *Nursing Research,* 35(3), 144-148.

32. Fitzpatrick, J., Whall, A., Johnston, R., & Floyd, J. (1982). *Nursing models and their psychiatric mental health application.* Bowie, MD: Brady.

33. Frank, D.I. & Lang, A.R. (1990). Disturbances in sexual role performance of chronic alcoholics: An analysis using Roy's adaptation model. *Issues in Mental Health Nursing,* 11(3), 243-254.

34. Galligan, A.C. (1979, Jan.). Using Roy's concept of adaptation to care for young children. *American Journal of Maternal Child Nursing,* 4, 24-28.

35. Gallagher, M.S. (1998). Urogenital distress and the psychosocial impact of urinary incontinence on elderly women. *Rehabilitation Nursing,* 23(4), 192-197.

36. Giger, J.N., Davidhizar, R., & Miller, S.W. (1990). Nightingale & Roy: A comparison of nursing models. *Today's OR Nurse,* 12(4), 25-28.

37. Gless, P.A. (1995). Applying the Roy adaptation model to the care of clients with quadriplegia. *Rehabilitation Nursing,* 20(1), 11-16, 66.

38. Hamner, J.B. (1989). Applying the Roy adaptation model to the CCU. *Critical Care Nurse,* 9(3), 51-52.

39. Hartley, B. & Campion-Fuller, C. (1994). Juvenile dermatomyositis: A Roy nursing perspective. *Journal of Pediatric Nursing: Nursing Care of Children and Families,* 9(3), 175-182.

40. Haunt, C., Peddicord, K., & O'Brien, E. (1994). Supporting bonding in the NICU: A care plan for nurses. *Neonatal Network: Journal of Neonatal Nursing,* 13(8), 19-25.

41. Hill, B.J. & Roberts, C.S. (1981). Formal theory construction: An example of the process. In C. Roberts & S.L. Roberts (Eds.), *Theory construction in nursing: An adaptation model.* Englewood Cliffs, NJ: Prentice-Hall.

42. Ingram, L. (1995). Roy's adaptation model and accident and emergency nursing. *Accidental and Emergency Nursing,* 3(3), 150-153.

43. Keen, M., Breckenridge, D., Frauman, A.C., Hartigan, M.F., Smith, L., Butera, E., Hooper, S.T., Mapes, D., Neff, M., & Fawcett, J. (1998). Nursing assessment and intervention for adult hemodialysis patients: Application of Roy's Adaptation Model. *American Nephrology Nurses' Association Journal,* 25(3), 311-319.

44. Kurek-Ovshinsky, C. (1991). Group psychotherapy in an acute inpatient setting: Techniques that nourish self-esteem. *Issues in Mental Health Nursing,* 12(1), 81-88.

45. Lankester, K. & Sheldon, L.M. (1999). Health visiting with Roy's model: A case study. *Journal of Child Health Care,* 3(10), 28-34.

46. Levesque, L., Ricard, N., Ducharme, F., Duquette, A., & Bonin, J.P. (1998). Empirical verification of a theoretical model derived from the Roy adaptation model: Findings form five studies. *Nursing Science Quarterly,* 11(1), 31-339.

47. Limadri, B.J. (1986). Research and practice with abused women, use of the Roy model as an explanatory framework. *Advances in Nursing Science,* 8(4), 52-61.

48. Logan, M. (1986). Palliative care nursing: Applicability of the Roy model. *Journal of Palliative Care,* 1(2), 18-24.

49. Lutjens, L.R.J. (1992). Derivation and testing of tenets of a theory of social organizations as adaptive systems. *Nursing Science Quarterly,* 5(2), 62-71.

50. Mastal, M. & Hammond, H. (1980, July). Analysis and expansion of the Roy model: A contribution to holistic nursing. *Advances in Nursing Science,* 3, 7-78.

51. Mastal, M., Hammond, H., & Roberts, M. (1982, June). Theory into hospital practice: A pilot implementation. *Journal of Nursing Administration,* 12, 9-15.

52. Meleis, A.I. (1986). *Theoretical nursing development and process* (pp. 206-218). Philadelphia: J.B. Lippincott.

53. Mitchell, G.J. & Pilkington, B. (1990). Theoretical approaches in nursing practice: A comparison of Roy and Parse. *Nursing Science Quarterly,* 3(2), 81-87.

54. Mock, V., Burke, M.B., Sheehan, P., Creaton, E.M., Winningham, M.L., McKenney-Tedder, S., Schwager, L.P., & Liebman, M. (1994). A nursing rehabilitation program for women with breast cancer receiving adjuvant chemotherapy. *Oncology Nursing Forum,* 21(5), 899-908.

55. Modrcin-McCarthy, M.A., McCue, S., & Walker, J. (1997). Preterm infants and STRESS: A tool for the neonatal nurse. *Journal of Perinatal and Neonatal Nursing,* 10(4), 62-71.

56. Modrcin-Talbott, M.A., Pullen, L., Ehrenberger, H., Zandstra, K., & Muenchen, B. (1998). Self-esteem in adolescents treated in an outpatient mental health setting. *Issues in Comprehensive Pediatric Nursing,* 21(3), 159-171.

57. Modrcin-Talbott, M.A., Pullen, L., Zandstra, K., Ehrenberger, H., & Muenchen, B. (1998). A study of self-esteem among well adolescents: Seeking a new direction. *Issues in Comprehensive Pediatric Nursing,* 21(4), 229-241.

58. Morales-Mann, E.T. & Logan, M. (1990). Implementing the Roy model: Challenges for nurse educators. *Journal of Advanced Nursing*, 15(2), 142-147.

59. Newman, D.M.L. (1997). The inventory of functional status-caregiver of a child in a body cast. *Journal of Pediatric Nursing*, 12(3), 142-147.

60. Nuamah, I.F., Cooley, M.E., Fawcett, J., McCorkle, R. (1999). Testing a theory for health-related quality of life in cancer patients: A structural equation approach. *Research in Nursing and Health*, 22(3), 231-242.

61. Phillips, K.D. (1994). Biobehavioral adaptation in persons living with AIDS. Unpublished doctoral dissertation, The University of Tennessee, Knoxville.

62. Phillips, K.D. (1997). Roy's adaptation model in nursing practice. In M. Alligood & A. Marriner Tomey (Eds.), *Nursing theory utilization and application* (pp. 175-200). St. Louis: Mosby.

63. Piazza, D. & Foote, A. (1990). Roy's adaptation model: A guide for rehabilitation nursing practice. *Rehabilitation Nursing*, 15(5), 254-259.

64. Piazza, D., Foote, A., Holcombe, J., Harris, M.G., & Wright, P. (1992). The use of Roy's adaptation model applied to a patient with breast cancer. *European Journal of Cancer Care*, 1(4), 17-22.

65. Pittman, K.P. (1992). *A Q-analysis of the enabling characteristics of chronically ill school age children for the promotion of personal wellness.* Unpublished doctoral dissertation, University of Alabama, Birmingham.

66. Pollock, S.E. (1993). Adaptation to chronic illness: A program of research for testing nursing theory. *Nursing Science Quarterly*, 6(2), 86-92.

67. Rambo, B. (1983). *Adaptation nursing: Assessment and intervention.* Philadelphia: W.B. Saunders.

68. Randell, B., Tedrow, M.P., & Van Landingham, J. (1982). *Adaptation nursing: The Roy conceptual model applied.* St. Louis: Mosby.

69. Reynolds, P.D. (1971). *A primer in theory construction.* Indianapolis: Bobbs-Merrill.

70. Riehl, J.P. & Roy, C. (Eds.). (1980). *Conceptual models for nursing practice* (2nd ed.). New York: Appleton-Century-Crofts.

71. Roy, C. (1970, March). Adaptation: A conceptual framework in nursing. *Nursing Outlook,* 18, 42-45.

72. Roy, C. (1971, April). Adaptation: A basis for nursing practice. *Nursing Outlook,* 19, 254-257.

73. Roy, C. (1973, March). Adaptation: Implications for curriculum change. *Nursing Outlook,* 21, 163-168.

74. Roy, C. (1975, Feb.). A diagnostic classification system for nursing. *Nursing Outlook,* 23, 90-94.

75. Roy, C. (1976, Summer). The impact of nursing diagnosis. *Nursing Digest,* 4, 67-69.

76. Roy, C. (1976). *Introduction to nursing: An adaptation model.* Englewood Cliffs, NJ: Prentice-Hall.

77. Roy, C. (1976, Nov.). The Roy adaptation model: Comment. *Nursing Outlook,* 24, 690-691.

78. Roy, C. (1979, Feb.). Relating nursing theory to nursing education: A new era. *Nurse Educator,* 4, 16-21.

79. Roy, C. (1980). The Roy adaptation model. In J.P. Riehl & C. Roy (Eds.), *Conceptual models for nursing practice* (2nd ed., pp. 179-188). New York: Appleton-Century-Crofts.

80. Roy, C. (1983). Theory development in nursing: A proposal for direction. In N. Chaska (Ed.), *The nursing profession: A time to speak* (pp. 453-467). New York: McGraw-Hill.

81. Roy, C. (1984). *Introduction to nursing: An adaptation model* (2nd ed.). Englewood Cliffs, NJ: Prentice-Hall.

82. Roy, C. (1987). Responses to "Needs of spouses of surgical patients, a conceptualization within the Roy adaptation model." *Scholarly Journal for Nursing Practice,* 1(1), 45-50.

83. Roy, C. (1991). Senses. In C. Roy & H. Andrews (Eds.), *The Roy adaptation model: The definitive statement* (pp. 165-189). Norwalk, CT: Appleton & Lange.

84. Roy, C. (1997). Future of the Roy adaptation model: Challenge to redefine adaptation. *Nursing Science Quarterly,* 10(1), 42-48.

85. Roy, C. & Andrews, H. (1991). *The Roy adaptation model: The definitive statement.* Norwalk, CT: Appleton & Lange.

86. Roy, C. & Andrews, H. (1999). *The Roy adaptation model* (2nd ed.). Stamford, CT: Appleton & Lange. Quotes reprinted by permission of Pearson Education, Inc., Upper Saddle River, NJ.

87. Roy, C. & Corliss, C.P. (1993). The Roy adaptation model: Theoretical update and knowledge for practice. In M.E. Parker (Ed.), *Patterns of nursing theories in practice* (pp. 215-229). New York: National League for Nursing.

88. Roy, C. & McLeod, D. (1981). Theory of the person as an adaptive system. In C. Roy & S.L. Roberts (Eds.), *Theory construction in nursing: An adaptation model.* Englewood Cliffs, NJ: Prentice-Hall.

89. Roy, C. & Obloy, M. (1978, Oct.). The practitioner movement. *American Journal of Nursing,* 78, 1698-1702.

90. Roy, C. & Roberts, S. (1981). *Theory construction in nursing: An adaptation model.* Englewood Cliffs, NJ: Prentice-Hall.

91. Samarel, N., Fawcett, J., Krippendorf, K., Piacentino, J.C., Eliasof, B., Hughes, P., Kowitski, C., & Ziegler, E. (1998). Women's perceptions of group support and adaptation to breast cancer. *Journal of Advanced Nursing,* 28(6), 1259-1268.

92. Samarel, N., Fawcett, J., Tulman, L., Rothman, H., Spector, I., Spillane, P.A., Dickson, M.A., & Toole, J.H. (1998). A resource kit for women with breast cancer: Development and evaluation. *Oncology Nursing Forum,* 26(3), 611-618.

93. Schmitz, M. (1980). The Roy adaptation model: Application in a community setting. In J.P. Riehl & C. Roy (Eds.), *Conceptual models for nursing practice* (2nd ed.). New York: Appleton-Century-Crofts.

94. Silva, M.C. (1986). Research testing theory: State of the art. *Advanced Nursing Science,* 9(1), 1-11.

95. Silva, M.C. (1987). Needs of spouses of surgical patients, a conceptualization within the Roy adaptation model. *Scholarly Inquiry for Nursing Practice,* 1(1), 29-44.

96. Smith, C.E., Garvis, M.S., & Martinson, M.I. (1983, Aug.). Content analysis of interviews using a nursing model: A look at parents adapting to the impact of childhood cancer. *Cancer Nursing,* 6, 269-275.

97. Sr. Callista Roy to assume nurse theorist post at Boston College. (1987). *Nursing and Health Care,* 8(9), 536.

98. Swimme, B. & Berry, T. (1992). *The universe story.* San Francisco: Harper.

99. Thornbury, J.M. & King, L.D. (1992). The Roy adaptation model and care of persons with Alzheimer's disease. *Nursing Science Quarterly,* 5(3), 129-133.

100. Tiedeman, M.E. (1983). The Roy adaptation model. In J. Fitzpatrick & A. Whall (Eds.), *Conceptual models of nursing: Analysis and application* (pp. 157-180). Bowie, MD: Brady.

101. Tulman, L. (1990). Changes in functional status after childbirth. *Nursing Research,* 39(2), 70-75.

102. Tulman, L. & Fawcett, J. (1988). Return of functional ability after childbearing. *Nursing Research,* 37(2), 77-78.

103. Tulman, L. & Fawcett, J. (1990). A framework for studying functional status after diagnosis of breast cancer. *Cancer Nursing,* 13(2), 95-99.

104. Tulman, L. & Fawcett, J. (1990). Functional status during pregnancy and the postpartum: A framework for research. *Image: The Journal of Nursing Scholarship,* 22(3), 191-194.

105. Tulman, L. & Fawcett, J. (1990). Maternal employment following childbirth. *Research in Nursing and Health,* 13(3), 181-188.

106. Tulman, L., Fawcett, J., Groblewski, L., & Silverman, L. (1990). Changes in functional status after childbirth. *Nursing Research,* 39(2), 70-75.

107. Tulman, L., Fawcett, J., & McEvoy, M.D. (1991). Development of the inventory of functional status-cancer. *Cancer Nursing,* 14(5), 254-260.

108. Tulman, L., Fawcett, J., & Weiss, M. (1993). The Inventory of functional status-fathers: Development and psychometric testing. *Journal of Nurse Midwifery,* 38(5), 276-282.

109. Tulman, L., Higgins, K., Fawcett, J., Nunno, C., Vansickel, C., Haas, M.B., & Speca, M.M. (1991). The Inventory of functional status-antepartum period: Development and testing. *Journal of Nurse Midwifery,* 36(2), 117-123.

110. Wagner, P. (1976, Nov.). The Roy adaptation model: Testing the adaptation model in practice. *Nursing Outlook,* 24, 682-685.

111. Walker, L.O. & Avant, K.C. (1983). *Strategies for theory construction in nursing.* Norwalk, CT: Appleton-Century-Crofts.

112. Wright, P.S., Holcombe, J., Foote, A., & Piazza, D. (1993). The Roy adaptation model used a guide for the nursing care of an 8-year-old child with leukemia. *Journal of Pediatric Oncology Nursing,* 10(2), 68-74.

113. Wright, P.S., Piazza, D., Holcombe, J., & Foote, A. (1994). A comparison of three theories of nursing used as a guide for the nursing care of an 8-year-old child with leukemia. *Journal of Pediatric Oncology Nursing,* 11(1), 14-19.

114. Zhan, L. & Shen, C. (1994). The development of an instrument to measure self-consistency. *Journal of Advanced Nursing,* 20(3), 509-516.

BIBLIOGRAPHY
Primary Sources
Books

Andrews, H. & Roy, C. (1986). *Essentials of the Roy adaptation model.* Norwalk, CT: Appleton-Century-Crofts.

Riehl, J.P. & Roy, C. (Eds.). (1974). *Conceptual models for nursing practice.* Englewood Cliffs, NJ: Prentice-Hall.

Riehl, J.P. & Roy, C. (Eds.). (1980). *Conceptual models for nursing practice* (2nd ed.). New York: Appleton-Century-Crofts.

Roy, C. (1976). *Introduction to nursing: An adaptation model.* Englewood Cliffs, NJ: Prentice-Hall.

Roy, C. (1982). *Introduction to nursing: An adaptation model.* (Japanese translation by Yuriko Kanematsu.) Tokyo, Japan: UNI Agency.

Roy, C. (1984). *Introduction to nursing: An adaptation model* (2nd ed.). Englewood Cliffs, NJ: Prentice-Hall.

Roy, C. & Andrews, H.A. (1991). *The Roy adaptation model: The definitive statement.* Norwalk, CT: Appleton & Lange.

Roy, C. & Andrews, H.A. (1999). *The Roy adaptation model* (2nd ed.). Stamford, CT: Appleton & Lange.

Roy, C. & Roberts, S. (1981). *Theory construction in nursing: An adaptation model.* Englewood Cliffs, NJ: Prentice-Hall.

Book Chapters

Barone, S.H. & Roy, C. (1996). The Roy adaptation model in research: Rehabilitation nursing. In P.H. Walker & B. Neuman (Eds.), *Blueprint for use of nursing models: Education, research, practice, and administration* (pp. 64-87). New York: National League for Nursing.

Gortner, S., Ellis, R., Roy, C., Williams, C., Benner, P., & Mercer, R. (1984). Explanation in nursing science. Symposium abstract. *Community Nursing Research, 17,* 101-103.

Pollock, S.E., Frederickson, K., Carson, M.A., Massey, V.H., & Roy, C. (1994). Contributions to nursing science: Synthesis of findings from adaptation model research. *Scholarly Inquiry for Nursing Practice,* 8(4), 361-374.

Roy, C. (1974). The Roy adaptation model. In J.P. Riehl & C. Roy (Eds.), *Conceptual models for nursing practice.* New York: Appleton-Century-Crofts.

Roy, C. (1975, June). Adaptation framework. In *Curriculum innovation through framework application.* Loma Linda, CA: Loma Linda University.

Roy, C. (1978). The stress of hospital events: Measuring changes in level of stress. In M.V. Batey (Ed.), *Symposium on stress* (Vol. 11). Boulder, CO: Western Interstate Commission on Higher Education.

Roy, C. (1979). Health-illness (powerlessness) questionnaire and hospitalized patient decision-making. In M.J. Ward & C.A. Linderman (Eds.), *Instruments for measuring practice and other health care variables* (Vol. 1). Hyattsville, MD: U.S. Department of Health, Education, and Welfare.

Roy, C. (1980). The Roy adaptation model. In J.P. Riehl & C. Roy (Eds.), *Conceptual models for nursing practice* (2nd ed.). New York: Appleton-Century-Crofts.

Roy, C. (1981). A systems model of nursing care and its effect on the quality of human life. *Proceedings of the International Congress on Applied Systems Research and Cybernetics.* London: Pergamon.

Roy, C. (1983). Foreword. In B.J. Rambo (Ed.), *Adaptation nursing: Assessment and intervention.* Philadelphia: W.B. Saunders.

Roy, C. (1983). The expectant family: Analysis and application of the Roy adaptation model, and the family in primary care—Analysis and application of the Roy adaptation model. In I.W. Clements & F. Roberts (Eds.), *Family health: A theoretical approach to nursing care.* New York: John Wiley & Sons.

Roy, C. (1983). The family in primary care: Analysis and application of the Roy adaptation model. In I.W. Clements & F.B. Roberts (Eds.), *Family health: A theoretical approach to nursing care.* New York: John Wiley & Sons.

Roy, C. (1984). Framework for classification systems development: Progress and issues. *Proceedings of the Fifth National Conference on the Classification of Nursing Diagnosis.* St. Louis: Mosby.

Roy, C. (1984). The Roy adaptation model: Applications in community health nursing. *Proceedings of the Eighth Annual Community Health Nursing Conference.* Chapel Hill, NC: University of North Carolina.

Roy, C. (1984, May). The Roy adaptation model: Applications in community health nursing. *Proceedings of the Annual Community Health Nursing Conference.* Chapel Hill, NC: University of North Carolina.

Roy, C. (1985). The future of the nursing science: Response of the Academy. *Scientific Session of the American Academy of Nursing.* Kansas City, MO: American Academy of Nursing.

Roy, C. (1987). Roy's adaptation model. In R.R. Parse (Ed.), *Nursing science: Major paradigms, theories, and critiques.* Philadelphia: W.B. Saunders.

Roy, C. (1987). The influence of nursing models on clinical decision making II. In K.J. Hannah, M. Reimer, W.C. Mills, & S. Letourneau (Eds.), *Clinical judgment and decision making: The future with nursing diagnosis* (pp. 42-47). New York: John Wiley & Sons.

Roy, C. (1988). An explication of the philosophical assumptions of the Roy adaptation model. *Nursing Science Quarterly,* 1(10), 26-34.

Roy, C. (1988). Human information processing and nursing research. In J. Fitzpatrick & R.L. Tauton (Eds.), *Annual Review of Nursing Research 6.* New York: Springer.

Roy, C. (1988). Sister Callista Roy. In T.M. Schorr & A. Zimmerman (Eds.). *Making choices: Taking chances* (pp. 291-298). St. Louis: Mosby.

Roy, C. (1990). Strengthening the Roy adaptation model through conceptual clarification–response: Conceptual clarification. *Nursing Science Quarterly,* 3(2), 64-66.

Roy, C. (1991). Altered cognition: An information processing approach. In P.H. Mitchell, L.C. Hodges, M. Muwaswes, & C.A. Walleck (Eds.), *AANN's neuroscience nursing: Phenomenon and practice—Human responses to neurological health problems* (pp. 185-211). Norwalk, CT: Appleton & Lange.

Roy, C. (1991). Structure of knowledge: Paradigm, model, and research specifications for differentiated practice. In I.E. Goertzen (Ed.), *Differentiating nursing practice: Into the twenty-first century* (pp. 31-39). Kansas City, MO: American Academy of Nursing.

Roy, C. (1992). Vigor, variables, and vision: Commentary of Florence Nightingale. In F. Nightingale (Ed.), *Notes on nursing: What it is, and what it is not.* Philadelphia: J.B. Lippincott.

Roy, C. & Anway, J. (1988). Roy's adaptation model: Theories for nursing administration. In B. Henry, C. Arndt, M. DiVincenti, & A. Marriner Tomey (Eds.), *Dimensions of nursing administration.* Boston: Blackwell Scientific.

Roy, C. & Corliss, C.P. (1993). The Roy adaptation model: Theoretical update and knowledge for practice. In M.E. Parker (Ed.), *Patterns of nursing theories in practice* (pp. 215-229). New York: National League for Nursing.

Roy, C. & McLeod, D. (1981). Theory of the person as an adaptive system. In C. Roy & S.L. Roberts (Eds.), *Theory construction in nursing: An adaptation model.* Englewood Cliffs, NJ: Prentice-Hall.

Roy, S.C. (1983). A conceptual framework for clinical specialist practice. In A. Harris & J. Spross (Eds.), *The clinical nurse specialist in theory and practice.* New York: Grune & Stratton.

Roy, S.C. (1983). Roy's adaptation model and application to family case studies. In I. Clements & F. Roberts (Eds.), *Theoretical approaches to family health.* New York: Wiley.

Roy, S.C. (1983). Theory development in nursing: A proposal for direction. In N. Chaska (Ed.), *The nursing profession: A time to speak.* New York: McGraw-Hill.

Roy, S.C. (1985). Practice in action: Clinical research. In K.E. Barnard & G.R. Smith (Eds.), *Faculty practice in action: Annual symposium on nursing faculty practice 2* (pp. 192-200). New York: American Academy of Nursing.

Journal Articles

Roy, C. (1967, Feb.). Role cues and mothers of hospitalized children. *Nursing Research, 16,* 178-182.

Roy, C. (1970, March). Adaptation: A conceptual framework in nursing. *Nursing Outlook, 18,* 42-45.

Roy, C. (1971, April). Adaptation: A basis for nursing practice. *Nursing Outlook, 19,* 254-257.

Roy, C. (1973). Adaptation: Implications for curriculum change. *Nursing Outlook, 21,* 163-168.

Roy, C. (1975, Feb.). Adaptation: Implications for curriculum change. *Nursing Outlook, 21,* 163-168.

Roy, C. (1975, Feb.). A diagnostic classification system for nursing. *Nursing Outlook, 23,* 90-94.

Roy, C. (1975, May). The impact of nursing diagnosis. *AORN Journal, 21,* 1023-1030.

Roy, C. (1976). Comment. *Nursing Outlook, 24,* 690-691.

Roy, C. (1976, Summer). The impact of nursing diagnosis. *Nursing Digest,* 467-469.

Roy, C. (1976, Nov.). The Roy adaptation model: Comment. *Nursing Outlook, 24,* 690-691.

Roy, C. (1979, Feb.). Relating nursing theory to nursing education: A new era. *Nurse Educator, 4,* 16-21.

Roy, C. (1979, Dec.). Nursing diagnosis from the perspective of a nursing model. *Nursing Diagnosis Newsletter,* p. 6.

Roy, C. (1980). Exposé de Callista Roy sur theories. Exposé de Callista Roy sur l'utilisation de sa theories au nouveau de la recherche. *Acta Nursological,* 3, Ecole Genevoise D. Infirmieres Le Bon Secours, Geneva.

Roy, C. (1983). To the editor. *Nursing Research, 23,* 320.

Roy, C. (1985). Acoustic neuroma: Notes. *Acoustic Neuroma Association, 13,* 8-9.

Roy, C. (1985). Nursing research makes a difference. *Newsletter of Nurses Educational Fund, Inc.* 4(1), 2-3.

Roy, C. (1987). Response to "Needs of spouses of surgical patients, a conceptualization within the Roy adaptation model." *Scholarly Journal for Nursing Practice,* 1(1), 45-50.

Roy, C. (1988). An explication of the philosophical assumptions of the Roy adaptation model. *Nursing Science Quarterly,* 1(1), 26-34.

Roy, C. (1990). Case reports can provide a standard for care in nursing practice. *Journal of Professional Nursing,* 6(3), 179-180.

Roy, C. (1990). Strengthening the Roy adaptation model through conceptual clarification. *Nursing Science Quarterly,* 3(2), 64-66.

Roy, C. (1997). Future of the Roy model: Challenge to redefine adaptation. *Nursing Science Quarterly,* 10(1), 42-48.

Roy, C. (2000). A theorist envisions the future and speaks to nursing administrators. *Nursing Administration Quarterly,* 24(2), 1-12.

Roy, C. & Obloy, M. (1978, Oct.). The practitioner movement. *American Journal of Nursing,* 78, 1698-1702.

Dissertation

Roy, C. (1977). *Decision-making by the physically ill and adaptation during illness.* Unpublished doctoral dissertation, University of California, Los Angeles.

Booklet

Roy, S.C. (1978). The future of nursing. In Forum of Nursing Service, *Administrators in the West* (Pub. No. 52-1805). San Diego: National League for Nursing.

Audiotapes

Roy, C. (1978, Dec.). *Paper presented at the second annual nurse educator conference* [Audiotape]. Available: Teach 'em Inc., 160 E. Illinois Street, Chicago, IL 60611.

Roy, C. (1984, May). *Nurses' theorist conference at Edmonton, Alberta* [Audiotape]. Available: Kennedy Recordings, R.R. 5, Edmonton, Alberta, Canada TSP 4B7.

Correspondence

Roy, S.C. (1984, March 26), Curriculum vitae.

Roy, S.C. (1988, March 8). Curriculum vitae.

Interviews

Professional profile: "Sister Callista Roy: Influencing the direction of nursing." (1985). *Focus on Critical Care Nursing,* 12(3), 45-46.

Roy, S.C. (1984, March 25). Telephone interview.

Secondary Sources
Book Reviews

[Review of the book *Conceptual models for nursing practice*]. (1975, July). *Nursing Outlook,* 23, 457.

[Review of the book *Conceptual models for nursing practice*]. (1975, July/Aug.). *Nursing Research,* 24, 306-307.

[Review of the book *Introduction to nursing: An adaptation model*]. (1977, Aug.). *American Journal of Nursing,* 77, 1359.

[Review of the book *Introduction to nursing: An adaptation model*]. (1977, Oct.). *Nursing Outlook,* 25, 658.

[Review of the book *Theory construction in nursing*]. (1982, Feb.). *Nursing Outlook,* 30, 141.

Books

Chinn, P.L. & Jacobs, M.K. (1987). *Theory and nursing: A systematic approach.* St. Louis: Mosby.

Fitzpatrick, J.J. & Whall, A.L. (1983). *Conceptual models of nursing: Analysis and application.* Bowie, MD: Robert J. Brady.

Fitzpatrick, J.J., Whall, A., Johnson, R., & Floyd, J. (1982). *Nursing models and their psychiatric mental health applications.* Bowie, MD: Robert J Brady.

Kim, H.S. (1983). *The nature of theoretical thinking in nursing.* Norwalk, CT: Appleton-Century-Crofts.

Lutjens, L.R.J. (1991). *Callista Roy: An adaptation model.* Newbury Park, CA: Sage.

Nicoll, L.H. (1986). *Perspectives on nursing theory.* Boston: Little, Brown.

Potter, D.O. (Ed.). (1984). *Practice nurses' reference library.* Springhouse, PA: Springhouse.

Rambo, B. (1983). *Adaptation nursing: Assessment and intervention.* Philadelphia: W.B. Saunders.

Randell, B., Tedrow, M.P., & Van Landingham, J. (1982). *Adaptation nursing: The Roy conceptual model applied.* St. Louis: Mosby.

Reynolds, P.D. (1971). *A primer in theory construction.* Indianapolis: Bobbs-Merrill.

Torres, G. (1986). *Theoretical foundations of nursing* (pp. 151-165). Norwalk, CT: Appleton-Century-Crofts.

Walker, L.O. & Avant, K.C. (1983). *Strategies for theory construction in nursing.* Norwalk, CT: Appleton-Century-Crofts.

Book Chapters

Blue, C.L., Brubaker, K.M., Fine, J.M., Kirsch, M.J., Papazian, K.R., Rieser, C.M., & Sobiech, M.A. (1989). Sister Callista Roy: Adaptation model. In A. Marriner Tomey (Ed.), *Nursing theorists and their work* (2nd ed., pp. 325-344). St. Louis: Mosby.

Blue, C.L., Brubaker, K.M., Fine, J.M., Kirsch, M.J., Papazian, K.R., Rieser, C.M., & Sobiech, M.A. (1994). Sister Callista Roy: Adaptation model. In A. Marriner Tomey (Ed.), *Nursing theorists and their work* (3rd ed., pp. 246-268). St. Louis: Mosby.

Blue, C.L., Brubaker, K.M., Papazian, K.R., & Riester, C.M. (1986). Sister Callista Roy: Adaptation model. In A. Marriner (Ed.), *Nursing theorists and their work* (pp. 297-312). St. Louis: Mosby.

Fawcett, J. (1981). Assessing and understanding the cesarean father. In C.F. Kehoe (Ed.), *The cesarean experience: Theoretical and clinical perspectives for nurses* (pp. 371-376). New York: Appleton-Century-Crofts.

Fawcett, J. (1984). Roy's adaptation model. In J. Fawcett (Ed.), *Analysis and evaluation of conceptual models of nursing* (pp. 247-285). Philadelphia: F.A. Davis.

Fawcett, J. (1995). Roy's adaptation model. In J. Fawcett (Ed.), *Analysis and evaluation of conceptual models of nursing* (pp. 437-515). Philadelphia: F.A. Davis.

Fitzpatrick, J.J., Whall, A., Johnson, R., & Floyd, J. (1982). *Nursing models: Applications to psychiatric mental health nursing.* Bowie, MD: Robert J. Brady.

Galbreath, J.G. (1980). Sister Callista Roy. In Nursing Theories Conference Group, J.B. George (Chairperson), *Nursing theories: The base for professional nursing practice* (pp. 199-212). Englewood Cliffs, NJ: Prentice-Hall.

Galbreath, J.G. (1985). Sister Callista Roy. In J.B. George (Ed.), *Nursing theories* (2nd ed., pp. 300-318). Englewood Cliffs, NJ: Prentice-Hall.

Gordon, J. (1974). Nursing assessment and care plan for a cardiac patient. In J.P. Riehl & C. Roy (Eds.), *Conceptual models for nursing practice.* New York: Appleton-Century-Crofts.

Hill, B.J. & Roberts, C.S. (1981). Formal theory construction: An example of the process. In C. Roy & S.L. Roberts (Eds.), *Theory construction in nursing: An adaptation model* (pp. 30-39). Englewood Cliffs, NJ: Prentice-Hall.

Idle, B.A. (1978). SPAL: A tool for measuring self-perceived adaptation level appropriate for an elderly population. In E.E. Bauwens (Ed.), *Clinical nursing research: Its strategies and findings. Monograph series 1978: Two* (pp. 56-63). Indianapolis: Sigma Theta Tau.

Kehoe, C.F. (1981). Identifying the nursing needs of the postpartum cesarean mother. In C.F. Kehoe (Ed.), *The cesarean experience: Theoretical and clinical perspectives for nurses* (pp. 85-141). New York: Appleton-Century-Crofts.

Kehoe, C.F. & Fawcett, J. (1981). An overview of the Roy adaptation model. In C.F. Kehoe (Ed.), *The cesarean experience: Theoretical and clinical perspectives for nurses* (pp. 79-84). New York: Appleton-Century-Crofts.

Leddy, S. & Pepper, J.M. (1985). Sister Callista Roy's adaptation model. In S. Leddy & J.M. Pepper (Eds.), *Conceptual bases of professional nursing* (pp. 142-144). Philadelphia: J.B. Lippincott.

Levesque, L. (1980, Oct.). Rehabilitation of the chronically ill elderly: A method of operationalizing a conceptual model for nursing. In R.C. MacKay & E.G. Zilm (Eds.), *Research for practice: Proceedings of the National Nursing Research Conference,* Halifax, Nova Scotia, Canada.

Lewis, F. (1978). Measuring adaptation of chemotherapy patients. In J.C. Krueger, A.H. Nelson, & M. Opal (Eds.), *Nursing Research: Development, collaboration, utilization.* Rockville, MD: Aspen Systems.

Meleis, A.I. (1985). Sister Callista Roy. In A.I. Meleis (Ed.), *Theoretical nursing: Development and progress* (pp. 206-218). Philadelphia: J.B. Lippincott.

Phillips. K.D. (1997). Roy's adaptation model in nursing practice. In M. Alligood & A. Marriner Tomey (Eds.), *Nursing theory utilization and application* (pp. 175-200). St. Louis. Mosby.

Sato, M. (1986). The Roy adaptation model. In P. Winsted-Fry (Ed.), *Case studies in nursing theory* (pp. 103-125). New York: National League for Nursing.

Schmitz, M. (1980). The Roy adaptation model: Application in a community setting. In J.P. Riehl & C. Roy (Eds.), *Conceptual models for nursing practice* (2nd ed., pp. 193-206). New York: Appleton-Century-Crofts.

Starr, S.L. (1980). Adaptation applied to the dying patient. In J.P. Riehl & C. Roy (Eds.), *Conceptual models for nursing practice* (2nd ed., pp. 189-192). New York: Appleton-Century-Crofts.

Tiedman, M.E. (1983). The Roy adaptation model. In J. Fitzpatrick & A. Whall (Eds.), *Conceptual models of nursing: Analysis and application* (pp. 157-180). Bowie, MD: Robert J. Brady.

Journal Articles

Aggleton, P. & Chalmers, H. (1984, Oct.). The Roy adaptation model. *Nursing Times,* 80, 45-48.

Andreoli, K.G. & Thompson, C.E. (1977, June). The nature of science in nursing. *Image,* 9(2), 33-37.

Baker, A.C. (1993). The spouse's positive effect on the stroke patient's recovery. *Rehabilitation Nursing,* 18(1), 30-33, 67-68.

Barnfather, J.S., Swain, M.A.P., & Erickson, H.C. (1989). Evaluation of two assessment techniques for adaptation to stress. *Nursing Science Quarterly,* 2(4), 172-182.

Beckstrand, J. (1980). A critique of several conceptions of practice theory in nursing. *Research in Nursing and Health,* 3, 69-79.

Brower, H.T.F. & Baker, B.J. (1976, Nov.). The Roy adaptation model: Using the adaptation model in a practitioner curriculum. *Nursing Outlook,* 24, 686-689.

Calvert, M.M. (1989). Human-pet interaction and loneliness: A test of concepts from Roy's adaptation model. *Nursing Science Quarterly,* 2(4), 194-202.

Calvillo, E.R. & Flaskerud, J.H. (1993). The adequacy of Roy's adaptation model to guide cross-cultural pain research. *Nursing Science Quarterly,* 6(3), 118-129.

Camooso, C., Green, M., & Reilly, P. (1981). Students' adaptation according to Roy. *Nursing Outlook,* 29, 108-109.

Carveth, J.A. (1987). Conceptual models in nurse-midwifery. *Journal of Nurse-Midwifery,* 32(1), 20-25.

Chance, K.S. (1982). Nursing models: A requisite for professional accountability. *Advances in Nursing Science,* 4(2), 57-65.

Chen, H. (1994). Hearing in the elderly: Relation of hearing loss, loneliness, and self-esteem. *Journal of Gerontological Nursing,* 20(6), 22-28.

Coleman, P.M. (1993). Depression during the female climacteric period. *Journal of Advanced Nursing,* 18(10), 1540-1546.

Cottrel, B.H. & Shannaha, M.D. (1987). Effect of the birth chair in duration of second stage labor and maternal outcome. *Nursing Research,* 35(6), 364-367.

Dickoff, J., James, P., & Wiedenbach, E. (1968, May). Theory in a practice discipline. Part I. Practice oriented theory. *Nursing Research,* 17, 413-435.

Farkas, L. (1981, March). Adaptation problems with nursing home application for elderly persons: An application of the Roy adaptation nursing model. *Journal of Advanced Nursing,* 6, 363-368.

Fawcett, J. (1981). Needs of cesarean birth parents. *Journal of Obstetric, Gynecologic, and Neonatal Nursing,* 10, 371-376.

Fawcett, J. (1990). Preparation for cesarean childbirth: Derivation of a nursing intervention from the Roy adaptation model. *Journal of Advanced Nursing,* 15(12), 1418-1425.

Fawcett, J. & Buritt, J. (1985). An exploratory study of antenatal preparation for cesarean birth. *Journal of Obstetric, Gynecologic, and Neonatal Nursing,* 14, 224-230.

Florence, M.E., Lutzen, K., & Alexius, B. (1994). Adaptation of heterosexually infected HIV-positive women: A Swedish pilot study. *Health Care for Women International,* 15(4), 265-273.

Friedmann, M. & Andrews, M. (1990). Family support and child adjustment in single-parent families . . . secondary analysis. *Issues in Comprehensive Pediatric Nursing,* 13(14), 289-301.

Frederickson, K., Jackson, B.S., Strauman, T., & Strauman, J. (1991). Testing hypotheses derived from the Roy adaptation model. *Nursing Science Quarterly,* 4(4), 168-174.

Galligan, A.C. (1979, Jan.). Using Roy's concept of adaptation to care for young children. *American Journal of Maternal Child Nursing,* 4, 24-28.

Gamble, N. & Devanev, S. (1985). Application of the adaptation framework in an LPN program: A project. *Missouri Nurse,* 54(6), 10-13.

Gartner, S.R. & Nahm, H. (1977, Jan./Feb.). An overview of nursing research in the United States. *Nursing Research,* 26, 10-29.

Germain, C.P. (1984). Sheltering abused women: A nursing perspective. *Journal of Psychological Nursing,* 22(9), 24-31.

Gerrish, C. (1989). From theory to practice: Applied Roy's model while caring for a woman with Hodgkin's disease. *Nursing Times,* 85(35), 42-45.

Glasper, A. (1986). Spotlight on children: Scaling down a model. *Nursing Times,* 82(43), 53-58.

Goodwin, J.O. (1980). A cross-cultural approach to integrating nursing theory and practice. *Nurse Educator,* 5(6), 15-20.

Gunderson, L.P. & Kenner, C. (1987, Aug.). Neonatal stress: Physiologic adaptation and nursing implications. *Neonatal Network,* 6(1), 37-42.

Harrison, L.L., Leeper, J.D., & Yoon, M. (1990). Effects of early parent touch on preterm infants' heart rates and arterial oxygen saturation levels. *Journal of Advanced Nursing,* 15(8), 877-885.

Heinrich, K. (1989). Growing pains: Faculty stages in adopting a nursing model. *Nurse Educator,* 14(1), 3-4.

Hoon, E. (1986). Game playing: A way to look at nursing models. *Journal of Advanced Nursing,* 11(4), 421-427.

Jackson, D.A. (1990). Roy in the postanesthesia care unit. *Journal of Post Anesthesia Nursing,* 5(3), 143-148.

Jackson, B.S., Strauman, J., Frederickson, K., & Strauman, T.J. (1991). Long-term biopsychosocial effects of interleukin-2 therapy. *Oncology Nursing Forum,* 18(4), 683-690.

Janelli, L.M. (1980). Utilizing Roy's adaptation model from a gerontological perspective. *Journal of Gerontological Nursing,* 6(3), 140-150.

Johnston, D.E. (1974, Sept./Oct.). Development of theory: A requisite for nursing as a primary health profession. *Nursing Research,* 23, 372-377.

Kasemwatana, S. (1982). An application of Roy's adaptation model. *Thai Journal of Nursing,* 31(1), 25-46.

Kurek-Ovshinsky, C. (1991). Group psychotherapy in an acute inpatient setting: Techniques that nourish self-esteem. *Issues in Mental Health Nursing,* 12(1), 81-88.

Laros, J. (1977). Deriving outcome criteria from a conceptual model. *Nursing Outlook,* 25, 333-336.

LeMone, P. (1995). Assessing psychosexual concerns in adults with diabetes: Pilot project using Roy's modes of adaptation. *Issues in Mental Health Nursing,* 16(1), 67-78.

Lewis, F.M., Firsich, S.C., & Parsell, S. (1979). Clinical tool development for adult chemotherapy patients: Process and content. *Cancer Nursing,* 2, 99-108.

Limandri, B.J. (1986). Research and practice with abused women: Use of the Roy model as an explanatory framework. *Advanced Nursing Science,* 8(4), 52-61.

Logan, M. (1990). The Roy adaptation model: Are nursing diagnoses amendable to independent nurse functions? *Journal of Advanced Nursing,* 15(4), 468-470.

Mason, T. (1990). Nursing models in a special hospital: A critical analysis of efficacy. *Journal of Advanced Nursing,* 15(6), 667-673.

Mastal, M. & Hammond, H. (1980, July). Analysis and expansion of the Roy adaptation model: A contribution to holistic nursing. *Advances in Nursing Science,* 2, 71-81.

Mastal, M., Hammond, H., & Roberts, M. (1982, June). Theory into hospital practice: A pilot implementation. *Journal of Nursing Administration,* 12, 9-15.

McGill, J.S. & Paul, P.B. (1993). Functional status and hope in elderly people with and without cancer. *Oncology Nursing Forum,* 20(8), 1207-1213.

Meek, S.S. (1993). Effects of slow stroke back massage on relaxation in hospice clients. *Image: The Journal of Nursing Scholarship,* 25(1), 17-21.

Miller, F. (1991). Using Roy's model in a special hospital. *Nursing Standard,* 5(27), 29-32.

Newman, D.M.L. & Fawcett, J. (1995). Caring for a young child in a body cast: Impact on the care giver. *Orthopedic Nursing,* 14(1), 41-46.

Norris, S., Campbell, L., & Brenkert, S. (1982). Nursing procedures and alterations in transcutaneous oxygen tension in premature infants. *Nursing Research,* 31, 330-336.

Park, K.O. (1982). Study of Roy's adaptation model. *Trehan Kanho,* 21(3), 49-58.

Pepin, J., Ducharme, F., Kerouac, S., Levesque, L., Ricard, N., & Duquette, A. (1994). Development of a research program based on a conceptual model of the nursing discipline. *Canadian Journal of Nursing Research,* 26(1), 41-53.

Pollock, S.E., Frederickson, K., Carson, M.A., Massey, V.H., & Roy, C. (1994). Contributions to nursing science: Synthesis of findings from Adaptation Model research. *Scholarly Inquiry for Nursing Practice,* 8(4), 361-374.

Porth, C.M. (1977). Physiological coping: A model for teaching pathophysiology. *Nursing Outlook,* 25, 781-784.

Richard, L. (1982). Roy's adaptation model. *Infirmiere Canadienne,* 24(9), 12-13.

Robinson, J.H. (1995). Grief responses, coping processes, and social support of widows: Research with Roy's model. *Nursing Science Quarterly,* 8(4), 158-164.

Robitaille-Tremblay, M. (1983). Les soins infirmiers en psychiatrie a l'ere d'un modele conceptuel. *L'infirmiere Canadienne,* 6, 37-40.

Robitaille-Tremblay, M. (1984, Aug.). A data collection tool for the psychiatric nurse. *Canadian Nurse,* 31(7), 26-31.

Rogers, M., Paul, L.J., Clarke, J., MacKay, C., Potter, M., & Ward, W. (1991). The use of the Roy adaptation model in nursing administration. *Canadian Journal of Nursing Administration,* 4(2), 21-26.

Samarel, N. & Fawcett, J. (1992). Enhancing adaptation to breast cancer: The addition of coaching to support groups. *Oncology Nursing Forum,* 19(4), 591-596.

Selman, S.W. (1989). Impact of total hip replacement on quality of life. *Orthopedic Nursing,* 8(5), 43-49.

Sheppard, V.A. & Cunnie, K.L. (1996). Incidence of diuresis following hysterectomy. *Journal of Post Anesthesia Nursing,* 11, 20-28.

Short, J.D. (1994). Interdependence needs and nursing care of the new family. *Issues in Comprehensive Pediatric Nursing,* 17(1), 1-14.

Silva, M.C. (1977, Oct.). Philosophy science theory: Interrelationships and implications for nursing research. *Image,* 9(3), 59-63.

Silva, M.C. (1986). Research testing nursing theory, state of the art. (Published erratum appears in ANS1987, Jan. 9(2): ix.) *Advanced Nursing Science,* 9(1), 1-11.

Silva, M.C. (1987). Needs of spouses of surgical patients: A conceptualization within the Roy adaptation model. *Scholarly Inquiry for Nursing Practice,* 1(1), 29-44.

Smith, C.E., Garvis, M.S., & Martinson, I.M. (1983, Aug.). Content analysis of interviews using a nursing model: A look at parents adapting to the impact of childhood cancer. *Cancer Nursing,* 6, 269-275.

Strohmyer, L.L., Noroian, E.L., Patterson, L.M., & Carlin, B.P. (1993). Adaptation six months after multiple trauma: A pilot study. *Journal of Neuroscience Nursing,* 25(1), 270-276.

Torosian, L.C., DeStefano, M., & Deitrick-Gallager, M. (1985). Day gynecologic chemotherapy unit: An innovative approach to changing health care systems. *Cancer Nursing,* 8, 221-227.

Tulman, L. (1990). Maternal employment after birth. *Research in Nursing and Health,* 13(3), 181-188.

Vicenzi, A.E. & Thiel, R. (1992). AIDS education on the college campus: Roy's adaptation model in practice: Nurses' perspectives. *Nursing Science Quarterly,* 7(2), 80-86.

Wagner, P. (1976, Nov.). The Roy adaptation model: Testing the adaptation model in practice. *Nursing Outlook,* 24(11), 682-685.

Weiss, M.E., Hastings, W.J., Holly, D.C., & Craig, D.I. (1994). Using Roy's adaptation model in practice: Nurses' perspectives. *Nursing Science Quarterly,* 7(2), 80-86.

Weiss, M.E. & Teplick, F. (1993). Linking perinatal standards, documentation, and quality monitoring. *Journal of Perinatal and Neonatal Nursing,* 7(2), 18-27.

Other Sources

Coombs, A. & Snygg, D. (1959). *Individual behavior: A perceptual approach to behavior.* New York: Harper Brothers.

Dohrendwend, B.P. (1961). The social psychological nature of stress: A framework for causal inquiry. *Journal of Abnormal and Social Psychology,* 62(2), 294-302.

Driever, M.J. (1976). Theory of self-concept. In C. Roy (Ed.), *Introduction to nursing: An adaptation model.* Englewood Cliffs, NJ: Prentice-Hall.

Ellis, R. (1968, May/June). Characteristics of significant theories. *Nursing Research,* 17, 217-223.

Epstein, S. (1973, May). The self-concept revisited or a theory of a theory. *American Psychologist,* 28(5), 404-416.

Erikson, E.H. (1963). *Childhood and society* (2nd ed.). New York: W.W. Norton.

Gardner, B.D. (1964). *Development in early childhood.* New York: Harper & Row.

Helson, H. (1964). *Adaptational-level theory: An experimental and systematic approach to behavior.* New York: Harper & Row.

Lazarus, R.S. (1966). *Psychological stress and the coping process.* New York: McGraw-Hill.

Lazarus, R.S., Averill, J.R., & Opton, E.M., Jr. (1974). The psychology of coping: Issues of research and assessment. In G.V. Coelho, D.A. Hamburg, & J.E. Adams (Eds.), *Coping and adaptation.* New York: Basic Books.

Malaznik, N. (1976). Theory of role function. In C. Roy (Ed.), *Introduction to nursing: An adaptation model.* Englewood Cliffs, NJ: Prentice-Hall.

Maslow, A.H. (1968). *Toward a psychology of being* (2nd ed.). New York: Van Nostrand Reinhold.

Mead, G.H. (1934). *Mind, self, and society.* Chicago: University of Chicago.

Mechanic, D. (1970). Some problems in developing a social psychology of adaptation to stress. In J. McGrath (Ed.), *Social and psychological factors in stress.* New York: Holt, Rinehart, & Winston.

Mechanic, D. (1974). Social structure and personal adaptation: Some neglected dimensions. In G.V. Coelho, D.A. Hamburg, & J.E. Adams (Eds.), *Coping and adaptation.* New York: Basic Books.

Miller, J.G. (1965, July). Living systems: Basic concepts. *Behavioral Science,* 10, 193-237.

Pousch, M. & Van Landingham, J. (1977). *Interdependence mode module* [Class handout]. Mount St. Mary's College, Los Angeles.

Randell, B. (1976). *Introduction to nursing: An adaptation model.* Englewood Cliffs, NJ: Prentice-Hall.

Reynolds, P.D. (1971). *A primer in theory construction.* Indianapolis: Bobbs-Merrill.

Selye, H. (1978). *The stress of life.* New York: McGraw-Hill.

Smith, B.J.A. (1989). *Caregiver burden and adaptation in middle-aged daughters of dependent elderly parents: A test of Roy's model* (p. 177). Unpublished a doctoral dissertation, University of Pittsburgh.

Sullivan, H.S. (1953). *The interpersonal theory of psychiatry.* New York: W.W. Norton.

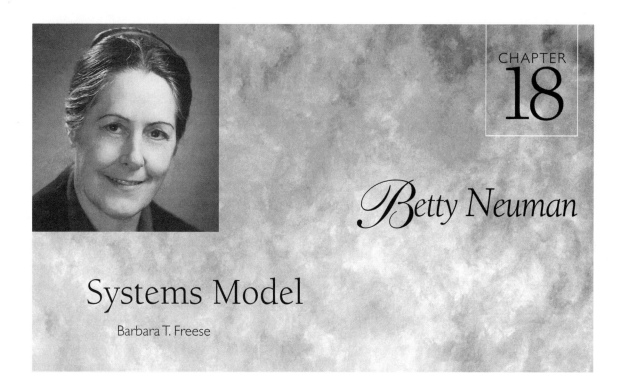

Betty Neuman

Systems Model

Barbara T. Freese

CREDENTIALS AND BACKGROUND OF THE THEORIST

Betty Neuman was born in 1924 on a farm near Lowell, Ohio. Her father was a farmer and her mother a homemaker. She developed a love for the land growing up in rural Ohio and this rural background developed her compassion for people in need. Neuman's initial nursing education was completed with double honors at Peoples Hospital School of Nursing (now General Hospital), Akron, Ohio in 1947. She then moved to Los Angeles to live with relatives. In California, she worked in a variety of nursing roles that included hospital staff and head nurse, school nurse, and industrial nurse. She was also involved in clinical teaching in what is now the University of Southern California Medical Center, Los Angeles, in the areas of medical-surgical, communicable disease, and critical

Previous authors: Barbara T. Freese, Sarah J. Beckman, Sanna Boxley-Harges, Cheryl Bruick-Sorge, Susan Matthews Harris, Mary E. Hermiz, Mary Meininger, and Sandra E. Steinkeler.

care. She had always been interested in human behavior; therefore she attended the University of California at Los Angeles (UCLA) with a double major in public health and psychology. She completed her baccalaureate degree with honors in nursing in 1957 and then helped establish and manage her husband's medical practice. In 1966, she received her master's degree in Mental Health, Public Health Consultation, from UCLA.[79,80] She received a doctoral degree in clinical psychology from Pacific Western University in 1985.[79]

Neuman was a pioneer of nursing involvement in mental health. She developed, taught, and refined a community mental health program for postmaster's level nurses at UCLA. Neuman and Donna Aquilina were the first two nurses to develop the nurse counselor role within Los Angeles-based community crisis centers.[86] She developed her first explicit teaching and practice model for mental health consultation in the late 1960s, before the creation of her systems model. This teaching and practice model is cited in her first book publication, *Consultation and Community Organization in Community Mental Health Nursing*,[92] in 1971. Neuman designed a conceptual model for nursing in 1970 in response to requests from UCLA graduate students who wanted a course emphasizing breadth rather than depth in understanding the variables in nursing. Initially, the model was developed to integrate students' understanding of client variables that extend nursing beyond the medical model.[93] The Neuman model included such behavioral science concepts as problem identification and prevention. Neuman[84,86] first published her model in 1972. She spent the following decade further defining and refining various aspects of the model in preparation for her book, *The Neuman Systems Model: Application to Nursing Education and Practice*.[78] Further development and revisions of the model are illustrated in the second (1989)[83] and third (1995)[88] editions. Neuman[91] states that the fourth edition will offer an integrative review of use of the model with guidelines for application of the model in practice, research, education, and administration.

Neuman has been involved in a wide variety of professional international activities since developing the Neuman Systems Model, including numerous publications, paper presentations, consultations, lectures, and conferences. Neuman has a wide range of teaching expertise and taught nurse continuing education at UCLA and in community agencies for 14 years. She is a Fellow of the American Association of Marriage and Family Therapy. She continues in active, private practice as a licensed clinical marriage and family therapist, with an emphasis on Christian counseling. Neuman lives in Ohio and maintains a leadership role in the Neuman Systems Model Trustees Group, Inc. She serves as a consultant internationally for nursing schools and with practice agencies adopting the model for theory-based practice.[83,85,87,91]

THEORETICAL SOURCES

The Neuman Systems Model is based in general system theory and reflects the nature of living organisms as open systems.[116] General system theory states that all elements in a complex organization are in interaction.[78] Within the model, Neuman synthesizes knowledge from several disciplines and incorporates her own philosophical beliefs and clinical nursing expertise, particularly in mental health nursing.

The model draws from Gestalt theory,[78] which describes homeostasis as the process by which an organism maintains its equilibrium, and consequently its health, under varying conditions. Neuman describes adjustment as the process by which the organism satisfies its needs. Many needs exist and each may disrupt client balance or stability; therefore the adjustment process is dynamic and continuous. All life is characterized by this ongoing interplay of balance and imbalance within the organism. When the stabilizing process fails to some degree, or when the organism remains in a state of disharmony for too long and is consequently unable to satisfy its needs, illness may develop. When illness as a compensatory process fails completely, the organism may die.[93] The Gestalt approach considers the individual within the organism-environmental field and views behavior as a reflection of relatedness within that field.[94]

The model is also derived from the philosophical views of deChardin and Marx.[78] Marxist philosophy suggests that the properties of parts are determined partly by the larger wholes within dynamically organized systems. With this view, Neuman[78] confirms that the patterns of the whole influence awareness of the part, which is drawn from deChardin's philosophy of the wholeness of life.

Neuman used Selye's definition of *stress*, which is the nonspecific response of the body to any demand made on it.[107] Stress increases the demand for readjustment. This demand is nonspecific; it requires adaptation to a problem, irrespective of the nature of the problem. Therefore the essence of stress is the nonspecific demand for activity.[107] Stressors are the tension-producing stimuli that result in stress; they may be positive or negative.

Neuman adapts the concept of levels of prevention from Caplan's conceptual model[23] and relates these prevention levels to nursing. Primary prevention is used to protect the organism before it encounters a harmful stressor. Primary prevention involves reducing the possibility of encountering the stressor or strengthening the organism to decrease its reaction to the stressor.[23] Secondary and tertiary prevention are used following the organism's encounter with a harmful stressor. Secondary prevention attempts to reduce the effect or possible effect of stressors through early diagnosis and effective treatment of illness symptoms. Tertiary prevention attempts to reduce the residual stressor effects after treatment.[23]

USE OF EMPIRICAL EVIDENCE

Neuman conceptualized the model from sound theories rather than from nursing research. She evaluated the utility of the model by submitting a tool to her nursing students at UCLA who were beginning their master's program. The outcome data were published in the Spring 1972 issue of *Nursing Research*.[93] The tool was for student evaluation rather than statistical evidence; therefore the model originally lacked empirical support. However, during the past decade, nursing research has produced considerable empirical evidence in support of the Neuman Systems Model.[102,104,108] A research survey published in 1995 identified nearly 100 studies conducted between 1989 and 1993 for which the model provided the organizing framework.[59] Over 50 additional studies (dissertations, theses, and journal articles) published between 1996 and 2000 are listed in the bibliography of this chapter.

Text continued on p. 305

MAJOR CONCEPTS & DEFINITIONS

The major concepts identified in the model (Figure 18-1) are wholistic client approach, open system, basic structure, environment, created environment, stressors, lines of defense and resistance, degree of reaction, prevention as intervention, and reconstitution.[78] Neuman's second edition included further development of the concepts of scholastic approach, content, process, input and output, feedback, negentropy, entropy, stability, wellness, and illness.[72,82,86]

WHOLISTIC CLIENT APPROACH

The Neuman Systems Model is a dynamic, open, systems approach to client care originally developed to provide a unifying focus for nursing problem definition and for best understanding the client in interaction with the environment. The client as a system may be defined as a person, family, group, community, or issue.[82]

WHOLISTIC CONCEPT

Clients are viewed as wholes whose parts are in dynamic interaction. The model considers all variables simultaneously affecting the client system: physiological, psychological, sociocultural, developmental, and spiritual. Neuman[82] included the spiritual variable in the second book edition. She changed the spelling of the term *holistic* to *wholistic* in the second edition to enhance understanding of the term as referring to the whole person.[82]

OPEN SYSTEM

A system is open when its elements are exchanging information energy within its complex organization. Stress and reaction to stress are basic components of an open system.[82]

ENVIRONMENT

Internal and external forces affecting and being affected by the client at any time comprise the environment.[82]

CREATED ENVIRONMENT

The created environment is the client's unconscious mobilization of all system variables toward system integration, stability, and integrity.[34]

CONTENT

The five variables (physiological, psychological, sociocultural, developmental, and spiritual) of man in interaction with the environment comprise the whole system of the client.[82]

Continued

MAJOR CONCEPTS & DEFINITIONS—cont'd

BASIC STRUCTURE

"The core structure consists of basic survival factors common to the species, such as innate or genetic features . . ."[88:26] The inner circle of the diagram (see Figure 18-1) represents the basic survival factors or energy resources of the client.

PROCESS OR FUNCTION

"The client is a system capable of both input and output related to . . . environmental influences, interacting with the environment by adjusting to it; or as a system, adjusting the environment to itself."[88:22]

INPUT AND OUTPUT

Matter, energy, and information that are exchanged between the client system.[82]

FEEDBACK

System output in the form of matter, energy, and information serves as feedback for future input for corrective action to change, enhance, or stabilize the system.[88]

NEGENTROPY

A process of energy utilization that assists system progression toward stability or wellness.[82]

ENTROPY

A process of energy depletion and disorganization that moves the system toward illness or possible death.[82,94]

STABILITY

The client system successfully copes with stressors; it is able to maintain an adequate level of health. Functional harmony or balance preserves the integrity of the system.[82]

STRESSORS

Stressors are tension-producing stimuli occurring within the boundaries of the client system. They may be:

1. Intrapersonal forces occurring within the individual, such as conditioned responses.
2. Interpersonal forces occurring between one or more individuals, such as role expectations.
3. Extrapersonal forces occurring outside the individual, such as financial circumstances.[88]

WELLNESS

Wellness exists when the parts of the client system interact in harmony. System needs are met.[82,86]

ILLNESS

Disharmony among the parts of the system is considered illness, which is the result of unmet needs in varying degrees.[82,86]

NORMAL LINE OF DEFENSE

The normal line of defense is the model's outer solid circle. It represents a stability state for the individual or system. It is maintained over time and serves as a standard to assess deviations from the client's usual wellness. It includes system variables and behaviors such as the individual's usual coping patterns, lifestyle, and developmental stage.[88]

FLEXIBLE LINE OF DEFENSE

The model's outer broken ring is called the flexible line of defense. It is dynamic and can be rapidly altered over a short time. It is perceived as a protective buffer for preventing stressors from breaking through the usual wellness state as represented by the normal line of defense. The relationship of the variables (physiological, psychological, sociocultural, developmental, and spiritual) can

MAJOR CONCEPTS & DEFINITIONS—cont'd

affect the degree to which individuals are able to use their flexible line of defense against possible reaction to a stressor or stressors, such as loss of sleep.[82,88]

LINES OF RESISTANCE

The series of broken rings surrounding the basic core structure are called the lines of resistance. These rings represent resource factors that help the client defend against a stressor. An example is the body's immune response system.[78,86]

DEGREE OF REACTION

The degree of reaction is the amount of energy required for the client to adjust to the stressor(s).[88]

PREVENTION AS INTERVENTION

Interventions are purposeful actions to help the client retain, attain, and/or maintain system stability. They can occur before or after protective lines of defense and resistance are penetrated in both reaction and reconstitution phases. Neuman[78] supports beginning intervention when a stressor is either suspected or identified. Interventions are based on possible or actual degree of reaction, resources, goals, and the anticipated outcome. Neuman identifies three levels of intervention: (1) primary, (2) secondary, and (3) tertiary.

Primary Prevention

Primary prevention is carried out when a stressor is suspected or identified. A reaction has not yet occurred, but the degree of risk is known. Neuman[78:15] states, "The actor or intervener would perhaps attempt to reduce the possibility of the individual's encounter with the stressor or in some way attempt to strengthen the individual's encounter with the stressor or attempt to strengthen the individual's flexible line of defense to decrease the possibility of a reaction."

Secondary Prevention

Secondary prevention involves interventions or treatment initiated after symptoms from stress have occurred. Both the client's internal and external resources are used toward system stabilization to strengthen internal lines of resistance, reduce the reaction, and increase resistance factors.[78]

Tertiary Prevention

Tertiary prevention occurs after the active treatment or secondary prevention stage. It focuses on readjustment toward optimal client system stability. A primary goal is to strengthen resistance to stressors to help prevent recurrence of reaction or regression. This process leads back in a circular fashion toward primary prevention. An example would be avoidance of stressors known to be hazardous to the client.[78,86]

RECONSTITUTION

Reconstitution is the state of adaptation to stressors in the internal and external environment.[78] It can begin at any degree or level of reaction and may progress beyond or stabilize somewhat below the client's previous normal line of defense. Included in reconstitution are interpersonal, intrapersonal, extrapersonal, and environmental factors interrelated with client system variables (physiological, psychological, sociocultural, developmental, and spiritual).[78,82]

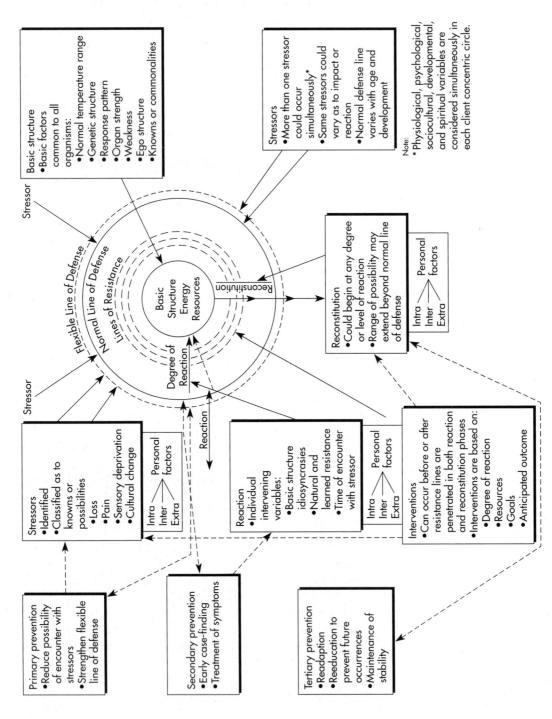

Figure 18-1 **The Neuman Systems Model.** (Original copyright © 1970 by Betty Neuman. Used with permission.)

MAJOR ASSUMPTIONS

Nursing

Neuman believes nursing is concerned with the whole person. She views nursing as a "unique profession in that it is concerned with all of the variables affecting an individual's response to stress."[78:14] The nurse's perception influences the care given; therefore Neuman states that the perceptual field of the caregiver and the client must be assessed. She has developed an assessment and intervention tool to help with this task.

Person

The Neuman Systems Model presents the concept of person as a client/client system that may be an individual, family, group, community, or social issue. The client system is a dynamic composite of interrelationships among physiological, psychological, sociocultural, developmental, and spiritual factors. The client system is viewed as being in constant change or motion and is seen as an open system in reciprocal interaction with the environment.[33,34,37,78]

Health

Neuman considers her work as a wellness model. She views health as a continuum of wellness to illness that is dynamic in nature and constantly subject to change. "Optimal wellness or stability indicates that total system needs are being met. A reduced state of wellness is the result of unmet system needs. The client is in a dynamic state of either wellness or illness, in varying degrees, at any given point in time."[88:46]

Environment

Environment and person are identified as the basic phenomena of the Neuman Systems Model, with the relationship between environment and person being reciprocal. Environment is defined as being all the internal and external factors that surround or interact with person and client. Stressors (intrapersonal, interpersonal, and extrapersonal) are significant to the concept of environment and are described as environmental forces that interact with and potentially alter system stability.

Neuman has identified three relevant environments: (1) internal, (2) external, and (3) created. The internal environment is intrapersonal, with all interaction contained within the client. The external environment is interpersonal or extrapersonal with all interactions occurring outside the client. The created environment is unconsciously developed and used by the client to support protective coping. It is primarily intrapersonal. The created environment is dynamic in nature and mobilizes all system variables to create an insulating effect that helps the client cope with the threat of environmental stressors by changing the self or the situation. Examples are the use of denial (psychological variable) and life-cycle continuation of survival patterns (developmental variable).[88] The created environment perpetually influences and is influenced by changes in the client's perceived state of wellness.[16,34,88]

THEORETICAL ASSERTIONS

Theoretical assertions are the relationships among the essential concepts of a model.[97,115] The Neuman model depicts the nurse as an active participant with the client and as "concerned with all the variables affecting an individual's response to stressors."[78:14] The client is in a reciprocal relationship with the environment in that "he interacts with this environment by adjusting himself to it or adjusting it to himself."[78:14] Neuman links the four essential concepts of person, environment, health, and nursing in her statements regarding primary, secondary, and tertiary prevention. Earlier publications by Neuman stated basic assumptions that linked essential concepts of the model. These statements, listed in Box 18-1, have also been identified as propositions and serve to define, describe, and link the concepts of the model.

LOGICAL FORM

Neuman used both deductive and inductive logic in developing her model. As previously discussed, Neuman derived her model from other theories and

Box 18-1

Basic Assumptions of the Neuman Systems Model

1. Although each individual client or group as a client system is unique, each system is a composite of common known factors or innate characteristics within a normal, given range of response contained within a basic structure.

2. Many known, unknown, and universal environmental stressors exist. Each differs in its potential for disturbing a client's usual stability level, or normal line of defense. The particular interrelationships of client variables—physiological, psychological, sociocultural, developmental, and spiritual—at any point in time can affect the degree to which a client is protected by the flexible line of defense against possible reaction to a single stressor or a combination of stressors.

3. Each individual client/client system has evolved a normal range of response to the environment that is referred to as a normal line of defense, or usual wellness/stability state. The normal line of defense can be used as a standard from which to measure health deviation.

4. When the cushioning, accordian-like effect of the flexible line of defense is no longer capable of protecting the client/client system against an environmental stressor, the stressor breaks through the normal line of defense. The interrelationships of variables—physiological, psychological, sociocultural, developmental, and spiritual—determine the nature and degree of system reaction or possible reaction to the stressor.

5. The client, whether in a state of wellness or illness, is a dynamic composite of the interrelationships of variables (physiological, psychological, sociocultural, developmental, and spiritual). Wellness is on a continuum of available energy to support the system in an optimal state of system stability.

6. Implicit within each client system are internal resistance factors known as lines of resistance, which function to stabilize and return the client to the usual wellness state (normal line of defense) or possibly to a higher level of stability following an environmental stressor reaction.

7. Primary prevention relates to general knowledge that is applied in client assessment and intervention in identification and reduction or mitigation of possible or actual risk factors associated with environmental stressors to prevent possible reaction. The goal of health promotion is included in primary prevention.

8. Secondary prevention relates to symptomatology following a reaction to stressors, appropriate ranking of intervention priorities, and treatment to reduce their noxious effects.

9. Tertiary prevention relates to the adjustive processes taking place as reconstitution begins and maintenance factors move the client back in a circular manner toward primary prevention.

10. The client as a system is in dynamic, constant energy exchange with the environment.

disciplines. The model is also a product of her philosophy and of observations made in teaching mental health nursing and clinical counseling.[38]

ACCEPTANCE BY THE NURSING COMMUNITY

Neuman's model has been described by Walker and Avant[117] as a grand nursing theory. A grand theory consists of a global conceptual framework that defines broad perspectives for practice and includes diverse ways of viewing nursing phenomena based on these perspectives. As a grand theory, the Neuman Systems Model provides a comprehensive foundation for scientific nursing practice, education, and research.

The Neuman model has attained acceptance throughout the world and provides an ideal framework for health initiatives to address the World Health Organization's goal of health for the world community.[120] The model is used extensively in the United States, Canada, Australia, Brazil, Costa Rica, Denmark, Egypt, England, Finland, Ghana, Hong Kong, Iceland, Japan, Korea, New Zealand, Portugal, Puerto Rico, The Republic of China, Spain, Sweden, Taiwan, Wales, and Yugoslavia. As an example, the model was used to structure the World Health Organization's Collaborative Center for Primary Health Care Nursing in Maribor, Yugoslavia (Slovenia).[87]

The model has been adapted equally well to all levels of nursing education and to a wide variety of practice areas. It adapts well transculturally and is used extensively for public health nursing in other countries. The model is the most widely accepted model for community health nursing in the United States and Canada.[63]

Ongoing development and universal appeal of the model are reflected in the biennial International Symposia of the Neuman Systems Model. The first symposium was held at Neumann College in Aston, Pennsylvania (1986).[70,72,81] Subsequent symposia have been held in Kansas City, Missouri (1988), Dayton, Ohio (1990), Rochester, New York (1993), Orlando (1995), Boston (1997), Vancouver, British Columbia (1999), and Salt Lake City, Utah (2001). The ninth symposium is scheduled for 2003 in Pennsylvania. Each symposium shows increased participation from more countries of the world and other disciplines beyond nursing.

Practice

The Neuman Systems Model has broad relevance for current and future nursing practice. Use of the model by nurses facilitates goal-directed, unified, wholistic approaches to client care, yet it is also appropriate for multidisciplinary use to prevent fragmentation of client care. The model delineates a client system and classification of stressors that can be understood and used by all members of the healthcare team.[73] Increasingly, other health disciplines are finding the work beneficial.

Neuman has developed several instruments to facilitate use of the model. These instruments include an assessment and intervention tool to assist nurses in collecting and synthesizing client data, a format for prevention as intervention, and a format for application of the nursing process within the framework of the Neuman Systems Model.[8] The Neuman Nursing Process Format consists of three steps: (1) nursing diagnosis, (2) nursing goals, and (3) nursing outcomes.[8] Nursing diagnosis involves obtaining a broad, comprehensive database from which variances from wellness can be determined. Goals are then established by negotiation with the client for desired prescriptive changes to correct variances from wellness. Nursing outcomes are determined by nursing intervention through the use of one or more of the three prevention-as-intervention modes. Evaluation then takes place either to confirm the desired outcome goals or to reformulate subsequent nursing goals.

Fawcett[38] has incorporated Neuman's Nursing Process Format and Prevention as Intervention Format into an outline (Box 18-2) to illustrate steps of the nursing process based on the Neuman Systems Model.

The breadth of the Neuman model has resulted in its application and adaptation in a variety of nursing practice settings with individuals, families, groups, and communities. Numerous examples are cited in Neuman's books.[77,78,83,88] The model has been used

Box 18-2

The Neuman Systems Model: Nursing Process Format

I. Nursing diagnosis
A. Establish database that includes the simultaneous consideration of the dynamic interactions of physiological, psychological, sociocultural, developmental, and spiritual variables
   1. Identify client/client system's perceptions
     a. Assess condition and strength of basic structure factors and energy resources
     b. Assess characteristics of the flexible and normal lines of defense, lines of resistance, degree of potential or actual reaction, and potential for reconstitution following a reaction
     c. Assess internal and external environments
       (1) Identify and evaluate potential or actual stressors that pose a threat to the stability of the client/client system
       (2) Classify stressors that threaten stability of client/client system
         (a) Deprivation
         (b) Excess
         (c) Change
         (d) Intolerance
     d. Identify, classify, and evaluate potential and/or actual intrapersonal, interpersonal, and extrapersonal interactions between the client/client system and the environment, considering all five variables
     e. Assess the created environment
       (1) Discover the nature of client/client system's created environment
         (a) Assess client/client system's perception of stressors
         (b) Identify client/client system's major problem, stress areas, or areas of concern
         (c) Identify client/client system's perception of how present circumstances differ from usual pattern of living
         (d) Identify ways in which client/client system handled similar problems in the past
         (e) Identify what client/client system anticipates for self in the future as a consequence of the present situation
         (f) Determine what client/client system is doing and what he or she can do to help himself or herself
         (g) Determine what client/client system expects caregivers, family, friends, or others to do for him or her
       (2) Determine degree of protection provided
       (3) Uncover cause of client/client system's created environment
     f. Evaluate influence of past, present, and possible future life process and coping patterns on client/client system stability
     g. Identify and evaluate actual and potential internal and external resources for optimal state of wellness
   2. Identify caregiver's perceptions (repeat 1 a, b, c, d, e, f, g from caregiver's perspective)

From Fawcett, J. (1995). *Analysis and evaluation of conceptual models of nursing* (3rd ed.). Philadelphia: F.A. Davis. (Adapted from Neuman, B. [1989]. *The Neuman systems model* [pp. 18-21]. Norwalk, CT: Appleton & Lange, © 1980, rev. 1987 Betty Neuman; Neuman, B.M. [1990]. Health as a continuum based on the Neuman systems model. *Nursing Science Quarterly,* 3, 129-135.)

Box 18-2

The Neuman Systems Model: Nursing Process Format—cont'd

      3. Compare client/client system's and caregiver's perceptions
        a. Identify similarities and differences in perceptions
        b. Facilitate client awareness of major perceptual distortions
        c. Resolve perceptual differences
   B. Variances from wellness
      1. Synthesize client database with relevant theories from nursing and adjunctive disciplines
      2. State a comprehensive nursing diagnosis
      3. Prioritize goals
        a. Consider client/client system wellness level
        b. Consider system stability needs
        c. Consider total available resources
      4. Postulate outcome goals and interventions that will facilitate the highest possible level of client/client system stability or wellness (maintain the normal line of defense and retain the flexible line of defense)
II. Nursing goals
   A. Negotiate desired prescriptive changes or outcome goals to correct variances from wellness with the client/client system
      1. Consider needs identified in I.B.3.b.
      2. Consider resources identified in I.B.3.c.
   B. Negotiate prevention as intervention modalities and actions with client/client system
III. Nursing outcomes
   A. Implement nursing interventions through use of one or more of three prevention modalities
      1. Primary prevention nursing action to retain system stability
        a. Prevent stressor invasion
        b. Provide information to retain or strengthen existing client/client system strengths
        c. Support positive coping and functioning
        d. Desensitize existing or possible noxious stressors
        e. Motivate toward wellness
        f. Coordinate and integrate interdisciplinary theories and epidemiological input
        g. Educate or reeducate
        h. Use stress as a positive intervention strategy
      2. Secondary prevention nursing actions to attain system stability
        a. Protect basic structure
        b. Mobilize and optimize internal/external resources to attain stability and energy conservation
        c. Facilitate purposeful manipulation of stressors and reactions to stressors
        d. Motivate, educate, and involve client/client system in healthcare goals
        e. Facilitate appropriate treatment and intervention measures

Continued

Box 18-2

The Neuman Systems Model: Nursing Process Format—cont'd

   f. Support positive factors toward wellness
   g. Promote advocacy by coordination and integration
   h. Provide primary prevention intervention as required
  3. Tertiary prevention nursing actions to maintain system stability
   a. Attain and maintain highest possible level of wellness and stability during reconstitution
   b. Educate, reeducate, and/or reorient as needed
   c. Support client/client system toward appropriate goals
   d. Coordinate and integrate health service resources
   e. Provide primary and/or secondary preventive intervention as required
 B. Evaluate outcome goals
  1. Confirm attainment of outcome goals
  2. Reformulate goals
 C. Set intermediate and long-range goals for subsequent nursing action that are structured in relation to short-term goal outcomes

From Fawcett, J. (1995). *Analysis and evaluation of conceptual models of nursing* (3rd ed.). Philadelphia: F.A. Davis. (Adapted from Neuman, B. [1989]. *The Neuman systems model* [pp. 18-21]. Norwalk, CT: Appleton & Lange, © 1980, rev. 1987 Betty Neuman; Neuman, B.M. [1990]. Health as a continuum based on the Neuman systems model. *Nursing Science Quarterly, 3*, 129-135.)

successfully with clients in many settings, including hospitals, nursing homes, rehabilitation centers, hospices, and childbirth centers. The model was selected for a comprehensive community nursing center in Rochester, New York because it facilitates client-centered care and also because it has proven strengths as a model for community practice.[21,63]

The model's wholistic approach makes it particularly applicable for clients experiencing complex stressors that affect multiple client variables.[112] Black, Deeny, and McKenna[12] used the model as a framework to guide nurses in preventing and alleviating sensoristrain in intensive care patients. Bowman[14] studied sleep satisfaction, perceived pain, and psychological concerns in elderly patients having hip surgery. One group had planned hip replacement and the other group had unplanned emergency surgery following hip fracture. Black, Deeny, and McKenna found differences between the groups although they had similar treatments and similar postoperative care. Schlentz[105] applied the model as the organizing framework to plan care at primary, secondary, and tertiary levels for patients in a long-term care facility.

Neuman's model provides a systems perspective that enables nurses to assess and care for the family unit as a client. Issel[50] used it as the theoretical framework for a comprehensive case management program for obstetrical client families. Within the broader context of the caregiver unit as a system, Jones[52] identified the intrapersonal, interpersonal, and extrapersonal stressors of primary caregivers of persons with traumatic head injuries. Jones found positive correlations between both intrapersonal stressors and interpersonal stressors and the caregiver's changing stress level. Lin, Ku, Leu, Chen, and Lin[57] described the interrelationships among stress, coping behavior, and health status in family caregivers of hepatoma patients. They reported that the greatest stress among family caregivers was related to characteristics of the disease. Reed[100] used the model to describe the family as a client system based on clinical data and the experiences of practicing family nurses. Picton[98] used the model with emergency care patients to assist nurses to view them wholistically as part of a family system.

The Neuman Systems Model is used in community-based practice with groups and in public health nursing.[3] Anderson, McFarland, and Helton[2] adapted the model to develop a community health needs assessment in which they identified violence toward women as a major community health concern. Mannina[67] used the model as the conceptual framework for a study to define an effective testing protocol for elementary school-aged children. Taggart and Mattson[113] surveyed white, Hispanic, and African-American women in public health and low-income clinics to determine whether battering during pregnancy resulted in a delay in seeking prenatal care. They found that women in the battered group sought care 6.5 weeks later than did women in the nonabused group, with a similar delay in each ethnic group. Wilson[120] used the comprehensive community health needs assessment based on the Neuman Systems Model to determine that cardiovascular disease was identified as the priority health concern among residents of a small Midwestern city.

The Neuman Systems Model is used effectively in advanced practice nursing.[6] Barker, Robinson, and Brautigan[7] used the model in evaluating whether psychiatric nurse home visits could decrease hospital readmission rates of patients with depression. They found a substantial reduction in readmissions in the group that received psychiatric nurse home follow-up. Dwyer, Walker, Suchman, and Coggiola[31] used it as the basis for a collaborative practice by nurse practitioners and physicians at the University of Rochester community nursing center. Hassell[47] integrated the Neuman Systems Model and medical perspectives to improve the management of depression by nurse practitioners. Martin[69] applied the model to the practice of nurse anesthesia using specific examples of the nurse anesthetist's role.

The model is being studied and applied in other disciplines, such as physical therapy.[9,114] Further research continues to validate its applicability beyond nursing.

Education

The model has been accepted in academic circles and is used widely as a curriculum guide oriented toward wellness. It is used at all levels of nursing education throughout the United States and in other countries, including Australia, Canada, Denmark, England, Korea, Kuwait, Portugal, Taiwan, Holland, and Japan.*

The model's wholistic perspective provides an effective framework for the education of generic nursing students from diploma, associate, and baccalaureate programs. Lowry and Newsome[66] reported on a study of 12 associate degree programs that use the model as a conceptual framework for curriculum development. The results indicated that graduates use the model most often in the roles of teacher and care provider and that they tend to continue practice from a Neuman Systems Model-based perspective following graduation.

Neuman's model has been selected for baccalaureate programs on the basis of its theoretical and comprehensive perspectives for a wholistic curriculum and of its potential for use with the individual, family, small groups, and community. Neuman College Division of Nursing was the first school to select the Neuman Systems Model as its conceptual base for its curriculum and approach to client care in 1976. The faculty has developed an assessment and intervention tool based on Neuman's framework and has developed clinical evaluation tools based on Neuman's model and Bondy's Evaluation Format.[66] Mirenda[72] has formulated a set of questions related to graduates' perceptions and continued use of the model. The University of Pittsburgh in Pennsylvania had one of the first baccalaureate nursing programs to implement the model in an integrated curriculum.[55,82] The model has been used at Lander University in Greenwood, South Carolina as the framework for baccalaureate nursing education since 1987.[40] Its selection by the faculty was based on its wholistic perspective and on its potential for use with community aggregate populations. The model is used as a comprehensive framework to organize data collected from maternity patients by undergraduate nursing students at the University of South Florida.[63] At the University of Texas-Tyler, the model is used as the unifying construct for the Bachelor of Science in Nursing program. Neuman's levels of prevention as intervention are used to level content in courses across the curriculum.[54] The Minnesota Intercollegiate Nursing Consortium (MINC), composed of

_____

*References 9, 56, 58, 76, 79, 89, 92.

three private church-related colleges, has developed a cooperative baccalaureate nursing program that uses the Neuman Systems Model as its organizing curriculum framework. Over time, MINC faculty have engaged in the evaluation of the utility of the model, affirming its value.[44]

The model has demonstrated its effectiveness in supporting the conceptual transition among levels of nursing education. Hilton and Grafton[48] discussed its application as the framework for the transition from diploma to associate degree education at the Los Angeles County Medical Center School of Nursing. Sipple and Freese[108] described the transition from associate degree to Neuman Systems Model-based baccalaureate education at Lander College in Greenwood, South Carolina. At the University of Tennessee at Martin, the model provided the curriculum framework for a Bachelor of Science in Nursing degree program initiated in 1988; Strickland-Seng[111] described its use as the basis for clinical evaluation of students in their Bachelor of Science in Nursing degree program.

The Neuman Systems Model has been used effectively in postbasic nursing education and beyond. Bunn[19] described the development and implementation of a community mental health nursing course based on Canadian healthcare principles for registered nurses enrolled in a Bachelor of Science in Nursing program at the University of Ottawa. The model enabled students to study selected client populations, such as elderly Chinese, as a high-risk aggregate and to plan culturally relevant health prevention activities at primary, secondary, and tertiary levels. Martin[69] stated that the transition of nurse anesthesia education into graduate nursing programs will require incorporation of advanced nursing theory and applied the Neuman Systems Model to the practice of nurse anesthesia.

Multidisciplinary use of the model continues to grow. For example, the model is currently being implemented beyond nursing in Kuwait and Jordan.[89] The model's emphasis on wholism, systems, prevention, and wellness prompted the Commission on Accreditation in Physical Therapy Education (CAPTE) to adapt it to conceptualize sections of the CAPTE evaluative criteria that address the organization and resources required for a physical therapy program.[114] Lowry, Burns, Smith, and Jacobson[64] described an interdisciplinary approach to training health professionals based on experiences with a multidisciplinary team of faculty from four disciplines.

The model's inclusion of both client perception and nurse perception makes it particularly relevant for teaching culture concepts. The model is used at California State University, Fresno to study the significance of culture and how culture influences each of the five client system variables.[110] Bloch and Bloch[13] described a format that uses the model to assist students to assess clients and provide culturally appropriate care across cultural barriers. Capers[22] stated that the model can foster the delivery of culturally relevant care because its wholistic perspective includes the cultural aspects of client systems.

The Neuman Systems Model is used to provide the conceptual framework for multiple levels of nursing and health-related curricula around the world. Acceptance by the nursing community is clearly evident.

Research

Testing the efficacy and usefulness of nursing models through controlled research is imperative for nursing to advance as a scientific discipline. Research on the components of the model for additional explication and generation of testable nursing theories through research are examples of the Neuman model's potential contribution to research activity and nursing knowledge.[35,36,73,101,103] Rules for Neuman Systems Model-based nursing research have been specified by Fawcett, a Neuman model trustee, based on the content of the model and related literature.[90]

Neuman[85,90] reports that her model is one of the three most frequently used models for nursing research. Increasing empirical use of the model is evident from research conducted in the nursing community. In the third edition of *The Neuman Systems Model*,[88] Louis[58,59,60] discussed the model's use in nursing research and identified recent published studies using the model. The third edition also contains an annotated bibliography of selected studies conducted from 1989 to 1993, with an appendix listing of research studies published in journals, dissertations, and masters' theses.

The Neuman Systems Model has provided the conceptual framework for recently published research on clients across the life span, on nurses and lay persons as caregivers, and on nursing education and administration. Additional research studies using the model are listed in the bibliography following this chapter.

Nursing research using the model has advanced the level of knowledge of women's health issues. Marlett[68] examined the history of breast-feeding experiences in women with breast cancer; the results supported previously reported risk factors for developing breast cancer. Monahan[74] studied 140 pregnant drug-using females to develop a profile of social and demographic characteristics, STD risk behaviors, and use of prenatal care and substance abuse treatment. Gigliotti[42] studied role stress in women who are both mothers and students and found that mothers-as-students experience multiple role stresses.

Several studies have been reported on the influence of ethnic differences on women's health and healthcare needs.[75] Doherty[30] explored spousal abuse from an African-American female perspective; the results identified five stages of abuse and coping. The five stages were: (1) transference of rules, when the victim learns rules of intimate behavior from her family of origin; (2) beginning abusive period, when the couple has begun living together and violence begins; (3) rage and reality, when attempts to stop the violence have failed and anger predominates; (4) transition, when the victim leaves the relationship; (5) stabilization and integration, when the victim stabilizes her life. Jennings[51] explored predictors of intention to obtain pap smears in African-American and Hispanic women. Hanson[46] studied beliefs about smoking behavior in African-American, Puerto Rican, and white women. The findings indicated differences between smokers and nonsmokers and some differences among ethnic groups. Taggart and Mattson[113] studied the impact of battering on seeking prenatal care in white American, Hispanic, and African-American women. They found that the incidence of abuse was not significantly different among the ethnic groups and women in the battered group sought prenatal care 6.5 weeks later than did women in the nonabused group.

The model has been used extensively to guide research to enhance the nursing care of clients with specific physiological stressors.[29,32,53] Flannery[39] reported a study using the model as a framework to adapt a cognitive functioning assessment tool for patients with traumatic brain injury; the purpose is to provide a tool for planning appropriate nursing care. Bowman[14] studied pain and sleep in elderly orthopedic surgery patients within the context of the surgery experience (as planned or unplanned).

The aging population and the shift from hospital-based care to home-based care has resulted in the need for research on the stressors and special needs of caregivers of the patients who require complex care in nonhospital settings. Researchers have used the model to study selected variables in the caregivers of dependent elderly[96] and in patients with traumatic head injury[52] and hepatoma.[57]

The biennial Neuman Systems Model Symposia provides a forum for presentation of research (completed and in progress) using the model.[26,27,45] At the sixth (1997) and seventh (1999) symposia, five studies were reported on women's health issues.[11,20,43,65,74] Four studies were reported on use of the model in nursing education.[1,5,10,24] Two studies were reported that dealt with nursing management issues[4,25] and two on chronic illness management and long-term care.[17,18] In response to earlier identification of the spiritual variable as an area for further development, five studies on this component of the model were reported.* Research projects that were reported at the fourth (1993) and fifth (1995) symposia are cited in the previous edition of this chapter.

Fawcett[37] has set forth guidelines for research studies based on the Neuman Systems Model. Synthesizing the results of such studies will increase understanding of the model's effectiveness in enhancing client system stability.

*References 9, 61, 95, 99, 118, 119.

FURTHER DEVELOPMENT

A conceptual model identifies relevant phenomena and describes the interrelationships in general and abstract terms, representing the initial step in the development of theoretical statements.[38] In 1983, the Neuman Systems Model was described as being at a very early stage of theory development.[117] However, findings from Louis and Koertvelyessy's 1987 study[62] and from subsequent research[16,36] support increasing utility of the model for theory development in nursing.

The model diagram has remained unchanged because Neuman has received continuous positive feedback on its completeness. The breadth of the model appeals to those in nursing because it allows for much creativity within its structure.[86]

Most nursing models have not been researched sufficiently to establish their validity fully. Although the Neuman Systems Model has proved itself empirically, additional research is indicated to clarify and validate several components of the model.

Earlier evaluation of the model stated that two components needed further development: (1) the spiritual variable and (2) the created environment.[9] Neuman views the spiritual variable as an innate component of the basic structure; consideration of the spiritual variable is necessary for a wholistic perspective and for caring concern for the client.[88] Description of the spiritual variable was expanded significantly in *The Neuman Systems Model,* third edition,[28,41] and more recent research studies were reported at the Seventh and Eighth Neuman Systems Model Symposia.

Neuman's concept of health and her view of the relationship between client and environment are two of the areas identified for further development and clarification. Fawcett[37] suggests clarification of the concept of health by identification of wellness and illness as polar ends of a continuum rather than as dichotomous conditions. Further, Fawcett[37] states that viewing client-environment interactions as a dynamic equilibrium, as a steady state, and as homeostasis is logically incompatible and that Neuman should specify which view best represents her conceptualization of client-environment interaction.

Further research is also indicated regarding the lines of defense and resistance, vulnerable aggregate client populations, providing culturally sensitive nursing care across cultural barriers, and development and evaluation of primary prevention programs.[80,81,82,89]

Future validity of the model depends on extending the development and testing of middle-range theory from the model. Neuman and Koertvelyessy[37] have identified two theories being generated from the model: (1) the Theory of Optimal Client System Stability and (2) the Theory of Prevention as Intervention. Breckenridge[16] has described the use of the model to develop middle-range theory through research based on practice with nephrology patients.

A Neuman Systems Model Trustee Group was established in 1988 to preserve, protect, and perpetuate the integrity of the model for the future of nursing. Its international members, personally selected by Neuman, are dedicated professionals.[82] The home of the Neuman Archives has been established at Neumann College Library at Aston, Pennsylvania.[71,72] Smith and Edgil[109] have proposed the creation of an Institute for the Study of the Neuman Systems Model to formulate and test theories within the model. A website has been placed on the Internet on the Neumann College home page at www. neumann.edu, Undergraduate Programs, Nursing.

CRITIQUE

Neuman developed a comprehensive nursing conceptual model that operationalizes systems concepts for nursing relevant to the breadth of nursing phenomena. It should also remain relevant to future nursing needs as identified by the American Nurses Association and the World Health Organization. The model's wholistic perspective allows for a wide range of nurse creativity in its use. Neuman's own critique notes that prior criticisms, such as those claiming its concepts are too broad, have been discounted. The model is congruent with the general trend toward wholistic systemic thinking in nursing. Its comprehensive and flexible nature will allow for future structuring of all nursing activities "as it has proven to do in the past."[86]

Clarity

Neuman presents abstract concepts that are familiar to nurses. The model's concepts of client, environment, health, and nursing are congruent with traditional nursing values. Concepts defined by Neuman and those borrowed from other disciplines are used consistently throughout the model.

Simplicity

Multiple interactions and interrelationships comprise this broad systems-based model; they are organized in a complex, yet logical manner and variables tend to overlap to some degree. The concepts coalesce, but a loss of theoretical meaning would occur if they were completely separated. Neuman[82] states that the concepts can be separated for analysis, specific goal setting, and interventions. The model can be used to delineate further the systems concept for nursing and also to describe various other healthcare systems. It can be used to explain the client's dynamic state of equilibrium and the reaction or possible reaction to stressors. Using the prevention concept within the framework, the origin of stressors can be predicted. The model can be used to describe, explain, or predict nursing phenomena. The model is complex in nature; therefore it cannot be described as a simple framework, yet nurses using the model describe it as easy to understand and use across cultures and in a wide variety of practice settings.

Generality

The Neuman Systems Model has been used in a wide variety of nursing situations; it is readily adaptable and comprehensive enough to be useful in all healthcare settings, including administration and research. Other related health fields can use this framework because it is systemic and it emphasizes the client system as a whole. The social goals and utility of the model are congruent with present social values (for example, wholistic care, prevention, and systems concepts).

Some concepts are broad and represent the phenomena of one person as a client or a larger system

and others are more definitive and identify specific modes of action, such as primary prevention. The subgoals can be identified as broad nursing actions. The broad scope of this model allows it to be considered general enough to be useful to nurses and other healthcare professionals in working with individuals, families, groups, or communities in all healthcare settings.

Empirical Precision

Although the model has not been completely tested to date, nursing scientists are demonstrating major interest in and use of the model to guide nursing research. Early work by Hoffman[49] described a list of variables and selected operational definitions that were derived from the model. Louis and Koertvelyessy's 1989 survey[62] on the use of the model in nursing research and subsequent research reports provides further documentation of increasing empiricism with the model. Continued testing and refinement will increase the model's empirical precision as the research process, analysis, and synthesis of findings from multiple studies are completed.[43]

Derivable Consequences

Neuman's conceptual model provides the professional nurse with important guidelines for assessment of the client system, utilization of the nursing process, and implementation of preventive intervention. The focus on primary prevention and interdisciplinary care facilities is futuristic and improves quality of care. The Neuman nursing process fulfills current health mandates by involving the client actively in negotiating the goals of nursing care.[86]

Another derivable consequence of the model is its potential to generate nursing theory; for example, the theories of optimal client stability and prevention as intervention.[37] The model concepts are relevant to twenty-first century health professional trends. Through continued theory development and research with the model, nursing can expand its scientific knowledge. According to Fawcett,[33,34,37] the model meets social considerations of congruence, significance, and utility. The model is broad and systemically based. It lends itself well to a comprehensive view within which nursing can be responsive to the world's rapidly changing healthcare needs.

The Neuman Systems Model provides an appropriate nursing framework and a comprehensive approach to contemporary and future goal phenomena and concerns facing nursing and healthcare delivery in the twenty-first century.[73] A Trustee member, Linda Drew (now deceased), wrote a letter to Neuman, which appropriately draws closure to this chapter and shares some of the excitement that is felt as the nursing profession advances the scientific foundation of its knowledge base:

> In my opinion, the Neuman model is not only alive and well, but will have a very long shelf life because it is so adaptable and continues to provide a very pragmatic framework for dealing with a whole host of issues in nursing practice, education, administration and research. This along with the bold commitment of nurses and other healthcare providers to continue using this framework will guarantee a very healthy, exciting future for the model.[21:4,89]

CRITICAL THINKING *Activities*

1. **Case study:** Martina is a middle-aged Hispanic woman who brings her family to a local free clinic to obtain medical care. She works part time in a restaurant for minimum wage. She lives in a small apartment with her daughter and four preschool children; her daughter is not employed. Martina and her daughter speak only very broken English. Martina's medical diagnoses are hypertension, arthritis, and depression. Use the Neuman Systems Model as a conceptual framework to respond:
   - Describe the family as a system.
   - How does the dominant Anglo culture impact on the family's stability as a system?
   - What stressors (actual and potential) threaten the family?

   - What additional assessment data are needed related to Martina's medical diagnoses?
   - Related to the family's health status?
   - How will cultural differences influence planning for prevention as intervention at primary, secondary, and tertiary levels?

2. **Organizational planning:** Use the Neuman Systems Model as a conceptual framework to analyze your employing organization and to support organizational planning:
   - What is the basic structure (core)? What factors in the lines of resistance support the status quo? What factors in the lines of defense support healthy organizational functioning?
   - What stressors can you identify that may disrupt the system and result in organizational change?
   - What is the employees' perception of goals that would be appropriate for this change?
   - What is the administration's perception of goals that would be appropriate for this change?
   - If these perceptions differ, how can the differences be resolved for mutual goal setting that will be beneficial for the organization?
   - What prevention as intervention strategies will support the organization in making the changes successfully?

3. **Patient care conference:** Organize a patient care conference in your workplace to deal with a patient situation that has been difficult to manage. Involve caregivers from nursing and at least one other discipline to discuss each of the following, using the Neuman Systems Model as a conceptual framework:
   - What factors comprise the patient's normal and flexible lines of defense and lines of resistance?
   - What stressors are causing the problem(s) with this patient? What is the patient's re-

action to the stressors? What is each discipline's perspective on the problems or issues that are involved?

- How is the situation influenced by the patient's family system? By the patient's environment?
- What would be the *ideal* outcome to this situation from each discipline's perspective? From the patient's perspective?
- What goals would be appropriate to negotiate with the patient?
- What primary, secondary, and tertiary prevention-as-interventions would support attainment of these goals?

REFERENCES

1. Agren, C., Froistedt, M., & Olsson, H. (1999, April). *Identifying stress in trainee psychiatric care nurses using the Neuman systems model.* Paper presented at the Seventh Biennial Neuman Systems Model Symposium, Vancouver, BC.
2. Anderson, E., McFarland, J., & Helton, A. (1986). Community-as-client: A model for practice. *Nursing Outlook,* 34(5), 220-224.
3. Babcock, P. (1984, June 10). Telephone interview.
4. Backe, H. & Olsson, H. (1997, March). *Stressors which might affect supervision in nursing practice using the Neuman systems model as reference.* Paper presented at the Sixth Biennial International Neuman Systems Model Symposium, Boston, MA.
5. Backe, H. & Olsson, H. (1999, April). *Stress amongst student nurses: An application of the Neuman systems model.* Paper presented at the Seventh Biennial Neuman Systems Model Symposium, Vancouver, BC.
6. Baker, N.A. (1982). Use of the Neuman model in planning for the psychological needs of the respiratory disease patient. In B. Neuman (Ed.), *The Neuman systems model: Application to nursing education and practice* (pp. 241-256). Norwalk, CT: Appleton-Century-Crofts.
7. Barker, E., Robinson, D., & Brautigan, R. (1999). The effect of psychiatric home nurse follow-up on readmission rates of patients with depression. *Journal of American Psychiatric Nurses Association,* 5(4), 111-6.
8. Barnes, K.M. (1993, April). *The relationship between mistreatment of the elderly, quality of care, and demographic characteristics.* Paper presented at the Fourth International Neuman Systems Model Symposium, Rochester, NY.
9. Beckman, S.J., Boxley-Harges, S., Bruick-Sorge, C., Harris, S.M., Hermiz, M.E., Meininger, M., & Steinkeler, S.E. (1994). Betty Neuman systems model. In A. Marriner Tomey (Ed.), *Nursing theorists and their work* (3rd ed., pp. 269-304). St. Louis: Mosby.
10. Beckman, S.J. & Bruick-Sorge, C. (1997, March). *Assessment of program outcomes: A longitudinal study using the Neuman systems model.* Paper presented at the Sixth Biennial International Neuman Systems Model Symposium, Boston, MA.
11. Bemker, M. & Edgil, A. (1997, March). *Adolescent female substance abuse: Risk and resiliency factors.* Paper presented at the Sixth Biennial International Neuman Systems Model Symposium, Boston, MA.
12. Black, P., Deeny, P., & McKenna, H. (1997). Sensoristrain: An exploration of nursing interventions in the context of the Neuman systems theory. *Intensive and Critical Care Nursing,* 13(5), 249-258.
13. Bloch, C. & Bloch, C. (1995). Teaching content and process of the Neuman systems model. In B. Neuman (Ed.), *The Neuman systems model* (3rd ed., pp. 175-182). Norwalk, CT: Appleton & Lange.
14. Bowman, A.M. (1997). Sleep satisfaction, perceived pain and acute confusion in elderly clients undergoing orthopaedic procedures. *Journal of Advanced Nursing,* 26(3), 550-64.
15. Breckenridge, D. (1992). A brief update on the Neuman systems model. *Neuman News,* 3(1), 2.
16. Breckenridge, D.M. (1995). Nephrology practice and directions for nursing research. In B. Neuman (Ed.), *The Neuman systems model* (3rd ed., pp. 499-507). Norwalk, CT: Appleton & Lange.
17. Breckenridge, D.M. (1997, March). *Clients' perceptions of why, how, and by whom treatment modality was chosen.* Paper presented at the Sixth Biennial International Neuman Systems Model Symposium, Boston, MA.
18. Breckenridge, D.M. (1999, April). *Patient participation in treatment decisions for prostate cancer.* Paper presented at the Seventh Biennial Neuman Systems Model Symposium, Vancouver, BC.
19. Bunn, H. (1995). Preparing nurses for the challenge of the new focus on community mental health nursing. *The Journal of Continuing Education in Nursing,* 26(2), 55-59.
20. Cagle, R.H. (1997, March). *The relationship between health care provider advice and the initiation of breast-feeding.* Paper presented at the Sixth Biennial International Neuman Systems Model Symposium, Boston, MA.
21. Capers, C. (Ed.). (1992). The Neuman Trustee Group, Inc. *Neuman News,* 3(1), 1-8.

22. Capers, C.F. (1996). The Neuman systems model: A culturally relevant perspective. *ABNF Journal, 7*(5), 113-7.

23. Caplan, G. (1964). *Principles of preventive psychiatry.* New York: Basic Books.

24. Carras, C. & Olsson, H. (1999, April). *Exploratory study of student nurse attitudes to humor using Neuman systems model analysis.* Paper presented at the Seventh Biennial Neuman Systems Model Symposium, Vancouver, BC.

25. Chiverton, P. & Cornwell, C. (1997, March). *Bridging the gap between psychiatric hospitalization and community care: A Neuman systems model pilot project.* Paper presented at the Sixth Biennial International Neuman Systems Model Symposium, Boston, MA.

26. Craig, D. (1993, April). *An interdisciplinary high risk assessment tool for older adults' use of nursing services, life stress, ways of coping and health, mood and energy for living.* Paper presented at the Fourth International Neuman Systems Model Symposium, Rochester, NY.

27. Craig, D. & Timmings, C. (1995, Feb.). *Health promotion for older adults: Does it make a difference?* Paper presented at the Fifth International Neuman Systems Model Symposium, Orlando, FL.

28. Curran, G. (1995). The Neuman systems model revisited. In B. Neuman (Ed.), *The Neuman systems model* (3rd ed., pp. 93-99). Norwalk, CT: Appleton & Lange.

29. Darland, W. (1986). Congenital adrenocortical hyperplasia: Supportive nursing interventions. *Journal of Pediatric Nursing,* 1(2):117-123.

30. Doherty, D.C. (1997). Spousal abuse: An African-American female perspective. *Dissertations Abstracts International,* 58, 04B, 1798.

31. Dwyer, C.M., Walker, P.H., Suchman, A., & Coggiola, P. (1995). Opportunities and obstacles: Development of a true collaborative practice with physicians. In B. Murphy (Ed.), *Nursing centers: The time is now* (pp. 134-55, NLN Pub. No. 41-2629). New York: National League for Nursing.

32. Echlin, J.D. (1982). Palliative care and the Neuman model. In B. Neuman (Ed.), *The Neuman systems model: Application to nursing education and practice* (pp. 257-259). Norwalk, CT: Appleton-Century-Crofts.

33. Fawcett, J. (1989). *Analysis and evaluation of conceptual models of nursing.* Philadelphia: F.A. Davis.

34. Fawcett, J. (1989). Analysis and evaluation of conceptual models of nursing (2nd ed., pp. 172-177). Philadelphia: F.A. Davis.

35. Fawcett, J. (1990, Nov.). *Neuman systems model: Directions for research.* Keynote address presented at the Third International Neuman Systems Model Symposium, Dayton, OH.

36. Fawcett, J. (1995). Constructing conceptual-theoretical-empirical structures for research. In B. Neuman (Ed.), *The Neuman systems model* (3rd ed., pp. 459-471). Norwalk, CT: Appleton & Lange.

37. Fawcett, J. (1995). *Neuman's systems model: Analysis and evaluation of conceptual models of nursing* (3rd ed., pp. 217-275). Philadelphia: F.A. Davis.

38. Fawcett, J., Carpenito, L.J., Efinger, J., Goldblum-Graff, D., Groesbeck, M., Lowry, L.W., McCreary, C.S., & Wolf, Z.R. (1982). A framework for analysis and evaluation of conceptual models of nursing with an analysis of the Neuman systems model. In B. Neuman (Ed.), *The Neuman systems model: Application to nursing education and practice* (pp. 30-43). Norwalk, CT: Appleton-Century-Crofts.

39. Flannery, J. (1995). Cognitive assessment in the acute care setting: Reliability and validity of the levels of cognitive function assessment scale (LOCFAS). *Journal of Nursing Measurement,* 3(1), 43-58.

40. Freese, B.T. & Lander University Faculty (1995, Feb.). *Application of the Neuman systems model to education: Baccalaureate workshop.* Paper presented at the Fifth International Neuman Systems Model Symposium, Orlando, FL.

41. Fulton, R.A.B. (1995). The spiritual variable: Essential to the client system. In B. Neuman (Ed.), *The Neuman systems model* (3rd ed., pp. 77-92). Norwalk, CT: Appleton & Lange.

42. Gigliotti, E. (1997, March). *The relations among maternal and student role involvement, perceived social support and perceived multiple role stress in mothers attending college: A study based on Betty Neuman's systems model.* Paper presented at the Sixth Biennial International Neuman Systems Model Symposium, Boston, MA.

43. Gigliotti, E. (1999). Women's multiple role stress: Testing Neuman's flexible line of defense. *Nursing Science Quarterly,* 12(1), 36-44.

44. Glazebrook, D.S. (1995). The Neuman systems model in cooperative baccalaureate nursing education: The Minnesota Intercollegiate Nursing Consortium experience. In B. Neuman (Ed.), *The Neuman systems model* (3rd ed., pp. 227-230). Norwalk, CT: Appleton & Lange.

45. Hamilton, E.M. & Schwieterman, I. (1995, Feb.). *The Neuman systems model in research data integration.* Paper presented at the Fifth International Neuman Systems Model Symposium, Orlando, FL.

46. Hanson, M.J.S. (1999). Cross-cultural study of beliefs about smoking among teenaged females . . . including commentary by Laffrey S.C. with author response. *Western Journal of Nursing Research,* 21(5), 635-51.

47. Hassell, J.S. (1996). Improved management of depression through nursing model application and critical thinking. *Journal of the American Academy of Nurse Practitioners, 8*(4), 161-6.

48. Hilton, S.A. & Grafton, M.D. (1995). Curriculum transition based on the Neuman systems model: Los Angeles County Medical Center School of Nursing. In B. Neuman (Ed.), *The Neuman systems model* (3rd ed., pp. 163-174). Norwalk, CT: Appleton & Lange.

49. Hoffman, M.K. (1982). From model to theory construction: An analysis of the Neuman health-care system model. In B. Neuman (Ed.), *The Neuman systems model: Application to nursing education and practice* (pp. 44-54). Norwalk, CT: Appleton-Century-Crofts.

50. Issel, L.M. (1995). Evaluating case management programs. *Maternal/Child Nursing Journal, 29,* 67-74.

51. Jennings, K.M. (1997). Predicting intention to obtain a pap smear among African-American and Latina women. *Dissertation Abstracts International,* 58-07B, 3557.

52. Jones, W.R. (1996). Stressors in the primary caregivers of traumatic head injured persons. *AXON,* 18(1), 9-11.

53. Kiernan, B.S. & Scoloveno, M.A. (1986). Assessment of the neonate. *Topics in Clinical Nursing,* 8(1), 1-10.

54. Klotz, L.D. (1995). Integration of the Neuman systems model into the BNS curriculum at the University of Texas at Tyler. In B. Neuman (Ed.), *The Neuman systems model* (3rd ed., pp. 183-190). Norwalk, CT: Appleton & Lange.

55. Knox, J.E., Kilchenstein, L., & Yakulis, I.M. (1982). Utilization of the Neuman model in an integrated baccalaureate program: University of Pittsburgh. In B. Neuman (Ed.), *The Neuman systems model: Application to nursing education and practice* (pp. 117-124). Norwalk, CT: Appleton-Century-Crofts.

56. Lebold, M.M. & Davis, L.H. (1982). A baccalaureate nursing curriculum based on the Neuman systems model: Saint Xavier College. In B. Neuman (Ed.), *The Neuman systems model: Application to nursing education and practice* (pp. 124-129). Norwalk, CT: Appleton-Century-Crofts.

57. Lin, M., Ku, N., Leu, J., Chen, J., & Lin, L. (1996). An exploration of the stress aspects, coping behaviors, health status, and related aspects in family caregivers of hepatoma patients. *Nursing Research (China),* 4(2), 171-85.

58. Louis, M. (1988, Jan. 10). Personal communication.

59. Louis, M. (1995). The Neuman model in nursing research: An update. In B. Neuman (Ed.), *The Neuman systems model* (3rd ed., pp. 473-495). Norwalk, CT: Appleton-Lange.

60. Louis, M. (1995, Feb.). *Preferred other relationships, perceived health, and quality of life of elders.* Paper presented at the Fifth International Neuman Systems Model Symposium, Orlando, FL.

61. Louis, M. & Alpert, P. (1999, April). *Comparison of nurses' use of spirituality to Neuman systems model concepts.* Paper presented at the Seventh Biennial Neuman Systems Model Symposium, Vancouver, BC.

62. Louis, M. & Koertvelyessy, A. (1989). Neuman model: Use in research. In B. Neuman (Ed.), *The Neuman systems model* (2nd ed., pp. 93-114). Norwalk, CT: Appleton & Lange.

63. Lowry, L. (1992, June 4). Personal communication.

64. Lowry, L.W., Burns, C.M., Smith, A.A., & Jacobson, H. (2000). Compete or complement? An interdisciplinary approach to training health professionals. *Nursing and Health Care Perspectives,* 21(2), 76-80.

65. Lowry, L.W., Callahan, A., Tapas, D., & Philippi, T. (1999, April). *Development of a model for delivery of improved prenatal care: Phase 2.* Paper presented at the Seventh Biennial Neuman Systems Model Symposium, Vancouver, BC.

66. Lowry, L.W. & Newsome, G.G. (1995). Neuman-based associate degree programs: Past, present, and future. In B. Neuman (Ed.), *The Neuman systems model* (3rd ed., pp. 197-214). Norwalk, CT: Appleton & Lange.

67. Mannina, J. (1997). Finding an effective hearing testing protocol to identify hearing loss and middle ear disease in school-aged children. *Journal of School Nursing,* 13(5), 23-8.

68. Marlett, L.A. (1998). The breast feeding practices of women with a history of breast cancer. *Masters Abstracts International,* 37-04, 1180.

69. Martin, S.A. (1996). Applying nursing theory to the practice of nurse anesthesia. *American Association of Nurse Anesthetists Journal,* 64(4), 369-372.

70. Mirenda, R. (1988, Jan. 10). Personal communication.

71. Mirenda, R. (1992, March 17). Personal communication.

72. Mirenda, R. (1992, June 16). Personal communication.

73. Mirenda, R.M. (1986). The Neuman systems model: Description and application. In P. Winstead-Fry (Ed.), *Case studies in nursing theory* (pp. 127-167). New York: National League for Nursing.

74. Monahan, G.L. (1996). A profile of pregnant drug-using female arrestees in California: The relationships among sociodemographic characteristics, reproductive and drug addiction histories, HIV/STD risk behaviors, and utilization of prenatal care services and substance abuse programs. *Dissertations Abstracts International,* 57, 09B, 5576.

75. Monahan, G., Anglin, M.D., Lewis, M.A., & Annon, K. (1997, March). *Profile of pregnant drug using female arrestees in California.* Paper presented at the Sixth Biennial International Neuman Systems Model Symposium, Boston, MA.

76. Moxley, P.A. & Allen, M.H. (1982). The Neuman systems model approach in a master's degree program: Northwestern State University. In B. Neuman (Ed.), *The Neuman systems model: Application to nursing education and practice* (pp. 168-175). Norwalk, CT: Appleton-Century-Crofts.

77. Neuman, B. (1977, Jan.). *An explanation of the Betty Neuman nursing model.* Paper presented at Indiana University-Purdue University at Fort Wayne, IN.

78. Neuman, B. (1982). *The Neuman systems model: Application to nursing education and practice.* Norwalk, CT: Appleton-Century-Crofts.

79. Neuman, B. (1983). Curriculum vitae.

80. Neuman, B. (1984, June 3). Personal communication.

81. Neuman, B. (1988, Jan. 10). Personal communication.

82. Neuman, B. (1988, Jan. 20). Personal communication.

83. Neuman, B. (1989). *The Neuman systems model* (2nd ed.). Norwalk, CT: Appleton & Lange.

84. Neuman, B. (1992, March). *Current status of the Neuman systems model.* Paper presented at Neuman Systems Model Theory Conference, Toledo, OH.

85. Neuman, B. (1992, June 17). Personal communication.

86. Neuman, B. (1992, June 21). Personal communication.

87. Neuman, B. (1995). In conclusion—Toward new beginnings. In B. Neuman (Ed.), *The Neuman systems model* (3rd ed., pp. 671-703). Norwalk, CT: Appleton & Lange.

88. Neuman, B. (1995). *The Neuman systems model* (3rd ed.). Norwalk, CT: Appleton & Lange.

89. Neuman, B. (1996, July 18). Personal communication.

90. Neuman, B. (1996). The Neuman systems model in research and practice. *Nursing Science Quarterly,* 9(2), 67-70.

91. Neuman, B. (2000, July 19). Personal communication.

92. Neuman, B., Deloughery, G.W., & Gebbie, M. (1971). *Consultation and community organization in community mental health nursing.* Baltimore: Williams & Wilkins.

93. Neuman, B. & Young, R.J. (1972, May/June). A model for teaching total person approach to patient problems. *Nursing Research,* 21, 264-269.

94. Perls, F. (1973). *The Gestalt approach: Eye witness to therapy.* Palo Alto, CA: Science and Behavior Books.

95. Peterson, G.A. (1999, April). *Nursing perceptions of the spiritual dimensions of patient care: The Neuman systems model in curricular formations.* Paper presented at the Seventh Biennial Neuman Systems Model Symposium, Vancouver, BC.

96. Picot, S.J.F., Zauszniewski, J.A., Debanne, S.M., & Holston, E.C. (1999). Mood and blood pressure in black female caregivers and noncaregivers. *Nursing Research,* 48(3), 150-61.

97. Reynolds, P.D. (1971). *A primer in theory construction.* Indianapolis: Bobbs-Merrill.

98. Picton, C.E. (1995). An explanation of family-centered care in Neuman's model with regard to the care of the critically ill adult in an accident and emergency setting. *Accident and Emergency Nursing,* 3, 33-37.

99. Potter, M.L. (1997, March). *Spirituality, learned resourcefulness, and health perception in the older adult with a chronic illness.* Paper presented at the Sixth Biennial International Neuman Systems Model Symposium, Boston, MA.

100. Reed, K.S. (1993). Adapting the Neuman systems model for family nursing. *Nursing Science Quarterly,* 6(2), 93-97.

101. Ross, M.M. & Bourbannais, F.F. (1985). The Neuman systems model in nursing practice: A case study approach. *Journal of Advanced Nursing,* 10, 199-207.

102. Rowles, C.J. (1993, April). *The relationship between selected personal and organizational variables and the tenure of directors in nursing homes.* Paper presented at the Fourth International Neuman Systems Model Symposium, Rochester, NY.

103. Russell, J. (1988, Jan. 10). Personal communication.

104. Schlentz, M.D. (1993). The minimum data set and levels of prevention in the long term care facility. *Geriatric Nursing,* 14, 79-83.

105. Schlentz, M.D. (1993, April). *The Neuman systems model in long term care.* Paper presented at the Fourth International Neuman Systems Model Symposium, Rochester, NY.

106. Schwieterman, I., Hamilton, E.M., & Braun, J.W. (1995, Feb.). *The Neuman systems model as a framework for describing physical mobility among the elderly.* Paper presented at the Fifth International Neuman Systems Model Symposium, Orlando, FL.

107. Selye, H. (1974). *Stress without distress.* Philadelphia: J.B. Lippincott.

108. Sipple, J.A. & Freese, B.T. (1989). Transition from technical to professional level education. In B. Neuman (Ed.), *The Neuman systems model* (2nd ed., pp. 193-200). Norwalk, CT: Appleton & Lange.

109. Smith, M.C. & Edgil, A.E. (1995). Future directions for research with the Neuman systems model. In B. Neuman (Ed.), *The Neuman systems model* (3rd ed., pp. 509-517). Norwalk, CT: Appleton & Lange.

110. Stittich, E.M., Flores, F.C., & Nuttall, P. (1995). Cultural considerations in a Neuman-based curriculum. In B. Neuman (Ed.), *The Neuman systems model* (3rd ed., pp. 147-162). Norwalk, CT: Appleton & Lange.

111. Strickland-Seng, V. (1995). The Neuman systems model in clinical evaluation of students. In B. Neuman (Ed.), *The Neuman systems model* (3rd ed., pp. 215-223). Norwalk, CT: Appleton & Lange.

112. Sullivan, J. (1986). Using Neuman's model in the acute phase of spinal cord injury. *Focus on Critical Care,* 13(5), 34-41.

113. Taggart, L. & Mattson, S. (1996). Delay in prenatal care as a result of battering in pregnancy: Cross-cultural implications. *Health Care for Women International,* 17(1), 25-34.

114. Toot, J.L. & Schmull, B.J. (1995). The Neuman systems model and physical therapy educational curricula. In B. Neuman (Ed.), *The Neuman systems model* (3rd ed., pp. 231-246). Norwalk, CT: Appleton & Lange.

115. Torres, G. (1986). *Theoretical foundations of nursing.* Norwalk, CT: Appleton-Century-Crofts.

116. Von Bertalanffy, L. (1968). *General system theory.* New York: George Braziller.

117. Walker, L.O. & Avant, K. (1983). *Strategies for theory construction in nursing.* Norwalk, CT: Appleton-Century-Crofts.

118. Weber, R.C. & Carrigg, K.C. (1997, March). *The spiritual care scale: Measurement of the spiritual variable.* Paper presented at the Sixth Biennial International Neuman Systems Model Symposium, Boston, MA.

119. Westrick, G.J. (1999, April). *Addiction and spiritual well being in the health perspective of the Neuman systems model.* Paper presented at the Seventh Biennial Neuman Systems Model Symposium, Vancouver, BC.

120. Wilson, L.C. (2000). Implementation and evaluation of church-based health fairs. *Journal of Community Nursing,* 17(1), 39-48.

121. World Health Organization & United Nations Children's Fund. (1978). *Primary health care: A joint report.* Geneva: World Health Organization.

BIBLIOGRAPHY
Primary Sources
Books

Neuman, B. (1982). *The Neuman systems model: Application to nursing education and practice.* Norwalk, CT: Appleton-Century-Crofts.

Neuman B. (1989). *The Neuman systems model* (2nd ed.). Norwalk, CT: Appleton & Lange.

Neuman B. (1995). *The Neuman systems model* (3rd ed.). Norwalk, CT: Appleton & Lange.

Neuman, B., Deloughery, G.W., & Gebbie, M. (1971). *Consultation and community organization in community mental health nursing.* Baltimore: Williams & Wilkins.

Neuman, B.M. & Walker, P.H. (1996). *Blueprint for use of nursing models: Education, research, practice, and administration.* New York: National League for Nursing Press.

Book Chapters

Neuman, B. (1974). The Betty Neuman health care systems model: A total person approach to patient problems. In J.P. Riehl & C. Roy (Eds.), *Conceptual models for nursing practice* (pp. 94-104). New York: Appleton-Century-Crofts.

Neuman, B. (1980). The Betty Neuman health care systems model: A total person approach to patient problems. In J.P. Riehl & C. Roy (Eds.), *Conceptual models for nursing practice* (pp. 119-134). New York: Appleton-Century-Crofts.

Neuman, B. (1983). Analysis and application of Neuman's health care model. In I.W. Clements & F.B. Roberts (Eds.), *Family health: A theoretical approach to nursing care* (pp. 239-254, 353-367). New York: John Wiley & Sons.

Neuman, B. (1986). The Neuman systems model explanation: Its relevance to emerging trends toward wholism in nursing. In I.B. Engberg & K. Kuld (Eds.), *Omvårdnad 1986* [Nursing Care Book]. Omvårdnad's Forum HB. Mullsjö: Sweden.

Neuman, B. (1989). The Neuman nursing process format: Adapted to a family case study. In J.P. Riehl & C. Roy (Eds.), *Conceptual models for nursing practice* (pp. 49-62). Norwalk, CT: Appleton & Lange.

Neuman B. (1989). The Neuman nursing process format: Family. In J.P. Riehl-Sisca (Ed.), *Conceptual models for nursing practice* (3rd ed., pp. 49-62). Norwalk, CT: Appleton & Lange.

Neuman, B. (1990). The Neuman systems model: A theory for practice. In M.E. Parker (Ed.), *Nursing theories in practice* (pp. 24-26). New York: National League for Nursing.

Neuman, B. (1995). In conclusion—Toward new beginnings. In B. Neuman (Ed.), *The Neuman systems model* (3rd ed., pp. 671-703). Norwalk, CT: Appleton & Lange.

Neuman, B. (1995). The Neuman systems model. In B. Neuman (Ed.), *The Neuman systems model* (3rd ed., pp. 3-62). Norwalk, CT: Appleton & Lange.

Neuman, B. & Wyatt, M. (1980). The Neuman stress/adaptation systems approach to education for nurse administrators. In J.P. Riehl & C. Roy (Eds.), *Conceptual models for nursing practice* (2nd ed., pp. 142-150). New York: Appleton-Century-Crofts.

Journal Articles

Neuman, B. (1985, Sept.). The Neuman Systems Model: Its importance for nursing. *Senior Nurse*, 3, 3.

Neuman, B. (1990). Health: A continuum based on the Neuman systems model. *Nursing Science Quarterly*, 3, 129-135.

Neuman, B. (1996). The Neuman systems model in research and practice. *Nursing Science Quarterly*, 9(2), 67-70.

Neuman, B., Chadwick, P.L., Beynon, C.E., Craig, D.M., Fawcett, J., Chang, N.J., Freese, B.T., & Hinton-Walker, P. (1997). The Neuman systems model: Reflections and projections. *Nursing Science Quarterly*, 10(1), 18-21.

Neuman, B.M., Deloughery, G.W., & Gebbie, K.M. (1970, Jan./Feb.). Levels of utilization: Nursing specialists in community mental health. *Journal of Psychiatric Nursing and Mental Health Services*, 8(1), 37-39.

Neuman, B.M., Deloughery, G.W., & Gebbie, K.M. (1970). Changes in problem solving ability among nurses receiving mental health consultation: A pilot study. *Communicating Nursing Research*, 3, 41-52.

Neuman, B.M., Deloughery, G.W., & Gebbie, K.M. (1971, Oct.). Nurses in community mental health: An informative interpretation for employees of professional nurses. *Public Personnel Review*, 32(4).

Neuman, B.M., Deloughery, G.W., & Gebbie, K.M. (1972, Feb.). Mental health consultation as a means of improving problem solving ability in work groups: A pilot study. *Comparative Group Studies*, 3(1), 81-97.

Neuman, B., Deloughery, G.W., & Gebbie, K.M. (1974, Jan.). Teaching organizational concepts to nurses in community mental health. *Journal of Nursing Education*, 13, 1.

Neuman, B.M. & Martin, K.S. (1998). Neuman systems model and the omaha system. *Image: Journal of Nursing Scholarship*, 30(1), 8.

Neuman, B., Newman, D.M.L., & Holder, P. (2000). Leadership-scholarship integration: Using the Neuman systems model for 21st-century professional nursing practice. *Nursing Science Quarterly*, 13(1), 60-3.

Neuman, B.M. & Young, R.J. (1972, May/June). A model for teaching total person approach to patient problems. *Nursing Research*, 21, 264-269.

Neuman, B. & Wyatt, M.A. (1981, Jan.). Prospects for change: Some evaluative reflections by faculty members from one articulated baccalaureate program. *Journal of Nursing Education*, 20, 40-46.

Secondary Sources
Books

Berkey, K.M. & Hanson, S.M.H. (1991). *Pocket guide to family assessment and intervention*. St. Louis: Mosby.

Lowry, Lois W. (1998). The Neuman Systems Model and nursing education: teaching strategies and outcomes. Indianapolis, IN: Sigma Theta Tau International: Center Nursing Press.

Mirenda, R.M. (1986). The Neuman systems model: Description and application. In P. Winsted Fry (Ed.), *Case studies in nursing theory* (pp. 127-166). New York: National League for Nursing.

Reed, K.S. (1993). Betty Neuman: The Neuman systems model. Newbury Park, CA: Sage.

Book Reviews

Hawkins, J. (1983). [Review of the book *The Neuman systems model: Application to nursing education and practice*]. *Western Journal of Nursing Research*, 5, 182-183.

Varicchio, C.G. (1983). [Review of the book *The Neuman systems model: Application to nursing education and practice*]. *American Journal of Nursing*, 83, 963-964.

Book Chapters

Arndt, C. (1982). Systems concepts for management of stress in complex health-care organizations. In B. Neuman (Ed.), *The Neuman systems model: Application to nursing education and practice* (pp. 107-116). Norwalk, CT: Appleton-Century-Crofts.

Arndt, C. (1982). Systems theory and educational programs for nursing service administration. In B. Neuman (Ed.), *The Neuman systems model: Application to nursing education and practice* (pp. 182-187). Norwalk, CT: Appleton-Century-Crofts.

Baker, N.A. (1982). The Neuman systems model as a conceptual framework for continuing education in the work place. In B. Neuman (Ed.), *The Neuman systems model: Application to nursing education and practice* (pp. 260-266). Norwalk, CT: Appleton-Century-Crofts.

Baker, N.A. (1982). Use of the Neuman model in planning for the psychological needs of the respiratory disease patient. In B. Neuman (Ed.), *The Neuman systems model: Application to nursing education and practice* (pp. 241-256). Norwalk, CT: Appleton-Century-Crofts.

Balch, C. (1974). Breaking the lines of resistance. In J.P. Riehl & C. Roy (Eds.), *Conceptual models for nursing practice* (pp. 130-134). New York: Appleton-Century-Crofts.

Beckman, S.J., Boxley-Harges, S., Bruick-Sorge, C., & Eichenaur, J. (1998). Critical thinking, the Neuman systems model, and associate degree education. In L. Lowry (Ed.), *The Neuman systems model and nursing education: Teaching strategies and outcomes* (pp. 53-58). Indianapolis, IN: Center Nursing Press.

Beckman, S.J., Boxley-Harges, S., Bruick-Sorge, C., & Eichenaur, J. (1998). Evaluation modalities for assessing student and program outcomes. In L. Lowry (Ed.), *The Neuman systems model and nursing education: Teaching strategies and outcomes* (pp. 149-60). Indianapolis, IN: Center Nursing Press.

Beckman, S.J., Boxley-Harges, S., Bruick-Sorge, C., Harris, S.M., Hermiz, M.E., Meininger, M., & Steinkeler, S.E. (1994). Betty Neuman systems model. In A. Marriner Tomey (Ed.), *Nursing theorists and their work* (3rd ed., pp. 269-304). St. Louis: Mosby.

Beddome, G. (1995). Community-as-client assessment: A Neuman-based guide for education and practice. In B. Neuman (Ed.), *The Neuman systems model* (3rd ed., pp. 567-580). Norwalk, CT: Appleton & Lange.

Beitler, B., Tkachuck, B., & Aamodt, D. (1980). The Neuman model applied to mental health, community health, and medical-surgical nursing. In J.P. Riehl & C. Roy (Eds.), *Conceptual models for nursing practice* (2nd ed., pp. 170-178). New York: Appleton-Century-Crofts.

Benedict, M.B. & Sproles, J.B. (1982). Application of the Neuman model to public health nursing practice. In B. Neuman (Ed.), *The Neuman systems model: Application to nursing education and practice* (pp. 223-240). Norwalk, CT: Appleton-Century-Crofts.

Beynon, C.E. (1995). Neuman-based experiences of the Middlesex-London health unit. In B. Neuman (Ed.), *The Neuman systems model* (3rd ed., pp. 537-549). Norwalk, CT: Appleton & Lange.

Bloch, C. & Bloch, C. (1995). Teaching content and process of the Neuman systems model. In B. Neuman (Ed.), *The Neuman systems model* (3rd ed., pp. 175-182). Norwalk, CT: Appleton & Lange.

Bonner, Sr. M. (1988). *Proceedings.* First Individual Nursing Symposium: Neuman Systems Model. Aston, PA: Neumann College Nursing Program.

Bower, F.L. (1982). Curriculum development and the Neuman model. In B. Neuman (Ed.), *The Neuman systems model: Application to nursing education and practice* (pp. 223-240). Norwalk, CT: Appleton-Century-Crofts.

Bowman, G.E. (1982). The Neuman assessment tool adapted for child day-care centers. In B. Neuman (Ed.), *The Neuman systems model: Application to nursing education and practice* (pp. 324-334). Norwalk, CT: Appleton-Century-Crofts.

Breckenridge, D.M. (1982). Adaptation of the Neuman systems model for the renal client. In B. Neuman (Ed.), *The Neuman systems model: Application to nursing education and practice* (pp. 267-277). Norwalk, CT: Appleton-Century-Crofts.

Breckenridge, D.M. (1995). Nephrology practice and directions for nursing research. In B. Neuman (Ed.), *The Neuman systems model* (3rd ed., pp. 499-507). Norwalk, CT: Appleton & Lange.

Bueno, M.M. & Sengin, K.K. (1995). The Neuman systems model for critical care nursing: A framework for practice. In B. Neuman (Ed.), *The Neuman systems model* (3rd ed., pp. 275-292). Norwalk, CT: Appleton & Lange.

Busch, P. & Lynch, M. (1998). Creative teaching strategies in a Neuman-based baccalaureate curriculum. In L. Lowry (Ed.), *The Neuman systems model and nursing education: Teaching strategies and outcomes* (pp. 59-70). Indianapolis, IN: Center Nursing Press.

Campbell, V. (1989). The Betty Neuman health care systems model: An analysis. In J.P. Riehl-Sisca (Ed.), *Conceptual models for nursing practice* (3rd ed., pp. 63-72). Norwalk, CT: Appleton & Lange.

Cardona, V.D. (1982). Client rehabilitation and the Neuman model. In B. Neuman (Ed.), *The Neuman systems model: Application to nursing education and practice* (pp. 178-290). Norwalk, CT: Appleton-Century-Crofts.

Chang, N.J. & Freese, B.T. (1998). Teaching culturally competent care: A Korean-American experience. In L. Lowry (Ed.), *The Neuman systems model and nursing education: Teaching strategies and outcomes* (pp. 85-90). Indianapolis, IN: Center Nursing Press.

Chiverton, P. & Flannery, J.C. (1995). Cognitive impairment: Use of the Neuman systems model. In B. Neuman (Ed.), *The Neuman systems model* (3rd ed., pp. 249-262). Norwalk, CT: Appleton & Lange.

Clark, F. (1982). The Neuman systems model: A clinical application for psychiatric nurse practitioners. In B. Neuman (Ed.), *The Neuman systems model: Application to nursing education and practice* (pp. 335-354). Norwalk, CT: Appleton-Century-Crofts.

Clark, V.L. (1982). Teaching the Neuman systems model: An approach to student and faculty development. In B. Neuman (Ed.), *The Neuman systems model: Application to nursing education and practice* (pp. 176-181). Norwalk, CT: Appleton-Century-Crofts.

Conners, V., Harmon, V.M., & Langford, R.W. (1982). Course development and implementation using the Neuman systems model as a framework: Texas Woman's University (Houston campus). In B. Neuman (Ed.), *The Neuman systems model: Application to nursing education and practice* (pp. 153-158). Norwalk, CT: Appleton-Century-Crofts.

Cookfair, J.M. (1996). Community as client. In J.M. Cookfair (Ed.), *Nursing care in the community* (2nd ed., pp. 19-37). St. Louis: Mosby.

Craddock, R.B. & Stanhope, M.K. (1980). The Neuman health care systems model: Recommended adaptation. In J.P. Riehl & C. Roy, (Eds.), *Conceptual models for nursing practice* (2nd ed., pp. 159-169). New York: Appleton-Century-Crofts.

Craig, D.M. (1995). Community/public health nursing in Canada: Use of the Neuman systems model in a new paradigm. In B. Neuman (Ed.), *The Neuman systems model* (3rd ed., pp. 521-528). Norwalk, CT: Appleton & Lange.

Craig, D. & Beynon, C. (1996). Nursing administration and the Neuman Systems model. In P.H. Walker (Ed.), *Blueprint for use of nursing models: Education, research, practice, and administration* (pp. 251-74). New York: National League for Nursing Publications.

Craig, D.M. & Morris-Coulter, C. (1995). Neuman implementation in a Canadian psychiatric facility. In B. Neuman (Ed.), *The Neuman systems model* (3rd ed., pp. 397-406). Norwalk, CT: Appleton & Lange.

Cross, J. (1985). Betty Neuman. In J. George (Ed.), *Nursing theories: The base for professional nursing practice* (pp. 258-285). Englewood Cliffs, NJ: Prentice-Hall.

Cross, J. (1990). Betty Neuman. In J. George (Ed.), *Nursing theories: The base for professional nursing practice* (3rd ed., pp. 259-278). Norwalk, CT: Appleton & Lange.

Cunningham, S.G. (1982). The Neuman model applied to an acute care setting: Pain. In B. Neuman (Ed.), *The Neuman systems model: Application to nursing education and practice* (pp. 291-296). Norwalk, CT: Appleton-Century-Crofts.

Curran, G. (1995). The Neuman systems model revisited. In B. Neuman (Ed.), *The Neuman systems model* (3rd ed., pp. 93-99). Norwalk, CT: Appleton & Lange.

Curran, G. (1995). The spiritual variable: A world view. In B. Neuman (Ed.), *The Neuman systems model* (3rd ed., pp. 581-590). Norwalk, CT: Appleton & Lange.

Damant, M. (1995). Community nursing in the United Kingdom: A case for reconciliation using the Neuman systems model. In B. Neuman (Ed.), *The Neuman systems model* (3rd ed., pp. 607-620). Norwalk, CT: Appleton & Lange.

Davies, P. & Proctor, H. (1995). In Wales: Using the model in community mental health nursing. In B. Neuman (Ed.), *The Neuman systems model* (3rd ed., pp. 621-628). Norwalk, CT: Appleton & Lange.

Davis, L.H. (1982). Aging: A social and preventive perspective. In B. Neuman (Ed.), *The Neuman systems model: Application to nursing education and practice* (pp. 197-307). Norwalk, CT: Appleton-Century-Crofts.

Dunbar, S.B. (1982). Critical care and the Neuman model. In B. Neuman (Ed.), *The Neuman systems model: Application to nursing education and practice* (pp. 297-307). Norwalk, CT: Appleton-Century-Crofts.

Dwyer, C.M., Walker, P.H., Suchman, A., & Coggiola, P. (1995). *In Nursing centers: The time is now* (pp. 135-155, NLN Pub. No. 41-2629). New York: National League for Nursing.

Echlin, D.J. (1982). Palliative care and the Neuman model. In B. Neuman (Ed.), *The Neuman systems model: Application to nursing education and practice* (pp. 257-259). Norwalk, CT: Appleton-Century-Crofts.

Engberg, I.B. (1995). Brief abstracts: Use of the Neuman systems model in Sweden. In B. Neuman (Ed.), *The Neuman systems model* (3rd ed., pp. 653-656.) Norwalk, CT: Appleton & Lange.

Engberg, I.B., Bjalming, E., & Bertilson, B. (1995). A structure for documenting primary health care in Sweden using the Neuman systems model. In B. Neuman (Ed.), *The Neuman systems model* (3rd ed., pp. 637-654). Norwalk, CT: Appleton & Lange.

Evans, B. (1998). Fourth-generation evaluation and the Neuman Systems model. In L. Lowry (Ed.), *The Neuman Systems model and nursing education: Teaching strategies and outcomes* (pp. 117-28). Indianapolis, IN: Center Nursing Press.

Fawcett, J. (1984). Neuman systems model. In J. Fawcett (Ed.), *Analysis and evaluation of conceptual models of nursing* (pp. 154-174). Philadelphia: F.A. Davis.

Fawcett, J. (1989). Neuman systems model. In J. Fawcett, *Analysis and evaluation of conceptual models of nursing* (2nd ed., pp. 169-204). Philadelphia: F.A. Davis.

Fawcett, J. (1995). Constructing conceptual-theoretical-empirical structures for research: Future implications for use of the Neuman systems model. In B. Neuman (Ed.), *The Neuman systems model* (3rd ed., pp. 459-472). Norwalk, CT: Appleton & Lange.

Fawcett, J. (1995). Neuman's systems model. In J. Fawcett (Ed.), *Analysis and evaluation of conceptual models of nursing* (3rd ed., pp. 217-275). Philadelphia: F.A. Davis.

Fawcett, J., Carpenito, L., Epinger, J., Goldblum-Graff, D., Groesbeck, M., Lowry, L., McCreary, C., & Wolf, Z. (1982). A framework for analysis and evaluation of conceptual models of nursing with an analysis and evaluation of the Neuman systems model. In B. Neuman (Ed.), *The Neuman systems model: Application to nursing education and practice* (pp. 30-43). Norwalk, CT: Appleton-Century-Crofts.

Felix, M., Hinds, C., Wolfe, Sr. C., & Martin, A. (1995). The Neuman systems model in a chronic care facility: A Canadian experience. In B. Neuman (Ed.), *The Neuman systems model* (3rd ed., pp. 549-566). Norwalk, CT: Appleton & Lange.

Freese, B.T. & Scales, C.J. (1998). NSM-based care as an NLN program evaluation outcome. In L. Lowry (Ed.), *The Neuman Systems model and nursing education: Teaching strategies and outcomes* (pp. 135-39). Indianapolis, IN: Center Nursing Press.

Frieburger, O.A. (1998). Overview of strategies that integrate the Neuman Systems model, critical thinking, and cooperative learning. In L. Lowry (Ed.), *The Neuman systems model and nursing education: teaching strategies and outcomes* (pp. 31-26). Indianapolis, IN: Center Nursing Press.

Frieburger, O.A. (1998). The Neuman Systems model, critical thinking, and cooperative learning in a nursing issues course. In L. Lowry (Ed.), *The Neuman systems model and nursing education: Teaching strategies and outcomes* (pp. 79-84). Indianapolis, IN: Center Nursing Press.

Frioux, T.D., Roberts, A.G., & Butler, S.J. (1995). Oklahoma state public health nursing: Neuman-based. In B. Neuman (Ed.), *The Neuman systems model* (3rd ed., pp. 407-414). Norwalk, CT: Appleton & Lange.

Fulton, R.A.B. (1995). The spiritual variable: Essential to the client system. In B. Neuman (Ed.), *The Neuman systems model* (3rd ed., pp. 77-92). Norwalk, CT: Appleton & Lange.

Glazebrook, D.S. (1995). The Neuman systems model in cooperative baccalaureate nursing education: The Minnesota intercollegiate nursing consortium experience. In B. Neuman (Ed.), *The Neuman systems model* (3rd ed., pp. 227-230). Norwalk, CT: Appleton & Lange.

Goldblum-Graff, D. & Graff, H. (1982). The Neuman model adapted to family therapy. In B. Neuman (Ed.), *The Neuman systems model: Application to nursing education and practice* (pp. 217-222). Norwalk, CT: Appleton-Century-Crofts.

Gunter, L.M. (1982). Application of the Neuman systems model to gerontic nursing. In B. Neuman (Ed.), *The Neuman systems model: Application to nursing education and practice* (pp. 196-210). Norwalk, CT: Appleton-Century-Crofts.

Harty, M.B. (1982). Continuing education in nursing and the Neuman model. In B. Neuman (Ed.), *The Neuman systems model: Application to nursing education and practice* (pp. 100-106). Norwalk, CT: Appleton-Century-Crofts.

Hassell, J.S. (1998). Critical thinking strategies for family and community client systems. In L. Lowry (Ed.), *The Neuman systems model and nursing education: Teaching strategies and outcomes* (pp. 71-78). Indianapolis, IN: Center Nursing Press.

Hermiz, M.E. & Meininger, M. (1986). Betty Neuman: Systems model. In A. Marriner (Ed.), *Nursing theorists and their work* (pp. 313-331). St. Louis: Mosby.

Hilton, S.A. & Grafton, M.D. (1995). Curriculum transition based on the Neuman systems model: Los Angeles County Medical Center School of Nursing. In B. Neuman (Ed.), *The Neuman systems model* (3rd ed., pp. 163-174). Norwalk, CT: Appleton & Lange.

Hinton-Walker, P. & Raborn, M. (1989). Application of the Neuman model in nursing administration and practice. In B. Henry, C. Arndt, M. DiVencenti, & A. Marriner Tomey (Eds.), *Dimensions of nursing administration* (pp. 711-723). Boston: Blackwell Scientific Publications.

Hoffman, M.K. (1982). From model to theory construction: An analysis of the Neuman health-care systems model. In B. Neuman (Ed.), *The Neuman systems model: Application to nursing education and practice* (pp. 44-54). Norwalk, CT: Appleton-Century-Crofts.

Johnson, M., Vaughn-Wrobel, B., Ziegler, S.M., Hugh, L., Bush, H.A., & Kurtz, P. (1982). Use of the Neuman health-care systems model in the Master's curriculum: Texas Woman's University. In B. Neuman (Ed.), *The Neuman systems model: Application to nursing education and practice* (pp. 130-152). Norwalk, CT: Appleton-Century-Crofts.

Kelley, J.A. & Sanders, N.F. (1995). A systems approach to the health of nursing and health care organizations. In B. Neuman (Ed.), *The Neuman systems model* (3rd ed., pp. 347-364). Norwalk, CT: Appleton & Lange.

Klotz, L.C. (1995). Integration of the Neuman systems model into the BSN curriculum at the University of Texas at Tyler. In B. Neuman (Ed.), *The Neuman systems model* (3rd ed., pp. 183-190). Norwalk, CT: Appleton & Lange.

Knox, J.E., Kilchenstein, L., & Yakulis, I.M. (1982). Utilization of the Neuman model in an integrated baccalaureate program: University of Pittsburgh. In B. Neuman (Ed.), *The Neuman systems model: Application to nursing education and practice* (pp. 117-123). Norwalk, CT: Appleton-Century-Crofts.

Lebold, M. & Davis, L. (1980). A baccalaureate nursing curriculum based on the health systems model. In J.P. Riehl & C. Roy (Eds.), *Conceptual models for nursing practice* (2nd ed., pp. 151-158). New York: Appleton-Century-Crofts.

Leddy, S. & Pepper, J.M. (1985). Models of nursing. In S. Leddy & J.M. Pepper (Eds.), *Conceptual bases of professional nursing* (pp. 135-149). Philadelphia: J.B. Lippincott.

Louis, M. (1989). An intervention to reduce anxiety levels for nurses working with long-term care clients using Neuman's model. In J.P. Riehl-Sisca (Ed.), *Conceptual models for nursing practice* (3rd ed., pp. 95-103). Norwalk, CT: Appleton & Lange.

Louis, M. (1995). The Neuman model in nursing research: An update. In B. Neuman (Ed.), *The Neuman systems model* (3rd ed., pp. 473-495). Norwalk, CT: Appleton & Lange.

Louis, M. & Koertvelyessy, A. (1989). Neuman model: Use in research. In B. Neuman (Ed.), *The Neuman systems model: Applications in nursing education and practice* (2nd ed.) Norwalk, CT: Appleton & Lange.

Lowry, L.W. (1998). Creative teaching and effective evaluation. In L. Lowry (Ed.), *The Neuman systems model and nursing education: Teaching strategies and outcomes* (pp. 17-30). Indianapolis, IN: Center Nursing Press.

Lowry, L.W. (1998). Efficacy of the Neuman systems model as a curriculum framework: A longitudinal study. In L. Lowry (Ed.), *The Neuman systems model and nursing education: Teaching strategies and outcomes* (pp. 139-48). Indianapolis, IN: Center Nursing Press.

Lowry, L.W. (1998). Vision, values, and verities. In L. Lowry (Ed.), *The Neuman systems model and nursing education: Teaching strategies and outcomes* (pp. 167-74). Indianapolis, IN: Center Nursing Press.

Lowry, L.W., Bruick-Sorge, C., Freese, B.T., & Sutherland, R. (1998). Development and renewal of faculty for Neuman-based teaching. In L. Lowry (Ed.), *The Neuman systems model and nursing education: Teaching strategies and outcomes* (pp. 161-66). Indianapolis, IN: Center Nursing Press.

Lowry, L.W. & Newsome, G.G. (1995). Neuman-based associate degree programs: Past, present, and future. In B. Neuman (Ed.), *The Neuman systems model* (3rd ed., pp. 197-214). Norwalk, CT: Appleton & Lange.

Lowry, L.W., Walker, P.H., & Mirenda, R. (1995). Through the looking glass back to the future. In B. Neuman (Ed.), *The Neuman systems model* (3rd ed., pp. 63-76). Norwalk, CT: Appleton & Lange.

Mayers, M.A. & Watson, A.B. (1982). Nursing care plans and the Neuman systems model. In B. Neuman (Ed.), *The Neuman systems model: Application to nursing education and practice* (pp. 69-84). Norwalk, CT: Appleton-Century-Crofts.

McCulloch, S.J. (1995). Utilization of the Neuman systems model: University of South Australia. In B. Neuman (Ed.), *The Neuman systems model* (3rd ed., pp. 591-598). Norwalk, CT: Appleton & Lange.

McGee, M. (1995). Implications for use of the Neuman systems model in occupational health nursing. In B. Neuman (Ed.), *The Neuman systems model* (3rd ed., pp. 657-668). Norwalk, CT: Appleton & Lange.

McInerey, K.A. (1982). The Neuman systems model applied to critical care nursing of cardiac surgery clients. In B. Neuman (Ed.), *The Neuman systems model: Application to nursing education and practice* (pp. 308-315). Norwalk, CT: Appleton-Century-Crofts.

Meleis, A.I. (1995). Theory testing and theory support: Principles, challenges, and a sojourn into the future. In B. Neuman (Ed.), *The Neuman systems model* (3rd ed., pp. 447-458). Norwalk, CT: Appleton & Lange.

Mirenda, R.M. (1986). The Neuman systems model: Description and application. In P. Winstead-Fry (Ed.), *Case studies in nursing theory* (pp. 127-167). New York: National League for Nursing.

Mischke-Berkey, K., Warner, P., & Hanson, S. (1989). Family health assessment and intervention. In P. Bomar (Ed.), *Nurses and family health promotion: Concepts, assessment, and interventions* (pp. 115-154). Baltimore: Williams & Wilkins.

Moxley, P.A. & Allen, L.M.H. (1982). The Neuman systems model approach in a master's degree program: Northwestern State University. In B. Neuman (Ed.), *The Neuman systems model: Application to nursing education and practice* (pp. 168-175). Norwalk, CT: Appleton-Century-Crofts.

Moynihan, M.M. (1993). Implementation of the Neuman systems model in an acute care nursing department. In M.E. Parker (Ed.), *Nursing theories in practice* (pp. 263-273). New York: National League for Nursing.

Mrkonich, D.E., Hessian, M., & Miller, M.W. (1989). A cooperative process in curriculum development using the Neuman health-care systems model. In J.P. Riehl-Sisca (Ed.), *Conceptual models for nursing practice* (3rd ed., pp. 87-94). Norwalk, CT: Appleton & Lange.

Neal, M.C. (1982). Nursing care plans and the Neuman systems model: II. In B. Neuman (Ed.), *The Neuman systems model: Application to nursing education and practice* (pp. 85-93). Norwalk, CT: Appleton-Century-Crofts.

Newsome, G.G. & Lowry, L.W. (1998). Evaluation in nursing: History, models, and Neuman's framework. In L. Lowry (Ed.), *The Neuman systems model and nursing education: Teaching strategies and outcomes* (pp. 37-52). Indianapolis, IN: Center Nursing Press.

Nuttall, P.R., Stittich, E.M., & Flores, F.C. (1998). The Neuman systems model in advanced practice nursing. In L. Lowry (Ed.), *The Neuman systems model and nursing education: Teaching strategies and outcomes* (pp. 109-116). Indianapolis, IN: Center Nursing Press.

Pierce, A.G. & Fulmer, T.T. (1995). Application of the Neuman systems model to gerontological nursing. In B. Neuman (Ed.), *The Neuman systems model* (3rd ed., pp. 293-308). Norwalk, CT: Appleton & Lange.

Pinkerton, A. (1974). Use of the Neuman model in a home health-care agency. In J.P. Riehl & C. Roy (Eds.), *Conceptual models for nursing practice* (pp. 122-129). New York: Appleton-Century-Crofts.

Poole, V.L. & Flowers, J.S. (1995). Care management of pregnant substance abusers using the Neuman systems model. In B. Neuman (Ed.), *The Neuman systems model* (3rd ed., pp. 377-386). Norwalk, CT: Appleton & Lange.

Proctor, N.G. (1995). Nurses' role in world catastrophic events: War dislocation effects on Serbian Australians. In B. Neuman (Ed.), *The Neuman systems model* (3rd ed., pp. 119-132). Norwalk, CT: Appleton & Lange.

Purushotham, D. & Walker, G. (1994). The Neuman systems model: A conceptual framework for clinical teaching/learning process. In R.M. Carroll-Johnson & M. Paquette (Eds.), *Classification of nursing diagnosis: Proceedings of the tenth conference* (pp. 271-273). Philadelphia: J.B. Lippincott.

Reed, K. (1982). The Neuman systems model: A basis for family psychosocial assessment and intervention. In B. Neuman (Ed.), *The Neuman systems model: Application to nursing education and practice* (pp. 188-195). Norwalk, CT: Appleton-Century-Crofts.

Rice, M.J. (1982). The Neuman systems model applied in a hospital medical unit. In B. Neuman (Ed.), *The Neuman systems model: Application to nursing education and practice* (pp. 310-323). Norwalk, CT: Appleton-Century-Crofts.

Rodriguez, M.L. (1995). The Neuman systems model adapted to a continuing care retirement community. In B. Neuman (Ed.), *The Neuman systems model* (3rd ed., pp. 431-442). Norwalk, CT: Appleton & Lange.

Russell, J., Hileman, J.W., & Grant, J.S. (1995). Assessing and meeting the needs of home caregivers using the Neuman systems model. In B. Neuman (Ed.), *The Neuman systems model* (3rd ed., pp. 331-342). Norwalk, CT: Appleton & Lange.

Scicchitani, B., Cox, J., Heyduk, L.J., Maglicco, P.A., & Sargent, N.A. (1995). Implementing the Neuman model in a psychiatric hospital. In B. Neuman (Ed.), *The Neuman systems model* (3rd ed., pp. 387-396). Norwalk, CT: Appleton & Lange.

Seng, V.S. (1998). Clinical evaluation: The heart of clinical performance. In L. Lowry (Ed.), *The Neuman systems model and nursing education: Teaching strategies and outcomes* (pp. 129-34). Indianapolis, IN: Center Nursing Press.

Seng, V.S., Mirenda, R., & Lowry, L.W. (1996). The Neuman systems model in nursing education. In P.H. Walker, (Ed.), *Blueprint for use of nursing models: Education, research, practice, and administration* (pp. 91-140). New York: National League for Nursing Publications.

Sipple, J.A. & Freese, B.T. (1989). Transition from technical to professional level education. In B. Neuman (Ed.), *The Neuman systems model* (2nd ed., pp. 193-200). Norwalk, CT: Appleton & Lange.

Smith, M.C. & Edgil, A.E. (1995). Future directions for research with the Neuman systems model. In B. Neuman (Ed.), *The Neuman systems model* (3rd ed., pp. 509-517). Norwalk, CT: Appleton & Lange.

Sohier, R. (1995). Nursing care for the people of a small planet: Culture and the Neuman systems model. In B. Neuman (Ed.), *The Neuman systems model* (3rd ed., pp. 101-118). Norwalk, CT: Appleton & Lange.

Sohier, R. (1997). Neuman's systems model in nursing practice. In M.R. Alligood & A. Marriner Tomey (Eds.). *Nursing theory: Utilization and application* (pp. 109-127). St. Louis: Mosby.

Stittich, E.M., Flores, F.C., & Nuttall, P. (1995). Cultural considerations in a Neuman-based curriculum. In B. Neuman (Ed.), *The Neuman systems model* (3rd ed., pp. 147-162). Norwalk, CT: Appleton & Lange.

Strickland-Seng, V. (1995). The Neuman systems model in clinical evaluation of students. In B. Neuman (Ed.), *The Neuman systems model* (3rd ed., pp. 215-223). Norwalk, CT: Appleton & Lange.

Stuart, G.W. & Wright, L.K. (1995). Applying the Neuman systems model to psychiatric nursing practice. In B. Neuman (Ed.), *The Neuman systems model* (3rd ed., pp. 263-274). Norwalk, CT: Appleton & Lange.

Sutherland, R. & Forrest, D.L. (1998). Primary prevention in an associate of science curriculum. In L. Lowry (Ed.), *The Neuman systems model and nursing education: Teaching strategies and outcomes* (pp. 99-108). Indianapolis, IN: Center Nursing Press.

Thibodeau, J.A. (1983). A systems model: The Neuman model. In J.A. Thibodeau (Ed.), *Nursing models: Analysis and evaluation* (pp. 105-123). Monterey, CA: Wadsworth.

Tollett, S.M. (1982). Teaching geriatrics and gerontology: Use of the Neuman systems model. In B. Neuman (Ed.), *The Neuman systems model: Application to nursing education and practice* (pp. 157-164). Norwalk, CT: Appleton-Century-Crofts.

Tomlinson, P.S. & Anderson, K.S. (1995). Family health and the Neuman systems model. In B. Neuman (Ed.), *The Neuman systems model* (3rd ed., pp. 133-144). Norwalk, CT: Appleton & Lange.

Toot, J.L. & Schmull, B.J. (1995). The Neuman systems model and physical therapy educational curricula. In B. Neuman (Ed.), *The Neuman systems model* (3rd ed., pp. 231-246). Norwalk, CT: Appleton & Lange.

Torres, G. (1986). Systems-oriented theories. In G. Torres (Ed.), *Theoretical foundations of nursing* (pp. 112-165). Norwalk, CT: Appleton-Century-Crofts.

Trepanier, M.J., Dunn, S.J., & Sprague, A.E. (1995). Application of the Neuman systems model to perinatal nursing. In B. Neuman (Ed.), *The Neuman systems model* (3rd ed., pp. 309-329). Norwalk, CT: Appleton & Lange.

Vaughn, B. & Gough, P. (1995). Use of the Neuman systems model in England: Abstracts. In B. Neuman (Ed.), *The Neuman systems model* (3rd ed., pp. 599-606). Norwalk, CT: Appleton & Lange.

Venable J. (1974). The Neuman health-care systems model: An analysis. In J.P. Riehl & C. Roy (Eds.), *Conceptual models for nursing practice* (pp. 115-121). New York: Appleton-Century-Crofts.

Venable, J.F. (1980). The Neuman health-care systems model: An analysis. In J.P. Riehl & C. Roy (Eds.), *Conceptual models for nursing practice* (2nd ed., pp. 135-141). New York: Appleton-Century-Crofts.

Verbeck, F. (1995). In Holland: Application of the Neuman model in psychiatric nursing. In B. Neuman (Ed.), *The Neuman systems model* (3rd ed., pp. 629-636). Norwalk, CT: Appleton & Lange.

Vokaty, D.A. (1982). The Neuman systems model applied to the clinical nurse specialist role. In B. Neuman (Ed.), *The Neuman systems model: Application to nursing education and practice* (pp. 165-167). Norwalk, CT: Appleton-Century-Crofts.

Walker, P.H. (1995). Neuman-based education, practice, and research in a community nursing center. In B. Neuman (Ed.), *The Neuman systems model* (3rd ed., pp. 415-430). Norwalk, CT: Appleton & Lange.

Walker, P.H. (1995). TQM and the Neuman systems model: Education for health care administration. In B. Neuman (Ed.), *The Neuman systems model* (3rd ed., pp. 365-376). Norwalk, CT: Appleton & Lange.

Walker, L.O. & Avant, K.C. (1983). Theory analysis: The Betty Neuman health care systems model: A total person approach to patient problems. In L.A. Walker & K.C. Avant (Eds.), Strategies for theory construction in nursing (pp. 133-143). Norwalk, CT: Appleton-Century-Crofts.

Ware, L.A. & Shannahan, M.K. (1995). Using Neuman for a stable support group in neonatal intensive care. In B. Neuman (Ed.), *The Neuman systems model* (3rd ed., pp. 321-330). Norwalk, CT: Appleton & Lange.

Weitzel, A.R. & Wood, K.C. (1998). Community health nursing: Keystone of baccalaureate education. In L. Lowry (Ed.), *The Neuman systems model and nursing education: Teaching strategies and outcomes* (pp. 91-98). Indianapolis, IN: Center Nursing Press.

Wesley, R.L. (1992). Neuman systems model. In R.L. Wesley (Ed.), *Springhouse notes: Nursing theories and models—a study and learning tool* (pp. 84-93). Springhouse, PA: Springhouse Corp.

Whall, L.O. & Avant, K.C. (1983). The Betty Neuman health care systems model. In J. Fitzpatrick & A.L. Whall (Eds.), *Conceptual models of nursing analysis and application* (pp. 204-219). Bowie, MD: Robert J. Brady.

Ziegler, S.M. (1982). Taxonomy for nursing diagnosis derived from the Neuman systems model. In B. Neuman (Ed.), *The Neuman systems model: Application to nursing education and practice* (pp. 55-68). Norwalk, CT: Appleton-Century-Crofts.

Journal Articles

Aggleton, P. & Chalmers, H. (1989). Neuman's systems model. *Nursing Times,* 85(51), 27-29.

Ali, N.S. & Khalil, H.Z. (1989). Effect of psychoeducational intervention on anxiety among Egyptian bladder cancer patients. *Cancer Nursing,* 12, 236-242.

Anderson, E., McFarland, J., & Helton, A. (1986). Community-as-client: A model for practice. *Nursing Outlook,* 34(5), 220-224.

Baerg, K.L. (1991). Using Neuman's model to analyze a clinical situation. *Rehabilitation Nursing,* 16, 38-39.

Barker, E., Robinson, D., & Brautigan, R. (1999). The effect of psychiatric home nurse follow-up on readmission rates of patients with depression. *Journal of American Psychiatric Nurses Association,* 5(4), 111-6.

Barrett, M. (1991). A thesis is born. *Image: Journal of Nursing Scholarship,* 23, 261-262.

Beckingham, A.C. & Baumann, A. (1990). The aging family in crisis: Assessment decision-making models. *Journal of Advanced Nursing,* 15, 782-787.

Bennett, S., Hulkes, C., Jones, J., Marden, B., Richards, A., Stone, A., Warren, D., & Lawson, L. (1998). Models of care: Developing a trust-wide philosophy. *Community Practitioner,* 71(10), 334, 336.

Beyea, S. & Matzo, M. (1989). Assessing elders using the functional health pattern assessment model. *Nurse Educator,* 14(5), 32-37.

Beynon, C. (1993). Theory-based practice: Attitudes of nursing managers before and after educational sessions. *Public Health Nursing,* 10(3), 183-188.

Biley, F. (1990). The Neuman model: An analysis. *Nursing (London),* 4(4), 25-28.

Biley, F.C. (1989). Stress in high dependency units. *Intensive Care Nursing,* 5, 134-141.

Black, P., Deeny, P., & McKenna, H. (1997). Sensoristrain: An exploration of nursing interventions in the context of the Neuman systems theory. *Intensive and Critical Care Nursing,* 13(5), 249-58.

Blank, J.J., Clark, L., Longman, A.J., & Atwood, J.R. (1989). Perceived home care needs of cancer patients and their caregivers. *Cancer Nursing,* 12, 78-84.

Bowdler, J.E. & Barrell, L.M. (1987). Health needs of homeless persons. *Public Health Nursing,* 4, 135-140.

Bowles, L., Oliver, N., & Stanley, S. (1995, Jan.). A fresh approach. *Nursing Times,* 91(1), 40-41.

Bowman, A.M. (1997). Sleep satisfaction, perceived pain, and acute confusion in elderly clients undergoing orthopaedic procedures. *Journal of Advanced Nursing,* 26(3), 550-64.

Breckenridge, D.M. (1997). Decisions regarding dialysis treatment modality: A holistic perspective. *Holistic Nursing Practice,* 12(1), 54-61.

Breckenridge, D.M. (1997). Patients' perceptions of why, how, and by whom dialysis treatment modality was chosen . . . including commentary by Whittaker, A.A. and Locking-Cusolito, H. with author response. *American Nephrology Nurses Association Journal,* 24(3), 313-21.

Breckenridge, D.M., Cupit, M.C., & Raimond, J.N. (1982, Jan./Feb.). Systematic nursing assessment tool for the CAPD client. *Nephrology Nurse,* 24, 26-27, 30-31.

Brown, M.W. (1988). Neuman's systems model in risk factor reduction. *Cardiovascular Nursing,* 24(6), 43.

Buchanan, B.F. (1987). Human-environment interaction: A modification of the Neuman systems model for aggregates, families, and the community. *Public Health Nursing,* 4(1), 52-64.

Bullock, L.F. (1993). Nursing interventions for abused women on obstetrical units. *AWHONN'S Clinical Issues in Perinatal and Women's Health Nursing,* 4(3), 371-377.

Bunn, H. (1995). Preparing nurses for the challenge of the new focus on community mental health nursing. *The Journal of Continuing Education in Nursing,* 26(2), 55-59.

Burke, S.O. & Maloney, R. (1986). The women's value orientation questionnaire: An instrument revision study. *Nursing Papers,* 18(1), 32-44.

Cantin, B. & Mitchell, M. (1989). Nurses' smoking behavior. *The Canadian Nurse,* 85(1), 20-21.

Capers, C.F. (1991). Nurses' and lay African Americans' views about behavior. *Western Journal of Nursing Research,* 13, 123-135.

Capers, C.F. (1996). The Neuman systems model: A culturally relevant perspective. *ABNF Journal,* 7(5), 113-117.

Carrigg, K.C. & Weber, R. (1997). Development of the spiritual care scale. *Image: Journal of Nursing Scholarship,* 29(3), 293.

Carroll, T.L. (1989). Role deprivation in baccalaureate nursing students pre and post curriculum revision. *Journal of Nursing Education,* 28, 134-139.

Cheung, Y.L. (1997). Student forum. The application of the Neuman system model to nursing in Hong Kong? *Hong Kong Nursing Journal,* 33(4), 17-21.

Chiverton, P., Tortoretti, D., LaForest, M., & Walker, P.H. (1999). Bridging the gap between psychiatric hospitalization and community care: Cost and quality outcomes. *Journal of the American Psychiatric Nurses Association,* 5(2), 46-53.

Clark, C.C., Cross, J.R., Deane, D.M., & Lowry, L.W. (1991). Spirituality: Integral to quality care. *Holistic Nursing Practice,* 5, 67-76.

Collins, M.A. (1996). The relation of work stress, hardiness, and burnout among full-time hospital staff nurses. *Journal of Nursing Staff Development,* 12(2), 81-85.

Courchene, V.S., Patalski, E., & Martin, J. (1991). A study of the health of pediatric nurses administering cyclosporine A. *Pediatric Nursing,* 17, 497-500.

Cowperthwaite, B., LaPlante, K., Mahon, B., & Markowski, T. (1997). Latex allergy in the nursing population. *Canadian Operating Room Nursing Journal,* 15(2), 23-4.

Dale, J.L. & Savala, S.M. (1990). A new approach to the senior practicum. *Nursing Connections,* 3(1), 45-51.

Darland, N.W. (1986). Congenital adrenocortical hyperplasia: Supportive nursing interventions. *Journal of Pediatric Nursing,* 1(2), 117-123.

Delunas, L.R. (1990). Prevention of elder abuse: Betty Neuman health care systems approach. *Clinical Nurse Specialists,* 4, 54-58.

Evely, L. (1994). A model for successful breastfeeding. *Modern Midwife,* 4(12), 25-27.

Flanders-Stepans, M.B. & Fuller, S.G. (1999). Physiological effects of infant exposure to environmental tobacco smoke: A passive observation study. *Journal of Perinatal Education,* 8(1), 10-21.

Flannery, J. (1991). FAMLI-RESCUE: A family assessment tool for use by neuroscience nursing in the acute care setting. *Journal of Neuroscience Nursing,* 23, 111-115.

Flannery, J. (1995). Cognitive assessment in the acute care setting: Reliability and validity of the levels of cognitive function assessment scale (LOCFAS). *Journal of Nursing Measurement,* 3(1), 43-58.

Foote, A.W., Piazza, D., & Schultz, M. (1990). The Neuman systems model: Application to a patient with a cervical spinal cord injury. *Journal of Neuroscience Nursing,* 22, 302-306.

Fowler, B.A. & Risner, P.B. (1994). A health promotion program evaluation in a minority industry. *ABNF Journal,* 5(3), 72-76.

Galloway, D.A. (1993). Coping with a mentally and physically impaired infant: A self-analysis. *Rehabilitation Nursing,* 18(1), 34-36.

Gavin, C.A.S., Hastings-Tolsma, M.T., & Troyan, P.J. (1988). Explication of Neuman's model: A holistic systems approach to nutrition for health promotion in the life process. *Holistic Nursing Practice,* 3(1), 26-38.

Gellner, P., Landers, S., O'Rouke, D., & Schlegal, M. (1994). Community health nursing in the 1990's: Risky business? *Holistic Nursing Practice,* 8(2), 15-21.

George, J. (1997). Nurses' perceived autonomy in a shared governance setting. *Journal of Shared Governance,* 3(2), 17-21.

Gibson, M. (1996). Health promotion for a group of elderly clients. *Perspectives,* 20(3), 2-5.

Gifford, D.K. (1997). Monthly incidence of stroke in rural Kansas. *Kansas Nurse,* 71(5), 3-4.

Gigliotti, E. (1997). Use of Neuman's lines of defense and resistance in nursing research: Conceptual and empirical considerations. *Nursing Science Quarterly,* 10(3), 136-143.

Gigliotti, E. (1998). You make the diagnosis. Case study: Integration of the Neuman systems model with the theory of nursing diagnosis in postpartum nursing . . . including commentary by Lunney, M. *Nursing Diagnosis: The Journal of Nursing Language and Classification,* 9(1), 14.

Gigliotti, E. (1999). Women's multiple role stress: Testing Neuman's flexible line of defense. *Nursing Science Quarterly,* 12(1), 36-44.

Goodman, H. (1995). Patients' views count as well. *Nursing Standard,* 9(40), 55.

Grant, J.S., Kinney, M.R., & Davis, L.D. (1993). Using conceptual frameworks or models to guide nursing research. *Journal of Neuroscience Nursing,* 25(1), 52-56.

Gries, M. & Fernsler, J. (1988). Patient perceptions of the mechanical ventilation experience. *Focus on Critical Care,* 15, 52-59.

Haggart, M. (1993). A critical analysis of Neuman's systems model in relation to public health nursing. *Journal of Advanced Nursing,* 18(2), 1917-1922.

Hainsworth, D.S. (1996). Research briefs. The effect of death education on attitudes of hospital nurses toward care of the dying. *Oncology Nursing Forum,* 23(6), 963-967.

Hanson, M.J.S. (1999). Cross-cultural study of beliefs about smoking among teenaged females . . . including commentary by Laffery S.C. with author response. *Western Journal of Nursing Research,* 21(5), 635-651.

Hassell, J.S. (1996). Improved management of depression through nursing model application and critical thinking. *Journal of the American Academy of Nurse Practitioners,* 8(4), 161-166.

Heffline, M.S. (1991). A comparative study of pharmacological versus nursing interventions in the treatment of postanesthesia shivering. *Journal of Post Anesthesia Nursing,* 6, 311-320.

Herrick, C.A. & Goodykoonts, L. (1989). Neuman's systems model for nursing practice as a conceptual framework for a family assessment. *Journal of Child and Adolescent Psychiatric and Mental Health Nursing,* 2, 61-67.

Herrick, C.A., Goodykoonts, L., Herrick, R.H., & Kracket, B. (1991). Planning a continuum of care in child psychiatric nursing: A collaborative effort. *Journal of Child and Adolescent Psychiatric and Mental Health Nursing,* 4, 41-48.

Hinds, C. (1990). Personal and contextual factors predicting patients' reported quality of life: Exploring congruency with Betty Neuman's assumptions. *Journal of Advanced Nursing,* 15, 456-462.

Hitz, D. (1990). The Neuman systems model: An analysis of clinical situation. *Rehabilitation Nursing,* 15, 330-332.

Hoch, C.C. (1987). Assessing delivery of nursing care. *Journal of Gerontological Nursing,* 13(1), 10-17.

Hoeman, S.P. & Winters, D.M. (1990). Theory-based case management: High cervical spinal cord injury. *Home Healthcare Nurse,* 8, 25-33.

Huch, M.H. (1991). Perspective of health. *Nursing Science Quarterly,* 4, 33-40.

Issel, L.M. (1995). Evaluating case management programs. *Maternal/Child Nursing Journal,* 29, 67-74.

Johns, C. (1991). The Burford nursing development unit holistic model of nursing practice. *Journal of Advanced Nursing,* 16, 1090-1098.

Johnson, P.T. (1983). Black hypertension: A transcultural case study using the Betty Neuman model of nursing care. *Issues in Health Care,* 4, 191-210.

Jones, W.R. (1996). Stressors in the primary caregivers of traumatic head injured persons. *AXON,* 18(1), 9-11.

Kiernan, B.S. & Scoloveno, M.A. (1986). Assessment of the neonate. *Topics in Clinical Nursing,* 8(1), 1-10.

Knight, J.B. (1990). The Betty Neuman systems model applied to practice: A client with multiple sclerosis. *Journal of Advanced Nursing,* 15, 447-455.

Leja, A.M. (1989). Using guided imagery to combat post-surgical depression. *Journal of Gerontological Nursing,* 15(4), 6-11.

Lile, J.L., Pace, N.M., Hoffman, R.G., & Mace, M.K. (1994). The Neuman systems model as applied to the terminally ill client with pressure ulcers. *Advances in Wound Care,* 7(4), 44-48.

Lin, M., Ku, N., Leu, J., Chen, J., & Lin, L. (1996). An exploration of the stress aspects, coping behaviors, health status, and related aspects in family caregivers of hepatoma patients. *Nursing Research (China),* 4(2), 171-85.

Lindell, J. & Olsson, H. (1991). Can combined oral contraceptives be made more effective by means of a nursing care model? *Journal of Advanced Nursing,* 16, 475-479.

Loescher, L.J., Clark, L., Attwood, J.R., Leigh, S., & Lamb, G. (1990). The impact of the cancer experience on long-term survivors. *Oncology Nursing Forum,* 17(2), 223-229.

Lowry, L. (1986). Adapted by degrees. *Senior Nurse,* 5(3), 25-26.

Lowry, L.W. (1988). Operationalizing the Neuman systems model: A course in concepts and process. *Nursing Educator,* 13(3), 19-22.

Lowry, L. & Anderson, B. (1993). Neuman's framework and ventilator dependency: A pilot study. *Nursing Science Quarterly,* 6(4), 195-199.

Lowry, L.W., Burns, C.M., Smith, A.A., & Jacobson, H. (2000). Compete or complement? An interdisciplinary approach to training health professionals. *Nursing and Health Care Perspectives,* 21(2), 76-80.

Lowry, L.W., Saeger, J., & Barnett, S. (1997). Client satisfaction with prenatal care and pregnancy outcomes. *Outcomes Management for Nursing Practice,* 1(1), 29-35.

Mackenzie, S. & Spence-Laschinger, H.K. (1995). Correlates of nursing diagnosis quality in public health nursing. *Journal of Advanced Nursing,* 21, 800-808.

Maligalig, R.M.L. (1994). Parents' perceptions of the stressors of pediatric ambulatory surgery. *Journal of Post Anesthesia Nursing,* 9(5), 278-282.

Mann, A.H., Hazel, C., Geer, C., Hurley, C.M., & Podrapovic, T. (1993). Development of an orthopaedic case manager role. *Orthopaedic Nursing,* 12(4), 23-27.

Mannina, J. (1997). Finding an effective hearing testing protocol to identify hearing loss and middle ear disease in school-aged children. *Journal of School Nursing,* 13(5), 23-28.

Marsh, V., Beard, M.T., & Adams, B.N. (1999). Job stress and burnout: The mediational effect of spiritual well-being and hardiness among nurses. *Journal of Theory Construction and Testing,* 3(1), 13-19.

Martin, S.A. (1996). Applying nursing theory to the practice of nurse anesthesia. *American Association of Nurse Anesthetists Journal,* 64(4), 369-372.

Martsolf, D.S. & Mickley, J.R. (1998). The concept of spirituality in nursing theories: Differing world-views and extent of focus. *Journal of Advanced Nursing,* 27(2), 294-303.

McHolm, F.A. & Geib, K.M. (1998). Application of the Neuman systems model to teaching health assessment and nursing process. *Nursing Diagnosis: The Journal of Nursing Language and Classification,* 9(1), 23-33.

Mill, J.E. (1997). The Neuman systems model: Application in a Canadian HIV setting. *British Journal of Nursing,* 6(3), 163-166.

Miner, J. (1995). Incorporating the Betty Neuman systems model into HIV clinical practice. *AIDS Patient Care,* 9(1), 37-39.

Mirenda, R.M. (1986). The Neuman model in practice. *Senior Nurse,* 5(3), 26-27.

Molassiotis, A. (1997). A conceptual model of adaptation to illness and quality of life for cancer patients treated with bone marrow transplants. *Journal of Advanced Nursing,* 26(3), 572-579.

Moody, N.B. (1996). Nurse faculty job satisfaction: A national survey. *Journal of Professional Nursing,* 12(5), 277-288.

Moore, S.L. & Munro, M.F. (1990). The Neuman systems model applied to mental health nursing of older adults. *Journal of Advanced Nursing,* 15, 293-299.

Mynatt, S.L. & O'Brien, J. (1993). A partnership to prevent chemical dependency in nursing using Neuman's systems model. *Journal of Psychosocial Nursing and Mental Health Services,* 31(4), 27-34.

Mytka, S. & Beynon, C. (1994). A model for public health nursing in the Middlesex-London, Ontario, schools. *Journal of School Health,* 64(2), 85-86.

Narsavage, G.L. (1997). Promoting function in clients with chronic lung disease by increasing their perception of control. *Holistic Nursing Practice,* 12(1), 17-26.

Orr, J.P. (1993). An adaptation of the Neuman systems model to the care of the hospitalized preschool child. *Curationis: South African Journal of Nursing,* 16(3), 37-44.

Owens, M. (1995). Care of a woman with Down's syndrome using the Neuman systems model. *British Journal of Nursing,* 4(13), 752-758.

Parr, M.S. (1993). The Neuman health care systems model: An evaluation. *British Journal of Theatre Nursing,* 3(8), 20-27.

Peternelj-Taylor, C.A. & Johnson, R. (1996). Custody and caring: Clinical placement of student nurses in a forensic setting. *Perspectives in Psychiatric Care: The Journal for Nurse Psychotherapists,* 32(4), 23-29.

Picot, S.J.F., Zauszniewski, J.A., Debanne, S.M., & Holston, E.C. (1999). Mood and blood pressure in black female caregivers and noncaregivers. *Nursing Research,* 48(3), 150-161.

Picton, C.E. (1995). An explanation of family-centered care in Neuman's model with regard to the care of the critically ill adult in an accident and emergency setting. *Accident and Emergency Nursing,* 3, 33-37.

Reed, K.S. (1993). Adapting the Neuman systems model for family nursing. *Nursing Science Quarterly,* 6(2), 93-97.

Ridgell, N.H. (1993). Home apnea monitoring: A systems approach to the family's home care needs. *Caring,* 12(2), 34-37.

Roberts, A.G. (1994). Effective inservice education process. *Oklahoma Nurse,* 39(4), 11.

Rodrigues-Fisher, L., Bourguignon, C., & Good, B.V. (1993). Dietary fiber nursing intervention: Prevention of constipation in older adults. *Clinical Nursing Research,* 2(4), 464-477.

Roggensack, J. (1994, Jun./Aug.). The influence of perioperative theory and clinical in a baccalaureate nursing program on the decision to practice perioperative nursing. *Prairie Rose,* 63(2), 6-7.

Ross, M. & Bourbannais, F. (1985). The Neuman systems model in nursing practice: A case study approach. *Journal of Advanced Nursing,* 10, 199-207.

Ross, M.M., Bourbonnais, F.F., & Carroll, G. (1987). Curriculum design and the Betty Neuman systems model: A new approach to learning. *International Nursing Review,* 34(3), 75-79.

Russell, J. & Hezel, L. (1994). Role analysis of the advanced practice nurse using the Neuman health care systems model as a framework. *Clinical Nurse Specialist,* 8(4), 215-220.

Sabo, C.E. & Michael, S.R. (1996). The influence of personal message with music on anxiety and side effects associated with chemotherapy. *Cancer Nursing,* 19(4), 283-289.

Schare, B.L. (1993). A comparison of family needs based on the presence or absence of DNR orders. *DCCN: Dimensions of Critical Care Nursing Journal,* 11(5), 286-292.

Schlentz, M.D. (1993). The minimum data set and levels of prevention in the long term care facility. *Geriatric Nursing,* 14, 79-83.

Schorr, J. (1993). Music and pattern change in chronic pain. *Advances in Nursing Science,* 15(4), 27-36.

Smith, M.C. (1989). Neuman's model in practice. *Nursing Science Quarterly,* 2, 116-117.

Speck, B.J. (1990). The effect of guided imagery upon first semester nursing students performing their first injections. *Journal of Nursing Education,* 29, 346-350.

Story, E.L. & DuGas, B.W. (1988). A teaching strategy to facilitate conceptual model implementation in practice. *Journal of Continuing Education in Nursing,* 19, 244-247.

Sullivan, J. (1986). Using Neuman's model in the acute phase of spinal cord injury. *Focus on Critical Care,* 13(5), 34-41.

Taggart, L. & Mattson, S. (1996). Delay in prenatal care as a result of battering in pregnancy: Cross-cultural implications. *Health Care for Women International,* 17(1), 25-34.

Tlaskund, J.H. (1980). Areas in theory development. *Advances in Nursing Science,* 3, 1-7.

Torkington, S. (1988). Nourishing the infant. *Senior Nurse,* 8(2), 24-25.

Utz, S.W. (1980). Applying the Neuman model to nursing practice with hypertensive clients. *Cardiovascular Nursing,* 16, 29-34.

Vaughn, M., Cheatwood, S., Sirles, A.T., & Brown, K.C. (1989). The effect of progressive muscle relaxation on stress among clerical workers. *American Association of Occupational Health Nursing Journal,* 37, 302-306.

Waddell, K.L. & Demi, A.S. (1993). Effectiveness of an intensive partial hospitalization program for treatment of anxiety disorders. *Archives of Psychiatric Nursing,* 7(1), 2-10.

Walker, P.H. (1994). Dollars and sense in health reform: Interdisciplinary practice and community nursing centers. *Nursing Administration Quarterly,* 19(1), 1-11.

Wallingford, P. (1989). The neurologically impaired and dying child: Applying the Neuman systems model. *Issues in Comprehensive Pediatric Nursing,* 12, 139-157.

Waters, T. (1993). Self-efficacy, change, and optimal client stability. *Addictions Nursing Network,* 6(2), 48-51.

Weinberger, S.L. (1991). Analysis of a clinical situation using the Neuman systems model. *Rehabilitation Nursing,* 16, 278-281.

Wilson, L.C. (2000). Implementation and evaluation of church-based health fairs. *Journal of Community Nursing,* 17(1), 39-48.

Wormald, L. (1995). Samuel—The boy with tonsillitis: A care study. *Intensive and Critical Care Nursing,* 11(3), 157-160.

Wright, P.S., Piazza, D., Holcombe, J., & Foote, A. (1994). A comparison of three theories of nursing used as a guide for the nursing care of an 8-year-old child with leukemia. *Journal of Pediatric Oncology Nursing,* 11(1), 14-19.

Newsletters

Neuman News. (1992-present). The Neuman Systems Model Trustee Group, Inc. Available: Neumann College, c/o Director of Library Media and Archives, One Neumann Drive, Aston, PA, 19014.

Dissertations and Theses

Allen, K.S. (1997). The effect of cancer diagnosis information on the anxiety of patients with an initial diagnosis of first cancer. *Masters Abstracts International,* 30-04, 0996.

Al-Nagshabandi, E.A.H. (1993). An exploration of the physical and psychological responses of surgically-induced menopausal Saudi women using the Neuman systems model. *Dissertation Abstracts International,* 55-04B, 1374.

Ark, P.D. (1997). *Health risk behaviors and coping strategies of African-American sixth graders.* Unpublished doctoral dissertation, The University of Tennessee Center for the Health Sciences.

Averill, J.B. (1988). The impact of primary prevention as an interventions strategy. *Masters Abstracts International,* 27-01, 89.

Barnes, M.E. (1993). Knowledge, experiences, attitudes, and assessment practices of nurse practitioners with regard to stressors related to childhood sexual abuse. *Masters Abstracts International,* 32-01, 0223.

Barnes-McDowell, B.M. (1997). Home apnea monitoring: Family functioning, concerns, and coping. *Dissertation Abstracts International,* 58-03B, 1205.

Baskin-Nedzelski, J. (1991). Job stressors among visiting nurses. *Masters Abstracts International,* 30-01, 0079.

Bemker, M.A. (1996). *Adolescent female substance abuse: Risk and resiliency factors.* Unpublished doctoral dissertation, University of Alabama at Birmingham.

Bittinger, J.P. (1995). Case management and satisfaction with nursing care of patients hospitalized with congestive heart failure. *Dissertation Abstracts International,* 56-07B, 3688.

Blount, K.R. (1988). The relationship between the parent's and five- to six-year-old child's perception of life events as stressors within the Neuman health care systems framework. *Masters Abstracts International,* 27-04, 0487.

Brown, F.A. (1994). The effects of an eight-hour affective education program on fear of AIDS and homophobia in student nurses. *Masters Abstracts International,* 33-05, 1487.

Burritt, J.E. (1988). The effects of perceived social support on the relationship between job stress and job satisfaction and job performance among registered nurses employed in acute care facilities. *Dissertation Abstracts International,* 49, 2123B.

Butts, M.J. (1998). Outcomes of comfort touch in institutionalized elderly female residents. *Dissertation Abstracts International,* 59-07B, 3344.

Cagle, R. (1996). The relationship between health care provider advice and the initiation of breast-feeding. *Dissertation Abstracts International,* 57-08B, 4974.

Capers, C.F. (1986). Perceptions of problematic behavior as held by lay black adults and registered nurses. *Dissertation Abstracts International,* 47-11B, 4467.

Chilton, L.L.A. (1996). *The influence of behavioral cues on immunization practices of elders.* Unpublished doctoral dissertation, The University of Alabama at Birmingham.

Collins, A.S. (1991). *Effects of positional changes on selected physiological and psychological measurements in clients with atrial fibrillation.* Unpublished doctoral dissertation, University of Alabama at Birmingham.

Collins, C.R. (1999). *The older widow-adult child relationship as an influence upon health promoting behaviors.* Unpublished doctoral dissertation, The Catholic University of America.

Cullen, L.M. (1993). Nurses' perceptions of humor as a preventive intervention to promote the health of clients in a health care setting. *Masters Abstracts International,* 32-02, 0592.

Doherty, D.C. (1997). Spousal abuse: An African-American female perspective. *Dissertation Abstracts International,* 58-04B, 1798.

Fields, W.L. (1987). The effects of the 12-hour shift on fatigue and critical thinking performance in critical care nurses. *Masters Abstracts International,* 26-02, 0237.

Flannery, J.C. (1988). Validity and reliability of levels of cognitive functioning assessment scale for adults with closed head injuries. *Dissertation Abstracts International,* 48, 3248B.

Fulton, B.J. (1992). *Evaluation of the effectiveness of the Neuman systems model as a theoretical framework for baccalaureate nursing programs.* Unpublished doctoral dissertation, University of Massachusetts.

Geiger, P.A. Participation in a phase II cardiac rehabilitation program and perceived quality of life. *Masters Abstracts International,* 34-04, 1548.

Gigliotti, E. (1997). *The relations among maternal and student role involvement, perceived social support and perceived multiple role stress in mothers attending college: A study based on Betty Neuman's systems model.* Unpublished doctoral dissertation, New York University.

Goble, D.S. (1991). A curriculum framework for the prevention of child sexual abuse. *Dissertation Abstracts International,* 52-06A, 2004.

Gray, R. (1998). The lived experience of children, ages 8-12 years, who witness family violence in the home. *Masters Abstracts International,* 36-05, 1327.

Gullivar, K.M. (1997). Hopelessness and spiritual well-being in persons with HIV infection. *Masters Abstracts International,* 35-05, 1374.

Hanson, M.J.S. (1995). Beliefs, attitudes, subjective norms, perceived behavioral control, and cigarette smoking in white, African-American, and Puerto Rican-American teenage women. *Dissertation Abstracts International,* 56-08B, 4240.

Hanson, P.A. (1997). An application of Bowen family systems theory: Triangulation, differentiation of self and nurse manager job stress. *Dissertation Abstracts International,* 58-11B, 5889.

Harbin, P.D.O. (1990). A Q-analysis of the stressors of adult female nursing students enrolled in baccalaureate schools of nursing. *Dissertation Abstracts International,* 50, 3919B.

Harper, B. (1992). Nurses' beliefs about social support and the effect of nursing care on cardiac clients' attitudes in reducing cardiac risk factors. *Masters Abstracts International,* 31-01, 0273.

Hayes, K.V.D. (1994). Diagnostic content validation and operational definitions of risk factors for the nursing diagnosis high risk for disuse syndrome. *Dissertation Abstracts International,* 55-12B, 5284.

Heaman, D.J. (1991). *Perceived stressors and coping strategies of parents with developmentally disabled children.* Unpublished doctoral dissertation, University of Alabama at Birmingham.

Henze, R.L. (1993). The relationship among selected stress variables and white blood count in severely head injured patients. *Dissertation Abstracts International,* 55-02B, 03365.

Herald, P.A. (1993). Relationship between hydration status and renal function in patients receiving aminoglycoside antibiotics. *Dissertation Abstracts International,* 55-02B, 0365.

Higgs, K.T. (1994). Preterm labor risk factors identified in an ambulatory perinatal setting with home uterine activity monitoring support. *Masters Abstracts International,* 33-05, 1490.

Holloway, C. (1995). Stress perceived among nurse managers in community health settings. *Masters Abstracts International,* 33-05, 1490.

Hood, L.J. (1997). The effects of nurse faculty hardiness and sense of coherence on perceived stress, scholarly productivity, and job satisfaction. *Dissertation Abstracts International,* 58-09B, 4720.

Jennings, K.M. (1997). Predicting intention to obtain a pap smear among African-American and Latina women. *Dissertation Abstracts International,* 58-07B, 3557.

Kazakoff, K.J. (1990). The evaluation of return to work and retention of employment of cardiac patients following cardiac rehabilitation programs. *Masters Abstracts International,* 29-03, 0450.

Lamb, K.A. (1998). Baccalaureate nursing students' perception of empathy and stress in their interactions with clinical instructors: Testing a theory of optimal student system stability according to the Neuman systems model. *Dissertation Abstracts International,* 60-03B, 1028.

Lancaster, D.R.N. (1991). *Coping with appraised threat of breast cancer: Primary prevention coping behaviors utilized by women at increased risk.* Unpublished doctoral dissertation, Wayne State University.

Landry, K.A. (1994). *Relationship of serum levels of total cholesterol and selected risk factors in clients diagnosed with a cerebrovascular accident.* Unpublished master's thesis, Northwestern State University of Louisiana.

Larino, E.A. (1997). Determining the level of care provided by a family nurse practitioner during deployment. *Masters Abstracts International,* 35-05, 1376.

Lee, P.L. (1995). Caregiver stress as experienced by wives of institutionalized and in-home dementia husbands. *Dissertation Abstracts International,* 56-08B, 4241.

Lijauco, C.C. (1997). Factors related to length of stay in coronary artery bypass graft patients. *Masters Abstracts International,* 36-02, 0512.

Marlett, L.A. (1998). The breast feeding practices of women with a history of breast cancer. *Masters Abstracts International,* 37-04, 1180.

Marsh, V. (1997). Job stress and burnout among nurses: The mediational effect of spiritual well-being and hardiness. *Dissertation Abstracts International,* 58-08B, 4142.

McDaniel, G.M.S. (1990). The effects of two methods of dangling on heart rate and blood pressure in postoperative abdominal hysterectomy patients. *Dissertation Abstracts International,* 50, 3923B.

McMillan, D.E. (1995). Impact of therapeutic support of inherent coping strategies on chronic low back pain: A nursing intervention study. *Masters Abstracts International,* 35-02, 0520.

Micevski, V. (1996). Gender differences in the presentation of physiological symptoms of myocardial infarction. *Masters Abstracts International,* 35-02, 0520.

Mirenda, R.M. (1995). A conceptual-theoretical strategy for curriculum development in baccalaureate nursing programs. *Dissertation Abstracts International,* 56-10B, 5421.

Monahan, G.L. (1996). A profile of pregnant drug-using female arrestees in California: The relationships among sociodemographic characteristics, reproductive and drug addiction histories, HIV/STD risk behaviors, and utilization of prenatal care services and substance abuse programs. *Dissertation Abstracts International,* 57-09B, 5576.

Moody, N.B. (1991). *Selected demographic variables, organizational characteristics, role orientation, and job satisfaction among nurse faculty.* Unpublished doctoral dissertation, University of Alabama at Birmingham.

Morris, D.C. (1991). Occupational stress among home care first line managers. *Masters Abstracts International,* 29-03, 0443.

Murphy, N.G. (1989). Factors associated with breastfeeding success and failure: A systematic integrative review. *Masters Abstracts International,* 28-02, 0275.

Neabel, B. (1998). A comparison of family needs perceived by nurses and family members of acutely brain-injured patients. *Masters Abstracts International,* 37-02, 0592.

Nicholson, C.H. (1995). Clients' perceptions of preparedness for discharge home following total hip or knee replacement surgery. *Masters Abstracts International,* 33-03, 0873.

Norman, S.E. (1991). The relationship between hardiness and sleep disturbances in HIV-infected men. *Dissertation Abstracts International,* 51, 4780B.

Norris, E.W. (1990). Physiologic response to exercise in clients with mitral valve prolapse syndrome. *Dissertation Abstracts International,* 50, 5549B.

O'Neal, C.A.S. (1993). Effects of BSE on depression/anxiety in women diagnosed with breast cancer. *Masters Abstracts International,* 31-04, 1747.

Parodi, V.A. (1997). Neuman based analysis of women's health needs aboard a deployed navy ship: Can nursing make a difference? *Dissertation Abstracts International,* 58-12B, 6491.

Peoples, L.T. (1990). *The relationship between selected client, provider, and agency variables and the utilization of home care services.* Unpublished doctoral dissertation, University of Alabama at Birmingham.

Peters, M.R. (1997). An exploratory study of job stress and stressors in hospice administration. *Masters Abstracts International,* 36-02, 0502.

Peterson, G.A. (1997). Nursing perceptions of the spiritual dimensions of patient care: The Neuman systems model in curricular formations. *Dissertation Abstracts International,* 59-02B, 0605.

Petock, A.M. (1990). Decubitus ulcers and physiological stressors. *Masters Abstracts International,* 29-02, 0267.

Pothiban, L. (1993). *Risk factor prevalence, risk status, and perceived risk for coronary heart disease among Thai elderly.* Unpublished doctoral dissertation, University of Alabama at Birmingham.

Ramsey, B.A. (1999). Can a multidisciplinary team decrease hospital length of stay for elderly trauma patients? *Masters Abstracts International,* 37-04, 1182.

Robinson, C.A. (1998). The difference in perception of quality of life in patients one year after an infrainguinal bypass for critical limb ischemia. *Masters Abstracts International,* 37-03, 0914.

Rowe, M.L. (1989). *The relationship of commitment and social support to the life satisfaction of caregivers to patients with Alzheimer's disease.* Unpublished doctoral dissertation, The University of Texas at Austin.

Rowles, C.J. (1992). *The relationship of selected personal and organizational variables and the tenure of directors of nursing in nursing homes.* Unpublished doctoral dissertation, University of Alabama at Birmingham.

Scalzo Tarrant, T. (1992). Improving the frequency and proficiency of breast self examination. *Masters Abstracts International,* 31-03, 1211.

Schlosser, S.P. (1985). The effect of anticipatory guidance on mood state in primiparas experiencing unplanned cesarean delivery. *Dissertation Abstracts International,* 46-08B, 2627.

Sipple, J.E.A. (1990). A model for curriculum change based on retrospective analysis. *Dissertation Abstracts International,* 50, 1927A.

Tarmina, M.S. (1992). *Self-selected diet of adult women with families.* Unpublished doctoral dissertation, University of Utah.

Terhaar, M.F. (1989). The influence of physiologic stability, behavior stability, and family stability on the preterm infant's length of stay in the neonatal intensive care unit. *Dissertation Abstracts International,* 50, 1328B.

Thomas, Y.M. (1996). *Measuring the diabetes knowledge of senior nursing students attending a bachelor of science in nursing program.* Unpublished master's thesis, Pittsburgh State University.

Vincent, J.L.M. (1988). A Q analysis of the stressors of fathers with an infant in an intensive care unit. *Dissertation Abstracts International,* 49, 3111B.

Vitthuhn, K.M. (1999). Delivery of analgesics for the postoperative thoracotomy patient. *Masters Abstracts International,* 37-04, 1185.

Watson, L.A. (1991). Comparison of the effects of usual, support, and informational nursing interventions on the extent to which families of critically ill patients perceive their needs were met. *Dissertation Abstracts International,* 52-06B, 2999.

Webb, C.A. (1989). A cross-sectional study of hope, physical status, cognitions and meaning and purpose of pre- and post-retirement adults. *Dissertation Abstracts International,* 50, 1922A.

Whatley, J.H. (1988). Effects of health locus of control and social network on risk-taking in adolescents. *Dissertation Abstracts International,* 50-01B, 0129.

Wilkey, S.F. (1990). The effects of an eight-hour continuing education course on the death anxiety levels of registered nurses. *Masters Abstracts International,* 28-04, 0480.

Williamson, J.W. (1989). *The influence of self-selected monotonous sounds on the night sleep pattern of postoperative open heart surgery patients.* Unpublished doctoral dissertation, University of Alabama at Birmingham.

Wright, J.G. (1996). The impact of preoperative education on health locus of control, self-efficacy, and anxiety for patients undergoing total joint replacement surgery. *Masters Abstracts International,* 35-01, 0216.

Computer Software

Fuld Institute for Technology in Nursing Education. (1997). Betty Neuman: Neuman systems model [Computer software]. In Fuld Institute for Technology in Nursing Education, *The nurse theorists, portraits of excellence.* Athens, OH: The Institute.

$\mathcal{I}$mogene King

Interacting Systems Framework and Theory of Goal Attainment

Christina L. Sieloff

CREDENTIALS AND BACKGROUND OF THE THEORIST

Imogene King earned a diploma in nursing from St. John's Hospital of Nursing in St. Louis, Missouri, in 1945. While working in a variety of staff nurse roles, she began course work toward a Bachelor of Science in Nursing Education, which she received from St. Louis University in 1948. From 1947 to 1958, King worked as an instructor in medical-surgical nursing

Previous authors: Chistina L. Sieloff, Mary Lee Ackermann, Sallie Anne Brink, Jo Anne Clanton, Cathy Greenwell Jones, Ann Marriner Tomey, Sandra L. Moody, Gwynn Lee Perlich, Debra L. Price, and Beth Bruns Prusinski.
The author wishes to thank Dr. Imogene King for her past review of this chapter. The author and Dr. King strongly encourage all readers to read Dr. King's original materials in conjunction with this chapter.

and as an assistant director at St. John's Hospital School of Nursing. She earned an M.S.N. (1957) from St. Louis University and a Doctor of Education (1961) from Teachers College, Columbia University, New York. King was awarded an honorary Ph.D. from Southern Illinois University in 1980.

From 1961 to 1966, King was an associate professor of nursing at Loyola University in Chicago, where she developed a masters degree program in nursing based on a nurse's conceptual framework. Her first theory article appeared in 1964 in the journal *Nursing Science* edited by Dr. Martha Rogers.[28] Between 1966 and 1968, King served as Assistant Chief of Research Grants Branch, Division of Nursing, in the United States Department of Health, Education, and Welfare. While she was in Washington,

DC, her article "A Conceptual Frame of Reference for Nursing" was published in *Nursing Research.*[29]

From 1968 to 1972, King was the director of the School of Nursing at The Ohio State University in Columbus. While at Ohio State, her book *Toward a Theory for Nursing*[30] was published. In this early work, King[30:129] concluded, "a systematic representation of nursing is required ultimately for developing a science to accompany a century or more of art in the everyday world of nursing." Her book subsequently was awarded the American Journal of Nursing Book of the Year Award in 1973.[39]

King returned to Chicago in 1972 as a professor in the Loyola University graduate program. She also served as the Coordinator of Research in Clinical Nursing at the Loyola Medical Center, Department of Nursing from 1978 to 1980.

From 1972 to 1975, she was a member of the Defense Advisory Committee on Women in the Services for the United States Department of Defense. She was elected Alderman in Ward 2, Wood Dale, Illinois in 1975 and served until 1979.

In 1980, King moved to Tampa, Florida, where she was appointed professor at the University of South Florida College of Nursing. The manuscript for her second book, *A Theory for Nursing: Systems, Concepts, Process,*[34] was published in 1981. In addition to her first two books, she has authored multiple book chapters and articles in professional journals, and a third book, *Curriculum and Instruction in Nursing,*[38] was published in 1986.

King retired in 1990 and is currently professor emeritus at the University of South Florida, where she continues to lecture. She also continues to provide community service and help plan care through her framework and theory at various healthcare organizations. She keynoted two Sigma Theta Tau theory conferences in 1992 and continues to present at local, national, and international nursing education conferences. She consults with doctoral and masters students who are developing theories within the interacting systems framework. She has contributed to the development of instruments to measure the power of a nursing group within an organization[56] and patient satisfaction with professional nursing care.[27]

King has been an active member of the American Nurses Association, the Florida Nurses' Association, and Sigma Theta Tau International. She has held offices in various organizations and has frequently served as a delegate from the Florida Nurses' Association to the American Nurses Association House of Delegates. In 1994, she was inducted into the American Academy of Nursing. Currently, she is one of the founding members of a nursing organization, the King International Nursing Group (KING), established to facilitate the dissemination and utilization of her interacting systems framework, Theory of Goal Attainment, and related theories. In 1996, she received the Jessie M. Scott Award at the American Nurses Association convention.

THEORETICAL SOURCES

King[30:ix] describes the purpose of her first book as:

> propos[ing] a conceptual frame of reference for nursing. It is intended to be utilized specifically by students and teachers, and also by researchers and practitioners to identify and analyze events in specific nursing situations. The framework suggests that the essential characteristics of nursing are those properties that have persisted in spite of environmental changes.

King[30:125] also identifies that the framework served:

> several purposes . . . . It is a way of thinking about the real world of nursing; . . . an approach for selecting concepts perceived to be fundamental for the practice of professional nursing; [and] shows a process for developing concepts that symbolize experiences within the physical, psychological, and social environment in nursing.

King clearly identifies and references theoretical sources throughout her 1981 book.[34]

USE OF EMPIRICAL EVIDENCE

King[30:11-12] speaks of concepts as "abstract ideas that give meaning to our sense perceptions, permit generalizations, and tend to be stored in our memory for recall and use at a later time in new and different situations." King[35:11] defines theory as "a set of concepts, which, when defined, are interrelated and observable in the world of nursing practice." Theory serves to build "scientific knowledge for nursing."[40:24]

King[31] identifies at least two methods for developing theory: (1) a theory can be developed and then tested in research and (2) research can provide data from which a theory may be developed. King's opinion[33] is that "in today's world of building knowledge for a complex profession such as nursing, one must consider these two strategies."

King[34] cites many research studies in her 1981 book, especially regarding the development of her concepts. Within the personal system, King examines studies related to *perception* by Allport,[3] Kelley and Hammond,[25] Ittleson and Cantril,[21] and others. In developing her definition of *space,* she uses studies from Sommer[57] and Ardrey[4] and notes Minckley's research.[46] For the concept of *time,* she acknowledges Orme's work.[48]

Within the interpersonal system, King presents communication theories and models, citing the studies of Watzlawick, Beavin, and Jackson[58] and Krieger.[42] She examines studies by Whiting,[59] Orlando,[47] and Diers and Schmidt[11] for information on *interaction.* She also notes Dewey and Bentley's Theory of Knowledge,[10] which addresses selfaction, interaction, and transaction in Knowing and the Known, and Kuhn's work[43] on transactions.

Commenting on research existing at that time, particularly operations research regarding patient care, King[32:9] notes that, "most studies have centered on technical aspects of patient care and of the health care systems rather than on patient aspects directly. . . . Few problems have been stated that begin with what the patient's condition demands or what the patient wants." In her 1981 book, King[34:151-152] further discusses that "several theoretical formulations about interpersonal relations and nursing process have been described in nursing situations," citing studies by Peplau,[50] Orlando,[47] Paterson and Zderad,[49] Yura and Walsh,[62] and herself.

Development of the Interacting Systems Framework

In preparation of her 1971 book, King[30,39] posed several questions:
1. What is the goal of nursing?
2. What are the functions of nurses?
3. How can nurses continue to expand their knowledge to provide quality care?

As a result of a review of 20 years of nursing literature (before 1971), King identified multiple concepts used by nurses to describe nursing.

Figure 19-1 demonstrates the interacting systems framework that provides "one approach to studying systems as a whole rather than as isolated parts of a system,"[39:18] and is "designed to explain (the) organized wholes within which nurses are expected to function."[40:23]

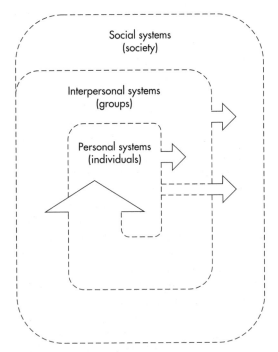

Figure **19-1** Dynamic interacting systems. (From King, I. [1981]. *A theory for nursing: Systems, concepts, process* [p. 11]. New York: Delmar. Used with permission from I. King.)

King[34:10] used a systems approach in the development of her interacting systems framework and the subsequent Theory of Goal Attainment because systems have been used in the past to comprehend and respond to "changes and complexity in health care organizations." She adds that "some scientists who have been studying systems have noted that the only way to study human beings interacting with the environment is to design a conceptual framework of interdependent variables and interrelated concepts."[34:10] King[39:21] believes that her "framework differs from other conceptual schema in that it is concerned not with fragmenting human beings and the environment but with human transactions in different kinds of environments."

"An awareness of the complex dynamics of human behavior in nursing situations prompted [King's] formulation of a conceptual framework that represents personal, interpersonal and social systems as the domain of nursing."[34:130] Each of the three systems identifies human beings as the basic element in the system. In addition, "the unit of analysis in [the] framework is human behavior in a variety of social environments."[39:18]

Individuals exist within personal systems, and King provides an example of a *total system* as being a patient or a nurse. King believes that it is necessary to understand the concepts of body image, growth and development, perception, self, space, and time to comprehend human beings as persons.

Interpersonal systems are formed when two or more individuals interact, forming dyads (two people) or triads (three people). The dyad of a nurse and a patient is one type of interpersonal system. Families, when acting as small groups, can also be considered as interpersonal systems. Comprehension of the interpersonal system requires an understanding of the concepts of communication, interaction, role, stress, and transaction.

A comprehensive interacting system consists of groups that make up society and is referred to as a *social system*. Religious, educational, and healthcare systems are examples of social systems. The influential behavior of an extended family on an individual's growth and development in society is another example of the influence of a social system. Within a social system, the concepts of authority, decision making, organization, power, and status are essential for understanding of this system.

"The concepts in the framework are the organizing dimensions and represent knowledge essential for understanding the interactions between the three systems."[39:18] Concepts were placed in the personal system because they primarily related to individuals, whereas concepts were placed in the interpersonal system because they "emphasized interactions between two or more persons."[39:18] Concepts were placed in the social system because they "provided knowledge for nurses to function in larger systems."[39:18] However, King[39:19] clearly identifies that "the concepts in the framework are not limited to only one of the dynamic interacting systems but cut across all three systems." See Table 19-1 for the location of concepts from the Systems Framework and the Theory of Goal Attainment in King's 1981 text, *A Theory for Nursing: Systems, Concepts, Process.*[34]

Development of the Theory of Goal Attainment

In 1981, King[34] derived the Theory of Goal Attainment from her interacting systems framework. The question that "motivated [King] to develop a theory was, what is the nature of nursing?"[40:25] The answer, "the way in which nurses, in their role, do with and for individuals that differentiates nursing from other health professionals," guided the development of the Theory of Goal Attainment.[40:26]

King[40] used the following criteria to develop the theory:

1. What are the philosophical assumptions?
2. Are the concepts clearly identified and defined?
3. Are the concepts related in propositional statements or models?
4. Does the theory generate questions to be answered or hypotheses to be tested in research to generate knowledge and affirm the theory?

"The human process of interactions formed the basis for designing a model of transactions

[Figure 19-2] that depicts theoretical knowledge used by nurses to help individuals and groups attain goals."[39:27]

Mutual goal setting [between a nurse and a client] is based on (a) nurses' assessment of a client's concerns, problems, and disturbances in health; (b) nurses' and client's perceptions of the interfer-ence; and (c) their sharing of information whereby each functions to help the client attain the goals identified. In addition, nurses interact with family members when clients cannot verbally participate in the goal setting.[40:28]

To test her theory, King[34:153] conducted research, identifying that her study varied from previous

Table **19-1**

Location of Concept Definitions in I.M. King's A Theory for Nursing: Systems, Concepts, Process*

CONCEPTS	FROM SYSTEMS FRAMEWORK	FROM THEORY OF GOAL ATTAINMENT
Authority	p. 124	
Body image	p. 33	
Communication		p. 146
Decision making	p. 132	
Growth and development		p. 148
Interaction	p. 32	p. 145
Nursing situation	p. 2	
Organization (operational)	p. 119	
Perception	p. 24	p. 146
Power	p. 127	
Role	p. 93	
Space	pp. 37-38	
Status	p. 129	
Stress	p. 32	
Time	p. 44	
Transaction	p. 82	p. 147

*New York: John Wiley & Sons, 1981.

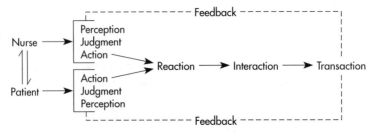

Figure **19-2** A process of human interactions that lead to transactions: A model of transaction. (From King, I. [1981]. *A theory for nursing: Systems, concepts, process* [p. 61]. New York: Delmar. Used with permission from I. King.)

studies in that it "described the nurse-patient interaction process that leads to goal attainment." King's research describes a process that leads to goal attainment and studied nurse-patient interactions to determine whether nurses made transactions. King used a method of nonparticipant observation to collect information of nurse-patient interactions in a patient care unit in a hospital setting. Patients and nurses volunteered to participate in the study. King then trained graduate students in the nonparticipant observation technique before collecting data. She examined multiple interactions and recorded verbal and nonverbal behaviors as raw data. King[41] developed a classification system that nurses can use to determine if they are making transactions that lead to goal attainment.

MAJOR CONCEPTS & DEFINITIONS

"Concepts give meaning to our sense perceptions and permit generalizations about persons, objects, and things."[39:16] A limited number of definitions based on the systems framework are listed below. The remainder of King's definitions can be found in her 1981 book.[34] To assist the reader, those concepts, the pages where the definitions can be found from the interacting systems framework, and the theory are listed alphabetically in Table 19-1.

HEALTH

"Health is defined as dynamic life experiences of a human being, which implies continuous adjustment to stressors in the internal and external environment through optimum use of one's resources to achieve maximum potential for daily living."[34:5]

NURSING

"Nursing is defined as a process of action, reaction, and interaction whereby nurse and client share information about their perceptions in the nursing situation."[34:2]

SELF

"The self is a composite of thoughts and feelings which constitute a person's awareness of his [/her] individual existence, his [/her] conception of who and what he [/she] is. A person's self is the sum total of all he [/she] can call his [/hers]. The self includes, among other things, a system of ideas, attitudes, values, and commitments. The self is a person's total subjective environment. It is a distinctive center of experience and significance. The self constitutes a person's inner world as distinguished from the outer world consisting of all other people and things. The self is the individual as known to the individual. It is that to which we refer when we say 'I.'"[22:9-10]

MAJOR ASSUMPTIONS

King's personal philosophy about human beings and life influenced her assumptions, including those related to the environment, health, nursing, individuals, and nurse-patient interactions. Her interacting systems framework and Theory of Goal Attainment are "based on an overall assumption that the focus of nursing is human beings interacting with their environment leading to a state of health for individuals, which is an ability to function in social roles."[34:143]

Nursing

"Nursing is an observable behavior found in the health care systems in society."[30:125] The goal of nursing "is to help individuals maintain their health so they can function in their roles."[34:3-4] Nursing is an interpersonal process of action, reaction, interaction, and transaction. Perceptions of a nurse and a patient also influence the interpersonal process.

Person

Specific assumptions relating to persons or individuals are detailed in *A Theory for Nursing: Systems, Concepts, Process.*[34] In addition, the following assumptions are detailed in King's subsequent works:
1. Individuals are spiritual beings.[41]
2. Individuals have the capacity to think, know, make choices, and select alternative courses of action.[34]
3. Individuals have the ability through their language and other symbols to record their history and preserve their culture.[38]
4. Individuals are open systems in transaction with the environment. Transaction connotes that no separateness exists between human beings and the environment.[34]
5. Individuals are unique and holistic, are of intrinsic worth, and are capable of rational thinking and decision making in most situations.[40]
6. Individuals differ in their needs, wants, and goals.[40]

Health

Health is a dynamic state in the life cycle; illness is an interference in the life cycle. Health "implies continuous adjustment to stress in the internal and external environment through optimum use of one's resources to achieve maximum potential for daily living."[34:5]

Environment

King[34:2] believes that "an understanding of the ways that human beings interact with their environment to maintain health is essential for nurses." Open systems imply that interactions occur between the system and the system's environment, inferring that the environment is constantly changing. "Adjustments to life and health are influenced by [an] individual's interactions with environment. . . . Each human being perceives the world as a total person in making transactions with individuals and things in the environment."[34:141]

THEORETICAL ASSERTIONS

King's Theory of Goal Attainment[34] focuses on the interpersonal system and the interactions that take place between individuals, specifically in the nurse-patient relationship. In the nursing process, each member of the dyad perceives the other, makes judgments, and takes actions. Together these activities culminate in reaction. Interaction results and, if perceptual congruence exists and disturbances are conquered, transactions occur. The system is open to permit feedback because each phase of the activity potentially influences perception.

King[34] developed eight propositions in her Theory of Goal Attainment. These propositions are detailed in Box 19-1 and describe the relationships between concepts. Diagrams follow each proposition. When the propositions were analyzed, 23 relationships were not specified; 22 relationships were positive and no relationship was negative (Figure 19-3). In addition, King[34] derived seven hypotheses from the Theory of Goal Attainment, which are found in *A Theory for Nursing: Systems, Concepts, Process.*

LOGICAL FORM

In the initial framework suggested in her 1968 article, King[29] identified four comprehensive concepts that center around human beings: (1) health, (2) interpersonal relationships, (3) perceptions, and (4) social systems. She viewed individuals as open systems and energy exchange takes place within and external to human beings. Although King's original framework[30:128] was abstract and dealt with "only a few elements of concrete situations," she believes that her four "universal ideas, social systems, health, perception, and interpersonal relations, are relevant in every nursing situation."

Later, in 1975, King[31:36] identified that her "personal approach to synthesizing knowledge for nursing was to use data and information available from research in nursing and related fields, and from 25 years in active practice, teaching, and research. From all the knowledge available, a theoretical framework relevant for nursing was formulated." In 1978, King[33] indicated that theory development is composed of inductive and deductive reasoning, with the theory's primary purpose being the generation of knowledge through research.

King[34:142] then began further development of her interacting systems framework and proposed the Theory of Goal Attainment to describe "the nature of nurse-client interactions that lead to achievement of goals."

> Nurses purposely interact with clients to mutually establish goals and to explore and agree on means to achieve goals. Mutual goal setting is based on nurses' assessment of clients' concerns, problems, and disturbances in health, their perceptions of problems, and their sharing information to move toward goal attainment.[34:142-143]

King's 1981 publication[34] indicates less dichotomy between health and illness and she referred to illness as an interference in the life cycle. Through reformulation, King provided a more open system relationship between person and environment. King also revised her terminology, using *adjustment* instead of *adaptation,* and *person, human being,* and *individual* rather than *man.*

A logical progression of development existed in the framework from 1971[30] to 1981[34] with King deriving her Theory of Goal Attainment from her interacting systems framework. Her theory "organize[d] elements in the process of nurse-client interactions that result in outcomes, that is, goals attained."[34:143]

King initially stated:

> [i]f nurses are to assume the roles and responsibilities expected of them, . . . the discovery of knowledge must be disseminated in such a way that they are able to use it in their practice. . . . Descriptive data collected systematically provide cues for generating hypotheses for research in human behavior in nursing situations.[30:128]

During a 1978 nursing theorist conference, King[33] indicated that if nurses were taught this process, they

Box **19-1**

Propositions Within King's Theory of Goal Attainment

1. If perceptual accuracy (PA) is present in nurse-client interactions (I), transactions (T) will occur.
$$PA\ (I) \xrightarrow{+} T$$
2. If nurse and client make transactions (T), goals will be attained (GA).
$$T \xrightarrow{+} GA$$
3. If goals are attained (GA), satisfactions (S) will occur.
$$GA \xrightarrow{+} S$$
4. If goals are attained (GA), effective nursing care (NC_e) will occur.
$$GA \xrightarrow{+} NC_e$$
5. If transactions (T) are made in nurse-client interactions (I), growth and development (GD) will be enhanced.
$$(I)T \xrightarrow{+} GD$$
6. If role expectations and role performance as perceived by nurse and client are congruent (RCN), transactions (T) will occur.
$$RCN \xrightarrow{+} T$$
7. If role conflict (RC) is experienced by nurse and client or both, stress (ST) in nurse-client interactions (I) will occur.
$$RC(I) \xrightarrow{+} ST$$
8. If nurses with special knowledge and skills communicate (CM) appropriate information to clients, mutual goal setting (T) and goal attainment (GA) will occur. [Mutual goal setting is a step in transaction and thus has been diagrammed as transaction.]
$$CM \xrightarrow{+} T \xrightarrow{+} GA$$

Reprinted from Austin, J.K. & Champion, V.L. (1983). King's theory of nursing: Explication and evaluation. In P.L. Chinn (Ed.), *Advances in nursing theory development* (p. 55). Rockville, MD: Aspen. Used with permission of Aspen Publishers, Inc., © 1983.

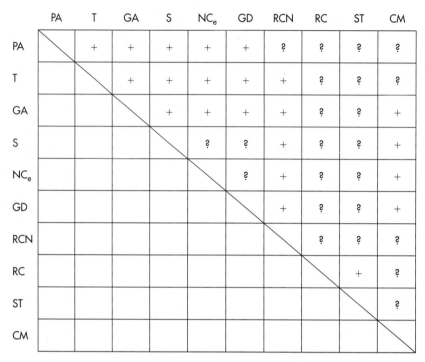

Figure 19-3 Relationship table. *PA*, Perceptional accuracy; *T*, transactions; *GA*, goals attained; *S*, satisfactions; *NC$_e$*, effective nursing care; *GD*, growth and development; *RCN*, role congruency; *RC*, role conflict; *ST*, stress; *CM*, communicate. (From Austin, J.K. & Champion, V.L. [1983]. King's theory for nursing: Explication and evaluation. In P.L. Chinn [Ed.]., *Advances in theory development* [p. 58]. Rockville, MD: Aspen. Used with permission of Aspen Publishers, copyright © 1983.)

could begin to predict outcomes in nursing. Later, in 1981, she added, "This theory should serve as a standard of practice related to nurse-patient interactions, and is in this sense a normative theory."[34:145] Clements and Roberts[8] expanded on these ideas in 1983 to show the process of the theory in relation to various nursing situations, including the health of families.

ACCEPTANCE BY THE NURSING COMMUNITY

Practice

King's early publication[30] led to nursing curriculum development and practice application at Ohio State and other universities. In her 1981 book, King[34:157]

identifies that "theory, because it is abstract, cannot be immediately applied to nursing practice or to concrete nursing education programs. When empirical referents are identified, defined and described, . . . theory is useful and can be applied in concrete situations." However, "knowledge of the concepts can be applied in concrete situations."[41]

Professionals in most specialty areas have used the concepts of King's Theory of Goal Attainment[34] in nursing practice. Its relationship to practice is obvious because the profession of nursing functions primarily through interactions with individuals and groups within the environment.[17] Even before King's interacting systems framework was published, Brown[7:469] stated that "this proposed intrasystems model provides an approach for stimulating continued learning, for establishing innovative foundations for nursing practice, and for generating inquiry through research." King[35:12] believes that "nurses, who have knowledge of the concepts of this theory of goal attainment, are able to accurately perceive what is happening to patients and family members and are able to suggest approaches for coping with the situations."

King also developed a documentation system, the Goal Oriented Nursing Record (GONR), to accompany the Theory of Goal Attainment and to record goals and outcomes. The GONR is a method of collecting data, identifying problems, and implementing and evaluating care that has been used effectively in patient settings. The Theory and the GONR are useful in practice because nurses have the ability to provide individualized plans of care while encouraging active participation from patients in the decision-making phase.[35]

Nurses can also use the GONR approach to document the effectiveness of nursing care. "The major elements in this record system are: (a) data base, (b) nursing diagnosis, (c) goal list, (d) nursing orders, (e) flow sheets, (f) progress notes, and (g) discharge summary."[40:30-31]

Healthcare professionals have implemented King's interacting systems framework and Theory of Goal Attainment[34] in various national and international practice settings. The following briefly identifies some of the settings and the bibliography details additional settings. Jolly and Winker[23] described the application of the Theory of Goal Attainment within the context of nursing administration. Benedict and Frey[6] reported the implementation of theory-based practice in an emergency department. Alligood[1] applied the Theory of Goal Attainment to adult patients within orthopedic nursing settings. Laben, Sneed, and Seidel[44] used goal attainment in short-term group psychotherapy. Messmer[45] detailed the implementation of theory-based nursing practice in a large urban teaching hospital. Coker and colleagues[9] used the framework to implement nursing diagnoses in a Canadian community hospital and Fawcett, Vaillancourt, and Watson[13] used the framework within a large Canadian tertiary care hospital.

Education

Nursing faculty at several universities (Ohio State, Loyola in Chicago, and University of Texas in Houston) have used King's interacting systems framework to design curricula in nursing programs.[36] In 1980, Brown and Lee[7:468] reported that King's concepts were useful in developing a framework for "use in nursing education, nursing practice, and for generating hypotheses for research . . . [They] provide a systematic means of viewing the nursing profession, organizing a body of knowledge for nursing, and clarifying nursing as a discipline." King's framework and theory also have application for nursing education internationally as described by Rooke[51] for a Swedish educational setting. Additional publications detail the application of King's work in core curricula (Gold, Haas, and King[19]).

Research

Many researchers have used King's work as a theoretical base. Several studies are mentioned here and others are listed in the Bibliography.

Many researchers have used concepts from King's interacting systems framework. Winker[61] developed a system's view of health. Rooke[52] identified the implications of space for nursing. Sieloff[54] defined the health of a social system.

Other researchers have used King's framework[34] as a theoretical base. This group of research includes the following studies:

1. Kemppainen[26] analyzed a case study of a patient who had HIV and was also experiencing psychotic symptoms.
2. Alligood, Evans, and Wilt[2] developed the concept of empathy within King's framework.
3. Hobdell[20] used King's framework[33] to work with parents of children with neural tube defects.
4. Sharts-Hopko[53] explored the perceived health status of women during the transition to menopause.
5. Doornbos[12] used King's framework to explore the health of families with young people who are chronically mentally ill.

Researchers have also developed middle-range theories using King's interacting systems framework.[33] These include Frey's Theory of Families,

Children, and Chronic Illness,[15] Killeen's Theory of Patient Satisfaction with Professional Nursing Care,[27] Sieloff's Theory of Departmental Power,[55] and Wicks' Theory of Family Health.[60]

Researchers have also performed studies using the concepts of the Theory of Goal Attainment.[34] Hanucharurnkui and Vinya-nguag[19] used goal attainment to study the outcomes of self-care on postoperative patients' recovery and satisfaction. Froman[16] studied the perceptual congruency between nurses and patients experiencing medical-surgical conditions. Hanna's use[18] of the Theory of Goal Attainment promoted the health behavior of adolescents, and Kameoka[24] analyzed nurse-patient interactions.

FURTHER DEVELOPMENT

King has consistently demonstrated her belief in the need for further testing of the Theory of Goal Attainment as early as 1971. "Any profession that has as its primary mission the delivery of social services requires continuous research to discover new knowledge that can be applied to improve practice. . . . The basis for the practice of nursing is knowledge; its activity is guided by the intellect, and applied in the practical realm."[30:112-113] "Because [the interacting] systems framework has been synthesized from basic elements in nursing, it will persist into the 21st century despite professional and social changes."[39:15]

Fawcett and Whall[14] identified five major areas in which further development of King's work would be helpful:

1. The concept of environment will benefit from additional definition and clarification. Additional work remains to be done in this area.
2. King's views of illness, health, and wellness will benefit from additional clarification and discussion.
3. Middle-range theories that are currently implied rather than explicit, such as those of Alligood, Evans, and Wilt[2] and Rooke,[51] will benefit from development into formal theories. Additional work is still needed.
4. Future linkages between King's interacting systems framework[34] and other existing middle-range theories should continue to be done in a

manner that ensures congruency between the framework and the specific middle-range theory. Further linkages continue to be needed.
5. Empirical testing should continue for the Theory of Goal Attainment[34] and other middle-range theories developed within King's interacting systems framework. Such testing will "add to the evidence regarding the empirical adequacy of the theories and their generalizability across various situations and client populations."[14:332]

CRITIQUE
Simplicity

King maintains that her definitions are clear and conceptually derived from research literature that existed at the time the definitions were published. King's Theory of Goal Attainment[33] presents 10 major concepts, making the theory complex. However, these concepts are easily understood and, with the exception of the concept of self, they have been derived from the research literature.

Generality

King's Theory of Goal Attainment[34] has been criticized for having limited application in areas of nursing in which patients are unable to competently interact with the nurse. King has responded that 70% of communication is nonverbal and describes the following:

> Try observing a good nurse interact with a baby or a child who has not yet learned the language. If you systematically recorded your observations, you would be able to analyze the behaviors and find many transactions at a nonverbal level. I have a beautiful example of that when I was working side by side with a graduate student in a neuro unit with a comatose patient. I was talking to the patient, explaining everything that was happening and showing the graduate student what I believe to be important in nursing care. When the patient regained consciousness a few days later, she asked the nurse in the unit to find that wonderful nurse who was the only one who explained what was happening to her. She wanted to thank her. I made transactions. I

could observe her muscle movement. She was trying to help us as a physician poked a tube down her throat.

A nurse midwife reports observing transactions between mothers and newborns. Psychiatric nurses have reported to me the value of my theory in their practice. So the need in nursing is to broaden nurses' knowledge of communication and that is what my theory is all about.[37]

Healthcare professionals have documented additional examples of the application of the Theory of Goal Attainment with psychiatric patients,[26,44] patients with acute and chronic orthopedic problems,[1] and developmentally disabled patients.[45]

King believes that critics are assuming that a theory will address every person, event, and situation, which is clearly impossible. She reminded critics that even Einstein's Theory of Relativity could not be tested completely until space travel made testing possible.[37]

Empirical Precision

King gathered empirical data on the nurse-patient interaction process that leads to goal attainment. A descriptive study was conducted to identify the characteristics of transaction and whether nurses made transactions with patients. From a sample of 17 patients, goals were attained in 12 cases (70% of the sample). King[34] believes that if nursing students are taught the Theory of Goal Attainment and it is used in nursing practice, goal attainment can be measured and the effectiveness of nursing care can be demonstrated.

King continues to serve as a consultant to researchers who test hypotheses derived from her theory. Since the publication of her theory in 1981,[34] multiple research studies provide additional and ongoing evidence of the empirical precision of the Theory of Goal Attainment.

Froman[16] tested perceptual congruency between nurses and patients who were experiencing medical-surgical problems. Hanna[18] tested the Theory of Goal Attainment in promoting health behaviors of adolescents. Using the Theory of Goal Attainment, Kameoka[24] analyzed interactions between nurses and

patients. Additional research projects are currently ongoing and others are listed in the Bibliography.

Derivable Consequences

King's Theory of Goal Attainment focuses on all aspects of the nursing process: assessment, planning, implementation, and evaluation. King believes that nurses must assess to set mutual goals, plan to provide alternative means to achieve goals, and evaluate to determine if the goal was attained. King[37] has stated that she is "the only [nurse theorist] who has provided a theory that deals with choice, alternatives, participation of all individuals in decision making and specifically deals with outcomes of nursing care."

Healthcare professionals have used and continue to use King's interacting systems framework and Theory of Goal Attainment to implement theory-based practice in various nursing practice settings in Canada, Japan, Sweden, and the United States. In addition, King's work has been demonstrated over time to be a comprehensive frame for curriculum development at various education levels. King and other nurse scientists and researchers have used her framework for theory testing and theory development at the grand and middle-range levels.

CRITICAL THINKING *Activities*

1. Think about and write your personal definitions of *environment, health, nursing,* and *person.* Compare your definitions with King's definitions. How are they similar? How are they different? Are they more alike than different? If they are more alike, develop a plan to use King's framework and theory more extensively in your practice.

2. Analyze an interaction you have had with a patient. Were you able to achieve a transaction as King describes it? If so, think about what you did differently with this person? If not, think about the interaction and try to identify why the transaction was not achieved?

3. Does the philosophy of one of the agencies in which you have practiced encourage the involvement of the patients in their care? If so, does mutual goal setting occur? If not, what changes would you suggest to more actively involve patients in their own care?

4. Analyze the goal-setting process that occurs between the direct care staff and nursing management and administration in an agency where you have practiced. Does mutual goal setting occur? Discuss changes that could be made in the organizational culture to facilitate mutual goal setting and goal attainment between nurse managers, administrators, and registered nurses.

5. Develop a quality improvement plan to review patient outcomes based on whether mutual goal setting and attainment of patient goals occur. Document changes in the effectiveness and efficiency of the care provided based on King's interacting systems framework and related theories.

REFERENCES

1. Alligood, M.R. (1995). Theory of goal attainment: Application to adult orthopedic nursing. In M.A. Frey & C.L. Sieloff (Eds.), *Advancing King's systems framework and theory of nursing* (pp. 209-222). Thousand Oaks, CA: Sage.

2. Alligood, M.R., Evans, G.W., & Wilt, D.L. (1995). King's interacting systems and empathy. In M.A. Frey & C.L. Sieloff (Eds.), *Advancing King's systems framework and theory of nursing* (pp. 66-78). Thousand Oaks, CA: Sage.

3. Allport, F.H. (1955). *Theories of perception and the concept of structure.* New York: John Wiley & Sons.

4. Ardrey, R. (1966). *The territorial imperative.* New York: Atheneium.

5. Austin, J.K. & Champion, V.L. (1983). King theory for nursing: Explication and evaluation. In P. Chinn (Ed.), *Advances in nursing theory development* (pp. 49-61). Rockville, MD: Aspen.

6. Benedict, M. & Frey, M.A. (1995). Theory-based practice in the emergency department. In M.A. Frey & C.L. Sieloff (Eds.), *Advancing King's systems framework and theory of nursing* (pp. 317-324). Thousand Oaks, CA: Sage.

7. Brown, S.T. & Lee, B.T. (1980). Imogene King's conceptual framework: A proposed model for continuing nursing education. *Journal of Advanced Nursing,* 5(5), 467-473.

8. Clements, I.W. & Roberts, F.B. (1983). *Family health: A theoretical approach to nursing care.* New York: John Wiley & Sons.

9. Coker, E., Fridley, T., Harris, J., Tomarchio, D., Chan, V., & Caron, C. (1995). Implementing nursing diagnoses within the context of King's conceptual framework. In M.A. Frey & C.L. Sieloff (Eds.), *Advancing King's systems framework and theory of nursing* (pp. 161-175). Thousand Oaks, CA: Sage.

10. Dewey, J. & Bentley, A. (1949). *Knowing and the known.* Boston: Beacon Press.

11. Diers, D. & Schmidt, R. (1977). Interaction analysis in nursing research. In P. Verhonick (Ed.), *Nursing research II* (pp. 77-132). Boston: Little, Brown.

12. Doornbos, M.M. (1995). Using King's systems framework to explore family health in the families of the young chronically mentally ill. In M.A. Frey & C.L. Sieloff (Eds.), *Advancing King's systems framework and theory of nursing* (pp. 192-205). Thousand Oaks, CA: Sage.

13. Fawcett, J.M., Vaillancourt, V.M., & Watson, C.A. (1995). Integration of King's framework into nursing practice. In M.A. Frey & C.L. Sieloff (Eds.), *Advancing King's systems framework and theory of nursing* (pp. 176-191). Thousand Oaks, CA: Sage.

14. Fawcett, J.M. & Whall, A.L. (1995). State of the science and future directions. In M.A. Frey & C.L. Sieloff (Eds.), *Advancing King's systems framework and theory of nursing* (pp. 327-334). Thousand Oaks, CA: Sage.[*]

15. Frey, M.A. (1995). Toward a theory of families, children, and chronic illness. In M.A. Frey & C.L. Sieloff (Eds.), *Advancing King's systems framework and theory of nursing* (pp. 109-125). Thousand Oaks, CA: Sage.

16. Forman, D. (1995). Perceptual congruency between clients and nurses: Testing King's theory of goal attainment. In M.A. Frey & C.L. Sieloff (Eds.), *Advancing King's systems framework and theory of nursing* (pp. 223-238). Thousand Oaks, CA: Sage.

17. Gonot, P.J. (1989). Imogene M. King: A theory for nursing. In J. Fitzpatrick & A. Whall, *Conceptual model of nursing: Analysis and application.* Bowie, MD: Robert J. Brady.

18. Hanna, K.M. (1995). Use of King's theory of goal attainment to promote adolescents' health behavior. In M.A. Frey & C.L. Sieloff (Eds.), *Advancing King's systems framework and theory of nursing* (pp. 239-250). Thousand Oaks, CA: Sage.

19. Hanucharurnkui, S. & Vinya-nguag, P. (1991). Effects of promoting patients' participation in self-care on postoperative recovery and satisfaction with care. *Nursing Science Quarterly,* 4(1), 14-20.

20. Hobdell, E.F. (1995). Using King's interacting systems framework for research on parents of children with neural tube defect. In M.A. Frey & C.L. Sieloff (Eds.), *Advancing King's systems framework and theory of nursing* (pp. 126-136). Thousand Oaks, CA: Sage.

21. Ittleson, W. & Cantril, H. (1954). *Perception: A transactional approach.* Garden City, NY: Doubleday.

22. Jersild, A.T. (1952). *In search of self.* New York: Teachers College Press.

23. Jolly, M.L. & Winker, C.K. (1995). Theory of goal attainment in the context of organizational structure. In M.A. Frey & C.L. Sieloff (Eds.), *Advancing King's systems framework and theory of nursing* (pp. 305-316). Thousand Oaks, CA: Sage.

24. Kameoka, T. (1995). Analyzing nurse-patient interactions in Japan. In M.A. Frey & C.L. Sieloff (Eds.), *Advancing King's systems framework and theory of nursing* (pp. 251-260). Thousand Oaks, CA: Sage.

25. Kelley, K.J. & Hammond, K.R. (1964). An approach to the study of clinical inference. *Nursing Research,* 13(4), 314-322.

26. Kemppainen, J.K. (1990). Imogene King's theory: A nursing case study of a psychotic client with human immunodeficiency virus infection. *Archives of Psychiatric Nursing,* 4(6), 384-388.

27. Killeen, M.B. (1996). *Patient-consumer perceptions and responses to professional nursing care: Instrument development.* Unpublished doctoral dissertation, Wayne State University, Detroit.

28. King, I.M. (1964). Nursing theory: Problems and prospects. *Nursing Science,* 1(3), 394-403.

29. King, I.M. (1968). A conceptual frame of reference for nursing. *Nursing Research,* 17(1), 27-31.

30. King, I.M. (1971). *Toward a theory for nursing: General concepts of human behavior.* New York: John Wiley & Sons.

31. King, I.M. (1975). A process for developing concepts for nursing through research. In P. Verhonick (Ed.), *Nursing research.* Boston: Little, Brown.

32. King, I.M. (1975). Patient aspects. In L.J. Schumann, R.D. Spears, Jr., & J.P. Young (Eds.), *Operations research in health care: A critical analysis.* Baltimore: Johns Hopkins University Press.

33. King, I.M. (Speaker). (1978). *Speech presented at Second Annual Nurse Educators' Conference.* Chicago: Teach 'Em.

34. King, I.M. (1981). *A theory for nursing: Systems, concepts, process.* New York: John Wiley & Sons.

35. King, I.M. (1984). Effectiveness of nursing care: Use of a goal oriented nursing record in end stage renal disease. *American Association of Nephrology Nurses and Technicians Journal,* 11(2), 11-17, 60.

36. King, I.M. (1984). Telephone interview.

37. King, I.M. (1985). Personal correspondence.

38. King, I.M. (1986). *Curriculum and instruction in nursing: Concepts and process.* Norwalk, CT: Appleton-Century-Crofts.

39. King, I.M. (1995). A systems framework for nursing. In M.A. Frey & C.L. Sieloff (Eds.), *Advancing King's systems framework and theory of nursing* (pp. 14-22). Thousand Oaks, CA: Sage.*

40. King, I.M. (1995). The theory of goal attainment. In M.A. Frey & C.L. Sieloff (Eds.), *Advancing King's systems framework and theory of nursing* (pp. 23-32). Thousand Oaks, CA: Sage.†

41. King, I.M. (1996, July 11). Personal communication.

42. Krieger, D. (1975). Therapeutic touch: The imprimatur of nursing. *American Journal of Nursing,* 75(5), 784-787.

43. Kuhn, A. (1975). *Unified social science.* Homewood, IL: Dorsey.

44. Laben, J.K., Sneed, L.D., & Seidel, S.L. (1995). Goal attainment in short-term group psychotherapy settings: Clinical implications for practice. In M.A. Frey & C.L. Sieloff (Eds.), *Advancing King's systems framework and theory of nursing* (pp. 261-277). Thousand Oaks, CA: Sage.

45. Messmer, P.R. (1995). Implementation of theory-based nursing practice. In M.A. Frey & C.L. Sieloff (Eds.), *Advancing King's systems framework and theory of nursing* (pp. 294-304). Thousand Oaks, CA: Sage.

46. Minckley, B.B. (1968). Space and place in patient care. *American Journal of Nursing,* 68(3), 510-516.

47. Orlando, I.J. (1961). *The dynamic nurse-patient relationship: Functions, process, principles.* New York: G.P. Putnam's Sons.

48. Orme, J.E. (1969). *Time, experience and behavior.* New York: American Elsevier.

49. Paterson, J. & Zderad, L. (1976). *Humanistic nursing.* New York: John Wiley & Sons.

50. Peplau, H.E. (1952). *Interpersonal relations in nursing.* New York: G.P. Putnam's Sons.

51. Rooke, L. (1995). Focusing on King's theory and systems framework in education by using an experiential learning model: A challenge to improve the quality of nursing care. In M.A. Frey & C.L. Sieloff (Eds.), *Advancing King's systems framework and theory of nursing* (pp. 278-293). Thousand Oaks, CA: Sage.

52. Rooke, L. (1995). The concept of space in King's systems framework: Its implications for nursing. In M.A. Frey & C.L. Sieloff (Eds.), *Advancing King's systems framework and theory of nursing* (pp. 79-96). Thousand Oaks, CA: Sage.

53. Sharts-Hopko, N.C. (1995). Using health, personal, and interpersonal system concepts within the King's systems framework to explore perceived health status during the menopause transition. In M.A. Frey & C.L. Sieloff (Eds.), *Advancing King's systems framework and theory of nursing* (pp. 147-160). Thousand Oaks, CA: Sage.

54. Sieloff, C.L. (1995). Defining the health of a social system within Imogene King's framework. In M.A. Frey & C.L. Sieloff (Eds.), *Advancing King's systems framework and theory of nursing* (pp. 137-146). Thousand Oaks, CA: Sage.

55. Sieloff, C.L. (1995). Development of a theory of departmental power. In M.A. Frey & C.L. Sieloff (Eds.), *Advancing King's systems framework and theory of nursing* (pp. 46-65). Thousand Oaks, CA: Sage.

56. Sieloff, C.L. (1996). *Development of an instrument to estimate the actualized power of a nursing department.* Unpublished doctoral dissertation, Wayne State University, Detroit.

57. Sommer, R. (1969). *Personal space.* Englewood Cliffs, NJ: Prentice-Hall.

58. Watzlawick, P., Beavin, J.W., & Jackson, D.D. (1967). *Pragmatics of human communication.* New York: Norton.

59. Whiting, J.F. (1955). Q-sort technique for evaluating perceptions of interpersonal relationship. *Nursing Research,* 4, 71-73.

60. Wicks, M.N. (1995). Family health as derived from King's framework. In M.A. Frey & C.L. Sieloff (Eds.), *Advancing King's systems framework and theory of nursing* (pp. 97-108). Thousand Oaks, CA: Sage.

61. Winker, C.K. (1995). A systems view of health. In M.A. Frey & C.L. Sieloff (Eds.), *Advancing King's systems framework and theory of nursing* (pp. 35-45). Thousand Oaks, CA: Sage.

62. Yura, H. & Walsh, M. (1978). *The nursing process.* New York: Appleton-Century-Crofts.

BIBLIOGRAPHY
Primary Sources
Books

Fawcett, J. & King, I. (Eds.). (1997). *The language of nursing theory and metatheory.* Indianapolis, IN: Sigma Theta Tau International Center Press.

King, I.M. (1971). *Toward a theory for nursing: General concepts of human behavior.* New York: John Wiley & Sons.

King, I.M. (1976). *Toward a theory of nursing: General concepts of human behavior* (Sugimori, M., Trans.). Tokyo: Igaku-Shoin.

King, I.M. (1981). *A theory for nursing: Systems, concepts, process.* New York: John Wiley & Sons.

King, I.M. (1985). *A theory for nursing: Systems, concepts, process* (Sugimori, M., Trans.). Tokyo: Igaku-Shoin.

King, I.M. (1986). *Curriculum and instruction in nursing: Concepts and process.* Norwalk, CT: Appleton-Century-Crofts.

Book Chapters

King, I.M. (1968). Toward the future of nursing research. In M.V. Batey (Ed.), *Communicating nursing research: The research critique* (Vol. 1). Boulder, Colorado: Western Interstate Commission for Higher Education.

King, I.M. (1975). A process for developing concepts for nursing through research. In P. Verhonick (Ed.), *Nursing research I.* Boston: Little Brown and Company.

King, I.M. (1975). The decision maker's perspective: Patient care aspects. In L. Schuman, R. Dixon Spears, & J.P. Young (Eds.). *Health research: The systems approach.* New York: Springer.

King. I.M. (1976). The health care systems: Nursing intervention subsystem. In H.H. Werley, A. Zuzick, M.N. Zaikowski, & A.D. Zagornik (Eds.), *Health research: The systems approach* (pp. 51-60). New York: Springer.

King, I.M. (1978). How does the conceptual framework provide structure for the curriculum? In National League for Nursing, *Curriculum process for developing or revising baccalaureate nursing programs* (pp. 23-34). New York: National League for Nursing.

King, I.M. (1978). The "why" of theory development. In National League for Nursing, *Theory development: What, why, how?* (pp. 11-16). New York: National League for Nursing.

King, I.M. (1983). King's theory of nursing. In I.W.R. Clements & F.B. Roberts (Eds.), *Family health: A theoretical approach to nursing care* (pp. 177-188). New York: John Wiley & Sons.

King, I.M. (1983). The family coping with a medical illness: Analysis and application of King's theory of goal attainment. In I.W.R. Clements & F.B. Roberts (Eds.), *Family health: A theoretical approach to nursing care* (pp. 383-385). New York: John Wiley & Sons.

King, I.M. (1983). The family with an elderly member: Analysis and application of King's theory of goal attainment. In I.W.R. Clements & F.B. Roberts (Ed.), *Family health: A theoretical approach to nursing care* (pp. 341-345). New York: John Wiley & Sons.

King, I.M. (1984). A theory for nursing: King's conceptual model applied in community health nursing. In M.K. Asay & C.C. Ossler (Eds.), *Proceedings of the Eighth Annual Community Health Nursing Conference: Conceptual models of nursing applications in community health nursing.* Chapel Hill: University of North Carolina.

King, I.M. (1986). King's goal attainment theory. In P. Winfred Fry (Ed.), *Case studies in nursing theories* (pp. 197-213). New York: National League for Nursing.

King, I.M. (1988). Imogene M. King. In T.A. Schorr & A. Zimmerman (Eds.), *Making choices, taking chances* (pp. 146-153). St. Louis: Mosby.

King, I.M. (1988). King's system framework for nursing administration. In B. Henry, C. Arndt, M. DiVincenti, A. Marriner Tomey (Eds.), *Dimensions of nursing administration* (pp. 35-45). Boston: Blackwell Scientific.

King, I.M. (1988). Measuring health goal attainment in patients. In C.F. Waltz & O.L. Strickland (Eds.), *Measurement of nursing outcomes: Vol. 4. Measuring client outcomes* (pp. 108-127). New York: Springer.

King, I.M. (1988). Research: The basis for excellence. In J.F. Wang, P.S. Simoni, & C.L. Nath (Eds.), *Nursing: Power through excellence* (pp. 3-4). Charleston, WV: University of West Virginia.

King, I.M. (1989). King's general systems framework and theory. In J.P. Riehl-Sisca (Ed.), *Conceptual models for nursing practice* (3rd ed., pp. 149-166). Norwalk, CT: Appleton & Lange.

King, I.M. (1989). King's systems framework for nursing administration. In B. Henry, C. Arndt, M. Vincenti, & A. Marriner Tomey (Eds.), *Dimensions of nursing administration: Theory, research, education, practice* (pp. 25-46). Cambridge, MA: Blackwell Scientific Publications.

King, I.M. (1990). King's conceptual framework and theory of goal attainment. In M.E. Parker (Ed.), *Nursing theories in practice* (pp. 73-84). New York: National League for Nursing.

King, I.M. (1995). A systems framework for nursing. In M.A. Frey & C.L. Sieloff (Eds.), *Advancing King's systems framework and theory of nursing* (pp. 14-22). Thousand Oaks, CA: Sage.

King, I.M. (1995). The theory of goal attainment. In M.A. Frey & C.L. Sieloff (Eds.), *Advancing King's systems framework and theory of nursing* (pp. 23-32). Thousand Oaks, CA: Sage.

Journal Articles

Daubenmire, M.J. & King, I.M. (1973). Nursing process models: A systems approach. *Nursing Outlook, 21*(8), 512-517.

Gold, C., Haas, S., & King, I. (2000). Conceptual frameworks: Putting the nursing focus into core curricula. *Nurse Educator, 25*(2), 95-98.

Gulitz, E.A. & King, I.M. (1988, Aug.). King's general systems model: Application to curriculum development. *Nursing Science Quarterly, 1*(3), 128-132.

Heller, M.P. & King, I.M. (1965). Team teaching. *Nursing Outlook, 13*(10), 50-51.

King, I.M. (1963). Junior college education for nursing: An urgent necessity. *Illness Medical Journal, 123*(1), 88-89.

King, I.M. (1964). Nursing theory—problems and prospect. *Nursing Science, 2*(5), 394-403.

King, I.M. (1968). Conceptual frame of reference for nursing. *Nursing Research, 17*(1), 27-31.

King, I.M. (1969). Symposium on neurologic and neurosurgical nursing. *Nursing Clinics of North America, 4*(2), 179-180.

King, I.M. (1970). A conceptual frame of reference for nursing. *Japanese Journal of Nursing Research, 3,* 199-204.

King, I.M. (1970). Planning for change. *Ohio Nurses Review, 45,* 4-7.

King, I.M. (1975). [Review of the book *Conceptual Models for Nursing*], *Nursing Research, 24*(4), 306-307.

King, I.M. (1984). Effectiveness of nursing care: Use of a goal-oriented nursing record in end-stage renal disease. *American Association of Nephrology Nurses and Technicians Journal, 11*(2),11-17, 60.

King, I.M. (1984). Philosophy of nursing education: A national survey. *Western Journal of Nursing Research, 6*(4), 387-406.

King, I.M. (1985). Circadian rhythm: Screening for fever. *Nursing Research, 34*(6), 377-379.

King, I.M. (1985). Collaborative relationship in nursing research. *Florida Nurse, 33*(2), 3, 15.

King, I.M. (1985). Patient education: Barriers and gateways. *Florida Nurse, 33*(5), 4, 15.

King, I.M. (1987). Concepts: Essential elements of theories. *Nursing Science Quarterly, 1*(1), 22-25.

King, I.M. (1987). Translating nursing research into practice. *Journal of Neuroscience Nursing, 19*(1), 44-48.

King, I.M. (1990, Fall). Health as the goal for nursing. *Nursing Science Quarterly, 3*(3), 123-128.

King, I.M. (1992). King's theory of goal attainment. *Nursing Science Quarterly, 5*(1), 19-26.

King, I.M. (1993). Quality of life and goal attainment. *Nursing Science Quarterly, 7*(1), 29-32.

King, I.M. (1994). Quality of life and goal attainment. *Nursing Science Quarterly, 7*(1), 29-32.

King, I.M. (1996). The theory of goal attainment in research and practice. *Nursing Science Quarterly, 9*(2), 61-66.

King, I.M. (1997). King's theory of goal attainment in practice. *Nursing Science Quarterly, 10*(4), 180-185.

King, I.M. (1997). Reflections on the past and a vision for the future. *Nursing Science Quarterly, 10*(1), 15-17.

King, I.M. (1998). Nursing informatics: A universal nursing language. *Florida Nurse, 46*(1), 1-3, 5, 9.

King, I.M. (1998). The Bioethics Focus Group Report. *Florida Nurse, 46*(8), 24.

King, I.M. (1999). A theory of goal attainment: Philosophical and ethical implications. *Nursing Science Quarterly, 12*(4), 292-296.

King, I.M. & Tarsitano, B. (1982). The effect of structured and unstructured preop teaching: A replication. *Nursing Research,* 31(6), 324-329.

Quigley, P., Janzen, S.K., King, I.M., & Goucher, E. (1999). Nurse staffing patient outcomes from one acute care setting within the Department of Veteran's Affairs. *Florida Nurse,* 47(2), 34.

Samples, J., Vancott, M.L., Long, C., King, I.M., & Kersenbrock, A. (1985). Circadian rhythms: Basis for screening for fever. *Nursing Research,* 34(6), 377-379.

Letter to the Editor

King, I.M. (1975). Reaction to "The patient rights advocate," by G.J. Annas & J. Healey [Letter to the Editor]. *Journal of Nursing Administration,* 5(1), 40-41.

Forewords

King, I.M. (1969). Symposium on neurologic and neurosurgical nursing. *Nursing Clinics of North America,* 4(2), 199-200.

King, I.M. (1991). Foreword. In C.L. Sieloff Evans, *Imogene King: A conceptual framework for nursing* (pp. vii-viii). Newbury Park, CA: Sage.

Audiotapes

King, I.M. (1978, Dec.). *Nursing theory* [Audiotape]. Wakefield, MA: Nursing Resources, Inc.

King, I.M. (1978). Second Annual Nurse Educators' Conference, held in New York City [Audiotape]. Available: Teach 'em, Inc., 160 E. Illinois Street, Chicago, IL 60611.

King, I.M. (1984, 1986). Nurse Theorist Conference held at Edmonton, Alberta [Audiotape]. Available: Kennedy Recording, R.R. 5, Edmonton, Alberta, T5P 487 Canada.

King, I.M. (1985, 1987). *King's theory* [Audiotape]. Nurse Theorist Conference held in Pittsburgh, PA. Available: Meetings International, 1200 Delor Ave., Louisville, KY 40217.

Videotapes

King, I.M. (1987). *King's theory* [Videotape]. Nurse Theorist Conference held in Pittsburgh, PA. Available: Meetings International, 1200 Delor Ave., Louisville, KY 40217.

King, I.M. (1989). *The nurse theorist: Portraits of excellence* [Videotape]. Oakland: Studio III. Available: Fuld Video Project, 370 Hawthorne Ave., Oakland, CA 94609.

Presented Papers

King, I.M. (1968). *Trends in doctoral program.* Presentation at the Proceedings of the Southern Regional Education Board, Atlanta.

King, I.M. (1980, April). *Theory development in nursing.* Paper presented at Georgia State University, Atlanta.

King, I.M. (1984). *A theory for nursing: King's conceptual model applied in community health nursing.* Paper presented at the Conceptual Models of Nursing, Application in Community Health Nursing: Proceedings of the Eighth Annual Community Health Nursing Conference, Chapel Hill, NC.

King, I. M. (1989, May). *Health as a goal for nursing.* Paper presented at an International Theory Conference, Pittsburgh.

King, I.M. (1989, May). *Nursing in the 21st century.* Paper presented for Nurses' Week at Tampa VA Hospital, Tampa, FL.

King, I.M. (1989, Nov.). *Graduate education in nursing for the 21st century.* Paper presented at the 25th Anniversary of the Graduate Program, Loyola University, Chicago.

King, I.M. (1989, Nov.). *Humor in nursing.* Paper presented at the Florida Nurses Association, 13th district.

King, I.M. (1989, Nov.). *Theory: What it is and what it is not.* Paper presented at the Biennial Convention of Sigma Theta Tau International, Indianapolis.

King, I.M. (1990, April). *Transactions: The key to health family dynamics.* Paper presented at the 2nd Annual Conference on Family Health, University of South Florida College of Nursing, Tampa, FL.

King, I.M. (1990, May). *Together in caring.* Paper presented at Nurses' Day Celebration, Tampa General Hospital, Tampa, FL.

King, I.M. (1990, Sept.). *Enhancing nursing research visibility.* Presentation at the Council of Nursing Research, Florida Nurses' Association.

King, I.M. (1990, Oct.). *Nursing practice with King's framework and knowledge development with King's framework.* Seminars at the University of Tennessee College of Nursing, Knoxville, TN.

King, I.M. (1990, Oct.). *Theory-based quality assurance in nursing.* Conference presented in Sedona, Arizona.

King, I.M. (1990, Nov.). *Relationship of theory, research and nursing practice.* Paper presented at the 7th District Florida Nurses Association.

King, I.M. (1991, March). *Application of King's theory to nursing practice.* Keynote paper presented at Sigma Theta Tau Chapter, Erie, PA.

King, I.M. (1991, July). *Conceptual system and general system theory of goal attainment.* Paper presented at International Nursing Theory Conference, Tokyo.

King, I.M. (1992, March). *The research process: Past, present, and future.* Presentation at three Sigma Theta Tau Chapters, Valdosta, GA.

King, I.M. (1992, March). *Update on nursing theory.* Keynote presentation at Sigma Theta Tau, Pittsburgh, PA.

King, I.M. (1992, April). *Update on nursing theory.* Keynote presentation at Sigma Theta Tau Conference, Wilkes-Barre, PA.

King, I.M. (1992, May). *Another goal achieved.* Commencement presentation at University of Tampa, Department of Nursing, Tampa, FL.

King, I.M. (1995, June). *Jessie M. Scott award presentation.* Paper presented at the 100th American Nurses Association Convention, Washington, DC.

King, I.M. (1997, May). *Nursing and the future of health care.* Paper presented at District V of the Florida Nurses Association.

King, I.M. (1997, July). *Theoretical basis for nursing informatics.* Paper presented at the University of Maryland Summer Institute on Nursing Informatics.

King, I.M. (1997, Sept.). *Nursing's vision for the future.* Paper presented at the American Operating Room Nurses Convention, Sarasota, FL.

King, I.M. (1997, Sept./Oct.). *A theoretical basis for nursing informatics.* Paper presented at the International Nursing Informatics Conference, Stockholm.

King, I.M. (1997, Oct.). *Nursing and health care in the twenty-first century.* Keynote presented at the Idaho Nurses Association convention.

King, I.M. (1999, Oct.). *Reflections of the past: Visions of the Future.* Paper presented at the Inaugural Conference of the King International Nursing Group, Troy, MI.

King, I.M. (1999, Nov.). *Discovery, controversy, self-actualization.* Paper presented at the Ethics Conference, Loyola University, Chicago.

King, I.M. (1999, Nov.). *High tech, high touch: Nursing in the new millenium.* Paper presented at the Florida Nursing Student Association Annual Convention, St. Petersburg, FL.

King, I.M. (1999, Dec.). *Implementing a research program in a large medical center.* Paper presented at the Department of Nursing, Clearwater, FL.

King, I.M. & Fawcett, J. (1999, Oct.). *Charting the course for the new millenium.* Paper presented at the Inaugural Conference of the King International Nursing Group, Troy, MI.

King, I.M. & Killeen, M. (1999, Oct.). *Interaction, transaction, and new technology.* Paper presented at the Inaugural Conference of the King International Nursing Group, Troy, MI.

Secondary Sources
Book Reviews

[Review of the book *Toward a theory for nursing: General concepts of human behavior*]. (1971). *Canadian Nurse, 67,* 40.

[Review of the book *Toward a theory for nursing: General concepts of human behavior*]. (1971). *Nursing Outlook, 19,* 513.

[Review of the book *Toward a theory for nursing: General concepts of human behavior*]. (1971). *Nursing Research, 20,* 462.

[Review of the book *Toward a theory for nursing: General concepts of human behavior*]. (1972). *American Journal of Nursing, 72,* 1153.

[Review of the book *Toward a theory for nursing: General concepts of human behavior*]. (1972). *Journal of Nursing Administration, 2,* 63.

[Review of the book *Toward a theory for nursing: General concepts of human behavior*]. (1973). *South African Nursing Journal, 40,* 32.

[Review of the book *A theory for nursing: Systems, concepts, process*]. (1982). *Nursing Mirror, 154,* 32.

[Review of the book *A theory for nursing: Systems, concepts, process*]. (1982). *Nursing Outlook, 30,* 414.

[Review of the book *A theory for nursing: Systems, concepts, process*]. (1982). *Nursing Times, 78,* 331.

[Review of the book *A theory for nursing: Systems, concepts, process*]. (1982). *Research in Nursing and Health, 5,* 166-167.

[Review of the book *A theory for nursing: Systems, concepts, process*]. (1982). *Today's OR Nurse, 4,* 62.

[Review of the book *A theory for nursing: Systems, concepts, process*]. (1982). *Western Journal of Nursing Research, 4,* 103-104.

[Review of the book *A theory for nursing: Systems, concepts, process*]. (1983). *Australian Nurses Journal, 12*(7), 33-34.

Books

Barnum, B.J. (1994). *Nursing theory: Analysis, application, evaluation* (4th ed.). Philadelphia: J.B. Lippincott.

Bevis, E.O. (1982). *Curriculum building in nursing: A process.* St. Louis: Mosby.

Chinn, P.L. (Ed.). (1983). *Advances in nursing theory development.* Rockville, MD: Aspen.

Chinn, P.L. & Jacobs, M.K. (1995). *Theory and nursing: A systematic approach.* St. Louis: Mosby.

Fitzpatrick, J.J. & Whall, A.L. (1995). *Conceptual models of nursing: Analysis and application.* Bowie, MD: Robert J. Brady.

Fitzpatrick, J.J., Whall, A., Johnston, R., & Floyd, J. (1982). *Nursing models and their psychiatric mental health applications.* Bowie, MD: Robert J. Brady.

Frey, M.A. & Sieloff, C.L. (1995). *Advancing King's systems framework and theory of nursing.* Thousand Oaks, CA: Sage.

George, J.B. (1995). *Nursing theories: The base for professional nursing practice.* Englewood Cliffs, NJ: Prentice-Hall.

Polit, D. & Hungler, B. (1995). *Nursing research: Principles and methods* (5th ed.). Philadelphia: J.B. Lippincott.

Steele, S. (1981). *Child health and the family: Nursing concepts and management.* New York: Masson.

Walker, L.O. & Avant, K.C. (1995). *Strategies for theory construction in nursing.* Norwalk, CT: Appleton-Century-Crofts.

Who's who in America. (43rd ed.). (1984). Chicago: Marquis.

Who's who in American nursing. (1987, 1988). Chicago: Marquis.

Who's who in American women. (1986). Chicago: Marquis.

Who's who in the Midwest. (1984). Chicago: Marquis.

Book Chapters

Alligood, M.R. (1995). Theory of goal attainment: Application to adult orthopedic nursing. In M.A. Frey & C.L. Sieloff (Eds.), *Advancing King's systems framework and theory of nursing* (pp. 209-222). Thousand Oaks, CA: Sage.

Alligood, M.R., Evans, G.W., & Wilt, D.L. (1995). King's interacting system and empathy. In M.A. Frey & C.L. Sieloff (Eds.). *Advancing King's systems framework and theory of nursing* (pp. 66-78). Thousand Oaks, CA: Sage.

Austin, J.K. & Champion, V.L. (1983). King theory for nursing: Explication and evaluation. In P. Chinn, *Advances in nursing theory development* (pp. 49-61). Rockville, MD: Aspen.

Benedict, M. & Frey, M.A. (1995). Theory-based practice in the emergency department. In M.A. Frey and C.L. Sieloff (Eds.). *Advancing King's systems framework and theory of nursing* (pp. 317-324). Thousand Oaks, CA: Sage.

Chinn, P.L. & Jacobs, M.K. (1983). Theory in nursing: A current overview. In P.L. Chinn & M.K. Jacobs (Eds.), *Theory and nursing: A systematic approach* (pp. 190-191). St. Louis: Mosby.

Coker, E.B. & Schreiber, R. (1990). Implementing King's conceptual framework at the bedside. In M.E. Parker (Ed.), *Nursing theories in practice* (pp. 85-102). New York: National League for Nursing.

Daubenmire, M.J. (1989). A baccalaureate nursing curriculum based on King's conceptual framework. In J.P. Riehl-Sisca (Ed.), *Conceptual models for nursing practice* (3rd ed., pp. 167-178). Norwalk, CT: Appleton & Lange.

DiNardo, P.B. (1989). Evaluation of the nursing theory of Imogene M. King. In J.P. Riehl-Sisca (Ed.), *Conceptual models for nursing practice* (3rd ed., pp. 159-166). Norwalk, CT: Appleton & Lange.

Doornbos, M.M.(1995). Using King's systems framework to explore family health in the families of the young chronically mentally ill. In M.A. Frey & C.L. Sieloff (Eds.), *King's systems framework and theory of nursing* (pp. 192-205). Thousand Oaks, CA: Sage.

Elberson, E. (1989). Applying King's model to nursing administration. In B. Henry, C. Arndt, M. DiVincenti, & A. Marriner Tomey (Eds.), *Dimensions of nursing administration* (pp. 47-53). Boston: Blackwell Scientific.

Fawcett, J. (1995). King's open systems model. In *Analysis and evaluation of conceptual models of nursing* (3rd ed., pp. 109-163). Philadelphia: F.A. Davis.

Fawcett, J. & Whall, A.L.(1995). State of the science and future directions. In M.A. Frey & C.L. Sieloff (Eds.), *King's systems framework and theory of nursing* (pp. 327-334). Thousand Oaks, CA: Sage.

Fawcett, J.M., Vaillancourt, V.M. & Watson, C.A. (1995). Integration of King's framework into nursing practice. In M.A. Frey & C.L. Sieloff (Eds.), *Advancing King's systems framework and theory of nursing* (pp. 176-191). Thousand Oaks, CA: Sage.

Fitzpatrick, J., Whall, A., Johnston, R., & Floyd, J. (1982). Nursing models. In *Nursing models and their psychiatric mental health application* (pp. 62-64). Bowie, MD: Robert J. Brady.

Frey, M.A. (1993). A theoretical perspective of family and child health derived from King's conceptual framework of nursing: A deductive approach to theory building. In S.L. Feetham, S.B. Meister, J.M. Bell, & C.L. Gillis (Eds.), *The nursing of families: theory/research/education/practice* (pp. 30-37). Newbury Park, CA: Sage.

Frey, M.A. (1995). From conceptual framework to nursing knowledge. In M.A. Frey & C.L. Sieloff (Eds.), *Advancing King's framework and theory for nursing* (pp. 3-13). Thousand Oaks, CA: Sage.

Frey, M.A. & Norris, D. (1997). King's systems framework and theory in nursing practice. In M.R. Alligood & A. Marriner Tomey (Eds.), *Nursing theory: Utilization and application* (pp. 71-88). St. Louis: Mosby.

Froman, D. (1995). Perceptual congruency between clients and nurses: Testing King's theory of goal attainment. In M.A. Frey & C.L. Sieloff (Eds.), *Advancing King's systems framework and theory of nursing* (pp. 223-238). Thousand Oaks, CA: Sage.

George, J.B. (1980). Imogene M. King. In J.B. George (Ed.), *Nursing theories: The base for professional nursing practice* (pp. 184-198). Englewood Cliffs, NJ: Prentice-Hall.

Gonot, P.J. (1983). Imogene M. King: A theory for nursing. In J. Fitzpatrick & A. Whall (Eds.), *Conceptual models of nursing: Analysis and application* (pp. 221-243). Bowie, MD: Robert J. Brady.

Gonot, P.J. (1986). Family therapy as derived from King's conceptual model. In A.L. Whall (Ed.), *Family therapy theory for nursing: Four approaches* (pp. 33-48). Norwalk, Connecticut: Appleton-Century-Crofts.

Hanchett, E.S. (1988). Community assessment: King's conceptual framework—dynamic interacting systems. In *Nursing frameworks and community as client: Bridging the gap* (pp. 89-107). Norwalk, CT: Appleton & Lange.

Hanchett, E.S. (1988). King's general system framework. In *Nursing frameworks and community as client: Bridging the gap* (pp. 83-87). Norwalk, CT: Appleton & Lange.

Hanna, K.M. (1995). Use of King's theory of goal attainment to promote adolescents' health behavior. In M.A. Frey & C.L. Sieloff (Eds.), *Advancing King's systems framework and theory of nursing* (pp. 239-250). Thousand Oaks, CA: Sage.

Hobdell, E.F. (1995). Using King's interacting systems framework for research on parents of children with neural tube defects. In M.A. Frey & C.L. Sieloff (Eds.), *Advancing King's systems framework and theory of nursing* (pp. 126-136). Thousand Oaks, CA: Sage.

Jolly, M.L. & Winker, C.K. (1995). Theory of goal attainment in the context of organizational structure. In M.A. Frey & C.L. Sieloff (Eds.). *Advancing King's systems framework and theory of nursing* (pp. 305-316). Thousand Oaks, CA: Sage.

Kameoka, T. (1995). Analyzing nurse-patient interactions in Japan. In M.A. Frey & C.L. Sieloff (Eds.), *Advancing King's systems framework and theory of nursing* (pp. 251-260). Thousand Oaks, CA: Sage.

Laben, J.K., Sneed, L.D., & Seidel, S.L. (1995). Goal attainment in short-term group psychotherapy settings: Clinical implications for practice. In M.A. Frey & C.L. Sieloff (Eds.), *Advancing King's systems framework and theory of nursing* (pp. 261-277). Thousand Oaks, CA: Sage.

Meleis, A.I. (1991). Imogene King. In *Theoretical nursing: development and progress* (2nd ed.) (pp. 327-338). Philadelphia: J.B. Lippincott.

Messmer, P.R. (1995). Implementation of theory-based nursing practice. In M.A. Frey & C.L. Sieloff (Eds.). *Advancing King's systems framework and theory of nursing* (pp. 294-304). Thousand Oaks, CA: Sage.

Myks Babb, B.A., Fouladbakhsh, J.M., & Hanchett, E.S. (1988). Interactions on main street. In E.S. Hanchett (Ed.), *Nursing frameworks and community as client: Bridging the gap* (pp. 109-115). Norwalk, CT: Appleton & Lange.

Rooke, L. (1995). Focusing on King's theory and systems framework in education by using an experiential learning model: A challenge to improve the quality of nursing care. In M.A. Frey & C.L. Sieloff (Eds.), *Advancing King's systems framework and theory of nursing* (pp. 278-293). Thousand Oaks, CA: Sage.

Rooke, L. (1995). The concept of space in King's systems framework: Its implications for nursing. In M.A. Frey & C.L. Sieloff (Eds.), *Advancing King's systems framework and theory of nursing* (pp. 79-96). Thousand Oaks, CA: Sage.

Sharts-Hopko, N.C. (1995). Using health, personal and interpersonal system concepts within the King's systems framework to explore perceived health status during the menopause transition. In M.A. Frey & C.L. Sieloff (Eds.), *Advancing King's systems framework and theory of nursing* (pp. 147-160). Thousand Oaks, CA: Sage.

Sieloff, C.L. (1995). Defining the health of a social system within Imogene King's framework. In M.A. Frey & C.L. Sieloff (Eds.), *Advancing King's systems framework and theory of nursing* (pp. 137-146). Thousand Oaks, CA: Sage.

Sieloff, C.L. (1995). Development of a theory of departmental power. In M.A. Frey & C.L. Sieloff (Eds.), *Advancing King's systems framework and theory of nursing* (pp. 46-65). Thousand Oaks, CA: Sage.

Thibodeau, J.A. (1983). History of the development of nursing models. In *Nursing models: Analysis and evaluation* (pp. 37-38). Monterey, CA: Wadsworth.

Wicks, M.N. (1995). Family health as derived from King's framework. In M.A. Frey & C.L. Sieloff (Eds.), *Advancing King's systems framework and theory of nursing* (pp. 97-108). Thousand Oaks, CA: Sage.

Winker, C.K. (1995). A systems view of health. In M.A. Frey & C.L. Sieloff (Eds.), *Advancing King's systems framework and theory of nursing* (pp. 35-45). Thousand Oaks, CA: Sage.

Journal Articles

Alligood, M.R. & May, B.A. (2000). A nursing theory of personal system empathy: Interpreting a conceptualization of empathy in King's Interacting Systems. *Nursing Science Quarterly,* 13(3), 243-247.

Bramlett, M.H., Gueldner, S.H., & Sowell, R.L. (1989). Consumer-centric advocacy: Its connection to nursing frameworks. *Nursing Science Quarterly,* 3(4), 156-161.

Brooks, E.M. & Thomas, S. (1997). The perception and judgement of senior baccalaureate student nurses in clinical decision making. *Advances in Nursing Science,* 19(3), 50-69.

Brown, S.T. & Lee, B.T. (1980). Imogene King's conceptual framework: A proposed model for continuing nursing education. *Journal of Advanced Nursing,* 5(5), 467-473.

Bunting, S.M. (1988, Nov.). The concept of perception in selected nursing theories. *Nursing Science Quarterly,* 1(4), 168-174.

Burney, M.A. (1992). King and Neuman: In search of the nursing paradigm. *Journal of Advanced Nursing,* 17, 601-603.

Byrne, E. & Schreiber, R. (1989, Feb.). Concept of the month: Implementing King's conceptual framework at the bedside [tables/charts]. *Journal of Nursing Administration,* 19(2), 28-32.

Byrne-Coker, E., Fradley, T., Harris, J., Tomarchio, D., Chan, V., & Caron, C. (1990, July/Sept.). Implementing nursing diagnoses within the context of King's conceptual framework. *Nursing Diagnosis,* 1(3), 107-114.

Byrne-Coker, E. & Schreiber, R. (1990, Jan.). King at the bedside. *Canadian Nurse,* 86(1), 24-26.

Calladine, M.L. (1996). Nursing process for health promotion using King's theory. *Journal of Community Health Nursing,* 13(1), 51-57.

Caris-Verhallen, W.M.C.M., Kerkstra, A., van der Heijden, P.G.M., & Bensing, J.M. (1998). Nurse-elderly patient communication in home care and institutional care: An explorative study. *International Journal of Nursing Studies,* 35 1/2, 95-108.

Carter, K.F. & Dufour, L.T. (1994). King's theory: A critique of the critiques. *Nursing Science Quarterly,* 7(3), 128-133.

Chance K.S. (1982). Nursing models: A requisite for professional accountability. *Advances in Nursing Science,* 4(2), 46-65.

Connelly, C.E. (1986). Replication research in nursing. *American Operating Room Nurses Journal,* 23(1), 71-77.

Craig, S. (1980). Theory development and its relevance for nursing. *Journal of Advanced Nursing,* 5(4), 349-355.

Crossan, F. & Robb, A. (1998). Role of the nurse: Introducing theories and concepts. *British Journal of Nursing,* 7(10), 608-612.

Daubenmier, M.J. & King, I.M. (1973). Nursing process models: A systems approach. *Nursing Outlook,* 21, 512-517.

Daubenmire, M.J., Searles, S.S., & Ashton, C.A. (1978). A methodologic framework to study nurse-patient communication. *Nursing Research,* 27(5), 303-310.

Davis, D.C. (1987). A conceptual framework for infertility. *Journal of Obstetric, Gynecologic, and Neonatal Nursing,* 16, 30-35.

Davis, D.C. & Dearman, C.N. (1991). Coping strategies of infertile women. *Journal of Obstetric, Gynecologic, and Neonatal Nursing,* 20, 221-228.

DeFeo, D.J. (1990, Summer). Change: A central concern of nursing. *Nursing Science Quarterly,* 3(2), 88-94.

DeHowitt, M.C. (1992). King's conceptual model and individual psychotherapy. *Perspectives in Psychiatric Care,* 28(4), 11-14.

Fitch, M., Rogers, M., Ross, E., Shea, H., Smith, I., & Tucker, D. (1991). Developing a plan to evaluate the use of nursing conceptual frameworks. *Canadian Journal of Nursing Administration,* 4(1), 22-28.

Flaskerud, J.H. (1986). On "Toward a theory of nursing action: Skills and competency in nurse-patient interaction." *Nursing Research,* 35(7), 250-252.

Frey, M.A. (1989, Fall). Social support and health: A theoretical formulation derived from King's conceptual framework [research, tables/charts]. *Nursing Science Quarterly,* 2(2), 138-148.

Frey, M.A. (1996). Behavioral correlates of health and illness in youths with chronic illness. *Advanced Nursing Research,* 9(4), 167-176.

Frey, M.A. (1997). Health promotion in youth with chronic illness: Are we on the right track? *Quality Nursing,* 3(5), 13-18.

Frey, M.A. & Fox, M.A. (1990). Assessing and teaching self-care to youths with diabetes mellitus. *Pediatric Nursing,* 16, 597-599.

Frey, M.A., Rooke, L., Sieloff, C.L., Messmer, P., & Kameoka, T. (1995). King's framework and theory in Japan, Sweden, and the United States. *Image: Journal of Nursing Scholarship,* 27(2), 127-130.

Funashima, N. (1990). King's goal attainment theory. *Knago MOOK,* 35, 56-62.

Gill, J., Hopwood-Jones, L., Tyndall, J., Gregoroff, S., LeBlanc, P., Lovett, C., Rasco, L., & Ross, A. (1995). Incorporating nursing diagnosis and King's theory in the O.R. documentation. *Canadian Operating Room Nursing Journal,* 13(1), 10-14.

Gortner, S.R. & Nahm, H. (1977). An overview of nursing research in the U.S. *Nursing Research,* 26(1), 10-33.

Hampton, D.C. (1994). King's theory of goal attainment as a framework for managed care implementation in a hospital setting. *Nursing Science Quarterly,* 7(4), 170-173.

Hanchett, E.S. (1990, Summer). Nursing models and community as client . . . public health/community health nursing. *Nursing Science Quarterly,* 3(2), 67-72.

Hanna, K. (1993). Effect of nurse-client transaction on female adolescents' oral contraceptive use. *Image: Journal of Nursing Scholarship,* 25(4), 285-290.

Hanucharurnkul, S. (1989, May). Comparative analysis of Orem's and King's theories. *Journal of Advanced Nursing,* 14(5), 365-72.

Hanucharurnkui, S. & Vinya-nguag, P. (1991, Spring). Effects of promoting patients' participation in self-care on postoperative recovery and satisfaction with care [research, tables/charts]. *Nursing Science Quarterly,* 4(1), 14-20.

Hawks, J.H. (1991). Power: A concept analysis. *Journal of Advanced Nursing,* 16, 754-762.

Heggie, M. & Gangar, E. (1992). A nursing model for menopause clinics. *Nursing Standard,* 6(21), 32-34.

Houfek, J.F. (1992). Nurses' perceptions of the dimensions of nursing care episodes. *Nursing Research,* 41, 280-285.

Hughes, M.M. (1983). Nursing theories and emergency nursing. *Journal of Emergency Nursing,* 9, 95-97.

Husband, A. (1988, July). Application of King's theory of nursing to the care of the adult with diabetes. *Journal of Advanced Nursing,* 13(4), 484-488.

Husting, P.M. (1997). A transcultural critique of Imogene King's theory of goal attainment. *The Journal of Multicultural Nursing & Health,* 3(3), 15-20.

Jackson, A.L., Pokorny, M.E., & Vincent, P. (1993). Relative satisfaction with nursing care of patients with ostomies. *Journal of ET Nursing,* 20(6), 233-238.

Jacono, J., Hicks, G., Antonioni, C., O'Brien, K., & Rasi, M. (1990). Comparison of perceived needs of family members between registered nurses and family members of critically ill patients in intensive care and neonatal intensive care units. *Heart & Lung: Journal of Critical Care,* 19(1), 72-78.

Jonas, C.M. (1987). King's goal attainment theory: Use in gerontological nursing practice. *Perspectives,* 11(4), 9-12.

Jones, S., Clark, V.B., Merker, A., & Palau, D. (1995). Changing behaviors: Nurse educators and clinical nurse specialists design a discharge planning program. *Journal of Nursing Staff Development,* 11(6), 291-295.

Kasch, C.R. (1986). Toward a theory of nursing action: Skills and competency in nurse-patient interaction. *Nursing Research,* 35(4), 226-230.

Kenny, T. (1990). Erosion of individuality in care of elderly people in hospital—an alternative approach. *Journal of Advanced Nursing,* 15(5), 571-576.

Kneeshaw, M.F. (1990). Nurses' perception of co-worker responses to smoking cessation attempts. *Journal of the New York State Nurses Association,* 21(1), 9-13.

Kobayashi, F.T. (1970). A conceptual frame of reference for nursing. *Japanese Journal of Nursing Research,* 3(3), 199-204.

Kohler, P. (1988). Model of shared control. *Journal of Gerontological Nursing,* 14(7), 21-25, 37-38.

Kusaka, T. (1991). Application to the King's goal attainment theory in Japanese clinical setting. *Journal of the Japanese Academy of Nursing Education,* 1(1), 30-31.

Laben, J.K., Dodd, D., & Sneed, L. (1991). King's theory of goal attainment applied in group therapy for inpatient juvenile sexual offenders, maximum security state offenders, and community parolees, using visual aids. *Issues in Mental Health Nursing,* 12(1), 51-64.

LaFontaine, P. (1989). Alleviating patient's apprehension and anxieties. *Gastroenterology Nursing,* 11, 256-257.

Levine, C.D., Wilson, S.F., & Guido, G.W. (1988, July). Personality factors of critical care nurses. *Heart & Lung: Journal of Critical Care,* 17(4), 392-398.

Long, J.M., Kee, C.C., Graham, M.V., Saethan, T.B., & Dames, F.D. (1998). Medication compliance and the older hemodialysis patient. *American Nephrology Nurses Association Journal,* 25(1), 43-49.

Martin, J.P. (1990). Male cancer awareness: Impact of an employee education program [research, tables/charts]. *Oncology Nursing Forum,* 17(1), 59-64.

McGirr, M., Rukholm, E., Salmoni, A., O'Sullivan, P., & Koren, I. (1990). Perceived mood and exercise behaviors of cardiac rehabilitation program referrals. *Canadian Journal of Cardiovascular Nursing,* 1(4), 14-19.

McKinney, N. & Frank, D.I. (1998). Nursing assessment of adult females who are alcohol dependent and victims of sexual abuse. *Clinical Excellence for Nurse Practitioners,* 2(3), 152-158.

Messmer, P.R. (1992). Implementing theory based nursing practice. *Florida Nurse,* 40(3), 8.

Messner, R. & Smith, M.N. (1986). Neurofibromatosis: Relinquishing the masks; a quest for quality of life. *Journal of Advanced Nursing,* 11, 459-464.

Murray, R.L.E. & Baier, M. (1996). King's conceptual framework applied to a transitional living program. *Perspectives in Psychiatric Care,* 32(1), 15-19.

Nagano, M. & Funashima, N. (1995). Analysis of nursing situations in Japan: Using King's goal attainment theory. *Quality Nursing,* 1(1), 74-78.

Norgan, G.H., Ettipio, A.M., & Lasome, C.E.M. (1995). A program plan addressing carpal tunnel syndrome: The utility of King's goal attainment theory. *American Association of Occupational Health Nurses Journal,* 43(8), 407-411.

Norris, D.M. & Hoyer, P.J. (1993). Dynamism in practice: Parenting within King's framework. *Nursing Science Quarterly,* 6(2), 79-85.

Olsson, H. & Forsdahl, T. (1996). Expectations and opportunities of newly employed nurses at the University Hospital, Tromso, Norway. *Social Sciences in Health: International Journal of Research and Practice,* 2(1), 14-22.

Porteous, A. & Tyndall, J. (1994). Yes, I want to walk to the OR. *Canadian Operating Room Nursing,* 12(2), 15-16, 18-19.

Porter, H. (1991). A theory of goal attainment and ambulatory care oncology nursing: An introduction. *Canadian Oncology Nursing,* 1(4), 124-126.

Rawlins, P.S., Rawlins, T.D., & Horner, M. (1990). Development of the family needs assessment tool. *Western Journal of Nursing Research,* 12(2), 201-214.

Reed, P.G. (1986). A model for constructing a conceptual framework for education in clinical specialty. *Journal of Nursing Education,* 25(7), 295-329.

Richard-Hughes, S. (1997). Attitudes and beliefs of Afro-Americans related to organ and tissue donation. *International Journal of Trauma Nursing,* 3(4), 119-123.

Rooda, L.A. (1992). The development of a conceptual model for multicultural nursing. *Journal of Holistic Nursing,* 10(4), 337-347.

Rooke, L. & Norberg, A. (1988). Problematic and meaningful situations in nursing interpreted by concepts from King's nursing theory and four additional concepts. *Scandinavian Journal of Caring Sciences,* 2(2), 80-87.

Rosendahl, P.B. & Ross, V. (1982). Does your behavior affect your patient's response? *Journal of Gerontological Nursing,* 8, 572-575.

Rossi, K. & Heikkinen, M. (1990). A view of occupational health nursing practice: Current trends and future prospects. *Recent Advances in Nursing,* 26, 1-34.

Rundell, S. (1991). A study of nurse-patient interaction in a high dependency unit. *Intensive Care Nursing, 7,* 171-178.

Schreiber, R. (1991). Psychiatric assessment—"A la King." *Nursing Management,* 22(5), 90.

Scott, L.D. (1998). Perceived needs of parents of critically ill children. *Journal of the Society of Pediatric Nurses,* 3(1), 4-12.

Sirles, A.T. & Selleck, C.S. (1989). Cardiac disease and the family: Impact, assessment, and implications. *Journal of Cardiovascular Nursing,* 3(2), 23-32.

Smith, M.C. (1988). King's theory in practice. *Nursing Science Quarterly,* 1(4), 145-146.

Smith, M.J. (1988). Perspectives on nursing science. *Nursing Science Quarterly,* 1(2), 80-85.

Sorrentino, E.A. (1991). Making theories work for you. *Nursing Administration Quarterly,* 15(3), 54-59.

Sowell, R.L. & Lowenstein, A. (1994). King's theory: A framework for quality; linking theory to practice. *Nursing Connections,* 7(2), 19-31.

Spees, C.M. (1991). Knowledge of medical terminology among clients and families. *Image: Journal of Nursing Scholarship,* 23(4), 225-229.

Spratlen, L.P. (1976). Introducing ethnic-cultural factors in models of nursing: Some mental health care applications. *Journal of Nursing Education,* 15(2), 23-29.

Strauss, S.S. (1981). Abuse and neglect of parents by professionals. *Maternal/Child Nursing,* 6, 157-160.

Swindale, J.E. (1989). The nurse's role in giving preoperative information to reduce anxiety in patients admitted to hospital for elective minor surgery. *Journal of Advanced Nursing,* 14(11), 899-905.

Symanski, M.E. (1991, March). Use of nursing theories in the care of families with high-risk infants: Challenges for the future. *Journal of Perinatal & Neonatal Nursing,* 4(4), 71-77.

Takahashi, T. (1992). Perspectives on nursing knowledge. *Nursing Science Quarterly,* 5(2), 86-91.

Temple, A. & Fawdry, K. (1992). King's theory of goal attainment: Resolving filial caregiver role strain. *Journal of Gerontological Nursing,* 18(3), 11-15.

Tripp-Reimer, T., Woodworth, G., McCloskey, J.C., & Bulechek, G. (1996). The dimensional structure of nursing interventions. *Nursing Research,* 45(1), 10-17.

Tritsch, J.M. (1996). Application of King's theory of goal attainment and the Carondelet St. Mary's case management model. *Nursing Science Quarterly,* 11(2), 69-73.

Villeneuve, M.J. & Ozolins, P.H. (1991, March). Sexual counseling in the neuroscience setting: Theory and practical tips for nurses. *AXON,* 12(3), 63-67.

Weikel, C. (1987). Informed consent: An ethical dilemma . . . the nurse's role. *Today's OR Nurse,* 9(1), 10-15.

West, P. (1991). Theory implementation: A challenging journey. *Canadian Journal of Nursing Administration,* 4(1), 29-30.

Wheeler, K. (1989). Self-psychology's contributions to understanding stress and implications for nursing. *Journal of Advanced Medical-Surgical Nursing,* 1(4), 1-10.

Woods, E.C. (1994). King's theory in practice with elders. *Nursing Science Quarterly,* 7(2), 65-69.

Masters Theses

Allan, N.J. (1995). Goal attainment and life satisfaction among frail elderly. *Masters Abstracts International,* 35-05, 1486.

Aramburu-Drury, C.M. (1996). Exploring the association between body weight and health care avoidance. *Masters Abstracts International,* 35-03, 0725.

Arbeiter, N.A. (1998). The effect of a formal class on advance directives on nurses' perceptions. *Masters Abstracts International,* 36-04, 1059.

Batchelor, S.G. (1994). Relationship of budgetary knowledge and staff nurses' attitudes towards cost-effectiveness. *Masters Abstracts International,* 32-05, 1365.

Binder, B.K. (1992). King's transaction elements identified in adolescents' interactions with health care providers. *Masters Abstracts International,* 54-01B, 0163.

Davis, S.M. (1992). Patient outcome documentation: Development and implementation. *Masters Abstracts International,* 30-04, 1288.

Dawson, B.W. (1996). The relationship between functional social support, social network and the adequacy of prenatal care. *Masters Abstracts International,* 35-01, 0361.

Dispenza, J.M. (1990). Relationship of husband and wife perceptions of the coping responses of the female spouse of males in high level stress. *Masters Abstracts International,* 28-03, 407.

Genzel, M.C. (1998). Job satisfaction of the nursing staff development educator. *Masters Abstracts International,* 36-04, 1063.

Kahn, R. (1997). The number and types of interventions developed and employed for a population of ADHD students by an advanced nurse practitioner in a middle-sized urban school district in Michigan Title I Health Program during the 1995-1996 school year. *Masters Abstracts International,* 36-01, 0158.

Kaminski, L.A. (1999). Perceptions of home care nurses as facilitators of discussions and advance directives. *Masters Abstracts International,* 37-04, 1179.

Leonard, B.M. (1996). Team building using group and peer initiating processes within Imogene King's systems to facilitate CQI (Continuous Quality Improvement). *Masters Abstracts International,* 34-06, 2346.

Monti, A. (1992). Members' perceptions of the transactions within their psychosocial club. *Masters Abstracts International,* 30-04, 1296.

O'Shall, M.L. (1989). The relationship congruency of role conception between head nurse and staff nurse and staff nurse job satisfaction. *Masters Abstracts International, 27-03, 379.*

Phillips, E.L. (1995). Diploma nursing students' attitudes toward poverty. *Masters Abstracts International, 33-06, 1846.*

Pinnock-Philp, B.E. (1998). Attitudes toward restricting food in labor: Differences between caregivers in a tertiary care perinatal center and a birthing center. *Masters Abstracts International, 36-06, 1600.*

Six, D.M. (1998). Patient satisfaction with prenatal care services in a rural setting: Time. *Masters Abstracts International, 36-06, 1591.*

Sperry, E.J. (1999). Physician perceptions of behaviors associated with the nurse practitioner role. *Masters Abstracts International, 37-06, 1821.*

Tawil, T.M.P. (1993). Gender differences in frequency of assistance and perceived elderly patients' level of need by spouse primary caregivers with the activities of daily living: Dressing and bathing. *Masters Abstracts International, 32-04, 1172.*

Villanueva-Noble, N.S. (1998). Cross-cultural analysis of perceptions of health in children's drawings: A replicate study (Phillipines, Canada). *Masters Abstracts International, 36-04, 1070.*

White-Linn, V.M. (1994). Perceived quality of life of adults aged 30-50 years with type I and type II diabetes. *Masters Abstracts International, 33-05, 1496.*

Doctoral Dissertations

Brooks, E. (1995). Exploring the perception and judgment of senior baccalaureate student nurses in clinical decision-making from a nursing theoretical perspective. *Dissertation Abstracts International, 56-12B, 6667.*

duMont, Phyllis.(1998). *The effects of early menarche on health risk behaviors.* Unpublished doctoral dissertation, University of Tennessee, Knoxville.

Ehrenberger, H.E. (1998). Testing a theory of decision making derived from King's systems framework in women eligible for a cancer clinical trial. *Dissertation Abstracts International, 60-07B, 3201.*

Giovinco, G. (1985). Using patient care situations to apply Kohlberg's moral development theory to nursing. *Dissertation Abstracts International, 46-08A, 2333.*

Glenn, C.J. (1989). The development of autonomy in nurses. *Dissertation Abstracts International, 50, 1852B.*

Hanna, K.M. (1991). Effect of nurse-client transaction on female adolescents' contraceptive perceptions and adherence. *Dissertation Abstracts International, 51-07B, 3323.*

Killeen, M. (1996). Patient-consumer perceptions and responses to professional nursing care: Instrument development. *Dissertation Abstracts International, 57-04B, 2479.*

Krassa, T.J. (1994). A study of political participation by registered nurses in Illinois. *Dissertation Abstracts International, 56-02B, 0743.*

Lockhart, J.S. (1992). Female nurses' perceptions regarding the severity of facial disfigurement in patients following surgery for head and neck cancer: A comparison based on experience in head and neck oncology. *Dissertation Abstracts International, 54-02B, 0745.*

May, B.A. (2000). *Relationships among basic empathy, self-awareness, and learning styles of baccalaureate pre-nursing students within King's personal system.* Unpublished doctoral dissertation, University of Tennessee, Knoxville.

McKay, T. (1999). *An examination of case management nurses' role strain, participative decision making, and their relationships to patient satisfaction: Utilization of King's theory of goal attainment in a managed care environment.* Unpublished doctoral dissertation, University of Tennessee, Knoxville.

O'Connor, P. (1990). Service in nursing: Correlates of patient satisfaction. *Dissertation Abstracts International, 50-11B, 4985.*

Omar, M.A. (1990). Relationship of family processes to family life satisfaction in stepfamilies and biological families during pregnancy. *Dissertation Abstracts International, 51-03B, 1196.*

Rooke, L. (1990). Nursing and theoretical structures of nursing: A didactic attempt to develop the practice of nursing. *Dissertation Abstracts International, 51-04C, 579.*

Sieloff, C.L. (1996). Development of an instrument to estimate the actualized power of a nursing department. *Dissertation Abstracts International, 57-04B, 2484.*

Whelton, B.T.B. (1996). A philosophy of nursing practice: An application of the Thomistic-Aristotelian concept of nature to the science of nursing. *Dissertation Abstracts International, 57-03A, 1176.*

Winker, C. (1996). A descriptive study of the relationship of interaction disturbance to the organizational health of a metropolitan general hospital. *Dissertation Abstracts International, 57-07B, 4306.*

Zurakowski, T.L. (1990). Interpersonal factors and nursing home resident health (anomia). *Dissertation Abstracts International, 51-07B, 4281.*

Other Sources

Allport, F.H. (1955). *Theories of perception and the concept of structure.* New York: John Wiley & Sons.

Bruner, J., Goodnow, J., & Austin, G. (1956). *A study in thinking.* New York: John Wiley & Sons.

Bruner, J.S. & Krech, W. (Eds.). (1968). *Perception and personality.* New York: Greenwood Press.

Buber, M. (1970). *I and thou.* New York: Scribner.

Churchman, C.W. (1968). *The systems approach.* New York: Delacorte Press.

Churchman, C.W., Ackoff, R., & Arnoff, E.L. (1957). *Introduction to operations research.* New York: John Wiley & Sons.

Dewey, J. & Bentley, A. (1949). *Knowing and the known.* Boston: Beacon Press.

Dubin, R. (1978). *Theory building.* New York: Free Press.

Dubos, R. (1961). *Mirage of health: Utopias, progress and biological change.* Garden City, NY: Doubleday.

Dubos, R. (1965). *Man adapting.* New Haven: Yale University Press.

Erikson, E. (1950). *Childhood and society.* New York: Norton.

Fawcett, J. (1978). The "what" of theory development. In National League for Nursing, *Theory development: What, why, how?* (pp. 17-33). New York: Author.

Feigl, H. & Brodbeck, M. (Eds.). (1953). *Readings in the philosophy of science.* New York: Appleton-Century-Crofts.

Freud, S. (1965). *Introductory lectures on psychoanalysis.* New York: Norton.

Gesell, A.L. (1952). *Infant development: The embryology of early human behavior.* New York: Harper.

Hall, J.E. & Weaver, B.R. (1977). *Distributive nursing: A system approach to community health.* Philadelphia: J.B. Lippincott.

Ittleson, W.H. & Cantril, H. (1954). *Perception: A transactional approach.* Garden City, NY: Doubleday.

Kelley, K.J. & Hammond, K.R. (1964). An approach to the study of clinical inference. *Nursing Research,* 13(4), 314-322.

Knutson, A. (1965). *The individual, society, and health behavior.* New York: Russell Sage Foundation.

Linton, R. (1936). *The study of man: An introduction.* New York: Appleton-Century-Crofts.

Orlando, I.J. (1972). *The discipline and teaching of nursing process.* New York: G.P. Putnam's Sons.

Parsons, T. (1964). *The social system.* New York: Free Press of Glencoe.

Seyle, H. (1974). *Stress without distress.* Philadelphia: J.B. Lippincott.

Spiegel, J.P. (1971). *Transactions: The interplay between individual, family, and society.* New York: Science House.

von Bertalanffy, L. (1968). *General system theory: Foundations, development, application* (rev. ed.). New York: Braziller.

Weed, L.L. (1969). *Medical records, medical education, and patient care.* Cleveland: Press of Case Western Reserve University.

Wiener, N. (1967). *The human use of human beings: Cybernetics and society.* New York: Avon Books.

Woods, E.C. (1994). King's theory in practice with elders. *Nursing Science Quarterly,* 7(2): 65-69.

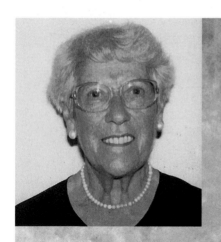

Nancy Roper

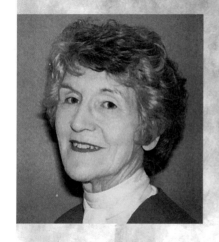

Winifred W. Logan

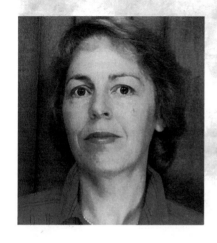

Alison J. Tierney

The Elements of Nursing: A Model for Nursing Based on a Model of Living

Ann Marriner Tomey

CREDENTIALS AND BACKGROUND OF THE THEORISTS

Nancy Roper

Nancy Roper was born in the United Kingdom on September 29, 1918. After completing a general education program, she left school in 1936 and became a student nurse for three years at a hospital for sick children, thereby gaining the qualification Registered Sick Children's Nurse (R.S.C.N.). During training, she acknowledged her commitment to nursing by joining the Students' Association of the Royal College of Nursing.

World War II was declared as Roper moved into a three-year program for general nursing and she gained the qualification Registered General Nurse (R.G.N.). Career options were curtailed because conscription to the armed services was in force, but a teaching post was reserved and the principal invited Roper to accept the post as a staff nurse. After two years, she was able to pursue the usual career of staff nurse posts in a variety of wards, followed by posts as a ward sister.

Previous author: Ann Marriner Tomey.
The author wishes to thank Nancy Roper, Winifred W. Logan, and Alison J. Tierney for reviewing the chapter.

In 1950, Roper gained the London University's Teaching Diploma; thereafter, she taught for 15 years. During this period, she acted as an examiner for the General Nursing Council and won a scholarship to investigate nurse education in the United States and Canada. Also during this time, she edited *Churchill Livingstone Nurses' Dictionary*[27] and *Churchill Livingstone Pocket Medical Dictionary*.[25] During this period, Roper wrote a book in which she integrated subjects, titled *Man's Anatomy, Physiology, Health and Environment*.[22] Toward the end of 1963, she had to make a choice between teaching and writing. In January 1964, Roper became self-employed as a writer; she was the first British nurse to do this.

For more than 30 years, Roper has enjoyed the privilege of spending her time reading, writing, and thinking about nursing and observing the ever-changing scene related to practice, education, management, and research. The first edition of *Principles of Nursing*[23] was published in 1967 and the fourth edition, *Principles of Nursing in Process Context*,[26] was published in 1988.

In 1970, she was awarded a fellowship, which she used to pursue an M.Phil. at the University of Edinburgh. She investigated whether patients require a core of nursing wherever the patients are located. She defined this core of nursing and designed a Model of Living and a Model for Nursing. Her research monograph, *Clinical Experience in Nurse Education,* was published in 1976.[24] It is now out of print; therefore Roper[28] has provided a synopsis of the recommendations, updating words where necessary:

> The model could be used for curriculum planning. Knowledge about each AL [activity of living] could be taught in the context of healthy people in a healthy environment. Knowledge about "the normal" would be assimilated before introduction to "the abnormal." The gap between theory and practice would be reduced if the model informed nursing education in such a way that it could guide nursing practice.
>
> The purpose of education programs is to help students to think in the way of the particular subject (discipline), for example, theologically. Our subject is nursing, and the suffix-ology means the study of, so logically the study of nursing is nursingology, and the objective of education programs should be to encourage nurses to think nursingologically.
>
> The literature refers to nursing as a practice discipline, and the two major components of practice disciplines are theory and practice. The practice of assessing, planning, implementing, and evaluating related to each patient needs to be supported by nursing's body of knowledge, a characteristic of a discipline, and this could be structured using the framework of the ALs.

From 1974 to 1978, Roper was employed by the Scottish Home and Health Department in a newly created post of Nursing Research Officer. This enabled her to carry out several short-term assignments for the World Health Organization (WHO) European Office in Copenhagen and the Eastern Mediterranean Office in Alexandria, which gave an international dimension to her nursing experience. She continues to collaborate with Winifred Logan and Alison Tierney in refining the Roper-Logan-Tierney (R-L-T) Model for Nursing based on a Model of Living.[28]

Winifred W. Logan

Winifred Logan qualified as a nurse at the Royal Infirmary, Edinburgh. She had previously gained an M.A. degree at the University of Edinburgh and returned there in 1961 to take a teaching qualification. In 1966, on a WHO Fellowship, she completed an M.A. in Nursing and Allied Fields at Columbia University, New York. She was greatly influenced by her studies at Columbia; she was actively involved in discussions of concepts, models, definitions of nursing, and the nursing process, all of which she incorporated into her later work.

Logan has enjoyed a varied career. Her nursing experience included periods in a diabetic unit and in thoracic and general surgery in the United Kingdom, Canada, and the United States.

While working in a thoracic surgery unit in Canada, the importance of considering the patient's psychological and sociocultural circumstances made a profound impact when about 200 Eskimos (often whole families including grandparents) were airlifted from Baffin Island, Canada to Hamilton, Ontario, Canada to have treatment for tuberculosis. Inevitably, there was considerable culture shock coming from igloos and skin tents to a modern hospital and returning home to resume a nomadic existence in their arctic environment after a two-year stay. Staff became aware of the Eskimos' psychological reactions not only to illness, but also to illness treated in an alien environment. Also, nurses had to be responsive to the sociocultural differences between the Eskimos and the other patients and staff at the hospital. Shortly after, when Logan wrote the final year dissertation for a teaching qualification, this experience certainly contributed to her choice of the subject "Psychological and Sociocultural Aspects of Nursing." Later experiences reinforced these interests.

In 1956, a novel development in the United Kingdom was the creation of the Department of Nursing Studies at the University of Edinburgh. Logan was appointed to the staff in 1962 and became course coordinator for the first basic degree in Europe that included nursing as a graduating subject (almost 50 years after the first such course in the United States). She also taught and was a course organizer for the postbasic programs to prepare nurse educators and administrators, some of whom were recruited to the International School, which was located in the department and sponsored by WHO. As a member of the staff over a 12-year period, she was involved in promoting master's degrees and research degrees within the department.

During 1971 and 1972, Logan was granted a leave of absence from the University to take an appointment as the first Director of Nursing Services in the newly created Ministry of Health in Abu Dhabi, where she was responsible for setting up the Nursing Division.

In 1974, she moved to the Scottish Office to take a newly created position as Nursing Officer for Education and Research. Later in the year, the research commitment became a separate post, to which Roper was appointed. In 1978, Logan was appointed as Executive Director to the International Council of Nurses in Geneva, which permitted invaluable communication and cooperation with nurses on a worldwide scale. Her final post before retirement was as Head of Department of Health and Nursing at what is now Glasgow Caledonian University. At different points in her career, she was invited to act as a WHO Short-Term Consultant in various countries, such as Malaysia, Iraq, Finland, Denmark, and Germany.

Logan has written a number of articles in a variety of journals and, as coauthor with Roper and Tierney, she has written several textbooks and articles. She has given lectures in various countries, participated in many nursing conferences nationally and internationally, and served on a number of nursing and academic committees. In recognition of her contributions to nursing nationally and internationally, she was awarded an honorary degree from the University of Surrey and an honorary Doctor of Science from Glasgow Caledonian University; in 1996, she was made an honorary Fellow of the University of Edinburgh.[12]

Alison J. Tierney

At an early age, Alison Tierney decided that she wanted to become a nurse. Like many Scottish girls, she liked the idea of going to London to train at one of the most famous schools of nursing. However, her parents persuaded her to go to a university because she had done well academically and they thought she could do better than nursing. In the mid1960s, nursing was still perceived as old fashioned and nurses were poorly paid. Her father learned that the University of Edinburgh combined university study with nurse training; therefore Tierney started as an undergraduate student in the Department of Nursing Studies at the University of Edinburgh in the autumn of 1966. Logan was one of the lecturers who taught Tierney.

The four and a half-year integrated degree-nursing course contained enough clinical experience to satisfy Tierney's interest in *real* nursing. She found that the academic aspects opened up new and challenging perspectives on nursing. Tierney found that, compared to other subjects that she studied as part of her integrated Social Sciences-Nursing degree (such as psychology and social anthropology), nursing was very underdeveloped in terms of its own literature and research. After graduating in 1969 with a degree with distinction (B.Sc.:Soc.Sc.) and registering as a general nurse (R.G.N.) early in 1971, Tierney worked as a Staff Nurse in London, where she quickly became frustrated by the highly routinized approach to patient care and the lack of opportunity to apply theoretical knowledge to practice.

Tierney returned home later that year to get married and move to central Scotland, where her husband was pursuing his Ph.D. in the area of psychology at the University of Stirling. She had the opportunity to pursue a government-funded Nursing Research Training Fellowship. The Department of Nursing Studies at the University of Edinburgh was the only academic nursing center in Scotland. Consequently, Tierney registered there as a postgraduate research student to obtain supervision for her research. She commuted to Edinburgh for academic supervision and study while performing her research fieldwork near her home. She was exploring the application of behavioral therapy in nursing practice.

When her fellowship period expired in the autumn of 1973, Tierney was appointed to a junior lectureship in the department. She also continued working on a doctoral thesis and, in 1976, was awarded a Ph.D., thereby becoming one of the

United Kingdom's first few graduate nurses to obtain this higher research degree. At this time, Tierney began working with Roper and Logan to further develop the Roper model. Tierney found this a valuable opportunity because she was revising the first-year undergraduate nursing curriculum and was finding it difficult in the absence of a conceptual framework.

Tierney and her husband moved back to Edinburgh and during the process of writing *The Elements of Nursing*,[29] she gave birth to their son. Soon after the publication of the book in 1980, she gave birth to their daughter. Tierney took a career break while both children were small and returned to work in 1984 as the Director of the Nursing Research Unit at the University of Edinburgh. When first established in 1971, the unit was the first government-funded center for nursing research in Europe. After 10 years, Tierney was tenured and then promoted to Reader in Nursing Studies in 1995. Tierney was also honored that year with a Fellowship of the Royal College of Nursing (F.R.C.N.) and elected to this position in recognition of her outstanding contribution to nursing research. She was appointed to a Personal Chair of Nursing Research at the University of Edinburgh.

Tierney's extensive and varied involvement in nursing and health services research in the United Kingdom is evident in the many journal articles she has published and is reflected in the many invitations to present papers at international nursing research conferences. On account of her research background, her contribution to new editions of *The Elements of Nursing*[33,34,35] are most concerned with the research content of the book. Tierney does not focus her own writing or conference presentations on the model. Roper is the group's ambassador. However, in 1997, Tierney[39] presented a paper at a major International Conference on Nursing Theories in Germany, using the occasion for a critical appraisal of the relevance and role of the R-L-T model in Europe's fast-changing healthcare systems.

THEORETICAL SOURCES

The original Roper models were based on research and an extensive review of the literature. They are now of historical interest only; they have been su-

perseded by the R-L-T models: first edition published in 1980,[29] second edition in 1985,[33] third edition in 1990,[34] fourth edition in 1996,[35] and the monograph in 2000.[31]

USE OF EMPIRICAL EVIDENCE

When Roper was a principal of a teaching department preparing students for general registration, she arranged for various medical consultants to give lectures in their specialty. The nurse teachers then gave lectures about and practical demonstrations of the nursing procedures relevant to each consultant's lectures. Discussions with students who had practiced on each of the consultants' wards revealed there were more similarities than differences in the nursing activities on the various awards. Roper noticed that the similarities seemed to center around the patient's personal living, which was not medically prescribed. She began to see *nursing* and *doctoring* as complementary with distinct identities. She felt challenged to identify *nursing* and in 1964 became self-employed to pursue this identification.

In 1970, she initiated a research project to investigate whether there was a core of nursing. A literature review revealed a few projects about a core of nursing, but they had not collected data about actual patients; therefore a Patient Profile was used to collect data about patients in all the clinical areas to which one college of nursing allocated its students. Seven hundred seventy-four profiles were analyzed and revealed a core of everyday living activities. From the data and the literature review, she developed a Model of Living and a Model of Nursing.[24]

In 1976, she invited Logan and Tierney to refine and develop the models. Each member of the trio contributed her particular experiences of nursing practice, education, management, and research and, after frequent discussions and numerous drafts, the first combined R-L-T models were revised and published in 1980 in *The Elements of Nursing*.[29] The title did not include the word *model*, so library searches related to models for nursing did not retrieve this publication. For the third and forth editions of the book, however, the title was expanded to *The Elements of Nursing: A Model for Nursing Based on a Model of Living*.[34,35]

At the time of the first edition (1980),[29] discussions of death and dying, environmental issues, and sociocultural factors were just beginning. The inclusion of politicoeconomic factors in the first edition[29] was made to look less cluttered for the third edition (1990)[34] and left unchanged for the fourth edition (1996)[35] with the exception of changing *physical* to *biological*. The monograph (2000)[31] is their final publication and is a lasting account of the model of nursing that has been the core of the R-L-T publications since 1980.

MAJOR CONCEPTS & DEFINITIONS

A diagram of the Model of Living is presented in Figure 20-1 and a diagram of the Model for Nursing is presented in Figure 20-2. A comparison of the main concepts of the Model of Living and the Model for Nursing is presented in Table 20-1. Four major concepts are common to both models:
- Factors influencing ALs
- ALs
- Lifespan
- Dependence/independence continuum
Five groups of factors influencing these:
- Biological
- Psychological
- Sociocultural (including spiritual, religious, and ethical)
- Environmental
- Politicoeconomic (including legal)

The interaction of these concepts produces the fifth main concept, which in the Model of Living is *individuality in living*. To individualize nursing, nurses need to know about the patient's individuality in living, which is accomplished by using the four phases of the nursing process dynamically and interactively. Furthermore, beginning students can imagine themselves at the center of the model and explore how the five concepts relate to their own lifestyle. Such knowledge about their own individuality in living can then influence their nursing practice.[34,35]

ACTIVITIES OF LIVING

The person at the center of the models is characterized by 12 activities of living (ALs), namely:[34,35]
- Maintaining a safe environment
- Communicating
- Breathing
- Eating and drinking
- Eliminating
- Personal cleansing and dressing
- Controlling body temperature
- Mobilizing
- Working and playing
- Expressing sexuality
- Sleeping
- Dying

Each AL has many dimensions and it can be likened to a compound that comprises many elements.[34,35] The more the ALs are analyzed, the complexity of each AL becomes more apparent. Compounding this complexity is the fact that the ALs are so closely related; individuals prioritize them in daily living and the concept of priority is of prime importance in nursing. The concept of relevance is also important, especially when people are being treated in day surgery units and short-stay wards. Consequently, data about all 12 ALs may not need to be collected for every patient/client. Only relevant ALs need to be considered.[34,35] The experienced nurse can make decisions about relatedness, priorities, and relevance with speed and relative ease. However, the student must learn to blend knowledge and reflection on practice experience before being able to make such professional judgments.

LIFESPAN

The lifespan is defined as the temporal span of life on this earth from birth to death. Most countries have registry offices where births, deaths, and causes of death must be recorded; from these data

MAJOR CONCEPTS & DEFINITIONS—cont'd

several predictions can be made about the population.[34] The relevance of the lifespan to nursing in general is discussed in the fourth edition of *The Elements of Nursing*;[35:37] its relevance to each particular AL is discussed in the same book in the chapter about that AL.

DEPENDENCE/INDEPENDENCE CONTINUUM

The dependence/independence continuum ranges from total dependence to total independence. Applying the continuum to the person as a whole is too broad, so it is directly applied to each AL. It acknowledges that there are stages when a person cannot yet (or can no longer) perform certain ALs independently.[34,35] Therefore the continuum is bidirectional, an important concept in its application to nursing.[34,35] Its relevance to a particular AL is discussed in the appropriate chapter of *The Elements of Nursing*.[29,34,35]

FACTORS INFLUENCING ALS

There are many factors that have influenced or continue to influence the way in which an individual enacts the ALs. For the purpose of this model, they are grouped under five headings:[34,35]

- Biological
- Psychological
- Sociocultural
- Environmental
- Politicoeconomic

In the Model of Living, they are discussed in *The Elements of Nursing*.[34,35] In the Model for Nursing, they are discussed in the same book.[34,35] They are applied to each particular AL in the appropriate chapter.

INDIVIDUALITY IN LIVING

Individuality in living is manifested by the style in which individuals attend to each of their ALs according to the achieved stage on the lifespan and place on the dependence/independence continuum, which have all been, and still are being, influenced by the interacting five groups of factors. A schema of questions is proposed in *The Elements of Nursing*[34,35] to help the beginning student conceptualize individuality in living.

MAJOR ASSUMPTIONS

- Living can be described as an amalgam of ALs.
- The way ALs are carried out by each person contributes to individuality in living.
- The individual is valued at all stages of the lifespan.
- Throughout the lifespan until adulthood, the individual tends to become increasingly independent in the ALs.
- While independence in the ALs is valued, dependence should not diminish the dignity of the individual.
- An individual's knowledge, attitudes, and behavior related to the ALs are influenced by a variety of factors, which can be categorized broadly as biological, psychological, sociocultural, environmental, and politicoeconomic factors.
- The way in which an individual carries out the ALs can fluctuate within a range of normal for that person.
- When the individual is "ill," there may be problems (actual or potential) with the ALs.
- During the lifespan, most individuals experience significant life events, which can affect the way they carry out ALs and may lead to problems, actual or potential.

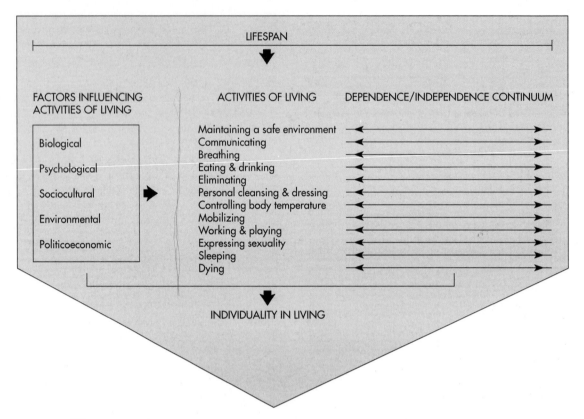

Figure **20-1 Diagram of the Model of Living.** (From Roper, N., Logan, W.W., & Tierney, A.J. [1996]. *The elements of nursing: A model for nursing based on a model of living* [4th ed., p. 20]. Edinburgh: Churchill Livingstone. Used with permission of Churchill Livingstone.)

- The concept of potential problems incorporates the promotion and maintenance of health, the prevention of disease, and identifies the role of the nurse as a health teacher, even in illness settings.
- Within a health care context, nurses work in partnership with the client/patient, who, except for special circumstances, is an autonomous, decision-making person.
- Nurses are part of a multiprofessional healthcare team who work in partnership for the benefit of the client/patient and for the health of the community.
- The specific function of nursing is to assist the individual to prevent, alleviate or solve, or cope

positively with problems (actual or potential) related to the ALs.[35:34-35]

Nursing

Nursing is defined as helping people to:
- Prevent potential problems related to their ALs, becoming actual problems. (This is particularly applicable to the work of midwives, health visitors, and school and occupational health nurses.)
- Alleviate or solve problems.
- Prevent recurrence of treated problems.
- Cope in a positive way with any problems including death, dying, and bereavement.[35:35]

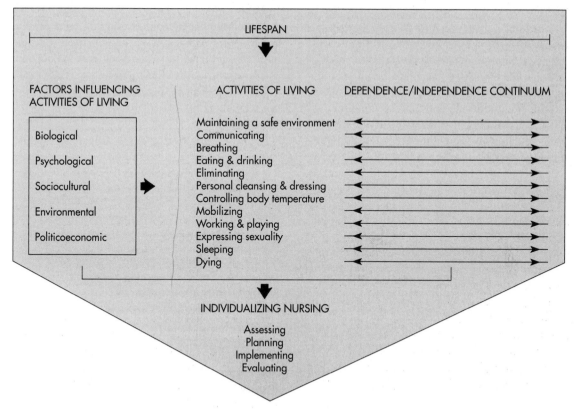

Figure 20-2 **Diagram of the Model for Nursing.** (From Roper, N., Logan, W.W., & Tierney, A.J. [1996]. *The elements of nursing: A model for nursing based on a model of living* [4th ed., p. 34]. Edinburgh: Churchill Livingstone. Used with permission of Churchill Livingstone.)

Table 20-1

Comparison of the Main Concepts in the Model of Living and the Model for Nursing	
MODEL OF LIVING	**MODEL FOR NURSING**
12 ALs	12 ALs
Lifespan	Lifespan
Dependence/independence continuum	Dependence/independence continuum
Factors influencing the ALs	Factors influencing the ALs
Individuality in living	Individualizing nursing

From Roper, N., Logan, W.W., & Tierney, A. (1996). *The elements of nursing: A model for nursing based on a model of living* (4th ed., p. 33). Edinburgh: Churchill Livingstone. Used with permission of Churchill Livingstone.

Person

An individual person is central to both models and is conceptualized as attending to the 12 ALs according to dependence/independence status for each of them and stage on the lifespan against the contextual background of biological, psychological, sociocultural, environmental, and politicoeconomic factors. The terms *person, patient,* and *client* are used interchangeably and sometimes include the family and significant others, who are also individuals.[35]

Health

The question, "What is health?," is discussed by describing the WHO definition of health, health/illness continuum, lay perceptions of health, health as coping, personal responsibility for health, and current health targets.[35] Aided independence is also discussed; a person may feel healthy even when he or she has a significant disability, which may be mental or physical.[35]

Obviously, the expected outcome when preventing potential problems from becoming actual ones is the acquisition and maintenance of a positive health status. At appropriate places throughout the text, activities to prevent such conditions as dental caries, lung cancer, malnutrition, and sexually transmitted disease are discussed.

Environment

The environment is conceptualized in a broad dimension and includes all that is physically external to a person.[35] This includes other people in the environment, highlighting the interaction of psychological and sociocultural factors with environmental factors. The environment is so important that maintaining a safe environment is featured as one of the 12 ALs and is discussed in each of the other ALs in the appropriate chapter of *The Elements of Nursing.*[35]

THEORETICAL ASSERTIONS

Individuality in living is a product of the constant interaction of the model's other four main con-

cepts: (1) the 12 ALs, (2) the lifespan, (3) the dependence/independence continuum, and (4) the five groups of factors influencing all of these.[35] People have to go on living while they require nursing; consequently, nurses need to know about a person's individuality in living before individualized nursing can be planned, implemented, and evaluated with the objectives of:[35]

- Preventing potential problems from becoming actual ones.
- Alleviating or solving actual problems.
- Coping in a positive way with problems that cannot be solved.
- Preventing recurrence of treated problems.
- Coping in a positive way with death, dying, and bereavement.

LOGICAL FORM

Roper, Logan, and Tierney have used inductive logic by observing particular care situations and analyzing them to develop general theoretical statements.

ACCEPTANCE BY THE NURSING COMMUNITY

The Model for Nursing based on a Model of Living is used widely throughout Europe in a wide range of clinical areas. Nursing communities have asked for translation of *The Elements of Nursing*[29,33,35] into Dutch, Estonian, Finnish, German, Italian, Lithuanian, Portuguese, and Spanish. Whittam[41] has described use of the model and Smith[37,38] has received grants to produce a booklet about providing nursing care based on the R-L-T model for people with Huntington's disease.

The model has provoked some negative criticism. When the first edition was published in 1980, expressing sexuality was still a taboo subject in the United Kingdom, whereas now it is discussed freely, even in lay magazines. The 1980 version was also criticized as retaining the medical model flavor. In fact, psychological, sociocultural, environmental, and politicoeconomic factors were discussed in addition to the biological or physical factor, but their importance was underscored as long ago as the second edition (1985),[33] when the five factors were presented as a separate concept in the diagram of the model and discussed as such within each AL chapter.

Practice

The Model for Nursing can be used by nurses in any specialty. The model is only a guideline and a reflection of reality. Nurses must make it real for each patient/client. There are numerous instances in the United Kingdom and in other countries where ward documentation has been based on the R-L-T model. Rowe[36] used the model to explore the uniqueness of patients who had suffered from a myocardial infraction and the uniqueness of the family members. Davis[5] adapted the model in orthopaedic nursing and Ramsden[21] used it to care for a dying patient in a nursing home. Pullen[20] used the ALs to help patients with stoma acquire or restore and maintain maximum independence. Jones[10] used the ALs of eating, drinking, and communicating regarding the needs of a patient undergoing pharyngeal surgery. Griffiths[9] documented a ward using the R-L-T model.

Education

The models are used widely in the United Kingdom in nursing education programs. McCaugherty[13] reported use of the model as the basis of an educational tool.

Research

Whittam[41] (Bolton Hospitals NHS Trust, the Royal Bolton Hospital, Minerva Road, Farnworth, Bolton, Lancashire, UK, BL4, OJR) conducted current studies related to the models in nursing practice and education. Bellman[4] addresses action research related to the model.

FURTHER DEVELOPMENT

The models can continue to be enlarged, changed, and refined. Concepts that are no longer useful in nursing practice can and should be deleted. The current pace of change in healthcare and in nursing motivated the trio to prepare a monograph about the R-L-T model (rather than produce further editions) to provide a lasting account of the conceptual model of nursing, which has been at the core of all the R-L-T publications since the first edition of *The Elements of Nursing*.[29] In the monograph, there is no attempt to include the many examples of the model's applications in various health settings with the many supporting references. Only the conceptual model is presented, leaving users to apply the concepts, which are relevant to the patient/client circumstances they encounter. In the process, users may wish to enlarge, change, or refine certain aspects of the model. As Roper, Logan, and Tierney have repeatedly emphasized, they would not wish their model, or any model, to be set in stone. A model is a growing point for further reflection on nursing practice and they hope there will continue to be creative use and further development of the R-L-T model in the future.[30]

CRITIQUE
Simplicity

The model appears to be simple because it uses everyday language, but the concepts are complex. Although Mitchell[15] has criticized the related complicated documentation, Walsh[40] criticized the over simplicity and lack of novelty. Bailey[3] criticized the lack of fresh conceptualization, and Lister[11] criticized the preservation of status quo. Ruskin indicated that it is more difficult to be simple than to be complex.[31] Parr[19] has given an unfavorable comparison to American models. Aggleton and Chalmers,[1] Fraser,[6] Lister,[11] Walsh,[40] and Minschull, Rose, and Turner[14] have criticized the model for being too physically oriented. However, Girot,[8] Newton,[16] Page,[17] and Parker[18] indicate that other dimensions are possible.

Generality

The models can be adapted to any nursing situation, including but not limited to:[16]
- Health promotion
- Health maintenance

- Prevention of disease
- In relation to illness, acute or chronic
- In relation to relationships
- Helping to die with dignity
- Any age group
- Irrespective of dependence or independence status
- Irrespective of culture, social class, environmental conditions, or politicoeconomic circumstances

Two publications, *Learning to Use the Process of Nursing*[30] and *Using a Model for Nursing*,[32] illustrate the application of the first R-L-T models[29] when providing nursing care for people of different age groups in different health settings (in the home or in medical, surgical, psychiatric, and maternity units) who have a variety of health problems (actual and potential), such as postnatal management, diabetes mellitus, the aftermath of head injury, or coping with lung cancer. Articles by other nurse authors also demonstrate the use of the R-L-T models (in some instances, the more recent versions) in a range of settings.

Empirical Precision

The model initially looks simple, but the concepts are complex and may be difficult to measure. However, the concept of *ALs* was selected in preference to *needs* because ALs are observable, they can be explicitly described, and, in some instances, they can be objectively measured.[16]

Derivable Consequences

It is not necessary for a model to attempt to exhaust every aspect of a discipline. It is a guideline amenable to the creativity of the user. These models can be used in any nursing situation.

CRITICAL THINKING *Activities*

1. Identify the four major concepts common to both the Model of Living and the Model for Nursing.

2. List the 12 ALs down the side of a piece of paper and the five factors influencing ALs across the top of the page to form a grid. Create a case study addressing the items on the grid.

3. Plan care based on the case study you developed, one that classmates developed, or a real situation using the Model for Nursing.

REFERENCES

1. Aggleton, P. & Chalmers, H. (1986). *Nursing models and the nursing process.* Basingstoke, UK: Macmillan Educational.
2. Aggleton, P. & Chalmers, H. (2000). *Nursing models and the nursing process* (2nd ed.). Basingstoke, UK: Macmillan Educational.
3. Bailey, F. (1992). Nursing models redundant in practice. *British Journal of Nursing, 1*(5), 219.
4. Bellman, L.M. (1996). Changing practice through reflection on the Roper, Logan and Tierney model: The enhancement approach to action research. *Journal of Advanced Nursing, 24,* 129-138.
5. Davis, P. (1997). Using models and theories in orthopaedic nursing. *Journal of Orthopaedic Nursing, 1,* 41-47.
6. Fraser, M. (1990). *Using conceptual nursing in practice: A research-based approach.* London: Harper & Row.
7. Fraser, M. (1996). *Using conceptual nursing in practice: A research-based approach* (2nd ed.). London: Harper & Row.
8. Girot, E. (1990). Discussing nursing theory. *Senior Nurse, 10*(6), 16-19.
9. Griffiths, P. (1998). An investigation into the description of patients' problems by nurses using two different needs-based nursing models. *Journal of Advanced Nursing, 28*(5), 969-977.
10. Jones, E. (1998). Surgical excision of a pharyngeal pouch. *Professional Nurse, 13*(6), 378-381.
11. Lister, P.E. (1991). Approaching models of nursing from a postmodernist perspective. *Journal of Advanced Nursing, 16,* 206-212.
12. Logan, W. (1996). Personal correspondence.
13. McCaugherty, D. (1992). The Roper nursing model as an educational and research tool. *British Journal of Nursing, 1*(9), 455-459.
14. Minshull, J., Rose, K., & Turner, J. (1986). The human needs model of nursing. *Journal of Advanced Nursing, 11,* 643-649.
15. Mitchell, J.R.A. (1984). Is nursing any business of doctors? A simple guide to the 'nursing process.' *British Medical Journal, 288,* 216-219.

16. Newton, C. (1992). *The Roper-Logan-Tierney in action.* Hampshire, UK: Macmillan.

17. Page, M. (1995). Tailoring nursing models to clients' needs: Using the Roper-Logan-Tierney model after discharge. *Professional Nurse,* 10(5), 284-288.

18. Parker, D. (1997). Nursing art and science: Literature and debate. In D. Marks-Maran & P. Rose (Eds.), *Reconstructing nursing: Beyond art and science.* London: Balliere Tindall.

19. Parr, M.S. (1993). The Newman health care systems model: An evaluation. *British Journal of Theatre Nursing,* 3(8), 20-27.

20. Pullen, M. (1998). Support role. *Nursing Times,* 94(47), 57.

21. Ramsden, J. (1997). Objective analysis of a critical incident. *Nursing Times,* 93(34), 43-45.

22. Roper, N. (1963). *Man's anatomy, physiology, health and environment.* Edinburgh: Churchill Livingstone.

23. Roper, N. (1967). *Principles of nursing.* Edinburgh: Churchill Livingstone.

24. Roper, N. (1976). *Clinical experience in nurse education* [Research monograph]. Edinburgh: Churchill Livingstone.

25. Roper, N. (1987). *Churchill Livingstone pocket medical dictionary* (14th ed.). Edinburgh: Churchill Livingstone.

26. Roper, N. (1988). *Principles of nursing in process context* (4th ed.). Edinburgh: Churchill Livingstone.

27. Roper, N. (1989). *Churchill Livingstone nurses' dictionary* (16th ed.). Edinburgh: Churchill Livingstone.

28. Roper, N. (1996). Personal correspondence.

29. Roper, N., Logan, W., & Tierney, A. (1980). *The elements of nursing.* Edinburgh: Churchill Livingstone.

30. Roper, N., Logan, W., & Tierney, A. (1981). *Learning to use the process of nursing.* Edinburgh: Churchill Livingstone.

31. Roper, N., Logan, W., & Tierney, A. (2000). *The Roper-Logan-Tierney model of nursing.* Edinburgh: Churchill Livingstone.

32. Roper, N., Logan, W., & Tierney, A. (Eds.). (1983). *Using a model for nursing.* Edinburgh: Churchill Livingstone.

33. Roper, N., Logan, W., & Tierney, A. (1985). *The elements of nursing* (2nd ed.). Edinburgh: Churchill Livingstone.

34. Roper, N., Logan, W., & Tierney, A. (1990). *The elements of nursing: A model for nursing based on a model of living* (3rd ed.). Edinburgh: Churchill Livingstone.

35. Roper, N., Logan, W., & Tierney, A. (1996). *The elements of nursing: A model for nursing based on a model of living* (4th ed.). Edinburgh: Churchill Livingstone.

36. Rowe, K. (1995). Nursing a person who had suffered a myocardial infarction. *British Journal of Nursing,* 4(3), 148-154.

37. Smith, S. (1983). Grant from National Board for Nursing Midwifery and Health Visiting Scotland, Education Fund to investigate Huntington's disease.

38. Smith, S. (1994). Grant from The Borders Health Board Research and Development to study Huntington's disease.

39. Tierney, A. (1996). Nursing models: Extant or extinct? *Journal of Advanced Nursing,* 28(1), 77-85.

40. Walsh, M. (1991). *Models in clinical: The way forward.* London: Balliere Tindall.

41. Whittam, S. (1993). *Introduction Roper/Logan/Tierney model into practice.* Unpublished manuscript.

BIBLIOGRAPHY
Primary Sources
Books

Roper, N. (1976). *Clinical experience in nurse education* [Research monograph]. Edinburgh: Churchill Livingstone.

Roper, N. (1976). *Man's anatomy, physiology, health and environment* (5th ed.). Edinburgh: Churchill Livingstone.

Roper, N. (1987). *Churchill Livingstone pocket medical dictionary* (14th ed.). Edinburgh: Churchill Livingstone.

Roper, N. (1988). *New American pocket medical dictionary* (2nd ed.). Edinburgh: Churchill Livingstone.

Roper, N. (1988). *Principles of nursing in process context* (4th ed.). Edinburgh: Churchill Livingstone.

Roper, N. (1989). *Churchill Livingstone nurses' dictionary* (16th ed.). Edinburgh: Churchill Livingstone.

Roper, N., Logan, W., & Tierney, A. (1980). *The elements of nursing.* Edinburgh: Churchill Livingstone.

Roper, N., Logan, W., & Tierney, A. (1981). *Learning to use the process of nursing.* Edinburgh: Churchill Livingstone.

Roper, N., Logan, W., & Tierney, A. (Eds.). (1983). *Using a model for nursing.* Edinburgh: Churchill Livingstone.

Roper, N., Logan, W., & Tierney, A. (1985). *The elements of nursing* (2nd ed.). Edinburgh: Churchill Livingstone.

Roper, N., Logan, W., & Tierney, A. (1990). *The elements of nursing: A model for nursing based on a model of living* (3rd ed.). Edinburgh: Churchill Livingstone.

Roper, N., Logan, W., & Tierney, A. (1996). *The elements of nursing: A model for nursing based on a model of living* (4th ed.). Edinburgh: Churchill Livingstone.

Roper, N., Logan, W., & Tierney, A. (2000). *The Roper-Logan-Tierney model of nursing.* Edinburgh: Churchill Livingstone.

Book Chapters

Roper, N. (1979). Nursing based on a model of living. In M. College & D. Jones (Eds.), *Readings in nursing.* Edinburgh: Churchill Livingstone.

Roper, N., Logan, W., & Tierney, A. (1986). Nursing models: A process of construction and refinement. In B. Kershaw & J. Salvage (Eds.), *Models for nursing.* Chichester, UK: John Wiley.

Roper, N., Logan, W., & Tierney, A. (1996). The Roper-Logan-Tierney model: A model in nursing practice. In P. Hinton-Walker & B. Newman (Eds.), *Blueprint for use of nursing models.* New York: National League for Nursing Press.

Journal Articles

Kilgour, D. & Logan, W. (1985). A model for health: Its use in an undergraduate nursing programme. *Nurse Education Today,* 82(35), 215-220.

Logan, W. (1981). A model for imitation [Janforum: The nursing process and standards of care]. *Journal of Advanced Nursing,* 6, 505-506.

Logan, W. (1987). Part of the plan: A degree programme in India (based on the R-L-T model). *Senior Nurse,* 6(6), 30-32.

Roper, N. (1976, April/May). An image of nursing for the 1970s. *Nursing Times [Occasional papers],* 72, 17, 18.

Roper, N. (1976, May). A model for nursing and nursology. *Journal of Advanced Nursing,* 1(3), 219-227.

Roper, N. (1983, Nov.). A model for nursing. *Nursing Mirror,* 157(22), 21-23.

Roper, N. (1986). The Roper/Logan/Tierney model for nursing: Part II. *Irish Nursing Forum and Health Sciences,* 3(4), 32-34.

Roper, N. (1994, April). Definition of nursing . . . Part 1. *British Journal of Nursing,* 3(7), 355-357.

Roper, N. (1994, May). Definition of nursing . . . Part 2. *British Journal of Nursing,* 3(9), 460-462.

Roper, N., Logan, W., & Tierney, A. (1983, March). A model for nursing. *Nursing Times,* 79(9), 24-27.

Roper, N., Logan, W., & Tierney, A. (1983, May). A nursing model: Nursing process 1. *Nursing Mirror,* 156(21), 17-19.

Roper, N., Logan, W., & Tierney, A. (1983, June 1). Is there a danger of "processing" patients? Nursing process 2. *Nursing Mirror,* 156(22), 32-33.

Roper, N., Logan, W., & Tierney, A. (1983, June 8). Problems or needs? Nursing process 3. *Nursing Mirror,* 156(23), 43-44.

Roper, N., Logan, W., & Tierney, A. (1983, June 15). Identifying the goals: Nursing process 4. *Nursing Mirror,* 156(24), 22-23.

Roper, N., Logan, W., & Tierney, A. (1983, June 22). Endless paperwork: Nursing process 5. *Nursing Mirror,* 156(25), 34-35.

Roper, N., Logan, W., & Tierney, A. (1983, June 29). Unity—with diversity: Nursing process 6. *Nursing Mirror,* 156(26), 35.

Roper, N., Logan, W., & Tierney, A. (1985, July). The Roper-Logan-Tierney model. *Senior Nurse,* 3(2), 20-26.

Tierney, A. (1984). A response to Professor Mitchell's "Simple guide to the nursing process." *British Medical Journal,* 288, 835-838.

Tierney, A. (1984, May). Defending the process. *Nursing Times,* 80(20), 38-41.

Tierney, A. (1998). Nursing models: Extant or extinct? Journal of Advanced Nursing 28(1), 77-85.

Secondary Sources
Books

Aggleton, P. & Chalmers, H. (1986). *Nursing models and the nursing process.* Basingstoke, UK: Macmillan Educational.

Aggleton, P. & Chalmers, H. (2000). *Nursing models and the nursing process* (2nd ed.). Basingstoke, UK: Macmillan Educational.

Fraser, M. (1990). *Using conceptual nursing in practice: A research-based approach.* London: Harper & Row.

Fraser, M. (1996). *Using conceptual nursing in practice: A research-based approach* (2nd ed.). London: Harper & Row.

Hinton-Walder, R. & Neuman, B. (1997). *Blueprint for use of nursing models.* New York: National League for Nursing Press.

Jamieson, E., McCall, J., Blythe, R., & Logan, W. (Consultant). (1992). *Guidelines for clinical nursing practices: Related to a nursing model* (2nd ed.). Edinburgh: Churchill Livingstone.

Jamieson, E., McCall, J., Blythe, R., & Whyte, L. (1997). *Clinical nursing practices* (3rd ed.). Edinburgh: Churchill Livingstone.

Marriner Tomey, A. & Alligood M.R. (1998). *Nursing theorists and their work* (4th ed.). St. Louis: Mosby.

Newton, C. (1991). *The Roper-Logan-Tierney model in action.* Basingstoke, Hampshire: Macmillan.

Pearson, A. & Vaughan, B. (Eds.). (1986). *Nursing models for practice.* London; Heinemann.

Pearson, A. & Vaughan, B. (Eds.). (1996). *Nursing models for practice* (2nd ed.). London: Heinemann.

Book Chapters

Chew, A. & Williams, A.P.M. (1988). Care plan for a woman with cardiac failure using Roper's activities of living model. In H. Chalmers (Ed.), *Choosing a model: Caring for patients with cardiovascular and respiratory problems* (pp. 57-69). London: Edward Arnold.

Pearson, A., Vaughn, B., & Fitzgerald, M. (1996). The activities of living model for nursing. In A. Pearson, B. Vaughn, & M. Fitzgerald (Eds.), *Nursing models for practice* (2nd ed., pp. 72-89). Oxford: Butterworth-Heinemann.

Journal Articles

Allan, D. (1986, Oct.). Nursing the unconscious patient. *The Professional Nurse,* 1, 15-17.

Allan, S. (1987). Arms extended (development of a tool to measure dependence/independence in people with multiple sclerosis). *Nursing Times,* 83(43), 44-45.

Bagnall, P. & Heslop, A. (1987, June). Chronic respiratory disease: Educating patients at home. *The Professional Nurse,* 2(9), 293-296.

Barr, A. (1992, Nov.). Care of a patient with breathing difficulties. *British Journal of Nursing,* 1(13), 660-665.

Bellman, L.M. (1996, July). Changing nursing practice through reflection on the Roper, Logan, and Tierney model. *Journal of Advanced Nursing,* 24(1), 129-138.

Davis, M. (1993, Jan.). Two contrasting nursing models. *Nursing Times,* 89(Suppl. 4), 1-8.

Dunn, C. (1986, Aug.). A holistic approach to intensive care. *Nursing Times,* 82(33), 36-38.

Ford, S. (1987). Into the outside. (Preparation of a mentally handicapped man to be discharged from hospital into the community.) *Nursing Times,* 83(20), 40-42.

Harrison, A. (1986, June). Compression fractures of the thoracic vertebrae. *Nursing Times,* 82(26), 40-42.

Heslop, A.P. & Bagnall, P. (1988). A study to evaluate the intervention of a nurse visiting patients with disabling chest disease in the community. *Journal of Advanced Nursing,* 13, 71-77.

James, G. (1986, April). Planning for terminal care. *Nursing Times,* 23, 24-27.

Jukes, M. (1987, March). Assessing the whole person (mental handicap). *Senior Nurse,* 6(3), 14-16.

Ledger, S.D. (1986). Management of a patient in respiratory failure due to chronic bronchitis. *Intensive Care Nursing,* 2, 30-43.

Mantle, F. (1996, Feb.). Safe practices. *Nursing Times,* 92(6), 36-38.

McCaugherty, D. (1992, Sept.). The Roper nursing model as an educational and research tool. *British Journal of Nursing,* 1(9), 455-459.

Mitchell, J.R.A. (1984). Is nursing any business of doctors? A simple guide to the nursing process. *British Medical Journal,* 288, 216-219.

Moir, S. (1986, May/June). Introducing a model for nursing to the community. *Irish Nursing Forum and Health Services,* 4(3), 26-28.

Page, M. (1995, Feb.). Tailoring nursing models to clients' needs. *Professional Nurse,* 10(5), 284-288.

Rhodes, K. (1990, May). Parkinson's disease using the Roper model. *Nursing Times,* 86(21), 36-39.

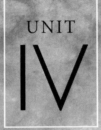
Theories and Middle-Range Theories

- *Nursing theories have been derived from works in other disciplines related to nursing and from earlier works in nursing, such as philosophies, nursing conceptual models, and grand theories.*

- *Middle-range nursing theories propose outcomes that are less abstract than grand theories and more specific to practice.*

- *Middle-range nursing theories are specific to nursing practice and specify the area of practice, age range of the patient, nursing action or intervention, and proposed outcome.*

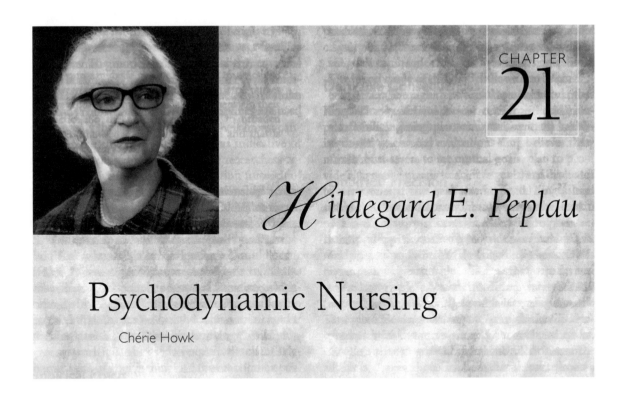

Hildegard E. Peplau

Psychodynamic Nursing

Chérie Howk

CREDENTIALS AND BACKGROUND OF THE THEORIST

Hildegard E. Peplau was born September 1, 1909 in Reading, Pennsylvania. She died peacefully in her sleep 89 years later on March 17, 1999 in her home in Sherman Oaks, California. She was the second daughter of six children born to immigrant parents, Gustav and Ottylie Peplau. Peplau began her nursing career in 1931 after graduating from Pottstown, Pennsylvania School of Nursing. She received a B.A. in interpersonal psychology from Bennington College, Vermont, in 1943; an M.A. in psychiatric nursing from Teachers College, Columbia, New York, in 1947; and an Ed.D. in curriculum development from Columbia University in 1953.[6] Peplau received honorary doctoral degrees during her prestigious career from the following universities: Alfred, Duke,

Previous authors: Chérie Howk, Gail H. Brophy, Elizabeth T. Carey, John Noll, LyNette Rasmussen, Bryn Searcy, and Nancy L. Stark. The author wishes to express appreciation to Hildegard E. Peplau for critiquing the original chapter.

Indiana, Ohio State, Rutgers, and the University of Ulster in Ireland.

Hildegard Peplau is considered to be the mother of psychiatric nursing; however, her contributions to the professionalization of nursing transcends her psychiatric nursing specialty. She influenced the advancement of professional, educational, and practice standards in nursing. A pioneer in her field, she emphasized the importance of professional self-regulation through credentialing and introduced the concept of advanced nursing practice. Peplau's most significant contribution to nursing science, professional nursing, and the psychiatric nursing specialty may be the development of the Theory of Interpersonal Relations, a midrange theory focusing on the relationship between the nurse and the patient.

It has been suggested that Peplau's work has created a paradigm change in the nature of the relationship between the nurse and the patient.[51] Before Peplau's seminal 1952 book, *Interpersonal Relations in Nursing*,[39] nursing practice involved acting on, to,

379

or for the patient. The patient was considered to be the object of nursing action and nurses were to do to or for the patient. Peplau's work forever changed the character of nursing by conceptualizing the patient as a partner in the nursing process.

Peplau's life work was built upon her personal and practice experiences. Peplau's understanding of the influence of illness and death on individuals and families was influenced by her early experiences during the great influenza epidemic.[2] Peplau's theorizing was largely inductive and based on keen observations of her clinical work and her environment. Her professional and teaching experiences have been broad and varied. She was the operating room supervisor at Pottstown Hospital and later headed the staff of the Bennington infirmary while pursuing her undergraduate degree.

Peplau practiced at the Bellevue and White Institute psychiatric facilities, during which time she studied with renowned psychiatrists Eric Fromm, Frieda Fromm-Reichman, and Harry Stack Sullivan. As a member of the Army Nurse Corps during World War II, Peplau worked in a neuropsychiatric hospital in England where she met and worked with leading figures in British and American psychiatry. After the war, Peplau again worked with many of these same men as they worked to reshape the mental health system in the United States through the passage of the National Mental Health Act of 1946. Peplau vigorously advocated for nurses to become further educated so that they could provide truly therapeutic care to patients rather than the custodial care that was prevalent in the mental hospitals of that era.

Peplau greatly contributed to the profession of nursing, in particular the specialty of psychiatric nursing, with the publication of *Interpersonal Relations in Nursing*.[39] Throughout the 1950s and 1960s, Peplau[40,31:123] conducted workshops based on analyzed notes of sessions with medical and psychiatric patients, "abundantly sharing her knowledge and clinical skills . . . [and] encouraged nurses to use their competence . . . in a continuous, experiential and educative process."

Peplau obtained her master's degree at Columbia University in New York and was invited to develop and teach in the graduate program in psychiatric nursing. She remained on the faculty at Columbia

for five years. In 1954, Peplau went to Rutgers, where she developed and chaired the graduate psychiatric nursing program until her retirement in 1974. While at Rutgers, Peplau created the first graduate-level program for the preparation of clinical specialists in psychiatric nursing.[21] After her retirement from Rutgers, Peplau served as a visiting professor at the University of Leuven in Belgium where she helped establish the first graduate-nursing program in Europe.

In 1969, Peplau became executive director of the American Nurses Association. She served as president of the American Nurses Association from 1970 to 1972 and as second vice president from 1972 to 1974.[47] Peplau is the only nurse to have been both the executive director and the president of the American Nurses Association. She has also served as director of the New Jersey State Nurses' Association; a member of the Expert Advisory Council of the World Health Organization (WHO); the National Nurse Consultant to the Surgeon General of the Air Force; and a nursing consultant to the United States Public Health Service, the National Institute of Mental Health, and various foreign countries.[3] She chaired the editorial board of *Perspectives in Psychiatric Care* when the journal was founded and served as chief advisor of *Nursing 74*. She has served on the editorial board of the *Journal of Psychosocial Nursing* and the *Journal of Psychiatric and Mental Health Nursing*. In 1987, the *Journal of Psychosocial Nursing* honored her as the first psychosocial nurse of the year.

In 1994, Peplau's career was highlighted by her induction into the American Academy of Nursing Living Legends Hall of Fame. In 1995, Peplau was selected as one of the 50 Great Americans chosen to be included in the Fiftieth Edition of *Who's Who in America*. She was an elected fellow of the American Academy of Nurses and Sigma Theta Tau, the national nursing honorary society. Peplau continued to lecture occasionally and present her work throughout the United States, Canada, Africa, and South America until her death in 1999. Peplau's publications[47] continued consistently from 1952 to 1996 in which she continued to enhance and develop her work.

The nursing profession has much reason to thank Hildegard Peplau. Her contributions to the profession emanated from her reasons for making nursing her career. Malone[28] reported that Peplau once stated that her reasons for becoming a nurse were largely irrelevant, but that her reasons for staying and making a career of it were paramount. Her reasons for staying included her intense interest in the work, the practice of nursing, the opportunity to develop her capabilities, and the opportunity to help advance the profession in the public interest.

William E. Field, Jr. perpetuated Peplau's work by publishing *The Psychotherapy of Hildegard E. Peplau*.[10] In this book, Field compiled copious notes on the numerous lectures that Peplau delivered to psychiatric nurses. Ultimately, Field's book presented Peplau's theory and method of investigative psychotherapy as it was developed from 1948 to 1974.

Peplau's archives are deposited in the Arthur and Elizabeth Schlesinger Library on the History of Women in America at Radcliffe College in Cambridge, Massachusetts.

THEORETICAL SOURCES

Peplau was committed to incorporating established knowledge into her conceptual framework, developing a theory-based nursing model. Peplau's Theory of Interpersonal Relations integrated existing theories into her model at a time when nursing theory development was relatively new.

The nature of science in nursing refers to the "body of verified knowledge found within the discipline of nursing . . . [that is] mainly knowledge from the biological and behavioral sciences."[1:35] The "synthesis, reorganization, or extension of concepts drawn from the basic and applied sciences, which in their reformation tend to become new concepts," have led to the growth of nursing science.[25:292]

Peplau used knowledge borrowed from behavioral science and what can be termed the *psychological model* to develop her Theory of Interpersonal Relations. Borrowing from the psychological model "enabled the nurse to begin to move away from a disease orientation to one whereby the psychologic meaning of events, feelings, and behaviors could be explored and incorporated into nursing interventions. It gave nurses an opportunity to teach patients how to experience their feelings and to explore with clients how to

bear their feelings."[47:6] The conceptual framework of interpersonal relations seeks to develop the nurse's skill in using these concepts. Sullivan,[54] Symonds,[55] Maslow and Mittleman,[29] and Miller[31] are some of the major sources Peplau used in developing her conceptual framework. Some of the therapeutic conceptions that these theorists devised arose directly from the works of Freud[17] and Fromm.[18]

USE OF EMPIRICAL EVIDENCE

Theories that were available when Peplau developed her theory described behavior within the perspectives of psychoanalytical theory, the principles of social learning, the concept of human motivation, and the concept of personality development. Peplau combined the various ideas of Maslow, Sullivan, Miller, and Symonds. The genius of Freud, Fromm, Adler, and Pavlov[34] initiated these theories.

Although Peplau found Freud's theory not very useful by itself, particularly in clinical work with patients, Freud's hypotheses were a rich source of research study. Freud emphasized the importance of motivation, conflict, and the role of the family in early childhood and discovered the significance of the unconscious. Freudian principles have been tested extensively, and his influence on later theorists' hypotheses is obvious.

Maslow's theory of human motivation is well known and a great deal of sound research has followed its publication. Maslow theorized that people are motivated to attain their inherent potential, a process referred to as *self-actualization*. Miller's work focused on personality theory, adjustment mechanisms, psychotherapy, and principles of social learning. Pavlov's stimulus-response model influenced Miller's principles of social learning. Miller assisted in translating psychoanalytical theory and practice into learning theory terms, laying the foundation for behaviorists to enter the field of therapy.

Sullivan was a pioneer in the field of modern psychiatry. With other prominent theorists and therapists, he broadened basic Freudian psychoanalytics. Sullivan worked toward including cultural and social determiners into the Freudian view and emphasized the development of interpersonal relationships as necessary extensions of the psychoanalytical view.[20]

MAJOR CONCEPTS & DEFINITIONS

PSYCHODYNAMIC NURSING

Peplau defines *psychodynamic nursing* because her model evolves through this type of nursing. "Psychodynamic nursing is being able to understand one's own behavior to help others identify felt difficulties, and to apply principles of human relations to the problems that arise at all levels of experience."[39:xiii] Peplau develops the model by describing the structural concepts of the interpersonal process, which are the phases of the nurse-patient relationship. She holds this to be basic to psychodynamic nursing.

NURSE-PATIENT RELATIONSHIP

Peplau describes four phases of the nurse-patient relationship. Although separate, they overlap and occur over the time of the relationship[39] (Figure 21-1):

Orientation

During the orientation phase, the individual has a *felt need* and seeks professional assistance. The nurse helps the patient recognize and understand his or her problem and determine his or her need for help.[39]

Identification

The patient identifies with those who can help him or her (relatedness). The nurse permits exploration of feelings to aid the patient in undergoing illness as an experience that reorients feelings and strengthens positive forces in the personality and provides needed satisfaction.[39]

Exploitation

During the exploitation phase, the patient attempts to derive full value from what he or she is offered through the relationship. The nurse can project new goals to be achieved through personal effort and power shifts from the nurse to the patient as the patient delays gratification to achieve the newly formed goals.[39]

Resolution

The patient gradually puts aside old goals and adopts new goals. This is a process in which the patient frees himself or herself from identification with the nurse.[39]

NURSING ROLES

Peplau[39] describes six nursing roles that emerge in the various phases of the nurse-patient relationship: (1) role of the stranger, (2) role of the resource person, (3) teaching role, (4) leadership role, (5) surrogate role, and (6) counseling role.

Role of the Stranger

Peplau states that because the nurse and patient are strangers to each other, the nurse should treat the patient with ordinary courtesy. In other words, the nurse should not prejudge the patient, but accept him or her as a person. During this nonpersonal phase, the nurse should treat the patient as emotionally able unless evidence indicates otherwise. This coincides with the identification phase.[39]

Role of the Resource Person

The nurse provides specific answers to questions, especially health information, and interprets to the patient the treatment or medical plan of care. These questions often arise within the context of a larger problem. The nurse determines what type of response is appropriate for constructive learning, either giving straightforward factual answers or providing counseling.[39]

Teaching Role

The teaching role is a combination of all roles and "always proceeds from what the patient knows and . . . develops around his interest in wanting and ability to use . . . information."[39:48] Peplau[42] expands on the role of teacher in later writings. She separates teaching into two categories: (1) instructional, which consists largely of giving information and is the form explained in educational literature, and (2) experiential, which is "using the

MAJOR CONCEPTS & DEFINITIONS—cont'd

experience of the learner as a basis from which learning products are developed."[42:98] The products of learning are generalizations and appraisals that the patient makes about his or her experiences. This concept of learning used in the teaching role overlaps with the nurse counselor role because the nurse carries out the concept of learning through psychotherapeutic techniques.[40]

Leadership Role

The leadership role involves the democratic process. The nurse helps the patient meet the tasks at hand through a relationship of cooperation and active participation.[39]

Surrogate Role

The patient casts the nurse in the surrogate role. The nurse's attitudes and behaviors create feeling tones in the patient that reactivate feelings generated in a previous relationship. The nurse's function is to help the patient recognize similarities between the nurse and the person recalled by the patient. The nurse then helps the patient see the differences between the nurse's role and that of the recalled person. In this phase, the patient and

nurse define areas of dependence, independence, and interdependence.[39]

Counseling Role

Peplau[41] believes that the counseling role has the greatest emphasis in psychiatric nursing. Counseling functions in the nurse-patient relationship by the way nurses respond to patients' demands. Peplau[39:64] says that the purpose of interpersonal techniques is to help "the patient remember and understand fully what is happening to him in the present situation, so that the experience can be integrated rather than dissociated from other experiences in life" (Figure 21-2).

PSYCHOBIOLOGICAL EXPERIENCES

Peplau describes four psychobiological experiences: (1) needs, (2) frustration, (3) conflict, and (4) anxiety. These experiences provide energy that is transformed into some form of action. Peplau uses nonnursing theoretical concepts to identify and explain these experiences that compel destructive or constructive responses from nurses and patients. This understanding provides a basis for goal formation and nursing interventions.[39]

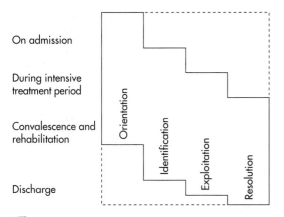

Figure **21-1** Overlapping phases in nurse-patient relationships. (From Peplau, H.E. [1952]. *Interpersonal relations in nursing.* New York: G.P. Putnam's Sons. Used with permission.)

MAJOR ASSUMPTIONS

Peplau[39:xii] identifies two explicit assumptions:
1. "The kind of person that the nurse becomes makes a substantial difference in what each patient will learn as he or she receives nursing care."
2. "Fostering personality development toward maturity is a function of nursing and nursing education. Nursing uses principles and methods that guide the process toward resolution of interpersonal problems."

One implicit assumption was that "the nursing profession has legal responsibility for the effective use of nursing and for its consequences to patients."[39:6]

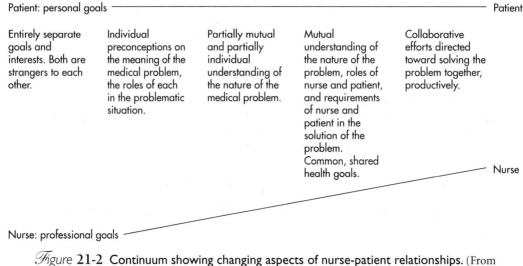

Figure 21-2 Continuum showing changing aspects of nurse-patient relationships. (From Peplau, H.E. [1952]. *Interpersonal relations in nursing.* New York: G.P. Putnam's Sons. Used with permission.)

Nursing

Peplau describes nursing as "a significant, therapeutic, interpersonal process. It functions cooperatively with other human processes that make health possible for individuals in communities."[39:16] When professional health teams offer health services, nurses participate in the organization of conditions that facilitate natural ongoing tendencies in human organisms. "Nursing is an educative instrument, a maturing force that aims to promote forward movement of personality in the direction of creative, constructive, productive, personal, and community living."[39:16]

Person

Peplau defines *person* in terms of a man. Man is an organism that lives in an unstable equilibrium.[39]

Health

Peplau[39:12] defines *health* as "a word symbol that implies forward movement of personality and other ongoing human processes in the direction of creative, constructive, productive, personal, and community living."

Environment

Peplau[39:163] implicitly defines the environment in terms of "existing forces outside the organism and in the context of culture," from which mores, customs, and beliefs are acquired. "However, general conditions that are likely to lead to health always include the interpersonal process."[39:14]

THEORETICAL ASSERTIONS

Peplau makes theoretical relationships throughout her book. In summarizing these relationships, Peplau addresses the patient-nurse relationship, the patient and his or her awareness of feelings, and the nurse and his or her awareness of feelings. She presents nursing as a maturing educative force that uses the experiential learning method for both patient and nurse (Figure 21-3).

LOGICAL FORM

The process that Peplau uses is an inductive approach to theory building. She inductively establishes empirical generalizations. "Induction is a type of relationship in which . . . one observes empirical events and

Nurse:	Stranger	Unconditional Surrogate mother		Counselor Resource person Leadership Surrogate: Mother Sibling	Adult person
Patient:	Stranger	Infant	Child	Adolescent	Adult person
Phases in nursing relationship:	Orientation ——— Identification ———				
			Exploitation ———		
		———			Resolution

Figure **21-3 Phases and changing roles in nurse-patient relationships.** (From Peplau, H.E. [1952]. *Interpersonal relations in nursing.* New York: G.P. Putnam's Sons. Used with permission.)

generalizes from specific events to all similar events."[24:8] According to Peplau,[44:37] "nursing situations provide a field of observations from which unique nursing concepts can be derived and used for the improvement of the professional's work." The selected concepts that Peplau uses are organized into a larger component, forming relationships that are logical and complete. The relationships describe behaviors that occur in the nurse-patient interaction.

ACCEPTANCE BY THE NURSING COMMUNITY

Practice

Sills[50:123] recalls that Peplau brought "a new perspective, a new approach, a theoretically based foundation for nursing practice for therapeutic work with patients." She states that "Peplau's work is responsible for a second order change in the nursing culture."[50:123] Peplau's ideas provide a design for the practice of psychiatric nursing with explication of the design in usable form.

Some of Peplau's ideas were not accepted in the early years, such as the concept of experiential learning for the patient and students.[50] In a panel discussion on psychotherapeutic strategies, Mertz, Mereness, and Mellow disagreed with Peplau on the methodology of psychotherapeutic functions and the role of the nurse as a surrogate.[43] Later criticisms of Peplau's model indicate the lack of development of social systems that would broaden the knowledge base for understanding the patient's problems.

Peplau[39] used the interpersonal and intrapersonal theories of Sullivan and Freud as the theoretical base for her model and did not take into consideration interrelationships between man and society. von Bertalanffy[59] later developed these concepts in general systems theory and included them in the curriculum of the Rutgers graduate program in psychiatric nursing of which Peplau chaired.

Clinicians continue to use Peplau's model extensively. Several researchers stand out in their use of Peplau's theory to guide a program of study that applies this theory to clinical practice. In her article, "Peplau's Therapy: An Application to Short-Term Individual Therapy," Thompson[56] uses Peplau's model to analyze short-term individual therapy. She states, "In working with individuals with psychological problems, the development of the interpersonal process is of the utmost importance. Without the development of a therapeutic relationship, little work could be accomplished by the nurse-counselor."[56:32]

In 1992, Forchuk[14] initiated a prolific program of study that tested Peplau's theory in clinical settings. Forchuk and Brown[13] tested Peplau's conceptualization of the nurse-patient relationship in their development of an instrument to measure the phases of the relationship. Furthermore, Forchuk and colleagues[12] incorporated Peplau's theory into a case-management model, which emphasized the importance of the interactive interpersonal relationship between the patient and the practitioner. Forchuk, Jewell, Schofield, Sircelj, and Valledor[16] used Peplau's Theory of Interpersonal Relations to investigate therapeutic relationships. Forchuk and colleagues[15] identified factors that influence movement of nurse-patient dyads from Peplau's orientation phase to the working phase. They found that nurses can facilitate this movement by remaining available and consistent and acting in a way that promotes trust.

Peden[35,36,37] used Peplau's process of practice-based theory development to direct a program of research in the area of depression. Using Peplau's theory, Peden[35,36,37] completed initial studies that investigated the recovery process in depressed women. More recently, Peden[38] used Peplau's process of practice-based theory development to guide a descriptive and exploratory study of negative thoughts in women with depression. In this research, Peden found that women were able to describe interpersonal patterns that resulted from negative thinking and identified strategies to manage them.

Education

Peplau's wrote the book *Interpersonal Relations in Nursing*[39] specifically as an aid to graduate nurses and nursing students. It was originally a hardback edition; a paperback edition was printed by Macmillan in 1988.

Few early critiques of Peplau's model exist in the literature. She designed and published her model in 1952,[39] 1957,[40] and 1962[41] with a particular emphasis on psychiatric nursing. The specialty journals in psychiatric nursing did not begin publication until 1963, 11 years after her model was first published. However, psychiatric nursing authors did write textbooks. Smoyak and Rouslin[52] state that after 1952, no psychiatric nursing text could ignore Peplau's work. Peplau's influence was reflected in books in the 1950s and 1960s, such as Burton's *Personal, Im-personal, and Interpersonal Relations*[8] in 1958, Burd and Marshall's *Some Clinical Approaches to Psychiatric Nursing*[7] in 1963, Hofling and Leininger's *Basic Psychiatric Concepts in Nursing*[23] in 1960, and Orlando's *The Dynamic Nurse-Patient Relationship*[32] in 1961. Most comments on Peplau and her work were written 25 years or more after her published model. O'Toole and Welt compiled Peplau's unpublished notes and lectures on the interpersonal theory in the book *Interpersonal Theory in Nursing Practice: Selected Works of Hildegard E. Peplau*.[33] They state that "Peplau's theoretical ideas, particularly her definition of nursing and nursing process, elaboration of anxiety and learning, and her psychotherapeutic methods, have become a part of the collective culture of the discipline of nursing."[33:365]

Research

Sills[49] states that Peplau's work influenced the direction of clinical work and studies. Initial efforts to use research as a tool to develop a body of nursing knowledge were uneven in quality and quantity and often did not explicitly recognize underlying assumptions. Early research followed the assumption that patient problems were within-the-person phenomena and were explored in nurse-patient relationship studies. This followed Peplau's conceptual model. Since the 1960s, research has shifted to within-the-social-system point of view, as studies have examined broader sets of relationships.

For more than 30 years, Peplau's model has formed the basis for numerous applications of research methods. Thomas, Baker, and Estes[57] used Peplau's concept of anxiety as a means to constructively resolve angry feelings through experiential learning within the nurse-patient relationship. Hays,[22] a Rutgers graduate student in psychiatric nursing and one of Peplau's students, describes a study teaching the concept of anxiety that is predominantly based on Peplau's concept of anxiety and used her conceptual model. This study is one example of Peplau's influence on new nursing leaders with graduate education in the field of psychiatric nursing. Topf and Dambacher[58] interpret the findings in their study using Peplau's role of the nurse as a stranger. Garrett, Manuel, and Vincent[19] cite Peplau's concept of anxiety for their operational definition of stress and its relationship to learning. Spring and Turk[53] developed a behavior scale using Peplau's conceptual framework and her assumption that therapeutic behavior in the nurse-patient relationship promotes experiential learning. Spring and Turk conclude that their behavior score was objective, reliable, and valid. Methven and Schlotfeldt,[30] who developed a tool to evaluate verbal responses, based their study on Peplau's assumption that therapeutic communication can be used to reduce or redirect anxiety.

Assumptions from Peplau's model continue to be used in current research. La Monica[26] devised an empathy instrument using Peplau's model (and work from other theorists) as a theoretical framework. She states, "The primary goal of nurses . . . is to provide services that assist in moving clients to their optimum health levels . . . and involves a helping relationship."[26:389]

Recent use of Peplau's theoretical model focuses on the concept of pattern integrations. Beeber and Caldwell[3] piloted a program that consisted of a collaborative relationship between primary care providers, two psychiatric-mental health clinical nurse specialists, and young women suffering with the symptoms of depression. They placed particular emphasis on creat-ing a "learning laboratory out of everyday experiences."[3:157] Peplau's model was ideal in this setting, offering a cost-effective alternative to more expensive treatment interventions. The researchers found that interpersonal intervention structures allow patients to achieve maximum quality of life by enlisting the support of others. Beeber[4,5] went on to examine Peplau's work as it would apply to interpersonal change strategies that occur in real relations between patients and their significant others and in primary care settings. Beeber encouraged nursing interventions to be guided by theory and was able to demonstrate how this could be done using Peplau's theory in her work.

Lego[27] best describes the influence and significance of Peplau's conceptual model in a thorough discussion of the history, trends, patterns, and assessment of published research that notes the direction of the one-to-one nurse-patient relationship. She states that ambiguity about the nurse-patient relationship abruptly ended in the literature as a result of Peplau's *Interpersonal Relations in Nursing*.[39] As she would continue to

do for the next 22 years, Peplau pulled together loose, ambiguous data and put them into systematic, scientific terms that could be tested, applied, and integrated into the practice of psychiatric nursing.[27] Lego[27] states that most of the published literature describing the one-to-one nurse-patient relationship is based on theoretical concepts inspired principally by Peplau.

Peplau made a significant contribution to the nursing community through the research done to evaluate, validate, and make more precise the Theory of Interpersonal Relations.

FURTHER DEVELOPMENT

As nursing broadens its scope, a need has arisen for further development of Peplau's theory for use with the healthy patient, group, and community. Further development is also indicated for patients who are unable to use their communication skills effectively. Increased use of Peplau's theory in practice is needed. Continued research is needed to further refine the theory and to build on nursing's knowledge base.

Before her death, Peplau[45,46] continued to write about the expansion and development needed to test her Theory of Interpersonal Relations and to offer explanations of such constructs as concepts, processes, patterns, problems, energy, and anxiety. Furthermore, she suggested that the constructs of focal attention, dissociation, forbidding gestures, and personification deserve additional study.

CRITIQUE
Simplicity

The major focus of Peplau's theory, interpersonal relations between patient and nurse, is easily understood. She clearly defines the theory's basic assumptions and key concepts. Of the assumptions Peplau listed, two are explicit and one is implicit. Peplau sequentially describes her four phases of the interpersonal process. She clearly indicates the roles of the nurse and the four psychobiological experiences. Her logic is based on inductive reasoning. She takes ideas from observations of the specific and applies them to the general. Peplau draws from other disciplines' theories. She is consistent with established theories and principles, such as those of Sullivan, Freud, and Maslow. Peplau deals with the relationships of the interpersonal process, nurse, patient, and psychobiological experiences. She then develops each of these relationships, within the theory, in an understandable way. Peplau's theory can be described as meeting the evaluative quality of simplicity.

Generality

Peplau[39] believed that her theory of interpersonal relationship met the criteria of generality. She felt that nurses could apply these principles in any area of their lives. The one drawback to the theory's generality is that an interpersonal relationship must exist. The theory is adaptable only to nursing settings in which communication can occur between the patient and nurse. Its use is limited in working with the comatose, senile, or newborn patient. In such situations, the nurse-patient relationship is often one-sided. The nurse and the patient cannot work together to become more knowledgeable, develop goals, and mature. Even Peplau[39:41] admits, "Understanding of the meaning of the experience to the patient is required in order for nursing to function as an educative, therapeutic, maturing force." Peplau's theory cannot be applied to all patients; therefore the quality of generality is not met.

Empirical Precision

Peplau provides a theory based on reality. The relationship between the theory and empirical data allows other scientists to validate and verify the theory. The definitions described by Peplau are in a middle range on a connotative-denotative continuum. Peplau operationally defines the four phases of the interpersonal process, the nurse with regard to his or her roles, and the patient with regard to his or her state of dependence. According to Duffey and Mullencamp,[9:573] "Peplau relates behavior to theory by naming and categorizing, operationalizing definitions of behavior, thematic abstractions of interaction phenomena, and diagnosis of problems and principles guiding nursing interactions." Peplau's theory can be considered empirically precise. With

further research and development, the degree of precision will increase.

Derivable Consequences

In historical perspective, Peplau is one of the first theorists since Nightingale to present a theory for nursing. Therefore her work can be considered pioneering in the nursing field. "She provided nursing with a meaningful method of self-directed practice at a time when medicine dominated the health care field."[11:44]

Peplau's work, thoughts, and ideas have touched many nurses, from students to practitioners. Although her book was published in 1952, five decades ago, it continues to provide direction for nursing practice, education, and research. Peplau's work has provided a significant contribution to nursing's knowledge base. The evaluative criteria of derivable consequences are unquestionably met.

CRITICAL THINKING *Activities*

1. Describe how the six subroles of the psychiatric nurse would be used during a therapeutic relationship with an acutely psychotic schizophrenic patient. For example, the nurturing needs of the patient when the patient is unable to carry out simple tasks would be met by the subrole of mother surrogate.

2. During the therapeutic relationship, patients may distort their perceptions of others. Therefore they may relate to the nurse not on the basis of the nurse's realistic attributes, but wholly or chiefly on the basis of interpersonal relationships existing in their environment. With the patient and nurse roles you have described in question #1, discuss how these distorted perceptions may affect the patient's care and the nurse-patient relationship.

3. Considering the nurse-patient relationship created in question #2, discuss the phases and changing roles that would be consid-

ered when working with this patient. Consider experiences in which you would and would not be able to accomplish the appropriate goals of each phase.

REFERENCES

1. Andreoli, R. & Thompson, C. (1977). The nature of science in nursing. *Image*, 9(2), 32-37.
2. Barker, P. (2000). Hildegard Peplau: Home thoughts from abroad. *Journal of the American Psychiatric Nurses Association*, 6(2), 63-64.
3. Beeber, L. & Caldwell, C. (1996). Pattern integrations in young depressed women: Part II. *Archives of Psychiatric Nursing*, 10(3), 157-164.
4. Beeber, L. & Charlie, M. (1998). Depressive symptom reversal for women in a primary care setting: A pilot study. *Archives of Psychiatric Nursing*, 12(5), 247-254.
5. Beeber, L. (2000). Hildahood: Taking the interpersonal theory of nursing to the neighborhood. *Journal of the American Psychiatric Nurses Association*, 6(2), 49-55.
6. Belcher, J.R. & Fish, L.J. (1980). Hildegard E. Peplau. In Nursing Theories Conference Group & J.B. George (Chairperson), *Nursing theories: The base for professional nursing practice*. Englewood Cliffs, NJ: Prentice Hall.
7. Burd, S.F. (1963). The development of an operational definition using the process of learning as a guide. In S.F. Burd & A. Marshall (Eds.), *Some clinical approaches to psychiatric nursing*. New York: Macmillan.
8. Burton, G. (1958). Personal, impersonal, and interpersonal relations. Cited by S.A. Smoyak & S. Rouslin (Eds.). (1982). *A collection of classics in psychiatric nursing literature*. Thorofare, NJ: Slack Inc.
9. Duffey, M. & Mullencamp, A.F. (1974, Sept.). A framework for theory analysis. *Nursing Outlook*, 22, 570-574.
10. Field, W.E., Jr. (Ed.). (1979). *The psychotherapy of Hildegard E. Peplau*. New Brunfels, TX: PSF Publications.
11. Fitzpatrick, J.J. & Whall, A.L. (1983). *Conceptual models of nursing, analysis, and application*. Bowie, MD: Robert J. Brady.
12. Forchuk, C., Beaton, S., Crawford, L., Ide, L., Voorberg, N., & Bethune, J. (1989). Incorporating Peplau's theory and case management. *Journal of Psychosocial Nursing*, 27(2), 35-38.
13. Forchuk, C. & Brown, B. (1989). Establishing a nurse-client relationship. *Journal of Psychosocial Nursing*, 27(2), 30-34.
14. Forchuk, C. (1992). *The orientation phase of the nurse-client relationship: Testing Peplau's theory*. Unpublished doctoral Dissertation, Wayne State University, Detroit.
15. Forchuk, C., Westwell, J., Martin, M., Azzapardi, W., Kosterewa Tolman, D., & Hux, M. (1998). Factors influencing movement of chronic psychiatric patients from the orientation to the working phase of the nursing-client relationship on an inpatient unit. *Psychotherapists*, 34(1), 36-44.
16. Forchuk, C., Jewell, J., Schofield, R., Sircelj, M., & Valledor, T. (1998). From hospital to community: Bridging therapeutic relationships. *Journal of Psychiatric and Mental Health Nursing*, 5(3), 197-202.
17. Freud, S. (1936). The problem of anxiety. Cited by H.E. Peplau. (1952). *Interpersonal relations in nursing*. New York: G.P. Putnam's Sons.
18. Fromm, E. (1947). Man for himself. Cited by H.E. Peplau. (1952). *Interpersonal relations in nursing*. New York: G.P. Putnam's Sons.
19. Garrett, A., Manuel, D., & Vincent, C. (1976, Nov.). Stressful experiences identified by student nurses. *Journal of Nursing Education*, 15(6), 9-21.
20. Gilliland, B., James, R., & Bowman, J. (1989). *Theories and strategies in counseling and psychotherapy*. Boston: Allyn and Bacon.
21. Gregg, D.E. (1978). Hildegard E. Peplau: Her contributions. *Psychiatry Care*, 16, 118-121.
22. Hays, D. (1961, Spring). Teaching a concept of anxiety. *Nursing Research*, 10(2), 108-113.
23. Hofling, C.K. & Leininger, M.M. (1960). Basic psychiatric concepts in nursing. Cited by S.A. Smoyak & S. Rouslin (Eds.). (1982). *A collection of classics in psychiatric nursing literature*. Thorofare, NJ: Slack Inc.
24. Jacox, A. (1974, Jan./Feb.). Theory construction in nursing: An overview. *Nursing Research*, 23, 4-12.
25. Johnson, D.E. (1959). The nature of a science of nursing. *Nursing Outlook*, 7, 292.
26. La Monica, E. (1981). Construct validity of an empathy instrument. *Research in Nursing and Health*, 4, 389-400.
27. Lego, S. (1980). The one-to-one nurse-patient relationship. *Perspectives in Psychiatric Care*, 18(2), 67-89. (Reprinted from *Psychiatric nursing 1946-1974: A report on the state of the art*. American Journal of Nursing Co.)
28. Malone, B. (2000). Tribute to Hildegard Peplau, RN, PhD, FAAN. *Journal of American Psychiatric Nurses Association*, 6(2), 72-73.
29. Maslow, A.H. & Mittleman, B. (1941). *Principles in abnormal psychology*. New York: Harper & Brothers.
30. Methven, D. & Schlotfeldt, R.M. (1962, Spring). The social intervention inventory. *Nursing Research*, 11(2), 83-88.d

31. Miller, N.E. & Dollard, J. (1941). *Social learning and initiation.* New Haven, CT: Yale University Press.

32. Orlando, I. (1961). The dynamic nurse-patient relationship. Cited by S.A. Smoyak & S. Rouslin (Eds.). (1982). *A collection of classics in psychiatric nursing literature.* Thorofare, NJ: Slack Inc.

33. O'Toole, A. & Welt, S. (1989). *Interpersonal theory in nursing practice: Selected works of Hildegard E. Peplau.* New York: Springer.

34. Pavlov, I. (1927). *Conditioned reflexes: An investigation of the physiological activity of the cerebral cortex.* London: Oxford University Press.

35. Peden, A. (1993). Recovering in depressed women: Research with Peplau's theory. *Nursing Science Quarterly, 6,* 140-146.

36. Peden, A. (1994). Up from depression: Strategies used by women recovering from depression. *Journal of Psychiatric and Mental Health Nursing, 2,* 77-84.

37. Peden, A. (1996). Recovering from depression: A one-year follow-up. *Journal of Psychiatric and Mental Health Nursing, 3,* 289-295.

38. Peden, A. (2000). Negative thoughts of women with depression. *Journal of American Psychiatric Nurses Association, 6*(2), 41-48.

39. Peplau, H.E. (1952). *Interpersonal relations in nursing.* New York: G.P. Putnam's Sons.

40. Peplau, H.E. (1957). Therapeutic concepts. In S.A. Smoyak & S. Rouslin (Eds.). (1982). *A collection of classics in psychiatric nursing literature.* Thorofare, NJ: Slack Inc. (Reprinted from National League for Nursing League Exchange No. 26: Aspects of psychiatric nursing.)

41. Peplau, H.E. (1962). Interpersonal techniques: The crux of psychiatric nursing. *American Journal of Nursing, 62*(6), 50-54.

42. Peplau, H.E. (1964). *Basic principles of patient counseling* (2nd ed.). Philadelphia: Smith, Kline, & French Laboratories.

43. Peplau, H.E. (1968). Psychotherapeutic strategies. Current concepts in psychiatric care: The implications for psychiatric nursing practice. Proceedings of the Institute on Psychiatric Nursing, cosponsored by Yale School of Nursing, Department of Psychiatric Nursing and the Community Mental Health Center Department of Nursing. In *Perspectives of Psychiatric Care, 6*(6), 271-289.

44. Peplau, H.E. (1969). Theory: The professional dimension. In C. Norris (Ed.), *Proceedings of the first nursing theory conference (March 21-28).* University of Kansas Medical Center, Department of Nursing Education, Kansas City.

45. Peplau, H.E. (1989). Future directions in psychiatric nursing from the perspective of history. *Journal of Psychosocial Nursing, 27*(2), 18-28.

46. Peplau, H.E. (1992). Interpersonal relations: A theoretical framework for application in nursing practice. *Nursing Science Quarterly, 5*(1), 13-18.

47. Peplau, H.E. (1996, July). Personal correspondence.

48. Phillips, J.R. (1977, Feb.). Nursing systems and nursing models. *Image: Journal of Nursing Scholarship, 9*(1), 6.

49. Sills, G.M. (1977, May/June). Research in the field of psychiatric nursing 1952-1977. *Nursing Research, 28*(3), 201-207.

50. Sills, G.M. (1978). Hildegard E. Peplau: Leader, practitioner, academician, scholar, and theorist. *Perspectives in Psychiatric Care, 16*(3), 122-128.

51. Sills, G.M. (2000). The Peplau web grows. *Journal of the American Psychiatric Nurses Association, 6*(2), 39-40.

52. Smoyak, S.A. & Rouslin, S. (Eds.). (1982). *Introduction. A collection of classics in psychiatric nursing literature.* Thorofare, NJ: Slack Inc.

53. Spring, F.E. & Turk, H. (1962, Fall). A therapeutic behavior scale. *Nursing Research, 11*(4), 214-218.

54. Sullivan, H.S. (1947). Conceptions of modern psychiatry. Cited by H.E. Peplau. (1952). *Interpersonal relations in nursing.* New York: G.P. Putnam's Sons.

55. Symonds, P. (1946). *The dynamics of human adjustments.* New York: Appleton-Century-Crofts.

56. Thompson, L. (1986, Aug.). Peplau's therapy: An application to short-term individual therapy. *Journal of Psychosocial Nursing, 24*(8), 26-31.

57. Thomas, M.D., Baker, J.M., & Estes, N.J. (1970, Dec.). Anger: A tool for developing self-awareness. *American Journal of Nursing, 70*(12), 2586-2590.

58. Topf, M. & Dambacher, B. (1979). Predominant source of interpersonal influence in relationships between psychiatric patients and nursing staff. *Research in Nursing and Health, 2*(1), 35-43.

59. von Bertalanffy, L. (1968). *General systems theory: Foundations, development, applications.* New York: G. Braziller.

BIBLIOGRAPHY
Primary Sources
Books

Peplau, H.E. (1952). *Interpersonal relations in nursing.* New York: G.P. Putnam's Sons.

Peplau, H.E. (1964). *Basic principles of patient counseling* (2nd ed.). Philadelphia: Smith, Kline, & French Laboratories.

Peplau, H.E. (1991). *Interpersonal relations in nursing: A conceptual framework of reference for psychodynamic nursing.* New York: Springer.

Book Chapters

Peplau, H.E. (1959). Principles of psychiatric nursing. In *American Handbook of Psychiatry* (Vol. 2). New York: Basic Books.

Peplau, H.E. (1963). Counseling in nursing practice. In E. Harms & P. Schreiber (Eds.), *Handbook of counseling techniques*. New York: Pergamon.

Peplau, H.E. (1966). Interpersonal techniques: The crux of psychiatric nursing. In D. Mereness, *Psychiatric nursing: developing psychiatric nursing skills,* (Vol. 1). (2nd ed.). Dubuque, IA: WM. C. Brown Company Publishers.

Peplau, H.E. (1966). Loneliness. In D. Mereness (Ed.), *Psychiatric nursing: Understanding the nurse's role in psychiatric patient care* (Vol. 2, 2nd ed.). Dubuque, IA: WM. C. Brown Company Publishers.

Peplau, H.E. (1966). Talking with patients. In D. Mereness (Ed.), *Psychiatric nursing: developing psychiatric nursing skills,* (Vol. 1, 2nd ed.). Dubuque, IA: WM. C. Brown Company Publishers.

Peplau, H.E. (1966). Themes in nursing situations—Power. In D. Mereness (Ed.), *Psychiatric nursing: developing psychiatric nursing skills,* (Vol. 1, 2nd ed.). Dubuque, IA: WM. C. Brown Company Publishers.

Peplau, H.E. (1966). Themes in nursing situations—Safety. In D. Mereness (Ed.), *Psychiatric nursing: developing psychiatric nursing skills,* (Vol. 1, 2nd ed.). Dubuque, IA: WM. C. Brown Company Publishers.

Peplau, H.E. (1966). Utilizing themes in nursing situations. In D. Mereness (Ed.), *Psychiatric nursing: developing psychiatric nursing skills,* (Vol. 1, 2nd ed.). Dubuque, IA: WM. C. Brown Company Publishers.

Peplau, H.E. (1967). Psychiatric nursing. In A.M. Freedman & A.I. Kaplan (Eds.), *Comprehensive textbook of psychiatry*. New York: Williams & Wilkins.

Peplau, H.E. (1968). Operational definitions and nursing practice. In L.T. Zderad & H.C. Belcher (Eds.), *Developing behavioral concepts in nursing*. Atlanta: Southern Regional Education Board.

Peplau, H.E. (1969). Pattern perpetuation in schizophrenia. In D. Sankar, *Schizophrenia: Current concepts and research*. Hicksville, NY: PJD.

Peplau, H.E. (1969). Theory: The professional dimension. In C. Norris (Ed.), *Proceedings of the first nursing theory conference (March 21-28)*. University of Kansas Medical Center, Department of Nursing Education, Kansas City.

Peplau, H.E. (1971). A working definition of anxiety. In S.F. Burd & M.A. Marshall (Eds.), *Some clinical approaches to psychiatric nursing* (pp. 323-327). London: The MacMillian Co.

Peplau, H.E. (1971). Process and concept of learning. In S.F. Burd & M.A. Marshall (Eds.), *Some clinical approaches to psychiatric nursing* (pp. 333-336). London: The MacMillian Co.

Peplau, H.E. (1982). Historical development of psychiatric nursing: A preliminary statement of some facts and trends. In S.A. Smoyak & S. Rouslin (Eds.), *A collection of classics in psychiatric nursing literature* (pp. 10-46). Thorofare, NJ: Slack Inc.

Peplau, H.E. (1982). The work of clinical specialists in psychiatric nursing. In S.A. Smoyak & S. Rouslin (Eds.), *A collection of classics in psychiatric nursing literature* (pp. 47-49). Thorofare, NJ: Slack Inc.

Peplau, H.E. (1987). Nursing science: A historical perspective. In R. Parse (Ed.), *Nursing science: Major paradigms, theories, critiques*. Philadelphia: W.B. Saunders.

Peplau, H.E. (1989). Anxiety, self, and hallucinations. In A.W. O'Toole & S. R. Welt (Eds.), *Interpersonal theory in nursing practice: Selected works of Hildegard E. Peplau* (pp. 278-295). New York: Springer.

Peplau, H.E. (1989). Investigative counseling. In A.W. O'Toole & S. R. Welt (Eds.), *Interpersonal theory in nursing practice: Selected works of Hildegard E. Peplau* (pp. 220-229). New York: Springer.

Peplau, H.E. (1989). Pattern interactions. In A.W. O'Toole & S.R. Welt (Eds.), *Interpersonal theory in nursing practice: Selected works of Hildegard E. Peplau* (pp. 108-119). New York: Springer.

Peplau, H.E. (1989). Theory: The professional dimensions. In A.W. O'Toole & S.R. Welt (Eds.), *Interpersonal theory in nursing practice: Selected works of Hildegard E. Peplau* (pp. 21-30). New York: Springer.

Peplau, H.E. (1992). Notes on Nightingale. In F. Nightingale, *Notes on nursing: What it is, and what it is not* (pp. 48-57). Philadelphia: J.B. Lippincott.

Journal Articles

Peplau, H.E. (1942). Health program at Bennington College. *Public Health Nursing*, 34(10), 573-575, 581.

Peplau, H.E. (1947). Discussion: A democratic participation technique. *American Journal of Nursing*, 47(5), 334-336.

Peplau, H.E. (1951). Toward new concepts in nursing and nursing education. *American Journal of Nursing*, 52(12), 722-724.

Peplau, H.E. (1952). The psychiatric nurses' family group. *American Journal of Nursing*, 52(12), 1475-1477.

Peplau, H.E. (1953). The nursing team in psychiatric facilities. *Nursing Outlook*, 1(2), 90-92.

Peplau, H.E. (1953). Themes in nursing situations: Power. *American Journal of Nursing*, 53(10), 1221-1223.

Peplau, H.E. (1953). Themes in nursing situations: Safety. *American Journal of Nursing*, 53(11), 1343-1346.

Peplau, H.E. (1954). Utilizing themes in nursing situations. *American Journal of Nursing*, 54 (3), 325-328.

Peplau, H.E. (1955). Loneliness. *American Journal of Nursing*, 55(12), 1476-1481.

Peplau, H.E. (1956). An undergraduate program in psychiatric nursing. *Nursing Outlook*, 4, 400-410.

Peplau, H.E. (1956). Present day trends in psychiatric nursing. *Neuropsychiatry*, 111(4), 190-204.

Peplau, H.E. (1957). What is experiential teaching? *American Journal of Nursing*, 57(7), 884-886.

Peplau, H.E. (1958). Public health nurses promote mental health. *Public Health Reports*, 73(9), 828.

Peplau, H.E. (1960). Anxiety in the mother-infant relationship. *Nursing World*, 134(5), 33-34.

Peplau, H.E. (1960). Must laboring together be called teamwork? Problems in team treatment of adults in state mental hospitals. *American Journal of Orthopsychiatry*, 30, 103-108.

Peplau, H.E. (1960). Talking with patients. *American Journal of Nursing*, 60, 964-967.

Peplau, H.E. (1962). Interpersonal techniques: The crux of psychiatric nursing. *American Journal of Nursing*, 62, 629-633.

Peplau, H.E. (1962). The crux of psychiatric nursing. *American Journal of Nursing*, 62, 50-54.

Peplau, H.E. (1963). Interpersonal relations and the process of adaptations. *Nursing Science*, 1(4), 272-279.

Peplau, H.E. (1964). Psychiatric nursing skills and the general hospital patient. *Nursing Forum*, 3(2), 28-37.

Peplau, H.E. (1965). Specialization in professional nursing. *Nursing Science*, 3(4), 268-287.

Peplau, H.E. (1965). The 91st day: A challenge to professional nursing. *Perspectives in Psychiatric Care*, 3(2), 20-24.

Peplau, H.E. (1965). The heart of nursing: Interpersonal relations. *Canadian Nurse*, 61(4), 273-275.

Peplau, H.E. (1965). The nurse in the community mental health program. *Nursing Outlook*, 13(11), 68-70.

Peplau, H.E. (1966). Nurse-doctor relationships. *Nursing Forum*, 5(1), 60-75.

Peplau, H.E. (1966). Nursing's two routes to doctoral degrees. *Nursing Forum*, 5(2), 57-67.

Peplau, H.E. (1967). Interpersonal relations and the work of the industrial nurse. *Industrial Nurse Journal*, 15(10), 7-12.

Peplau, H.E. (1968). Psychotherapeutic strategies. *Perspectives in Psychiatric Care*, 6(6), 264-289.

Peplau, H.E. (1969). Professional closeness as a special kind of involvement with a patient, client, or family group. *Nursing Forum*, 8(4), 342-360.

Peplau, H.E. (1969). The American Nurses' Association and nursing education. *Utah Nurse*, 20(3), 6.

Peplau, H.E. (1970). ANA's new executive director states her views. *American Journal of Nursing*, 70, 84-88.

Peplau, H.E. (1970). ANA: Who needs it? *Nursing News*, 43, 5-8.

Peplau, H.E. (1970). Changed patterns of practice. *Washington State Journal of Nursing*, 42, 4-6.

Peplau, H.E. (1970). Keynote address at the 68th annual convention of the New Jersey State Nurses' Association. *New Jersey Nurse*, 26, 3-10.

Peplau, H.E. (1970). What it means to be a professional nurse today. *Alabama Nurse*, 24, 8-17.

Peplau, H.E. (1970, Summer). Professional closeness as a special kind of involvement with a patient, client or family group. *Comprehensive Nurse Quarterly*, 5(3), 66-81.

Peplau, H.E. (1970, Dec.). The road ahead. *Maine Nurse*, 1(3), 3-8.

Peplau, H.E. (1971). ANA: Who needs it? 2. *Nursing News*, 44(1), 12-14.

Peplau, H.E. (1971). Communication in crisis intervention. *Psychiatric Forum*, 2, 1-7.

Peplau, H.E. (1971). Dilemmas of organizing nurses. *Image: Journal of Nursing Scholarship*, 4, 4-8.

Peplau, H.E. (1971). In support of nursing research. *Journal of the New York State Nurses' Association*, 2, 5.

Peplau, H.E. (1971). Responsibility, authority, evaluation, and accountability of nursing in patient care. *Michigan Nurse*, 44, 5-7.

Peplau, H.E. (1971). The now nurse in nursing: Some problems of diversity. *Oklahoma Nurse*, 46, 1.

Peplau, H.E. (1971). The task ahead. *American Journal of Nursing*, 71, 1800-1802.

Peplau, H.E. (1971). What it means to be a professional nurse in today's society. *Kansas Nurse*, 46, 1-3.

Peplau, H.E. (1971). Where do we go from here? *Pelican News*, 27, 14-16.

Peplau, H.E. (1972). Some issues and developments that should be of concern to nurses. *New Jersey State Nurses' Association News*, 2, 14-16.

Peplau, H.E. (1972). The independence of nursing. *Imprint*, 9, 11.

Peplau, H.E. (1972). The nurse's role in health care delivery systems. *Pelican News*, 28, 12-14.

Peplau, H.E. (1972). The president challenges nurses in address to delegates. *Kansas Nurse*, pp. 2-4.

Peplau, H.E. (1973). Meeting the challenge. *Mississippi RN*, 35, 1-6.

Peplau, H.E. (1974). Creativity and commitment in nursing. *Image: Journal of Nursing Scholarship*, 6, 3-5.

Peplau, H.E. (1974). Is health care a right? Affirmative response. *Image: Journal of Nursing Scholarship*, 7, 4-10.

Peplau, H.E. (1974). Nurses: Collaborate or isolate. *Pennsylvania Nurse*, 29, 2-5.

Peplau, H.E. (1974). Talking with patients. *Comprehensive Nursing Quarterly*, 9(3), 30-39.

Peplau, H.E. (1975). An open letter to a new graduate. *Nursing Digest*, 3, 36-37.

Peplau, H.E. (1975). Midlife crisis. *American Journal of Nursing*, 75, 1761-1765.

Peplau, H.E. (1977). The changing view of nursing. *International Nursing Review*, 24, 43-45.

Peplau, H.E. (1978). Psychiatric nursing: Role of nurses and psychiatric nurses. *International Nursing Review,* 25, 41-47.

Peplau, H.E. (1980). New statement defines scope of practice. *American Nurse,* 12(4), 1, 8, 24.

Peplau, H.E. (1980). The psychiatric nurses: Accountable? to whom? for what? *Perspectives in Psychiatric Care,* 18, 128-134.

Peplau, H.E. (1982). Some reflections on earlier days in psychiatric nursing. *Journal of Psychosocial Nursing Mental Health Services,* 20, 17-24.

Peplau, H.E. (1984). Internal versus external regulation. *New Jersey Nurse,* 14, 12-14.

Peplau, H.E. (1985). Is nursing self-regulatory power being eroded? *American Journal of Nursing,* 85(2), 140-143.

Peplau, H.E. (1986). The nurse counselor. *Journal of American College Health,* 35(11), 11-14.

Peplau, H.E. (1987). American Nurses Association social policy statement: Part I. *Archives of Psychiatric Nursing,* 1(5), 301-307.

Peplau, H.E. (1987). Interpersonal constructs for nursing practice. *Nurse Education Today,* 7 (5), 201-208.

Peplau, H.E. (1987). Is nursing's self-regulatory power being eroded? *Journal of the New York State Nurses Association,* 18(1), 13-17.

Peplau, H.E. (1987). Psychiatric skills: Tomorrow's world. *Nursing Times,* 83(1), 29-32.

Peplau, H.E. (1988). Peplau responds. *Pacesetter Newsletter of the American Nurses Association Council on Psychiatric and Mental Health Nursing,* 15(1), 1-4.

Peplau, H.E. (1988). The art and science of nursing: Similarities, differences, and relations. *Nursing Science Quarterly,* 1(1), 8-15.

Peplau, H.E. (1989). Future direction in psychiatric nursing from the perspective of history. *Journal of Psychosocial Nursing,* 27(2), 18-28.

Peplau, H.E. (1992). Interpersonal relations: A theoretical framework for application in nursing practice. *Nursing Science Quarterly,* 5(1), 13-18.

Peplau, H.E. (1994). Psychiatric mental health nursing. Challenge and change. *Journal of Psychiatric and Mental Health Nursing,* 1(1), 3-7.

Peplau, H.E. (1994). Quality of life: Remembrance of a life: Dr. Catherine M. Norris. *Journal of the American Psychiatric Nurses Association,* 1(1), 36.

Peplau, H.E. (1995). Encounters along a career line. *Journal of the American Psychiatric Nurses Association,* 1(6), 1.

Peplau, H.E. (1995). Encounters along a career line . . . people's perceptions change. *Journal of the American Nurses Association,* 1(2), 38.

Peplau, H.E. (1995). Hildegard Peplau in a conversation with Mark Welch. Part I. *Nursing Inquiry,* 2(1), 53-56.

Peplau, H.E. (1995). Hildegard Peplau in a conversation with Mark Welch. Part II. *Nursing Inquiry,* 2(2), 115-116.

Peplau, H.E. (1995). Some unresolved issues in era of biopsychosocial nursing. *Journal of the American Psychiatric Nurses Association,* 1(3), 92-96.

Peplau, H.E. (1995). Transitions in psychosocial nursing. Catherine M. Norris leaves a legacy of excellence in scholarship for psychiatric nurses. *Journal of Psychosocial Nursing and Mental Health Services,* 32(2), 40.

Peplau, H.E. (1996). Commentary. *Archives of Psychiatry Nursing,* 10(1), 14-15.

Peplau, H.E. (1996). Fundamental and special—the dilemma of psychiatric mental health nursing—commentary. *Archives of Psychiatric Nursing,* 10(1), 14-15.

Peplau, H.E. (1997). Peplau's theory of interpersonal relations. *Nursing Science Quarterly,* 10(4), 162-167.

Peplau, H.E. (1997). Some unresolved issues in the era of biopsychosocial nursing. *Journal of the American Psychiatric Nurses Association,* 1, 92-96.

Peplau, H.E., Holzberg, J.D., Williams, T.G., Schwartz, M.S., & Padula, H. (Panel). (1960). Problems on the team treatment of adults in state mental hospitals. *American Journal of Orthopsychiatry,* 30, 87-112.

Peplau, H.E. & Lego, S. (1994). The "Bridges of Madison County" has been on the best-seller list for more than 1 year. From a psychosocial perspective, what is the appeal of this popular book? *Journal of Psychosocial Nursing and Mental Health Services,* 32(6), 57-58.

Peplau, H.E., Merlz, H., Mereuess, D., Mellow, J., & Dumes, R. (Chairman). (1968). Discussion: Panel members. *Perspectives in Psychiatric Care,* 6(6), 271-289.

Peplau, H.E. & Reinkemeyer, A.G. (1976). What future for nursing? *AORN,* 24, 217-235.

Interviews

Peplau, H.E. (1975). Interview with Dr. Peplau: Future of nursing. *Japanese Journal of Nursing,* 39(10), 1046-1050.

Peplau, H.E. (1985, May). Help the public maintain mental health [Interview]. *Nursing Success Today,* 2(5), 30-34.

Peplau, H.E. (1985, Aug.). The power of the dissociative state [Interview]. *Journal of Psychosocial Nursing,* 23(8), 31-33.

Peplau, H.E. (1990). ANA honors Peplau with new award [Interview]. *American Nurse,* 22(6), 20.

Peplau, H.E. (1993). Nursing pioneers: The Peplau legacy (Interview by Phil Barker). *Nursing Times,* 89(11), 48-51.

Pamphlets, Proceedings, and Reports

Peplau, H.E. (1951). *Understanding ourselves. Fifty-seventh annual report.* New York: National League for Nursing Education.

Peplau, H.E. (1952). *The responsibility of professional nursing in psychiatry. Fifty-eighth annual report.* New York: National League for Nursing Education.

Peplau, H.E. (1954). *Some problems of the psychiatric nursing team.* Second Annual Psychiatric Institute, New Jersey Neuropsychiatric Institute.

Peplau, H.E. (1956). *Discussion. The League Exchange No. 18: Psychology and psychiatric nursing research* (pp. 20-22). New York: National League for Nursing Education.

Peplau, H.E. (1956). *The yearbook of modern nursing.* New York: G.P. Putnam's Sons.

Peplau, H.E. (1958). *Current concepts of psychiatric nursing care.* ANA Proceedings.

Peplau, H.E. (1958). *Educating the nurse to function in psychiatric services* (pp. 37-42). Nursing Personnel for Mental Health Programs, Southern Regional Educational Board, Atlanta.

Peplau, H.E. (1960). A personal responsibility: A discussion of anxiety in mental health. *Rutgers Alumni Monthly,* 14-16.

Peplau, H.E. (1960). Ward atmosphere: Cliche or task. In *Nursing papers.* Illinois State Psychiatric Institute.

Peplau, H.E. (1962). *Will automation change the nurse, nursing, or both? Technical innovations in health care: Nursing implications.* (Pamphlet 5). New York: American Nurses Association.

Peplau, H.E. (1963). A personal challenge for immediate action. In AHA Conference Group, *Psychiatric nursing practice.* National Institute Proceedings, Kansas City.

Peplau, H.E. (1963). *An approach to research in psychiatric nursing. Training for clinical research in psychiatric-mental health nursing* (pp. 5-44). Washington, DC: The Catholic University of America.

Peplau, H.E. (1963). Leadership responsibility in toleration of stress: The leader's role in helping staff to tolerate stress. In *Conferences on preparation for leadership in psychiatric nursing service.* Department of Nursing Education, Teachers College, Columbia University, New York.

Peplau, H.E. (1964). Professional and social behavior: Some differences worth the notice of professional nurses. *Quarterly Magazine,* 50(4), 23-33. (Published by the Columbia University-Presbyterian Hospital School of Nursing Alumni Association, New York.)

Peplau, H.E. (1966). An interpretation of the ANA position. *New Jersey State Nurses Association-News Letter,* 22(2), 6-10.

Peplau, H.E. (1966). Trends in nursing and nursing education. *New Jersey State Nurses Association-News Letter,* 22(3), 17-27.

Peplau, H.E. (1967). The work of psychiatric nurses. *Psychiatric Opinion,* 4(1), 5-11.

Peplau, H.E. (1969). *Theory: The professional dimension.* Presented at the Nursing Theory Conference, University of Kansas Medical Center, Kansas City.

Peplau, H.E. (1971). Time of decision. *Nevada Nurses' Association Quarterly Newsletter,* pp. 1-3.

Peplau, H.E. (1974). ANA and the professional nurse. *National League for Nursing Publications,* 23-1539, 26-28.

Peplau, H.E. (1974). *Associate degree education for nursing: Current issues, 1974. ANA and the professional nurse.* Pub. No. 23-1539. National League for Nursing, Department of Associate Degree Programs.

Peplau, H.E. (1986). Credentialing in nursing: Contemporary developments and trends. Internal vs. external regulation. *American Nurses Association Publications,* G-172B, 10.

Peplau, H.E. (1992). Notes on Nightingale. In F. Nightingale, *Notes on nursing: What it is, and what it is not.* Philadelphia: J.B. Lippincott.

Peplau, H.E. (1995). *Another look at schizophrenia from a nursing standpoint. Psychiatric Nursing 1946 to 1994: A report on the state of the art.* St. Louis: Mosby.

Peplau, H.E. (1995). *Preface: Psychiatric nursing 1946 to 1974: A report on the state of the art. Psychiatric nursing 1946 to 1994: A report on the state of the art.* St. Louis: Mosby.

Peplau, H.E. & Smoyak, S. (1968). *Pattern perpetuation and intellectual competencies in schizophrenia.* Paper presented at Conference on Schizophrenia: Current concepts and research. Waldorf Astoria, New York.

Videotape

The nurse theorist: Portraits of excellence: Hildegard Peplau [Videotape]. (1988). Oakland, CA: Studio III. Available: Fuld Video Project, Studio III, 370 Hawthorne Avenue, Oakland, CA 94609.

Thesis

Peplau, H.E. (1953). *An exploration of some process elements which restrict or facilitate instructor-student interaction in a classroom, Type B.* Doctoral Project, Teachers College, Columbia University, New York.

Forewords

Peplau, H.E. (1963). Foreword. In S. Armstrong & S. Rouslin, *Group psychotherapy in nursing practice.* New York: Macmillan.

Peplau, H.E. (1963). Foreword. In S.F. Burd & M.A. Marshall (Eds.), *Some clinical approaches to psychiatric nursing.* New York: Macmillan.

Peplau, H.E. (1987). Foreword. In P. Martin, *Psychiatric nursing: A therapeutic approach.* London: Macmillan Education Ltd.

Editorial Statements, Letters, Reactions

[Letter to Editor]. (1962). *American Journal of Nursing,* 62(3), 16, 25, 26.

Peplau, H.E. (1963.). Nursing has lost its way [Letter to Editor]. *Journal RN,* 25(9), 103-105.

Peplau, H.E. (1963). On semantics [Letter to Editor]. *Perspectives in Psychiatric Care,* 1, 10-11.

Reviews

Peplau, H.E. (1955). [Review of the book *The psychiatric interview*]. *American Journal of Nursing,* 55(5), 614.

Peplau, H.E. (1957). [Review of the book *Beyond laughter*]. *American Journal of Nursing,* 57(10), 1349-1450.

Peplau, H.E. (1957). [Review of the book *The foundation of human behavior*]. *Mental Hygiene,* 41(2), 285-286.

Peplau, H.E. (1963). [Review of the book *The management of the anxious patient*]. *Perspectives in Psychiatric Care,* 2(1) [1964]: 46-47.

Peplau, H.E. (1964). [Review of the book *Attitudes of nursing students toward direct patient care*]. *Journal of Nursing Research,* 13(4), 348-349.

Peplau, H.E. (1964). [Review of the book *More for the mind: A study of psychiatric services in Canada*]. *Perspectives in Psychiatric Care,* 11(3), 39-42.

Williams, C. (1989). Perspective on the hallucinatory process [Book Review]. *Issues in Mental Health Nursing,* 10 (2), 99-119.

Correspondence

Peplau, H.E. (1992, June). Personal correspondence.

Peplau, H.E. (1996, July). Personal correspondence.

Secondary Sources
Books

Chinn, P.L. & Jacobs, M.K. (1983). *Theory and nursing: A systematic approach.* St. Louis: Mosby.

Field, W.E., Jr. (Ed.). (1979). *The psychotherapy of Hildegard E. Peplau.* New Brunfels, TX: PSF Publications.

Field, W. & Ruelke, W. (1973). *The psychotherapy of Hildegard Peplau.* New Brunfels, TX: PSF Publications.

Fitzpatrick, J.J. & Whall, A.L. (1983). *Conceptual models of nursing: Analysis and application.* Bowie, MD: Robert J. Brady.

Miller, N.E. & Dollard, J. (1941). *Social learning and imitation.* New Haven, CT: Yale University Press.

Nursing Theories Conference Group & J.B. George (Chairperson). (1980). *Nursing theories: The base for professional nursing practice.* Englewood Cliffs, NJ: Prentice-Hall.

Orlando, I. (1961). The dynamic nurse-patient relationship. Cited by S.A. Smoyak & S. Rouslin (Eds.). (1982). *A collection of classics in psychiatric nursing literature.* Thorofare, NJ: Slack Inc.

O'Toole, A. & Welt, S. (1989). *Interpersonal theory in nursing practice: Selected works of Hildegard E. Peplau.* New York: Springer.

Book Chapters

Belcher, J.R. & Fish, L.J. (1980). Hildegard E. Peplau. In Nursing Theories Conference Group & J.B. George (Chairperson), *Nursing theories: The base for professional practice.* Englewood Cliffs, NJ: Prentice-Hall.

Burd, S.F. (1963). The development of an operational definition using the process of learning as a guide. In S.F. Burd & A. Marshall, *Some clinical approaches to psychiatric nursing.* New York: Macmillan.

Burton, G. (1958). Personal, impersonal, and interpersonal relations. Cited by S.A. Smoyak & S. Rouslin (Eds.). (1982). *A collection of classics in psychiatric nursing literature.* Thorofare, NJ: Slack Inc.

Journal Articles

Aggleton, P. & Chalmers, H. (1990). Peplau's development model. Part 4. *Nursing Times,* 86(2), 38-40.

American Nurses Association new executive director states her views. (1970). *American Journal of Nursing,* 70(1), 84-88.

Anonymous. (1985). Help the public maintain mental health: Hildegard Peplau, EdD, RN, *Nursing Success Today,* 2(5), 30-34.

Anonymous. (1985). The power of the dissociative state . . . first hand experience with empathic transmission of anxiety . . . Hildegard Peplau. *Journal of Psychosocial Nursing and Mental Health Services,* 23(8), 31-33.

Anonymous. (1986). Hildegard Peplau: Grande dame of psychiatric nursing . . . 70 plus and going strong. *Geriatric Nursing—American Journal of Care for the Aging,* 7(6), 328-330.

Anonymous. (1996). News in mental health nursing. *Journal of Psychosocial Nursing and Mental Health Services,* 34(9), 7.

Armstrong, M. & Kelly, A. (1993). Enhancing staff nurses' interpersonal skills: Theory to practice. *Clinical Nurse Specialist,* 7(6), 313-317.

Armstrong, M. & Kelly, A. (1995). More than the sum of their parts: Martha Rogers and Hildegard Peplau. *Archives of Psychiatric Nursing,* 9(1), 40-44.

Barker, P. (1993). The Peplau legacy . . . Hildegard Peplau. *Nursing Times,* 89(11), 48-51.

Barker, P., Reynolds, W., & Stevenson, C. (1997). The human science basis of psychiatric nursing theory and practice. *Journal of Advanced Nursing,* 25, 660-667.

Barron, C., Foxall, M., Von Dollen, K., Shull, K., & Jones, P. (1992). Loneliness in low-vision older women. *Issues in Mental Health Nursing,* 13(4), 387-401.

Beeber, L. (1989). Enacting corrective interpersonal experiences with the depressed client: An intervention model. *Archives of Psychiatric Nursing,* 3(4), 211-217.

Beeber, L. (1996). Pattern integration in young depressed women. 1. *Archives of Psychiatric Nursing,* 10(3), 151-156.

Beeber, L. (1998). Treating depression through the therapeutic nurse-client relationship. *Nursing Clinics of North America, 33*(1), 153-157.

Beeber, L. (2000). Hildahood: Taking the interpersonal theory of nursing to the neighborhood. *Journal of American Psychiatric Nurses Association, 6*(2), 49-55.

Beeber, L., Anderson, C., & Sills, G. (1990). Peplau's theory in practice. *Nursing Science Quarterly, 3*(1), 6-8.

Beeber, L. & Bourbonniere, M. (1998). The concept of interpersonal pattern in Peplau's theory of nursing. *Journal of Psychiatric and Mental Health Nursing, 5*, 187-192.

Beeber, L. & Caldwell, C. (1996). Pattern integrations in young depressed women: Part II. *Archives of Psychiatric Nursing, 10*(3), 157-164.

Buswell, C. (1997). A model approach to care of a patient with alcohol problems . . . Peplau's model. *Nursing Times, 93*(3), 34-35.

Chan, L., Forchuk, C., Jewell, J., Martin, M., Overby, B., Sircell, M., Schofield, R., Valledor, T. & Woodcox, V. (1998). Bridging the discharge process. *The Canadian Nurse, 94*(3), 22-26.

Comley, A. (1994). A comparative analysis of Orem's self-care model and Peplau's interpersonal theory. *Journal of Advanced Nursing, 20*(4), 755-760.

Dennis, S. (1996). Implementing a nursing model for ward-based students. *Nursing Standard, 11*(11), 33-35.

Doncliff, B. (1994). Putting Peplau to work. *Nursing New Zealand, 2*(1), 20-22.

Feely, M. (1997). Using Peplau's theory in nurse-client relations. *International Nursing Review, 44*(4), 115-120.

Forchuk, C. (1991). A comparison of the works of Peplau and Orlando. *Archives of Psychiatric Nursing, 5*(1), 38-45.

Forchuk, C. (1991). Conceptualizing the environment of the individual with a chronic mental illness. *Issues in Mental Health Nursing, 12*, 159-170.

Forchuk, C. (1991). Peplau's theory: Concepts and their relations. *Nursing Science Quarterly, 4*(2), 54-60.

Forchuk, C. (1992). The orientation phase of the nurse-client relationship: How long does it take? *Perspectives in Psychiatric Care, 28*(4), 7-10.

Forchuk, C. (1994). Preconceptions in the nurse-client relationship. *Journal of Psychiatric and Mental Health Nursing, 1*(3), 145-149.

Forchuk, C. (1994). The orientation phase of the nurse-client relationship: Testing Peplau's theory. *Journal of Advanced Nursing, 20*(3), 532-537.

Forchuk, C. (1995). Development of nurse-client relationships: What helps? *Journal of the American Psychiatric Nurses Association, 1*, 146-153.

Forchuk, C., Beaton, S., Crawford, I., Voorberg, N., & Bethune, J. (1989). Incorporating Peplau's theory and case management. *Journal of Psychosocial Nursing, 27*(2), 35-38.

Forchuk, C. & Brown, B. (1989). Establishing a nurse-client relationship. *Journal of Psychosocial Nursing, 27*(2), 30-34.

Forchuk, C. & Dorsay, J. (1995). Hildegard Peplau meets family systems nursing: Innovation in theory-based practice. *Journal of Advanced Nursing, 21*(1), 110-115.

Forchuk, C. & Dorsay, J. (1998). Guest editorial—Interpersonal theory of nursing practice: The Peplau legacy. *Journal of Psychiatric and Mental Health Nursing, 5*, 165-166.

Forchuk, C., Jewell, J., Sircell, M., Schofield, R., Valledor, T., & Woodcox, V. (1997). Evaluation of Bridging Institution and Housing: A joint consumer-care provider initiative. *Journal of Psychosocial Nursing, 35*(10), 9-14.

Forchuk, C. & Voorberg, N. (1991). Evaluation of a community mental health program. *Canadian Journal of Nursing Administration, 4*(2), 16-20.

Forchuk, C., Westwell, J., Martin, M., Azzapardi, W., Kosterewa-Tolman, D., & Hux, M. (1998). Factors influencing movement of chronic psychiatric patients from the orientation to the working phase of the nurse-client relationship. *Perspectives in Psychiatric Care: The Journal for Psychotherapists, 34*(1), 36-44.

Fowler, J. (1994). A welcome focus on a key relationship: Using Peplau's model in palliative care. *Professional Nurse, 10*(3), 194-197.

Fowler, J. (1995). Taking theory into practice: Using Peplau's model in the care of patients. *Professional Nurse, 10*(4), 226-230.

Garrett, A., Manuel, D., & Vincent, C. (1976). Stressful experiences identified by student nurses. *Journal of Nursing Education, 15*(6), 9-21.

Gastmans, C. (1998). Interpersonal relations in nursing: A philosophical-ethical analysis of the work of Hildegard Peplau. *Journal of Advanced Nursing, 28*(6), 1312-1319.

Gregg, D.E. (1978). Hildegard E. Peplau: Her contributions. *Perspective Psychiatric Care, 16*(3), 118-121.

Hall, K. (1994). Peplau's model of nursing: Caring for a man with AIDS. *British Journal of Nursing, 3*(8), 418-422.

Hays, D. (1961). Teaching a concept of anxiety. *Nursing Research, 10*(2), 108-113.

Hays, R. & DiMatteo, M. (1987). A short-form measure of loneliness. *Journal of Personality Assessment, 51*(1), 69-81.

Henderson, D. (1994). Commentary on recovering in depressed women: Research with Peplau's theory. *Association of Women's Health Obstetrical and Neonatal Nurse Women's Health Nursing Scan, 8*(2), 19-20.

Hofling, C.K. & Leininger, M.M. (1960). Basic psychiatric concepts in nursing. Cited by S.A. Smoyak & S. Rouslin (Eds.). (1982). *A collection of classics in psychiatric nursing literature.* Thorofare, NJ: Slack Inc.

Huch, M., (1995). Nursing and the next millennium. *Nursing Science Quarterly, 8*(1), 38-44.

Iveson, J. (1982). A two-way process . . . theories in nursing practice . . . Peplau's nursing model. *Nursing Mirror, 155*(18), 52.

Jewell, J. & Sullivan, E. (1996). Application of nursing theories in health education. *Journal of the American Psychiatric Nurses Association, 2,* 79-85.

Jones, A. (1995). Utilizing Peplau's psychodynamic theory for stroke patient care. *Journal of Clinical Nursing, 4*(1), 49-54.

Jones, A. (1996). Education and debate: The value of Peplau's theory for mental health nursing. *British Journal of Nursing, 5*(14), 877-881.

Kabiri, W. (1988). Peplau—A legend in her own time. *Southern California Nursing News, 1*(4).

Keda, A. (1970). From Henderson to Orlando to Wiedenback: Thoughts on completion of translation of basic principles of clinical nursing. *Comprehensive Nursing Quarterly, 5*(1), 85-94.

Kelley, S. (1996). "It's just me, my family, my treatments, and my nurse . . . oh yeah, and Nintendo." Hildegard Peplau's day with kids with cancer. *Journal of the American Psychiatric Nurses Association, 2*(1), 11-14.

LaMonica, E. (1981). Construct validity of an empathy instrument. *Research in Nursing and Health, 4,* 389-400.

Lego, S. (1980). The one-to-one nurse-patient relationship. *Perspectives in Psychiatric Care, 18*(2), 67-89. (Reprinted from *Psychiatric nursing 1946-1974: A report on the state of the art,* American Journal of Nursing Co.)

Lego, S. (1998). The application of Peplau's theory to group psychotherapy. *Journal of Psychiatric and Mental Health Nursing, 5,* 193-196.

Lund, V. & Frank, D. (1991). Helping the medicine go down: Nurse's and patients' perceptions about medication compliance. *Journal of Psychosocial Nursing, 29*(7), 7-9.

Marshall, J. (1963). Dr. Peplau's strong medicine for psychiatric nurses. *Smith, Kline & French Reporter, 7,* 11-14.

Martin, M., Forchuk, C., Scantopinto, M., & Butcher, H. (1992). Alternative approaches to nursing practice: Application of Peplau, Rogers, and Parse. *Nursing Science Quarterly, 5*(2), 80-85.

McCarter, P. (1980). New statement defines scope of practice discussion with Dr. Lane and Dr. Peplau. *American Nurse, 12*(4), 1, 8, 24.

Methven, D. & Schlotfeldt, R.M. (1962). The social interaction inventory. *Nursing Research, 11*(2), 83-88.

Morrison, E., Shealy, A., Kowalski, C., Lamont, J., & Range, B. (1996). Workroles of staff nurses in psychiatric settings. *Nurse Science Quarterly, 9*(1), 17-21.

Osborne, O. (1984). Intellectual traditions in psychiatric nursing. *Journal of Psychosocial Nursing, 22*(1), 27-32.

Peden, A. (1993). Recovering in depressed women: Research with Peplau's theory. *Nursing Science Quarterly, 6*(3), 140-146.

Peden, A. (2000). Negative thoughts of women with depression. *Journal of American Psychiatric Nurses Association. 6*(2), 41-48.

Peplau, H. (1968). Current concepts in psychiatric care: The implications for psychiatric nursing practice. Proceedings of the Institute on Psychiatric Nursing, cosponsored by Yale School of Nursing, Department of Psychiatric Nursing and the Community Mental Health Center Department of Nursing. In *Perspectives of Psychiatric Care, 6*(6), 271-289.

Perry, G. (1990). Loneliness and coping among tertiary-level adult cancer patients in the home. *Cancer Nursing, 13*(5), 293-302.

Price, B. (1998). Explorations in body image: Peplau and practice knowledge. *Journal of Psychiatric and Mental Health Nursing, 5,* 179-186.

Reed, P. (1996). Transforming practice knowledge into nursing knowledge—a revisionist analysis of Peplau. *Image: Journal of Nursing Scholarship, 28*(1), 29-33.

Reynolds, W. (1998). Peplau's theory in practice. *Nursing Science Quarterly, 10,* 168-170.

Ribeiro, V. (1989). The forgotten generation: Elderly women and loneliness. *Recent Advance in Nursing, 25,* 20-40.

Runtz, S. & Urtel, J. (1983). Evaluating your practice via a nursing model . . . the Orem self-care model and the Peplau interpersonal process model. *Nurse Practitioner: American Journal of Primary Health Care, 8*(3), 30, 32, 37-40.

Samhammer Hays, J. & Myers, J.B. (1964). Learning in the nurse-patient relationship. *Perspective in Psychiatric Care, 2*(3), 2-29.

Schroder, P. (1979). Nursing intervention with patients with thought disorders. *Perspective in Psychiatric Care, 17*(1), 32-39.

Sills, G.M. (1977). Research in the field of psychiatric nursing 1952-1977. *Nursing Research, 28*(3), 201-207.

Sills, G.M. (1978). Hildegard E. Peplau: Leader, practitioner, academician, scholar, and theorist. *Perspectives in Psychiatric Care, 16*(3), 122-128.

Smith, M. (1988). Perspective on nursing science. *Nursing Science Quarterly, 1*(2), 80-85.

Smoyak, S. (1990). Interview with Hildegard E. Peplau. *New Jersey, 20*(5), 10-11.

Smoyak, S. (1992). Conventions as prevention. *Journal of Psychosocial Nursing, 30*(12), 3-4.

Smoyak, S. (1994). Hildegard E. Peplau awarded honorary doctorate. *Journal of Psychosocial Nursing and Mental Health Services, 32*(11), 45-46.

Smoyak, S.A. & Rouslin, S. (Eds.). (1982). Introduction. In S.A. Smoyak & S. Rouslin (Eds.), *A collection of classics in psychiatric nursing literature.* Thorofare, NJ: Slack Inc.

Spring, F.E. & Turk, H. (1962). A therapeutic behavior scale. *Nursing Research, 11*(4), 214-218.

Takahashi, T. (1992). Perspectives on nursing knowledge. *Nursing Science Quarterly, 5*(2), 86-91.

Thelander, B. (1997). The psychotherapy of Hildegard Peplau in the treatment of people with serious mental illness. *Perspectives in Psychiatric Care, 33*(3), 24-33.

Thomas, M.D., Baker, J.M., & Estes, N.J. (1970). Anger: A tool for developing self-awareness. *American Journal of Nursing, 70*(12), 2586-2590.

Thompson, L. (1986). Peplau's Theory: An application to short-term individual therapy. *Journal of Psychosocial Nursing, 24*(8), 26-31.

Topf, M. & Dambacher, B. (1979). Predominant source of interpersonal influence in relationships between psychiatric patients and nursing staff. *Research in Nursing and Health, 2*(1), 35-43.

Vardy, C. & Price, V. (1998). The utilization of Peplau's theory of nursing in working with a male survivor of sexual abuse. *Journal of Psychiatric and Mental Health Nursing, 5,* 149-155.

Welt, S. & O'Toole, A. (1989) Hildegard E. Peplau: Observation in brief. *Archives of Psychiatric Nursing, 3*(5), 254-264.

Yamashita, M. (1997). Family caregiving: Application of Newman's and Peplau's theories. *Journal of Psychiatric and Mental Health Nursing, 4,* 401-405.

Other Sources

Andreoli, R.G. & Thompson, C.E. (1977). The nature of science in nursing. *Image, 9*(2), 32-37.

Arnold, W. & Nieswiadomy, R. (1993). Peplau's theory with an emphasis on anxiety. In S.M. Ziegler (Ed.), *Theory-directed nursing practice.* New York: Springer.

Duffey, M. & Mullencamp, A.F. (1974). A framework for theory analysis. *Nursing Outlook, 22,* 570-574.

Forchuk, C. (1993). *Hildegard E. Peplau: Interpersonal nursing theory.* Newbury Park, CA: Sage.

Freud, S. (1936). The problem of anxiety. Cited by H.E. Peplau. (1952). *Interpersonal relations in nursing.* New York: G.P. Putnam's Sons.

Fromm, E. (1947). Man for himself. Cited by H.E. Peplau. (1952). *Interpersonal relations in nursing.* New York: G.P. Putnam's Sons.

Jacox, A. (1974). Theory construction in nursing: An overview. *Nursing Research, 23,* 4-12.

Johnson, D.E. (1959). The nature of a science of nursing. *Nursing Outlook, 7,* 272.

Maslow, A.H. (1943). A theory of human motivation. *Psychological Review, 50,* 370-396.

Maslow, A.H. & Mittleman, B. (1941). *Principles in abnormal psychology.* New York: Harper & Brothers.

Miller, N.E. & Dollard, J. (1941). *Social learning and imitation.* New Haven, CT: Yale University Press.

Mullahy, P. (1948). *Oedipus: Myth and complex.* New York: Hermitage House.

Pavlov, I. (1927). *Conditioned reflexes: An investigation of the physiological activity of the cerebral cortex.* London: Oxford University Press.

Phillips, J.R. (1977). Nursing systems and nursing models. *Image, 9*(1), 6.

Popper, K.R. (1963). *Conjectures and refutations: The growth of scientific knowledge.* New York: Basic Books.

Reynolds, P.D. (1971). *A primer in theory construction.* Indianapolis: Bobbs-Merrill.

Solomon, A.P. (1943). Rehabilitation of patients with psychologically protracted convalescence. *Archives of Physical Therapy, 24,* 270-273.

Sullivan, H.S. (1947). Concepts of modern psychiatry. Cited by H.E. Peplau. (1952). *Interpersonal relations in nursing.* New York: G.P. Putnam's Sons.

Sullivan, H.S. (1948). *The meaning of anxiety in psychiatry and in life.* Washington, DC: William Alanson White Psychiatric Foundation.

Symonds, P. (1946). *The dynamics of human adjustment.* New York: Appleton-Century-Crofts.

von Bertalanffy, L. (1968). *General systems theory: Foundations, development, applications.* New York: Braziller.

Wertheimer, M. (1945). *Productive thinking.* New York: Harper & Brothers.

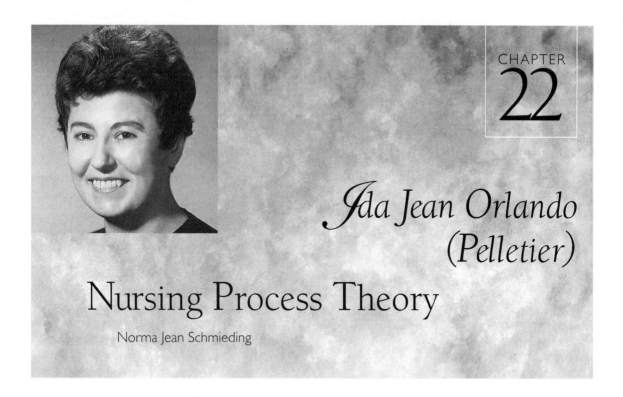

Ida Jean Orlando (Pelletier)

Nursing Process Theory

Norma Jean Schmieding

CREDENTIALS AND BACKGROUND OF THE THEORIST

Ida Jean Orlando was born August 12, 1926. In 1947, she received a diploma in nursing from New York Medical College, Flower Fifth Avenue Hospital School of Nursing, in New York. She received a B.S. in public health nursing from St. John's University in Brooklyn, New York in 1951 and an M.A. in mental health consultation from Columbia University Teachers College in 1954. While pursuing her education, Orlando worked intermittently, and sometimes concurrently, as a staff nurse in obstetrical, medical, surgical, and emergency nursing services. She also worked as a

Previous authors: Larry P. Schumacher, Susan Fisher, Ann Marriner Tomey, Deborah I. Mills, and Marcia K. Sauter.
The author expresses appreciation to Ida Jean Orlando (Pelletier) for her insightful contributions to this chapter. Orlando continually supports endeavors to extend the use of her theory and encouraged the author's interpretation of the theory. Patients, nurses, and the profession benefited from her theoretical contributions.

supervisor in a general hospital. In addition, as an assistant director of nursing, she was responsible for a general hospital's nursing service and for teaching several courses in the hospital's nursing school.

After receiving her master's degree in 1954, Orlando was employed for eight years at the Yale School of Nursing in New Haven, Connecticut. At Yale, she was a research associate and principal investigator of a federal project grant entitled "Integration of Mental Health Concepts in a Basic Curriculum" until 1958. The project focused on identifying factors influencing the integration of mental health principles in a basic nursing curriculum. Orlando conducted this project by observing and participating in student experiences with patients and medical, nursing, and instructional personnel throughout the students' basic curriculum. For three years, she recorded her observations and spent a fourth year analyzing the accumulated data. Orlando reported her findings in 1958 in her first book, *The Dynamic Nurse-Patient Relationship: Function, Process and Principles of*

399

Professional Nuring Practice.[50] Although written in 1958, this book was not published until 1961. Since then, there have been five foreign language editions of this book. The formulations in this publication provided the foundation for Orlando's nursing theory.[53] During the next four years (1958 to 1961) as an associate professor and then as director of the graduate program in mental health and psychiatric nursing, Orlando used her theory as the foundation of the program. She married Robert J. Pelletier and left Yale in 1961.

From 1962 through 1972, Orlando was Clinical Nursing Consultant at McLean Hospital in Belmont, Massachusetts. While at this position, she studied the interactions of nurses with patients, peers, and other staff members. She also studied how these interactions affected the processes that nurses used to help patients. Orlando convinced the hospital director that a training program for nurses was needed. As a result, the nursing service of McLean Hospital was reorganized and a training program based on her theory was implemented.[51] Orlando subsequently applied for and received federal funding to evaluate training in the nursing process discipline.

While at McLean Hospital, Orlando[55] published "The Patient's Predicament and Nursing Function" in a 1967 issue of *Psychiatric Opinion*. In 1972, she reported the 10 years of work at the hospital in her second book, *The Discipline and Teaching of Nursing Process: An Evaluative Study*.[51] This book has been printed, in full and in part, in Japanese and German.

From 1972 to 1981, Orlando lectured, served as a consultant, and conducted about 60 workshops about her theory throughout the United States and Canada. She served on the board of the Harvard Community Health Plan in Boston, Massachusetts from 1972 to 1984 and served on the hospital committee of the board from 1979 to 1985. Since then, she has served in various capacities, such as on the membership, program, and services committees. In 2001, the Massachusetts Nurse's Association will induct Orlando, and other outstanding nurses, into its newly established Hall of Fame.[46]

In 1981, Orlando accepted a position as Nurse Educator for Metropolitan State Hospital in Waltham, Massachusetts. From 1984 to 1987, she held various administrative nursing positions. In September 1987, Orlando[56] became the Assistant Director of Nursing for Education and Research at Metropolitan State Hospital. She retired from nursing in 1992.[57]

In 1990, the National League for Nursing (NLN) reprinted Orlando's 1961 publication.[53] In the preface to the NLN edition, Orlando[53:vii] states, "If I had been more courageous in 1961, when this book was first written, I would have proposed it as 'nursing process theory' instead of as a 'theory of effective nursing practice.'"

Orlando's nursing theory stresses the reciprocal relationship between patient and nurse. What the other says and does affects both nurse and patient. She was one of the first nursing leaders to identify and emphasize the elements of nursing process and the critical importance of the patient's participation in the nursing process. Orlando[34] viewed nursing as a distinct profession, separate from medicine. Orlando believed physicians' orders were for patients, not for nurses. However, the nurse helps the patient carry out the order or, if the patient is unable, the nurse does it for patient. Likewise, the nurse may help patients from adhering to physicians' orders if data supports it. The nurse would communicate the rationale for this to the physician.[55] Orlando may have facilitated the development of nurses as logical thinkers.[47] Orlando viewed nurses as determining nursing action rather than being prompted by physician's orders, organizational needs, and past personal experiences. Therefore nursing action is derived from the patient's immediate experience and immediate needs for help.

Orlando[56] states that her search for facts in observing nursing situations influenced her most before the development of her theory and that she derived her theory from the conceptualization of those facts. Her overall goal was to develop "a theory of effective nursing practice" that would identify a distinctive role for professional nurses that would provide "a foundation for systematic study of nursing."[50:viii]

Orlando made major contributions to nursing theory and practice. Her conceptualizations of the deliberative nursing process fulfill the criteria of a theory. In her theory, she: (1) presents interrelated concepts that represent a systematic view of nursing phenomena, (2) specifies relationships among the concepts, (3) explains what happens during the nursing process and why, (4) prescribes how nursing phenomena can be controlled, and (5) explains how the control leads to the prediction of outcome. Although nursing writers such as Fitzpatrick and Whall[23] note the debate about whether models are theory and conclude they are not, numerous other theorists such as Fawcett,[19] George,[25] and Walker and Avant[74] classify Orlando's theory at various levels of accepted theories. Despite these diverging views, Orlando's theory has considerable merit for its application to practice, research, education, and administration. Orlando's views[52] about nursing, nurses, and patients remain the same as when she developed her theory.

THEORETICAL SOURCES

Orlando does not acknowledge any theoretical sources for the development of her theory. None of her publications include a bibliography. However, Schmieding[66] traced similarities of her formulations to those of John Dewey and to some of the nurse colleagues and educators with whom Orlando was associated at Columbia.

USE OF EMPIRICAL EVIDENCE

Orlando was the first nurse to develop her theory from actual nurse-patient situations. Orlando recorded the content of 2000 nurse-patient contacts and constructed her theory based on the analysis of these data.[69] Orlando asserts that her theory was valid and she applied it in her work with patients and nurses and the teaching of students. She used a qualitative method to obtain data from which she developed her theory.[69] According to Meleis,[43:348] "Orlando used field methodology before it became a world view in research."

At McLean Hospital, Orlando implemented the nursing process theory that she had developed at Yale. During her last three years there, she received a research grant to do evaluative research of the training program to test her formulations. She published these results in her second book, *The Discipline and Teaching of Nursing Process: An Evaluative Study*.[51] In it, Orlando clearly and succinctly presents the components of her theory, describes a person's process of action, and specifies what types of action facilitate or hinder the nurse from finding out the patient's immediate need for help. Orlando's theory was used by several Yale faculty as a basis for discussing and developing a nursing practice theory.[33]

MAJOR CONCEPTS & DEFINITIONS

Orlando describes her model as revolving around five major interrelated concepts: (1) the function of professional nursing, (2) the presenting behavior of the patient, (3) the immediate or internal response of the nurse, (4) the nursing process discipline, and (5) improvement.[66]

NURSE'S RESPONSIBILITY

"Whatever help the patient may require for his needs to be met (i.e., for his physical and mental comfort to be assured as far as possible while he is undergoing some form of medical treatment or supervision)."[53:5] It is the nurse's responsibility to see that "the patient's needs for help are met, either directly by her own activity or indirectly by calling in the help of others."[50:29]

NEED

"Situationally defined as a requirement of the patient which, if supplied, relieves or diminishes his immediate distressor and improves his immediate sense of adequacy or well-being."[53:6]

Continued

MAJOR CONCEPTS *&* DEFINITIONS—cont'd

PRESENTING BEHAVIOR OF PATIENT

Any observable verbal or nonverbal behavior.[24]

IMMEDIATE REACTIONS

Include both the nurse and patient's individual perceptions, thoughts, and feelings.[24]

NURSING PROCESS DISCIPLINE

Includes the nurse communicating to the patient his or her own immediate reaction, clearly identifying that the item expressed belongs to the nurse, and then asking for validation or correction.[24] Nursing process discipline was called *deliberative nursing process* in Orlando's first book, *The Dynamic Nurse-Patient Relationship: Function, Process, and Principles of Professional Nuring Practice*,[50] and also called *nursing process* and *process discipline*.

IMPROVEMENT

"Means to grow better, to turn to profit, to use to advantage."[50:6]

PURPOSE OF NURSING

"Supply the help a patient requires in order for his needs to be met."[53:9]

AUTOMATIC NURSING ACTION

"Those (nursing actions) decided upon for reasons other than the patient's immediate need."[8:167]

DELIBERATIVE NURSING ACTION

Those actions decided upon after ascertaining a need and then meeting this need.[8]

MAJOR ASSUMPTIONS

Nearly all the assumptions in Orlando's theory are implicit. Meleis[42] thinks that one of the major problems with Orlando's assumptions is that it is not totally clear how they were derived because no documentation exists. However, Orlando, similar to other early theorists, did not specify assumptions. Various authors have extrapolated them. Schmieding[69] derived assumptions from Orlando's writings in four areas and elaborated on Orlando's view about each:

1. Assumptions about nursing:
   "Nursing is a distinct profession separate from other disciplines."[69:10]
   "Professional nursing has a distinct function and product (outcome)."[69:10]
   "There is a difference between lay and professional nursing."[69:11]
   "Nursing is aligned with medicine."[69:12]

2. Assumptions about patients:
   "Patients' needs for help are unique."[69:12]
   "Patients have an initial ability to communicate their needs for help."[69:12]

"When patients cannot meet their own needs they become distressed."[69:13]
"The patient's behavior is meaningful."[69:13]
"Patients are able and willing to communicate verbally (and non-verbally when unable to communicate verbally)."[69:13]

3. Assumptions about nurses:
   "The nurse's reaction to each patient is unique."[69:14]
   "Nurses should not add to the patient's distress."[69:14]
   "The nurse's mind is the major tool for helping patients."[69:14]
   "The nurse's use of automatic responses prevents the responsibility of nursing from being fulfilled."[69:15]
   "Nurse's practice is improved through self-reflection."[69:15]

4. Assumptions about the nurse-patient situation:
   "The nurse-patient situation is a dynamic whole."[69:15]
   "The phenomenon of the nurse-patient encounter represents a major source of nursing knowledge."[69:16]

The metaparadigm assumptions of Orlando's theory follow in the next section.

Nursing

Orlando's major assumption about nursing is that it should be a distinct profession that functions autonomously. Although nursing has been historically aligned with medicine and continues to have a close relationship with medicine, nursing and the practice of medicine are clearly separate professions.[50] These assumptions are reflected in Orlando's definition of the function of professional nursing.

Orlando[51:20] states that "the function of professional nursing is conceptualized as finding out and meeting the patient's immediate need for help." It is the nurse's responsibility to see that "the patient's needs for help are met, either directly by her own activity or indirectly by calling in the help of others."[50:22] This is more fully amplified by Orlando's approach[50:36] to nursing process discipline, which she proposes is composed of the following basic elements: "(1) the behavior of the patient, (2) the reaction of the nurse, and (3) the nursing actions, which are designed for the patient's benefit. The interaction of these elements with each other is nursing process."

Another assumption Orlando[51] makes is that nurses should help relieve physical or mental discomfort and should not add to the patient's distress. This assumption is evident in Orlando's concept of improvement in the patient's behavior as the intended outcome of nursing actions.

Orlando is concerned with providing direct assistance to individuals in whatever setting for the purpose of avoiding, relieving, diminishing, or curing the person's sense of helplessness.[24]

Person

Orlando assumes that persons behave verbally and nonverbally. Evidence of this assumption is found in Orlando's emphasis on behavior; namely, in observing changes in the patient's behavior. Orlando assumes that people are sometimes able to meet their own needs for help in some situations; however, they become distressed when they are unable to do so. This is the basis for Orlando's assertion[50] that professional nurses should be concerned only with those persons who are unable to meet their need for help independently. However, nurses observe and communicate with patients periodically to determine if there are new needs for help. She also states that each patient is unique and individual in his or her response; a professional nurse can recognize that the same behavior in different patients can signal quite different needs.[50]

Health

Orlando[50] does not define health, but she assumes that freedom from mental or physical discomfort and feelings of adequacy and well being cotribute to health. "Orlando implicitly assumed feelings of adequacy and well-being from fulfilled needs contribute to health."[36:4] Orlando[50:90] also notes that "repeated experiences of having been helped undoubtedly culminate over periods of time in greater degrees of improvement." Therefore these cumulative changes are fertile areas for further research.

Environment

Orlando does not define environment. She assumes that a nursing situation occurs when there is a nurse-patient contact and that both nurse and patient perceive, think, feel, and act in the immediate situation. However, she does point out that a patient may react with distress to any aspect of an environment that was designed for therapeutic and helpful purposes.[50] When the nurse observes any patient behavior, it needs to be viewed as a signal of distress. Any aspect of the environment, even though it is designed for therapeutic and helpful purposes, can cause the patient to become distressed.[50]

THEORETICAL ASSERTIONS

Orlando[50] views the professional function of nursing as finding out and meeting the patients' immediate needs for help. This function is fulfilled when the nurse finds out and meets a patient's immediate needs for help. Orlando's theory focuses on how to produce improvement in the patient's behavior. Evidence of relieving the patient's distress is determined by positive changes in the patient's observable behavior.

A person becomes a patient requiring nursing care when he or she has unmet needs for help that cannot be met independently because he or she has physical limitations, a negative reaction to an environment, or has an experience that prevents the patient from communicating his or her needs.[50] Orlando[50] asserts that these limitations on the patient's ability to meet his or her needs are most likely to occur while the patient is receiving medical care or supervision. The restrictions Orlando has frequently placed on the concept of patient can be viewed as a function of the impediments that people have in meeting their own needs.

Patients experience distress or feelings of helplessness as a result of unmet needs for help.[50] Orlando[50] believes there is a positive correlation between the length of time the patient experiences the unmet needs and the degree of distress. Therefore immediacy is emphasized throughout her theory. In Orlando's view,[50] when people are able to meet their own needs, they do not feel distress and do not require care from a professional nurse at that time. For a person who does have a need for help, it is crucial that the nurse obtain the patient's correction or verification of the nurse's perceptions, thoughts, and/or feelings to determine whether the patient is in need of help.[50]

Individuals in contact with each other go through an action process that involves the observation of the other's behavior, the resulting thought about this observation, a feeling originating from the person's thought, and an action chosen by each individual in response to the reaction.[51] When the nurse acts, an action process transpires. This action process by the nurse in a nurse-patient contact is called *nursing process*.[51] The nurse's action may be automatic or deliberative. Any patient behavior observed by the nurse must be viewed as a signal of distress because the patient may become distressed to any aspect of an environment that was designed for therapeutic and helpful purposes.[50] The nurse's perception of a pa-

tient's behavior produces thoughts that cause the nurse to experience a feeling. Orlando[50] identifies and defines the elements of this *immediate reaction* as: (1) perception, a physical stimulation of any one of a person's five senses; (2) the automatic thought about the perception that occurs in an individual's mind; and (3) a feeling stimulated by the thought that inclines a person toward or against a perception, thought, or feeling. The nurse's reaction then precipitates a nursing action.[50]

The nurse asking the patient about his or her perception of the patient's behavior rather than first exploring his or her own thoughts and feelings is more effective and less time consuming because the physical stimulus for perception has objective validity. Nursing actions that are not deliberative are automatic.[50] Automatic nursing actions are those having nothing to do with finding out and meeting the patient's needs for help. Deliberative nursing actions are those designed to identify and meet the patient's immediate need for help and to fulfill the professional nursing function. Deliberative nursing actions require that the nurse seek verification or correction of his or her thoughts and the origin of the feelings with the patient before the nurse and the patient can know what nursing action will meet the patient's need for help.[50]

In her second book, *The Discipline and Teaching of Nursing Process: An Evaluative Study*,[51] Orlando renamed deliberative nursing action a process discipline with three specific requirements. Application of the nursing *process discipline* qualifies as a *disciplined professional response*.[51] Despite this change in terminology, Orlando provides clear guidelines for nurses to find out and meet a patient's immediate needs for help. First, the nurse expresses to the patient any or all of the items contained in his or her reaction to the patient's behavior. Second, the nurse verbally states to the patient that the expressed item belongs to the nurse by use of the personal pronoun (an "I" message which indicates it is the nurse's perception). Finally, the nurse asks about the item expressed, attempting to verify or correct his or her perceptions, thoughts, or feelings.[67]

The value of the nursing process discipline is its accuracy in determining whether the patient experiences a distress and, if so, finding out what help is required to relieve the distress.[41] Without the investigation required by use of the nursing process discipline, the nurse does not have a reliable database for action.[51] When the nurse responds automatically, the perceptions, thoughts, and feelings of each person are not available to the other. When the nurse uses the nursing process discipline, the perceptions, thoughts, and feelings of the nurse are available to the patient and vice versa.[51] Orlando[50:67] views this latter type of response as a form of "continuous reflection as the nurse tries to understand the meaning to the patient of the behavior she observed and what he needs from her in order to be helped." The nurse evaluates his or her actions at the end of the contact by comparing the patient's verbal and nonverbal behavior with the patient's behavior that was present when the process started.[50]

LOGICAL FORM

Orlando's theory was developed inductively. She collected records of her observations of nurse-patient situations during a three-year period. After various attempts to categorize these data, Orlando recognized that they were either *good* or *bad* patient outcomes. Good outcomes were defined as those that improved the patient's behavior. Bad outcomes were defined as the absence of improvement. Orlando concluded that the nurse's use of the nursing process discipline was an effective means of achieving a good outcome. On this basis, Orlando formulated her nursing process theory from these qualitative data.[66]

If Walker and Avant's criteria[74] are used for theory analysis, Orlando's theory is logically adequate. Although inductive argument can produce false conclusions even when the premises are true, Orlando's conclusions are logically sound. The structure of relationships is clear and sufficiently precise; it is possible to represent the relationships schematically. The relationships progress from existence and conditional statement to prediction and control. The predictions Orlando makes are acceptable to the nursing profession because improvement in patient care is always considered valuable. There are no

logical fallacies within Orlando's theory because relationships are sufficiently developed.

ACCEPTANCE BY THE NURSING COMMUNITY

Henderson[31] accepted Orlando's theory early. Orlando's conclusions convinced her that "the most effective nursing involves a continuous analysis and validation of the nurse's interpretation of patient's needs."[31:65] Orlando's theory is readily applicable to nursing practice. Orlando's theory and the research by her students provided the foundation for behavioral and social practice in the late 1960s.[77] Likewise, Orlando's ideas were also evident in the writings of Dickoff and James.[9]

There is increasing evidence of its application in practice as indicated by the literature. Schmidt[64] reports using Orlando's theory as a basis for practice in 1972. Peitchinis[54] suggests that Orlando's nursing process discipline reflect the elements of the therapeutic relationship, which include expression of empathy, warmth, and genuineness. She proposes that nursing practice based on Orlando's theory would increase the therapeutic effectiveness of nursing.[54] Rosenthal[63] recommends Orlando's theory as the basis for perioperative nursing. She believes that because patients are in the operating room for a short duration of time, rapid accurate assessment is paramount. A case study illustrates application of the theory.

Individual nurses use Orlando's theory to guide their practice. Martha Brown, staff nurse, uses it with both English and nonEnglish speaking patients in the Public Health Department in Lincoln, Nebraska. Orlando[58] clarified how the nurse meets the requirements of the discipline process with non-English-speaking persons. Examples of Brown's work appear in Alligood and Marriner Tomey's second edition of *Nursing Theory: Utilization & Application*.[1] In the Boston area, Julie Felty,[21] a psychiatric nurse, uses Orlando's theory in private practice with patients who range in age from 17 to 96 and have various diagnoses. In 1993, Felty[21] and Susan Donaldson, MD, used Orlando's theory in establishing a 12-bed department of mental health unit in

Waltham, MA. The use of physical restraints were essentially eliminated.[21]

Orlando's theory was used successfully in psychiatric and general hospitals. Early examples of acceptance by the psychiatric nursing community includes the MidMissouri Mental Health Center and in a new psychiatric unit located within a general hospital in Antigonish, Nova Scotia.

More recently, Orlando's theory was used simultaneously in both practice and administration within the same setting. Schmieding[65] reports the advantages of adopting Orlando's theory throughout a nursing department. Implementation of Orlando's theory produced several benefits. Its use increased effectiveness in meeting patient needs; improved decision-making skills among staff nurses, particularly in determining what constituted nursing versus nonnursing functions; negotiated more effectively in resolving conflict among staff nurses and between staff and physicians; and influenced a more positive nursing identity and unity among staff.[65] Schmieding[67:435-436] discussed "how specific types of actions facilitate or thwart problem identification" and, using Orlando's theory, analyzed managerial responses in face-to-face contacts.

The New Hampshire Hospital Nursing Department also selected Orlando's theory for use in both nursing practice and nursing administration. Houle[35] describes the process of learning how to apply the theory in practice. Mimi Dye,[16] a student of Orlando's at Yale, serves as a consultant to the New Hampshire Hospital Orlando Project that involves educating people throughout the hospital. Additionally, as an advanced registered nurse practitioner, Dye[16] uses Orlando's theory with patients in her private practice.

The former Boston's Beth Israel Hospital Division of Nursing Statement of Philosophy and Purpose had based their nursing service on the formulations of Henderson, Wiedenbach, and Orlando. There is evidence that Orlando's theory is used at the patient care, managerial, and nursing division levels within organizations.

Although Orlando's theory has been used as an overall framework for practice, its predominate use is focused on immediate nurse-patient contacts. Observation of the patient's verbal and nonverbal behavior provides the nurse with immediate data for determining the patient's level of distress if the process discipline is used. With the patient, the nurse explores what action is to be taken to meet the patient's immediate need for help. Finally, the nurse investigates the patient's new behavior to determine whether the action actually relieved the patient's distress (evaluation). If the distress is not relieved, the process begins again until the patient's need for help is determined.

The process between the patient and the nurse is referred to as a *reflexive principle.*[4] The patient's input is required before the nurse's final judgment. Its reciprocal principle causes Orlando's theory to require four steps: "patient action, nurse reaction, nurse-patient validation, and nurse action."[4:206] Therefore it is more complicated than theories without specific guidelines. However, as an interaction theory, behaviors not previously recognized are brought to the forefront.[4] Orlando's theory continues to be used because it effectively facilitates inquiry and discovery in nurse-patient contacts. Therefore in both nursing practice and research, Oiler Boyd[48:18] recommends the "reconsideration of the centrality of the nurse-patient relationship."

Education

Orlando's nursing process theory is a conceptual framework by which professional nursing would be enhanced if it were taught and practiced. Orlando's process recording form has made a significant contribution to nursing education. Orlando[51] found that *training* in the nursing process discipline was necessary for the nurse to be able to control the nursing process and achieve improvement in the patient's behavior. Therefore she developed the process recording, a tool to facilitate self-evaluation of whether or not the nursing process discipline was used. This "systematic repetitious examination and study of the nursing process" was designed to facilitate students learning how to express their immediate reactions to patients and to ask for correction or verification.[51:32-33] The process recording is an educational tool still used in nursing education.[51] Larson's research[39] confirms the need for teaching student nurses to perceive patients as individuals rather than stereotyping them by categories.

The use of Orlando's theory permeates nursing education and practice.[43] However, acknowledgement that it originates from Orlando's theory is often not known or cited. To users of Orlando's theory, its creator remains unknown. In an e-mail communication, Greene[27] noted that, although she used this theory in teaching beginning students at Midwestern State University in Texas, when examining nursing theories in her doctoral program, she recognized that its origin was from Orlando's theory.

Serendipitously, it became known to Schmieding that for over 10 years, South Dakota State University has used Haggerty's communication model,[28] which is based on Orlando's theory, to teach beginning students. Orlando's theory is included in the junior mental health experience to reinforce communication skills.[22]

Orlando[50:viii] wrote her first book "to offer the professional nursing student a theory of effective practice." Since 1961, numerous psychiatric nursing texts have included Orlando's theory. Orlando deserves credit for providing clear guidelines for the nurse to use in contacts with patients. Orlando's theory was instrumental in the development of the interaction theory currently used in psychiatric nursing.[3]

Winder[75] identifies the need to provide a facilitating environment for implementing the caring process in the nursing curriculum. He suggests that Orlando's theory provides a model for such a training process, which is clearly presented in her book, *The Discipline and Teaching of Nursing Process: An Evaluative Study.*[51]

Studying student nurses, Haggerty[29] analyzed their responses to distressed patients based on Orlando's nursing process concept. She found that "emphasis on communication and psychosocial foundations in BSN curriculums may not translate into more effective exploratory skills in these students."[29:451] She recommends Orlando's model for teaching BSN students to conceptualize the interaction process and its goals.

In Sweden, Orlando's theory was considered useful for students in helping elderly patients cope with needs and maintaining the patient's identity and autonomy.[18] It is also used in Japan[37,38] and Germany.[44]

In 1982, Henderson[32] wrote that Orlando's insistence on validation was an important contribution to the practice of nursing. Recently, Mohr[45:1058] reiterated this insistence by Orlando, for "without this validation the nurse is working with an inadequate data base."

Research

Orlando's theory continues to have considerable acceptance in the area of nursing research and has been applied to a variety of research settings. Many of the studies provided empirical evidence that Orlando's theoretical assertions are valid. These are discussed later in this chapter, under "Empirical Precision."

Dracup and Breu[10] used Orlando's definition of the need for help in their study of the needs of grieving spouses. Hampe[30] used the definition in a similar study. In studying cancer patients, Pienschke[59] found adequacy of care enhanced by openness of approach, perception of patient needs, and congruity between patient and nurse on patient's need and adequacy of care.

Orlando's nursing process discipline has been designated the experimental approach in several studies to examine its effects on a patient's distress during admission and before surgery. Anderson, Mertz, and Leonard[2] found that deliberative nursing actions promoted stress reduction during admission. Wolfer and Visintainer[76] demonstrated this same result with both children and their parents. Dumas and Johnson[12] concluded that preoperative exploration with patients to determine the real source of distress permitted the nurse to take appropriate action to relieve the distress and that lower distress before surgery correlated with fewer postoperative complications. In their study of postoperative vomiting, Dumas and Leonard[13] used nursing process discipline as the experimental nursing action. Thibaudeau and Reidy[73] found that when nurses used deliberative nursing, mothers had more knowledge of illness and complications and complied more fully with treatments prescribed than did mothers who did not receive deliberative nursing.

Although Olson and Hanchett[49] considered five other nursing theories, they selected Orlando's theory because it was most suited for studying the relationship between nurse empathy and patient outcome. Results indicated support for the relationships proposed by the theory.

As was noted earlier, Haggerty[29] used Orlando's nursing process concept to conduct research on nursing students' responses to distressed patients. Princeton[62] tested the effects of using the nursing process discipline with breast-feeding mothers and their infants. These studies using the nursing process discipline can be considered both theory-testing studies and theory-generating studies. They provide empirical support for Orlando's theory (theory testing) and produced new principles for practice and education, especially in the area of pre-operative teaching and student nurse communication (theory generating).

Schmieding[68] used Orlando's theory to investigate the action process of nurse administrators to realistic hypothetical situations presented to them by their staff. The findings indicated the administrators' first thought was seldom about their staff's reaction to the situation and the majority of administrators would tell the nurse what to do rather than inquire about what the nurse thought about the situation. Schmieding[68] concludes that the quality of nursing is reflected in the quality of help nurses receive from their administrators in the problem-solving process. The results of this study indicate that the quality of this help may be less than optimal. In a review of this study, Sheafor[72] concludes that Orlando's theory should be included in a graduate program for nursing administrators. These studies also suggest that the use of Orlando's theory in the graduate education of advanced practice nurses is important. In a study of adult cancer patients, Ponte-Reid[60] examined the relationships among empathy and Orlando's nursing process discipline. A positive relationship was found between primary nurses' empathy skills and the use of nursing process discipline. Ponte-Reid[60] encourages further research in the area of nurses' interpersonal skills and patient outcomes.

In a Veterans Administration (VA) ambulatory psychiatric practice, Shea, McBride, Gavin, and Bauer[71] used Orlando's theoretical model with patients (N = 76) having a bipolar disorder. Their research results indicate that there was higher patient retention, reduced emergency services, decreased hospital stay, and increased satisfaction. They recommended its use throughout the VA system. Currently, Orlando's model is being used in a multimillion-dollar research study of patients with a bipolar disorder at 12 sites in the VA system.[40]

Recently, in a pilot study, Potter and Bockenhauer[61] found positive results after implementing Orlando's theory. These included positive, patient-centered outcomes; a model for staff to use to approach patients; and a decrease in patient's immediate distress. The study provides variable measurements that might be used in other research studies.

The diversity of the research using Orlando's theory attests to its breadth of application. It also indicates its utility for application of the findings.

FURTHER DEVELOPMENT

The nursing process discipline needs to be an integral part of student nurses' education so it can be implemented in any practice setting. Orlando's theory has provided the basis of both clinical and administrative practice in general and psychiatric settings. Its disciplined nursing process is also relevant to community and long-term nursing and in other areas where nursing is practiced. Orlando's study could be replicated to validate that the process discipline is directly related to the effectiveness of a nursing system.

Schmieding[70] expanded its development, incorporating criteria in a reflective inquiry framework for nurse administration. These theoretical formulations could be tested in both clinical and administrative practice and used in undergraduate and advanced practice nursing education.

Whereas nursing theories reflect distinct patterns of conceptual frameworks and theoretical perspectives, Cody[7] criticizes the mania of using borrowed theory only remotely connected to healthcare. He recommends that nursing theories be further developed, including Orlando's theory. Unquestionably, Orlando's theory, which is accepted by the nursing community, warrants continued development. Fawcett[20] agrees and notes that despite impressive evidence, continued study is needed to test Orlando's predictions of her theory.

CRITIQUE
Clarity

In her first book, *The Dynamic Nurse-Patient Relationship: Function, Process and Principles of Professional Nursing Practice,*[50] Orlando presents concepts clearly. She consistently used the same terms in her theory. In her second book, *The Discipline and Teaching of Nursing Process: An Evaluative Study,*[51] she redefines and renamed deliberative nursing process as nursing process discipline. Other than this change, Orlando consistently uses the same word for her major components and processes. Orlando's writing style involves defining concepts minimally at first and then developing them throughout the book. The evolution of the theory requires the reader to be familiar with both books to evaluate her theory thoroughly. Although her writing is clear and concise, some redundancy might facilitate easier comprehension.

Simplicity

As Orlando deals with relatively few concepts and their relationships with each other, her theory would be considered simple. However, it is elegant in its simplicity. Her theory may also be viewed as simplistic because she is able to make some predictive statements as opposed to only description and explanation. The simplicity of Orlando's theory has benefited research application.

Walker and Avant[74] use Orlando's theory as an example of grand nursing theory; however, not all grand theories are at the same level of abstraction. They state that grand nursing theories provide a global perspective, but by virtue of their generality and abstractness, most grand theories are untestable in their current form. Although Orlando's theory has undergone testing, its global perspective could support labeling this work as a grand theory. However, there is controversy among theorists in terms of its level. Orlando's theory has also been described as a practice theory. Practice theories provide a framework to specify when the guidelines should be applied, describe the means to be used, and specify the goals to be used for outcome evaluation.[24]

Generality

Orlando discusses and illustrates nurse-patient contacts in which the patient is conscious, able to communicate, and in need of help. Although she did not focus on unconscious patients and groups, application of her theory to unconscious patients or groups is feasible. Nonverbal behavior is an element of her formulations; therefore nurses would focus on this for determining the patient's need for help and observing for nonverbal behavioral changes after the nursing action.

It is possible that any other person could make use of the nursing process discipline with any other group if educated properly. Although Orlando's theory, at the time of development, focused on a moderate number of situations, their types are increasing. Conceivably, it could be adapted to other nursing situations and other professional fields whose focus is on identifying and finding out patients immediate needs for help.

Empirical Precision

Two thirds of Orlando's second book, *The Discipline and Teaching of Nursing Process: An Evaluative Study,*[51] is a report of a research project designed to test the validity of her nursing formulations. A training program based on her formulations had been in progress for three years before the project began.[51] Nurses were trained to use the nursing process discipline in nurse-patient contacts. Those nurses who became clinical nursing supervisors were trained to use the nursing process discipline in their supervisory contacts and with other contacts. The following is a brief description of the research methodology.

The purpose of the project was to evaluate the effectiveness of the nursing process discipline in the nurse's contacts at work and the effectiveness of the training program. However, these evaluations could not take place before hypothetical measures for the nursing process discipline and the effectiveness of the nursing process discipline were identified. A discipline variable was defined.[51] Effectiveness was determined by the presence or absence of a helpful outcome, as judged by two reliable outcome coders.

The outcome coders compared the beginning behavior of the subject with the behavior at the end of the record.[51] Testing the relationship of the nursing process discipline (in use) with the presence or absence of a helpful outcome in patient, staff, and supervisee contacts was also completed. Evaluation of the training program was performed by testing whether nurses increased their use of the nursing process discipline after being trained.[51]

Two groups of nurses were included in the study. The control group consisted of *veterans* (previously trained supervisors and staff nurses). The experimental group consisted of *novices* (untrained supervisors and staff nurses). Transcripts were made of the novices' and veterans' contacts at work from tape-recorded, 20-minute periods (six for each subject).

This report is extensive and detailed and may be difficult to read and interpret for those without a good understanding of statistics and research methodology. The study concludes that training in the nursing process discipline and its use achieves helpful outcomes in patients, supervisees, and staff contacts.

Although it requires precise understanding of Orlando's theory to develop research based on it, numerous studies by Orlando's first graduate students at Yale in the 1960s supported the validity of her theory.[2,5,6,11-17] Several studies that incorporated Orlando's nursing process discipline approach have previously been mentioned in this section on research application. Others who specifically tested the usefulness of the nursing process discipline approach included the following: Pienschke,[59] who also found that nursing intervention was more effective under conditions of open disclosure because patients' needs were perceived more accurately; Bochnak,[5] who found that the nursing process discipline was more effective in relieving patients' pain; Dye,[14] who controlled for staff-patient ratios and amount of nursing time and still demonstrated that deliberative nursing actions met patient needs effectively; and Cameron,[6] who revealed that the nursing process discipline led to the most consistent, effective results in verifying patient needs.

Orlando asserts that patient distress stems from a reaction to the environment that the patient cannot control alone. Dye[15] provides empirical evidence for this assertion in her study on clarifying patient needs. She found that patients experienced distress more as a reaction to the hospital setting than to their illness.[15]

Orlando also asserts that patient distress stems from the nurse's misinterpretation of the patient's experience or from the patient's initial inability to clearly communicate the need for help. Both necessitate the use of the nursing process discipline to find out the specific need for help. Two studies, one by Elder[17] and the other by Gowan and Morris,[26] provide support for this assertion. Both studies demonstrated that, although patients often did not express their needs clearly, deliberative nursing actions alleviated the problem.

Other research studies cited earlier in this chapter add to the empirical precision of Orlando's theory.

Derivable Consequences

Orlando's theory remains effective and efficient in achieving valued outcome. Identifying the patient's immediate needs for help and the nurse's ability to meet these needs are critically important to patient outcomes and the advancement of nursing practice.

Incorporating validation into the nursing process discipline, as Orlando suggests, allows for maximum participation by the patient in his or her care. Numerous researchers have also demonstrated that the use of a disciplined professional response enables the nurse to find out and meet the patient's immediate needs for help. The study of what nurses say and do in their practice, and the resulting effect manifested by the patient, is valuable content for use in nursing education and developing further research studies. The nursing process discipline allows nurses to view the patient from a nursing perspective rather than from a medical disease orientation. The use of Orlando's theory benefits the patient, enhances the nurse's professional identity, and helps to advance the nursing profession.

CRITICAL THINKING *Activities*

1. George is a 70-year-old patient who has been assigned to you as his community-based nurse case manager. George has severe congestive heart failure, peripheral vascular disease, and no family or social support. George had 15 admissions to the hospital and 35 visits to the emergency department this year from noncompliance with his medication and diet regimen. He receives a monthly Social Security check, which he spends on food, gambling (primarily bingo), and medications (in that order).

   a. Describe your immediate reactions to George, who really is uncertain of the need for a nurse.

   b. Place yourself in George's situation and describe the immediate reactions you would have as a nurse.

   c. What would your first interaction with George be like? Describe the dialogue.

   d. State your automatic nursing actions in relation to George.

   e. State your deliberative nursing actions in relation to George.

2. Select two situations in which a patient would not require medical interventions, but would require professional nursing action.

   a. List two deliberative nursing actions for each situation.

   b. List two automatic nursing actions for each situation.

3. Describe how Orlando's theory can be used in practice when the nurse-patient relationship is extremely short term, as in the extremely short lengths of stay experienced by hospitalized patients.

REFERENCES

1. Alligood, M.R. & Marriner Tomey, A. (2002). *Nursing theory: Utilization and application* (2nd ed.). St. Louis: Mosby.

2. Anderson, B., Mertz, H., & Leonard, R. (1965). Two experimental tests of a patient-centered admission process. *Nursing Research,* 14, 151-157.

3. Artinian, B. (1983). Implementation of the intersystem patient-care model in clinical practice. *Journal of Advanced Nursing,* 8, 117-124.

4. Barnum, B.J.S. (1994). *Nursing theory—Analysis, application, evaluation* (4th ed.). Philadelphia: J.B. Lippincott.

5. Bochnak, M. (1963). The effect of an automatic and deliberative process of nursing activity on the relief of patients' pain: A clinical experiment. *Abstract in Nursing Research,* 12, 191-192.

6. Cameron, J. (1963). An exploratory study of the verbal responses of the nurses in twenty nurse-patient interactions. *Abstract in Nursing Research,* 12, 192.

7. Cody, W.K. (1996). Drowning in eclecticism. *Nursing Science Quarterly,* 9(3), 86-88.

8. Crane, M. (1985). Ida Jean Orlando. In J.B. George (Ed.), *Nursing theories: The base for professional nursing practice* (pp. 158-179). Englewood Cliffs, NJ: Prentice-Hall.

9. Dickoff, J. & James, P. (1986). A theory of theories: A position paper. In L.H. Nicoll (Ed.), *Perspectives on nursing theory* (pp. 101-112). Boston: Little, Brown.

10. Dracup, K. & Breu, C. (1978). Using nursing research findings to meet the needs of grieving spouses. *Nursing Research,* 27, 212-216.

11. Dumas, R. (1963). Psychological preparation for surgery. *American Journal of Nursing,* 63, 52-55.

12. Dumas, R. & Johnson, B. (1972). Research in nursing practice: A review of five clinical experiments. *International Journal of Nursing Studies,* 9, 137-149.

13. Dumas, R. & Leonard, R. (1963). The effect of nursing on the incidence of postoperative vomiting. *Nursing Research,* 12, 12-15.

14. Dye, M. (1963). A descriptive study of conditions conducive to an effective process of nursing activity. *Abstract in Nursing Research,* 12, 194.

15. Dye, M. (1963). Clarifying patients' communications. *American Journal of Nursing,* 63, 56-59.

16. Dye, M. (2000, June 30). Telephone communication.

17. Elder, R. (1963). What is the patient saying? *Nursing Forum,* 11, 25-37.

18. Fagerberg, I. & Ekman, S. (1997). First-year Swedish nursing students' experiences with elderly patients. *Western Journal of Nursing Research,* 19(2), 177-189.

19. Fawcett, J. (1993). *Orlando's theory of the deliberative nursing process. Analysis and evaluation of nursing theories.* Philadelphia: F.A. Davis.

20. Fawcett, J. (2000). *Analysis and evaluation of contemporary nursing knowledge: Nursing models and theories* (pp. 603-626). Philadelphia: F.A. Davis.

21. Felty, J. (2000, June 27). E-mail communication.

22. Fjelland, J. (2000, June 12). E-mail communication.

23. Fitzpatrick, J. & Whall, A.L. (1989). *Conceptual models of nursing: Analysis and application* (2nd ed.). Norwalk, CT: Appleton & Lange.

24. Forchuk, C. (1991). A comparison of the works of Peplau and Orlando. *Archives of Psychiatric Nursing*, 5(1), 38-45.

25. George, J.B. (Ed.). (1995). *Nursing theories—The base for professional nursing practice* (4th ed.). Norwalk, CT: Appleton & Lange.

26. Gowan, N. & Morris, M. (1964). Nurses' responses to expressed patient needs. *Nursing Research*, 13, 68-71.

27. Greene, P. (2000, June 9). E-mail communication.

28. Haggerty, L.A. (1985). A theoretical model for developing students' communication skills. *Journal of Nursing Education*, 24(7), 296-298.

29. Haggerty, L.A. (1987). An analysis of senior nursing students' immediate responses to distressed patients. *Journal of Advanced Nursing*, 12, 451-461.

30. Hampe, S. (1975). Needs of the grieving spouse in a hospital setting. *Nursing Research*, 24, 113-120.

31. Henderson, V. (1964, Aug.). The nature of nursing. *American Journal of Nursing*, 64(8), 62-68.

32. Henderson, V. (1982). The nursing process—Is the title right? *Journal of Advanced Nursing*, 7, 103-109.

33. Henderson, V. (1987). Nursing process—A critique. *Holistic Nursing Practice*, 1(3), 7-18.

34. Hilton, P.A. (1997). Theoretical perspectives of nursing: A review of the literature. *Journal of Advanced Nursing*, 26, 1211-1220.

35. Houle, P. (1997). Ida in action. *BayState Nurse News*, 5(10), 12.

36. Jones, P.S. & Meleis, A.I. (1993). Health is empowerment. *Advance Nursing Science*, 15(3), 1-14.

37. Kobayshi, M. (1998). Skills of how to find out patients who have need for nurses' help in OPD nursing. *Kanko Gijutsu*, 44(13), 20-27.

38. Kumata, M. & Goto, H. (1984). What I learned from Orlando—Individuality and determination in actual interaction with a patient. *Gekkan Nursing*, 4(4), 129-133.

39. Larson, P., Sr. (1977). Nurse perceptions of patient characteristics. *Nursing Research*, 26, 416-421.

40. McBride, L. (2000, July 21). Telephone interview.

41. McCann-Flynn, J. & Heffron, B. (1984). *Nursing: From concept to practice*. Bowie, MD: Robert J. Brady.

42. Meleis, A.I. (1991). *Theoretical nursing: Development and progress* (2nd ed., pp. 343-379). New York: J.B. Lippincott.

43. Meleis, A.I. (1997). Ida Orlando theory description. In A.I. Meleis (Ed.), *Theoretical nursing: Development and progress* (3rd ed.). New York: J.B. Lippincott.

44. Mischo-Kelling, M. & Wittneben, K. (1995). *Ida Jean Orlando Pelletier: Zur bedeutungproblematischer situationen. Pfledgebidung und pflegetheorien* (pp. 184-187). Baltimore: Urban & Schwarzenberg.

45. Mohr, W.K. (1999). Deconstructing the language of psychiatric hospitalization. *Journal of Advanced Nursing*, 29(5), 1052-1059.

46. Moroney, S. (2000, June 13). Telephone communication.

47. Nursing Theories Conference Group & J.B. George (Chairperson). (1980). *Nursing theories: The base for professional practice*. Englewood Cliffs, NJ: Prentice-Hall.

48. Oiler Boyd, C. (1993). Toward a nursing practice research method. *Advanced Nursing Science*, 16(2), 9-25.

49. Olson, J. & Hanchett, E. (1997). Nurse-expressed empathy, patient outcomes, and development of a middle-range theory. *Image: Journal of Nursing Scholarship*, 29(1), 71-76.

50. Orlando, I.J. (1961). *The dynamic nurse-patient relationship: Function, process and principles of professional nursing practice*. New York: G.P. Putnam's Sons.

51. Orlando, I.J. (1972). *The discipline and teaching of nursing process: An evaluative study*. New York: G.P. Putnam's Sons.

52. Orlando, I.J. (2000, May 27). Personal interview.

53. Orlando, I.J. (1990). *The dynamic nurse-patient relationship: Function, process, and principles* (Pub. No. 15-2341). New York: National League for Nursing.

54. Peitchinis, L. (1972). Therapeutic effectiveness of counseling by nursing personnel. *Nursing Research*, 21, 138-148.

55. Pelletier, I.O. (1967). The patient's predicament and nursing function. *Psychiatric Opinion*, 4(1), 25-30.

56. Pelletier, I.O. (1984). Personal correspondence.

57. Pelletier, I.O. (1996). Telephone interview.

58. Pelletier, I.O. (2000). Telephone interview.

59. Pienschke, D., Sr. (1973). Guardedness or openness on the cancer unit. *Nursing Research*, 22, 484-490.

60. Ponte-Reid, P.A. (1992). Distress in cancer patients and primary nurses' empathy skills. *Cancer Nursing*, 15(4), 283-292.

61. Potter, M.L. & Bockenhauer, B.J. (2000). Implementing Orlando's nursing theory: A pilot study. *Journal of Psychosocial Nursing and Mental Health Services*, 38(3), 14-21.

62. Princeton, J. (1986). Incorporating a deliberative nursing care approach with breast-feeding mothers. *Health Care for Women International*, 7, 277-293.

63. Rosenthal, B.C. (1996). An interactionist's approach to perioperative nursing. *AORN Journal*, 64(2), 254-260.

64. Schmidt, J. (1972). Availability: A concept of nursing practice. *American Journal of Nursing*, 72, 1086-1089.

65. Schmieding, N. (1984). Putting Orlando's theory into practice. *American Journal of Nursing*, 84(6), 759-761.

66. Schmieding, N.J. (1986). Orlando's theory. In P. Winstead-Fry (Ed.), *Case studies in nursing theory* (pp. 1-36). New York: National League for Nursing.

67. Schmieding, N.J. (1987). Problematic situations in nursing: Analysis of Orlando's theory based on Dewey's theory of inquiry. *Journal of Advanced Nursing,* 12(4), 431-440.
68. Schmieding, N.J. (1988). Action process of nurse administrators to problematic situations based on Orlando's theory. *Journal of Advanced Nursing,* 13(1), 99-107.
69. Schmieding, N.J. (1993). *Ida Jean Orlando: A nursing process theory.* Newbury Park, CA: Sage Publications.
70. Schmieding, N.J. (1999). Reflective inquiry framework for nurse administrators. *Journal of Advanced Nursing,* 30(3), 631-639.
71. Shea, N.M., McBride, L., Gavin, C., & Bauer, M. (1997). The effects of an ambulatory collaborative practice model on process and outcome of care for bipolar disorder. *Journal of the American Psychiatric Nurses Association,* 3(2), 49-57.
72. Sheafor, M. (1991). Productive work groups in complex hospital units. *Journal of Nursing Administration,* 21(5), 25-30.
73. Thibaudeau, M. & Reidy, M. (1977). Nursing makes a difference: A comparative study of the health behavior of mothers in three primary care agencies. *International Journal of Nursing Studies,* 14, 97-107.
74. Walker, L.O. & Avant, K.C. (1995). *Strategies for theory construction in nursing* (3rd ed.). Norwalk, CT: Appleton & Lange.
75. Winder, A. (1984). A mental health professional looks at nursing care. *Nursing Forum,* 21, 184-188.
76. Wolfer, J. & Visintainer, M. (1975). Pediatric surgical patients' and parents' stress responses and adjustment. *Nursing Research,* 24, 244-255.
77. Wooldridge, P.J., Skipper, J.K., Jr., & Leonard, R.C. (1968). *Behavioral science, social practice, and the nursing profession.* Cleveland: The Case Western Reserve University.

BIBLIOGRAPHY
Primary Sources
Books

Orlando, I. (1961). *The dynamic nurse-patient relationship.* New York: G.P. Putnam's Sons.
Orlando, I. (1972). *The discipline and teaching of nursing process.* New York: G.P. Putnam's Sons.
Orlando, I.J. (1990). *The dynamic nurse-patient relationship* (Pub. No. 15-2341). New York: National League for Nursing.

Book Chapter

Orlando, I. (1962). *Function, process and principle of professional nursing practice. In Integration of mental health concepts in the human relations professions.* New York: Bank Street College of Education.

Journal Articles

Orlando, I. (1987). Nursing in the 21st century: Alternate path. *Journal of Advanced Nursing,* 12, 405-412.
Orlando, I.J. & Dugan, A. (1989, Feb.). Independent and dependent paths: The fundamental issue for the nursing profession. *Nursing and Health Care,* 2, 77-80.
Pelletier, I.O. (1967). The patient's predicament and nursing function. *Psychiatric Opinion,* 4, 25-30.

Video and CD

Ida Orlando the deliberative nursing process. (1997). In *The nurse theorists portraits of excellence* [CD]. Athens, OH: Fuld Institute for Technology in Nursing Education.
Pelletier, I.O. (1988). *The nurse theorist: Portraits of excellence. Ida Orlando Pelletier* [Videotape]. Athens, OH: Fuld Institute for Technology in Nursing Education.

Correspondence

Pelletier, I.O. (1984). Personal correspondence.
Pelletier, I.O. (1985). Personal correspondence.
Pelletier, I.O. (1988). Personal correspondence.

Interviews

McBride, L. (2000, July 21). Telephone interview.
Pelletier, I.O. (1984). Telephone interviews.
Pelletier, I.O. (1985). Telephone interviews.
Pelletier, I.O. (1988). Telephone interviews.
Pelletier, I.O. (1996). Telephone interviews.
Pelletier, I.O. (2000, June 5). Telephone interviews.

Secondary Sources
Book

Schmieding, N.J. (1993). *Ida Jean Orlando: A nursing process theory.* Newbury Park, CA: Sage.

Book Reviews

[Review of the book *The discipline and teaching of nursing process*]. (1973, Jan./Feb.). *Nursing Research,* 22, 10.
[Review of the book *The discipline and teaching of nursing process*]. (1973, Feb.). *Supervisor Nurse,* 4, 48-49.
[Review of the book *The discipline and teaching of nursing process*]. (1973, May). *American Journal of Nursing,* 73, 926.
[Review of the book *The discipline and teaching of nursing process*]. (1973, July). *Nursing Outlook,* 21, 432.
[Review of the book *The discipline and teaching of nursing process*]. (1974, Jan./Feb.). *Journal of Nursing Administration,* 4, 12.
[Review of the book *The dynamic nurse-patient relationship*]. (1962, March). *AAINJ,* 10, 41.

[Review of the book *The dynamic nurse-patient relationship*]. (1962, April). *Nursing Outlook, 10,* 221.

[Review of the book *The dynamic nurse-patient relationship*]. (1962, June). *Catholic Nurse, 10,* 54.

[Review of the book *The dynamic nurse-patient relationship*]. (1963, Jan.). *Journal of Psychiatric Nursing, 1,* 65.

Dissertations

Olson, J.K. (1993). *Relationships between nurse expressed empathy, patient perceived empathy and patient distress.* Unpublished doctoral dissertation, Wayne State University.

Ponte-Reid, P.A. (1988). *The relationships among empathy and the use of Orlando's deliberative process by the primary nurse and the distress of the adult cancer patient.* Unpublished doctoral dissertation. Boston University, Boston.

Schmieding, N. (1983). *A description and analysis of the directive process used by directors of nursing, supervisors, and head nurses in problematic situations based on Orlando's theory of nursing experience.* Unpublished doctoral dissertation, Boston University, Boston.

Sellers, S.C. (1991). *A philosophical analysis of conceptual models of nursing.* Unpublished doctoral dissertation, Iowa State University, Ames, Iowa.

Book Chapters

Andrews, C.M. (1983). Ida Orlando's model of nursing. In J. Fitzpatrick & A. Whall (Eds.), *Conceptual models of nursing: Analysis and application.* Bowie, MD: Robert J. Brady.

Andrews, C.M. (1989). Ida Orlando's model of nursing practice. In J.J. Fitzpatrick & A. L. Whall (Eds.), *Conceptual models of nursing—Analysis and application* (2nd ed.). Norwalk, CT: Appleton & Lange.

Crane, M.D. (1980). Ida Jean Orlando. In J.B. George (Ed.), *Nursing theories: The base for professional nursing practice.* Englewood Cliffs, NJ: Prentice-Hall.

Crane, M.D. (1985). Ida Jean Orlando. In J.B. George (Ed.), *Nursing theories: The base for professional nursing practice* (3rd ed.). Englewood Cliffs, NJ: Prentice-Hall.

Fawcett, J. (1993). Orlando's theory of the deliberative nursing process. In J. Fawcett (Ed.), *Analysis and evaluation of nursing theories.* Philadelphia: F.A. Davis.

Fawcett, J. (2000). *Analysis and evaluation of contemporary nursing knowledge: Nursing models and theories.* Philadelphia: F.A. Davis.

Fisher, S., Marriner Tomey, A., Mills, D.I., & Sauter, M.K. (1986). Ida Jean Orlando (Pelletier): Nursing process theory. In A. Marriner Tomey (Ed.), *Nursing theorists and their work.* St. Louis: Mosby.

Fisher, S., Marriner Tomey, A., Mills, D.I., & Sauter, M.K. (1994). Ida Jean Orlando (Pelletier): Nursing process theory. In A. Marriner Tomey (Ed.), *Nursing theorists and their work* (3rd ed.). St. Louis: Mosby.

Leonard, M.K. & Crane, M.D. (1990). Ida Jean Orlando. In J.B. George (Ed.), *Nursing theories—The base for professional nursing practice* (3rd ed.). Norwalk, CT: Appleton & Lange.

Leonard, M.K. & George, J.B. (1995). Ida Jean Orlando. In J.B. George (Ed.), *Nursing theories: The base for professional nursing practice* (4th ed.). Norwalk, CT: Appleton & Lange.

Marriner Tomey, A., Mills, D., & Sauter, M. (1989). Ida Jean Orlando (Pelletier): Nursing process theory. In A. Marriner Tomey (Ed.), *Nursing theorists and their work* (2nd ed.). St. Louis: Mosby.

Meleis, A.I. (1985). Ida Orlando theory description. In A.I. Meleis (Ed.), *Theoretical nursing: Development and progress.* Philadelphia: J.B. Lippincott.

Meleis, A.I. (1991). Ida Orlando theory description. In A.I. Meleis (Ed.), *Theoretical nursing: Development and progress* (2nd ed.). Philadelphia: J.B. Lippincott.

Meleis, A.I. (1997). Ida Orlando theory description. In A.I. Meleis (Ed.), *Theoretical nursing: Development and progress* (3rd ed.). New York: J.B. Lippincott.

Mertz, H. (1962). *Nurse actions that reduce stress in patients. In Emergency intervention by the nurse* (Monograph 1). New York: American Nurses Association.

Mischo-Kelling, M. & Wittneben, K. (1995). *Ida Jean Orlando Pelletier: Zur bedeutungproblematischer situationen. Pfledgebidung und pflegetheorien* (pp. 184-187). Baltimore: Urban & Schwarzenberg.

Schmieding, N.J. (1983). An analysis of Orlando's theory based on Kuhn's theory of science. In P.L. Chinn (Ed.), *Advances in nursing theory development.* Rockville, MD: Aspen.

Schmieding, N.J. (1986). Orlando's theory. In P. Winstead-Fry (Ed.), *Case studies in nursing theory.* New York: National League for Nursing.

Schmieding, N.J. (2000). Orlando's nursing process theory. In M.R. Alligood & A. Marriner Tomey (Eds.), *Nursing theory utilization and application* (2nd ed.). Philadelphia: Mosby.

Schumacher, L.P., Fisher, S., Marriner Tomey, A., Mills, D.I., & Sauter, M.K. (1998). Ida Jean Orlando (Pelletier)—Nursing process theory. In A. Marriner Tomey & M.R. Alligood (Eds.), *Nursing theorists and their work* (4th ed.). St. Louis: Mosby.

Wesley, R.L. (1995). Orlando's theory of the deliberative nursing process. In R.L. Wesley (Ed.), *Nursing theories and models* (2nd ed.). Springhouse, PA: Springhouse.

Journal Articles

Anderson, B., Mertz, H., & Leonard, R. (1965). Two experimental tests of a patient-centered admission process. *Nursing Research, 14,* 151-157.

Artinian, B. (1983). Implementation of the intersystem patient-care model in clinical practice. *Journal of Advanced Nursing, 8,* 117-124.

Beckstrand, J.A. (1980). A critique of several conceptions of practice model in nursing. *Research in Nursing and Health,* 3, 69-79.

Boschma, G. (1994). The meaning of holism in nursing: Historical shifts in holistic nursing ideas. *Public Health Nursing,* 11(5), 324-350.

de la Cuesta, C. (1983). The nursing process: From development to implementation. *Journal of Advanced Nursing,* 8, 365-371.

Diers, D. (1970). Faculty research development at Yale. *Nursing* Research, 19(1), 64-71.

Dixon, J., Dixon, J., & Spinner, J. (1989). Perceptions of life-pattern disintegrity as a link in the relationship between stress and illness. *Advances in Nursing Science,* 11(2), 1-11.

Dracup, K. & Breu, C. (1978). Using nursing research findings to meet the needs of grieving spouses. *Nursing Research,* 27, 212-216.

Dumas, R. (1963). Psychological preparation for surgery. *American Journal of Nursing,* 63, 52-55.

Dumas, R. & Johnson, B. (1972). Research in nursing practice: A review of five clinical experiments. *International Journal of Nursing Studies,* 9, 137-149.

Dumas, R. & Leonard, R. (1963). The effect of nursing on the incidence of postoperative vomiting. *Nursing Research,* 12, 12-15.

Dye, M. (1963). Clarifying patients' communications. *American Journal of Nursing,* 63, 56-59.

Eisler, J., Wolfer, J., & Diers, D. (1972). Relationship between need for social approval and postoperative recovery and welfare. *Nursing Research,* 21, 520-525.

Elder, R. (1963). What is the patient saying? *Nursing Forum,* 11, 25-37.

Elms, R. & Leonard, R. (1966). Effects of nursing approaches during admission. *Nursing Research,* 15, 39-48.

Forchuk, C. (1991). A comparison of the works of Peplau and Orlando. *Archives of Psychiatric Nursing,* 5(1), 38-45.

Gowan, N. & Morris, M. (1964). Nurses' responses to expressed patient needs. *Nursing Research,* 13, 68-71.

Haggerty, L. (1987). An analysis of senior nursing students' immediate response to distressed patients. *Journal of Advanced Nursing,* 12, 451-461.

Hampe, S. (1975). Needs of the grieving spouse in a hospital setting. *Nursing Research,* 24, 113-120.

Harrison, C. (1966). Deliberative nursing process versus automatic nurse action—The care of a chronically ill man. *Nursing Clinics of North America,* 1(3), 387-397.

Henderson, V. (1978). The concept of nursing. *Journal of Advanced Nursing,* 3, 113-130.

Huckabay, L. (1991). The role of conceptual frameworks in nursing practice, administration, education, and research. *Nursing Administration Quarterly,* 15(3), 17-28.

Johnson, J.L. (1994). A dialectical examination of nursing art. *Advances in Nursing Science,* 17(1), 1-14.

Kobayshi, M. (1998). Skills of how to find out patients who have need for nurses' help in OPD nursing. *Kanko Gijutsu,* 44(13), 20-27.

Kumata, M. & Goto, H. (1984). What I learned from Orlando—Individuality and determination in actual interaction with a patient. *Gekkan Nursing,* 4(4), 129-133.

Larson, P., Sr. (1977). Nursing perceptions of patient characteristics. *Nursing Research,* 26, 416-421.

Lego, S. (1999). The one-to-one nurse-patient relationship. *Perspectives in Psychiatric Care,* 35(4), 4-22.

Lipson, J.G. & Meleis, A.I. (1983). Issues in health care of Middle Eastern patients. *The Western Journal of Medicine,* 139, 854-861.

Madden, B. (1990). The hybrid model for concept development: Its value for the study of therapeutic alliance. *Advances in Nursing Science,* 12(4), 75-86.

McKenna, H. (1989). The selection by ward managers of an appropriate nursing model for long-stay psychiatric patient care. *Journal of Advanced Nursing,* 14, 762-775.

Meleis, A.I. (1998). Revisions in knowledge development: A passion for substance. *Scholarly Inquiry for Nursing Practice: An International Journal,* 12(1), 65-77.

Nagle, L.M. (1999). A matter of extinction or distinction. *Western Journal of Nursing Research,* 32, 71-82.

Nelson, B. (1978). A nursing approach to patients with long-term renal transplants—A practical application of nursing theory. *Nursing Clinics of North America,* 13(1), 157-169.

Peitchinis, L. (1972). Therapeutic effectiveness of counseling by nursing personnel. *Nursing Research,* 21, 138-148.

Pienschke, D., Sr. (1973). Guardedness or openness on the cancer unit. *Nursing Research,* 22, 484-490.

Pillar, B., Jacox, A., & Redman, B. (1990). A classification of nursing technology. *Nursing Outlook,* 38(2), 81-85.

Ponte-Reid, P.A. (1992). Distress in cancer patients and primary nurses' empathy skills. *Cancer Nursing,* 15(4), 283-292.

Powers, M. & Woldridge, P. (1982). Factors influencing knowledge, research, and compliance of hypertensive patients. *Research in Nursing and Health,* 5, 171-182.

Pride, L.F. (1968). An adrenal stress index as a criterion measure for nursing. *Nursing Research,* 17(4), 292-303.

Princeton, J. (1986). Incorporating a deliberative nursing approach with breast-feeding mothers. *Health Care for Women International,* 7, 277-293.

Reynolds, W.J. & Scott, B. (2000). Do nurses and other professional helpers normally display much empathy? *Journal of Advanced Nursing,* 31(1), 226-234.

Rhymes, J. (1964). A description of nurse-patient interaction in effective nursing activity. *Nursing Research,* 13, 365.

Schmidt, J. (1972). Availability: A concept of nursing practice. *American Journal of Nursing,* 72, 1086-1089.

Schmieding, N.J. (1970). Relationship of nursing to the process of chronicity. *Nursing Outlook,* 18(2), 58-62.

Schmieding, N.J. (1984). Putting Orlando's theory into practice. *American Journal of Nursing,* 83, 759-761.

Schmieding, N. (1986). Evaluation of nurse administrators' actions. *American Nurses Association Council of Nursing Administrators. Nurse Facilitator,* 10, 4.

Schmieding, N. (1987). Analyzing managerial responses in face-to-face contacts. *Journal of Advanced Nursing,* 12, 357-365.

Schmieding, N. (1987). Problematic situations in nursing: Analysis of Orlando's theory based on Dewey's theory of inquiry. *Journal of Advanced Nursing,* 12, 431-440.

Schmieding, N. (1988). Action process of nurse administrators to problematic situations based on Orlando's theory. *Journal of Advanced Nursing,* 13, 99-107.

Schmieding, N. (1990). A model for assessing nurse administrator's actions. *Western Journal of Nursing,* 12(3), 293-306.

Schmieding, N. (1990). An integrative nursing theoretical framework. *Journal of Advanced Nursing,* 15, 463-467.

Schmieding, N. (1990). Do head nurses include staff in problem solving? *Nursing Management,* 21(3), 58-60.

Schmieding, N. (1991). Relationship between head nurse responses to staff nurses and staff nurse responses to patients. *Western Journal of Nursing Research,* 13(6), 746-760.

Schmieding, N.J. (1993). Nurse empowerment through context, structure and process. *Journal of Professional Nursing,* 9(4), 239-245.

Schmieding, N.J. (1993). Successful superior-subordinate relationships require mutual management. *Health Care Supervisor,* 11(4), 52-63.

Schmieding, N.J. (1999). Reflective inquiry framework for nurse administrators. *Journal of Advanced Nursing,* 30(3), 631-639.

Sheafor, M. (1991). Productive work groups in complex hospital units. *Journal of Nursing Administration,* 21(5), 25-30.

Silva, M. (1979). Effects of orientation information on spouses' anxieties and attitudes toward hospitalization and surgery. *Research in Nursing and Health,* 2, 127-136.

Stevens, B. (1971). Analysis of structured forms used in nursing curricula. *Nursing Research,* 20, 388-397.

Thibaudeau, M. & Reidy, M. (1977). Nursing makes a difference: A comparative study of the health behavior of mothers in three primary care agencies. *International Journal of Nursing Studies,* 14, 97-107.

Tryon, P.A. (1963). An experiment of the effects of patients' participation in planning the administration of a nursing procedure. *Nursing Research,* 12, 262-265.

Tryon, P.A. & Leonard, R.C. (1964). The effect of patients' participation on the outcome of a nursing procedure. *Nursing Forum,* 3(2), 79-89.

Williamson, J. (1978). Methodologic dilemmas in tapping the concept of patient needs. *Nursing Research,* 27, 172-177.

Winder, A. (1984). A mental health professional looks at nursing care. *Nursing Forum,* 21, 184-188.

Wolfer, J. & Visintainer, M. (1975). Pediatric surgical patients' and parents' stress responses and adjustment. *Nursing Research,* 24, 244-255.

Books

Beck, C.M., Rawlins, R., & Williams, S. (1984). *Mental health: Psychiatric nursing.* St. Louis: Mosby.

Boyd, M.A. (1998). Theoretical basis of psychiatric nursing. In M.A. Boyd & M.A. Nihart (Eds.), *Psychiatric nursing—Contemporary practice.* Philadelphia: Lippincott.

Burgess, A.W. (1997). Psychiatric nursing. In A.W. Burgess (Ed.), *Psychiatric nursing: Promoting mental health.* Stamford, CT: Appleton & Lange.

Carter, F. (1981). *Psychosocial nursing.* New York: Macmillan.

Chaska, N. (1978). *The nursing profession: Views through the mist.* New York: McGraw-Hill.

Chinn, P.L. & Jacobs, M.K. (1983). *Theory and nursing: A systematic approach.* St. Louis: Mosby.

Chinn, P.L. & Kramer, M.K. (1991). *Theory and nursing: A systematic approach* (3rd ed., pp. 177-178). St. Louis: Mosby.

Chinn, P L. & Kramer, M.K. (1999). *Theory and nursing— Integrated knowledge development* (5th ed.). St. Louis: Mosby.

Diers, D. (1997). What is nursing? In J.C. McCloskey & H.K. Grace (Eds.), *Current issues in nursing* (5th ed., pp. 5-12). St. Louis: Mosby.

Joel, L. & Collins, D. (1978). *Psychiatric nursing: Model and application.* New York: McGraw-Hill.

Kim, H.S. & Kollack, I. (1999). *Nursing theories—Conceptual and philosophical foundations.* New York: Springer Publishing.

McBride, A.G. & Austin, A.G. (Eds.), *Psychiatric-mental health nursing—Integrating the behavioral and biological sciences.* Philadelphia: W.B. Saunders.

McCann-Flynn, J. & Heffron, B. (1984). *Nursing: From concept to practice.* Bowie, MD: Robert J. Brady.

Meleis, A. (1985). *Theoretical nursing: Development and progress.* Philadelphia: J.B. Lippincott.

Meleis, A. (1998). *Theoretical nursing: Development and progress* (3rd ed.). New York: J.B. Lippincott.

Murray, R. & Huelskoetter, M. (1983). *Psychiatric-mental health nursing: Giving emotional care.* Englewood Cliffs, NJ: Prentice-Hall.

Nursing Theories Conference Group & J.B. George (Chairperson). (1980). *Nursing theories: The base for professional nursing* practice. Englewood Cliffs, NJ: Prentice-Hall.

Stuart, G. & Sundeen, S. (1983). *Principles and practice of psychiatric nursing.* St. Louis: Mosby.

Torres, G. (1986). *Theoretical foundations in nursing.* Norwalk, CT: Appleton-Century-Crofts.

Wilson, H. & Kneisel, C. (1983). *Psychiatric nursing.* Reading, MA: Addison Wesley.

Research Abstracts

Barron, M.A. (1966). The effects varied nursing approaches have on patients' complaints of pain [Abstract]. *Nursing Research,* 15(1), 90-91.

Bochnak, M. (1963). The effect of an automatic and deliberative process of nursing activity on the relief of patients' pain: A clinical experiment [Abstract]. *Nursing Research,* 12, 191-192.

Cameron, J. (1963). An exploratory study of the verbal responses of the nurses in twenty nurse-patient interactions [Abstract]. *Nursing Research,* 12, 192.

Diers, D.K. (1966). The nurse orientation system: A method for analyzing the nurse-patient interactions [Abstract]. *Nursing Research,* 15(1), 91.

Dye, M. (1963). A descriptive study of conditions conducive to an effective process of nursing activity [Abstract]. *Nursing Research,* 12, 194.

Faulkner, S. (1963). A descriptive study of needs communicated to the nurse by some mothers on a postpartum service [Abstract]. *Nursing Research,* 12, 26.

Fichelis, M. (1963). An exploratory study of labels nurses attach to patient behavior and their effect on nursing activities [Abstract]. *Nursing Research,* 12, 195.

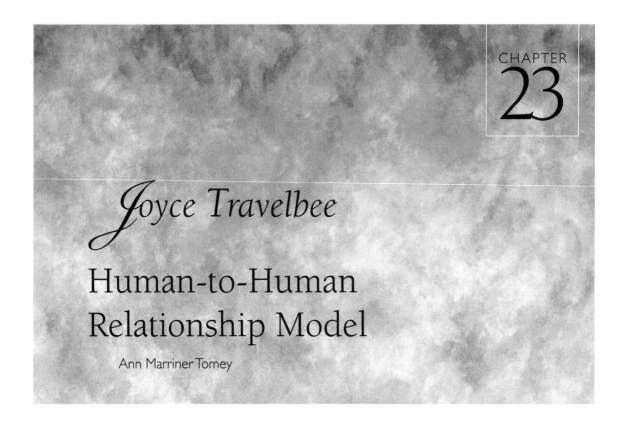

Joyce Travelbee

Human-to-Human Relationship Model

Ann Marriner Tomey

CREDENTIALS AND BACKGROUND OF THE THEORIST

Joyce Travelbee was a psychiatric nurse practitioner, educator, and writer. Born in 1926, she completed her basic nursing preparation in 1946 at Charity Hospital School of Nursing in New Orleans. She earned a B.S. degree in nursing education from Louisiana State University in 1956 and an M.S. degree in nursing from Yale in 1959. In the summer of 1973, Travelbee began a doctoral program in Florida; however, she was unable to complete the program because she died later that year.[3,4,12] She

Previous authors: Sheila Rangel, William H. Hobble, Theresa Lansinger, Jude A. Magers, and Nancy J. McKee.
The authors wish to express appreciation to Leigh DeNoon, Mary Ellen Doona, Joyce Lee, and Katharine Taylor for assistance with data collection. The authors have been unable to obtain a photograph of Joyce Travelbee.

died at the age of 47 after a brief illness, leaving no survivors.[8]

Travelbee began her career as a nursing educator in 1952, teaching psychiatric nursing at Depaul Hospital Affiliate School, New Orleans, while working on her baccalaureate degree. She also taught psychiatric nursing at Charity Hospital School of Nursing, Louisiana State University, New York University in New York City, and the University of Mississippi in Jackson. In 1970, she was named Project Director at Hotel Dieu School of Nursing in New Orleans. At the time of her death, Travelbee was the director of graduate education at Louisiana State University School of Nursing.[3,4,12]

Travelbee began publishing articles in nursing journals in 1963. Her first book, *Interpersonal Aspects of Nursing,* was published in 1966[14] and 1971.[16] A second book, *Intervention in Psychiatric Nursing:*

Process in the One-to-One Relationship,[15] was published in 1969. It was edited by Doona and published in 1979 as *Travelbee's Intervention in Psychiatric Nursing.*[4]

THEORETICAL SOURCES

Travelbee's experiences in her basic nursing education and initial practice in Catholic charity institutions greatly influenced the development of her theory. Travelbee believed that the nursing care given to patients in these institutions lacked compassion.[12] She felt that nursing needed "a humanistic revolution—a return to focus on the 'caring' function of the nurse—in the caring for (and) the caring about ill persons and predicted if this did not occur, consumers would demand the 'services of a new and different kind of health worker.'"[16:2]

Most likely, Travelbee was influenced by Ida Jean Orlando, one of her instructors during her graduate studies at Yale. Orlando's model possesses some similarities to the model that Travelbee proposes. Orlando[10:6] stated, "The nurse is responsible for helping the patient avoid and alleviate the distress of unmet needs." Orlando[10] also stated that the nurse and patient interact with each other. The similarities

between the two models are shown by Travelbee's assertion that the nurse and patient interact with each other and by her definition of the purpose of nursing. Travelbee[16:7] stated that the purpose of nursing is to assist "an individual, family, or community to prevent or cope with the experience of illness and suffering, and, if necessary, to find meaning in these experiences."

Travelbee also appears to have been influenced by Viktor Frankl, a survivor of Auschwitz and other Nazi concentration camps. As a result of his experiences, Frankl[5:153] proposed the theory of logotherapy, in which a patient "is actually confronted with and reoriented toward the meaning of his life." Travelbee[16] based the assumptions of her theory on the concepts of logotherapy.

USE OF EMPIRICAL EVIDENCE

Katharine Taylor,[12] a former student and colleague of Travelbee, remembers Travelbee as a prolific reader whose office was often crammed with files of bibliography cards. Apparently, Travelbee's theory is based on her cumulative nursing experiences and her readings rather than the evidence of a particular research study.

Major Concepts & Definitions

HUMAN BEING

"A human being is defined as a unique irreplaceable individual—a one-time being in this world—like yet unlike any person who has ever lived or ever will live."[16:26]

PATIENT

The term *patient* is a stereotype useful for communicative economy. "Actually there are no patients. There are only individual human beings in need of the care, services, and assistance of other human beings, whom, it is believed, can render the assistance that is needed."[16:32]

NURSE

The nurse is also a human being. "The nurse possesses a body of specialized knowledge and the ability to use it for the purpose of assisting other human beings to prevent illness, regain health, find meaning in illness, or to maintain the highest maximal degree of health."[16:40]

ILLNESS

Illness is "a category and a classification."[16:49] Travelbee did not use the term *illness* as a definition of being unhealthy, but rather explored the human experience of illness. Travelbee defined

Continued

illness by objective and subjective criteria. The objective criteria are determined by the outward effects of illness on the individual.[16] The subjective criteria refer to the way in which a human being perceives himself or herself as ill.[16]

SUFFERING

"Suffering is a feeling of displeasure which ranges from simple transitory mental, physical, or spiritual discomfort to extreme anguish, and to those phases beyond anguish, namely, the malignant phase of despairful 'not caring,' and the terminal phase of apathetic indifference."[16:62] Suffering can be placed on a continuum, which is illustrated in Figure 23-1.

PAIN

"Pain itself is not observable—only its effects are noted."[16:72] Pain is a lonely experience that is difficult to communicate fully to another individual.[16] The experience of pain is unique to each individual.

HOPE

"Hope is a mental state characterized by the desire to gain an end or accomplish a goal combined with some degree of expectation that what is desired or sought is attainable."[16:77] Hope is related to dependence on others, choice, wishing, trust and perseverance, and courage and is future oriented.[16]

HOPELESSNESS

Hopelessness is being devoid of hope.[16]

COMMUNICATION

"Communication is a process which can enable the nurse to establish a human-to-human relationship and thereby fulfill the purpose of nursing, namely, to assist individuals and families to prevent and to cope with the experience of illness and suffering and, if necessary, to assist them to find meaning in these experiences."[16:93]

INTERACTION

"The term *interaction* refers to any contact during which two individuals have reciprocal influence on each other and communicate verbally and/or nonverbally."[16:120]

NURSE-PATIENT INTERACTION

"The term *nurse-patient interaction* refers to any contact between a nurse and an ill person and is characterized by the fact that both individuals perceive the other in a stereotyped manner."[16:120]

NURSING NEED

"A nursing need is any requirement of the ill person (or family) which can be met by the professional nurse practitioner and which lies within the scope of the legal definition of nursing practice."[16:125]

THERAPEUTIC USE OF SELF

"The therapeutic use of self is the ability to use one's personality consciously and in full awareness in an attempt to establish relatedness and to structure nursing intervention."[16:19] It "requires self-insight, self-understanding, an understanding of the dynamics of human behavior, ability to interpret one's own behavior as well as the behavior of others, and the ability to intervene effectively in nursing situations."[16:19]

EMPATHY

"Empathy is a process wherein an individual is able to comprehend the psychological state of another."[16:143]

SYMPATHY

Sympathy implies a desire to help an individual who is undergoing stress.[13]

RAPPORT

"Rapport is a process, a happening, an experience, or series of experiences, undergone simultaneously by the nurse and the recipient of her care.

MAJOR CONCEPTS & DEFINITIONS—cont'd

It is composed of a cluster of interrelated thoughts and feelings, these thoughts, feelings and attitudes being transmitted, or communicated, by one human being to another."[16:150]

HUMAN-TO-HUMAN RELATIONSHIP

"A human-to-human relationship is primarily an experience or series of experiences between a nurse and the recipient of her care. The major characteristic of these experiences is that the nursing needs of the individual (or family) are met."[16:123] "The human-to-human relationship, in nursing situations, is the means through which the purpose of nursing is accomplished."[16:119] The human-to-human relationship is established when the nurse and the recipient of his or her care attain a rapport after having progressed through the stages of the original encounter, emerging identities, empathy, and sympathy (Figure 23-2).[16]

| Transitory feeling of displeasure | Extreme anguish | Malignant phase of despairful not caring | Terminal phase of apathetic indifference |

Figure **23-1 Continuum of suffering.** (Conceptualized by Theresa Lansinger based on Joyce Travelbee's definition.)

MAJOR ASSUMPTIONS

Nursing

Travelbee[16:7] defines *nursing* as an "interpersonal process whereby the professional nurse practitioner assists an individual, family, or community to prevent or cope with the experience of illness and suffering and, if necessary, to find meaning in these experiences." Nursing is an interpersonal process because it is an experience that occurs between the nurse and an individual or group of individuals.[13]

Person

The term *person* is defined as a human being. Both the nurse and patient are human beings. A human being is a unique, irreplaceable individual who is in the continuous process of becoming, evolving, and changing.[16]

Health

Travelbee defines *health* by the criteria of subjective and objective health. A person's subjective health status is an individually defined state of well being in accord with self-appraisal of physical-emotional-spiritual status.[16] Objective health is "an absence of discernible disease, disability, or defect as measured by physical examination, laboratory tests, assessment by a spiritual director, or psychological counselor."[16:10]

Environment

Travelbee does not explicitly define *environment* in the theory. She does define the human condition and life experiences encountered by all human beings as suffering, hope, pain, and illness. These conditions can be equated to the environment.

THEORETICAL ASSERTIONS

1. "The purpose of nursing is achieved through the establishment of a human-to-human relationship."[16:16]
2. The human condition is shared by all human beings and is dichotomous in nature.[16]

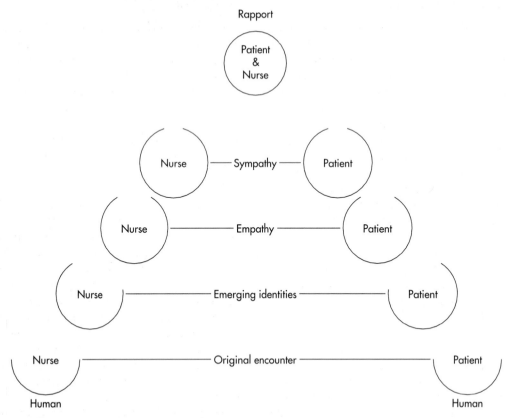

Figure **23-2** **Human-to-human relationship.** (Conceptualized by William Hobble and by Theresa Lansinger based on Joyce Travelbee's writings.)

3. Most people, at one time or another and in varying degrees, will experience joy, contentment, happiness, and love.[16]

4. "All persons, at some time in their lives, will be confronted by illness and pain (mental, physical, or spiritual suffering), and eventually they will encounter death."[16:29]

5. The nurse's perception of the patient greatly influences the quality and quantity of nursing care delivered to an ill human being.[16]

6. The terms *patient* and *nurse* are stereotypes and are only useful for communicative economy.[16]

7. The roles of the nurse and patient must be transcended to establish a human-to-human relatedness.[16]

8. Illness and suffering "are spiritual encounters as well as emotional-physical experiences."[16:61]

9. The communication process enables "the nurse to establish a human-to-human relationship and thereby fulfill the purpose of nursing."[16:93]

10. "Individuals can be assisted to find meaning in the experience of illness and suffering. The meanings can enable the individual to cope with the problems engendered by these experiences."[16:158]

11. "The spiritual and ethical values of the nurse, or her philosophical beliefs about illness and suffering, will determine the extent to which she will be able to assist individuals and families to find meaning (or no meaning) in these difficult experiences."[16:158]

12. "It is the responsibility of the professional nurse practitioner to assist individuals and families to find meaning in illness and suffering (if this be necessary)."[16:158]

Human-to-Human Relationship

The human-to-human relationship model, shown in Figure 23-2, represents the interaction between the nurse and patient. The half circles at the point of the original encounter indicate the possibility of and need for developing the encounter into a therapeutic relationship. As the interaction process progresses toward rapport, the circles join into one full circle, representing that the potential for a therapeutic relationship has been attained.

Original encounter. The original encounter is characterized by first impressions by the nurse of the ill person and by the ill person of the nurse. The nurse and patient perceive each other in stereotyped roles.[16]

Emerging identities. The emerging identities phase is characterized by the nurse and patient perceiving each other as unique individuals. The bond of a relationship is beginning to form.[16]

Empathy. The empathy phase is characterized by the ability to share in the other person's experience. The result of the empathic process is the ability to predict the behavior of the individual with whom he or she has empathized.[16] Travelbee[16] believed that two qualities that enhanced the empathy process were similarities of experience and the desire to understand another person.

Sympathy. Sympathy goes beyond empathy and occurs when the nurse desires to alleviate the cause of the patient's illness or suffering. "When one sympathizes, one is involved but not incapacitated by the involvement."[16:142] The nurse is to create helpful nursing action as a result of reaching the phase of sympathy. "This helpful nursing action requires a combination of the disciplined intellectual approach combined with the therapeutic use of self."[16:149]

Rapport. Rapport is characterized by nursing actions that alleviate a patient's distress. The nurse and ill person are relating as human being to human being. The ill person exhibits both trust and confidence in the nurse. "A nurse is able to establish rapport because she possesses the necessary knowledge and skills required to assist ill persons, and because she is able to perceive, respond to, and appreciate the uniqueness of the ill human being."[16:155]

LOGICAL FORM

Travelbee's theory is inductive. She has used specific nursing situations to create general ideas. Travelbee appears to follow a logical form by first defining the labels in her theory, then listing the assumptions, and finally establishing specific nursing goals.

ACCEPTANCE BY THE NURSING COMMUNITY
Practice

Travelbee believed that the condition of an individual who is exhibiting apathetic indifference is just as critical as that of an individual who is hemorrhaging. She believed that both people need emergency resuscitative measures. However, an examination of patient care given by nurses today indicates that the patient's physical needs still hold top priority. The current acceptance and use of nursing diagnosis appears to focus nursing care more on the total needs of the patient as compared with when Travelbee published her theory. However, nursing has not yet reached the humanistic revolution that Travelbee proposed.

Hospice is the one area of nursing practice in which the philosophy closely adheres to the tenets of Travelbee's theory. The hospice nurse attempts to develop a rapport with the patient and significant others. Most hospice nurses agree with Kübler-Ross[7:2] in "death does not have to be a catastrophic, destructive thing; indeed, it can be viewed as one of the most constructive, positive, and creative elements of culture and life." Travelbee[16] asserted that finding meaning in illness and suffering enables the patient not only to accept the illness, but also to use it as a self-actualizing life experience. An ill individual's perception of meaninglessness in his or her illness and suffering leads to nonacceptance of his or her illness and a feeling of hopelessness. One hospice nurse believes that the dying person must find meaning in his or her death before he or she can ever begin to accept the actuality of death, just as his or her loved ones must find meaning in death before they can complete the grieving process.[11]

Education

Nursing education appears to have identified the need to prepare nurses to address the emotional and spiritual needs of patients. The focus of nursing education has changed from the disease entity approach (signs, symptoms, and nursing interventions) to a more holistic care approach. However, basic nursing programs do not seem to prepare nurses adequately to help individuals find meaning in illness and suffering as Travelbee proposed. Travelbee's second book, *Intervention in Psychiatric Nursing: Process in the One-to-One Relationship*,[15] has been used in various nursing programs. However, this book alone does not adequately prepare nurses to help individuals find meaning in illness and suffering. Nursing programs need to offer a much broader background in communication techniques, values clarification, and thanatology. Courses in philosophy and religion would also be helpful in preparing nurses to fulfill the purpose of nursing adequately as stated in Travelbee's model.

Research

Several sources in research studies have cited some aspects of the one-to-one relationship proposed by Travelbee. One study by O'Connor, Wicker, and Germino,[9] which is closely related to some of Travelbee's ideas, explores how individuals who were recently diagnosed with cancer described their personal search for meaning. The researchers identified six major themes: (1) seeking an understanding of the personal significance of the cancer diagnosis; (2) looking at the consequences of the cancer diagnosis; (3) review of life; (4) change in outlook toward self, life, and others; (5) living with cancer; and (6) hope and two major sources of support: (1) faith and (2) social support. The findings of this study reveal that the search for meaning seems to be both a spiritual and psychosocial process. The researchers identified nursing interventions that would support this process. No other major research studies generated by Travelbee's specific theory, which could stimulate further development, are available. Gregory[6] used Travelbee's model to study suffering inherent in the cancer experience. Bennett[2] used the model in relation to immune deficiency and Baker[1] used it to study schizophrenia.

FURTHER DEVELOPMENT

The advent of diagnostic-related groups (DRGs) has created the need to produce the highest quality nursing care by the most economical method. Tools such as patient acuity systems determine nursing staffing patterns in accordance with the nursing needs of patients. Although this type of tool can account for the emotional needs of patients, emotional needs are not weighed as heavily as patients' physical needs. DRGs may shift the nursing focus back to meeting only the patient's physical needs. If nurses are to prevent this shift, they must prove to healthcare administrators and healthcare consumers that the time taken by the nurse to meet a patient's emotional and spiritual needs is a valuable investment. Travelbee's theory could be used to provide the research data to justify this time investment. However, Travelbee's theory does not currently contain the empirical precision to support such research data. To be more readily accepted, the theory's major assumptions must be assigned operational definitions. Then the theory could perhaps generate the data needed to facilitate further acceptance.

CRITIQUE
Clarity

All concepts of Travelbee's theory are defined in the Travelbee theory, but the definitions are not consistent with regard to origin and explicitness. Some of the definitions are Travelbee's own and she adopted others from Webster's dictionary. She explicitly presents some of the definitions, but derives others from contextual usage. None of the concepts are operationally defined. Travelbee also uses different terms for the same definition. The terms *rapport, human-to-human relationship,* and *human-to-human relatedness* all have the same definition.

The goal or purpose of nursing, as stated in Travelbee's definition of *nursing*,[16] is inconsistent with the emphasis of her presentation. Travelbee focuses on adult individuals who are ill and the nurse's role in helping them find meaning in their illness and suffering. She addresses families and their needs minimally and does not include communities.

Simplicity

Travelbee's theory does not possess simplicity because there are many variables. The theory is designed to help nurses appreciate not only the patient's humanness, but also the nurse's humanness. To be human is to be unique, so the variables present in each phase of the human-to-human relationship are numerous.

Generality

Travelbee's theory has a wide scope of application. She generated it primarily as a result of her experience with psychiatric patients, but it is not limited to use in this setting. It is applicable whenever the nurse encounters patients in distress. It seems to be most useful when working with those who are chronically ill, those who are undergoing long-term rehabilitation, or those who are terminally ill.

Empirical Precision

Travelbee's theory appears to have a low degree of empirical validity, most of which can be traced to the lack of simplicity in the theory. She defines concepts theoretically, but she does not define them operationally. The model has not been tested; therefore it has no empirical support.

Derivable Consequences

The usefulness of a theory is related to its ability to describe, explain, predict, and control phenomena. Travelbee's theory does describe some variables that may affect the establishment of a therapeutic relationship between the nurse and patient. However, the lack of empirical precision also creates a lack of derivable consequences. Travelbee's theory focuses on the development of the attribute of caring. In this respect, the theory can be useful because caring is a major characteristic of the nursing profession.

CRITICAL THINKING *Activities*

1. Review a clinical experience in which you, as a nurse, observed or provided clinical care to a patient. Identify the opportunities and/or potential topics for patient education (either patient or family) during routine care.

2. Conduct a comprehensive nursing assessment of a patient in a healthcare setting and do the following:
   a. Identify actual and potential patient needs.
   b. Categorize each need according to Maslow's hierarchy and rank the needs according to priorities.
   c. Describe conditions creating barriers to the patient's successful attainment of needs.
   d. Describe nursing actions to help the patient meet his or her individual needs.

3. Describe a parable or some type of story that might help a patient cope with a difficult diagnosis.

4. Design a nursing care plan for a patient, paying special attention to his or her spiritual needs.

REFERENCES

1. Baker, M. (1995). *The process of developing insight and finding meaning within persons with schizophrenia.* St. Louis: St. Louis University.
2. Bennett, J.A. (1993). *The effects of empathy, knowledge, and attitudes about sex, and homophobia on nurses' attitudes about AIDS care an exploration of Orem's concept of nursing agency using propositions from Travelbee's theory of interpersonal relations in nursing (immune deficiency).* New York: New York University.
3. Doona, M.E. (1984, Oct.). Telephone interview.
4. Doona, M.E. (1979). *Travelbee's intervention in psychiatric nursing.* Philadelphia: F.A. Davis.
5. Frankl, V. (1963). *Man's search for meaning: An introduction to logotherapy.* New York: Washington Square Press.
6. Gregory, D.M. (1994). *Narratives of suffering in the cancer experience.* Phoenix: University of Arizona.

7. Kübler-Ross, E. (1975). *Death: The final stage of growth*. Englewood Cliffs, NJ: Prentice-Hall.
8. Obituary for Joyce Travelbee. (1973, Sept.). *New Orleans Times-Picayune*, Section 1, p. 22.
9. O'Connor, A.P., Wicker, C.A., & Germino, B.B. (1990). Understanding the cancer patient's search for meaning. *Cancer Nursing*, 13(3), 167-175.
10. Orlando, I.J. (1961). *The dynamic nurse-patient relationship*. New York: G.P. Putnam's Sons.
11. Schoon, F. (1984, Oct.). Personal interview.
12. Taylor, K. (1984, Oct.). Telephone interview.
13. Travelbee, J. (1964, Jan.). What's wrong with sympathy? *American Journal of Nursing*, 64, 68-71.
14. Travelbee, J. (1966). *Interpersonal aspects of nursing*. Philadelphia: F.A. Davis.
15. Travelbee, J. (1969). *Intervention in psychiatric nursing: Process in the one-to-one relationship*. Philadelphia: F.A. Davis.
16. Travelbee, J. (1971). *Interpersonal aspects of nursing* (2nd ed.). Philadelphia: F.A. Davis.

BIBLIOGRAPHY
Primary Sources
Books

Travelbee, J. (1966). *Interpersonal aspects of nursing*. Philadelphia: F.A. Davis.

Travelbee, J. (1969). *Intervention in psychiatric nursing: Process in the one-to-one relationship*. Philadelphia: F.A. Davis.

Travelbee, J. (1971). *Interpersonal aspects of nursing* (2nd ed.). Philadelphia: F.A. Davis.

Travelbee, J. & Doona, M.E. (1979). *Travelbee's intervention in psychiatric nursing* (2nd ed.). Philadelphia: F.A. Davis.

Journal Articles

Travelbee, J. (1963, Feb.). Humor survives the test of time. *Nursing Outlook*, 11, 128.

Travelbee, J. (1963, Feb.). What do we mean by rapport? *American Journal of Nursing*, 63, 70-72.

Travelbee, J. (1964, Jan.). What's wrong with sympathy? *American Journal of Nursing*, 64, 68-71.

Secondary Sources
Book Reviews

[Review of the book *Interpersonal aspects of nursing*]. (1966, June). *Nursing Outlook*, 14, 77.

[Review of the book *Interpersonal aspects of nursing*]. (1966, July). *American Journal of Nursing*, 66, 1504.

[Review of the book *Interpersonal aspects of nursing*]. (1966, Aug.). *Nursing Mirror*, 122, 438.

[Review of the book *Interpersonal aspects of nursing*]. (1971, Dec.). *Supervisor Nurse*, 2, 44.

[Review of the book *Interpersonal aspects of nursing*]. (1972, April). *Nursing Outlook*, 20, 278.

[Review of the book *Interpersonal aspects of nursing*]. (1973, Jan./Feb.). *Journal of Nursing Administration*, 3, 14-15.

[Review of the book *Intervention in psychiatric nursing: Process in the one-to-one relationship*]. (1970, Jan.). *American Journal of Nursing*, 70, 101-102.

[Review of the book *Intervention in psychiatric nursing: Process in the one-to-one relationship*]. (1970, Aug.). *Nursing Outlook*, 18, 16.

[Review of the book *Intervention in psychiatric nursing: Process in the one-to-one relationship*]. (1970, Sept.). *Nursing Mirror*, 131, 31.

Book Chapters

Chinn, R. (1974). The utility of system models and development models for practitioners. In J. Riehl & C. Roy (Eds.), *Conceptual models for nursing practice* (pp. 46-53). New York: Appleton-Century-Crofts.

Meleis, A.I. (1985). Joyce Travelbee. In A.I. Meleis (Ed.), *Theoretical nursing: Development and progress* (pp. 254-262). Philadelphia: J.B. Lippincott.

Roy, C. (1974). Travelbee's developmental approach. In J.P. Riehl & C. Roy (Eds.), *Conceptual models for nursing practice* (pp. 267-268). New York: Appleton-Century-Crofts.

Thibodeau, J.A. (1983). An interaction model: The Travelbee model. In J.A. Thibodeau (Ed.), *Nursing models: Analysis and evaluation* (pp. 89-104). Belmont, CA: Wadsworth.

Wesley, R.L. & McHugh, M.K. (1992). Appendix B: Additional nursing theorists and the nursing metaparadigm. In R.L. Wesley & M.K. McHugh (Eds.), *Nursing theories and models*. Springhouse, PA: Springhouse.

Journal Articles

Aggleton, P. & Chalmers, H. (1987). Models of nursing, nursing practice and nurse education. *Journal of Advanced Nursing*, 12(5), 573-581.

Arnold, H.M. (1976). Working with schizophrenic patients: Guide to one-to-one relationships. *American Journal of Nursing*, 76, 941-943.

Axelsson, K., Norbert, A., & Asplund, K. (1986). Relearning to eat late after a stroke by systematic nursing intervention: A case report. *Journal of Advanced Nursing*, 11, 553-559.

Barker, P.J. (1989). The nursing care of people experiencing affective disorder: A review of the literature. *Journal of Advanced Nursing*, 14(8), 618-629.

Barker, P.J. & Reynolds, B. (1994). A critique: Watson's caring ideology: The proper focus of psychiatric nursing? *Journal of Psychosocial Nursing*, 32(5), 17-22.

Barker, P.J., Reynolds, W., & Ward, T. (1995). The proper focus of nursing: A critique of the "caring" ideology. *International Journal of Nursing Studies, 32*(4), 386-397.

Belcher, A.E., Dettmore, D., & Holzemer, S.P. (1989). Spirituality and sense of well-being in persons with AIDS. *Holistic Nursing Practice, 3*(4), 16-25.

Brumbach, A.E. (1994). What gives nurses hope? *Journal of Christian Nursing,* 11(4), 30-35.

Bullough, V.L. & Seidl, A. (1987). Attitudes on sexuality in nursing texts today and yesterday. *Holistic Nursing Practice,* 1(4), 84-92.

Carson, V., Soeken, K.L., & Grimm, P.M. (1988). Hope and its relationship to spiritual well-being. *Journal of Psychology and Theology,* 16(2), 159-167.

Cohen, M.Z. (1987). A historical overview of the phenomenologic movement. *Image: The Journal of Nursing Scholarship,* 19(1), 31-34.

Comp, H.D.R. (1995). Satisfying a hunger: A personal journey of self-discovery through further nursing education. *Nursing Practice in New Zealand,* 10(1), 12-21.

Criddle, L. (1993). Healing from surgery: A phenomenological study. *Image: The Journal of Nursing Scholarship,* 25(3), 208-213.

DiSalvo, V.S., Larsen, J.K., & Backus, D.K. (1986). The health care communicator: An identification of skills and problems. *Communication Education,* 35(3), 231-242.

Dobson, S.M. (1989). Conceptualizing for transcultural health visiting: The concept of transcultural reciprocity. *Journal of Advanced Nursing,* 14(2), 97-102.

Fenton, M.V. (1987). Development of the scale of humanistic nursing behaviors. *Nursing Research,* 36, 82-93.

Flaskerud, J.H. (1986). On "Toward a theory of nursing action: Skills and competency in nurse-patient interaction." *Nursing Research,* 35, 250-252.

Forbes, S.B. (1994). Hope: An essential human need in the elderly. *Journal of Gerontological Nursing,* 20(6), 5-10.

Forchuk, C. (1994). The orientation phase of the nurse-client relationship: Testing Peplau's theory. *Journal of Advanced Nursing,* 20(3), 532-537.

Freihofer, P. & Felton, G. (1976). Nursing behaviors in bereavement. *Nursing Research,* 25, 332-337.

Gould, D. (1990). Empathy: A review of the literature with suggestions for an alternative research strategy. *Journal of Advanced Nursing,* 15(10), 1167-1174.

Hagland, M.R. (1995). Nurse-patient communication in intensive care: A low priority? *Intensive Critical Care Nursing,* 11(2), 111-115.

Hall, J.M. & Stevens, P.E. (1991). Rigor in feminist research. *Advances in Nursing Science,* 13(3), 16-29.

Henault, M. (1985). Un obstacle de plus pour l'enfant qui eprouve des problemes psychosociaux. *Nursing Quebec,* 5(7), 24-27.

Herth, K. (1990). Fostering hope in terminally-ill people. *Journal of Advanced Nursing,* 15(11), 1250-1259.

Hinds, P.S. (1984). Introducing a definition of hope through the use of grounded theory methodology. *Journal of Advanced Nursing,* 9, 357-362.

Hinds, P.S. (1988). Adolescent hopefulness in illness and health. *Advances in Nursing Science,* 10(3), 79-88.

Holmes, C.A. (1990). Alternatives to natural-science foundations for nursing. *International Journal of Nursing Studies,* 27(3), 187-198.

Johnson, J. (1994). The communication training needs of registered nurses. *Journal of Continuing Education,* 25(5), 213-218.

Kasch, C.R. (1986). Skills and competency in nurse-patient interaction. *Nursing Research,* 35, 226-229.

Koshi, P.T. (1976). Cultural diversity in nursing curricula. *Journal of Nursing Education,* 15, 14-21.

Laine, L., Shulman, R.J., Bartholomew, K., Gardner, P., Reed, T., & Cole, S. (1989). An educational booklet diminishes anxiety in parents whose children receive total parenteral nutrition. *American Journal of Diseases of Children,* 143(3), 374-377.

Larson, P.A. (1977). Nurse perceptions of patient characteristics. *Nursing Research,* 26, 416-421.

Limandri, B.J. & Boyle, D.W. (1978). Instilling hope. *American Journal of Nursing,* 78, 78-80.

Marshall, C. (1994). The concept of advocacy. *British Journal of Theater Nursing,* 4(2), 11-13.

McBride, A.B. (1986). Theory and research: Present issues and future perspectives of psychosocial nursing. *Journal of Psychosocial Nursing,* 24(9), 29-32.

McKenna, H.P. (1989). The selection by ward managers of an appropriate nursing model for long-stay psychiatric patient care. *Journal of Advanced Nursing,* 14(9), 762-775.

McMahon, R. (1988). The 24-hour reality orientation type of approach to the confused elderly: A minimum standard for care. *Journal of Advanced Nursing,* 13(6), 693-700.

Mickley, J.R., Soeken, K., & Belcher, A. (1992). Spiritual well-being, religiousness and hope among women with breast cancer. *Image: The Journal of Nursing Scholarship,* 24(4), 267-272.

Moch, S.D. (1989). Health within illness: Conceptual evolution and practice possibilities. *Advances in Nursing Science,* 11(4), 23-31.

Moch, S.D. (1990). Health within the experience of breast cancer. *Journal of Advanced Nursing,* 15(12), 1426-1435.

Morse, B.W. & Vandenberg, E. (1978). Interpersonal relationships in nursing practice, interdisciplinary approach. *Communication Education,* 27, 158-163.

Morse, J.M., Anderson, G., Bottorff, J.L., Yonge, O., O'Brien, B., Solberg, S.M., & McIlveen, K.H. (1992). Exploring empathy: A conceptual fit for nursing practice? *Image: The Journal of Nursing Scholarship,* 24(4), 273-280.

Muxlow, J. (1995). The relationship between nurse and patient. *Professional Nurse*, 11(1), 63-65.

Narayanasamy, A. (1993). Nurses' awareness and educational preparation in meeting their patients' spiritual needs. *Nurse Education Today*, 13, 196-201.

Nix, J. & Dillon, K. (1986). Short-term nursing therapy: A conceptual model for inpatient psychiatric care. *Hospital and Community Psychiatry*, 37(5), 493-496.

Norberg, A. & Athlin, E. (1989). Eating problems in severely demented patients: Issues and ethical dilemmas. *Nursing Clinics of North America*, 24(3), 781-789.

Nowotny, M.L. (1989). Assessment of hope in patients with cancer: Development of an instrument. *Oncology Nursing Forum*, 16(1), 57-61.

Owen, D.C. (1989). Nurses' perspectives on the meaning of hope in patients with cancer: A qualitative study. *Oncology Nursing Forum*, 16(1), 75-79.

Paul, D., Hagan, L., & Lambert, J. (1985). Au-dela du malade. *Nursing Quebec*, 5(7), 18-23.

Peterson, E.A. & Nelson, K. (1987). How to meet your clients' spiritual needs. *Journal of Psychosocial Nursing*, 25(5), 34-39.

Pinch, W.J. & Spielman, M.L. (1989). Ethical decision-making for high-risk infants: The parents' perspective. *Nursing Clinics of North America*, 24(4), 1017-1023.

Podrasky, D.L. & Sexton, D.L. (1988). Nurses' reactions to difficult patients. *Image: The Journal of Nursing Scholarship*, 20(1), 16-21.

Ramos, M.C. (1992). The nurse-patient relationship: Theme and variations. *Journal of Advanced Nursing*, 17(4), 496-506.

Sarter, B. (1987). Evolutionary idealism. *Advanced Nursing Science*, 9(2), 1-9.

Scanlon, C. & Weir, W.S. (1997, Aug.). Learning from practice? Mental health nurses' perceptions and experiences of clinical supervision. *Journal of Advanced Nursing*, 26(2), 295-303.

Schweer, S.F. & Dayani, E.C. (1973). Extended role of professional nursing: Patient education. *International Nursing Review*, 20, 174.

Shelly, J. & Fish, S. (1995). Praying with patients: Why, when, and how. *Journal of Christian Nursing*, 12(1), 9-13.

Sodestrom, K.E. & Martinson, I.M. (1987). Patients' spiritual coping strategies: A study of nurse and patient perspectives. *Oncology Nursing Forum*, 14(2), 41-44.

Sorgen, L.M. (1979). Student learning following an educational experience at an alcohol rehabilitation center in Saskatoon, Saskatchewan, Canada. *International Journal of Nursing Studies*, 16, 41-50.

Spratlen, L.P. (1976). Introducing ethnic-cultural factors in models of nursing: Some mental health applications. *Journal of Nursing Education*, 15, 23-29.

Stephenson, C. (1991). The concept of hope revisited for nursing. *Journal of Advanced Nursing*, 16(12), 1456-1461.

Stetler, C.B. (1977). Relationship of perceived empathy to nurses' communication. *Nursing Research*, 26, 432-438.

Stoll, R.I. (1979). Guidelines for spiritual assessment. *American Journal of Nursing*, 79, 1574-1577.

Stuart, E.M., Deckro, J.P., & Mandle, C.L. (1989). Spirituality in health and healing: A clinical program. *Holistic Nursing Practice*, 3(3), 35-44.

Swanson, K.M. (1993). Nursing as informed caring for the well-being of others. *Image: The Journal of Nursing Scholarship*, 25(4), 352-357.

Sweeting, H.N. & Gilhooly, M.L.M. (1992). Doctor, am I dead: A review of social death in modern societies. *Omega: Journal of Death and Dying*, 24(4), 251-269.

Wallston, K.A. & Wallston, B.S. (1975). Role-playing simulation approach toward studying nurses' decisions to listen to patients. *Nursing Research*, 24, 16-22.

Wallston, K.A., Wallston, B.S., & Devellis, B.M. (1976). Effect of a negative stereotype on nurse's attitudes toward an alcoholic patient. *Journal of Studies on Alcohol*, 37, 659-665.

Webb, C. & Hope, K. (1994). What kind of nurses do patients want? *Journal of Clinical Nursing*, 4, 101-108.

Young, J.C. (1988). Rationale for clinician self-disclosure and research agenda. *Image: The Journal of Nursing Scholarship*, 20(4), 196-199.

Correspondence

Doona, M.E. (1984, Oct. 19). Personal communication.

Interviews

Doona, M.E. (1984, Oct.). Telephone interview.
Taylor, K. (1984, Oct.). Telephone interview.

Dissertations

Baier, M. (1995). *The process of developing insight and finding meaning within persons with schizophrenia.* Unpublished doctoral dissertation, St. Louis University, St. Louis.

Bennett, J.A. (1993). *The effects of empathy, knowledge, and attitudes about sex, and homophobia on nurses' attitudes about aids care an exploration of Orem's concept of nursing agency using propositions from Travelbee's theory of interpersonal relations in nursing (immune deficiency).* Unpublished doctoral dissertation, New York University, New York.

Gregory, D.M. (1994). *Narratives of suffering in the cancer experience.* Unpublished doctoral dissertation, University of Arizona, Phoenix.

Moses, M. (1995). *The process of developing insight and finding meaning within persons with schizophrenia.* Unpublished doctoral dissertation, St. Louis University, St. Louis.

Other Sources

Barrett-Lennard, G.T. (1962). Dimensions of therapist responses as causal factors in therapeutic change. *Psychological Monographs,* 76, 43 (Whole No. 562).

Cartwright, R.D. & Lerner, B. (1963). Empathy, need to change, and improvement with psychotherapy. *Journal of Consulting Psychology,* 27, 138-144.

Chinsky, J.M. & Rappaport, J. (1970). Brief critique of the meaning and reliability of "accurate empathy" ratings. *Psychological Bulletin,* 73, 379-382.

Frankl, V. (1963). *Man's search for meaning: An introduction to logotherapy.* New York: Washington Square Press.

Kurtz, R.R. & Grummon, D.L. (1972). Different approaches to the measurement of therapist empathy and their relationship to therapy outcomes. *Journal of Consulting and Clinical Psychology,* 30, 106-115.

May, R. (1953). *Man's search for himself.* New York: W.W. Norton.

McBride, M.A. (1967). Nursing approach, pain, and relief: An exploratory experiment. *Nursing Research,* 16(4), 337-341.

Critical Thinking Activities References
Books

Bandman, E. & Bandman, B. (1995). *Critical thinking in nursing.* Norwalk, CT: Appleton-Lange.

Hoover, K.G. (1993). *Study guide to accompany fundamentals of nursing.* St. Louis: Mosby.

LeFevre, R.A. (1995). *Critical thinking in nursing.* Philadelphia: W.B. Saunders.

Journal Articles

Adams, M.H., Whitlow, J.F., Stover, L.M., & Johnson, K.W. (1996). Critical thinking as an educational outcome: An evaluation of current tools of measurement. *Nurse Educator,* 21(3), 23-32.

Heiney, S.P. (1995). The healing power of story. *Oncology Nursing Forum,* 22(6), 899-903.

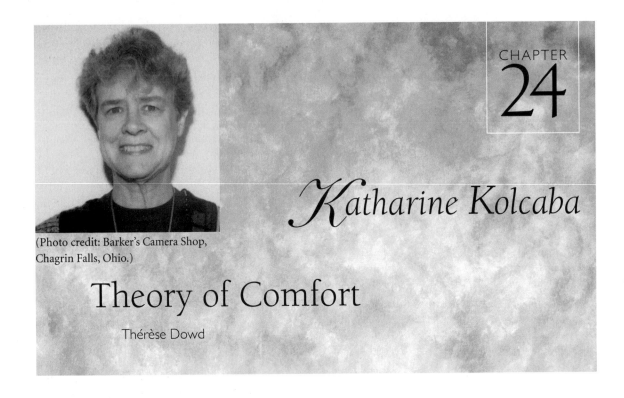

(Photo credit: Barker's Camera Shop, Chagrin Falls, Ohio.)

Katharine Kolcaba

Theory of Comfort

Thérèse Dowd

CREDENTIALS AND BACKGROUND OF THE THEORIST

Katharine Kolcaba was born in Cleveland, Ohio, where she spent most of her life. In 1965, she received a diploma in nursing from St. Luke's Hospital School of Nursing in Cleveland. She practiced part time for many years in medical-surgical nursing, long-term care, and home care before returning to school. In 1987, she graduated in the first RN to MSN class at the Frances Payne Bolton School of Nursing, Case Western Reserve University (CWRU), with a specialty in gerontology. While going to school, Kolcaba job shared a head nurse position on a dementia unit. In the context of that unit, she began theorizing about the outcome of comfort.

Following graduation with her master's degree in nursing, Kolcaba joined the faculty at The University of Akron College of Nursing. Since that time,

she has maintained American Nurses Association (ANA) Certification in Gerontology. She returned to CWRU to pursue her doctorate in nursing on a part-time basis while continuing to teach full time. Over the next ten years, she used course work from her doctoral program to develop and explicate her theory. During that time, Kolcaba published a concept analysis of comfort with her philosopher-husband,[21] diagrammed the aspects of comfort,[11] operationalized comfort as an outcome of care,[13] contextualized comfort in a midrange theory,[14] and tested the theory in an intervention study.[19]

Professors to whom Kolcaba is indebted include: Beverly Roberts, May Wykle, Wilma Phipps, Mary Adams, Betty Adams, Rosemary Ellis, Joanne Youngblut, Shirley Moore, and Jaclene Zauszniewski. She also wanted to thank her students who gave her valuable feedback over the years as they applied the Theory of Comfort in their gerontological nursing courses and assisted her in refining the

The author wishes to thank Katharine Kolcaba for her assistance.

theory, making it user friendly.[15] Ongoing presentations about comfort at research societies helped to refine her theory further. Her theory continues to evolve through personal and website interactions with colleagues and students.

Kolcaba received a Predoctoral Fellowship for Interdisciplinary Health from CWRU and an ANA scholarship to complete her dissertation. In 1995, she received the Honor a Researcher Award from the Midwest Nursing Research Society and the Lillian De Young Research Award from the University of Akron College of Nursing for outstanding merit in research in development. Kolcaba graduated with her Ph.D. in Nursing in 1997 and received her Certificate of Authority (Clinical Nurse Specialist) at that time. She also received the Marie Haug Student Award for excellence in aging studies from CWRU, is a member of the ANA Society of Scholars, and is in *Who's Who in American Nursing*[37] and *The Encyclopedia of Nursing Research.*[16]

Currently, Kolcaba is an associate professor of Nursing at the University of Akron College of Nursing, where she teaches nursing theory and nursing research. Her areas of interest include interventions and measurements for urinary incontinence (UI), measurement of comfort at end of life, and outcomes research. She continues to reside in the Cleveland area with her husband and she enjoys being near her grandchildren and her mother. She is founder and coordinator of her local parish nurse program and is a member of ANA, Sigma Theta Tau, Midwest Nursing Research Society, Health Ministries Association, and League of Women Voters.

THEORETICAL SOURCES

Kolcaba originally began her theoretical work when she diagrammed her nursing practice early in her doctoral work. This is described in detail later in this chapter. When Kolcaba presented her framework for dementia care,[12] an audience member asked, "Have you done a concept analysis of comfort?" Kolcaba's reply was, "No, but that is my next step." This began her long investigation into the concept of comfort.

The first step, the promised concept analysis, began with an extensive review of the literature about comfort from the disciplines of nursing, medicine, psychology, psychiatry, ergonomics, and English (specifically Shakespeare's use of comfort and the Oxford English dictionary, which traces origins of words). In different articles, she gives a historical account of the use of comfort in nursing. For example, in 1859, Nightingale[26:70] exhorted, "It must never be lost sight of what observation is for. It is not for the sake of piling up miscellaneous information or curious facts, but for the sake of saving life and increasing health and comfort."

From 1900 to 1929, comfort was the central goal of nursing and medicine because, through comfort, recovery was achieved.[23] The nurse was duty bound to attend to details influencing patient comfort. Aikens[1] stated that there was nothing concerning the comfort of the patient that was small enough to ignore. Comfort of the patient was the nurse's first and last consideration. A good nurse made patients comfortable and the provision of comfort was a primary determining factor of a nurse's ability and character.[1]

In 1926, Harmer[6:25] stated that nursing care was concerned with providing a "general atmosphere of comfort" and that personal care of patients included attention to "happiness, comfort, and ease, physical and mental" in addition to "rest and sleep, nutrition, cleanliness, and elimination." Goodnow[5] devoted a chapter in her book, *The Technique of Nursing*, to the patient's comfort. She wrote, "A nurse is judged always by her ability to make her patient comfortable. Comfort is both physical and mental, and a nurse's responsibility does not end with physical care."[5:95] In textbooks dated 1904, 1914, and 1919, emotional comfort was called *mental comfort* and was achieved mostly by providing physical comfort and modifying the environment for patients.[23]

In these examples, comfort is positive, it is achieved with the help of nurses, and, in some cases, it indicates an improvement from a previous state or condition. Intuitively, comfort is associated with a nurturing activity. From its origins, Kolcaba explicated its strengthening features and, from ergonomics, comfort's direct link to job performance. However, often its meaning is implicit, hidden in context, and ambiguous. The concept varies semantically as a verb, noun, adjective, adverb, process, and outcome.

Three early nursing theorists were used to synthesize or derive the types of comfort in Kolcaba's concept analysis.[21] Relief was synthesized from the work of Orlando,[28] who stated that nurses relieved the needs expressed by patients. Ease was synthesized from the work of Henderson,[8] who described 13 basic functions of human beings that had to be maintained in homeostasis. Transcendence was derived from Paterson and Zderad,[30] who believed that patients could rise above their difficulties with the help of nurses.

In her theory of caring, Watson[36] claimed that the patients' environment was critical for their mental and physical well being. Therefore when possible, nurses provided comfort through environmental interventions. Watson[36] identified comfort measures that nurses used in that regard. She used the term *comfort measures* synonymously with *interventions.*

USE OF EMPIRICAL EVIDENCE

The seeds of modern inquiry about comfort were sown in the 1980s, marking a period of collective, but separate, awareness about the concept of holistic comfort. Morse[24:6] began observing the comforting actions of nurses and described comfort as "the most important nursing action in the provision of nursing care for the sick." Hamilton[7] made a leap forward by exploring the meaning of comfort from the patients' perspective. She used interviews to ascertain how each patient in a long-term care facility defined comfort. The theme that most frequently emerged was *relief from pain*, but patients also identified good position in well-fitting furniture and a feeling of being independent, encouraged, worthwhile, and useful. At the end of the article, Hamilton[7:32] stated, "The clear message is that comfort is multi-dimensional, meaning different things to different people."

Morse continued to focus on comforting as a nursing action and believed that this action was central to nursing and must be described. She used a qualitative, observational approach to study nurses at work. The comforting actions that Morse[24] described consisted of touching and talking and, to a lesser extent, listening. Although she did not specify semantic senses or definitions and often used the terms *comfort, comforting, comfortable,* and *comforted* interchangeably, she was describing the process of comfort by nurses. In and of itself, this process can be called a *comfort measure* if the outcome of that process is enhanced comfort compared to a previous baseline.

After Kolcaba[19] developed her theory, she tested it in an experimental design for her dissertation. In this study, healthcare needs were those stressors (comfort needs) associated with a diagnosis of early breast cancer. The holistic intervention was guided imagery (GI), designed specifically for this population to meet their comfort needs, and the desired outcome was comfort. The findings revealed a significant difference in comfort over time between women receiving GI and the usual care group.[19] A second test of the theory was with persons with UI.[4] Cognitive strategies (CS) were designed to meet the specific comfort needs of persons with UI. Again, findings revealed a significant difference in comfort over time between persons receiving CS compared to the usual care group. Dowd, Kolcaba, and Steiner[4] credit the significant results of the above studies to the congruence between the design of the study, patient needs, interventions, and outcomes measures as guided by the Theory of Comfort.

The most recent evidence that has been published in support of the Theory of Comfort was a theoretical study that looked at four major tenets about the nature of holistic comfort: (1) comfort is generally state specific; (2) the outcome of comfort is sensitive to changes over time; (3) any consistently applied holistic nursing intervention with an established history for effectiveness enhances comfort over time; and (4) total comfort is greater than the sum of its parts.[22] The results of tests for each tenet, using data from Kolcaba and Fox's study of women with breast cancer,[19] supported each one.

MAJOR CONCEPTS & DEFINITIONS

In Kolcaba's Theory of Comfort, recipients of comfort measures are known in a variety of ways such as patients, students, prisoners, workers, older adults, communities, and institutions.

HEALTHCARE NEEDS

Kolcaba defines healthcare needs as needs for comfort, arising from stressful healthcare situations, that cannot be met by recipients' traditional support systems. These needs include physical, psychospiritual, social, and environmental needs made apparent through monitoring and verbal or nonverbal reports, needs related to pathophysiological parameters, needs for education and support, and needs for financial counseling and intervention.[14]

COMFORT MEASURES

Comfort measures are defined as nursing interventions designed to address specific comfort needs of recipients, including physiological, social, financial, psychological, spiritual, environmental, and physical.[14]

INTERVENING VARIABLES

Intervening variables are defined as interacting forces that influence recipients' perception of total comfort. These consist of variables such as past experiences, age, attitude, emotional state, support system, prognosis, finances, and the totality of elements in recipients' experience.[14]

COMFORT

Comfort is defined as the state that is experienced by recipients of comfort measures. It is the immediate and holistic experience of being strengthened through having the needs met for the three types of comfort (relief, ease, and transcendence) in four contexts of experience (physical, psychospiritual, social, and environmental).[14,19] Types of comfort are defined as:[18]

- Relief: the state of a recipient who has had a specific need met
- Ease: the state of calm or contentment
- Transcendence: the state in which an individual rises above his or her problems or pain

Kolcaba derived the contexts in which comfort is experienced from the literature on holism and she defined them as:

- Physical: pertaining to bodily sensations
- Psychospiritual: pertaining to internal awareness of self, including esteem, self-concept, sexuality, and meaning in life; relationship to a higher order or being
- Environmental: pertaining to external surroundings, conditions, and influences
- Social: pertaining to interpersonal, family, and societal relationships

HEALTH-SEEKING BEHAVIORS

The concept of health-seeking behaviors (HSBs) was synthesized by Dr. Rozella Schlotfeldt[33] and represents the broad category of subsequent outcomes related to the pursuit of health as defined by the recipient(s), in consultation with the nurse. Schlotfeldt stated that HSBs could be internal, external, or a peaceful death.

INSTITUTIONAL INTEGRITY

Kolcaba[17] provides the following technical definition of institutional integrity: corporations, communities, schools, hospitals, churches, reformatories, etc. that possess qualities or states of being complete, whole, sound, upright, appealing, honest, and sincere. This definition was derived from the literature on outcomes research and entails both normative and descriptive components. The institution can have, but does not need to have, walls. The relationship between comfort and institutional integrity is recursive.

MAJOR ASSUMPTIONS
METAPARADIGM CONCEPTS

Kolcaba[18] provides the following definitions:

Nursing

Nursing is the intentional assessment of comfort needs, design of comfort measures to address those needs, and reassessment of comfort levels after implementation compared to the previous baseline. Assessment and reassessment can be intuitive and/or subjective, such as when a nurse asks if the patient is comfortable, or objective, such as in observations of wound healing, changing lab values, or changes in behavior. Assessment can be achieved through the administration of visual analog scales or traditional questionnaires, both of which Kolcaba[18] has developed.

Patient

Recipients of care can be individuals, families, institutions, or communities in need of healthcare.

Environment

The environment is any aspect of patient, family, or institutional surroundings that can be manipulated by nurse(s) or loved one(s) to enhance comfort.

Health

Health is the optimum functioning, as defined by the patient or group, of a patient, family, or community.

ASSUMPTIONS

1. Human beings have holistic responses to complex stimuli.[14]
2. Comfort is a desirable holistic outcome that is germane to the discipline of nursing.[14]
3. Human beings strive to meet their basic comfort needs or to have them met. It is an active endeavor.[14]
4. Enhanced comfort strengthens patients to engage in HSBs of their choice.[21]

5. Patients who are empowered to actively engage in HSBs are satisfied with their healthcare.[17,18]
6. Institutional integrity is based on a value system oriented to the recipients of care.[17,18]

THEORETICAL ASSERTIONS

1. Nurses identify unmet comfort needs of their patients, design comfort measures to address those needs, and seek to enhance their patients' comfort, which is the immediate desired outcome.[14]
2. Enhanced comfort is directly and positively related to engagement in HSBs, which is the subsequent desired outcome.[14]
3. When persons have the proper support to engage fully in HSBs, such as their rehabilitation and/or recovery program or regimen, institutional integrity is enhanced as well.[17,18]

LOGICAL FORM

Kolcaba states that she developed the Theory of Comfort through three types of logical reasoning: (1) induction, (2) deduction, and (3) retroduction.

Induction

Induction occurs when generalizations are built from a number of specific observed instances.[2] When nurses are earnest about their practice and earnest about nursing as a discipline, they become familiar with implicit or explicit concepts, terms, propositions, and assumptions that underpin their practice. When nurses are in graduate school, they may be asked to diagram their practice (as Dr. Rosemary Ellis asked Kolcaba to do), which is a deceptively easy-sounding assignment.

Such was the scenario in the late 1980s. Kolcaba was head nurse on an Alzheimer's unit at the time and knew some of the current terms used to describe the practice of dementia care, such as *facilitative environment, excess disabilities,* and *optimum function.* When she drew relationships between them, she recognized that these three terms did not fully describe her practice. There was an important nursing piece that was missing and she pondered about what nurses were doing to prevent excess disabilities (later naming those actions *interventions*) and how to judge if the interventions were working. Optimum function had been conceptualized as the ability to engage in special activities on the unit, such as setting the table, preparing a salad, or going to a program and sitting through it. These activities made the residents feel good about themselves, as if it was the *right* activity at the *right* time. These activities did not happen more than twice a day because the residents couldn't tolerate much more than that. What were they doing in the mean time? What behaviors did the staff hope they would exhibit that would indicate an absence of excess disabilities? Should the term *excess disabilities* be further delineated for clarity?

Partial solutions to these questions were to: (1) divide excess disabilities into physical and mental, (2) introduce the concept of comfort to the original diagram because this word seemed to convey the desired state for patients to be in when they were not engaging in special activities, and (3) note the recursive relationship between comfort and optimum functioning. These efforts marked the first steps towards a theory of comfort and thinking about the complexities of the concept.[12]

Deduction

Deduction is a form of logical reasoning in which specific conclusions are inferred from more general premises or principles; it proceeds from the general to the specific.[2] The deductive stage of theory development resulted in comfort being related to other concepts to produce a theory. The work of three nursing theorists were entailed in the definition of comfort; therefore Kolcaba had to look elsewhere for the common ground that was needed to unify relief, ease, and transcendence. What was needed, she realized, was a more abstract and general conceptual framework that was congruent with comfort and contained a manageable number of highly abstract constructs.

The work of psychologist Henry Murray[25] in 1938 met these criteria for a framework upon which to hang Kolcaba's nursing concepts. His theory was about human needs; therefore it was applicable to patients who experience multiple stimuli in stressful healthcare situations. This was the deductive stage of theory development, beginning with an abstract, general theoretical construction and substructing downward to more specific levels that included concepts for nursing practice.

Murray's intent was to synthesize a grand theory for psychology from existing, lesser psychological theories of his time. His concepts are found in lines 1, 2, and 3 of Figure 24-1. Comfort was perceived by patients; therefore it was logically substructed under Murray's concept of *perception. Obstructing forces* were substructed for nursing as healthcare needs, *facilitating forces* were comfort measures, and *interacting forces* were intervening variables.

The second and practical part of the theory addressed the question, "Why comfort?" For nursing, *unitary trend* was substructed to health thema, which was further substructed to HSBs. Some examples of HSBs are decreased length of stay, improved functional status, better response (or effort) to therapy, faster healing, or increased patient satisfaction.[33]

Retroduction

Retroduction is a form of reasoning that originates ideas. It is useful for selecting phenomena that can be developed further and tested. This type of reasoning is applied in fields in which there are few available theories.[2] Such is the case with outcomes research, which, to date, is centered on collecting large databases for measuring selected outcomes and relating those outcomes to types of nursing, medical, institutional, or community protocols. Adding a nursing theoretical framework to outcomes research would enhance this area of nursing investigation because theory-based practice enables nurses to design interventions that are congruent with desired outcomes, increasing the likelihood of finding significant results (Figure 24-2). Significant results for desired outcomes would provide data to respective institutions and policy makers about the importance of nursing in the present competitive market.

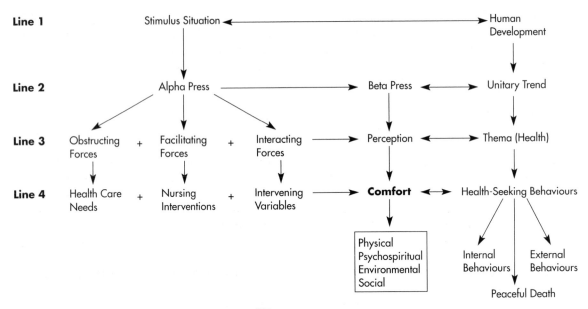

Figure **24-1 (Mid-Range) Theory of Comfort.** (From Kolcaba, K.Y. [1994]. A theory of holistic comfort for nursing. *Journal of Advanced Nursing,* 19, 1178-1184. Blackwell Science, Ltd.)

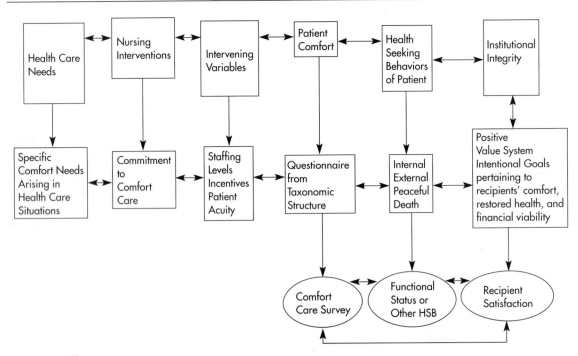

Figure **24-2 Comfort Theory adapted for outcomes research.** (From Kolcaba, K. [2001]. Evolution of the mid-range theory of comfort for outcomes research. *Nursing Outlook,* 49[2], 86-92.)

Murray's twentieth-century framework could not account for twenty-first-century emphasis on institutional and/or community outcomes. However, using retroduction, Kolcaba added the concept of institutional integrity to the midrange Theory of Comfort at the end of line 4. Adding the term to the Theory of Comfort extends the theory to considering relationships between HSBs and institutional integrity.

Line 4 of the diagram represents the midrange Theory of Comfort and can be further applied to any specific healthcare situation or research problem at the practice level. More narrow concepts congruent with a specific setting can be derived from line 4 to form a new line 5 (micro or practice level theories). These micro-level comfort theories can serve as conceptual frameworks for practice, education, and research and would be publishable as such. The Theory of Comfort can be tested in parts or as a whole.

ACCEPTANCE BY THE NURSING COMMUNITY

Practice

This theory is still quite new. It is being recognized increasingly by students who are choosing it as a guiding frame for their studies, such as in nurse midwifery,[34] cardiac catheterization,[9] critical care,[10,20] hospice,[35] infertility,[32] radiation therapy,[3,19] orthopedic nursing,[29] and UI.[4] Areas of study that are yet unpublished, but discussed with Kolcaba through her website, include burn units, nursing homes, home care, chronic pain, massage therapy, pediatrics, oncology, and perioperative.

Education

Following the guidelines for teaching comfort in baccalaureate nursing programs, the Theory of Comfort was applied to the nursing care of older adults and reported by Cox[3] in 1998. The theory proved to be easy to understand and apply for student nurses and provided an effective method to assess and address holistic comfort needs in elders in an acute-care setting. There is also a subchapter about comfort theory in *Core Concepts for Advanced Nursing Practice.*[31] The theory is not limited to gerontological or advanced practice education. It would be difficult to bring to mind a nursing setting or practice in which comfort would not be appropriate.

Research

An entry in the *Encyclopedia of Nursing Research*[16] speaks to the importance of measuring comfort as a nursing-sensitive outcome. Nurses can provide evidence to influence decision making at institutional, community, and legislative levels only through comfort studies that demonstrate the effectiveness of holistic nursing care. Recently, the measurement of comfort in large hospital and home care data sets has been advocated to add to the literature on outcomes research.[17,18]

Using the taxonomic structure of comfort (Figure 24-3) as a guide, Kolcaba[11,13,20,35] developed the General Comfort Questionnaire to measure holistic comfort in a sample of hospital and community participants. To do this, positive and negative items were generated for each cell in the grid. Twenty-four positive items and twenty-four negative items were compiled with a Likert-type format ranging from *strongly agree* to *strongly disagree*. Higher scores indicated higher comfort. At the end of the instrumentation study with 206 one-time participants from all types of units in two hospitals and 50 people from the community, the General Comfort Questionnaire demonstrated a Cronbach's alpha of .88.[13]

The taxonomic structure of comfort provides a map of the content domain of comfort so future researchers can use it to design their own comfort instruments. Kolcaba[18] has listed steps for adapting the General Comfort Questionnaire for new research problems on her web pages. Therefore it is very easy for researchers to generate comfort questionnaires specific to their area of research. Visual analog scales and other traditionally formatted questionnaires are also available for downloading from Kolcaba's website. Kolcaba believes that her Internet presence and responsiveness to inquiries that arise from her web pages has enhanced the popularity of her theory. In addition, it is very easy to ac-

Type of Comfort

	Relief	Ease	Transcendence
Physical			
Psychospiritual			
Environmental			
Social			

Context in Which Comfort Occurs

Type of Comfort:
Relief: The state of a patient who has had a specific need met.
Ease: The state of calm or contentment.
Transcendence: The state in which one rises above one's problems or pain.

Context in Which Comfort Occurs:
Physical: Pertaining to bodily sensations.
Psychospiritual: Pertaining to internal awareness of self, including esteem, concept, sexual
   and meaning in one's life; one's relationship to a higher order or being.
Environmental: Pertaining to the external surroundings, conditions, and influences.
Social: Pertaining to interpersonal, family, and societal relationships.

Figure **24-3** **Taxonomic structure of comfort.** (Reprinted with permission from Kolcaba, K. & Fisher, E. [©1996]. A holistic perspective on comfort care and an advance directive. *Critical Care Nursing Quarterly,* 18[4], 66-76. Aspen Publishers, Inc.)

quire and use existing questionnaires, or develop new questionnaires if necessary, given the instructions on the website. The theory may also be popular because comfort seems to be a universally desirable outcome of nursing care, at least for patients.

FURTHER DEVELOPMENT

Kolcaba has persisted in the development of her theory from its conception as the root of her practice, to the concept analysis that provided taxonomic structure of comfort, to the development of ways to measure the concept, and currently in its use for practice, education, and research. She has used a full array of approaches to develop her concept. Through qualitative work, Kolcaba identified the concept's historical use in nursing and strongly supported her rationale for her claim to its centrality for nursing. The three types of comfort that were synthesized from Orlando (relief), Henderson (ease), and Paterson and Zderad (transcendence) are integral to the theory and were validated through factor analysis of the instrument developed with the guidance of the taxonomic structure.[12,14]

The methodical development of the concept resulted in a strong, clearly organized and logical theory that is readily applied in many settings for education, practice, and research. Kolcaba has developed templates for instrument development so individuals can measure the concept in new settings. Kolcaba has also provided comfort care templates for use in practice settings. Students have identified how useful the concept is in practice. Research outcomes have shown the appropriateness of this concept for measuring whole-person changes that have been difficult to glean from standard, narrow measures such as those for UI.

So far, the first part of the Theory of Comfort has been standing up to empirical testing. When a comfort measure (intervention) is targeted to meet the holistic comfort needs of patients in specific healthcare situations, patients' comfort can be enhanced over a previous baseline measurement (given a strong study design and carefully adapted comfort instruments). Also, enhanced comfort has been correlated with engagement in HSBs.[33] Testing which of the variables come first (comfort or HSBs) can be, but has not yet been, tested with path analysis.

Currently, Kolcaba is developing ways to test the last part of the theory; that is, demonstrating if a relationship exists between patient comfort in an institutional or community setting, their engagement in HSBs, and the extent of their patient satisfaction with care as they are surveyed after discharge. It is postulated that an intentional emphasis on and support for comfort care by an institution or community will be rewarded by increased satisfaction because persons are healed, strengthened, and motivated to be healthier. If this scenario stands up to testing, institutions and communities will have more evidence that comfort care matters, not only for recipients of care, but for the viability of those institutions.

Extending the theory of comfort to the community is of current interest. It is well known that some communities are more comfortable to live in, grow old in, and go to school in than are others. Can the comfort of a community be enhanced with nursing interventions? Can the comfort of a community be measured? These are questions that Kolcaba is

mulling over; input on answers or insights regarding these questions are eagerly requested through her web pages or personal contact.

Another area of interest for further development is the universal nature of comfort. Currently, the General Comfort Questionnaire has been translated into Taiwanese and Spanish. A pending study is a translation into Norweigan. Kolcaba is also very interested in measuring comfort in children and is in negotiations with pediatric nurses and researchers to develop a comfort instrument for self-assessment by children. Trying to determine the age-appropriateness for understanding the complexities of comfort is a challenge to this line of research.

The Theory of Comfort has already made significant contributions to nursing and is poised for greatly expanded use in the discipline. Kolcaba's energy for disseminating her theory through presentations, publications, and websites is as great as her energy for developing and applying her theory. This committed theoretician is a model of excellence for the nursing community in her drive to further the discipline's domain of knowledge and to promote patient-focused care.

CRITIQUE
Clarity

Some of the early articles, such as the concept analysis piece, are difficult to read, but are consistent in terms of definitions, derivations, assumptions, and propositions. The seminal article explicating the Theory of Comfort is easier to read and, in subsequent articles, Kolcaba applies the theory to specific practices using academic, but understandable, language. All research concepts are theoretically and operationally defined.

Simplicity

The Theory of Comfort is simple because it goes back to basic nursing care and the traditional mission of nursing. It is low tech in language and application, but this does not preclude its usage in high-tech settings. There are few variables in the theory and not all of the variables have to be used for any research or educational project. The main thrust of the theory is to return nursing to a practice focused on needs of patients, inside or outside institutional walls. Its simplicity allows students and practicing nurses to learn and practice the theory easily.[15,29]

Generality

Kolcaba's theory has been applied in numerous research settings, cultures, and age groups. The only limiting factor for its application is how much commitment nurses and administrators are willing to make in meeting the comfort needs of patients. If both the nurse and the institution or community are committed to this type of nursing care, the Theory of Comfort enables nurses to practice in efficient, individualized, holistic patterns. The taxonomic structure of comfort allows researchers to develop their own comfort instruments for new settings.[11]

Empirical Precision

The first part of the theory, predicting that effective nursing interventions offered over time will demonstrate enhanced comfort, has been tested and supported with women with breast cancer[19] and persons with UI.[4] In the UI study, enhanced comfort was related to an increase in HSBs, supporting the second part of the comfort theory. The relationship between comfort and institutional integrity has yet to be tested.

For patients with breast cancer and UI and for those at end of life,[35] the adapted comfort instruments have demonstrated strong psychometric properties, which means that those questionnaires are good measurements of comfort and can reveal changes in comfort over time. These findings support the theoretical foundation for the taxonomic structure of comfort.

Derivable Consequences

The Theory of Comfort is able to describe a patient-centered practice and explain how to determine if comfort measures matter to patients, their health, and the viability of institutions. The theory can pre-

dict the benefits of effective comfort measures (interventions) for enhancing comfort and engagement in HSBs. The Theory of Comfort is dedicated to strengthening nursing while bringing the discipline back in contact with its roots.

CRITICAL THINKING *Activities*

1. Does the Theory of Comfort offer a comprehensive framework for practice? Why or why not?

2. Do you believe that comfort is a universal need? How could you demonstrate that comfort theory is transcultural?

3. How would you apply comfort theory in the community? A country? What types of interventions could you design to enhance comfort in an aggregate group? How would you measure if your intervention was effective compared to a baseline?

4. How can comfort theory influence policy change?

5. If you were asked to diagram your practice, what concepts would you include as desirable outcomes? As intervening variables? As nursing interventions? What would your diagram look like, including directional arrows and positive or negative relationships? Are there any concepts that need further exploration (do not have a nursing history)?

6. What should be added to Kolcaba's website? Is there anything you don't understand? Feel free to e-mail your suggestions to her.

REFERENCES

1. Aikens, C. (1908). Making the patient comfortable. *The Canadian Nurse,* 4(9), 422-424.
2. Bishop, S. (1998). Logical reasoning. In A. Marriner Tomey & M.A. Alligood (Eds.), *Nursing theorists and their work* (pp. 25-34). St. Louis: Mosby.
3. Cox, J. (1998). Assessing patient comfort in radiation therapy. *Radiation Therapist,* 5(2), 119-125.
4. Dowd, T., Kolcaba, K., & Steiner, R. (2000). Using cognitive strategies to enhance bladder control and comfort. *Holistic Nursing Practice,* 14(2), 91-103.

5. Goodnow, M. (1935). *The technique of nursing* (p. 95). Philadelphia: W.B. Saunders.

6. Harmer, B. (1926). *Methods and principles of teaching the principles and practice of nursing.* New York: MacMillan.

7. Hamilton, J. (1989). Comfort and the hospitalized chronically ill. *Journal of Gerontological Nursing,* 15(4), 28-33.

8. Henderson, V. (1966). *The nature of nursing.* New York: Macmillan.

9. Hogan-Miller, E., Rustad, D., Sendelbach, S., & Goldenberg, I. (1995). Effects of three methods of femoral site immobilization on bleeding and comfort after coronary angiogram. *American Journal of Critical Care,* 4(2), 143-148.

10. Jenny, J. & Logon, J. (1996). Caring and comfort metaphors used by patients in critical care. *Image: Journal of Nursing Scholarship,* 28(4), 349-352.

11. Kolcaba, K. (1991). A taxonomic structure for the concept comfort. *Image: Journal of Nursing Scholarship,* 23(4), 237-240.

12. Kolcaba, K. (1992). The concept of comfort in an environmental framework. *Journal of Gerontological Nursing,* 18(6), 33-38.

13. Kolcaba, K. (1992). Holistic comfort: Operationalizing the construct as a nurse-sensitive outcome. *Advances in Nursing Science,* 15(1), 1-10.

14. Kolcaba, K. (1994). A theory of holistic comfort for nursing. *Journal of Advanced Nursing,* 19, 1178-1184.

15. Kolcaba, K. (1995). The art of comfort care. *Image: Journal of Nursing Scholarship,* 27(4), 287-289.

16. Kolcaba, K. (1998). Comfort. In J. Fitzpatrick (Ed.), *The encyclopedia of nursing research* (pp. 102-104). New York: Springer.

17. Kolcaba, K. (2001). Evolution of the midrange theory of comfort for outcomes research. *Nursing Outlook,* 49(2), 86-92.

18. Kolcaba, K. (2001). *The comfort line* [Online]. Available: http://www.uakron.edu/comfort.

19. Kolcaba, K. & Fox, C. (1999). The effects of guided imagery on comfort of women with early stage breast cancer undergoing radiation therapy. *Oncology Nursing Forum,* 26(1), 67-92.

20. Kolcaba, K. & Fisher, E. (1996). A holistic perspective on comfort care as an advance directive. *Critical Care Nursing Quarterly,* 18(4), 66-76.

21. Kolcaba, K. & Kolcaba, R. (1991). An analysis of the concept of comfort. *Journal of Advanced Nursing,* 16, 1301-1310.

22. Kolcaba, K. & Steiner, R. (2000). Empirical evidence for the nature of holistic comfort. *Journal of Holistic Nursing,* 18(1), 46-62.

23. McIlveen, K. & Morse, J. (1995). The role of comfort in nursing care: 1900-1980. *Clinical Nursing Research,* 4(2), 127-148.

24. Morse, J. (1983). An enthonocentric analysis of comfort: A preliminary investigation. *Nursing Papers,* 15(4), 6-19.

25. Murray, H. (1938). *Explorations in personality.* New York: Oxford Press.

26. Nightingale, F. (1859). *Notes on nursing* (p. 70). London: Harrison.

27. Novak, B., Kolcaba, K., Steiner, R., & Dowd, T. (2001). Instrumentation study for end-of-life comfort questionnaires. *American Journal of Palliative Care,* 18(3), 170-180.

28. Orlando, I. (1961). *The dynamic nurse-patient relationship: Function, process, and principles.* New York: Putnam.

29. Panno, J., Kolcaba, K., & Holder, C. (2000). Acute care for elders (ACE): A holistic model for geriatric orthopaedic nursing care. *Journal of Orthopaedic Nursing,* 19(6), 53-60.

30. Paterson, J. & Zderad, L. (1975, 1988). *Humanistic nursing* (2nd ed.). New York: National League for Nursing.

31. Robinson, D. & Kish, C. (2001). *Core concepts in advanced nursing practice.* St. Louis: Mosby.

32. Schoerner, C. & Krysa, L. (1996). The comfort and discomfort of infertility. *Journal of Obstetrical, Gynecological, and Neonatal Nurses,* 25(2), 167-172.

33. Schlotfeldt, R. (1975). The need for a conceptual framework. In P. Verhovic (Ed.), *Nursing research* (pp. 3-25). Boston: Little & Brown.

34. Schuiling, K. & Sampselle, C. (1999). Comfort in labor and midwifery art. *Image: Journal of Nursing Scholarship,* 31(1), 77-81.

35. Vendlinski, S. & Kolcaba, K. (1997). Comfort care: A framework for hospice nursing. *The American Journal of Hospice and Palliative Care,* 14(6), 271-276.

36. Watson, J. (1979). *Nursing: The philosophy and science of caring.* Boulder, CO: Associated University Press.

37. *Who's who in American nursing.* (1991). Washington, DC: The Society of Nursing Professionals.

BIBLIOGRAPHY
Primary Sources

Journal Articles

Dowd, T., Kolcaba, K., & Steiner, R. (2000). Cognitive strategies to enhance comfort and decrease episodes of urinary incontinence. *Holistic Nursing Practice,* 14(2), 91-102.

Fox, C. & Kolcaba, K. (1996). Decision making in unsafe practice situations. *Revolution: The Journal of Nurse Empowerment,* Spring, 68-69.

Kinion, E. & Kolcaba, K. (1992). Plato's model of the psyche. *Journal of Holistic Nursing,* 10, 218-230.

Kolcaba, K. (1991). A taxonomic structure for the concept comfort: Synthesis and application. *Image: Journal of Nursing Scholarship, 23,* 237-240.

Kolcaba, K. (1992). Holistic comfort: Operationalizing the construct as a nurse-sensitive outcome. *Advances in Nursing Science, 15*(1), 1-10.

Kolcaba, K. (1992). The concept of comfort in an environmental framework. *Journal of Gerontological Nursing, 18*(6), 33-38.

Kolcaba, K. (1995). Process and product of comfort care, merged in holistic nursing art. *Journal of Holistic Nursing, 13*(2), 117-131.

Kolcaba, K. (1995). The art of comfort care. *Image: The Journal of Nursing Scholarship, 27,* 293-295.

Kolcaba, K. (2001). Evolution of the mid range theory of comfort for outcomes research. *Nursing Outlook, 49*(2), 86-92.

Kolcaba, K. & Fisher, E. (1996). A holistic perspective on comfort care as an advance directive. *Critical Care Nursing Quarterly, 18*(4), 66-76.

Kolcaba, K. & Fox, C. (1999). The effects of guided imagery on comfort of women with early-stage breast cancer going through radiation therapy. *Oncology Nursing Forum, 26*(1), 67-71.

Kolcaba, K. & Kolcaba, R. (1991). An analysis of the concept comfort. *Journal of Advanced Nursing, 16,* 1301-1310.

Kolcaba, K., Panno, J., & Holder, C. (2000). Acute care for elders (ACE): A holistic model for geriatric orthopaedic nursing care. *Journal of Orthopaedic Nursing, 19*(6), 53-60.

Kolcaba, K. & Miller, C. (1989). Geropharmacology: A nursing intervention. *Journal of Gerontological Nursing, 15*(5), 29-35.

Kolcaba, K. & Steiner, R. (2000). Empirical evidence for the nature of holistic comfort. *Journal of Holistic Nursing, 18*(1), 46-62.

Kolcaba, K. & Wykle, M. (1996). Comfort research: Spreading comfort around the world. *Reflections: Sigma Theta Tau International, 23*(2), 12-13.

Novak, B., Kolcaba, K., Steiner, R., & Dowd, T. (2001). Measuring comfort in families and patients during end of life care. *American Journal of Hospice and Palliative Care, 13*(3), 170-180.

Vendlinski, S. & Kolcaba, K. (1997). Comfort care: A framework for hospice nursing. *The American Journal of Hospice and Palliative Care, 11,* 271-276.

Book Chapters

Kolcaba, K. (1998). Comfort. In *The encyclopedia of nursing research* (pp. 102-104). New York: Springer Publishing.

Kolcaba, K. (2001). Holistic care: Is it feasible in today's health care environment? In Feldman, H. (Ed.), *Nursing leaders speak out* (p. 49-54). New York: Springer.

Kolcaba, K. (2001). Kolcaba's theory of comfort. In D. Robinson & C. Kish (Eds.), *Core concepts for advanced nursing practice* (pp. 418-422). St. Louis: Mosby.

Other

Fox, C. & Kolcaba, K. (1995). Unsafe practice: A lack of strategies for effective decision making. *Nurse Educator, 20*(5), 3-4.

Kolcaba, K. (1987). Reaching optimum function is realistic goal for elderly [Letter to the Editor]. *Journal of Gerontological Nursing, 13*(12), 36.

Kolcaba, K. (1988). A framework for the nursing care of demented patients. *Mainlines, 9*(6), 12-13.

Kolcaba, K. (1997). *The comfort line* [Online]. Available: www. uakron.edu/comfort/.

Kolcaba, K. & Dowd, T. (2000). Kegel exercises: Strengthening the weak pelvic floor muscles that cause urinary incontinence. *American Journal of Nursing, 100*(11), 59.

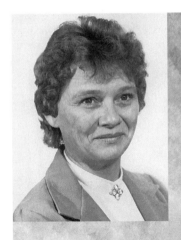

Helen C. Erickson

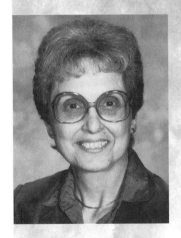

Evelyn M. Tomlin

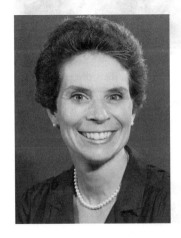

Mary Ann P. Swain

Modeling and Role-Modeling

Margaret E. Erickson

CREDENTIALS AND BACKGROUND OF THE THEORISTS

Helen C. Erickson

Helen C. Erickson received a diploma from Saginaw General Hospital, Saginaw, Michigan in 1957. Her degrees include a B.S.N in 1974, a M.S.N in Psychiatric Nursing in 1976, and a Doctor of Educational Psychology (D.Ed. Psych.) in 1984, all from the University of Michigan.

Erickson's professional experience began in the emergency room of the Midland Community Hospital in Midland, Texas, where she was the head nurse for two years. She then worked in Mount Pleasant, Michigan as night supervisor of nursing in the State Home for the Handicapped. She was then Director of Health Services at the Inter-American University in San German, Puerto Rico from 1960 to 1964. On her return to the United States, she worked as a staff nurse at both St. Joseph's Hospital and University Hospital in Ann Arbor, Michigan. Erickson later served as a psychiatric nurse consultant to the Pediatric Nurse Practitioner Program at

the University of Michigan and the University of Michigan Hospitals–Adult Care. Her academic career began as a teaching assistant in the RN Studies Program at the University of Michigan School of Nursing, where she later served as chairperson of the undergraduate program and Dean for Undergraduate Studies.

Erickson was an assistant professor of nursing at the University of Michigan from 1978 to 1986. In 1986, Erickson left Michigan to go to the University of South Carolina College of Nursing. Initially, she served as an associate professor and assistant dean for academic programs; later she held the position of Associate Dean for Academic Affairs. Since 1988, Erickson has been a professor of nursing and Chair of Adult Health at the University of Texas at Austin. She currently holds the additional title of Special Assistant to the Dean, Graduate Programs. Erickson has maintained an independent nursing practice since 1976.

Erickson is a member of the American Nurses Association, American Nurses' Foundation, the Charter Club, American Holistic Nurses' Association, Texas Nurses' Association, Sigma Theta Tau, and the Institute for the Advancement of Health. In addition, she has served as President of the Society for the Advancement of Modeling and Role-Modeling from 1986 to 1990. She was the chairperson of the First National Symposium on Modeling and Role-Modeling in 1986 and served on the

Previous authors: Margaret E. Erickson, Jane A. Caldwell-Gwin, Lisa A. Carr, Brenda Kay Harmon, Karen Hartman, Connie Rae Jarlsberg, Judy McCormick, and Kathryn W. Noone.
The authors wish to express appreciation to Helen C. Erickson, Evelyn M. Tomlin, and Mary Ann P. Swain for critiquing earlier editions of this chapter.

planning committee for the Second, Third, Fourth, Fifth, and Sixth National Conferences in 1988, 1990, 1992, 1994, and 1996, respectively.

Erickson has been listed in *Who's Who Among University Students* and is a member of Phi Kappa Phi. She received the Sigma Theta Tau Rho Chapter Award of Excellence in Nursing in 1980, the Amoco Foundation Good Teaching Award in 1982, and was accepted into ADARA (a University of Michigan honor society) in 1982. In 1990, she received the Faculty Teaching Award, University of Texas at Austin, School of Nursing.[27] She was nominated for the Sigma Theta Tau International Honor Society in Nursing, Excellence in Education Award by the Epsilon Theta Chapter in 1993; she received the Graduate Faculty Teaching Award, University of Texas at Austin School of Nursing in 1995; and she was accepted as a Fellow in the American Academy in 1996.[24]

Erickson is actively researching the Modeling and Role-Modeling Theory and has presented numerous seminars and papers on various aspects of the theory both nationally and internationally. She has served as a consultant in the implementation of the theory into clinical practice at the University of Michigan Medical Center in the surgical area, at Brigham and Women's Hospital, Boston, and at the University of Pittsburgh Hospitals. She has consulted with faculty members in various schools of nursing and service agencies who have adopted the theory into their curriculum and practice. Humboldt University School of Nursing in Arcata, California is the first school to be accredited by the National League for Nursing, which used the Modeling and Role-Modeling Theory as its conceptual base. Metropolitan State University at St. Paul, Minnesota has adopted the Modeling and Role-Modeling Theory for its RN/B.S.N. and M.S.N. programs. St. Catherine's College, St. Paul, Minnesota has also adopted it for their Associate Degree Nursing program. The University of Texas at Austin has adopted concepts as a foundation for their alternate entry program and the University of Texas at Galveston has adopted core concepts for the academic and service model at the University of Texas Medical Branch in Galveston.[24,25,27,28,32]

Erickson has been an invited speaker at multiple national and international conferences and has participated in numerous workshops, including several Congresses on Ericksonian Approaches to Hypnosis sponsored by the Erickson Foundation and several International Psychology of Health, Immunity, and Disease Conferences sponsored by the National Institute for the Clinical Application of Behavioral Medicine. Erickson has also been involved in activities sponsored by the American Association for Holistic Nursing. She served as a content expert for certification curricula and was included in a published book featuring nurse healers.[28] Although retired from The University of Texas at Austin, Erickson continues to be actively involved in the promotion of holistic nursing. She currently sits on the board of directors of the American Holistic Nurses' Certification Corporation as Chair-Elect, provides consultation and educational programs, and is actively involved in the Society for the Advancement of Modeling and Role-Modeling.[29]

Evelyn M. Tomlin

Evelyn M. Tomlin's nursing education began in Southern California. She attended Pasadena City College, Los Angeles County General Hospital School of Nursing, and the University of Southern California, where she received her Bachelor of Science in Nursing. She received a Master of Science in Psychiatric Nursing from the University of Michigan in 1976.

Tomlin's professional experiences are varied, beginning when she was a clinical instructor at Los Angeles County General Hospital School of Nursing in surgical nursing and maternal and premature infant nursing. She later lived in Kabul, Afghanistan, where she taught English at the Afghan Institute of Technology. In addition, she also served as a school nurse and practiced family nursing in the overseas American and European communities with which she was associated, a role that included attending more than 46 home deliveries with a certified nurse-midwife. After the establishment of medical services at the United States Embassy Hospital, Tomlin functioned as a relief staff nurse. After returning to the United States, she was employed by the Visiting Nurse Association as a staff nurse in Ann Arbor, Michigan. She was then the coordinator and clinical instructor for student practical nurses. She was a staff nurse in a coronary care unit for five years, worked in the respiratory intensive care unit, and was also the head nurse of the emergency department at St. Joseph's Mercy Hospital in Ann Arbor. She was also an assistant professor in the RN Studies Program at the University of Michigan School of Nursing. She served as the mental health consultant to the pediatric nurse practitioner program at the University of Michigan. For eight years, she was an assistant professor of nursing in the fundamentals at the University of Michigan.

Tomlin was among the first 16 nurses in the United States to be certified by the American Association of Critical Care Nurses. With several colleagues, she opened one of the first offices for independent nursing practice in Michigan. She continued her independent practice until 1993.

Tomlin is a member of Sigma Theta Tau Rho Chapter, the California Scholarship Federation, and the Philathian Society. She has presented programs incorporating a variety of nursing topics based on the Modeling and Role-Modeling Theory and paradigm, with an emphasis on clinical applications.

In late 1985, Tomlin moved with her husband to Big Rock, Illinois, where she enjoyed teaching small community and nursing groups and working with a community shelter serving the women and children of Fox Valley. Later she moved to Geneva, Illinois, where she currently resides with her husband. Tomlin has had inquiries from staff nurses for help in integrating the framework into practice. Tomlin believes that elements of the theory and paradigm can be introduced easily in many settings and can be very valuable for practicing nurses. Tomlin[64-68] was first editor for the newsletter of the Society for the Advancement of Modeling and Role-Modeling.

Tomlin currently identifies herself as a Christian in retirement from nursing for pay, but not from nursing practice. She is pursing her interest in the practice of healing prayer, stating that she has always been interested in the interface of the Modeling and Role-Modeling Theory and Judeo-Christian principles. She is on the board of directors and works as a volunteer at Wayside Cross Ministries in Aurora, Illinois, where she teaches and counsels homeless women, most of whom are single mothers. Her goal is to help them develop skills necessary to live healthier, happier lives.[64-68]

Mary Ann P. Swain

Mary Ann P. Swain's educational background is in psychology. She received her Bachelor of Arts in psychology from DePauw University in Greencastle, Indiana and her Master of Science and doctoral degrees from the University of Michigan, both in the field of psychology.

Swain has taught psychology research methods and statistics as a teaching assistant at DePauw University and later as a lecturer and an associate professor of psychology in nursing at the University of Michigan. She became the Director of the Doctoral Program in Nursing in 1975 and served in that capacity for one year. She was Chairperson of Nursing Research from 1977 to 1982 and is currently a professor of nursing research at the University of Michigan. In 1983, Swain[63] became Associate Vice President for Academic Affairs at the University of Michigan.

Swain is a member of the American Psychological Association and an associate member of the Michigan Nurses' Association. She has developed and taught classes in psychology, research, and nursing research methods. She has collaborated with nurse researchers on various projects, including health promotion among diabetics and influencing compliance among hypertensive patients, and has worked with Erickson to develop a model for assessing potential adaptation to stress, which is significant to the Modeling and Role-Modeling Theory.

Swain received the Alpha Lambda Delta, Psi Chi, Mortar Board, and Phi Beta Kappa awards while at DePauw University. In 1981, she was recognized by the Rho Chapter of Sigma Theta Tau for Contributions to Nursing and, in 1983, became an honorary member of Sigma Theta Tau.

Swain currently holds the position of Provost for the New York State University System and resides in Appalachia, New York with her husband.

THEORETICAL SOURCES

The theory and paradigm Modeling and Role-Modeling was developed using a retroductive process. The original model was derived inductively from the primary author's clinical and personal life experiences. The works of Maslow, Erikson, Piaget, Engel, Seyle, and M. Erickson were then integrated and synthesized into the original model to label, further articulate, and refine a holistic theory and paradigm for nursing. Erickson[21] argues that people have mind-body relations and have an identifiable resource potential that predicts their ability to contend with stress. She also articulates a relationship between needs status and developmental processes, satisfaction with needs and attachment objects, loss and illness, and health and need satisfaction. Tomlin and Swain validate and affirm Erickson's practice model and help to expand and articulate labeled phenomena, concepts, and theoretical relationships.

The authors used Maslow's Theory of Human Needs to label and articulate their personal observations that "all people want to be the best that they can possibly be; unmet basic needs interfere with holistic growth whereas satisfied needs promote growth."[33:45] The authors further integrated the model to state that unmet basic needs create need deficits, which can lead to initiation or aggravation of physical or mental distress or illness. At the same time, need satisfaction creates assets that provide resources needed to contend with stress and promote health, growth, and development.

Piaget's Theory of Cognitive Development provides a framework for understanding the development of thinking. On the other hand, integration of Erikson's work on the stages of psychosocial development through the life span provides a theoretical basis for understanding the psychosocial evolution of the individual. Each of his eight stages represent developmental tasks. As an individual resolves each

task, he or she gains strengths that contribute to character and health. Furthermore, as an outcome of each stage, people develop a sense of their own worth and therefore a projection of themselves into the future. "The utility of Erikson's theory is the freedom we may take to view aspects of people's problems as uncompleted tasks. This perspective provides a hopeful expectation for the individual's future since it connotes something still in progress."[33:62-63]

The works of Winnicott, Klein, Mahler, and Bowlby on object attachment were integrated with the original model to develop and articulate the concept of affiliated-individuation (AI). Object relations theory proposes that an infant initially forms an attachment to his or her caregiver after having repeated positive contacts. As the child grows and begins to move toward a more separate and individuated state, a sense of autonomy develops. During this time, he or she usually transfers some attachment to an inanimate object such as a cuddly blanket or a teddy bear. Later, the child may attach to a favorite baseball glove, doll, or pet and finally onto more abstract things in adulthood, such as an educational degree, professional role, or relationship. On the basis of the work of these individuals, a theoretical relationship was identified between object attachment and need satisfaction. According to the theorists, when an object repeatedly meets an individual's basic needs, attachment or connectedness to that object occurs. After further synthesis of these theoretical linkages and research findings, the authors identified a new concept, AI. They defined AI as the inherent need to be connected with significant others at the same time that there is a sense of separateness from them that enhances the uniqueness. AI runs across the life span from birth to death. Research supports that AI and object attachment is essential to need satisfaction, adaptive coping, and healthy growth and development.

The authors further state that "object loss results in basic need deficits."[33:88] Loss is real, threatened, or perceived; it may be a normal part of the developmental process; or it may be situational. Loss always results in grief; normal grief is resolved in approximately one year. When only inadequate or inappropriate objects are available to meet needs, morbid grief results. Morbid grief interferes with the individual's ability to grow and develop to maximum potential. The work of Selye and Engel, as cited by Erickson, Tomlin, and Swain,[33] provides additional conceptual basis for the beliefs the theorists hold regarding loss and an individual's stress response to that loss or losses. Seyle's theory pertains to an individual's biophysical responses to stress, whereas Engel's work explores the psychosocial responses to stressors.

The synthesis of these theories, with the integration of the primary author's clinical observations and lived experiences, resulted in the development of the Adaptive Potential Assessment Model (APAM). The focus of the APAM is the ability of the individual to mobilize resources when confronted with stressors rather than the adaptation process. This model was first developed by Erickson[21] and published by Erickson and Swain in 1982.[32]

Erickson credits M. Erickson with influencing her clinical practice and providing inspiration and direction in the development of this theory. Initially, M. Erickson articulated the formulation of the Modeling and Role-Modeling Theory when he urged Erickson to "model the client's world, understand it as they do, then role-model the picture the client has drawn—building a healthy world for them."[22]

USE OF EMPIRICAL EVIDENCE

Several studies have provided initial evidence for philosophical premises and theoretical linkages implied in the original book by Erickson, Tomlin, and Swain[33] and later specified by Erickson.[20] The APAM (Figures 25-1 and 25-2) has been tested as a classification model,[4,21,50] as a predictor for health status[5] and length of hospital stay,[32] and as it relates to basic need status.[6] Findings provide beginning evidence for the proposed three-state model across populations, a relationship between health and ability to mobilize resources, and ability to mobilize resources and needs status. Two other studies have

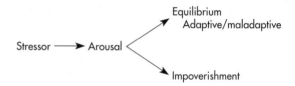

Figure 25-1 Adaptive Potential Assessment Model. (From Erickson, H.C., Tomlin, E.M., & Swain, M.A.P. [1983]. *Modeling and role-modeling: A theory and paradigm for nursing.* Englewood Cliffs, NJ: Prentice Hall. Reprinted with permission.)

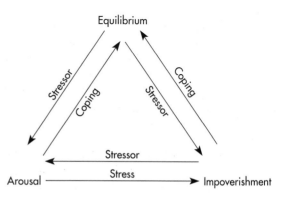

Figure 25-2 Dynamic relationship among the states of the Adaptive Potential Assessment Model. (From Erickson, H.C., Tomlin, E.M., & Swain, M.A.P. [1983]. *Modeling and role-modeling: A theory and paradigm for nursing.* Englewood Cliffs, NJ: Prentice Hall. Reprinted with permission.)

shown relationships between stressors (measured as life events) and propensity for accidents[3] and resource state and ability to take in and use new information.[14]

Relationships among self-care knowledge, resources, and activities have been demonstrated in several studies.[1,42,45,55] The self-care knowledge construct, first studied by Erickson,[18,24,27] was replicated and found to be significantly associated with perceived control.[10] Self-directedness, need for harmony (affiliation), and need for autonomy (individuation) were found when multidimensional scaling was used to explore relationships among self-care knowledge, resources, and actions. The author concluded that a positive attitude was a major factor when health-directed self-care actions were assessed.[60] Physical activity in postmyocardial infarction patients was shown to be affected by life satisfaction (not physical condition); life satisfaction was predicted by availability of self-care resources and resources needed. Furthermore, resources needed served as a suppresser for resources available.[2] In a sample of caregivers, social support predicted for stress level and self-worth and had an indirect effect on hope through self-worth,[42] whereas persons with diabetes with spiritual well being were better able to cope.[52]

When the Modeling and Role-Modeling Theory was used as a guideline, interviews were used to determine the client's model of the world. The following seven themes emerged:[20]

1. Cause of the problem, which was unique to the individual
2. Related factors (also unique to the individual)
3. Expectations for the future
4. Types of perceived control
5. Affiliation
6. Lack of affiliation
7. Trust in the caregiver

Each model was unique and each warranted individualized interventions. Other qualitative studies on self-care knowledge showed that postcardiac patients perceived monitoring, caring, presence, touch, and voice tones as comforting;[47] healthy adults sought need satisfaction from the nurse-practitioner in primary care;[8] and hospice patients benefited from nurse empathy.[57] Studies also showed relationships among mistrust and length of stay in hospitalized subjects;[37] perceived support, control, and well being in the elderly;[12] and loss, morbid grief, and onset of symptoms of Alzheimer's disease.[30,43]

Other studies addressed linkages between role-modeled interventions and outcomes.[30,39,42,47] College-level students who perceived need satisfaction were more successful in school; seven nursing students who perceived that they were supported were more able to attain their goals for advanced education;[62] the elderly who felt supported reported higher need satisfaction and were better able to cope;[46] those with a strong social network reported better health;[17] and persons con-

victed of sexual offenses and then provided with support to *remodel* their worlds were able to develop new behaviors and *move on* with their lives.[61] Families and postmyocardial infarction patients who were able to participate in planning their own care through contracting had less anxiety and more perceived control and perceived support[40] and caregivers of adults with dementia who experienced theory-based nursing using the Modeling and Role-Modeling Theory perceived that their needs were met and that they were healthier.[41] They also reported feeling that they were encouraged, which helped them accept the situation and transcend the experience of caregiving.[41] Self-care resources, measured as needs, have been found to be related to perceived support and coping in women with breast cancer,[46] physical well being in persons with chronic obstructive pulmonary disease,[51] and anxiety in hospitalized cardiac patients and their families.[40] When AI was tested as a buffer between stress and well being, a mediation effect[42] and maternal-attachment in adolescents[35] were found.

Other studies operationalizing self-care resources by measuring developmental residuals have shown that identity resolution in facially disfigured adolescents can be predicted by previous developmental residual;[56] trust predicts for adolescent clients' involvement in the prescribed medical regimen;[38] perceived support and adaptation are related to developmental residual in families with newborn infants;[16] mistrust predicts for hospital stay; and positive residual serves as a buffer.[36] Positive residual in the intimacy stage of healthy adults predicts for health behaviors;[53] developmental residual predicts for hope; trust-mistrust residual predicts for generalized hope; autonomy-shame and doubt residual predicts for particularized hope in the elderly;[15] and negative residual is related to speed and impatience behaviors in a healthy sample of military personnel.[49] Case study methods have been used to show relationships among needs, attachment, and developmental residual[48] and needs and coping[45] and two other unpublished studies have shown relationships between healthy adults and need status.[31] Studies have also been used to explore self-care knowledge in informants in the hospital,[18] the individual's ability to mobilize coping resources and basic needs,[7] and the human-environment relationship when healing from an episodic illness.[9]

Tools that have been developed to test the Modeling and Role-Modeling Theory include the Basic Needs Satisfaction Inventory,[51] the Erikson Psychosocial Stage Inventory,[16] the Perceived Enactment of Autonomy tool designed to measure a prerequisite to self-care actions,[39] the Self-Care Resource Inventory,[2] the Robinson Self-Appraisal Inventory designed to measure denial (the first stage in the grief process) in postmyocardial infarction patients,[58] the Erickson Maternal Bonding-Attachment Tool designed to measure self-care knowledge as motivational style (deficit or being motivation) and self-care resource,[34] and the Hopkins Clinical Assessment of the APAM.[40]

MAJOR CONCEPTS & DEFINITIONS

The theory and paradigm Modeling and Role-Modeling contains multiple concepts.

MODELING

"The act of Modeling, then, is the process the nurse uses as she develops an image and understanding of the client's world—an image and understanding developed within the client's framework and from the client's perspective. . . . The art of Modeling is the development of a mirror image of the situation from the client's perspective. . . . The science of Modeling is the scientific aggregation and analysis of data collected about the client's model."[33:95]

"Modeling occurs as the nurse accepts and understands her client."[33:96]

ROLE-MODELING

"The art of Role-Modeling occurs when the nurse plans and implements interventions that are unique for the client. The science of Role-Modeling occurs as the nurse plans interventions with respect to her theoretical base for the practice of nursing. . . . Role-Modeling is . . . the essence of nurturance. . . . Role-Modeling requires an unconditional acceptance of the person as the person is while gently encouraging the facilitating growth and development at the person's own pace and within the person's own model."[33:95]

"Role-Modeling starts the second the nurse moves from the analysis phase of the nursing process to the planning of nursing interventions."[33:95]

NURSING

"Nursing is the holistic helping of persons with their self-care activities in relation to their health. This is an interactive, interpersonal process that nurtures strengths to enable development, release, and channeling of resources for coping with one's circumstances and environment. The goal is to achieve a state of perceived optimum health and contentment."[33:49]

NURTURANCE

"Nurturance fuses and integrates cognitive, physiological and affective processes, with the aim of assisting a client to move toward holistic health. Nurturance implies that the nurse seeks to know and understand the client's personal model of his or her world and to appreciate its value and significance for that client from the client's perspective."[33:48]

UNCONDITIONAL ACCEPTANCE

"Being accepted as a unique, worthwhile, important individual—with no strings attached—is imperative if the individual is to be facilitated in developing his or her own potential. The nurse's use of empathy helps the individual learn that the nurse accepts and respects him or her as is. The acceptance will facilitate the mobilization of resources needed as this individual strives for adaptive equilibrium."[33:49]

PERSON

People are alike because they have holism, lifetime growth and development, and their need for AI. They are different because they have inherent endowment, adaptation, and self-care knowledge.

HOW PEOPLE ARE ALIKE
Holism

"Human beings are holistic persons who have multiple interacting subsystems. Permeating all subsystems are the inherent bases. These include genetic makeup and spiritual drive. Body, mind, emotion, and spirit are a total unit and they act together. They affect and control one another interactively. The interaction of the multiple subsystems and the inherent bases creates holism: Holism implies that the whole is greater than the sum of the parts."[33:44-45]

Basic Needs

"All human beings have basic needs that can be satisfied, but only from within the framework of the individual."[31:58] "Basic needs are only met when the individual perceives that they are met."[33:57]

Lifetime Development

Lifetime development evolves through psychological and cognitive stages.
Psychological Stages "Each stage represents a developmental task or decisive encounter resulting in a turning point, a moment of decision between alternative basic attitudes (for example, trust versus mistrust or autonomy versus shame and doubt). As a maturing individual negotiates or resolves each age-specific crisis or task, the individual gains enduring strengths and attitudes that contribute to the character and health of the individual's personality in his or her culture."[33:61]

Cognitive Stages "Consider how thinking develops rather than what happens in psychosocial or affective development. . . . Piaget believed that cognitive learning develops in a sequential manner and he has identified several periods in this process. Essentially, there are four periods: sensorimotor, preoperational, concrete operations, and formal operations."[33:63-64]

Affiliated-Individuation

"Individuals have an instinctual need for affiliated-individuation. They need to be able to be dependent on support systems while simultaneously maintaining independence from these support systems. They need to feel a deep sense of both the 'I' and the 'we' states of being and to perceive freedom and acceptance in both states."[33:47]

HOW PEOPLE ARE DIFFERENT
Inherent Endowment

"Each individual is born with a set of genes that will to some extent predetermine appearance, growth, development, and responses to life events. . . . Clearly, both genetic makeup and inherited characteristics influence growth and development. They might influence how one perceives oneself and one's world. They make individuals different from one another, each unique in his or her own way."[33:74-75]

Adaptation

Adaptation occurs as the individual responds to external and internal stressors in a health- and growth-directed manner. Adaptation involves mobilizing internal and external coping resources. No subsystem is left in jeopardy when adaptation occurs.[33]

The individual's ability to mobilize resources is depicted by the APAM. The APAM identifies three different coping potential states: (1) arousal, (2) equilibrium (adaptive and maladaptive), and

Continued

MAJOR CONCEPTS *&* DEFINITIONS—cont'd

(3) impoverishment. Each of these states represents a different potential to mobilize self-care resources.[33] "Movement among the states is influenced by one's ability to cope [with ongoing stressors] and the presence of new stressors."[33:80-81] Nurses can use this model to predict an individual's potential to mobilize self-care resources in response to stress.

Mind-Body Relationships

"We are all biophysical, psychosocial beings who want to develop our potential, this is, to be the best we can be."[33:70]

Self-Care

Self-care involves the use of knowledge, resources, and action.

Self-Care Knowledge "At some level a person knows what has made him or her sick, lessened his or her effectiveness, or interfered with his or her growth. The person also knows what will make him or her well, optimize his or her effectiveness or fulfillment (given circumstances), or promote his or her growth."[33:48]

Self-Care Resources Self-care resources are "the internal resources, as well as additional resources, mobilized through self-care action that help gain, maintain, and promote an optimum level of holistic health."[33:254-255]

Self-Care Action Self-care action is "the development and utilization of self-care knowledge and self-care resources."[33:254]

MAJOR ASSUMPTIONS

Nursing

"The nurse is a facilitator, not an effector. Our nurse-client relationship is an interactive, interpersonal process that aids the individual to identify, mobilize, and develop his or her own strengths."[33:48] Rogers[59] has defined this concept as *facilitative-affiliation.*

Person

A differentiation is made between patients and clients in this theory. A patient is given treatment and instruction; a client participates in his or her own care. "Our goal is for nurses to work with clients."[33:21] "A client is one who is considered to be a legitimate member of the decision-making team, who always has some control over the planned regimen, and who is incorporated into the planning and implementation of his or her own care as much as possible."[33:20]

Health

"Health is a state of physical, mental, and social well-being, not merely the absence of disease or infirmity. It connotes a state of dynamic equilibrium among the various subsystems [of a holistic person]."[33:46]

Environment

"Environment is not identified in the theory as an entity of its own. The theorists see environment in the social subsystems as the interaction between self and others both cultural and individual. Biophysical stressors are seen as part of the environment."[26]

THEORETICAL ASSERTIONS

The theoretical assertions of the Modeling and Role-Modeling Theory are based on the linkages between completion of developmental tasks and basic need satisfaction; among basic need satisfaction, object attachment and loss, and developmental tasks; and between the ability to mobilize coping resources and need satisfaction. Three generic theoretical assertions that constitute several theoretical linkages implied in the theory, but less specifically delineated are as follows:

1. "The degree to which developmental tasks are resolved is dependent on the degree to which human needs are satisfied."[33:87]
2. "The degree to which needs are satisfied by object attachment depends on the availability of those objects and the degree to which they provide comfort and security as opposed to threat and anxiety."[33:90]
3. "An individual's potential for mobilizing resources—the person's state of coping according to the APAM—is directly associated with the person's need satisfaction level."[33:91]

LOGICAL FORM

The Modeling and Role-Modeling Theory is formulated by the use of retroductive thinking. The theorists go through four levels of theory development and then recycle from inductive to deductive to inductive to deductive.[26] The theoretical sources were used to validate clinical observations. Clinical observations were tested in light of the theoretical bases. These sources were synthesized with their observations, which enabled Erickson, Tomlin, and Swain to develop a "multidimensional new theory and paradigm—Modeling and Role-Modeling."[23]

The theorists label Modeling and Role-Modeling as a theory and a paradigm. The Modeling and Role-Modeling Theory meets the five functions of a paradigm as identified by Merton,[54:70] who said that paradigms "provide a compact arrangement of central concepts and their interrelations that are utilized for description and analysis."

1. The theorists provide a clear presentation of their central concepts and build on the relationships as they described them.
2. "Paradigms lessen the likelihood of inadvertently introducing hidden assumptions and concepts, for each new assumption and concept must be either logically derived from previous components or explicitly introduced into it."[32:71] Erickson, Tomlin, and Swain build on previous components as their paradigm is developed, each component being logically derived from clinical observations or based in theory.
3. "Paradigms advance the cumulation of theoretical interpretation."[32:71] The assumptions and concepts allow for interpretation in multiple clinical and research situations in which the concepts may be applied, thereby expanding the theory base of nursing.
4. "Paradigms promote analysis rather than descriptions of concrete details."[32:71] The Modeling and Role-Modeling Theory promotes analysis of significant concepts. The interrelationships among the concepts can be empirically examined because they have broad applicability and lend themselves to multiple research questions.
5. "Paradigms make for codification of qualitative analysis in a way that approximates the logic if not the empirical rigor of quantitative analysis."[32:71] Erickson states that a qualitative approach has been used to form concepts. On the basis of that approach, scales were built with deductive logic to test those concepts.[23]

The methods used will become available for replication of studies as they are published.

ACCEPTANCE BY THE NURSING COMMUNITY
Practice

Publication of the book *Modeling and Role-Modeling: A Theory and Paradigm for Nursing,*[33] chapters in several nursing theory books, and research studies based on the theory have exposed practicing nurses to this theory. Nurses on surgical units at the University of Michigan Medical Center are using an assessment tool based on the Modeling and Role-Modeling Theory. The tool is used to gather information to identify the client's need assets, deficits, developmental residual, attachment-loss and grief status, and potential therapeutic interventions (see Appendix at the end of this chapter).[9,24]

The theorists have spoken on their theory and have held one-on-one consultations that exposed nurses from various practice and educational backgrounds to the theory. Nurses in critical care, adult health, mental health, and hospices are using the theory. Erickson[23] has noted that what seemed to be a revolutionary idea as recently as 11 to 12 years ago (calling for the client to be the head of the health-care team) is rapidly gaining acceptance, as is the notion that nurses can practice nursing independently. According to Erickson,[23] negative responses to the theory came from individuals who cannot accept the idea of listening to the client first or who do not take the concept of holism seriously.

Brigham and Women's Hospital in Boston has used the Modeling and Role-Modeling Theory as a theoretical basis for their professional practice model in the institution for the past several years. The nurses use the theory as a framework to structure care planning and conduct case conferences. James,[44] the former vice president for nursing, states that "consistency of language, the way care is talked about and planned" is one of the major advantages of using this theoretical basis. The basic fundamentals of the theory are easy to apply in practice and, with a small amount of knowledge, an individual can begin to apply the theory. Nurses at Brigham and Women's Hospital use an adaptation of the assessment tool developed at the University of Michigan Medical Center. At the Fourth National Conference on Modeling and Role-Modeling held in Boston in October 1992, information on the implementation of the professional practice model at Brigham and Women's Hospital and case studies were presented by staff nurses.[44] Nurses at the University of Pittsburgh Medical Center and other hospitals and state agencies across the United States have also adopted the Modeling and Role-Modeling Theory as a foundation for their professional practice model.

Education

The Modeling and Role-Modeling Theory is introduced into the curriculum in the sophomore year at the University of Michigan School of Nursing and is required for returning registered nursing students as well. Faculty members at several nursing schools have contacted Erickson regarding the use of the theory in their curricula. Many use the theory for specific courses. Others, such as Humboldt State University at Arcata, California, have selected modeling and role-modeling as a conceptual framework for their curriculum and have been accredited by the National League for Nursing.[28] Other nursing programs that use the Modeling and Role-Modeling Theory as a basis for curriculum include Metro State University at St. Paul, Minnesota and St. Catherine's University, St. Paul, Minnesota. Foo Yin College of Nursing and Medical Technology is developing a baccalaureate program based on this theory.

Research

Erickson and Swain continue to research the Modeling and Role-Modeling Theory. One study completed was entitled "Modeling and Role-Modeling: Testing Nursing Theory." Research activity continues to support and validate the self-care knowledge construct and the importance of support and control.[21,25] The initial study provided evidence that psychosocial factors are significantly related to physical health problems. A follow-up study in 1988 conducted by Erickson, Lock, and Swain[24] supported these findings, and subsequent research has provided for expansion and enrichment of the concepts. Key concepts include perceived support, perceived control, hope for the future, and satisfaction with daily life. The theorists identify several other research projects that are tests of the theory. Several doctoral students at the University of Michigan School of Nursing, the University of Texas at Austin, and other universities are pursuing various research questions based on the theory. Campbell, Finch, Allport, Erickson, and Swain[11] conducted a research study at the University of Michigan Medical Center and hypothesized that the length of hospital stay correlated with stages of development. They used a nursing assessment tool adapted from the assessment model to measure a patient's psychosocial development and to relate developmental status to the length of hospitalization and the number of health problems identified during hospitalization. Results indicate that the balance of trust-mistrust accounts for a large percentage of the variance in the length of hospitalization. No significant relationship was evident between psychosocial coping skills and the number of health problems identified.

Erickson was the principal investigator of a research project, Modeling and Role-Modeling with Alzheimer's Patients, funded by the National Institutes of Health, National Center for Nursing Research. This research project included 10 other investigators. Results supported the constructs of self-care knowledge and affiliated individuation.[28]

Numerous graduate students have also used the Modeling and Role-Modeling Theory as a basis for their theses and dissertations. In addition, extensive work has been published that substantiates many of the major constructs and theoretical linkages of the theory.[19] Baas[2] and Hertz[39] conducted an integrative review of all research using modeling and role-modeling (through 1992) as a theoretical basis. Empirical evidence has provided bases for validation, refinement, and revision of the theory. Research will continue to expand the Modeling and Role-Modeling Theory.

FURTHER DEVELOPMENT

This theory is in its adolescence; therefore much potential exists for further development. Currently, the theory is gaining national and international attention. One reason for this increased attention is the founding of the Society for the Advancement of Modeling and Role-Modeling. The society was formed to develop a network of colleagues who could advance the development and application of the Modeling and Role-Modeling Theory. One of the goals is to promote continued research related to the theory. The society held its first national symposium in 1986 and has met biennially thereafter. At the 1988 conference, held at Hilton Head, South Carolina, the membership chair announced that society members came from 12 different states.[24] By the time of the 1990 conference in Austin, members represented more than 33 states.[28] These confer-

ences are a forum for researchers, educators, and practitioners to disseminate knowledge pertaining to the Modeling and Role-Modeling Theory and paradigm.[24]

The Fourth National Conference on Modeling and Role-Modeling Theory and Paradigm for Professionals, held in Boston in October 1992, demonstrated the breadth and depth of the current use and research for the Modeling and Role-Modeling Theory. Presentations included studies based in critical care units and community-based practice, in multiple types of educational settings, and across the age span. The most recent conference was held in Minneapolis, Minnesota, June 8-11, 2000. The biennial conferences continue to provide an opportunity for nurses to discuss interrelationships among nursing practice, theory, research, and education.

Much of the research data related to the theory are yet to be published. Erickson[22] states, "Every part of it [the theory] needs further development. . . . There are a thousand research questions in that book. . . . You can take any one statement we make and ask a research question about it. . . . Modeling and Role Modeling has only begun."

CRITIQUE
Clarity

Erickson, Tomlin, and Swain present their theory clearly. Definitions in the theory are denotative, with the concepts explicitly defined. They use everyday language and offer many examples to illustrate their meaning. Their definitions and assumptions are consistent and there is a logical progression from assumptions to assertions.

Simplicity

The theory appears simple at first. However, on closer inspection it becomes complex. It is based on biological and psychological theories and several of the theorists' own assumptions. The interactions among the major concepts, assumptions, and assertions add depth to the theory and increase its complexity.

Generality

Major assumptions that deal with developmental tasks, basic needs satisfaction, object attachment and loss, and adaptive potential are broad enough to be applicable in multiple diverse nursing situations; therefore the theory is generalizable to all nursing and patient situations. The theorists cite many examples of the applicability of their concepts, both in clinical practice and research. Although it may be argued that the theory lacks applicability in the pediatric or comatose population, the theorists believe that the theory is also applicable in these situations, although it may take some creativity by the clinician. The Modeling and Role-Modeling Theory is generalizable to all aspects of professional nursing practice.

Empirical Precision

Empirical precision is increased if the theory has operationally defined concepts, identifiable subconcepts, and denotative definitions. The major concepts, modeling and role-modeling, are reality-based, which makes them more empirical than general. Definitions in the theory are denotative, making it possible to test the concepts identified empirically. The theorists provide an outline for collecting, analyzing, and synthesizing data and guidelines for implementing their theory based on the client's model. These explicit guidelines increase the empirical precision of the theory by allowing any practitioner to test the theory using these tools.

Chinn and Jacobs[13:42] state, "Empirical precision is necessarily increased with research testing." Data reflecting research testing of the theory are not currently readily available; however, as has been stated, studies are ongoing. The Modeling and Role-Modeling Theory will gain empirical precision when data become available for critical analysis. The theorists recognize the need for further research of their theory and encourage practicing nurses to do it.[8]

Derivable Consequences

One of the many challenges facing the profession of nursing is the development of a unique, scientific knowledge base. One aid in this process is the use of nursing theory as a basis for professional practice. The Modeling and Role-Modeling Theory can provide the stimulus to accomplish this goal.

Although this theory is relatively new, it is gaining recognition in the nursing community. As interest grows, additional research supporting its theoretical statements will be generated. Many nurses are engaged in research based on this theory. Publication of the findings will lend credence to the theoretical propositions.

Chinn and Jacobs[13] state that a theory should be evaluated in terms of its derivable consequences. The derivable consequences can be determined by examining whether the theory guides research, directs practice, generates new ideas, and differentiates the focus of nursing from other professions.[13] In terms of these criteria, this theory does appear to possess inherent value, although the scope is not determinable at this time. As the theory matures, the extent of its merit and worth will become evident; however, one thing can undoubtedly be said: Erickson, Tomlin, and Swain's Modeling and Role-Modeling Theory encourages and challenges nurses to practice theory-based nursing.

CRITICAL THINKING *Activities*

1. Interview a client and use the theory to interpret the data. Identify nursing diagnoses based on the interpretations.

2. Given the findings, propose a nursing plan of care. Identify what predictions can be made if the care is not given.

3. Assuming that the goal is to promote the client's health and development, predict the outcome on the basis of the proposed nursing plan of care.

4. Assess the client from primary, secondary, and tertiary sources. Compare for congruency among the three types of sources.

REFERENCES

1. Acton, G. (1993). *Relationships among stressors, stress, affiliated-individuation, burden, and well-being in caregivers of adults with dementia: A test of the theory*

and paradigm for nursing, modeling and role-modeling. Unpublished doctoral dissertation, University of Texas, Austin.

2. Baas, L.S. (1992). The relationships among self-care knowledge, self-care resources, activity level and life satisfaction in persons three to six months after a myocardial infarction. *Dissertation Abstracts International,* 53, 1780B.

3. Babcock, M. & Mueller, P. (1980). *Accidents and life stress.* Unpublished master's thesis, University of Michigan.

4. Barnfather, J.S. (1987). Mobilizing coping resources related to basic need status in healthy, young adults. *Dissertation Abstracts International,* 49/02-B, 0360.

5. Barnfather, J.S. (1990). Mobilizing coping resources related to basic need status. In C. Kinney & H. Erickson (Eds.), *Modeling and role-modeling: Theory, practice and research* (Vol. 1). Austin, TX: Society for the Advancement of Modeling and Role-Modeling.

6. Barnfather, J. (1993). Testing a theoretical proposition for modeling and role-modeling: A basic need and adaptive potential status. *Issues in Mental Health Nursing,* 13, 1-18.

7. Barnfather, J.S. (1990). An overview of the ability to mobilize coping resources related to basic needs. In H. Erickson & C. Kinney (Eds.), *Modeling and role-modeling: Theory, practice and research* (Monogragph 1). Austin, TX: Society for the Advancement of Modeling and Role-Modeling.

8. Boodley, C.A. (1990). The experience of having a healthy examination. In H. Erickson & C. Kinney (Eds.), *Modeling and role-modeling: Theory, practice and research* (Vol. 1). Austin, TX: Society for the Advancement of Modeling and Role-Modeling.

9. Bowman, S.S. (1998). *The human-environment relationship in self-care when healing from episodic illness.* Unpublished doctoral dissertation, University of Texas, Austin.

10. Cain, E. & Perzynski, K. (1986). *Utilization of the self care knowledge model with wife caregivers.* Unpublished master's thesis, University of Michigan.

11. Campbell, J., Finch, D., Allport, C., Erickson, H.C., & Swain, M.A. (1985). A theoretical approach to nursing assessment. *Journal of Advanced Nursing,* 10, 111-115.

12. Chen, Y. (1996). *Relationships among health control orientation, self-efficacy, self-care, and subjective well-being in the elderly with hypertension.* Unpublished doctoral dissertation, University of Texas, Austin.

13. Chinn, P.L. & Jacobs, M.K. (1983). *Theory and nursing: A systematic approach.* St. Louis: Mosby.

14. Clementino, D. & Lapinske, M. (1980). *The effects of different preparatory messages on distress from a bronchoscopy.* Unpublished master's thesis, University of Michigan.

15. Curl, E.D. (1992). Hope in the elderly: Exploring the relationship between psychosocial developmental residual and hope. *Dissertation Abstracts International,* 47, 992B.

16. Darling-Fisher, C. & Leidy, N. (1988). Measuring Eriksonian development of the adult: The modified Erikson psychosocial stage inventory. *Psychological Reports,* 62, 747-754.

17. Doornbos, M. (1983). *The relationship of the social network to emotional health in the aged.* Unpublished master's thesis, University of Michigan.

18. Erickson, H. (1985). Self-care knowledge: Relations among the concepts support, hope, control, satisfaction with life, and physical health. In Sigma Theta Tau International Proceedings, *Social support and health: New directions for theory development and research.* Rochester, NY: University of Rochester.

19. Erickson, H. (1990). Modeling and role-modeling with psychophysiological problems. In J.K. Zeig & S. Gilligan (Eds.), *Brief therapy: Myths, methods, and metaphors.* New York: Brunner/Mazel.

20. Erickson, H. (1990). Theory based nursing. In C. Kinney & H. Erickson (Eds.), *Modeling and role-modeling: Theory, practice and research* (Vol. 1). Austin, TX: Society for the Advancement of Modeling and Role-Modeling.

21. Erickson, H.C. (1976). *Identification of states of coping utilization physiological and psychological data.* Unpublished master's thesis, University of Michigan.

22. Erickson, H.C. (1984, Nov. 5). Telephone interview.

23. Erickson, H.C. (1984, Nov. 7). Telephone interview.

24. Erickson, H.C. (1988). Personal correspondence.

25. Erickson, H.C. (1988, Feb.). Curriculum vitae.

26. Erickson, H.C. (1988, March 30). Telephone interview.

27. Erickson, H.C. (1992, July). Curriculum vitae.

28. Erickson, H.C. (1992, July 1). Personal correspondence.

29. Erickson, H.C. (2000, June, 10). Personal correspondence.

30. Erickson, H.C., Kinney, C., Becker, H., Acton, G., Irvin, B., Hopkins, R., & Jensen, B. (1994). *Modeling and role-modeling with Alzheimer's patients* (National Institutes of Health funded grant). Unpublished manuscript, University of Texas, Austin.

31. Erickson, H.C., Kinney, C., Stone, D., & Acton, G. (1990). *Self-care activities, knowledge, and resources related to physical health.* Unpublished manuscript, University of Texas, Austin.

32. Erickson, H.C. & Swain, M.A. (1982). A model for assessing potential adaptation to stress. *Research in Nursing and Health,* 5, 93-101.

33. Erickson, H.C., Tomlin, E.M., & Swain, M.A. (1983). *Modeling and role-modeling: A theory and paradigm for nursing.* Englewood Cliffs, NJ: Prentice-Hall.

34. Erickson, M. (1996). *Relationships among support, needs satisfaction, and maternal attachment in the adolescent mother.* Unpublished doctoral dissertation, University of Texas, Austin.

35. Erickson, M. (2000). *Development of the Erickson bonding-attachment tool.* Manuscript under review.

36. Finch, D. (1987). *Testing a theoretically based nursing assessment.* Unpublished doctoral dissertation, University of Michigan.

37. Finch, D.A. (1990). Testing a theoretically based nursing assessment. In C. Kinney & H. Erickson (Eds.), *Modeling and role-modeling: Theory, practice and research* (Vol. 1). Austin, TX: Society for the Advancement of Modeling and Role-Modeling.

38. Hannan, J. & McLaughlin, K. (1983). *Relationship between interpersonal trust and compliance in the adolescent with diabetes.* Unpublished master's thesis, University of Michigan.

39. Hertz, J.E.G. (1991). The perceived enactment of autonomy scale: Measuring the potential for self-care action in the elderly. *Dissertation Abstracts International, 52,* 1953B.

40. Holl, R.M. (1992). The effect of role-modeled visiting in comparison to restricted visiting on the well-being of clients who had open heart surgery and their significant family members in the critical care unit. *Dissertation Abstracts International, 53,* 4030B.

41. Hopkins, B.A. (1995). *Adaptive potential of caregivers of adults with dementia.* Paper presented at the meeting of Sigma Theta Tau International, Detroit.

42. Irvin, B.L. (1993). Social support, self-worth and hope as self-care resources for coping with caregiver stress. *Dissertation Abstracts International, 54* (06), B2995.

43. Irvin, B.L. & Acton, G. (1996). Stress meditation in caregivers of cognitively impaired adults: Theoretical model testing. *Nursing Research, 45*(3), 160-166.

44. James, J. (1992, July 6). Telephone interview.

45. Jensen, B. (1995). *Caregiver responses to a theoretically based intervention program: Case study analysis.* Unpublished doctoral dissertation, University of Texas, Austin.

46. Keck, V.E. (1989). Perceived social support, basic needs satisfaction, and coping strategies of the chronically ill. *Dissertation Abstracts International, 50,* 3921B.

47. Kennedy, G.T. (1991). A nursing investigation of comfort and comforting care of the acutely ill patient. *Dissertation Abstracts International, 52,* 6318B.

48. Kinney, C.K. (1990). Facilitating growth and development: A paradigm case for modeling and role-modeling. *Issues in Mental Health Nursing, 11,* 375-395.

49. Kinney, C. (1992). *Psychosocial developmental correlates of coronary prone behavior in healthy adults.* Unpublished manuscript.

50. Kleinbeck, S. (1977). *Coping states of stress.* Unpublished master's thesis, University of Michigan.

51. Kline, N.W. (1988). Psychophysiological processes of stress in people with a chronic physical illness. *Dissertation Abstracts International, 49,* 2129B.

52. Landis, B.J. (1991). Uncertainty, spiritual well-being, and psychosocial adjustment to chronic illness. *Dissertation Abstracts International, 52,* 4124B.

53. MacLean, T.T. (1987). Erikson's development and stressors as factors in healthy lifestyle. *Dissertation Abstracts International, 48,* 1710A.

54. Merton, R.K. (1968). *Social theory and social structure.* New York: The Free Press.

55. Miller, E.W. (1994). *The meaning of encouragement and its connection to the inner-spirit as perceived by caregivers of the cognitively impaired.* Unpublished doctoral dissertation, University of Texas, Austin.

56. Miller, S.H. (1986). The relationship between psychosocial development and coping ability among disabled teenagers. *Dissertation Abstracts International, 47,* 4113B.

57. Raudonis, B. (1991). *A nursing study of empathy from the hospice patient's perspective.* Unpublished doctoral dissertation, University of Texas, Austin.

58. Robinson, K.R. (1992). Developing a scale to measure responses of clients with actual or potential myocardial infarctions. *Dissertation Abstracts International, 53,* 6226B.

59. Rogers, S. (1996). Facilitative affiliation: Nurse-client interactions that enhance healing. *Issues in Mental Health Nursing, 17,* 171-184.

60. Rosenow, D.J. (1991). Multidimensional scaling analysis of self-care actions for reintegrating holistic health after a myocardial infarction: Implications for nursing. *Dissertation Abstracts International, 53,* 1789B.

61. Scheela, R. (1991). *The remodeling process: A grounded study of adult male incest offenders' perceptions of the treatment process.* Unpublished doctoral dissertation, University of Texas, Austin.

62. Smith, K. (1980). *Relationship between social support and goal attainment.* Unpublished master's thesis, University of Michigan.

63. Swain, M.A.P. (1988, Feb.). Curriculum vitae.

64. Tomlin, E.M. (1984, Oct.). Curriculum vitae.

65. Tomlin, E.M. (1988, Feb.). Curriculum vitae.

66. Tomlin, E.M. (1992, July). Curriculum vitae.

67. Tomlin, E.M. (1992, July). Telephone interview.

68. Tomlin, E.M. (1996, July 10). Telephone interview.

BIBLIOGRAPHY
Primary Sources
Books

Erickson, H. & Kinney, C. (Eds.). (1990). *Modeling and role-modeling: Theory, practice and research.* Austin, TX: Society for the Advancement of Modeling and Role-Modeling.

Erickson, H.C., Tomlin, E.M., & Swain, M.A. (1990). *Modeling and role-modeling: A theory and paradigm for nursing.* Austin, TX: EST, Inc.

Book Chapters

Barnfather, J. (1990). An overview of the ability to mobilize coping resources related to basic needs. In H. Erickson & C. Kinney (Eds.), *Modeling and role-modeling: Theory, practice and research* (Vol. 1, pp. 156-169). Austin, TX: Society for the Advancement of Modeling and Role-Modeling.

Boodley, C.A. (1990). The experience of having a healthy examination. In H. Erickson & C. Kinney (Eds.), *Modeling and role-modeling: Theory, practice and research* (Vol. 1, pp. 1170-1177). Austin, TX: Society for the Advancement of Modeling and Role-Modeling.

Erickson, H. (1977). Communication in nursing. In *Professional nursing matrix: A workbook* (pp. 1-150). Ann Arbor, MI: Media Library, University of Michigan.

Erickson, H. (1985). Modeling and role modeling: Ericksonian approaches with physiological problems. In J. Zeig & S. Langton (Eds.), *Ericksonian psychotherapy: The state of the art.* New York: Brunner/Mazel.

Erickson, H. (1990). Modeling and role-modeling with psychophysiological problems. In J.K. Zeig & S. Gilligan (Eds.), *Brief therapy: Myths, methods, and metaphors* (pp. 473-491). New York: Brunner/Mazel.

Erickson, H. (1990). Self-care knowledge: An exploratory study. In C. Kinney & H. Erickson (Eds.), *Modeling and role-modeling: Theory, practice and research* (Vol. 1, pp. 178-202). Austin, TX: Society for the Advancement of Modeling and Role-Modeling.

Erickson, H. (1990). Theory based nursing. In C. Kinney & H. Erickson (Eds.), *Modeling and role-modeling: Theory, practice and research* (Vol. 1, pp. 1-27). Austin, TX: Society for the Advancement of Modeling and Role-Modeling.

Finch, D.A. (1990). Testing a theoretically based nursing assessment. In C. Kinney & H. Erickson (Eds.), *Modeling and role-modeling: Theory, practice and research* (Vol. 1, pp. 203-213). Austin, TX: Society for the Advancement of Modeling and Role-Modeling.

MacLean, T. (1990). Health behaviors, developmental residual and stressors. In C. Kinney & H. Erickson (Eds.), *Modeling and role-modeling: Theory, practice and research* (Vol. 1, pp. 147-155). Austin, TX: Society for the Advancement of Modeling and Role-Modeling.

Tomlin, E.M. (1983). Self-care. In J. Lindberg, M. Hunter, & A. Kruszewski (Eds.), *Introduction to person-centered nursing* (pp. 51-60). Philadelphia: J.B. Lippincott.

Journal Articles

Acton, G. & Miller, E. (1996). Affiliated-individuation in caregivers of adults with dementia. *Issues in Mental Health Nursing, 17,* 245-260.

Barnfather, J. (1993). Testing a theoretical proposition for modeling and role-modeling: A basic need and adaptive potential status. *Issues in Mental Health Nursing, 13,* 1-18.

Barnfather, J., Swain, M.A., Erickson, H. (1989). Construct validity of an aspect of the coping process: Potential adaptation to stress. *Issues in Mental Health Nursing, 10,* 23-40.

Barnfather, J., Swain, M.A., & Erickson, H. (1989). Evaluation of two assessment techniques. *Nursing Science Quarterly, 4,* 172-182.

Beery, T. & Baas, L. (1996). Medical devices and attachment: Holistic healing in the age of invasive technology. *Issues in Mental Health Nursing, 17,* 233-243.

Campbell, J., Finch, D., Allport, C., Erickson, H., & Swain, M. (1985). A theoretical approach to nursing assessment. *Journal of Advanced Nursing, 10,* 111-115.

Darling-Fisher, C. & Leidy, N. (1988). Measuring Eriksonian development of the adult: The modified Erikson psychosocial stage inventory. *Psychological Reports, 62,* 747-754.

Erickson, H. (1983, March). Coping with new systems. *Journal of Nursing Education,* 132-136.

Erickson, H. (1991). Modeling y role-modeling con psychophysiological problemas. Rapport. *Journal of Instituto de Hipnoterapia Ericksoniana.* Buenes Aires, Argentina.

Erickson, H. & Swain, M.A. (1982). A model for assessing potential adaptation to stress. *Research in Nursing and Health, 5,* 93-101.

Erickson, H. & Swain, M.A. (1990). Mobilizing self-care resources: A nursing intervention for hypertension. *Issues in Mental Health Nursing, 11,* 217-236.

Erickson, M. (1996). Factors that influence the mother-infant dyad relationships and infant well-being. *Issues in Mental Health Nursing, 17,* 185-200.

Hertz, J. (1996). Conceptualization of perceived enactment of autonomy in the elderly. *Issues in Mental Health Nursing, 17,* 261-273.

Irvin, B. & Acton, G. (1996). Stress mediation in caregivers of cognitively impaired adults: Theoretical model testing. *Nursing Research, 45(3),* 160-166.

Irvin, B. & Acton, G. (1997). Stress, hope and well-being of women caring for family members with Alzheimer's disease. *Holistic Nursing Practice, 11(2),* 69-79.

Kinney, C. (1996). Transcending breast cancer: Reconstructing one's self. *Issues in Mental Health Nursing, 17,* 201-216.

Kinney, C. & Erickson, H. (1990). Modeling the client's world: A way to holistic care. *Issues in Mental Health Nursing, 11,* 93-108.

Kinney, C.K. (1990). Facilitating growth and development: A paradigm case for modeling and role-modeling. *Issues in Mental Health Nursing, 11,* 375-395.

Landis, B.J. (1996). Uncertainty, spiritual well-being, and psychosocial adjustment to chronic illness. *Issues in Mental Health Nursing, 17,* 217-231.

Leidy, N. (1990). A structural model of stress, psychosocial resources and symptomatic experience in chronic physical illness. *Nursing Research, 39,* 230-236.

Leidy, N. (1994). Operationalizing Maslow's theory: Development and testing of the Basic Needs Satisfaction Inventory. *Issues in Mental Health Nursing, 15,* 277-295.

Leidy, N.K. (1989). A physiological analysis of stress and chronic illness. *Journal of Advanced Nursing, 14,* 868-876.

Leidy, N.K. & Traver, G.A. (1995). Psychophysiological factors contribution to functional performance in people with COPD: Are there gender differences? *Research in Nursing and Health, 18,* 535-546.

MacLean, T. (1992). Influence of psychosocial development and life events on the health practices of adults. *Issues in Mental Health Nursing, 13,* 403-414.

Miller, E.W. (1995). Encouraging Alzheimer's caregivers. *Journal of Christian Nursing, 12*(4), 7-12.

Ozbolt, J. (1987). Developing decision support systems for nursing—theoretical bases for advanced computer systems. *Computers in Nursing, 5,* 105-111.

Robinson, K.R. (1994). Developing a scale to measure denial levels of clients with actual or potential myocardial infarctions. *Heart and Lung, 23,* 36-44.

Rogers, S. (1990). Facilitative affiliation: Nurse-client interactions that enhance healing. *Issues in Mental Health Nursing, 17,* 171-184.

Sappington, J. & Kelley, J.H. (1996). Modeling and role-modeling theory: A case study of holistic care. *Journal of Holistic Nursing, 14*(2), 130-141.

Walsh, K.K., Vanden Bosch, T.M., & Boehm, S. (1989). Modeling and role-modeling: Integrating nursing theory into practice. *Journal of Advanced Nursing, 14,* 775-761.

Abstracts

Erickson, H. (1985). Self-care knowledge: Relations among the concepts support, hope, control, satisfaction with life, and physical health [Abstract]. In Sigma Theta Tau International Proceedings, *Social support and health: New directions for theory development and research* (pp. 208-212). Rochester, NY: University of Rochester.

Erickson, H. (1989). *Mind-body relationships as a factor in the care of people with diabetes* (p. 47) [Abstract]. Third Annual Conference of the Southern Nursing Research Society, Austin, TX.

Erickson, H. (1989). *Study of the self-care knowledge construct* (p. 10) [Abstract]. Third Annual Conference of the Southern Nursing Research Society, Austin, TX.

Erickson, H. (1990). *The McKennell model: using qualitative methods to guide instrument development* (p. 115)

[Abstract]. Fourth Annual Conference of the Southern Nursing Research Society, Orlando.

Erickson, H. (1991). *The relationships among self-care knowledge, self-care resources and physical health* [Abstract]. Proceedings of the Fifth Annual Conference of the Southern Nursing Research Society, Orlando.

Erickson, H. (1993). *Intervention research with cognitively impaired persons and their caregivers. Nursing's Challenge: Leadership in Changing Times* [Abstract]. Sigma Theta Tau International 32nd Biennial Convention, Indianapolis.

Erickson, H. (1995). *Caring, comforting and healing* [Abstract]. Conference Proceedings. Sixth National American Journal of Nursing Conference on Medical-Surgical and Geriatric Nursing.

Erickson, H., Acton, G., Baas, L., Robinson, K., & Rossi, L. (1992). *Strategies to humanize care in the ICU. Proceedings: Celebrating partnerships* [Abstract]. American Association of Critical Care Nursing National Technology Institute, New Orleans.

Erickson, H. & Kennedy, G. (1992). *Viewing the world through the patient's eyes. Proceedings: Celebrating partnerships* [Abstract]. American Association of Critical Care Nursing National Technology Institute, New Orleans.

Erickson, H., Kinney, C., Acton, G., Becker, H., Irvin, B., Jensen, B., & Miller, E. (1994). *An intervention study: Persons with Alzheimer's disease and their caregivers* [Abstract]. Conference Proceedings. The Fifth National Conference for the Theory of Modeling and Role-Modeling, Arcata, CA.

Erickson, H., Lock, S., & Swain, M. (1989). *Continuation of the study of the self-care knowledge construct in the modeling and role-modeling theory. Advances in International Nursing Scholarship. Sigma Theta Tau International Research Congress* (p. 84) [Abstract]. Taipei, Taiwan: Sigma Theta Tau International Honor Society.

Erickson, H.C. & Swain, M.A. (1977). The utilization of a nursing care model for treatment of essential hypertension [Abstract]. *Circulation, 56*(Suppl III), 145.

Theses

Babcock, M. & Mueller, P. (1980). *Accidents and life stress.* Unpublished master's thesis, University of Michigan.

Cain, E. & Perzynski, K. (1986). *Utilization of the self care knowledge model with wife caregivers.* Unpublished master's thesis, University of Michigan.

Calvin, A. (1991). *Personal control: Conceptual analysis and its role in the nursing theory of modeling and role-modeling.* Unpublished master's thesis, University of Texas, Austin.

Cehaich, K. & Nalski, J. (1984). *Life change events, self-concept, and the injury rate of female high school basketball players.* Unpublished master's thesis, University of Michigan.

Clementino, D. & Lapinske, M. (1980). *The effects of different preparatory messages on distress from a bronchoscopy.* Unpublished master's thesis, University of Michigan.

Doornbos, M. (1983). *The relationship of the social network to emotional health in the aged.* Unpublished master's thesis, University of Michigan.

Finch, D. (1987). *Testing a theoretically based nursing assessment.* Unpublished master's thesis, University of Michigan.

Hannan, J. & McLaughlin, K. (1983). *Relationship between interpersonal trust and compliance in the adolescent with diabetes.* Unpublished master's thesis, University of Michigan.

Kirk, L. (1996). *A descriptive study of level of hope in cancer patients.* Unpublished master's thesis, University of Texas, San Antonio.

Kleinbeck, S. (1977). *Coping states of stress.* Unpublished master's thesis, University of Michigan.

Merritt, J. & Swender, K. (1984). *Marital status and social support in elderly women.* Unpublished master's thesis, University of Michigan.

Smith, K. (1980). *Relationship between social support and goal attainment.* Unpublished master's thesis, University of Michigan.

Stein, K. (1986). *Beyond self-esteem: New dimensions in the relationship between the self concept and coping.* Unpublished preliminary examination, University of Michigan.

Walker, M. (1990). *Modeling and role-modeling and quantum physics.* Unpublished master's thesis, University of Texas, Austin.

Dissertations

Acton, G. (1993). *Relationships among stressors, stress, affiliated-individuation, burden, and well-being in caregivers of adults with dementia: A test of the theory and paradigm for nursing, Modeling and Role-modeling.* Unpublished doctoral dissertation, University of Texas, Austin.

Baas, L.S. (1992). The relationships among self-care knowledge, self-care resources, activity level and life satisfaction in persons three to six months after a myocardial infarction. *Dissertation Abstracts International, 53,* 1780B.

Barnfather, J.S. (1987). Mobilizing coping resources related to basic need status in healthy, young adults. *Dissertation Abstracts International, 49,* 360B.

Boodley, C.A. (1986). A nursing study of the experience of having a health examination. *Dissertation Abstracts International, 47,* 992B.

Chen, Y. (1996). *Relationships among health control orientation, self-efficacy, self-care, and subjective well-being in the elderly with hypertension.* Unpublished doctoral dissertation, University of Texas, Austin.

Curl, E.D. (1992). Hope in the elderly: Exploring the relationship between psychosocial developmental residual and hope. *Dissertation Abstracts International, 47,* 992B.

Daniels, R. (1994). *Exploring the self-care variables that explains a wellness lifestyle in spinal cord injured wheelchair basketball athletes.* Unpublished doctoral dissertation, University of Texas, Austin.

Darling-Fisher, C.S. (1987). The relationship between mothers' and fathers' Eriksonian psychosocial attributes, perceptions of family support, and adaptation to parenthood. *Dissertation Abstracts International, 48,* 1640B.

Erickson, M. (1996). *Relationships among support, needs satisfaction, and maternal attachment in the adolescent mother.* Unpublished doctoral dissertation, University of Texas, Austin.

Hertz, J.E.G. (1991). The perceived enactment of autonomy scale: Measuring the potential for self-care action in the elderly. *Dissertation Abstracts International, 52,* 1953B.

Holl, R.M. (1992). The effect of role-modeled visiting in comparison to restricted visiting on the well-being of clients who had open heart surgery and their significant family members in the critical care unit. *Dissertation Abstracts International, 53,* 4030B.

Hopkins, B. (1994). *Assessment of adaptive potential.* Unpublished doctoral dissertation, University of Texas, Austin.

Irvin, B.L. (1993). Social support, self-worth and hope as self-care resources for coping with caregiver stress. *Dissertation Abstracts International, 54*(06), B2995.

Jensen, B. (1995). *Caregiver responses to a theoretically based intervention program: Case study analysis.* Unpublished doctoral dissertation, University of Texas, Austin.

Kennedy, G.T. (1991). A nursing investigation of comfort and comforting care of the acutely ill patient. *Dissertation Abstracts International, 52,* 6318B.

Kline, N.W. (1988). Psychophysiological processes of stress in people with a chronic physical illness. *Dissertation Abstracts International, 49,* 2129B.

Landis, B.J. (1991). Uncertainty, spiritual well-being, and psychosocial adjustment to chronic illness. *Dissertation Abstracts International, 52,* 4124B.

MacLean, T.T. (1987). Erikson's development and stressors as factors in healthy lifestyle. *Dissertation Abstracts International, 48,* 1710A.

Miller, E.W. (1994). *The meaning of encouragement and its connection to the inner-spirit as perceived by caregivers of the cognitively impaired.* Unpublished doctoral dissertation, University of Texas, Austin.

Miller, S.H. (1986). The relationship between psychosocial development and coping ability among disabled teenagers. *Dissertation Abstracts International, 47,* 4113B.

Raudonis, B. (1991). *A nursing study of empathy from the hospice patient's perspective.* Unpublished doctoral dissertation, University of Texas, Austin.

Robinson, K.R. (1992). Developing a scale to measure responses of client with actual or potential myocardial infarctions. *Dissertation Abstracts International,* 53, 6226B.

Rosenow, D.J. (1991). Multidimensional scaling analysis of self-care actions for reintegrating holistic health after a myocardial infarction: Implications for nursing. *Dissertation Abstracts International,* 53, 1789B.

Scheela, R. (1991). *The remodeling process: A grounded study of adult male incest offenders' perceptions of the treatment process.* Unpublished doctoral dissertation, University of Texas, Austin.

Sofhauser, C. (1996). *The relationships among self-esteem, psychosocial residual, self-concept, and hostility in persons with coronary heart disease.* Unpublished doctoral dissertation, University of Texas, Austin.

Straub, H. (1993). *The relationship among intellectual, psychosocial, and ego development of nursing students in associate, baccalaureate, and baccalaureate-completion programs.* Unpublished doctoral dissertation, University of Texas, Austin.

Weber, G. (1995). *Employed mothers with pre-school aged children: An exploration of their lived experiences and the nature of their well-being.* Unpublished doctoral dissertation, University of Texas, Austin.

Correspondence

Erickson, H.C. (1984, Oct.). Curriculum vitae.
Erickson, H.C. (1988, Oct.). Personal correspondence.
Erickson, H.C. (1988, Feb.). Curriculum vitae.
Erickson, H.C. (1992, July). Curriculum vitae.
James, J. (1992, July). Curriculum vitae.
Swain, M.A. (1984, Oct.). Curriculum vitae.
Swain, M.A.P. (1988. Feb.). Curriculum vitae.
Tomlin, E.M. (1984, Oct.). Curriculum vitae.
Tomlin, E.M. (1988, Feb.). Curriculum vitae.
Tomlin, E.M. (1992, July). Curriculum vitae.

Interviews

Erickson, H. (1984, Nov. 5). Telephone interview.
Erickson, H. (1984, Nov. 7). Telephone interview.
Erickson, H.C. (1988, March 30). Telephone interview.
Erickson, H.C. (1992, July 1). Personal correspondence.
Erickson, H.C. (1996, July 9). Personal interview.
James, J. (1992, July 6). Telephone interview.
Tomlin, E.M. (1992, July 6). Telephone interview.
Tomlin, E.M. (1996, July 10). Telephone interview.

Secondary Sources

Book Reviews

[Review of the book *Modeling and role-modeling: A theory and paradigm for nursing*]. (1983, Sept.). *American Journal of Nursing,* 83, 1355.

[Review of the book *Modeling and role-modeling: A theory and paradigm for nursing*]. (1983, Sept.). *Nursing and Health Care,* 4, 413.

[Review of the book *Modeling and role-modeling: A theory and paradigm for nursing*]. (1984, Feb.). *Nursing Outlook,* 32, 116.

Correspondence

Barnfather, J.S. (1988, March). Personal correspondence.
Finch, D. (1988, March). Personal correspondence.

Other Sources

Adamson, J. & Schmale, A. (1965). Object loss, giving up, and the onset of psychiatric disease. *Psychosomatic Medicine,* 27(6), 557-576.

Bartholomew, K. (1990). Avoidance of intimacy: An attachment perspective. *Journal of Social and Personal Relationships,* 7, 147-178.

Bowlby, J. (1958). The nature of the child's tie to his mother. *International Journal of Psychoanalysis,* 39, 89-97.

Bowlby, J. (1960). Child care and the growth of love. In M. Haimowitz & N. Haimowitz (Eds.), *Human development* (2nd ed., pp. 155-166). New York: Thomas Y. Crowell.

Bowlby, J. (1961). Childhood mourning and its explications for psychiatry. *American Journal of Psychiatry,* 118, 481-498.

Bowlby, J. (1961). Process of mourning. *International Journal of Psychoanalysis,* 42, 317-340.

Bowlby, J. (1969). *Attachment.* New York: Basic Books.

Bowlby, J. (1973). *Separation.* New York: Basic Books.

Bowlby, J. (1980). *Loss.* New York: Basic Books.

Bowlby, J., Robertson, J., & Rosenbluth, D. (1952). A two-year-old goes to the hospital. *Psychoanalytic Study of the Child,* 7, 89-94.

Chinn, P.L. & Kramer, M.K. (1994). *Theory and nursing: A systematic approach* (3rd ed.). St. Louis: Mosby.

Engel, G. (1968). A life setting conducive to illness: The giving-up—given-up complex. *Annuals of Internal Medicine,* 69,(2), 293-300.

Engel, G.S. (1962). *Psychological development in health and disease.* Philadelphia: W.B. Saunders.

Erikson, E. (1960). Identity versus self-diffusion. In M. Haimowitz & N. Haimowitz (Eds.), *Human development* (2nd ed., pp. 766-770). New York: Thomas Y. Crowell.

Erikson, E. (1960). The case of Peter. In M. Haimowitz & N. Haimowitz, *Human development* (2nd ed.) (pp. 355-359). New York: Thomas Y. Crowell.

Erikson, E. (1963). *Childhood and society.* New York: W.W. Norton.

Erickson, H. (1986). *Synthesizing clinical experiences: A step in theory development.* Ann Arbor, MI: Biomedical Communications.

Haley, J. (1973). *Uncommon therapy: The psychiatric techniques of Milton H. Erickson, M.D.* New York: W.W. Norton.

Hassan, A. & Hassan, B.M. (1987). Interpersonal development across the life span: Communion and its interaction with agency in psychosocial development. In L.A. Meachem (Ed.), *Contributions to human development* (Vol. 18, pp. 102-127). Basel: Werner Druck AG.

Klein, M. (1952). Some theoretical conclusions regarding the emotional life of the infant. In J. Riviere (Ed.), *Developments in psycho-analysis* (pp. 198-236). London: Hogarth Press.

Mahler, M.S. (1967). On human symbiosis and the vicissitudes of individuation. *Journal of the American Psychoanalytic Association, 15,* 740-763.

Mahler, M.S. & Furer, M. (1968). *On human symbiosis and the vicissitudes of individuation (Vol. I). Infantile psychosis.* New York: International Universities Press.

Maslow, A.H. (1936). The need to know and the fear of knowing. *Journal of General Psychology, 68,* 111-125.

Maslow, A.H. (1968). *Toward a psychology of being* (2nd ed.). New York: D. Von Nostrand.

Maslow, A.H. (1970). *Motivation and personality* (2nd ed.). New York: Harper & Row.

Merton, R.K. (1968). *Social theory and social structure.* New York: The Free Press.

Montgomery, C. & Webster, D. (1993). Caring and nursing's metaparadigm: Can they survive the era of managed care? *Perspectives in Psychiatric Care, 29*(4), 5-12.

Piaget, J. (1952). *The origins of intelligence in children.* New York: International Universities Press.

Piaget, J. (1974). The pathway between subjects' recent life changes and their near-future illness reports: Representative results and methodological issues. In B.S. Dohrenwend & B.P. Dohrenwend (Eds.), *Stressful life events: Their nature and effects* (pp. 73-86). New York: John Wiley & Sons.

Piaget, J. & Inhelder, B. (1969). *The psychology of the child.* New York: Basic Books.

Rossi, E. (1986). *The psychobiology of mind-body healing.* New York: W.W. Norton.

Selye, H. (1974). *Stress without distress.* Philadelphia: J.B. Lippincott.

Selye, H. (1976). *The stress of life* (2nd ed.). New York: McGraw-Hill.

Selye, H. (1979). Further thoughts on stress without distress. *Resident and Staff Physician, 25,* 125-134.

Stoddard, J. & Stoddard, H.J. (1985). Affectional bonding and the impact of bereavement. *Advances: Institute for the Advancement of Health, 2*(2), 19-28.

Winnicott, D.W. (1953). Transitional objects and transitional phenomena: A study of the first not-me possession. *International Journal of Psychoanalysis, 34,* 89-97.

Winnicott, D.W. (1965). The theory of the parent-infant relationship. In D.W. Winnicott (Ed.), *The maturational processes and the facilitating environment.* London: Hogarth Press.

APPENDIX

ASSESSMENT TOOL BASED ON MODELING AND ROLE-MODELING*

1. Description of the situation
   a. Overview of the situation
   b. Etiology
      (1) Eustressors
      (2) Stressors
      (3) Distressors
   c. Therapeutic needs
2. Expectations
   a. Immediately
   b. Long term
3. Resource potential
   a. External
      (1) Social network
      (2) Support system
      (3) Healthcare system
   b. Internal
      (1) Strengths
      (2) Adaptive potential
         (a) Feeling states
         (b) Physiological parameters
4. Goals and life tasks
   a. Current
   b. Future

*Interview questions and thoughts that guide critical thinking are suggested in Erickson, H.C., Tomlin, E.M., & Swain, M.A. (1983). *Modeling and role-modeling: A theory and paradigm for nursing* (pp. 116-168). Englewood Cliffs, NJ: Prentice-Hall. Suggestions for interviewing techniques are found in Erickson, H.C. (1990). Self-care knowledge. In H.C. Erickson & C. Kinney (Eds.), *Modeling and role-modeling: Theory, practice and research.* Austin, TX: Society for the Advancement of Modeling and Role-Modeling.

Continued

APPENDIX—cont'd

DATA INTERPRETATION TOOL BASED ON MODELING AND ROLE-MODELING[†]

1. Interpret data for ability to mobilize resources (APAM)
2. Interpret data for needs status (assets and deficits related to type of need), attachment objects, loss, grief (normal or morbid), life tasks (developmental: actual and chronological)

DATA ANALYSIS TOOL BASED ON MODELING AND ROLE-MODELING[‡]

1. Step one
   a. Articulate relationships between stressors and needs status
   b. Articulate relationships between needs status and ability to mobilize resources
   c. Articulate relationships between needs status and loss of attachment
   d. Articulate relationships between loss and type of grief response
   e. Articulate relationships between type of need assets and deficits and developmental residual
   f. Articulate relationships between chronological developmental task and developmental residual
2. Step two
   a. Articulate relationships among stressors, resource potential, needs status, loss, grief status, developmental residual, chronological task, and attachment potential
   b. Articulate relationships among needs, status, potential resources, developmental residual, and personal goals

PLANNING TOOL BASED ON MODELING AND ROLE-MODELING[§]

1. Aims of interventions
   a. Build trust
   b. Promote positive orientation
   c. Promote client control
   d. Promote strengths
   e. Set health-directed goals
2. Intervention goals
   a. Develop a trusting and functional relationship between yourself and your client
   b. Facilitate a self-projection that is futuristic and positive
   c. Promote AI with the minimum degree of ambivalence possible
   d. Promote a dynamic, adaptive, and holistic state of health
   e. Promote and nurture a coping mechanism that satisfies basic needs and permits growth-need satisfaction
   f. Facilitate congruent actual and chronological developmental stages

[†]Critical thinking guidelines for data interpretation are suggested in Erickson, H.C., Tomlin, E.M., & Swain, M.A. (1983). *Modeling and role-modeling: A theory and paradigm for nursing* (pp. 148-166). Englewood Cliffs, NJ: Prentice-Hall; and Erickson, H.C. (1990). Theory based nursing. In H.C. Erickson & C. Kinney (Eds.), *Modeling and role-modeling: Theory, practice and research*. Austin, TX: Society for the Advancement of Modeling and Role-Modeling.

[‡]Critical thinking guidelines for data analysis are suggested in Erickson, H.C., Tomlin, E.M., & Swain, M.A. (1983). *Modeling and role-modeling: A theory and paradigm for nursing* (pp. 148-166). Englewood Cliffs, NJ: Prentice-Hall; and Erickson, H.C. (1990). Theory based nursing. In H.C. Erickson & C. Kinney (Eds.), *Modeling and role-modeling: Theory, practice and research*. Austin, TX: Society for the Advancement of Modeling and Role-Modeling.

[§]Critical thinking guidelines are suggested in Erickson, H.C., Tomlin, E.M., & Swain, M.A. (1983). *Modeling and role-modeling: A theory and paradigm for nursing* (pp. 169-220). Englewood Cliffs, NJ: Prentice-Hall; and Erickson, H.C. (1990). Theory based nursing. In H.C. Erickson & C. Kinney (Eds.), *Modeling and role-modeling: Theory, practice and research*. Austin, TX: Society for the Advancement of Modeling and Role-Modeling.

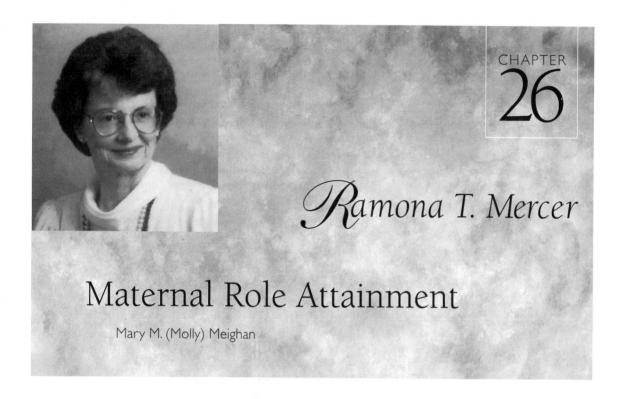

Ramona T. Mercer

Maternal Role Attainment

Mary M. (Molly) Meighan

CREDENTIALS AND BACKGROUND OF THE THEORIST

Ramona T. Mercer began her nursing career in 1950 when she received her diploma from St. Margaret's School of Nursing in Montgomery, Alabama. She graduated with the L.L. Hill Award for Highest Scholastic Standing. She returned to school in 1960 after working as a staff nurse, head nurse, and instructor in the areas of pediatrics, obstetrics, and contagious diseases. She completed a B.S.N. degree in 1962, graduating with distinction from the University of New Mexico, Albuquerque. She went on to earn an M.S.N. in maternal child nursing from Emory University in 1964 and completed a Ph.D. in maternity nursing from the University of Pittsburgh in 1973.

After receiving a Ph.D., Mercer moved to California and accepted the position of assistant professor

Previous authors: Mary M. (Molly) Meighan, Alberta M. Bee, Denise Legge, and Stephanie Oetting.

in the Department of Family Health Care Nursing at the University of California, San Francisco. She was promoted to associate professor in 1977 and in 1983, she accepted a position as professor. She remained in that role until her retirement in 1987. Currently, Dr. Mercer is Professor Emeritus in Family Health Nursing at the University of California, San Francisco. Today, she is active in writing, speaking engagements, and consultations.[23,29]

Throughout her career, Mercer has received several awards. In 1963, while working and pursuing studies in nursing, she received the Department of Health, Education, and Welfare Public Health Service Nurse Trainee Award at Emory University and was inducted into Sigma Theta Tau. She received this award again during her years at the University of Pittsburgh. She also received the Bixler Scholarship for Nursing Education and Research, Southern Regional Board for doctoral study. In 1982, she received the Maternal Child Health Nurse of the Year Award by the National Foundation of the March of

Dimes and American Nurses Association, Division of Maternal Child Health Practice. She was presented with the Fourth Annual Helen Nahm Lecturer Award at the University of California, San Francisco School of Nursing in 1984. Mercer's research awards include the American Society for Psychoprophylaxis in Obstetrics (ASPO)/Lamaze National Research Award in 1987; the Distinguished Research Lectureship Award, Western Institute of Nursing, Western Society for Research in Nursing in 1988; and the American Nurses Foundation's Distinguished Contribution to Nursing Science Award in 1990.[19,23,29]

Mercer has authored numerous articles, editorials, and commentaries. In addition, she has published six books and six book chapters. In early research efforts, Mercer focused on the behaviors and needs of breast-feeding mothers, mothers with postpartum illness, and mothers bearing infants with defects. The results were published in several articles and led to the writing of *Nursing Care for Parents at Risk,* which was published in 1977.[8] Her first book received an *American Journal of Nursing* Book of the Year Award in 1978. Preceding research led Mercer to study family relationships, antepartal stress as related to familial relationships and the maternal role, and mothers of various ages. A portion of that work concerning teenage mothers over the first year of motherhood, resulted in the book *Perspectives on Adolescent Health Care,*[9] which also received an *American Journal of Nursing* Book of the Year Award in 1980. In 1986, Mercer's work on mothers at various ages was drawn together in her third book, *First-Time Motherhood: Experiences From Teens to Forties.*[15] Mercer's fifth book, *Parents at Risk,*[21] published in 1990, also received an *American Journal of Nursing* Book of the Year Award. *Parents at Risk*[21] focuses on strategies for facilitating early parent-infant interactions and promoting parental competence in relation to specific risk situations. Mercer's sixth book, *Becoming a Mother: Research on Maternal Role Identity Since Rubin,*[26] was published by Springer Publishing Company of New York in 1995. This book contains a more complete description of Mercer's Theory of Maternal Role Attainment and her framework for studying variables that impact the maternal role.[26]

Since her first publication in 1968, Mercer has published numerous articles for both nursing and nonnursing journals and continues to write for *Nurseweek.* Some of her most recent writing is found on the Internet at the *Nurseweek* site (http://www.nurseweek.com)[27,28,32] and includes:
Adolescent sexuality and childbearing:
    (http://www.cyberchalk.com/nurse/courses/
    nurseweek/NW0520new/course.html)
The employed mother's challenges:
    (http://www.nurseweek.com/ce/ce250a.html)
Transitions to Parenthood:
    (http://nurse.cyberchalk.com/nurse/courses/
    nurseweek/nw/1850/menu.html)

Mercer has maintained membership in seven professional organizations, including the American Nurses Association and the American Academy of Nursing, and has been an active member on many national committees. From 1983 to 1990, she was the associate editor of *Health Care for Women International.* She has served on the review panel for *Nursing Research* and *Western Journal of Nursing Research* and was on the executive advisory board of *California Nursing* and *Nurseweek.* She has also served as a reviewer for numerous grant proposals. Additionally, she has been actively involved with regional, national, and international scientific and professional meetings and workshops.[25,29]

THEORETICAL SOURCES

Mercer's Theory of Maternal Role Attainment is based on her extensive research on the topic beginning in the late 1960s. The stimulus for both research and theory development came from Mercer's admiration of her professor and mentor, Reva Rubin, at the University of Pittsburgh. Rubin[42,43] is well known for her work in defining and describing maternal role attainment as a process of *binding-in* or being attached to the child and *maternal role identity* or seeing oneself in the role and having a sense of comfort about it. Mercer's framework and study variables clearly reflect many of Rubin's concepts.

In addition to Rubin's work, Mercer[11,17,26] relied on both role and developmental theories. She relied

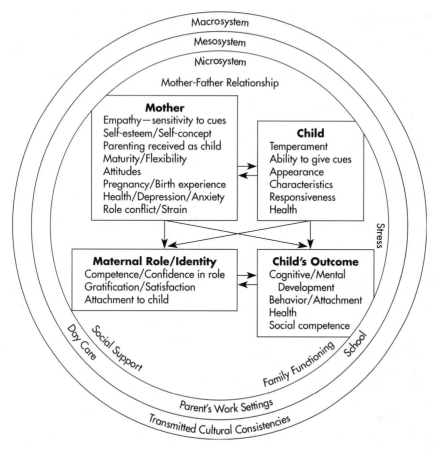

Figure **26-1 Proposed model of Maternal Role Attainment.** (Modified from a paper presented by Ramona T. Mercer at symposium, "Maternal Role: Models and Consequences," at the International Research Conference sponsored by the Council of Nurse Researchers and the American Nurses Association, Los Angeles, CA. Copyright © 1991 by Ramona T. Mercer. Reprinted with permission. Note: This figure has been modified based on personal communication with R.T. Mercer.[30] The word *exosystem* was replaced with the word *mesosystem* to be more consistent with Bronfenbrenner's model[1] on which it is based.)

heavily on an interactionist approach to role theory, using Mead's theory on role enactment and Turner's theory on the *core self*.[17] In addition, Thornton and Nardi's role acquisition process also helped shape Mercer's theory, as did the work of Burr, Leigh, Day, and Constantine.[11,17] Werner and Erikson's developmental process theories also contributed.[16,17] Mercer's work is also based on von Bertalanffy's General System Theory.[45] Her model of maternal role attainment depicted in Figure 26-1 uses Bronfenbrenner's nested circles as a general systems approach.[1]

The complexity of her research interest led Mercer to rely on many other theoretical sources to identify and study variables that affect maternal role attainment. Although much of her work was based on Rubin's theories, she also looked to Gottlieb's research on attachment and caretaking roles and the most current research on maternal-infant relationships.[11]

In her work with high-risk families, she examined the Life Span Developmental Models of Baltes, Reese, and Lipsitt and research on families by Rankin and Weekes.[20] Gloger-Tippelt's Process Model for the Course of Pregnancy also influenced Mercer to examine maternal role attainment as a process.[17]

USE OF EMPIRICAL EVIDENCE

Mercer selected both maternal and infant variables for her studies on the basis of her review of the literature and findings of researchers in several different disciplines. She found that many factors may have a direct or indirect influence on the maternal role, adding to the complexity of her studies. Maternal factors in Mercer's research included age at first birth, birth experience, early separation from the infant, social stress, social support, personality traits, self-concept, child-rearing attitudes, and health. She included the infant variables of temperament, appearance, responsiveness, health status, and ability to give cues. Mercer also noted the importance of the father's role and applied many of her previous findings in studying the paternal response to parenthood. Her research required the use of numerous instruments to measure the variables of interest.

Mercer has studied these variables in her research efforts over several intervals including the immediate postpartum period and one month, four months, eight months, and one year following birth. In addition, she has included adolescents, older mothers, ill mothers, mothers dealing with congenital defects, families experiencing antepartal stress, parents at high risk, mothers who had cesarean deliveries, paternal-infant attachment, and parental competence in her research.

Major Concepts & Definitions

Mercer bases her theory for Maternal Role Attainment on the following factors.

MATERNAL ROLE ATTAINMENT

An interactional and developmental process occurring over time in which the mother becomes attached to her infant, acquires competence in the care-taking tasks involved in the role, and expresses pleasure and gratification in the role.[15] "The movement to the personal state in which the mother experiences a sense of harmony, confidence, and competence in how she performs the role is the end point of maternal role attainment—maternal identity."[11:74]

MATERNAL AGE

Chronological and developmental.[17]

PERCEPTION OF BIRTH EXPERIENCE

A woman's perception of her performance during labor and birth.[21]

EARLY MATERNAL-INFANT SEPARATION

Separation from the mother after birth resulting from illness and/or prematurity.[21]

SELF-ESTEEM

"An individual's perception of how others view one and self-acceptance of the perceptions."[40:341]

SELF-CONCEPT (SELF-REGARD)

"The overall perception of self that includes self-satisfaction, self-acceptance, self-esteem, and congruence or discrepancy between self and ideal self."[15:18]

FLEXIBILITY

Roles are not rigidly fixed; therefore who fills the roles is not important.[21] "Flexibility of childrearing attitudes increases with increased development. . . . Older mothers have the potential to respond less

MAJOR CONCEPTS & DEFINITIONS—cont'd

rigidly to their infants and to view each situation in respect to the unique nuances."[15:43,21:12]

CHILDREARING ATTITUDES

Maternal attitudes or beliefs about childrearing.[15]

HEALTH STATUS

"The mother's and father's perception of their prior health, current health, health outlook, resistance-susceptibility to illness, health worry concern, sickness orientation, and rejection of the sick role."[40:342]

ANXIETY

"A trait in which there is specific proneness to perceive stressful situations as dangerous or threatening, and as situation-specific state."[40:342]

DEPRESSION

"Having a group of depressive symptoms, and in particular the affective component of the depressed mood."[40:342]

ROLE STRAIN

The conflict and difficulty felt by the woman in fulfilling the maternal role obligation.[14]

GRATIFICATION

"The satisfaction, enjoyment, reward, or pleasure that a woman experiences in interacting with her infant, and in fulfilling the usual tasks inherent in mothering."[16:296]

ATTACHMENT

A component of the parental role and identity. Attachment is viewed as a process in which an enduring affectional and emotional commitment to an individual is formed.[21]

INFANT TEMPERAMENT

An easy versus a difficult temperament; it is related to whether the infant sends hard-to-read cues,

leading to feelings of incompetence and frustration in the mother.[15]

INFANT HEALTH STATUS

Illness causing maternal-infant separation, interfering with the attachment process.[15]

INFANT CHARACTERISTICS

Temperament, appearance, and health status.[11]

FAMILY

"A dynamic system which includes subsystems—individuals (mother, father, fetus/infant) and dyads (mother-father, mother-fetus/infant, and father-fetus/infant) within the overall family system."[40:339]

FAMILY FUNCTIONING

The individual's view of the activities and relationships between the family and its subsystems and broader social units.[36]

STRESS

Positively and negatively perceived life events and environmental variables.[21]

SOCIAL SUPPORT

"The amount of help actually received, satisfaction with that help, and the persons (network) providing that help."[40:341]

Four areas of social support are the following:

Emotional Support

"Feeling loved, cared for, trusted, and understood."[15:14]

Informational Support

"Helps the individual help herself by providing information that is useful in dealing with the problem and/or situation."[15:14]

Physical Support

A direct kind of help.[39]

Continued

MAJOR CONCEPTS & DEFINITIONS—cont'd

Appraisal Support

"A support that tells the role taker how she is performing in the role; it enables the individual to evaluate herself in relationship to others' performance in the role."[15:14]

MOTHER-FATHER RELATIONSHIP

Perception of the mate relationship that includes intended and actual values, goals, and agreements between the two.[17]

MAJOR ASSUMPTIONS

For maternal role attainment, Mercer stated the following assumptions:

1. A relatively stable *core self,* acquired through lifelong socialization, determines how a mother defines and perceives events; her perceptions of her infant's and others' responses to her mothering, with her life situation, are the real world to which she responds.[15]

2. In addition to the mother's socialization, her developmental level and innate personality characteristics also influence her behavioral responses.[15]

3. The mother's role partner, her infant, will reflect the mother's competence in the mothering role through growth and development.[15]

4. The infant is considered an active partner in the maternal role-taking process, affecting and being affected by the role enactment.[11]

5. The father or mother's intimate partner contributes to role attainment in a way that cannot be duplicated by any other supportive person.[26,30]

6. Maternal identity develops with maternal attachment and each depends on the other.[24,42]

Nursing

Mercer[12:xii] does not define nursing, but refers to nursing as a science emerging from "a turbulent adolescence to adulthood." Nurses are the health professionals having the most "sustained and intense interaction with women in the maternity cycle."[10:xi] Nurses are responsible for promoting the health of families and children; nurses are *pioneers* in developing and sharing assessment strategies for these patients.[10]

In her writing, Mercer refers to the importance of nursing care. Although she does not specifically mention nursing care, Mercer[26] emphasizes that the kind of help or care a woman receives during pregnancy and over the first year following birth can have long-term effects for her and her child. Nurses in maternal-child settings play a sizable role in providing both care and information during this period.

Person

Mercer[14] does not specifically define person, but refers to the *self* or *core self.* She views the self as separate from the roles that are played. Through maternal individuation, a woman may regain her own *personhood* as she extrapolates her *self* from the mother-infant dyad.[15] The core self evolves from a culture context and determines how situations are defined and shaped.[14] The concepts of self-esteem and self-confidence are important in attainment of the maternal role.

The mother as a person is seen as separate, but in interaction with her infant and with the father or her significant other. She is both influential and is influenced by both of them.[26]

Health

In her theory, Mercer defines health status as the mother and father's perception of their prior health, current health, health outlook, resistance-susceptibility to illness, health worry or concern, sickness orientation, and rejection of the sick role. Health status of the newborn is the extent of disease present and infant health status by parental rating of overall health.[15] The health status of a family is negatively affected by antepartum stress. Health status is an important indirect influence on satisfaction with relationships in childbearing families.

Health is also viewed as a desired outcome for the child, influenced by both maternal and infant variables, and achieved through maternal role identity. Mercer[26] stresses the importance of healthcare during the childbearing and child-rearing process.

Environment

Mercer[26,31] defines the environment according to Bronfenbrenner's definition of the ecological environment on which her model in Figure 26-1 is based. The model illustrates the ecological environment in which maternal role attainment develops. Mercer[31] explains, "Development of a role/person cannot be considered apart from the environment; there is a mutual accommodation between the developing person and the changing properties of the immediate settings, relationships between the settings, and the larger contexts in which the settings are embedded." The ecological environment, according to Bronfenbrenner, may be viewed as a nested arrangement of systems within the next.[26] Mercer's model in Figure 26-1 shows this nesting of the mother and infant within the microsystem, mesosystem, and macrosystem.

Stresses within the environment influence both maternal and paternal role attainment and the developing child. Mercer's model as shown in Figure 26-1 indicates that environmental factors such as social support, stress, and family functioning within the microsystem and environmental factors such as work setting, school, and daycare impact role attainment.

THEORETICAL ASSERTIONS

Mercer's Theory of Maternal Role Attainment and Model was first introduced in 1991 during a symposium at the International Research Conference sponsored by the Council of Nursing Research and American Nurses Association in Los Angeles, California.[22] Since that time, it has been refined based on current studies and is more clearly presented in her latest book, *Becoming a Mother: Research on Maternal Role Identity Since Rubin.*[26]

Mercer's Model of Maternal Role Attainment is placed within Bronfenbrenner's nested circles of the microsystem, mesosystem, and macrosystem (see Figure 26-1).[1] The original model proposed by Mercer was altered based on Mercer's most recent writings and a personal communication with her on January 4, 2000.[26,30] The term *exosystem* originally found in the second circle was replaced with the term *mesosystem.* Mercer[30] explained that this change makes the model more consistent with Bronfenbrenner's model.

1. The immediate environment in which maternal role attainment occurs is the microsystem, which includes the family and factors such as family functioning, mother-father relationships, social support, and stress. The variables contained within the microsystem interact with one or more of the other variables in affecting the maternal role. The infant as an individual is embedded within the family system. The family is viewed as a semiclosed system maintaining boundaries and control over interchange between the family system and other social systems.[21]

   The microsystem is the most influential on maternal role attainment.[26,30] In 1995, Mercer[26:15] expanded her earlier concepts and model to emphasize the importance of the father on role attainment, stating that he helps "diffuse tension developing within the mother-infant dyad." Maternal role attainment is achieved within the microsystem through the interactions of father, mother, and infant. Figure 26-2, first introduced in Mercer's sixth book, *Becoming a Mother: Research on Maternal Role Identity Since Rubin*[26] depicts this interaction. In Figure 26-2, the layers *a* through *d* represent the stages of maternal role attainment from anticipatory to personal (role identity) and the infant's growth and developmental stages.[26]

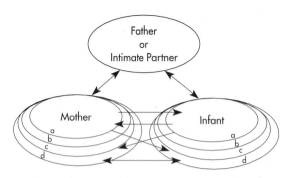

Figure **26-2** A microsystem within the evolving model of Maternal Role Attainment. (From Mercer, R.T. [©1995]. *Becoming a mother: Research on maternal role identity since Rubin.* New York: Springer Publishing Company, Inc., New York 10012 Used by permission.)

2. The mesosystem encompasses, influences, and delimits the microsystem. The mother-infant unit is not contained within the mesosystem, but the mesosystem may determine in part what happens to the developing maternal role and the child. It includes extended family, school, work, church and other entities within the mother's more immediate community. The *exosystem,* a term used in Mercer's first model, is an extension of the mesosytem, and it is defined as the interrelationships of two or more settings or subsystems that influence the mother more indirectly.[26,30] An example of the exosystem would be interactions between work setting, day care, local laws and rules, community, and church.

3. The macrosystem refers to the general prototypes existing in a particular culture or transmitted cultural consistencies. The macrosystem includes the social, political, and cultural influences on the other two systems. The healthcare environment and the impact of the current healthcare system on maternal role attainment originates in the macrosystem.[26]

Maternal role attainment is a process that follows four stages of role acquisition; these stages have been adapted from Thornton and Nardi's 1975 research.[21] As previously stated, these four stages are indicated in Figure 26-2 as the layers *a* through *d*.

a. Anticipatory: The anticipatory stage begins in pregnancy and includes the initial social and psychological adjustments to pregnancy. The mother learns the expectations of the role, fantasizes about the role, relates to the fetus in utero, and begins role play.

b. Formal: The formal stage begins with the birth of the infant and includes learning and taking on the role of mother. Role behaviors are guided by formal, consensual expectations of others in the mother's social system.

c. Informal: Begins as the mother develops unique ways of dealing with the role not conveyed by the social system. The woman makes her new role fit within her existing lifestyle based on past experiences and future goals.

d. Personal: The personal or role-identity stage occurs as the woman internalizes her role. The mother experiences a sense of harmony, confidence, and competence in the way she performs the role and the maternal role is achieved.

Stages of role attainment overlap and are altered as the infant grows and develops. The final stage of maternal role identity may be achieved in a month, or it can take several months.[26] The stages are influenced by social support, stress, family functioning, and the relationship between mother and father or significant other.

Traits and behaviors of both the mother and the infant may influence maternal role identity and child outcome. Maternal traits and behaviors included in Mercer's model are empathy, sensitivity to infant cues, self-esteem and self-concept, parenting received as a child, maturity and flexibility, attitude, pregnancy and birth experience, health, depression, and role conflict. Infant traits having an impact on maternal role identity include temperament, ability to send cues, appearance, general characteristics, responsiveness, and health.

According to Mercer, the maternal role is attained when the mother feels internal harmony with the role and its expectations. She describes three major components of the role: "(1) attachment to the infant, (2) gaining competence in mothering behaviors, and (3) expressing gratification in maternal-infant interactions."[15:6,26:13] Outcome for the child includes cognitive and mental development, attachment, health, and social competence.

LOGICAL FORM

Mercer used both deductive and inductive logic in developing the theoretical framework for studying factors that influence maternal role attainment in the first year of motherhood and in her theory. Deductive logic is demonstrated in Mercer's use of works from other researchers and disciplines. Role and developmental theories and the work of Rubin on maternal role attainment provided a base for the framework. Mercer also used inductive logic in the development of her Maternal Role Attainment Theory. Through practice and research, she observed adaptation to motherhood from a variety of circumstances. She noted that differences existed in adaptation to motherhood when maternal illness complicated the postpartum period, when a child with a defect was born, and when a teenager became a mother. These observations directed the research about those situations and subsequently the development of her theory.

ACCEPTANCE BY THE NURSING COMMUNITY

Practice

Mercer's theory is highly practice oriented. The concepts in her theory have been cited in many obstetrical textbooks and have been used in practice by nurses and those in other disciplines. Both the theory and the proposed model are capable of serving as a framework for assessment, planning, implementing, and evaluating nursing care of new mothers and their infants. The utility of Mercer's theory and its relationship to practice is described by Meighan in the second edition of *Nursing Theory: Utilization and Application* by Alligood and Marriner Tomey.[7]

Mercer's theory is also useful to practicing nurses across many maternal-child settings. In her book, *First-Time Motherhood: Experiences From Teens to Forties,*[15] Mercer links her research findings with nursing practice at each time interval from birth through the first year, making her theory applicable in a variety of pediatric settings.

In addition, Mercer's theory has been used in organizing patient care. Concepts in the research conducted by Neeson, Patterson, Mercer, and May, *Pregnancy Outcomes for Adolescents Receiving Prenatal Care by Nurse Practitioners in Extended Roles,*[41] were used in setting up a clinical practice.

Education

As previously stated, Mercer's work has appeared extensively in nursing texts, but not only as it relates to maternal role attainment; each individual piece of research is used and valued. Many of the current concepts in maternal child nursing texts are based on Mercer's research.

Mercer's theory and model help simplify a very complex process, enhancing understanding and making Mercer's contribution extremely valuable to nursing education.

Research

Mercer has advocated the involvement of students in faculty research. During her tenure at the University of California, San Francisco, she chaired committees and was a committee member for numerous graduate theses and dissertations. Her work has been used as the basis for several graduate students' topics of research.[18,19] Collaborative research with a graduate student and junior faculty member in 1977 and 1978 led to the development of a highly reliable, valid instrument to measure mothers' attitudes about the labor and delivery experience.[19] Numerous researchers have requested permission to use the instrument.

Mercer's numerous research and scholarly achievements are evidence of her great contribution to nursing research. Her work has served as a springboard for other researchers. Mercer's theoretical framework for a correlational study exploring differences between three age groups for first-time mothers (ages 15 to 19, 20 to 29, and 30 to 42) has been tested in part by others, including Walker, Crain, and Thompson;[46,47] University of Texas, Austin; and as reported in *Nursing*

Research. In 1991, Sank[44] used Mercer's theory in her doctoral dissertation research at the University of Texas, Austin, entitled *Factors in the Prenatal Period that Affect Parental Role Attainment During the Post-partum Period in Black American Mothers and Fathers.*

McBride[6:72] wrote, "Maternal role attainment has been a fundamental concern of nursing since the pioneering work of Mercer's mentor, Rubin, almost two decades ago. It is now becoming the research-based, theoretically sound construct that nurse researchers have been searching for in their analysis of the experience of new mothers."

FURTHER DEVELOPMENT

Mercer used her initial research as a building block for other studies. In later research, Mercer aimed at identifying predictors of maternal-infant attachment on the basis of maternal experience with childbirth and maternal risk status. She also examined paternal competence on the basis of experience with childbirth and pregnancy risk status. In another study, she developed and tested a causal model to predict partner relationships in high- and low-risk pregnancy. More work and refinement of the original model and theory has taken place in the past few years as described earlier. Based on more recent research, she included the importance of the father in maternal role attainment, adding this to her model and theory in a section of her most recent book, *Becoming a Mother: Research on Maternal Role Identity Since Rubin.*[26] Mercer is devoted to expanding and describing her theory more clearly. This is evidenced in that some of her original ideas have been abandoned. In her book, *First-Time Motherhood: Experiences From Teens to Forties,*[15] Mercer presents a model of four phases occurring in the process of maternal role attainment during the first year of motherhood. The four phases are labeled as follows: (1) the physical recovery phase, occurring from birth to one month; (2) the achievement phase from two to four or five months; (3) the disruptions phase, occurring from six to eight months; and (4) the reorganization phase, from after the eighth month and still in process at one year.[15] Additionally, adaptation to the maternal role is proposed to occur at three levels (biological, psychological, and social), which are interacting and interdependent throughout the phases. These phases and levels of adaptation are briefly described and have been applied to her research. This model appears logical and useful, but is in need of further explanation, exposure, and development.

According to Mercer, there are several areas in need of further research. More testing and revision of the proposed causal model, developed to predict partner relationships, are needed.[33,36-38] In addition, more information is needed about the antecedents and mediators of partner relationships when pregnancy is at high risk.[34,35,36] Mercer also emphasized the need for more research into sources of stress and anxiety that potentially interfere with maternal-infant attachment and role competence.[3,5]

In paternal-infant attachment and paternal role competence studies, Mercer noted higher rates of depression among inexperienced fathers.[3,5] She stresses the need for further research to develop interventions for depression among first-time fathers during the first year.[4] Continued testing of the application of Mercer's framework in a variety of perinatal situations, including multiple gestation, would be useful and investigation of theory beyond the first year is also warranted.

CRITIQUE
Clarity

The concepts, variables, and relationships are not always explicitly defined, but are described and implied. However, they are theoretically defined and operationalized. The operational and theoretical definitions are consistent. Some interchanging of terms and labels used to identify concepts, such as adaptation and attainment, social support, and support network, can create some confusion for the reader. Additionally, maternal role attainment is not consistently defined and obstructs clarity. *Maternal identity,* a term borrowed from Rubin, is sometimes substituted for *maternal role attainment.* However, Mercer has continued to work toward greater clarity. Overall, the concepts, assumptions, and goals are organized into a logical and coherent whole and understanding the interrelationships among the concepts is relatively easy.

Simplicity

Despite numerous concepts and relationships, the theoretical framework for maternal role attainment organizes a rather complex phenomenon into an easily understood and useful form. The theory is predictive in nature and readily lends itself to guide practice.[2] Concepts are not specific to time and place and are abstract, but they are described and operationalized to the extent that meanings are not easily misinterpreted. However, it should be noted that the research completed to define and support the theoretical relationships was very complex, which was due largely to the great number of concepts.

Generality

Maternal role attainment is a theory specific to parent-child nursing. The theory can be generalized to all women during pregnancy through the first year after birth, regardless of age, parity, or environment. It is among the few theories applicable to high-risk perinatal patients and their families. As previously mentioned, it can be applied to a variety of pediatric settings. Mercer[26] has also respecified her theory to study and predict parental attachment, including the pregnant woman's partner. Therefore it is useful in both studying and working with family members following birth.

Mercer's work has done much to broaden the range of application of previously existing theories on maternal role attainment because her studies have spanned various developmental levels and situational contexts, a quality that other studies do not share.

Empirical Precision

Mercer's work was derived from extensive research efforts. The concepts, assumptions, and relationships are grounded predominantly in empirical observations and are congruent. The degree of concreteness and the completeness of operational definitions fur-

ther increase the empirical precision.[2] The theoretical framework for exploring differences between age groups of first-time mothers lends itself well to further testing and is being used by others, as previously discussed in the acceptance section of this chapter.

Derivable Consequences

The theoretical framework for maternal role attainment in the first year has proved to be useful, practical, and valuable to nursing. Mercer's work is repeatedly used in research, practice, and education. The framework is also readily applicable to any discipline that works with mothers and children in the first year of motherhood. McBride[6:72] wrote, "Dr. Mercer is the one who developed the most complete theoretical framework for studying one aspect of parental experience, namely, the factors that influence the attainment of the maternal role in the first year of motherhood."

According to Chinn and Jacobs,[2:145] nursing theory should "differentiate the focus of nursing from other service professions." Mercer achieves this criterion by combining the social, psychological, and biological sciences.

Throughout her career, Mercer has consistently linked research to practice. Implications for nursing and/or nursing interventions are addressed and provide the bond between research and practice in most of her works. She believes that nursing research is the "bridge to excellence" in nursing practice.[13:47]

CRITICAL THINKING *Activities*

1. In your own practice, consider Mercer's Theory and Model of Maternal Role Attainment as a guide. In what ways is it useful?

2. High-risk families often continue to experience problems for years after the birth of a child with a congenital problem. Can Mercer's theory and proposed model be adapted to help in assessment and intervention for these mothers and their families beyond the first year? What areas need further research and development?

3. Consider the current healthcare environment. Does the model proposed by Mercer adequately address current changes in healthcare delivery and the impact on the family? What changes in Mercer's model, if any, would you suggest?

4. In the following high-risk perinatal case, Mercer's framework should be useful for nursing assessment and intervention to facilitate maternal role attainment. How would you use it as a guide in planning care for Susan?

Susan, a 19-year-old woman, prematurely delivered her first infant five days ago. Although her postpartum course has been relatively uneventful, the infant has had difficulty and must remain hospitalized. Susan and her young husband visit the nursery every afternoon to be with the baby, but they ask very few questions. In talking with the couple, the nurse learns that the only living grandparents of the baby live a great distance away. Susan will not have any family or friends to turn to when she takes the baby home.

REFERENCES

1. Bronfenbrenner, U. (1979). *The ecology of human development: Experiment by nature and design.* Cambridge, MA: Harvard University Press.
2. Chinn, P.L. & Jacobs, M.K. (1987). *Theory and nursing: A systematic approach.* St. Louis: Mosby.
3. Ferketich, S.L. & Mercer, R.T. (1995). Paternal-infant attachment of experienced and inexperienced fathers during infancy. *Nursing Research, 44,* 31-37.
4. Ferketich, S.L. & Mercer, R.T. (1995). Predictors of paternal role competence by risk status. *Nursing Research, 43,* 80-85.
5. Ferketich, S.L. & Mercer, R.T. (1995). Predictors of role competence for experienced and inexperienced fathers. *Nursing Research, 44,* 89-95.
6. McBride, A.B. (1984). The experience of being a parent. *Annual Review of Nursing Research, 2,* 63-81.
7. Meighan, M. (2001). Mercer's maternal role theory and nursing practice. In M.R. Alligood & A. Marriner Tomey (Eds.), *Nursing theory: Utilization and application* (2nd ed.). St. Louis: Mosby.
8. Mercer, R.T. (1977). *Nursing care for parents at risk.* Thorofare, NJ: Charles B. Slack.
9. Mercer, R.T. (1979). *Perspectives on adolescent health care.* Philadelphia: J.B. Lippincott.
10. Mercer, R.T. (1981). Foreword. In C. Kehoe (Ed.), *The cesarean experience.* New York: Appleton-Century-Crofts.
11. Mercer, R.T. (1981). A theoretical framework for studying factors that impact on the maternal role. *Nursing Research, 30,* 73-77.
12. Mercer, R.T. (1982). Foreword. In S. Humenick (Ed.), *Assessment evaluation: A clinical and technical review of selected assessment strategies for use in the health care of families in pregnancy and early parenting years.* New York: Appleton-Century-Crofts.
13. Mercer, R.T. (1984). Nursing research: The bridge to excellence in practice. *Image: The Journal of Nursing Scholarship, 16*(2), 47-51.
14. Mercer, R.T. (1985). The process of maternal role attainment over the first years. *Nursing Research, 34,* 198-204.
15. Mercer, R.T. (1986). *First-time motherhood: Experiences from teens to forties.* New York: Springer.
16. Mercer, R.T. (1985). The relationship of age and other variables to gratification in mothering. *Health Care for Women International, 6,* 295-308.
17. Mercer, R.T. (1986). The relationship of developmental variables to maternal behavior. *Research in Nursing and Health, 9,* 25-33.
18. Mercer, R.T. (1987, Feb.). Curriculum vitae.
19. Mercer, R.T. (1988). Curriculum vitae.
20. Mercer, R.T. (1989). Response to "Life-span development: A review of theory and practice for families with chronically ill members." *Scholarly Inquiry for Nursing Practice, 3,* 23-26.
21. Mercer, R.T. (1990). *Parents at risk.* New York: Springer.
22. Mercer, R.T. (1991). *Parenting models: Where are we? Where are we going? Symposium. Maternal role: Models and consequences* (p. 502) [Abstract]. 1991 International Nursing Research Conference Abstracts, Nursing Research: Global Health Perspectives, American Nurses' Association, Council of Nurse Researchers.
23. Mercer, R.T. (1992). Curriculum vitae.
24. Mercer, R.T. (1992, Feb.). Personal correspondence.
25. Mercer, R.T. (1992, March). Personal correspondence.
26. Mercer, R.T. (1995). *Becoming a Mother: Research on maternal role identity since Rubin.* New York: Springer.
27. Mercer, R.T. (1997, Aug 26). *The employed mother's challenge* [Online]. Nurseweek Continuing Education Article. Available: http://www.nurseweek.com/ce/ce250a.html.

28. Mercer, R.T. (1998). *Transitions to parenthood* [Online]. Nurseweek online course. Available: http://nurse.cyberchalk.com/nurse/courses/nurseweek/nw1850/menu.html.

29. Mercer, R.T. (2000). Curriculum vitae.

30. Mercer, R.T. (2000, Jan. 4). Personal correspondence.

31. Mercer, R.T. (2000, June 24). Personal correspondence.

32. Mercer, R.T. (2001). *Adolescent sexuality and childbearing* [Online]. Nurseweek online course. Available: http://www.cyberchalk.com/nurse/courses/nurseweek/NW0520new/course.htm.

33. Mercer, R.T. & Ferketich, S.L. (1990). Predictors of family functioning eight months following birth. *Nursing Research,* 39, 76-82.

34. Mercer, R.T. & Ferketich, S.L. (1990). Predictors of parental attachment during early parenthood. *Journal of Advanced Nursing,* 15, 268-280.

35. Mercer, R.T. & Ferketich, S.L. (1994). Maternal-infant attachment of experienced and inexperienced mothers during infancy. *Nursing Research,* 43, 344-350.

36. Mercer, R.T. & Ferketich, S.L. (1995). Experienced and inexperienced mothers' maternal competence during infancy. *Research in Nursing and Health,* 18, 333, 343.

37. Mercer, R.T., Ferketich, S.L., & DeJoseph, J.F. (1993). Predictors of partner relationships during pregnancy and infancy. *Research in Nursing and Health,* 16, 45-56.

38. Mercer, R.T., Ferketich, S.L., DeJoseph, J., May, K.A., & Sollid, D. (1988). Effects of stress on family functioning during pregnancy. *Nursing Research,* 37, 268-275.

39. Mercer, R.T., Hackley, K.C., & Bostrom, A. (1984). Social support of teenage mothers. *Birth Defects: Original Article Series,* 20(5), 245-290.

40. Mercer, R.T., May, K.A., Ferketich, S., & DeJoseph, J. (1986). Theoretical models for studying the effect of antepartum stress on the family. *Nursing Research,* 35, 339-346.

41. Neeson, J.D., Patterson, K.A., Mercer, R.T., & May, K.A. (1983). Pregnancy outcome for adolescents receiving prenatal care by nurse practitioners in extended roles. *Journal of Adolescent Health Care,* 4, 94-99.

42. Rubin, R. (1977). Binding in the postpartum period. *Maternal-Child Nursing Journal,* 6, 67-75.

43. Rubin, R. (1984). *Maternal identity and the maternal experience.* New York: Springer.

44. Sank, J.C. (1991). *Factors in the prenatal period that affect prenatal role attainment during the postpartum period in black American mothers and fathers.* Unpublished doctoral dissertation, University of Texas, Austin, Texas.

45. Von Bertalanffy, L. (1968). *General system theory.* New York: George Braziller.

46. Walker, L.O., Crain, H., & Thompson, E. (1986). Maternal role attainment and identity in the postpartum period: Stability and change. *Nursing Research,* 35(2), 68-71.

47. Walker, L.O., Crain, H., & Thompson, E. (1986). Mothering behavior and maternal role attainment during the postpartum period. *Nursing Research,* 35(6), 322-325.

BIBLIOGRAPHY
Primary Sources
Books

Mercer, R.T. (1977). *Nursing care for parents at risk.* Thorofare, NJ: Charles B. Slack.

Mercer, R.T. (1979). *Perspectives on adolescent health care.* Philadelphia: J.B. Lippincott.

Mercer, R.T. (1986). *First-time motherhood: Experiences from teens to forties.* New York: Springer.

Mercer, R.T. (1990). *Parents at risk.* New York: Springer.

Mercer, R.T. (1995). *Becoming a mother: Research on maternal role identity since Rubin.* New York: Springer.

Mercer, R.T., Nichols, E.G., & Doyle, G. (1989). *Transitions in a woman's life: Major life events in developmental context.* New York: Springer.

Journal Articles

Ferketich, S.L. & Mercer, R.T. (1989). Men's health status during pregnancy and early fatherhood. *Research in Nursing and Health,* 12, 137-148.

Ferketich, S.L. & Mercer, R.T. (1990). Effects of antepartal stress on health status during early motherhood. *Scholarly Inquiry for Nursing Practice: An International Journal,* 4(2), 127-149.

Ferketich, S.L. & Mercer, R.T. (1992). Focus on psychometrics: Aggregating family data. *Research in Nursing and Health,* 15, 313-317.

Ferketich, S.L. & Mercer, R.T. (1994). Predictors of paternal role competence by risk status. *Nursing Research,* 43, 80-85.

Ferketich, S.L. & Mercer, R.T. (1995). Paternal-infant attachment of experienced and inexperienced fathers during infancy. *Nursing Research,* 44, 31-37.

Ferketich, S.L. & Mercer, R.T. (1995). Predictors of role competence for experienced and inexperienced fathers. *Nursing Research,* 44, 89-95.

Highley, B.L. & Mercer, R.T. (1978). Safeguarding the laboring woman's sense of control. *MCN, The American Journal of Maternal-Child Nursing,* 4, 39-41.

Marut, J.S. & Mercer, R.T. (1979, Sept./Oct.). A comparison of primiparas' perception of vaginal and cesarean birth. *Nursing Research,* 28, 260-266.

Marut, J.S. & Mercer, R.T. (1981). The cesarean birth experience: Implications for nursing. *Birth Defects: Original Article Series,* 17, 129-152.

Mercer, R.T. (1973, Spring). One mother's use of negative feedback in coping with her infant with a defect. *Maternal-Child Nursing Journal,* 2, 29-37.

Mercer, R.T. (1974). A focus on field methodology as a method of research in nursing practice. *Occasional Papers in Nursing Research,* 2, 14-17.

Mercer, R.T. (1974). Two fathers' early responses to the birth of a daughter with a defect. *Maternal-Child Nursing Journal,* 3, 77-86.

Mercer, R.T. (1974, March/April). Mothers' responses to their infants with defects. *Nursing Research,* 23, 133-137.

Mercer, R.T. (1976). Mothering at sixteen. *MCN, The American Journal of Maternal-Child Nursing,* 1, 44-52.

Mercer, R.T. (1977, July). Postpartum illness and the acquaintance-attachment process. *American Journal of Nursing,* 77, 1174-1178.

Mercer, R.T. (1977, Nov.). Crisis: A baby is born with a defect. *Nursing,* 77, 7, 45-47.

Mercer, R.T. (1978). Internal and external constraints on teenage mothering. *Research in Education,* 13(8) 143.

Mercer, R.T. (1979, Sept./Oct.). She's a multip: She knows the ropes. *MCN, The American Journal of Maternal-Child Nursing,* 4, 301-304.

Mercer, R.T. (1980). Commentary on maternal identification and infant care: A theoretical perspective. *Western Journal of Nursing Research,* 2, 700-702.

Mercer, R.T. (1980, Jan./Feb.). Teenage motherhood: The first year. Part I: The teenage mothers' views and responses. Part II: How their infants fared. *Journal of Obstetric, Gynecologic, and Neonatal Nursing,* 9, 16-27.

Mercer, R.T. (1981). Factors impacting on the maternal role the first year. *Birth Defects: Original Article Series,* 17, 233-252.

Mercer, R.T. (1981, March/April). A theoretical framework for studying factors that impact on the maternal role. *Nursing Research,* 30, 73-77.

Mercer, R.T. (1981, Sept./Oct.). The nurse and maternal tasks of early postpartum. *MCN, The American Journal of Maternal-Child Nursing,* 6, 341-345.

Mercer, R.T. (1983, June). Assessing and counseling teenage mothers during the perinatal period. *Nursing Clinics of North America,* 8, 293-301.

Mercer, R.T. (1984). Commentary on subject mortality: Is it inevitable? *Western Journal of Nursing Research,* 6, 336-337.

Mercer, R.T. (1984). Student involvement in faculty research: A mentor's view. *Western Journal of Nursing Research,* 6(4), 433-437.

Mercer, R.T. (1985). Obstetrical nursing: Past, present, and future. *Birth Defects: Original Article Series,* 21(3), 29-70.

Mercer, R.T. (1985). Teenage pregnancy as a community problem. *Annual Review of Nursing Research,* 3, 49-76.

Mercer, R.T. (1985). The relationship of age and other variables to gratification in mothering. *Health Care for Women International,* 6, 295-308.

Mercer, R.T. (1985, July/Aug.). The process of maternal role attainment over the first year. *Nursing Research,* 34(4), 198-204.

Mercer, R.T. (1985, July/Aug.). The relationship of the birth experience to later mothering behavior. *Journal of Nurse Midwifery,* 30(4), 204-211.

Mercer, R.T. (1986). Predictors of maternal role attainment at one year post-birth. *Western Journal of Nursing Research,* 8(1), 9-32.

Mercer, R.T. (1986). The relationship of developmental variables to maternal behavior. *Research in Nursing and Health,* 9, 25-33.

Mercer, R.T. (1987). The mentor and research outcomes. *Search: Improved Nursing Care Through Research,* 11(2), 1-2.

Mercer, R.T. (1989). Responses to life-span development: A review of theory and practice for families with chronically ill members. *Scholarly Inquiry for Nursing Practice: An International Journal,* 3, 23-26.

Mercer, R.T. (1990). After surgery, patients and families still face difficulties. *California Nursing Review,* 12(4), 14.

Mercer, R.T. (1990). Allocating scarce resources. *California Nursing Review,* 12(4), 17-18.

Mercer, R.T. (1990). Caring for patients of infants with birth defects. *Nurseweek,* 3(18), 12-13.

Mercer, R.T. (1990). Caring for pregnant teens. *Nurseweek,* 3(21), 8-10.

Mercer, R.T. (1990). Commentary by Mercer (predicting paternal role enactment). *Western Journal of Nursing Research,* 12(2), 156-158.

Mercer, R.T. (1990). Fathers are parents, too! *Nurseweek,* 3(25), 810.

Mercer, R.T. (1990). Single-mother families require special care. *Nurseweek,* 3(14), 8-9.

Mercer, R.T. (1991). Caring for parents who have an infant in the NICU. *Nurseweek,* 4(8), 9-10.

Mercer, R.T. (1991). Commentary by Mercer (mother's perceptions of problem-solving competence for infant care). *Western Journal of Nursing Research,* 13(2), 176-178.

Mercer, R.T. (1991). Family adjustment after a child's death. *Nurseweek,* 4(25), 10-11, 14.

Mercer, R.T. (1991). Family adjustment to a chronically ill child. *Nurseweek,* 4(29), 8-9, 11.

Mercer, R.T. (1991). Helping parents handle a cesarean birth. *Nurseweek,* 4(5), 8-9, 19.

Mercer, R.T. (1991). Introduction. Adolescent pregnancy: Nursing perspectives on prevention. *March of Dimes Birth Defects Foundation Birth Defects: Original Article Series,* 27(1), 1-8.

Mercer, R.T. (1991). Postpartum depression. *Nurseweek,* 4(21), 10-11, 13.

Mercer, R.T. (1991). Second births: The myths and realities. *Nurseweek,* 4(8), 12-13, 11.

Mercer, R.T. (1991). Summary and challenge to nursing. *March of Dimes Birth Defects Foundation Birth Defects: Original Article Series,* 27(1), 271-275.

Mercer, R.T. (1991). Unexpected hospitalization during pregnancy. *Nurseweek,* 4(8), 11, 12-13.

Mercer, R.T. (1991). When parents suffer perinatal loss. *Nurseweek,* 4(20), 10-11, 13.

Mercer, R.T. (1992). Adolescent sexuality. *Nurseweek,* 5(18), 14-15, 19.

Mercer, R.T. (1992). Challenges in counseling adolescents. *Nurseweek,* 5(18), 12-13, 19.

Mercer, R.T. (1992). Facilitating parent-infant interaction. *Nurseweek,* 5(2), 10-12.

Mercer, R.T. (1992). Fostering growth of teen mothers and their infants. *Nurseweek,* 5(23), 16-17, 21.

Mercer, R.T. (1993). Commentary by Mercer (cross-cultural adaptation to cesarean birth). *Western Journal of Nursing Research,* 15(2), 295-296.

Mercer, R.T. (1993). Commentary by Mercer (development of the prenatal attachment inventory). *Western Journal of Nursing Research,* 15(2), 211-213.

Mercer, R.T. (1994). The evolution of maternity care: Driven by research or social change? *Association of Women's Health, Obstetric, Neonatal Nursing Women's Health Nursing Scan,* 8, 1-2.

Mercer, R.T. (1995). A tribute to Reva Rubin. *MCN,* 20, 184.

Mercer, R.T. (1997). Chronically ill children: How families adjust. *Nurseweek,* 10(9), 14-15, 17.

Mercer, R.T. (1997). The employed mother's challenges. *Nurseweek,* 10(17), 10-11, 15.

Mercer, R.T. & Ferketich, S.L. (1988). Stress and social support as predictors of anxiety and depression during pregnancy. *Advances in Nursing Science,* 10(2), 26-39.

Mercer, R.T. & Ferketich, S.L. (1990). Predictors of family functioning eight months following birth. *Nursing Research,* 29, 76-82.

Mercer, R.T. & Ferketich, S.L. (1990). Predictors of parental attachment during early parenthood. *Journal of Advanced Nursing,* 15, 268-280.

Mercer, R.T. & Ferketich, S.L. (1994). Maternal-infant attachment of experienced and inexperienced mothers during infancy. *Nursing Research,* 43, 344-350.

Mercer, R.T. & Ferketich, S.L. (1994). Predictors of maternal role competency by risk status. *Nursing Research,* 43, 38-43.

Mercer, R.T. & Ferketich, S.L. (1995). Experienced and inexperienced mothers' maternal competence during infancy. *Research in Nursing and Health,* 18, 333-343.

Mercer, R.T., Ferketich, S.L., & DeJoseph, J.F. (1993). Predictors of partner relationships during pregnancy and infancy. *Research in Nursing and Health,* 16, 45-56.

Mercer, R.T., Ferketich, S.L., DeJoseph, J., & Sollid, D. (1988, Sept./Oct.). Effect of stress on family functioning during pregnancy. *Nursing Research,* 37(5), 268-275.

Mercer, R.T., Ferketich, S.L., May, K., DeJoseph, J., & Sollid, D. (1988). Further exploration of maternal and paternal fetal attachment. *Research in Nursing and Health,* 11, 83-95.

Mercer, R.T., Hackley, K.C., & Bostrom, A.G. (1983, July/Aug.). Relationship of psychosocial and perinatal variables to perception of childbirth. *Nursing Research,* 32, 202-207.

Mercer, R.T., Hackley, K.C., & Bostrom, A.G. (1984). Adolescent motherhood: Comparisons of outcome with older mothers. *Journal of Adolescent Health Care,* 4, 7-13.

Mercer, R.T., Hackley, K.C., & Bostrom, A.G. (1984). Relationship of psychosocial and perinatal variables to perception of childbirth [Reprint]. *Taiwan Nursing Digest,* 106(21), 100-104.

Mercer, R.T., Hackley, K.C., & Bostrom, A. (1984). Social support of teenage mothers. *Birth Defects: Original Article Series,* 20(5), 245-290.

Mercer, R.T., Highley, B.L. (1978). Maternity specialization: Where are the challenges? In M.R. Spaulding (Ed.), *Report of conference on crisis in maternal-child nursing leadership* (pp. 63-75). Richmond, VA: Medical College of Virginia, School of Nursing.

Mercer, R.T., May, K.A., Ferketich, S., & DeJoseph, J. (1986, Nov./Dec.). Theoretical models for studying the effect of antepartum stress on the family. *Nursing Research,* 35(6), 339-346.

Mercer, R.T., Nichols, E., & Doyle, G. (1988). Transitions over the life cycle: A comparison of mothers and nonmothers. *Nursing Research,* 37, 144-151.

Mercer, R.T. & Stainton, M.C. (1984). Perceptions of the birth experience: A cross-cultural comparison. *Health Care for Women International,* 5, 28-27.

(Mercer) Evans, R.T., Thigpen, L., & Hamrick, M. (1969, Jan./Feb.). Exploration of factors involved in maternal physiological adaptation to breastfeeding. *Nursing Research,* 18(1), 28-33.

Neeson, J.D., Patterson, K.A., Mercer, R.T., & May, K.A. (1983, June). Pregnancy outcome for adolescents receiving prenatal care by nurse practitioners in extended roles. *Journal of Adolescent Health Care,* 4, 94-99.

Slavazza, K.L., Mercer, R.T., Marut, J.S., & Shnider, S.M. (1985, July/Aug.). Differences in maternal perceptions of anesthesia, analgesia for vaginal childbirth. *Journal of Obstetric, Gynecologic, and Neonatal Nursing,* 14(4), 321-329.

Book Chapters

Mercer, R.T. (1981). Potential effects of anesthesia and analgesia on mother-infant attachment process of cesarean mothers. In C. Kehoe (Ed.), *The cesarean experience.* New York: Appleton-Century-Crofts.

Mercer, R.T. (1981). Reaction of parents following cesarean delivery. In S. Rosno (Ed.), *A humanistic approach to cesarean childbirth.* San Jose, CA: Cesarean Birth Control International, Inc.

Mercer, R.T. (1983). Parent-infant attachment. In L.J. Sontegard, K.M. Kowalski, & B. Jennings (Eds.), *Women's health: Vol. II: Childbearing.* New York: Grune & Stratton.

Mercer, R.T. (1987). Adolescent pregnancy. In L.J. Sontegard, K.M. Kowalski, & B. Jennings (Eds.), *Women's health: Vol. III: Crisis and illness in childbearing.* Orlando, FL: Grune & Stratton.

Mercer, R.T. (1988). Theoretical perspectives on the family. In B. Gilliss, B. Highley, B. Roberts, & I. Martinson (Eds.), *Toward a science of family nursing.* Menlo Park, CA: Addison-Wesley.

Mercer, R.T., Ferketich, S.L., DeJoseph, J., & Sollid, D. (1991). Effect of stress on family functioning during pregnancy. In J. Fawcett & A. Whall (Eds.), *Family theory development in nursing: State of the science and art* (pp. 121-138). Philadelphia: F.A. Davis.

Mercer, R.T. & Marut, J.S. (1981). Comparative viewpoints: Cesarean versus vaginal birth. In D.D. Affonso (Ed.), *Impact of cesarean childbirth.* Philadelphia: FA Davis.

Correspondence

Mercer, R.T. (1988, Jan.). Curriculum vitae.

Mercer, R.T. (1988, Feb.). Revised curriculum vitae.

Mercer, R.T. (1992). Curriculum vitae.

Mercer, R.T. (1992, Feb.). Personal correspondence.

Mercer, R.T. (1992, March). Personal correspondence.

Mercer, R.T. (2000). Curriculum vitae.

Mercer, R.T. (2000, Jan. 4). Personal correspondence.

Mercer, R.T. (2000, June 24). Personal correspondence.

Continuing Education Courses

Mercer, R.T. (1998). *Adolescent sexuality and childbearing.* Sunnyvale, CA: Nurseweek.

Mercer, R.T. (1998). *Transition to parenthood.* Sunnyvale, CA: Nurseweek.

Mercer, R.T. (2000). *A nurses guide to helping parents at risk.* Sunnyvale, CA: Nurseweek.

Online Publications

Mercer, R.T. (1991). *Chronically ill children: How families adjust. Nurseweek* [Online]. Available: http://nurseweek.com/ce/ce565a.html.

Mercer, R.T. (1997, Aug. 26). *The employed mother's challenges. Nurseweek* [Online]. Available: http://nurseweek.com/ce/ce250a.html.

Mercer, R.T. (1998). *Transitions to parenthood. A continuing education offering 6.0 hours. Nurseweek* [Online]. Available: http://nurse.cyberchalk.com/nurse/courses/nurseweek/nu/850/menu.html.

Mercer, R.T. (2001). *Adolescent sexuality and childbearing* [Online]. Nurseweek Continuing Education Offering. Available: http://www.cyberchalk.com/nurse/courses/nurseweek/nw0520new/course.htm.

Grant Reports

Mercer, R.T., Ferketich, S.L, May, K.A., DeJoseph, J., & Sollid, D. (1987). *Antepartum stress: Effects on family health and functioning.* Grant No. R01-NR-01064. National Center for Nursing Research, National Institutes of Health, San Francisco: Department of Family Health Care Nursing, University of California, San Francisco.

Mercer, R.T., Hackley, K.C., & Bostrom, A. (1982). *Factors having an impact on maternal role attainment the first year of motherhood.* Grant No. MC-R-05-060435. Maternal and Child Health (Social Security Act, Title V), San Francisco: Department of Family Health Care Nursing, University of California, San Francisco.

Mercer, R.T. & Virden, S. (1978). *Selected materials from a review of the literature to identify instruments to measure maternal role attainment and related factors.* Nursing Graduate Research Support Grant.

Abstracts

Ferketich, S.L. & Mercer, R.T. (1993). *Predictors of paternal role competence* (p. 32) [Abstract]. The American Nurses Association's Council of Nurse Researchers 1993 Scientific Session, November 12-15, 1993. Washington, DC: American Nurses Association.

Ferketich, S.L. & Mercer, R.T. (1994). Experienced and inexperienced fathers' paternal role competence [Abstract]. *Communicating Nursing Research, 27,* 245.

Hackley, K. & Mercer, R.T. (1981). *Variables correlating with the mother's perception of her neonate early postpartum and at one month* [Abstract]. Proceedings Nurses' Association of American College of Obstetrics and Gynecologists, Third National Meeting, San Francisco, March 29-April 4, 1981. Libertyville, IL: Hollister.

Hackley, K.C., Mercer, R.T., & Bostrom, A. (1982). Motherhood in the 30s: A preview of their experiences [Abstract]. *Communicating Nursing Research, 15,* 61.

Hackley, K.C., Mercer, R.T., & Bostrom, A. (1982). Motherhood in the 30s: A preview of their experiences [Abstract]. *Western Journal of Nursing Research, 4(3),* 61.

Mercer, R.T. (1974). Responses of five multigravidae to the event of the birth of an infant with a defect [Abstract]. *Dissertation Abstracts International, 34(10).*

Mercer, R.T. (1979). Internal and external constraints on teenage mothering [Abstract]. Resources in Women's Educational Equity, ERIC Documents. *Research in Education, 13(8),* 143.

Mercer, R.T. (1980). Teenage mothering [Abstract]. *Perinatal Press,* 4(5), 71.

Mercer, R.T. (1982). *The changing family* [Abstract]. Proceedings Seventh Annual March of Dimes Perinatal Nursing Conference, March 22 & 23, 1982. Mead Johnson Nutritional Division.

Mercer, R.T. (1982). The early postpartum days: Expectations versus realities [Abstract]. *Pediatric Nursing Currents,* 29(1), 1-2.

Mercer, R.T. (1983). *Predictors of gratification for mothers 30 and older* [Abstract]. Proceedings Council on Nurse Researchers Conference, Minneapolis, September 21-23, American Nurses' Association.

Mercer, R.T. (1983). The relationship of attitudes toward the birth experience and mothering behaviors [Abstract]. *Journal of Adolescent Health Care,* 4, 212.

Mercer, R.T. (1984). Predictors of maternal role attainment at one year post birth [Abstract]. *Western Journal of Nursing Research,* 6(3), 62.

Mercer, R.T. (1986). Needs identified among breastfeeding mothers [Abstract]. *American Journal of Nursing,* 68, 1274-1275.

Mercer, R.T. (1991). *Parenting models: Where are we? Where are we going? Symposium. Maternal role: Models and consequences* (p. 502) [Abstract]. 1991 International Nursing Research Conference Abstracts, Nursing Research: Global Health Perspectives, American Nurses' Association, Council of Nurse Researchers.

Mercer, R.T. (1993). *Research forum: Attainment of maternal role identity* (pp.69-70) [Abstract]. The MCN Convention, March 6-9, 1994. Dallas, Texas.

Mercer, R.T. & Ferketich, S.L. (1993). *Predictors of maternal role competence* [Abstract]. The American Nurses Association Council of Nurse Researchers 1993 Scientific Session, November 12-15, 1993. Washington, DC.

Mercer, R.T. & Ferketich, S.L. (1994). Experienced and inexperienced mothers' maternal competence [Abstract]. *Communicating Nursing Research,* 27, 245.

Mercer, R.T., Ferketich, S., May, K., & DeJoseph, J. (1987). *A comparison of maternal and paternal responses during pregnancy* [Abstract]. Proceedings Council of Nurse Researchers Conference, Arlington, VA, October 13-16. American Nurses' Association.

Mercer, R.T., Ferketich, S., May, K., DeJoseph, J., & Sollid, D. (1987). *Maternal and paternal responses in high- and low-risk pregnancies* [Abstract]. Symposium. Proceedings Sigma Theta Tau International Biennial Conference, November 10, San Francisco, Sigma Theta Tau International.

Mercer, R.T. & Hackley, K. (1981). *Factors correlated with the primipara's perception of her labor and delivery experience* [Abstract]. Proceedings Nurses' Association of American College of Obstetrics and Gynecologists, Third National Meeting, San Francisco, March 29-April 4, 1981. Libertyville, IL: Hollister, Inc.

Mercer, R.T. & Hackley, K. (1982). Factors correlating with maternal age early postpartum [Abstract]. *Nursing Research,* 31, 188.

Mercer, R.T., Hackley, K., & Bostrom, A. (1980). *Maternal age and role attainment at one month postpartum. Nursing research advancing clinical practice for the 80's* [Abstract]. San Francisco: Department of Nursing Service, Stanford University Hospital, and Symposia Medicus.

Mercer, R.T., Hackley, K.C., & Bostrom, A., (1982). Adolescent mothers: Their assets and deficits [Abstract]. *Communicating Nursing Research,* 15, 59.

Mercer, R.T., Hackley, K.C., & Bostrom, A., (1982). Adolescent mothers: Their assets and deficits [Abstract]. *Western Journal of Nursing Research,* 4, 59.

Mercer, R.T., Hackley, K.C., & Bostrom, A. (1983). Impact on motherhood after thirty [Abstract]. *Communicating Nursing Research,* 16, 51-52.

Mercer, R.T., Hackley, K.C., & Bostrom, A. (1983, April). Comparison of mothering behaviors [Abstract]. *Maternal and Child Health Technical Information Series,* 8-9.

Mercer, R.T. & Hackley, K.C. (1984). A comparison of employed and unemployed mothers' responses and attitudes [Abstract]. *Western Journal of Nursing Research,* 6(3), 61.

Mercer, R.T., Nichols, E.G., & Doyle, G. (1987). *Transitions in the life cycle of women: Mothers and nonmothers* [Abstract]. Proceedings Sigma Theta Tau International Biennial Conference, San Francisco, November 10, Sigma Theta Tau International.

Audiovisual

Beland, J.W. & Mercer, R.T. (1975). *The crisis of loss, TIO: Psychiatric-mental-health nursing* [Filmstrip and audiotape]. New York: American Journal of Nursing Company, Educational Services Division.

Forewords

Mercer, R.T. (1981). Foreword. In C. Kehoe (Ed.), *Nursing management in cesarean births.* New York: Appleton-Century-Crofts.

Mercer, R.T. (1982). Foreword. In S. Humenick (Ed.), *Assessment evaluation: A clinical and technical review of selected assessment strategies for use in the health care of families in pregnancy and early parenting years.* New York: Appleton-Century-Crofts.

Mercer, R.T. (1986). Foreword. In J.D. Neeson & K.A. May (Eds.), *Comprehensive maternity nursing.* Philadelphia: J.B. Lippincott.

Mercer, R.T. (1990). Foreword. In K.A. May & L.R. Mahlmeister (Eds.), *Comprehensive maternity nursing: Nursing process and the childbearing family* (2nd ed.). Hagerstown, MD: J.B. Lippincott.

Published Letters to the Editor

Mercer, R.T. (1976). Preparation of the breast for breast-feeding [Letter to the Editor]. *Nursing Research, 25,* 222.

Mercer, R.T. (1977). Moving out of the nursing ghetto [Letter to the Editor]. *MCN, American Journal of Nursing, 2,* 65.

Mercer, R.T. (1984). Eight stages of a doctoral dissertation [Letter to the Editor]. *Nursing Research, 23,* 435-436.

Book Reviews

Mercer, R.T. (1983). [Review of the book *Parenting reassessed: A nursing perspective*]. *American Journal of Nursing, 83,* 963.

Mercer, R.T. (1985). [Review of the book *Maternal identity and the maternal experience*]. *American Journal of Nursing, 85,* 103-104.

Mercer, R.T. (1988). [Review of the book *Gay and lesbian parents*]. *Image: Journal of Nursing Scholarship, 20*(4), 234-235.

Secondary Sources

Barnard, K.E. & Neal, M.V. (1977). Maternal child nursing research: Review of the past and strategies for the future. *Nursing Research, 26,* 193-200.

Bee, A.M., Legge, D. & Oettinger, S. (1995). Ramona T. Mercer: Maternal role attainment. In A. Marriner Tomey & M.R. Alligood (Eds.), *Nursing theorists and their work* (3rd ed., pp. 390-405). St. Louis: Mosby.

Brouse, A.J. (1988). Easing the transition to the maternal role. *Journal of Advanced Nursing, 13*(2), 167-172.

Cranley, M.S., Hedahl, K.J., & Pegg, S.H. (1983). Women's perceptions of vaginal and cesarean deliveries. *Nursing Research, 32*(1), 10-15.

Crawford, G. (1982). A theoretical model of support network conflict experienced by new mothers. *Nursing Research, 34,* 100-102.

Curry, M.A. (1982). Maternal attachment behavior and the mother's self-concept: The effect of early skin-to-skin contact. *Nursing Research, 32*(2), 73-78.

Davis, C.E. (1994). Commentary on predictors of maternal role competence by risk status. *Nursing Research, 43*(1) 38-43.

Dunnington, R.M. & Glazer, G. (1991). Maternal identity and early mothering behavior in previously infertile and never infertile women. *Journal of Obstetric, Gynecologic and Neonatal Nursing, 20*(4), 309-318.

Gift, A.G. & Palmer, M.H. (1987). Planning clinical nursing research with a geriatric population. *Clinical Nurse Specialist, 1*(2), 56, 87.

Hawkins, J.W. (1986). Did we do all we could? *American Journal of Nursing, 86,* 158.

Lederman, R.P., Weingarten, C.T., & Lederman, E. (1981). Postpartum self-evaluation questionnaire: Measures of maternal adaptation. *Birth Defects: Original Article Series, 17*(6), 201-231.

Lin, R.C. (1986). A project for facilitating maternal adaptation with Chinese adolescent mothers in Taiwan. *Health Care For Women International, 7*(4), 311-327.

Lipson, J.G. & Tilden, V.P. (1980). Psychological integration of the cesarean birth experience. *American Journal of Orthopsychiatry, 50*(4), 598-609.

Majewski, J.L. (1986). Conflicts, satisfactions, and attitudes during transition to the maternal role. *Nursing Research, 35*(1), 10-14.

Meighan, M.M. (2002). Mercer's theory of maternal role attainment. In M.R. Alligood & A. Marriner Tomey (Eds.), *Nursing theory: Utilization and application* (2nd ed.). St. Louis: Mosby.

Meighan, M.M., Bee, A.M., Legge, D., & Oettinger, S. (1998). Ramona T. Mercer: Maternal role attainment. In A. Marriner Tomey & M.R. Alligood, (Eds.), *Nursing theorists and their work* (4th ed., pp. 407-422). St. Louis: Mosby.

Pridham, K.F., Lytton, D., Chang, A.S., & Rutledge, D. (1991). Early postpartum transition: Progress in maternal identity and role attainment. *Research in Nursing and Health, 14*(1), 21-31.

Proctor, S.E. (1986). A developmental approach to pregnancy prevention with early adolescent females. *Journal of School Health, 56*(8), 313-321.

Sadler, L.S. & Catrone, C. (1983). The adolescent parent: A dual developmental crisis. *Journal of Adolescent Health Care, 4*(2), 100-105.

Sank, J.C. (1991). *Factors in the prenatal period that affect parental role attainment during the postpartum period in black American mothers and fathers.* Unpublished doctoral dissertation, University of Texas, Austin.

Sims-Jones, N. (1986). Back to the theories: Another way to view mothers of prematures. *MCN, The Journal of Maternal-Child Nursing, 11*(6), 394-397.

Slager-Ernest, S.E., Hoffman, S.J., & Beckman, C.J.A. (1987). Effects of a specialized prenatal adolescent program on maternal and infant outcomes. *Journal of Obstetric, Gynecologic and Neonatal Nursing, 16*(6), 422-429.

Spivak, H. & Weitzman, M. (1987). Social barriers faced by adolescent parents and their children. *Journal of Adolescent Health Care, 258,* 1500-1504.

Walker, L.O. (1989). A longitudinal analysis of stress process among mothers of infants. *Nursing Research, 38*(6), 339-343.

Walker, L.O. (1989). Stress process among mothers of infants: Preliminary model testing. *Nursing Research, 38*(1), 10-16.

Walker, L.O. & Best, M.A. (1991). Well-being of mothers with infant children: A preliminary comparison of employed women and homemakers. *Women and Health,* 17(1), 71-89.

Walker, L.O., Crain, H., & Thompson, E. (1986). Maternal role attainment and identity in the postpartum period: Stability and change. *Nursing Research,* 35(2), 68-71.

Walker, L.O., Crain, H., & Thompson, E. (1986). Mothering behavior and maternal role attainment during the postpartum period. *Nursing Research,* 35(6), 322-355.

Wassermun, G.A. & Rhiasom, A. (1985). Maternal withdrawal from handicapped toddlers. *Journal of Child Psychology and Psychiatry and Allied Disciplines,* 26, 381-387.

White, M. & Dawson, C. (1981). Impact of the at-risk infant on family solidarity. *Birth Defects,* 17, 253-284.

Yonger, J.B. (1991). A model of parenting stress. *Research in Nursing and Health,* 14(3), 197-204.

Yoos, L. (1987). Perspectives on adolescent parenting: Effect of adolescent egocentrism on the maternal-child interaction. *Journal of Pediatric Nursing,* 2(3), 193-200.

Zahr, L.K. (1991). The relationship between maternal confidence and mother-infant behaviors in premature infants. *Research in Nursing and Health,* 14(4), 279-286.

Zuskar, D.M. (1987). The psychological impact of prenatal diagnosis of fetal abnormality: Strategies for investigation and intervention. *Women's Health,* 12, 91-103.

Other Sources

Baltes, P.B., Reese, H.W., & Lipsitt, L.P. (1980). Life-span developmental psychology. *Annual Review of Psychology,* 31, 65-110.

Bronfenbrenner, U. (1979). *The ecology of human development: Experiment by nature and design.* Cambridge, MA: Harvard University Press.

Burr, W.R., Leigh, G.K., Day, R.D. & Constantine, J. (1979). Symbolic interaction and the family. In W.R. Burr, R. Hill, F.I. Nye, & I.L. Reiss (Eds.), *Contemporary theories about the family* (Vol. 2, pp. 42-111). New York: Free Press.

Erikson, E.H. (1959). Identity and the life cycle [Monograph]. *Psychological Issues,* 1(1), 1-171.

Gloger-Tippelt, G. (1983). A process model of the pregnancy course. *Human Development,* 26, 134-138.

Gottlieb, L. (1978). Maternal attachment in primipara. *Journal of Obstetric Gynecologic Neonatal Nursing,* 7, 39-44.

Mead, G.H. (1934). *Mind, self and society.* Chicago: University of Chicago Press.

(Mercer) Evans, R.T. (1968). *Needs identified among breastfeeding mothers.* ANA clinical sessions (pp. 162-171). New York: Appleton-Century-Crofts.

Mercer, R.T. (1975). *Responses of mothers to the birth of an infant with a defect.* ANA clinical sessions (pp. 340-349). New York: Appleton-Century-Crofts.

Mercer, R.T. (1984). *Health of the children of adolescents* (pp. 60-66). Adolescent Family, Report of Fifteenth Ross Roundtable on Critical Approaches to Common Pediatric Problems. Columbus, OH: Ross Laboratories.

Mercer, R.T. (1984, June). *Challenges during the first year of motherhood.* The Fourth Helen Nahm Lecture. San Francisco: University of California, School of Nursing.

Mercer, R.T. (1988, Spring). *P's and q's of monitoring and maintaining a research career. Community nursing research, Vol. 21. Nursing: A socially responsible profession* (pp. 21-31). Boulder, CO: Western Institute of Nursing.

Rowe, G.P. (1966). The developmental conceptual framework to the study of the family. In F.I. Nye & F.M. Berardo (Eds.), *Emerging conceptual frameworks in family analysis* (pp. 198-222). New York: Macmillan.

Rubin, R. (1967). Attainment of the maternal role: Part I. Processes. *Nursing Research,* 16, 237-245.

Rubin, R. (1967). Attainment of the maternal role: Part II. Models and referrants. *Nursing Research,* 16, 342-346.

Rubin, R. (1977). Binding in the postpartum period. *Maternal-Child Nursing Journal,* 6, 67-75.

Rubin, R. (1984). *Maternal identity and the maternal experience.* New York: Springer.

Thornton, R. & Nardi, P.M. (1975). The dynamics of role acquisition. *American Journal of Sociology,* 80, 870-885.

Turner, J.H. (1978). *The structure of sociological theory* (Revised edition). Homewood, IL: Dorsey Press.

Von Bertalanffy, L. (1968). *General system theory.* New York: George Braziller.

Werner, H. (1957). The concept of development from a comparative and organismic point of view. In D.H. Harris (Ed.), *The concept of development* (pp. 125-148). Minneapolis: University of Minnesota.

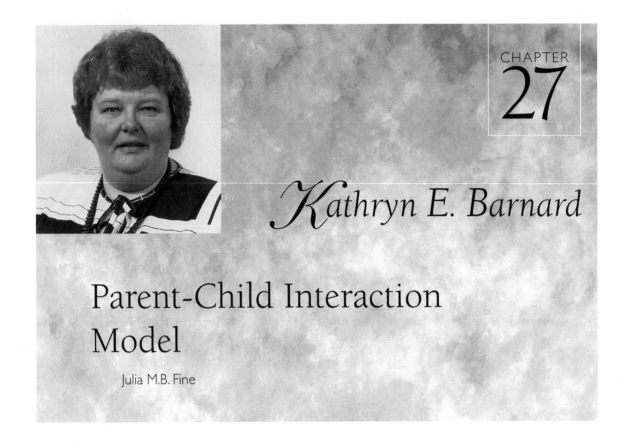

Kathryn E. Barnard

Parent-Child Interaction Model

Julia M.B. Fine

CREDENTIALS AND BACKGROUND OF THE THEORIST

Kathryn E. Barnard was born April 16, 1938 in Omaha, Nebraska. In 1956, she enrolled in a prenursing program at the University of Nebraska and graduated with a B.S.N. in June 1960. Upon graduation, she continued at the University of Nebraska in part-time graduate studies. That summer, she accepted an acting head nurse position and became an assistant instructor in pediatric nursing in the fall.[7] In 1961, Barnard moved to Boston, Massachusetts, where she enrolled in a Master's program

Previous authors: Julia M.B. Fine, Jill K. Baker, Debra A. Borchers, Debra Trnka Cochran, Karla G. Kaltofen, Nancy Orcutt, Jean A. Peacock, Elizabeth Godfrey Terry, Cynthia A. Wesolowski, and Lorraine A. Yeager.
The author wishes to thank Kathryn E. Barnard for reviewing the chapter.

at Boston University. She also worked as a private duty nurse. After earning her M.S.N. in June 1962 and a certificate of Advanced Graduate Specialization in Nursing Education, she accepted a position as an instructor in maternal and child nursing at the University of Washington in Seattle. In 1965, she was named assistant professor. She began consulting in the area of mental retardation and coordinated training projects for nurses in child development and the care of children with mental retardation and handicaps. Barnard became the project director for a research study to develop a method for nursing child assessment in 1971. The following year, she earned a Ph.D. in the ecology of early childhood development from the University of Washington.[7]

In 1972, Barnard accepted a position at the University of Washington as a professor in parent-child nursing. Since 1985, she has also served as adjunct professor of psychology at the University of Washington and served as Associate Dean for Academic Affairs for the School of Nursing from 1987 to 1992.[7] Since 1971, Barnard has served as the project director or principal investigator for more than 22 research grants and projects, including the evaluation of Early Head Start programs since 1996. From 1979 to the present, she has served as the principal researcher and advisor for the Nursing Child Assessment Satellite Training Project (NCAST).[7]

In addition to these research efforts, Barnard has provided consultation, presented lectures internationally, and served on multiple advisory boards for nursing and for state and national government. She has published articles in both nursing and nonnursing journals since 1966. Her books include a four-part series on child health assessment, two editions related to teaching the mentally retarded and developmentally delayed child, and work focusing on families of vulnerable infants.[7] Her most recent publications focus on the efficacy of hospital and home-visit interventions for improving interaction between caregivers and their children and the long-range effects of risk factors in either the caregiver or child.[6]

Barnard is a member of the American Nurses Association (ANA), where she has served on the Executive Committee for the Division of Maternal and Child Health Nursing. She is also an active member of nine other national organizations, including the Society for Research in Child Development, Sigma Theta Tau, American Public Health Association, and the World Association of Infant Mental Health.[7] She has served on numerous advisory boards and committees of these and other professional groups.[7]

In 1969, Barnard[7] was presented with the Lucille Perry Leone Award by the National League for Nursing for her outstanding contribution to nursing education. She was elected a Fellow of the American Academy of Nursing in 1975 and of the Institute of Medicine in 1985.[7] The ANA honored Barnard with the Maternal and Child Health Nurse of the Year Award in 1984 and named her the Nurse Scientist of the Year in 1987.[7] In May of 1992, the American Association for Care of Children's Health presented her with the T.B. Brazelton Lectureship Award. She

was the recipient of the Cameo Award from Sigma Theta Tau in 1993.[7]

THEORETICAL SOURCES

Although Barnard cites various nursing theorists, such as Florence Nightingale, Virginia Henderson, and Martha Rogers, their direct influence on her research and theory development is uncertain.

Barnard refers to the Neal Nursing Construct, which has four expressions of health and illness: (1) cognition, (2) sensation, (3) motion, and (4) affiliation. Neal worked on a construct for practice[11] and Barnard and her associates developed measures related to the period of infancy. Barnard[4:195-196] later stated, "In reviewing both the Maryland construct and the Washington research, we were impressed with how the design and results of the Nursing Child Assessment Project (NCAP) fit into the [Neal] construct."

Barnard credits Florence Blake for the beliefs and values making up the foundation of current nursing practice. She describes Blake as:

> a great pediatric nursing clinician and educator [who] turned our minds toward an orientation on the patient rather than the procedure. Blake saw the principal function of parenthood and nursing to be the capacity to establish and maintain constructive and satisfying relationships with others. She amplified for nursing important acts such as mother-infant attachment, maternal care, and separation of child from parents. She helped nursing understand the importance of the family.[4:194]

Many of Barnard's publications were coauthored by writers such as King and Pattullo, indicating a variety of influences. Barnard also coauthored the book, *Teaching the Mentally Retarded Child: A Family Care Approach*,[12] with Powell. Of greater influence were the coinvestigators and consultants of the NCAP.[20] Barnard and colleagues[4] state that they were influenced by child development theorists, such as Piaget, Brunner, Sander, and Brazelton, and *general systems' theory* in addition to nursing theorists. Barnard[5] states that Rubin's work was influential in crafting interventions during pregnancy.

USE OF EMPIRICAL EVIDENCE

Barnard used findings of many researchers, such as Brazelton, Ainsworth, and Bell, in the evolution of her model of parent-child interaction and adaptation.[20] The research findings contributed valuable knowledge for the task of developing tools to assess and measure the interaction between a caregiver and a child.

In addition to tapping others' research, Barnard conducted her own. She began her research in 1968 by studying mentally and physically handicapped children and adults. In the early 1970s, she studied the activities of the well child and later expanded her study to include methods of evaluating the growth and development of children. The majority of these research studies were funded by grants from the U.S. Department of Health, Education, and Welfare and later the Department of Health and Human Services.[7]

From 1976 to 1979, Barnard and colleagues from the University of Washington[4] initiated work to determine how research results could be communicated to practicing nurses across the nation. This led to the evolution of the NCAST. In 1977, Barnard began researching methods for disseminating information about newborns and young children to parents; in 1983, she commenced research with interventions for premature infants; and in 1996, she began projects to evaluate the national program, Early Head Start.[5,6,7]

Barnard[5] continues to study the mother-infant relationship, examining the nurses' role in relation to high-risk mothers and infants. The NCAP formed the basis for Barnard's Child Health Assessment Interaction Theory. This was a longitudinal study of 193 caregiver-child pairs continuing from the prenatal period to the second grade "to identify poor [child development] outcomes before they occur and to examine the variability of the screening and assessment measures over time."[9:16] As the project progressed, "the NCAP team realized that any comprehensive screening and assessment plan must look beyond the child to the transactions between the child and her social and physical environments."[20:3] From the findings of this project in 1979, Barnard refined the Nursing Child Assessment Feeding (NCAF) and Teaching (NCAT) scales.[20] After use in numerous research studies, the NCAST instruments remained "essentially unchanged" in the 1994 revised form.[20:4]

Researchers have used the NCAST instruments for research and as a basis for public health nursing intervention for families with problems including substance abusing, depressed, adolescent, and abusive parents.[20] Barnard and colleagues[10] developed and implemented the Nursing Systems Toward Effective Parenting-Preterm (NSTEP-P). Research using the NCAST instruments include populations of preterm infants, twins, infants with failure to thrive, infants with developmental disabilities, and infants exposed to human immunodeficiency virus (HIV).[13,20]

The NCAST instruments have been standardized and normed for several different ethnic groups including Caucasian, Hispanic, and African American.[15] The instruments were also used to assess urban Native Americans,[17,18] Alaskan Eskimos[16] and Hmong refugees.[15] These researchers found that the instruments were useful for both research and clinical use because the conceptual framework was universal,[18] but recommend comparing scores to appropriate group means and considering "the impact of culture and education."[15:243]

MAJOR CONCEPTS & DEFINITIONS

A major focus of Barnard's work was developing assessment tools to evaluate child health, growth, and development while viewing the parent and child as an interactive system. Barnard stated that the caregiver-child system was influenced by individual characteristics of each member and that the individual characteristics were also modified to meet the needs of the system. She defines modification as adaptive behavior. The interaction between parent and child is diagrammed in the Barnard model in Figure 27-1.

Barnard has defined the terms in the diagram as follows:

INFANT'S CLARITY OF CUES

To participate in a synchronous relationship, the infant must send cues to his or her caregiver signaling desires to engage or disengage in the interaction. The skill and clarity with which these cues are sent will make it either easy or difficult for caregivers to discern the cues and make modifications in their behavior. Ambiguous or confusing cues sent by an infant can interrupt a caregiver's adaptive abilities.[20]

INFANT'S RESPONSIVENESS TO THE CAREGIVER

"The infant's ability to respond to the caregiver's attempts to communicate and interact."[20:10] The child responds to the caregiver by stopping crying, by vocalizing, or by smiling. These behaviors reinforce the caregiving behaviors during an interaction.

CAREGIVER'S SENSITIVITY TO THE CHILD'S CUES

"The caregiver's ability to recognize and respond to the child's cues."[20:9] Caregivers modify their behavior and use "timing, force, rhythm, and duration. . . to set the tone of the interaction."[20:9]

CAREGIVER'S ABILITY TO ALLEVIATE THE INFANT'S DISTRESS

"The caregiver's ability to soothe or quiet a distressed child."[20:9] This ability involves the caregiver's recognition of distress cues, selection of appropriate action, and being available to recognize and respond.

CAREGIVER'S SOCIAL AND EMOTIONAL GROWTH-FOSTERING ACTIVITIES

"Includes the affective domain and communicates a positive feeling tone."[20:9] The caregiver supplies a supportive environment using voice, tone, touch and movement. This reinforces caregiver responsiveness.

PARENT'S COGNITIVE GROWTH-FOSTERING ACTIVITIES

"The type of learning experience the caregiver makes available to the child."[20:9] Caregiver verbalizations, encouraging child response, and allowing exploration are some examples of cognitive growth fostering.

"The break in the arrow (//) represents interference, an interruption in the adaptive process that causes the interaction to break down. This interference can originate in either the caregiver, the child or the environment."[20:8]

As the NCAP continued, Barnard's model became the foundation for her Child Health Assessment Interaction Theory. Three major concepts form the basis of this theory.

CHILD

In describing the child, Barnard used the personal characteristics of "physical appearance, temperament, feeding and sleeping patterns, and self regulation."[20:3]

CAREGIVER

The child's caregiver has characteristics, "including psychosocial assets, physical and mental health, life changes, expectation and concerns about the child, and most important—the caregiver's care giving style and adaptation skills."[20:3]

ENVIRONMENT

The environment affects both child and caregiver and includes "available (or the lack of) social and financial resources such as the presence of a supportive adult, adequate food and housing, a safe home, and community involvement."[20:3]

From Sumner, G. & Spietz, A. (Eds.). (1994). *NCAST caregiver/parent-child interaction teaching manual.* Seattle: NCAST Publications, University of Washington, School of Nursing. Used with permission.

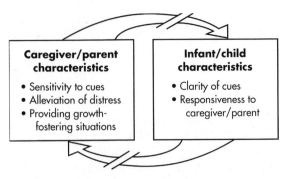

Figure **27-1 Barnard Model.** (From Sumner, G. & Spietz, A. [Eds.]. [1994]. *NCAST caregiver/parent-child interaction teaching manual* [p. 8]. Seattle: NCAST Publications, University of Washington, School of Nursing.)

MAJOR ASSUMPTIONS

Nursing

In 1966, Barnard defined nursing as "a process by which the patient is assisted in maintenance and promotion of his independence. This process may be educational, therapeutic, or restorative; it involves facilitation of change, most probably a change in the environment."[2:629] Fifteen years later, in a 1981 keynote address to the first International Nursing Research Conference, she defined nursing as "the diagnosis and treatment of human responses to health problems."[3:2] In the context of family-centered care, the role is to assist families in providing conditions that promote "growth and development of individual members."[21:127]

Person

When Barnard describes a person or a human being, she speaks of the ability to take part in an interaction to which both parts of the dyad bring qualities, skills, and responses that affect the interaction.[20] This term includes infants, children, and adults.

Health

As one of the six members of the Executive Committee of the ANA Maternal and Child Nursing Division in 1980, Barnard helped define health for the Scope of Practice Statement as:

Health is a dynamic state of being in which the developmental and behavioral potential of an individual is realized to the fullest extent possible. For purpose of this document, health is viewed as a continuum that includes wellness and illness. Each being possesses various strengths and limitations resulting from the interaction of environmental and hereditary factors. The relative dominance of the strengths and limitations determines an individual's place on the health continuum from wellness to illness.

During periods of illness, trauma, or disability, an individual or family may require varying degrees of personal assistance in coping with the manifest problem, with the treatment plan designed to alleviate the problem, or with the sequelae. During periods of wellness, an individual or family may require varying degrees of assistance to obtain information on matters of health, to receive anticipatory guidance and therapeutic counseling to resolve problems or to manage usual health practices when faced with a progressive or chronic health problem.[1:5]

Environment

Environment is an essential aspect of Barnard's theory. In *Child Health Assessment, Part II: The First Year of Life*,[9:53] she states, "In essence, the environment includes all experiences encountered by the child: people, objects, places, sounds, visual and tactile sensations." The environment includes social and financial resources, other persons, and adequacy of the home and the community, all qualities that also affect the caregiver.[4]

THEORETICAL ASSERTIONS

Barnard's Child Health Assessment Interaction Theory is based on the following 10 theoretical assertions:

1. In child health assessment, the ultimate goal is to identify problems at a point before they develop and when intervention would be most effective.

2. Social-environmental factors, as reflected by caregiver-child interaction, are important for determining child health outcomes.

3. Relatively brief observations of caregiver-infant interaction can provide a valid sample of a dyad's ongoing experiences and expectations.

4. Each adult caregiver brings to caregiving a basic personality and skill level that is the foundation upon which their caregiving skill is built. The enactment of caregiving depends on these characteristics and characteristics of the child and of the environment.

5. Through interaction, caregivers and children modify each other's behaviors. That is, the caregiver's behavior influences the child and, in turn, the child influences the caregiver so that both are changed.

6. The process of adaptation of caregiver to infant (and infant to caregiver) is more modifiable than the mother or infant's basic characteristics. Therefore in intervention, the professional should lend support to the way in which caregivers react to their children rather than trying to change caregivers' foundational characteristics.

7. An important way to promote learning is to respond and elaborate on child-initiated behaviors and reinforce the child's attempt to try new things.

8. A major task for the helping profession is to promote a positive early learning environment that includes a nurturing relationship.

9. Assessing the child's social environment, including the quality of caregiver-child interaction, is important in any comprehensive child health care model.

10. Assessing the child's physical environment is equally important in any child health assessment model.*

The Child Health Assessment Interaction Model was developed to illustrate Barnard's theory (Figure 27-2). "The smallest circle represents the child and his/her important characteristics. . . . The next

*From Sumner, G. & Spietz, A. (Eds.). (1994). NCAST *caregiver/ parent-child interaction teaching manual* (p. 5). Seattle: NCAST Publications, University of Washington, School of Nursing. Used with permission.

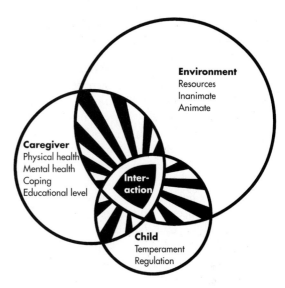

Figure **27-2 Child Health Assessment Model.** (From Sumner, G. & Spietz, A. [Eds.]. [1994]. *NCAST caregiver/parent-child interaction teaching manual* [p. 3]. Seattle: NCAST Publications, University of Washington, School of Nursing.)

largest circle represents the characteristics of the caregiver. . . . The largest circle represents the environment of both the child and the caregiver."[20:3]

Those portions of the model where the circles overlap represent interaction between any two concepts. The dark center area represents interaction among all three concepts. Barnard's theory focuses on this crucial mother-child-environment interactive process.[20]

LOGICAL FORM

According to Chinn and Kramer,[14:81] "With induction, people induce hypotheses and relationships by observing or experiencing an empiric reality and reaching some conclusions." Inductive logic is the form Barnard used in developing her Child Health Assessment Interaction Theory. This theory was an outcome of the investigation and findings of the NCAP. Barnard[8] states that all of the theoretical assertions are supported by evidence from research.

ACCEPTANCE BY THE NURSING COMMUNITY

Practice

The NCAST has prepared more than 20,000 nurses to use a series of standardized assessment tests and the *Keys to Caregiving* videos over a period of more than 30 years.[8] The scales are used to screen and plan individualized interventions with families. The scales also give measurable outcomes for both the caregiver and the child and form an ongoing assessment and basis for evaluation. "The Parent-Child Interaction Scales are used in most public health settings in the United States and have been introduced in many foreign countries, including Canada, England, Sweden, Portugal, Argentina, Korea, Japan, Taiwan, Australia."[8]

Education

The nursing satellite training project initially used satellite communications and later videotaped classes to teach nurses how to use a series of standard assessment instruments. Interrater reliability greater than 85% has encouraged nurses to share their knowledge and observations with co-workers. The explicitness of the observations has made the task of educating others easier.

Research

Barnard has continued to refine the assessment scales and continues to conduct research. She is well recognized for her work. She has received awards recognizing her work from several organizations, including the American Medical Association, the American Public Health Association, and Sigma Theta Tau International. The NCAST scales have been used in numerous research studies in both the United States and other countries. The University of Washington NCAST maintains a normative data bank with over 2100 observation records.[20]

FURTHER DEVELOPMENT

Barnard's model is a middle-range nursing theory, specifically targeting the caregiver-child relationship. The concepts are operationally defined and de-

tailed. In a series of research projects involving different levels of preventive interventions, Barnard[5:28] has become "more focused on the relationships among the parent, child, and intervenor." The model only includes the relationship between the parent and child, not the relationship of the intervenor with each. This is an area requiring further development.

In the Child Health Assessment Interaction Theory, the caregiver is identified as a major concept and all other humans are included in the description of the environment. Barnard[6] has noted the changes in primary caregivers in Western nations through the mother's employment and the contrast in selection of caregivers in nonWestern cultures. "Nursing scholarship and research have been focused on the nuclear family; we now need to broaden our lens—the young child is no longer primarily in the care of parents."[6:302] When there are multiple and nonparental caregivers, Barnard's model may need to be modified.

CRITIQUE

Clarity

"Clarity, in general, refers to how well the theory can be understood and how consistently the ideas are conceptualized."[14:101] Barnard identifies all and defines almost all of her model's concepts both semantically and operationally through the NCAST scales and uses the concepts consistently. "In a theory with structural clarity, . . . concepts are interconnected and organized into a coherent whole."[14:104] Conceptual interrelationships in Barnard's Child Health Assessment Interaction Model are relatively easy for the reader to understand. Barnard is consistent in the use of an inductive form of logic.

Simplicity

The Child Health Assessment Interaction Model is a simple way of communicating the main focus of Barnard's work as it relates to the caregiver-child interaction and the development of accurate assessment tools. However, how interventions affect the model is not easy to visualize. Seeking to clarify this relationship could cause the model to become more complex.

Generality

The original work involved interactions between the caregiver and child during the child's first 12 months of life. Subsequent work lengthened the period of the child assessment to 36 months. Currently, nurses can only generalize to caregiver-child interactions in the first three years of life. The parent-child interaction model approaches mid-range theory as defined by Chinn and Kramer.[14] Despite the narrow scope, Barnard's theory is applicable not only to nursing, but also to other disciplines that deal with the caregiver-child relationship. "The trainees have expanded from nurses to other professionals including psychologists, psychiatrists, social workers, nutritionists, occupational and physical therapists, early childhood educators, speech and hearing specialists and psychoanalysts."[8]

Empirical Precision

Much research was included in Barnard's original work. The scales were tested for reliability and established as reliable by studies of internal consistency and through test-retest procedures. By requiring certified NCAST training for clinicians or researchers to use the scales, Barnard and her colleagues have ensured a high degree of precision and reliability in the many research studies using the scales. The Feeding and Teaching scales were significantly correlated for each subscale concept.[20] Both criterion validity (including concurrent and predictive) and construct validity (including discriminant and intervention and evaluation) have also been addressed.[20]

Derivable Consequences

"NCAST Training in the Parent-Child Interaction Scales and *Keys to Caregiving* has reached over 20,000 individuals."[8] Nurses in the United States and in other countries use the observational skills in daily clinical practice. *Keys to Caregiving*, a series of six self-instructional tapes based on the Barnard model, assists nurses in communicating the knowledge about infant states, cues, and interaction to new parents.[19] "The Teaching Scale has been used in several national studies including the Comprehensive Child Development Program and the Early Head Start National Study both sponsored by the United States Administration of Children Youth and Families."[8]

In discussing research challenges, Barnard[6:303] states:

> The role of the early environment in developing the cortical feedback systems to regulate the aggression is emerging as one of the major issues in neuroscience. My challenge to nursing colleagues is to increase our attention to this critical area of human function, in the hope that nursing science will bring new insights into this dimension of human functioning—the formation of compassionate and caring relationships with one another.

The Barnard model and the Child Assessment Model, combined with the many research projects of Barnard and colleagues, furnish nursing with the tools to create these new insights.

CRITICAL THINKING *Activities*

1. You are a public health nurse in Alaska. You provide health services to a number of traditional Yup'ik Eskimo villages. The state Division of Public Health Nursing has urged use of the NCAST scales for assessment because there has been a recent statewide increase in child abuse and the need for early identification and intervention to prevent problems. You must gain the permission of the village councils to assess the village families. State the points you would cover and how you would explain Barnard's Child Health Assessment Interaction Model, the NCAST scales, and nursing interventions to the village councils.

2. Do you think it would be possible to adapt Barnard's Child Health Assessment

Interaction Model to other caregiver and care receiver situations, such as a wife caring for her husband with Alzheimer's disease? What changes in the concepts and definitions, assumptions, and theoretical assertions would be necessary?

3. Compare and contrast the Barnard Child Health Assessment Model and the Mercer Model of Maternal Health Attainment. What is the emphasis of each model? What are the major concepts of each and how do they overlap? What are the strengths and weaknesses? When would it be most appropriate to use each model? Could the models be used together?

4. Select one of the 10 theoretical assertions of the Barnard Child Health Assessment Interaction Theory. Find a research report from the last five years that supports or seems to refute the assertion.[8] Discuss your findings with your classmates.

REFERENCES

1. American Nurses Association, Division of Maternal and Child Health Nursing Practice. (1980). *A statement on the scope of maternal and child health nursing practice.* Kansas City, MO: The Association.
2. Barnard, K.E. (1966, Dec.). Symposium on mental retardation. *Nursing Clinics of North America,* 1, 629-630.
3. Barnard, K.E. (1982, Summer). The research cycle: Nursing, the profession, the discipline. *Western Journal of Nursing Research,* 4, 1-12.
4. Barnard, K.E. (Ed.). (1986). *Nursing child assessment satellite training: Learning resource manual.* Seattle, WA: NCAST Publications, University of Washington.
5. Barnard, K.E. (1998). Developing, implementing, and documenting interventions with parents and young children. *Zero to Three,* 18(4), 23-29.
6. Barnard, K.E. (1999). The developing family: How is it doing with nurturing young children? *Canadian Journal of Nursing Research,* 30, 299-304.
7. Barnard, K.E. (1999, Sept.). Curriculum vitae.
8. Barnard, K.E. (2000, June 20). Personal e-mail communication.
9. Barnard, K.E. & Eyres, S.J. (Eds.). (1979). *Child health assessment, part II: The first year of life.* Hyattsville, MD: U.S. Department of Health, Education, and Welfare.
10. Barnard, K.E., Hammond, M.A., Sumner, G.A., Kang, R., Johnson-Crowley, N., Snyder, C., Spietz, A., Blackburn, S., Brandt, P., & Magyary, D. (1987). Helping parents with preterm infants: Field test of a protocol. *Early Child Development and Care,* 27(2), 56-290.
11. Barnard, K.E. & Neal, M.V. (1977, May/June). Maternal-child nursing research: Review of the past and strategies for the future. *Nursing Research,* 26, 193-200.
12. Barnard, K.E. & Powell, M.L. (1972). *Teaching the mentally retarded child: A family care approach.* St. Louis: Mosby.
13. Byrne, M.W. (1998). Feeding interactions in a cross section of HIV-exposed infants... including commentary by Lobo, M.L. and Barnard, K.E. with author response. *Western Journal of Nursing Research,* 20(4), 409-430.
14. Chinn, P.L. & Kramer, M.K. (1999). *Theory and nursing: Integrated knowledge development* (5th ed.). St. Louis: Mosby.
15. Harney Boffman, J.L., MacDonald Clark, N.J., & Helsel, D. (1997). Can NCAST and HOME assessment scales be used with Hmong refugees? *Pediatric Nursing,* 23, 235-244.
16. MacDonald-Clark, N.J. & Boffman, J.L. (1995). Mother-child interaction among the Alaskan Eskimos. *Journal of Obstetric, Gynecologic, and Neonatal Nursing,* 24, 450-457.
17. Seideman, R.Y., Haase, J., Primeaux, M., & Burns, P. (1992). Using NCAST instruments with urban American Indians. *Western Journal of Nursing Research,* 14, 308-321.
18. Seideman, R.Y., Williams, R., Burns, T., Jacobson, S., Weatherby, R., & Primeaux, M. (1994). Culture sensitivity in assessing urban Native American parenting. *Public Health Nursing,* 11, 98-103.
19. Sherrard, K.R. (1998). Video review: Keys to caregiving: A self-instructional video series. *Canadian Journal of Nursing Research,* 30, 135-138.
20. Sumner, G. & Spietz, A. (Eds.). (1994). *NCAST caregiver/parent-child interaction teaching manual.* Seattle: NCAST Publications, University of Washington School of Nursing.
21. Thomas, R.B., Barnard, K.E., & Sumner, G.A. (1993). Family nursing diagnosis as a framework for family assessment. In S.L. Feetham, S.B. Meister, J.M. Bell, & C.L. Gilliss (Eds.). *The nursing of families: Theory, research, education, practice* (pp. 127-136). Newbury Park, CA: Sage.

BIBLIOGRAPHY
Primary Sources
Books

Barnard, K.E. (Ed.). (1983). *Structure to outcome: Making it work.* Kansas City, MO: American Academy of Nursing.

Barnard, K.E. (1984). *Social support and families of vulnerable infants.* White Plains, NY: March of Dimes Birth Defects Foundation.

Barnard, K.E. (Ed.). (1987). *Nursing child assessment satellite training: Learning resource manual.* Seattle, WA: Nursing Child Assessment Satellite Training Publications.

Barnard, K.E., Brandt, P.A., Raff, B.S., & Carroll, P. (Eds.). (1984). *Social support and families of vulnerable infants.* Birth Defects Original Article Series, Vol. 20, No. 5. White Plains, NY: March of Dimes Birth Defects Foundation.

Barnard, K.E. & Brazelton, T.B. (Chairpersons). (1984). *The many facets of touch.* Somerville, NJ: Johnson & Johnson.

Barnard, K.E. & Brazelton, T.B. (Eds.). (1990). *Touch: The foundation of experience* (Vol. 4). Clinical Infant Reports Series of the National Center for Clinical Infant Programs. Madison, CT: International Universities Press, Inc.

Barnard, K.E. & Douglas, H.B. (Eds.). (1974). *Child health assessment, part I: A literature review.* Bethesda, MD: U.S. Department of Health, Education, and Welfare.

Barnard, K.E. & Erickson, M.L. (1976). *Teaching children with developmental problems: A family care approach* (2nd ed.). St. Louis: Mosby.

Barnard, K.E. & Eyres, S.J. (Eds.). (1979). *Child health assessment, part II: The first year of life.* Hyattsville, MD: U.S. Department of Health, Education, and Welfare.

Barnard, K.E. & Powell, M.L. (1972). *Teaching the mentally retarded child: A family care approach.* St. Louis: Mosby.

Book Chapters

Barnard, K.E. (1973). Nursing. In J. Wortis (Ed.), *Mental retardation and developmental disabilities: An annual review.* New York: Brunner-Mazel.

Barnard, K.E. (1975). Infant programming. In R. Koch (Ed.), *Proceedings of confidence on Down's syndrome.* New York: Brunner-Mazel.

Barnard, K.E. (1976). The state of the art: Nursing and early intervention with handicapped infants. In T. Tjossem (Ed.), *Proceedings of 1974 president's committee on mental retardation meeting on infant intervention.* Baltimore, MD: University Park Press.

Barnard, K.E. (1978). Introduction to parent-infant interaction studies. In G.P. Sackett (Ed.), *Observing behavior (Vol. I): Theory and application in mental retardation.* Baltimore, MD: University Park Press.

Barnard, K.E. (1979). How focusing on the family changes the health care system. In T.B. Brazelton & V.C. Vaughan (Eds.), *The family: Setting priorities.* New York: Science & Medicine.

Barnard, K.E. (1980). How nursing care may influence prevention of development delay. In E.J. Sell (Ed.), *Follow-up of the high risk newborn: A practical approach.* Springfield, IL: Charles C Thomas.

Barnard, K.E. (1980). Sleep organization and motor development in prematures. In E.J. Sell (Ed.), *Follow-up of the high risk newborn: A practical approach.* Springfield, IL: Charles C. Thomas.

Barnard, K.E. (1981). An ecological approach to parent-child relations. In C.C. Brown (Ed.), *Infants at risk: Assessment and intervention.* Madison, CT: Johnson & Johnson Pediatric Round Table.

Barnard, K.E. (1981). A program of temporarily patterned movement and sound stimulation for premature infants. In V.L. Smeriglio (Ed.), *Newborns and parents: Parent-infant contact and newborn sensory stimulation* (pp. 31-48). Hillsdale, NJ: Lawrence Erlbaum Associates.

Barnard, K.E. (1981). General issues in parent-infant interaction during the first years of life. In D.L. Yeung (Ed.), *Essays of pediatric nutrition.* Ontario, Canada: The Canadian Science Committee on Food and Nutrition, Canadian Public Health Association.

Barnard, K.E. (1981). The nursing role in the promotion of child development. In M. Tudor (Ed.), *Child development.* New York: McGraw-Hill.

Barnard, K.E. (1984). Nursing research in relation to infants and young children. In H. Werley & J. Fitzpatrick (Eds.), *Annual review of nursing research* (Vol. 1, pp. 3-25). New York: Springer.

Barnard, K.E. (1985). Rituals that integrate nursing practice, education and research. In K.E. Barnard & G.R. Smith (Eds.), *The second annual symposium in nursing faculty practice.* Washington, DC: American Academy of Nursing.

Barnard, K.E. (1986). Major issues in program evaluation. In *Program evaluation: Issues, strategies and models.* Washington, DC: National Center for Clinical Infant Programs.

Barnard, K.E. (1987). Paradigms for intervention: Infant state modulation. In N. Gunzenhauser (Ed.), *Infant stimulation: For whom, what kind, when, and how much?* (pp. 129-136). Skillman, NJ: Johnson & Johnson Baby Products Company.

Barnard, K.E. (1992). Prenatal and infancy programs. In J.D. Hawkins, R.F. Catalano & Associates (Eds.), *Communities that care: Action for drug abuse prevention.* San Francisco, Jossey-Bass Publishers.

Barnard, K.E. (1994). What the NCAST feeding scale measures. In G. Sumner & A. Spietz (Eds.) *NCAST caregiver/child feeding manual.* Seattle: NCAST Publications, University of Washington.

Barnard, K.E. (1996). *Influencing parent-child interactions for children at risk.* In M.J. Guralnick (Ed.), *The effectiveness of early intervention* (pp. 249-265). New York: Brookes.

Barnard, K.E., Bee, H.L., & Hammond, M.A. (1984). Home environment and cognitive development in a health, low-risk sample: The Seattle study. In A.

Gottfried (Ed.), *Home environment and early cognitive development*. New York: Academic Press.

Barnard, K.E., Booth, C.L., Mitchell, S.K., & Telzow, R.W. (1988). Newborn nursing models: A test of early intervention to high-risk infants and families. In E. Hibbs (Ed.), *Children and families: Studies in prevention and intervention* (pp. 63-81). New York: International Universities Press.

Barnard, K.E. & Brazelton, T.B. (Eds.). (1990). *Touch: The foundation of experience* [Monograph No. 4]. Madison, CT: International Universities Press.

Barnard, K.E., Eyres, S.J., Lobo, M., & Snyder, C. (1983). An ecological paradigm for assessment and intervention. In T.B. Brazelton & B. Lester (Eds.), *New approaches to developmental screening of infants*. New York: Elsevier.

Barnard, K.E., Hammond, M.A., Booth, C.L., Bee, H.L., Mitchell, S.K., & Spieker, S.J. (1989). Measurement and meaning of parent-child interaction. In F.J. Morrison, C.E. Lord, & D.P. Keating (Eds.). *Applied developmental psychology* (Vol. III). New York: Academic Press.

Barnard, K.E., Hammond, M.A., Mitchell, S.K., Booth, C.L., Spietz, A., Snyder, C., & Elsas, T. (1985). Caring for high-risk infants and their families. In M. Green (Ed.), *The psychological aspects of the family*. Lexington, MA: Lexington Books.

Barnard, K. & Hoehn, R.E. (1978, Dec.). Nursing child assessment satellite training. In R.A. Duncan (Ed.), *Biomedical communications experiments*. Bethesda, MD: Lister Hill National Center for Biomedical Communications, Department of U.S. Health, Education, and Welfare, Public Health Service.

Barnard, K.E. & Kelly, J.F. (1988). Children with special needs—Early intervention. In H.M. Wallace, G. Ryan, & A.C. Oglesby (Eds.), *Maternal and child health practices* (3rd ed.). Oakland, CA: Third Party Publishing.

Barnard, K.E. & Kelly, J.F. (1990). Assessment of parent-child interaction. In S.J. Meisels & J.P. Shonkoff (Eds.), *Handbook of early childhood intervention* (pp. 278-302). New York: Cambridge University Press.

Barnard, K.E. & Kennell, L. (1980). Parmelee: Panel discussion. In E.J. Sell (Ed.), *Follow-up of the high risk newborn: A practical approach* (pp. 187-195). Springfield, IL: Charles C. Thomas.

Barnard, K.E. & Magary, D.L. (1987). Early identification. In H. Wallace, A. Oglesky, R. Biehl, & L. Taft (Eds.), *Handicapped children and youth: A comprehensive community and clinical approach* (pp. 99-110). New York: Human Science Press.

Barnard, K.E., Magary, D.L., Booth, C.L., & Eyres, S.J. (1987). Longitudinal design: Considerations and application to nursing research. In M. Cahoon (Ed.), *Recent advances in nursing: Research methodology*. Edinburgh: Churchill Livingstone.

Barnard, K.E. & Martell, L.K. (1995). Mothering. In M.H. Bornstein (Ed.), *Handbook of parenting, Vol. 3: Status and social conditions of parenting* (pp. 3-26). Hillsdale, NJ: Lawrence Erlbaum Associates.

Barnard, K.E. & Morisset, C.E. (1995). Preventive health and developmental care for children: Relationships as a primary factor in service delivery with at risk populations. In H.E. Fitzgerald, B.M. Lester, & B.S. Zuckerman (Eds.), *Children of poverty: Research, health, and policy issues. Reference books on family issues, Vol. 23. Garland reference library of social science, Vol. 968* (pp. 167-195). New York: Garland Publishing.

Barnard, K.E., Morisset, C.E., & Spieker, S. (1993). Preventive interventions: Enhancing parent-infant relationships. In C.H. Zeanah (Ed.), *Handbook of infant mental health* (pp. 386-401). New York: Guilford Press.

Barnard, K.E. & Sumner, G.A. (1981, June). The health of women with fertility-related needs. In L.V. Klerman (Ed.), *Research priorities in maternal and child health: Report of a conference* (pp. 49-102). Waltham, MA: Brandeis University.

Barnard, K.E., Wenner, W., Weber, B., Gray, C., & Peterson, A. (1977). Premature infant refocus. In P. Mittler (Ed.), *Research to practice in mental retardation: Biomedical aspects* (Vol. 3). Oxford, England: University Park.

Booth, C.L., Spieker, S.J., Barnard, K.E., & Morisset, C.E. (1992). Infants at risk: The role of preventive intervention in deflecting a maladaptive developmental trajectory. In J. McCord & R.E. Tremblay, (Eds.), *Preventing antisocial behavior: Interventions from birth through adolescence* (pp. 21-42). New York: Guilford Press.

Kang, R. & Barnard, K. (1979). Using the neonatal behavioral assessment scale to evaluate premature infants. In *Birth defects: Original article series* (Vol. 7, pp. 119-144). New York: National Foundation, Alan R. Liss.

Kelly, J.F. & Barnard, K.E. (in press). Assessment of parent-child interaction. In S.J. Meisels & J.P. Shonkoff (Eds.), *The handbook of early childhood intervention* (2nd ed.). Cambridge, MA: Syndicate of the Press of the University of Cambridge.

Magyary, D., Barnard, K., & Brandt, P. (1988). Biophysical considerations in the assessment of young children with a developmental disability. In T.D. Wachs & R. Sheehan (Eds.), *Assessment of young developmentally disabled children: Perspectives in developmental psychology* (pp. 347-370). New York: Plenum Press.

Magyary, D., Brandt, P., Barnard, K.E., & Hammond, M. (1992). School age follow-up of the development of preterm infants: Infant and family predictors. In M. Sigman (Ed.), *Advances in applied developmental psychology series: Low birth weight children*. New York: Ablex Press.

Mitchell, S.K., Barnard, K.E., Booth, C., Magyary, D., & Spieker, S. (1985). Prediction of school problems and behavior problems in children followed from birth to age eight. In W.K. Frankenburg, R.N. Emde, & J. Sullivan (Eds.). *Early identification of children at risk: An international perspective.* New York: Plenum Press.

Mitchell, S.K., Magyary, D.A., Barnard, K.E., Summer, G.A., & Booth, C.L. (1988). A comparison of home-based prevention programs for families of newborns. In L.A. Bond & B. Wagner (Eds.), *Families in transition: Primary prevention programs that work.* Beverly Hills, CA: Sage.

Solchany, J., Sligar, K., & Barnard, K.E. (in press). Promoting maternal role attainment and attachment in pregnancy: The parent-child communication program. In J.M. Maldonado Duran (Ed.), *Infant and early childhood mental health, models of clinical intervention.* American Psychiatric Press.

Spieker, S.J., Solchany, J., McKenna, M., DeKlyen, M., & Barnard, K.E. (1999). The story of mothers who are difficult to engage in prevention programs. In J.D. Osofsky & H.E. Fitzgerald (Eds.), *WAIMH handbook of infant mental health. Vol. 3: Parenting and child care.* Toronto, Canada: John Wiley and Sons.

Thomas, R.B., Barnard, K.E., & Sumner, G.A. (1993) Family nursing diagnosis as a framework for family assessment. In S.L. Feetham, S.B. Meister, J.M. Bell, & C.L. Gillis (Eds.), *The nursing of families: theory/research/education/practice.* Newbury Park, CA: Sage.

Journal Articles

Barnard, K.E. (1966, April/May). New four-part training project is developed. *Children Limited, 15,* 2.

Barnard, K.E. (1966, Dec.). Symposium on mental retardation. *Nursing Clinics of North America, 1,* 629-630.

Barnard, K.E. (1968, Feb.). Teaching the mentally retarded child is a family affair. *American Journal of Nursing, 68,* 305-311.

Barnard, K.E. (1969, Oct.). Are professionals educable? *Alabama Journal of Medical Sciences, 6,* 388-391.

Barnard, K.E. (1973, Dec.). The effect of stimulation on the sleep behavior of the premature infant. *Communicating Nursing Research, 6,* 12-33.

Barnard, K.E. (1975, Oct.). Trends in the care and prevention of developmental disabilities. *American Journal of Nursing, 75,* 1700-1704.

Barnard, K.E. (1976, Oct.). Predictive nursing: The baby and parents. *Health Care Dimensions, 3,* 185-202.

Barnard, K.E. (1977, Aug.). A challenge for nursing care. *American Nurse, 9,* 4.

Barnard, K.E. (1978, March/April). The family and you. *American Journal of Maternal Child Nursing, 3,* 82-83.

Barnard, K.E. (1979, Sept.). Child advocates must help parents, too. *American Nurse, 11,* 4.

Barnard, K.E. (1980, July). Knowledge for practice: Directions for the future. *Nursing Research, 29,* 208-212.

Barnard, K.E. (1981, May/June). The research question. *American Journal of Maternal Child Nursing, 6,* 211.

Barnard, K.E. (1981, July/Aug.). Breast-feeding is best for U.S. babies, too. *American Nurse, 13,* 44.

Barnard, K.E. (1981, July/Aug.). Research designs: Descriptive method. *American Journal of Maternal Child Nursing, 6,* 243.

Barnard, K.E. (1981, Sept./Oct.). Research designs: Experimental method. *American Journal of Maternal Child Nursing, 6,* 321.

Barnard, K.E. (1981, Nov./Dec.). Research designs: The historical method. *American Journal of Maternal Child Nursing, 6,* 391.

Barnard, K.E. (1982, Jan./Feb.). Research designs: Sampling. *American Journal of Maternal Child Nursing, 7,* 15.

Barnard, K.E. (1982, March/April). Measurements: Reliability. *American Journal of Maternal Child Nursing, 7,* 101.

Barnard, K.E. (1982, May/June). Measurement: Validity. *American Journal of Maternal Child Nursing, 7,* 165.

Barnard, K.E. (1982, Summer). The research cycle: Nursing, the profession, the discipline. *Communicating Nursing Research, 15,* 1-12.

Barnard, K.E. (1982, Summer). The research cycle: Nursing, the profession, the discipline. *Western Journal of Nursing Research, 4,* 1-12.

Barnard, K.E. (1982, July/Aug.). Measurement descriptive statistics. *American Journal of Maternal Child Nursing, 7,* 235.

Barnard, K.E. (1982, Sept./Oct.). Determining the focus of nursing research. *American Journal of Maternal Child Nursing, 7,* 299.

Barnard, K.E. (1982, Nov./Dec.). Determining the role of nursing. *American Journal of Maternal Child Nursing, 7,* 36.

Barnard, K.E. (1983, Jan.). Social policy statement can move nursing ahead. *American Nurse, 15,* 4, 14.

Barnard, K.E. (1983, Jan./Feb.). The case study method: A research tool. *American Journal of Maternal Child Nursing, 8,* 36.

Barnard, K.E. (1983, March/April). Identifying potential nursing research areas. *American Journal of Maternal Child Nursing, 8,* 117.

Barnard, K.E. (1983, May/June). Nursing diagnosis: A descriptive method. *American Journal of Maternal Child Nursing, 8,* 223.

Barnard, K.E. (1983, July/Aug.). Formulation of hypotheses. *American Journal of Maternal Child Nursing, 8,* 263.

Barnard, K.E. (1983, Aug.). Our concern for child health. NCAP follow-up at age two. *NCAST National News, 1,* 1.

Barnard, K.E. (1983, Sept./Oct.). Informed consent. *American Journal of Maternal Child Nursing, 8,* 327.

Barnard, K.E. (1983, Nov.). Child health screening indicators. *NCAST National News, 1,* 2.

Barnard, K.E. (1983, Nov./Dec.). Control groups. *Maternal Child Nursing*, 8, 431.

Barnard, K.E. (1984). Nursing research related to infants and young children. *Annual Review of Nursing Research*, 1, 3-25.

Barnard, K.E. (1984, Jan./Feb.). The family as a unit of measurement. *American Journal of Maternal Child Nursing*, 9, 21.

Barnard, K.E. (1984, Feb.). Home based intervention projects described. Newborn nursing models program study 1980-1983. Clinical nursing models study 1982-1987. *NCAST National News*, 1, 3.

Barnard, K.E. (1984, March/April). Children: Our greatest national resource. *Public Health Currents*, 24, 8-10.

Barnard, K.E. (1984, March/April). Commonly understood outcomes. *American Journal of Maternal Child Nursing*, 9, 99.

Barnard, K.E. (1984, May/June). Knowledge development. *American Journal of Maternal Child Nursing*, 9, 175.

Barnard, K.E. (1984, July/Aug.). Planning experiments. *American Journal of Maternal Child Nursing*, 9, 247.

Barnard, K.E. (1984, Sept./Oct.). Determining relationships. *American Journal of Maternal Child Nursing*, 9, 345.

Barnard, K.E. (1984, Dec.). Sleep behavior of infants—is it important? *NCAST National News*, 1, 6.

Barnard, K. (1985). Blending the art and science of nursing. *Maternal-Child Nursing*, 10(1), 63.

Barnard, K.E. (1985). Nursing systems toward effective parenting-premature. *NCAST National News*, 1, 9.

Barnard, K. (1985). Planning the analysis. *Maternal-Child Nursing*, 10(2), 139.

Barnard, K. (1985). Retention of research sample. *Maternal-Child Nursing*, 10(3), 214.

Barnard, K. (1985). Seeking approval of conducting research. *Maternal-Child Nursing*, 10(4), 292.

Barnard, K. (1985). Seeking funds for research. *Maternal-Child Nursing*, 10(6), 424.

Barnard, K. (1985). Studying patterns of behavior. *Maternal-Child Nursing*, 10(5), 358.

Barnard, K. (1985). Supportive measures for high-risk infants and families. *Birth Defects*, 20(5), 291-329.

Barnard, K.E. (1986). Research utilization: The clinician's role. *Maternal-Child Nursing*, 11(3), 224.

Barnard, K.E. (1986). Research utilization: The researcher's responsibilities. *Maternal-Child Nursing*, 11(2), 150.

Barnard, K.E. (1986). Writing a research proposal. *Maternal-Child Nursing*, 11(1), 76.

Barnard, K.E. (1986, April). Child health screening indicators. *NCAST National News*, 22, 2.

Barnard, K.E. (1986, Oct.). Parenting alterations. *NCAST National News*, 2, 4.

Barnard, K.E. (1987, Jan.). Systematic use of the NCAST scales. *NCAST National News*, 3, 1.

Barnard, K.E. (1987, Oct.). Clinical nursing models. *NCAST National News*, 3, 4.

Barnard, K.E. (1990). Developing superstars. *Journal of Professional Nursing*, 6(5), 250, 315.

Barnard, K.E. (1991, April). A construct for assessing families. *NCAST National News*, 7, 2.

Barnard, K.E. (1991, July). Family boundaries. *NCAST National News*, 7, 3.

Barnard, K.E. (1991, Oct.). Family communications. *NCAST National News*, 7, 4.

Barnard, K.E. (1995). NCAST feeding and teaching scales: Meaning and utilization. *NCAST National News*, 11(3), 1-3, 8.

Barnard, K.E. (1995). Practice dilemmas: Applying the step by step process when using the NCAST parent-child interaction scales. *NCAST National News*, 11(4), 1-3.

Barnard, K.E. (1996). Practice dilemmas. *NCAST National News*, 12(1), 7-8.

Barnard, K.E. (1996). Practice dilemmas—Parent-child interaction interventions. *NCAST National News*, 12(3), 6-7.

Barnard, K.E. (1997). Experiences promote brain development in the first year of life. *NCAST National News*, 13(3), 1-2, 10.

Barnard K.E. (1997). Practice dilemma: How to identify and address a parent's emotional availability. *NCAST National News*, 13(4), 1-2.

Barnard, K.E. (1997). Using NCAST parent-child interaction scales as evaluation tools leading to best practices. *NCAST National News*, 13(1), 1-4.

Barnard, K.E. (1998). Developing, implementing, and documenting interventions with parents and young children. *Zero to Three*, 18(4), 23-29.

Barnard, K.E. (1998). The developing family: How is it doing with nurturing young children? *Canadian Journal of Nursing Research*, 30(3), 7-12.

Barnard, K.E. (1999). The developing family: How is it doing with nurturing young children? . . . adapted from guest editorial in Canadian Journal of Nursing Research, 1998, Vol. 30, No. 3, 7-12. *Canadian Journal of Nursing Research*, 30(4), 299-304.

Barnard, K.E. & Bee, H.L. (1983). The impact of temporarily patterned stimulation on the development of preterm infants. *Child Development*, 54, 1156-1167.

Barnard, K.E. & Bee, H.L. (1984). Developmental changes in maternal interactions with term and preterm infants. *Infant Behavior and Development*, 7, 101-113.

Barnard, K.E., Bee, J.L., & Hammond, M.A. (1984). Developmental changes in maternal interactions with term and preterm infants. *Infant Behavior and Development*, 1, 101-113.

Barnard, K.E. & Blackburn, S. (1985). Making a case for studying the ecologic niche of the newborn. *Birth Defects*, 21(3), 71-88.

Barnard, K.E., Boothe, C., Johnson, C., & Crowley, N. (1985). Infant massage and exercise: Worth the effort? *Maternal-Child Nursing,* 10(3), 184-189.

Barnard, K.E. & Collar, B.S. (1973, Feb.). Early diagnosis, interpretation and intervention: A commentary on the nurse's role. *Annals of the New York Academy of Science,* 205, 373-382.

Barnard, K.E., Collar, B.S., Spietz, A., Snyder, C., & Kang, R. (1976). Predictive nursing: The baby and parents. *Health Care Dimensions,* 31(1), 185-202.

Barnard, K.E., Hammond, M.A., Sumner, G.A., Kang, R., Johnson-Crowley, N., Snyder, C., Spietz, A., Blackburn, S., Brandt, P., & Magyary, D. (1987). Helping parents with preterm infants: Field test of a protocol. *Early Child Development and Care,* 27(2), 56-290.

Barnard, K.E., Magyary, D., Sumner, G., Booth, C.L., Mitchell, S.K., & Spieker, S. (1988). Prevention of parenting alternations for women with low social support. *Psychiatry,* 51, 248-253.

Barnard, K.E. & Neal, M.V. (1977, May/June). Maternal-child nursing research: Review of the past and strategies for the future. *Nursing Research,* 26, 193-200.

Barnard, K., Osofsky, J., Beckwith, L., Hammond, M., & Appelbaum, M. (1996). A collaborative effort to study mother-child interaction in three risk groups: Social risk mother, adolescent mother, preterm infant. *Infant Mental Health Journal,* 17(4), 293-301.

Barnard, K.E., Snyder, C., & Spietz, A. (1984). Supportive measures for high-risk infants and families. In K.E. Barnard, P.A. Brandt, B.S. Raff, & P. Carroll (Eds.), Social support and families of vulnerable infants. *Birth Defects: Original Article Series,* 20(5), 291-329.

Bee, H.L., Barnard, K.E., Eyres, S.J., Gray, C.A., Hammond, M.A., Spitz, A.L., Snyder, C., & Clark, B. (1982). Prediction of IQ and language skill from perinatal status, child performance, family characteristics, and mother-infant interaction. *Child Development,* 53, 1134-1156.

Bee, H.L., Hammond, M.A., Eyres, J.J., Barnard, K.E., & Snyder, C. (1986). The impact of parental life change in the early development of children. *Research in Nursing and Health,* 9(1), 64-74.

Bee, H.L., Mitchell, S.K., Barnard, K.E., Eyres, S.J., & Hammond, M.A. (1984). Predicting intellectual outcomes: Sex differences in response to early environmental stimulation. *Sex Roles,* 10, 783-803.

Booth, C.L., Barnard, K.E., Mitchell, S.K., & Spieker, S.J. (1987). Successful intervention with multi-problem mothers: Effects on the mother-infant relationship. *Infant Mental Health Journal,* 9, 288-306.

Booth, C.L., Lyons, N.B., & Barnard, K.E. (1984). Synchrony in mother-infant interaction: A comparison of measurement methods. *Child Study Journal,* 14, 95-114.

Booth, C.L., Mitchell, S.K., Barnard, K.E., & Spieker, S.J. (1989). Development of maternal social skills in multi-problem families: Effects on the mother-child relationship. *Developmental Psychology,* 25(3), 403-412.

Brandt, P., Magyary, D., Hammond, M., & Barnard, K. (1992). Learning and behavioral-emotional problems of children born preterm at second grade. *Journal of Pediatric Psychology,* 17, 291-311.

Byrne, M.W. (1998). Feeding interactions in a cross section of HIV-exposed infants. . .including commentary by Lobo, M.L. and Barnard, K.E. with author response. *Western Journal of Nursing Research,* 20(4), 409-430.

Elliott, M.R., Drummond, J., & Barnard, K.E. (1996). Subjective appraisal of infant crying. *Clinical Nursing Research,* 5(2), 237-250.

Hammer, S.L. & Barnard, K.E. (1966, Nov.). The mentally retarded adolescent: A review of the characteristics and problems of 44 non-institutionalized adolescent retardates. *Pediatrics,* 38, 845-857.

Hann, D.M., Osofsky, J.D., Barnard, K.E., & Leonard, G. (1994). Dyadic affect regulation in three care giving environments. *American Journal of Orthopsychiatry,* 64, 263-269.

Hirose, T. & Barnard, K.E. (1997). Interactions between depressed mothers and their infants: Maternal verbal joint attention and its effect on the infant's cognitive development. *Early Child Development and Care,* 138, 83-95.

Houck, G.M., Booth, C.L., & Barnard, K.E. (1991). Maternal depression and locus of control orientation as predictors of dyadic play behavior. *Infant Mental Health Journal,* 12, 347-360.

Jacox, A., Lang, N., & Barnard, K.E. (1982, Oct.). Four nurses describe "dramatic" changes in education. *American Nurse,* 9, 8.

Kang, R. & Barnard, K. (1979). Using the neonatal behavioral assessment scale to evaluate premature infants. *Birth Defects: Original Article Series,* 15(7), 19-144.

Kang, R., Barnard, K., Hammond, M., Oshio, S., Spencer, C., Thibodeauz, B., & Williams, J. (1995). Preterm infant follow-up project: A multi-site test of a hospitalized and home intervention program for mothers and preterm infants. *Journal of Public Health Nursing,* 12(3), 171-180.

Kang, R., Barnard, K., & Oshio, S. (1994). Description of the clinical practice of advanced practice nurses in family-centered early intervention in two rural settings. *Public Health Nursing,* 11, 376-384.

Kelly, J.F., Morisset, C.E., Barnard, K.E., Hammond, M.A., & Booth, C.L. (1996). The influence of early mother-child interaction on preschool cognitive/linguistic outcomes in a high social risk group. *Infant Mental Health Journal,* 17(4), 310-321.

Kelly, J.F., Morisset, C.E., Barnard, K.E., & Patterson, D.L. (1996). Risky beginnings: Low maternal intelligence as a risk factor for children's intellectual development. *Infants and Young Children,* 8(3), 11-23.

King, D., Barnard, K.E., & Hoehn, R. (1981, March). Disseminating the results of nursing research. *Nursing Outlook, 29,* 164-169.

Lobo, M.L., Barnard, K.E., & Coombs, J.B. (1992). Failure to thrive: A parent-infant interaction perspective. *Journal of Pediatric Nursing, 7,* 251-261.

Mitchell, S.K., Barnard, K.E., Booth, C.L., Magyary, D., & Spieker, S. (1986). The natural alliance of psychology and nursing: Substance as well as practice (commentary). *American Psychologist, 41*(10), 1170.

Morisset, C.E., Barnard, K.E., & Booth, C.L. (1995). Toddlers' language development: Sex differences within social risk. *Developmental Psychology, 31,* 851-865.

Morisset, C.E., Barnard, K.E., Greenberg, M.T., Booth, C.L., & Spieler, S.J. (1990). Environmental influences on early language development: The context of social risk. *Development and Psychopathology, 2,* 127-149.

Murray, B.L. & Barnard, K.E. (1966, Dec.). The nursing specialist in mental retardation. *Nursing Clinics of North America, 1,* 631-640.

Patteson, D.M. & Barnard, K.E. (1990). Parenting of low birth weight infants: A review of issues and interventions. *Infant Mental Health Journal, 11,* 37-56.

Pattullo, A.W. & Barnard, K.E. (1968, Dec.). Teaching menstrual hygiene to the mentally retarded. Ame*rican Journal of Nursing, 12,* 2572-2575.

Snyder, C., Eyres, S.J., & Barnard, K.E. (1979, Nov./Dec.). New findings about mothers' antenatal expectations and their relationship to infant development. *American Journal of Maternal Child Nursing, 4,* 354-357.

Whitney, L. & Barnard, K.E. (1966, June). Implications of operant learning theory for nursing care of the mentally retarded. *Mental Retardation, 4,* 3.

Unpublished Papers

Barnard, K.E. (1967, April). *Nursing and mental retardation: A problem solving paper* (pp. 1-70). U.S. Public Health Service, Mental Retardation Division, Rockville, MD.

Barnard, K.E. (1967, April). *Planning for learning experiences in university affiliated centers.* Proceedings of the 4th National Workshop for Nurses in Mental Retardation, U.S. Children's Bureau, Washington, DC.

Barnard, K.E. (Principal Investigator). (1974, Sept./1981, April). *Premature infant refocus.* Grant No. MC-R-530348. Maternal and Child Health and Crippled Children's Services, Bureau of Community Health Services, Health Services Administration, Public Health Service, Department of Health and Human Resources.

Barnard, K.E. (1975). *Predictive nursing care.* Proceedings of Perinatal Nursing Conference, sponsored by University of Washington School of Nursing and Maternal and Child Health Services, Seattle, WA.

Barnard, K.E. (1976, Feb.). *A perspective on where we are in early intervention programs.* Adapted from a Keynote Address at a conference on "The Nursing Role in Early Intervention Programs for Developing Disabled Children," sponsored by the University of Utah College of Nursing Division of Continuing Education and Utah State Division of Health, Denver, CO.

Barnard, K.E. (1977). *Nursing child assessment satellite training fact sheet.* University of Washington School of Nursing, Seattle, WA.

Barnard, K.E. (Principal Investigator). (1979, July/1982, June). *Models of newborn nursing services.* Grant No. NU-00719. Division of Nursing, Bureau of Health Professions, Health Resources Administration, Public Health Service, Department of Health and Human Services.

Barnard, K.E. (1981). *Critical issues: Support of the caregiver. Maternal child nursing in the 80s: Nursing perspective.* Forum in honor of Katherine Kendall. School of Nursing, University of Maryland.

Barnard, K.E. (Principal Investigator). (1981, May). *Clinical nursing model for infants and their families.* National Institute of Mental Health, Alcohol, Drug Abuse, and Mental Health Administration, Public Health Service, Department of Health and Human Services. Grant submitted May 1981.

Barnard, K.E. (Ed.). (1983). *Structure to outcome—Making it work.* Papers of the First Faculty Practice Symposium, American Academy of Nursing. Kansas City, MO: American Nurses Association.

Barnard, K.E. & Bee, H.L. (1981, Sept.). *Premature infant refocus.* Final report on Grant No. MC-R-530348. Prepared for the Maternal and Child Health and Crippled Children's Services Research Grants Program, Bureau of Community Health Services, Health Services Administration, Public Health Service, Department of Health and Human Services.

Barnard, K.E., Booth, C.L., Mitchell, S.K., & Telzrow, R.W. (1983). *Newborn nursing models.* Final report on Grant No.R01-NU-00719. Prepared for the Division of Nursing, Bureau of Health Manpower, Health Resources Administration, Department of Health and Human Services.

Barnard, K.E. & Hoehn, R.E. (1978, Dec.). Nursing child assessment satellite training. In R.A. Duncan (Ed.), *Biomedical communications experiments.* Lister Hill National Center for Biomedical Communications, Department of Health, Education, and Welfare, Public Health Service.

Barnard, K.E. & Kelly, J.F. (1980, May). *Infant intervention: Parental consideration. State of art paper.* Guidelines for Early Intervention Programs. Based on a conference Health Issues in Early Intervention Programs, Washington, DC. Sponsored by College of Nursing, University of Utah, and School of Public Health, University of Hawaii. Office for Maternal and Child Health, Department of Health and Human Services.

Barnard, K.E., Lendzion, A., & Moser, J. (1974). *Final report on the measuring interactions project, technical report no. 3. The first three years: Programming for atypical infants and their families.* New York: United Cerebral Palsy Association.

Barnard, K.E. & Powell, M. (1967, April). *Planning for learning experiences in university affiliated centers.* Proceedings of the 4th National Workshop for Nurses in Mental Retardation, U.S. Children's Bureau.

Barnard, K.E. & Powell, M. (1969, Revised). *Washington guide to promoting development in the young child.* University of Washington, School of Nursing, mimeographed.

Barnard, K.E., Spietz, A.L., Snyder, C., Douglas, H.B., Eyres, S.J., & Hill, V. (1977). *The nursing child assessment satellite training study guide.* Unpublished program learning manual. University of Washington, Seattle, WA.

Barnard, K.E. & Summer, G.A. (1981, June). The health of women with fertility-related needs. In L.V. Klerman (Ed.), *Research priorities in maternal and child health: Report of a conference.* Brandeis University, Waltham, MA.

Bee, H.L., Disbrow, M.A., Johnson-Crowloy, N. (1981, April). *Parent-child interaction during teaching in abusing and nonabusing families.* Paper presented at the biennial meetings of the Society for Research in Child Development, Boston, MA.

Eyres, S.J., Barnard, K.E., & Gray, C.A. (1981). *Child health assessment, part III: 2-4 years.* University of Seattle, Seattle, WA.

Hammond, M.A., Bee H.L. Bernard, K.E. & Eyre, S.S. (1983, July). *Child health assessment, part IV: Follow-up at second grade.* Final report of Grant No. R01-NU-00816 prepared for Division of Nursing, Bureau of Health Professions, Health Resources and Services Administration, U.S. Public Health Service.

Interview

Barnard, K.E. (1984, Nov.). Cassette tape interview.

Correspondence

Barnard, K.E. (1999, Sept.). Curriculum vitae.

Barnard, K.E. (2000, June 20). Personal e-mail communication.

Videotapes

Barnard, K.E. (1990). *Keys to caregiving: Self-instructional video series. Nursing child assessment satellite training* [Videotape]. Available: University of Washington, School of Nursing, Seattle, WA, 98195. (206) 543-8528.

NAACOG invitational research conference, Indianapolis, Indiana [Videotape]. (1984, July). Available: Videotape

Services, Nursing Child Assessment Satellite Training, University of Washington.

Secondary Sources

Book Chapters

Disbrow, M.A. (1983). Conducting interdisciplinary research: Gratifications and frustrations. In N.L. Chaska (Ed.). *The nursing profession: A time to speak.* New York: McGraw-Hill.

Menke, E.M. (1983). Critical analysis of theory development in nursing. In N.L. Chaska (Ed.). *The nursing profession: A time to speak.* New York: McGraw-Hill.

Book Reviews

[Review of the book *Child health assessment, part I: A literature review*]. (1975, Sept.). *Registered Nurse,* 38, 122.

[Review of the book *Child health assessment, part I: A literature review*]. (1975, Oct.). *Nursing Mirror,* 141, 71.

[Review of the book *Child health assessment, part I: A literature review*]. (1975, Nov./Dec.). *Journal of Continuing Education in Nursing,* 6, 52.

[Review of the book *Teaching children with developmental problems: A family care approach* (2nd ed.).]. (1977, March). *American Journal of Nursing,* 77, 499.

[Review of the book *Teaching children with developmental problems: A family care approach* (2nd ed.).]. (1977, July). *Canadian Nurse,* 73, 46.

[Review of the book *Teaching the mentally retarded child: A family care approach*]. (1973, March). *Canadian Nurse,* 69, 54.

[Review of the book *Teaching the mentally retarded child: A family care approach*]. (1973, April). *American Journal of Nursing,* 73, 729.

Research Abstract

Barnard, K.E. (1972, Oct.). The effect of stimulation on the duration and amount of sleep and wakefulness in the premature infant. *Dissertation Abstracts International,* 33, 2167-2168.

News Releases

Kathryn E. Barnard named in directory of nurses with doctoral degrees. (1984). St. Louis: American Nurses Association.

Kathryn E. Barnard named in national nursing directory. (1982). Rockville, MD: Aspen Systems.

Kathryn E. Barnard named in Sigma Theta Tau directory of nurse researchers. (1983). Indianapolis: Sigma Theta Tau.

Kathryn E. Barnard presented with the Lucille Petry Leone award at NLN annual convention. (1969, May/June). *Washington State Journal of Nursing,* 41, 9.

Kathryn E. Barnard presented with the maternal and child health nurse of the year award for 1983 at ANA annual convention. (1984). *Nursing Outlook,* 32, 242.

Kathryn Elaine Barnard presented with the 1983 Martha May Eliot award of the American public health association, maternal and child health section. (1984, March/April). *Public Health Currents*, 24, 7-8.

Other Sources

(More than 122 articles document Barnard's work.)

Ainsworth, M.D.S. & Bell, S.M. (1974). Mother-infant interaction and development of competence (pp. 97-118). In K.J. Connolly & J. Bruner (Eds.), *The growth of competence.* New York: Academic Press.

Beckwith, L., Cohen, S.E., Kopp, C.B., Parmalee, A.H., & Marcy, T.G. (1976). Caregiver-infant interaction and early cognitive development in preterm infants. *Child Development*, 47, 579-587.

Brazelton, T.B. (1973). *The neonatal behavioral assessment scale.* London: William Heinemann

Brazelton, T.B. (1973). *The neonatal behavioral assessment scale.* Philadelphia: J.B. Lippincott.

Brazelton, T., Koslowski, B., & Main, M. (1974). The origins of reciprocity: The early mother-infant interaction. In M. Lewis & L. Rosenblum (Eds.), *The effect of the infant on its caregiver.* New York: John Wiley and Sons.

Brunner, J.S. (1956). *A study of thinking.* New York: John Wiley & Sons.

Brunner, J.S. (1966). *Studies in cognitive growth.* New York: John Wiley & Sons.

Caldwell, B.M. (1970). The rationale for early intervention. *Exceptional Children*, 36, 717-726.

Caldwell, B.M. (1971). Impact of interest in early cognitive stimulation. In H. Rie (Ed.), *Perspectives in psychopathology.* Chicago: Aldine-Atherton.

Caldwell, B.M., Hersher, L., Lipton, E., Richmond, J.B., Stern, G.A., Eddy, E., Drachman, R., & Rothman, A. (1963). Mother-infant interaction in monomatric and polymatric families. *American Journal of Orthopsychiatry*, 33, 653-664.

Caldwell, B.M. & Smith, L.E. (1970). Day care for the very young: Prime opportunity for primary prevention. *American Journal of Public Health*, 60, 690-697.

Caldwell, B.M., Wright, C.M., Honig, A.S., & Tannenbaum, B.S. (1970). Infant day care and attachment. *American Journal of Orthopsychiatry*, 40, 397-412.

Clarke-Stewart, K.A. (1973). Interactions between mothers and their young children: Characteristics and consequences. *Monographs of the Society for Research in Child Development*, 38(6-7), Serial No. 153.

Dubowitz, L.M.S., Dubowitz, V., & Goldberg, C. (1970). Clinical assessment of gestational age in the newborn infant. *Pediatrics*, 77, 1-10.

Piaget, J. (1962). *Judgment and reasoning in the child.* New York: Humanities. (Reproduction of 1928 edition.)

Robson, K.S. (1967). The role of eye to eye contact in maternal-infant attachment. *Journal of Child Psychology and Psychiatry*, 8, 13-25.

Sander, L.W. (1962). Issues in early mother child interaction. *Journal of American Academy of Child Psychiatry*, 3, 231-264.

Wachs, T.D., Uzgiris, I.C., & Hunt, J. McV. (1971). Cognitive development in infants of different age levels and from different environmental backgrounds: An explanatory investigation. *Merrill-Palmer Quarterly*, 17, 283-317.

Wesolowski, C. (1994, Oct.). Using keys to care giving in hospital-based nursing practice. *NCAST National News*, 10(4), 1-3.

Yarrow, L.J., Rubenstein, J.L., & Pederson, F.A. (1975). *Infant and environment: Early cognitive and motivational development.* Washington, DC: Hemisphere.

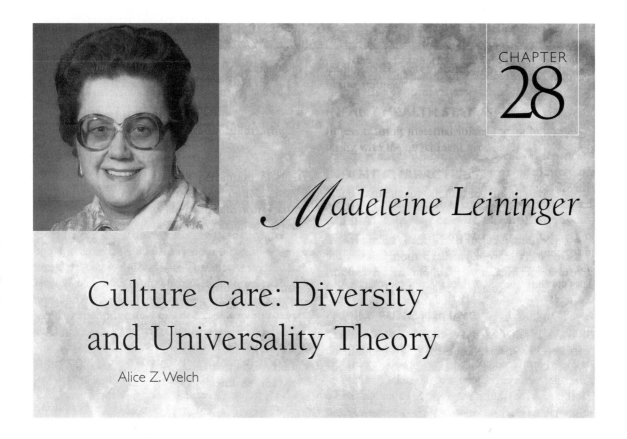

*M*adeleine Leininger

Culture Care: Diversity and Universality Theory

Alice Z. Welch

CREDENTIALS AND BACKGROUND OF THE THEORIST

Madeleine M. Leininger is the founder of transcultural nursing and a leader in transcultural nursing and human care theory. She is the first professional nurse with graduate preparation in nursing to hold a Ph.D. in cultural and social anthropology. She was born in Sutton, Nebraska and began her nursing career after graduating from a diploma program at St. Anthony's School of Nursing in Denver. She was a Cadet Corps nurse while pursuing the basic nursing program. In 1950, she obtained a B.S.

Previous authors: Alice Z. Welch, Sr. Judith E. Alexander, Carolyn J. Beagle, Pam Butler, Deborah A. Dougherty, Karen D. Andrews Robards, Kathleen C. Solotkin, and Catherine Velotta. The authors wish to express appreciation to Madeleine Leininger for critiquing the chapter and to librarians Melody Allison and Judy Tribble for locating obscure data.

degree in biological science from Benedictine College in Atchison, Kansas with a minor in philosophy and humanistic studies. After graduation, she served as an instructor, staff nurse, and head nurse on a medical-surgical unit and opened a new psychiatric unit as director of the nursing service at St. Joseph's Hospital in Omaha. During this time, she did advanced study in nursing, nursing administration, teaching and curriculum in nursing, and tests and measurements at Creighton University in Omaha.[22,26]

In 1954, Leininger obtained an M.S.N. in psychiatric nursing from the Catholic University of America in Washington, DC. She was then employed at the College of Health at the University of Cincinnati, where she began the first graduate clinical specialist program (M.S.N.) in child psychiatric nursing in the world. She also initiated and directed the first graduate-nursing program in psychiatric nursing at the University of Cincinnati and the Therapeutic Psychiatric Nursing Center at the University Hospital. During this time, she wrote one of the first basic psychiatric nursing texts with Hofling, *Basic Psychiatric Concepts in Nursing*,[2] which was published in 1960 in 11 languages and used worldwide.[23]

While working at the child guidance home in the mid1950s in Cincinnati, Leininger discovered the staff lacked an understanding of cultural factors influencing the behavior of children. Among these children of diverse cultural backgrounds, she observed differences that deeply concerned her in the care and psychiatric treatments of the children. Psychoanalytical theories and therapy strategies did not seem to reach children who were of different cultural backgrounds and needs. She became increasingly concerned that her nursing decisions and actions, and those of other staff, did not appear to help these children adequately. Leininger posed many questions to herself and the staff about cultural differences among children and therapy outcomes. She found few staff members were interested or knowledgeable about cultural factors in diagnosis and treatment of clients. A short time later, Margaret Mead became a visiting professor in the Department of Psychiatry, University of Cincinnati and Leininger discussed the potential interrelationships between nursing and anthropology with Mead. Although she did not get any direct help, encouragement, or solutions from Mead, Leininger decided to pursue her interests with doctoral (Ph.D.) focus on cultural, social, and psychological anthropology at the University of Washington, Seattle.

As a doctoral student, Leininger studied many cultures. She found anthropology fascinating and believed it was an area that should be of interest to all nurses. She focused on the Gadsup people of the Eastern Highlands of New Guinea, where she lived alone with the indigenous people for nearly two years and undertook an ethnographical and ethnonursing study of two villages.[22,26] Not only was she able to observe unique features of the culture, but she also observed a number of marked differences between Western and nonWestern cultures related to caring health and well-being practices. From her in-depth study and first-hand experiences with the Gadsup, she continued to develop her Theory of Culture Care and the ethnonursing method.[4,5,16,22] Her research and theory has helped nursing students understand cultural differences in human care, health, and illness. She has been the major nurse leader who has encouraged many students and faculty to pursue graduate foundational studies in anthropology and to relate this knowledge to transcultural nursing education and practice. Her enthusiasm and deep interests in developing this field of transcultural nursing with a human care focus has sustained her for four decades.

During the 1950s and 1960s, Leininger[3,4] identified several common areas of knowledge and theoretical research interests between nursing and anthropology, formulating transcultural nursing concepts, theory, principles, and practices. The book *Nursing and Anthropology: Two Worlds to Blend*,[3] which was the first beginning book in transcultural nursing, laid the foundation for developing the field of transcultural nursing, her theory, and culturally based healthcare. Her next book, *Transcultural Nursing: Concepts, Theories, and Practice*,[4] identified major concepts, theoretical ideas, and practices in transcultural nursing and was the first definitive publication on transcultural nursing in practice. In her writings, she has shown that transcultural nursing and anthropology are complementary to each other, but different from each other. Her theory and the conceptual framework for Culture Care Diversity and Universality were laid in *Transcultural Nursing: Concepts, Theories, and Practice*.[4] During the past 45 years, Leininger has established, explicated, and used the Theory of Culture Care to study many cultures within and outside the United States. She developed the ethnonursing qualitative research method to fit the theory, but especially to grasp the insider (emic) view of cultures.[16,22] The ethnonursing research method was the first nursing research method developed in nursing for nurses to examine complex care and cultural phenomena. In the past four decades, approximately 40 doctoral nurses and many masters and baccalaureate students have been prepared in transcultural nursing and have used the Leininger Theory of Culture Care.[12,16,27]

The first course offered in transcultural nursing was in 1966 at the University of Colorado, where Leininger was a professor of nursing and anthropology. This marked the first joint appointment of a professor of nursing and another discipline in the United States. She also initiated and served as the director of the first nurse-scientist program (Ph.D.) in the United States. In 1969, Leininger was appointed Dean and Professor of Nursing and Lecturer in Anthropology at the University of Washington, Seattle. There she established the first academic nursing department on comparative nursing care systems to support masters and doctoral programs in transcultural nursing. Under her leadership, the Research Facilitation Office was established in 1968 and 1969. She initiated several transcultural-nursing courses and guided the first nurses in a special Ph.D. program in transcultural nursing. She initiated the Committee on Nursing and Anthropology with the American Anthropological Association in 1968.[4]

In 1974, Leininger was appointed Dean and Professor of Nursing at the College of Nursing and Adjunct Professor of Anthropology at the University of Utah in Salt Lake City. At this institution, she initiated the first masters and doctoral programs in transcultural nursing and established the first doctoral program offerings at this institution.[4] The transcultural nursing courses were the first with substantive courses and research focused specifically on transcultural nursing in the world. She also initiated and was director of a new research facilitation office at the University of Utah.

In 1981, Leininger was recruited to Wayne State University in Detroit, where she was Professor of Nursing and Adjunct Professor of Anthropology and Director of Transcultural Nursing Offerings until her semiretirement in 1995. She was also Director of the Center for Health Research at this university for five years. While at Wayne State, she again developed several courses and seminars in transcultural nursing, caring, and qualitative research methods for baccalaureate, master, doctoral, and postdoctoral students. Currently, this doctoral program has the largest number of masters and doctoral students studying transcultural nursing in the world.[4] In addition to directing the transcultural offerings at

Wayne State University, Leininger taught and mentored many students and nurses in field research in transcultural nursing. As one of the first nurse leaders to use qualitative research methods in the early 1960s, she has continued to teach these methods at different universities within and outside the United States. To date, she has studied 14 cultures and continues to be a consultant to many research projects and institutions, especially those that are using her Theory of Culture Care.

With the growing interest in transcultural nursing and healthcare, Leininger[23] has delivered keynote addresses annually and conducted workshops and conferences both nationally and internationally since 1965. Her academic vitae records nearly 600 such conferences, keynote addresses, workshops, and consultant services in the United States, Canada, Europe, Pacific Islands, Asia, Africa, Australia, and the Scandinavian countries. She has been an invited guest specialist in most cultures and countries in the world. Educational and service settings continue to request her consultation to focus on transcultural nursing, humanistic caring, ethnonursing research, her Theory of Culture Care, and futuristic trends in healthcare worldwide.

As the first professional nurse to complete a doctoral degree in anthropology and to initiate several masters and doctoral nursing education programs, Leininger has many areas of expertise and interests. She has studied 14 major cultures in depth and has had experience with many different additional cultures. Besides transcultural nursing with care as a central focus, her other areas of interest are comparative education and administration, nursing theories, politics, ethical dilemmas of nursing and healthcare, qualitative research methods, the future of nursing and healthcare, and nursing leadership. Her Theory of Culture Care is now used worldwide and is growing in relevance and importance to obtain grounded cultural data from diverse cultures.

In 1974, she initiated the National Transcultural Nursing Society organization and has been an active leader in this society since its inception. She also initiated the National Research Care Conference in 1978 to help nurses focus specifically on the study of human care phenomena.* She initiated the *Journal of Transcultural Nursing* in 1989 and served as its editor through 1995. The *Journal of Transcultural Nursing* remains the only publication focusing primarily on transcultural nursing phenomena.

Leininger has gained international recognition in nursing and related fields through her transcultural nursing and care writings, theory, research, consultation, courses, and dynamic addresses. She has enthusiastically worked to persuade nurse educators and practitioners to incorporate transcultural nursing and culture-specific care concepts with research findings into nursing curricula and clinical practice as the new and futuristic direction of all aspects of nursing.[16,22,27] She has found time to give lectures to anthropologists, physicians, social workers, pharmacists, and educators and to do research with other colleagues. She is one of the few nurses who has kept active in two disciplines and has continued to contribute to both fields in national and international transcultural conferences and association meetings. Currently, Leininger resides in Omaha, Nebraska and is semiretired, but still active in worldwide consulting, writing, and lecturing. Her present interest is to establish transcultural-nursing institutes to educate and do research on transcultural nursing and health phenomena.

Leininger has authored or edited more than 27 books. Some of her books include: *Nursing and Anthropology: Two Worlds to Blend;*[3] *Transcultural Nursing: Concepts, Theories and Practice;*[4] *Caring: An Essential Human Need;*[5] *Care: The Essence of Nursing and Health;*[6] *Qualitative Research Methods in Nursing;*[9] *Ethical and Moral Dimensions of Care;*[12] *The Caring Imperative in Education;*[27] and *Culture Care Diversity and Universality: A Theory of Nursing,*[16] which is a full account of her theory with the method. She has published more than 200 articles and 45 chapters, plus numerous films and research reports focused on transcultural nursing, human care and health phenomena, the future of nursing, and related topics relevant in nursing and anthropology. She serves on eight editorial boards

*References 5, 6, 8, 12, 16, 27.

and several referee publications. She is known as one of the most creative, productive, innovative, and futuristic authors in nursing, always providing new and substantive research-based nursing content and ideas to advance nursing as a discipline and profession.

Leininger has received many awards and honors for her lifetime professional and academic accomplishments. She is listed in *Who's Who of American Women, Who's Who in Health Care, Who's Who in Community Leaders, World's Who's Who of Women in Education, International Who's Who in Community Service, Who's Who in International Women,* and other such listings. Her name appears on the *National Register of Prominent Americans and International Notables, International Women,* and the *National Register of Prominent Community Leaders.* She has received several honorary degrees, such as an L.H.D. from Benedictine College, a Ph.D. from the University of Kuopio (Finland), and a D.S. from the University of Indiana. In 1976 and 1995, she was recognized for her unique and significant contribution to the American Association of Colleges of Nursing as its first full-time president. Leininger received the Russell Sage Outstanding Leadership Award in 1995. Leininger is a Fellow in the American Academy of Nursing, a Fellow of the American Anthropology Society, and a Fellow of the Society for Applied Anthropology. Other affiliations include Sigma Theta Tau, the National Honor Society of Nursing, Delta Kappa Gamma, the National Honorary Society in Education, and the Scandinavian College of Caring Science in Stockholm. She has served as distinguished visiting scholar or lecturer in 85 universities in this country and abroad and was recently visiting professor at six universities in Sweden, Wales, Japan, China, Australia, Finland, and New Zealand. While at Wayne State University, she received the Board of Regents' Distinguished Faculty Awards, Distinguished Research Award, the President's Excellence in Teaching, and the Outstanding Graduate Faculty Mentor Award. In 1996, Madonna University honored her with the dedication of the Leininger Book Collection and a special Leininger Reading Room for her outstanding contributions to nursing and the social sciences and humanities.

THEORETICAL SOURCES

Leininger's theory[16,22] is derived from the disciplines of anthropology and nursing. She has defined transcultural nursing as a major area of nursing that focuses on a comparative study and analysis of different cultures and subcultures in the world with respect to their caring values, expression, and health-illness beliefs and pattern of behavior with the goal to develop a scientific and humanistic knowledge to provide culture-specific nursing care practice and/or culture-universal nursing care practice.[16,22]

Transcultural nursing goes beyond an awareness state to that of using culture care nursing knowledge to practice culturally congruent and responsible care.[16,22] Leininger has stated that in time, there will be a new kind of nursing practice that reflects different nursing practices that are culturally defined and grounded and specific to guide nursing care to individuals, families, groups, and institutions. She contends that because culture and care are the broadest and the most holistic means to conceptualize and understand people, this knowledge is central to and imperative to nursing education and practice.[16,22] In addition, she states that transcultural nursing has become one of the most important, relevant, and highly promising areas of formal study, research, and practice because people live in a multicultural world.[6,8,22] Leininger[16,22,24,26] predicts that for nursing to be meaningful and relevant to clients and other nurses in the world, transcultural nursing knowledge and competencies will be imperative to guide all nursing decisions and actions for effective and successful outcomes.

Leininger makes a distinction between transcultural nursing and cross-cultural nursing. The former refers to nurses prepared in transcultural nursing who are committed to develop knowledge and practice in transcultural nursing, whereas cross-cultural nursing refers to nurses using applied or medical anthropological concepts, with many nurses not committed to developing transcultural

nursing theory and research-based practices.[22] She also identifies that international nursing and transcultural nursing are different. International nursing focuses on nurses functioning between two cultures and transcultural nursing focuses on several cultures with a comparative theoretical and practice base.[22]

Leininger[10,11,17,22] describes the transcultural nurse as a nurse prepared at the baccalaureate level who is able to apply general transcultural nursing concepts, principles, and practices that are generated by transcultural nurse-specialists. The transcultural nurse-specialist prepared in graduate programs receives in-depth preparation and mentorship in transcultural nursing knowledge and practice. This specialist has acquired competency skills through postbaccalaureate education. "This specialist has studied selected cultures in sufficient depth (values, beliefs, lifeways) and is highly knowledgeable and theoretically based about care, health and environmental factors related to transcultural nursing perspectives."[7:252] The transcultural nurse-specialist serves as an expert field practitioner, teacher, researcher, and/or consultant with respect to select cultures. This individual also values and uses transcultural nursing theory to develop and advance knowledge within the discipline of transcultural nursing, the field Leininger[22] predicts must be the focus of all nursing education and practice.

Leininger[25] holds and promotes a new and different theory from the traditional theory in nursing, which usually defines theory as a set of logically interrelated concepts and hypotheses propositions that can be tested for the purpose of explaining or predicting an event, phenomenon or situation. Instead, Leininger defines theory as the systematic and creative discovery of knowledge about a domain of interest or a phenomenon that appears important to understand or account for some unknown phenomenon. She believes that nursing theory must take into account the creative discovery about individuals, families, and groups and their caring, values, expressions, beliefs, and actions or practices based on their cultural lifeways to provide effective, satisfying, and culturally congruent nursing care. If nursing practices fail to recognize the cultural care aspects of human needs, there will be signs of less beneficial or efficacious nursing care practices and even evidence of dissatisfaction with nursing services, which limits healing and well being.[16,20,22]

Leininger developed her Theory of Culture Care Diversity and Universality, which is based on the belief that people of different cultures can inform and are capable of guiding professionals to receive the kind of care they desire or need from others. Culture is the patterned and valued lifeways of people that influence their decisions and actions; therefore the theory is directed toward nurses to discover and document the world of the client and to use their emic viewpoints, knowledge, and practices, with appropriate etic (professional knowledge), as bases for making culturally congruent professional actions and decisions.[16,22] Indeed, culture care is the broadest holistic nursing theory because it takes into account the totality and holistic perspective of human life and existence over time, including the social structure factors, world view, cultural history and values, environmental context,[5] language expressions, and folk (generic) and professional patterns. These are some of the critical and essential bases to discover grounded care knowledge as the essence of nursing that can lead to the health and well being of clients and guide therapeutic nursing practice. The Theory of Culture Care can be inductive and deductive, derived from emic (insider) and etic (outsider) knowledge. However, Leininger encourages obtaining grounded emic knowledge from the people or the culture because such knowledge is most credible. The theory is not necessarily middle range nor macro theory, but must be viewed holistically or with specific domains of interest. Leininger[16,22] believes the terms *middle range* and *macro* are outdated in theory development and uses.

USE OF EMPIRICAL EVIDENCE

For more than four decades, Leininger[3,5,8,16] has held that care is the essence of nursing and the dom-

inant, distinctive, and unifying feature of nursing. She states that care is complex, illusive, and often embedded in social structure and other aspects of culture. She holds that there are different forms, expressions, and patterns of care that are diverse and some are universal.[16]

Leininger[9,13] favors qualitative ethnomethods, especially ethnonursing, to study care. These methods are directed toward discovering the people's *truth,* views, beliefs, and patterned lifeways. Ethnoscience is one of the rigorous ethnomethods used in anthropology to discover nursing knowledge. However, in the 1960s, Leininger developed the ethnonursing methods to study transcultural-nursing phenomena specifically and systematically. Ethnonursing focuses on the systematic study and classification of nursing care beliefs, values, and practices as cognitively or subjectively known by a designated culture (or cultural representatives) through their local emic people-centered language, experiences, beliefs, and value system about actual or potential nursing phenomena such as care, health, and environmental factors.[16,22] Although nursing has used the words *care* and *caring* for more than a century, the definitions and usage have been vague and used as clichés without specific meanings to the culture of the client or nurse.[5,6] "Indeed, the concepts about caring have been some of the least understood and studied of all human knowledge and research areas within and outside of nursing."[4:33] With the transcultural culture care theory and ethnonursing method based on emic (insider views) beliefs, a person gets close to the discovery of grounded or people-based care because it is primarily data centered from the informants and is not derived from the researcher's etic (outsider views) beliefs and practices. An important purpose of the theory is to document, know, predict, and explain systematically, by field-generated data, what is diverse and universal about generic and professional care of the cultures being studied within the broad Sunrise Model components. The purpose of transcultural nursing theory is to discover the cultural views or people's emic views about care as they know, believe, and practice care and then use this knowledge with appropriate etic professional knowledge to guide care practices. The goal of the theory is to provide culturally congruent and responsible care that reasonably fits with the client's culture needs, values, beliefs, and lifeway realities.[16,22]

Leininger[6,8] holds that detailed and culturally based caring knowledge and practices should distinguish nursing from the contributions of other disciplines. The first reason for studying care theory is that the construct of care appears to be critical to human growth, development, and survival for human beings from the beginning of human species.[5,6] The second reason is to explicate and fully understand the cultural knowledge and the roles of caregivers and care recipients in different cultures to provide culturally congruent care. Third, care knowledge is discovered and can be used as essential to promote the healing and well being of clients, to face death, or to ensure the survival of human cultures through time.[5,6,16] Fourth, the nursing profession needs to study systematic care from a broad and holistic cultural perspective to discover the expressions and meanings of care, health, illness, and well being as nursing knowledge. Leininger finds that care is largely an elusive phenomenon often embedded in cultural lifeways and values.

However, this knowledge is a sound basis for nurses to guide their practice for culturally congruent care and specific therapeutic ways to maintain health, prevent illness, heal, or to help people face death.[18] A central thesis of the theory is, if the meaning of culture care can be fully grasped, the well being or healthcare of individuals, families, and groups can be predicted and culturally congruent care can be provided. Leininger views care as one of the most powerful constructs and the central phenomena of nursing. However, such care constructs and patterns must be fully documented, understood, and used to ensure that culturally based care becomes the major guide to transcultural nursing therapy and is used to explain or predict nursing practices.

To date, Leininger has studied several cultures in depth and has studied many cultures with undergraduate and graduate students and faculty through the use of qualitative research methods. She has explicated 130 different care constructs in 56 cultures in which each culture has different meanings, cultural experiences, and uses by the people of diverse and similar cultures.[16,22] A new body of knowledge continues to be discovered by transcultural nurses in the development of transcultural care practices with diverse and similar cultures. In time, Leininger believes that both diverse and universal features of care and health will be documented as the essence of nursing knowledge and practice.

Leininger stated that the goal of the care theory is to provide culturally congruent care. She believes nurses must work toward explicating care use and meanings so culture care, values, beliefs, and lifeways can provide accurate and reliable bases for planning and effectively implementing culture-specific care and to identify any universal or common features about care. She maintains that nurses cannot separate worldviews, social structure, and cultural beliefs (folk and professional) from health, wellness, illness, or care when working with cultures because these factors are closely linked. Social structure factors such as religion, politics, culture, economics, and kinship are significant forces affecting care and influencing well being and illness patterns. She also emphasizes the importance of discovering generic (folk, local, and indigenous) care from the cultures and comparing it with professional care.

Leininger finds that today, cultural blindness, shock, imposition, and ethnocentrism by nurses still greatly reduce the quality of care to clients of different cultures.[15,18,22] Moreover, nursing diagnoses and medical diagnoses that are not culturally based and known are serious problems for cultures that lead to unfavorable and sometimes serious outcomes.[14] Providing culturally congruent care is what makes clients satisfied that they receive *good care;* it is a powerful healing force for quality healthcare. Quality care is what clients seek most when they come for services from nurses and it can only be realized when culturally derived care is known and used.

MAJOR CONCEPTS & DEFINITIONS

Leininger has developed many terms relevant to the theory; the major ones are defined here. The reader can study her full theory from her definitive book on the theory.[16]*

CARE (NOUN)

Refers to abstract and concrete phenomena related to assisting, supporting, or enabling experiences or behaviors toward or for others with evident or anticipated needs to ameliorate or improve a human condition or lifeway.

CARING (GERUND)

Refers to actions and activities directed toward assisting, supporting, or enabling another individual or group with evident or anticipated needs to ameliorate or improve a human condition or lifeway, or to face death.

CULTURE

Refers to the learned, shared, and transmitted values, beliefs, norms, and lifeways of a particular group that guides their thinking, decisions, and actions in patterned ways.

CULTURAL CARE

Refers to the subjectively and objectively learned and transmitted values, beliefs, and patterned lifeways that assist, support, facilitate, or enable another individual or group to maintain their well being and health, to improve their human condition and lifeway, or to deal with illness, handicaps, or death.

CULTURAL CARE DIVERSITY

Refers to the variabilities and/or differences in meanings, patterns, values, lifeways, or symbols of care within or between collectivities that are related to assistive, supportive, or enabling human care expressions.

CULTURAL CARE UNIVERSALITY

Refers to the common, similar, or dominant uniform care meanings, patterns, values, lifeways, or symbols that are manifest among many cultures and reflect assistive, supportive, facilitative, or enabling ways to help people. (The term *universality* is not used in an absolute way or as a significant statistical finding.)

NURSING

Refers to a learned humanistic and scientific profession and discipline that is focused on human care phenomena and activities to assist, support, facilitate, or enable individuals or groups to maintain or regain their well being (or health) in culturally meaningful and beneficial ways, or to help people face handicaps or death.

WORLDVIEW

Refers to the way people tend to look out on the world or their universe to form a picture or a value stance about their life or world around them.

CULTURAL AND SOCIAL STRUCTURE DIMENSIONS

Refers to the dynamic patterns and features of interrelated structural and organizational factors of a particular culture (subculture or society), which includes religious, kinship (social), political (and legal), economic, educational, technological, and cultural values and ethnohistorical factors, and how these factors may be interrelated and function to influence human behavior in different environmental contexts.

ENVIRONMENTAL CONTEXT

Refers to the totality of an event, situation, or particular experience that gives meaning to human expressions, interpretations, and social interactions, particularly physical, ecological, sociopolitical, and/or cultural settings.

*Used with permission from National League for Nursing, New York, NY.

MAJOR CONCEPTS & DEFINITIONS—cont'd

ETHNOHISTORY

Refers to those past facts, events, instances, and experiences of individuals, groups, cultures, and institutions that are primarily people centered (ethno) and that describe, explain, and interpret human lifeways within particular cultural contexts and over short or long periods.

GENERIC (FOLK OR LAY) CARE SYSTEM

Refers to culturally learned and transmitted, indigenous (or traditional), folk (home based) knowledge and skills used to provide assistive, supportive, enabling, or facilitative acts toward or for another individual, group, or institution with evident or anticipated needs to ameliorate or improve a human lifeway or health condition (or well being), or to deal with handicaps and death situations.

PROFESSIONAL CARE SYSTEM(S)

Refers to formally taught, learned, and transmitted professional care, health, illness, wellness, and related knowledge and practice skills that prevail in professional institutions usually with multidisciplinary personnel to serve consumers.

HEALTH

Refers to a state of well being that is culturally defined, valued, and practiced and reflects the ability of individuals (or groups) to perform their daily role activities in culturally expressed, beneficial, and patterned lifeways.

CULTURAL CARE PRESERVATION OR MAINTENANCE

Refers to those assistive, supporting, facilitative, or enabling professional actions and decisions that help people of a particular culture to retain and/or preserve relevant care values so that they can maintain their well being, recover from illness, or face handicaps and/or death.

CULTURAL CARE ACCOMMODATION OR NEGOTIATION

Refers to those assistive, supporting, facilitative, or enabling creative professional actions and decisions that help people of a designated culture to adapt to, or to negotiate with, others for a beneficial or satisfying health outcome with professional care providers.

CULTURAL CARE REPATTERNING OR RESTRUCTURING

Refers to those assistive, supporting, facilitative, or enabling professional actions and decisions that help clients reorder, change, or greatly modify their lifeways for new, different, and beneficial healthcare patterns while respecting the clients' cultural values and beliefs and still providing a beneficial or healthier lifeway than before the changes were coestablished with the clients.

CULTURAL CONGRUENT (NURSING) CARE

Refers to those cognitively based assistive, supportive, facilitative, or enabling acts or decisions that are tailor made to fit with individual, group, or institutional cultural values, beliefs, and lifeways to provide or support meaningful, beneficial, and satisfying healthcare or well-being services.

MAJOR ASSUMPTIONS

Major assumptions to support Leininger's Culture Care Diversity and Universality Theory follow. The definitions were taken from Leininger's definitive book on the theory.[16:44-45]

"1. Care is the essence of nursing and a distinct, dominant, central, and unifying focus.

2. Care (caring) is essential for well-being, health, healing, growth, survival, and to face handicaps or death.

3. Culture care is the broadest holistic means to know, explain, interpret, and predict nursing care phenomena to guide nursing care practices.

4. Nursing is a transcultural humanistic and scientific care discipline and profession with the central purpose to serve human beings worldwide.

5. Care (caring) is essential to curing and healing, for there can be no curing without caring.

6. Culture care concepts, meanings, expressions, patterns, processes, and structural forms of care are different (diversity) and similar (towards commonalities or universalities) among all cultures of the world.

7. Every human culture has generic (lay, folk, or indigenous) care knowledge and practices and usually professional care knowledge and practices, which vary transculturally.

8. Cultural care values, beliefs, and practices are influenced by and tend to be embedded in the world view, language, religious (or spiritual), kinship (social), political (or legal), educational, economic, technological, ethnohistorical, and environmental context of a particular culture.

9. Beneficial, healthy, and satisfying culturally based nursing care contributes to the well-being of individuals, families, groups, and communities within their environmental context.

10. Culturally congruent or beneficial nursing care can occur only when the individual, group, family, community, or culture care values, expressions, or patterns are known and used appropriately and in meaningful ways by the nurse with the people.

11. Culture care differences and similarities between professional caregiver(s) and client (generic) care-receiver(s) exist in any human culture worldwide.

12. Clients who experience nursing care that fails to be reasonably congruent with the client's beliefs, values, and caring lifeways will show signs of cultural conflicts, noncompliance, stresses, and ethical or moral concerns.

13. The qualitative paradigm provides new ways of knowing and different ways to discover epistemic and ontological dimensions of human care transculturally."

THEORETICAL ASSERTIONS

Leininger developed several predictive formulations from her Transcultural Nursing Culture Care Theory as examples to stimulate nursing research. These formulations are based on her ongoing inquiry, research studies, and other anthropological and nursing investigations from mainly qualitative investigations. A major prediction of her theory is that health or well being can be predicted from the epistemic and ontological dimensions of culture care. Predictive statements have also been formulated on the basis of field studies.

From her many articles and books, several predictions, such as the following, have been made by qualitative methods:

1. Identifiable differences in cultural caring values and patterns between and among cultures will lead to major differences in the nursing care expectations and practices.

2. Differences in cultural caring values, norms, and beliefs between technologically dependent and nontechnologically dependent societies will show marked comparative differences.

3. As professional nurses work in strange cultures with different values about nursing care or caring expectations, there will be overt signs of cultural conflicts, clashes, and stresses between the nurse and the client.

4. The greater the evidence of dependence of nursing personnel on technological tasks and activities, the greater the signs of interpersonal distance and fewer client satisfactions.

5. Nursing care interventions that provide culture-specific caring practices to clients will show positive signs of client satisfaction and well being.

6. From the study and use of cultures, care, beliefs, values, and practices, signs of health or well being of clients will be discovered.

In *Care: The Essence of Nursing and Health*[6] Leininger identified the following theoretical statements and a few hypotheses, with some added revisions since the book was published in 1984:

1. Intercultural differences in care beliefs, values, and practices will reflect identifiable differences and some commonalities for nursing care practices.

2. Cultures that highly value individualism with independence modes will show signs of self-care practices and values, whereas cultures that do not value individualism and independence will show limited signs of self-care practices and more signs of other-care practices.

3. If there is a close relationship between caregiver's beliefs and care receiver's beliefs and practices, client care outcomes will be health promoting and satisfying.

4. Clients from different cultures can identify their caring and noncaring values and beliefs with ethnonursing enablers.

5. The greater the differences between folk or generic care values and professional care values, the greater the signs of cultural conflict and stresses between professional caregivers and clients.

6. Technological caring acts, techniques, and practices differ transculturally and have different outcomes for the health and well being of clients.

7. The greater the signs of dependency on technology of the nurse, the greater the signs of depersonalized humanistic nursing care to clients.

8. Symbolic forms and ritual functions of nursing care behaviors and practices have different meanings and outcomes in different cultures.

9. Political, religious, economic, kinship, and cultural values and environmental contexts greatly influence cultural practices and the well being of individuals, families, and groups.

A sample of other predictive statements to be discovered from Leininger's *Transcultural Nursing: Concepts, Theories, and Practice* in 1978[4] and 1995[22] include the following:

1. Cultures that perceived illness to be largely a personal and internal body experience (caused by physical, genetic, and intrabody stresses) tend to use more technical and physical self-care methods (pills and physical techniques) than do cultures that view illness as cultural beliefs and extrapersonal and direct cultural experiences.

2. Cultures that strongly emphasize caring values, behaviors, and processes tend to have more females than males in caring roles.

3. Cultures that emphasize curing behaviors and treatment processes tend to have more male curers than female curers.

4. Clients in need of caring services tend to seek their caring persons first (local folk or generic healers), such as family members or friends, and only seek professional caregivers later if the folk remedies are not effective, if the condition worsens, or if death is feared.

5. Ritualized ethnocaring activities that have therapeutic benefits to clients and their families tend to be largely unknown or are less valued by Western professional nurses and physicians.

6. Where there is marked evidence of nurturant caring behaviors in a culture, there will be less need for professional services and curers.

7. Marked differences in generic and professional care practices lead to cultural conflicts and imposition practices.

8. Transculturally prepared nurses can make a major difference in client healthcare outcomes.

9. Healthcare reform will be unsuccessful unless cultural values, beliefs, and practices are explicitly known and used.

LOGICAL FORM

Leininger's theory[22] is derived from anthropology and nursing, but is reformulated to be transcultural nursing with human care perspective. She developed the ethnonursing research method and has emphasized the importance of studying people from their emic or local knowledge and experiences and later contrasting them with etic (outsider) beliefs and practices. Her book, *Qualitative Research Methods in Nursing*,[9] and related articles[16,22] provide substantive knowledge about qualitative methods in nursing.

In her own research, Leininger is skilled in using ethnonursing, ethnography, life histories, life stories, photography, and phenomenological methods that provide a holistic approach to study cultural behavior in diverse environmental contexts. With these qualitative methods, the researcher moves with the people in their daily living activities to grasp their world and the nurse researcher inductively obtains data of documented descriptive and interpretive accounts from informants through observations and participation or in other ways explicating care as a major challenge within the method. The qualitative approach is important to develop basic and substantive grounded data-based knowledge about cultural care to guide nurses in their work. From the beginning, ethnonursing has been primarily grounded in data from the cultures under study, which is different from grounded theory of Glasser and Strauss.[1]

Leininger[9] has also used the ethnoscience method as a formal and rigorous method to study nursing and human phenomena. Ethnoscience refers to the systematic study of the way of life of a designated cultural group to obtain an accurate account of the people's behavior and how they perceive and know their universe. This method involves a logical, semantic classifying of data as they reflect the people's views in their words through confirming the credibility of these data with the people. The ethnoscience method provides data that will help nurses understand the meanings of care for whatever phenomena are studied and to explain and predict human behavior within a cultural context. Emic data are largely obtained through ethnoscientific research; the research analyzes both emic and etic data. An emic analysis reveals the native's or a local culture's way of knowing and classifying their world. An etic analysis searches for common or more universal (outsider) features that may be found in more than one culture. Both emic and etic data are also used in ethnonursing and to discover universal and diverse features.[9] Although other methods of research, such as hypothesis testing and experimental quantitative methods, can be used to study transcultural care, the method of choice depends on the researcher's purposes, the goals of the study, and the phenomena to be studied. Creativity and the willingness of the nurse researcher to use different research methods to discover nursing knowledge are encouraged. However, Leininger holds that qualitative methods are important to establish meanings and accurate cultural knowledge. Quantitative methods have generally been of limited value to study cultures and care. Combining both qualitative and quantitative methods tends to obscure the findings and is a misuse of both paradigms.[16,22]

Leininger developed the Sunrise Model (Figure 28-1) in the 1970s to depict the essential components of the theory. She has refined the model since the late 1950s, but today the model is definitive and valuable to accurately study the diverse elements or its components of the theory and to make culturally logical clinical assessments. This model and the full theory of cultural care diversity and universality are not addressed here. Only selected ideas are offered to introduce the reader to Leininger's pioneering and creative work of evolving theory through time. The Sunrise Model symbolizes the rising of the sun (care).[16,22] The upper half of the circle depicts components of the social structure and worldview factors that influence care and health through language, ethnohistory, and environmental context. These factors also influence the folk, professional, and nursing system(s), which are in the middle part of the model. The two halves together form a full sun, which represents the universe that nurses must consider to appreciate human care and health.[16,22] According to Leininger, nursing acts as a bridge between the folk generic and the professional system. Three kinds of nursing care and decisions and actions are predicted in the theory: (1) cultural care preservation and maintenance, (2) cultural care accommodation and/or negotiation, and (3) cultural care repatterning and/or restructuring.[16,22]

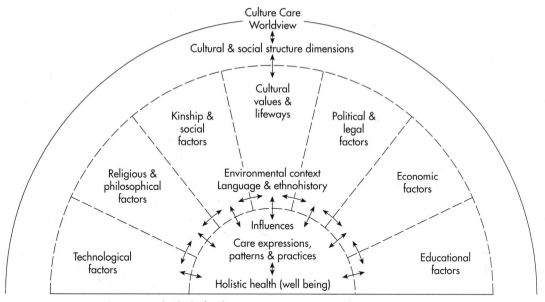

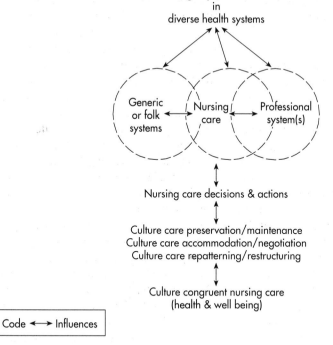

Figure **28-1** Leininger's Sunrise Model to depict Theory of Cultural Care Diversity and Universality. (Modified by Madeleine Leininger in personal correspondence of 1996 from Leininger, M.M. [1991]. *Culture care: Diversity and universality* [p. 43]. New York: National League for Nursing. Used with permission.)

The Sunrise Model depicts human beings as inseparable from their cultural background and social structure, worldview, history, and environmental context as a basic tenet of Leininger's theory.[16,22] Gender, race, age, and class are embedded in social structure factors and are studied. Biological, emotional, and other dimensions are studied from a holistic view and not fragmented or separate. Theory generation from this model may occur at multiple levels from the micro range (small-scale specific individuals) or to study groups, families, communities, or large-scale phenomena (several cultures). Leininger also describes two phases of generating research knowledge: (phase 1) discovering substantive knowledge and (phase 2) applying the knowledge to practice situations.[16,22]

Leininger has also developed a computer software program based on her theory, the Leininger-Templin-Thompson Ethnoscript Qualitative Software Program, to assist with detailed analysis of qualitative ethnodata. She has also developed several enablers to study phenomena with four phases of qualitative data analysis. Most important, the qualitative criteria are used to analyze the data: (1) credibility, (2) confirmability, (3) meaning in context, (4) saturations, (5) repatterncy, and (6) transferability.[12,16] Quantitative criteria should not be used with qualitative methods because the former have specific criteria to measure data outcomes.

ACCEPTANCE BY THE NURSING COMMUNITY

Practice

Leininger identifies several factors related to the slowness of nurses to recognize and value transcultural nursing and cultural factors in nursing practices and education. First, the theory was conceptualized in the 1950s, when virtually no nurses were prepared in anthropology or cultural knowledge to understand transcultural concepts, models, or her theory. In the early days, most nurses had no idea about the nature of anthropology and how anthropological knowledge might contribute to human care and health behaviors or serve as background knowledge to understand nursing phenomena or problems. Second, although people had long standing and inherent cultural needs, many clients were reluctant to push health personnel to meet their cultural needs and therefore did not demand that their cultural and social needs be recognized or met.[3,4,22] Third, until the past decade, transcultural nursing articles submitted for publication were often rejected because editors did not know, value, or understand the relevance of cultural knowledge to transcultural nursing or as essential to nursing. Fourth, the concept of care was of limited interest to nurses until the late 1970s, when Leininger began promoting the importance of nurses studying human care, obtaining background knowledge in anthropology, and obtaining graduate preparation in transcultural nursing, research, and practice. Fifth, Leininger contends that nursing tends to remain too ethnocentric and far too involved in following medicine's interest and directions. Sixth, nursing has been slow to make substantive progress in the development of its distinct body of knowledge because many nurse-researchers have been far too dependent on quantitative research methods to get measurable outcomes rather than qualitative data outcomes. The recent acceptance and use of qualitative research methods in nursing will provide new insights and knowledge related to nursing and transcultural nursing.[16,22] There is growing interest in using transcultural nursing knowledge, research, and practice by nurses worldwide.

Nurses are now realizing the importance of transcultural nursing, human care, and qualitative methods. Leininger[25] states:

> We are entering a new phase of nursing as we value and use transcultural nursing knowledge with a focus on human caring, health and illness behaviors focus. With the migration of many cultural groups and the rise of the consumer cultural identity, and demands in culturally based care, nurses are realizing the need for culturally sensitive and competent practices. Most countries and communities of the world are multicultural today, and so health personnel are expected to understand and respond to clients of diverse and similar cultures. Immigrants and people from unfamiliar cultures expect nurses to respect and respond to values, beliefs, lifeways, and needs. No longer can nurses practice unicultural nursing.

As our world becomes more culturally diverse, nurses will find the urgent need to be prepared to provide culturally competent care. Some nurses are experiencing culture shock, conflict, and clashes as they move from one area to another and from rural to urban communities without transcultural nursing preparation. As cultural conflicts arise, families are less satisfied with nursing and medical services.[16] Nurses who travel and seek employment in foreign lands are experiencing immigrant status. Transcultural nursing education has become imperative for all nurses worldwide.

Certification of transcultural nurses by the Transcultural Nursing Society has provided a major step toward protecting the public from unsafe and culturally incompetent nursing practices.[15] Accordingly, more nurses are seeking transcultural certification to protect themselves and their clients. The *Journal of Transcultural Nursing* has also provided transcultural nurses with research and theoretical perspectives of over 100 cultures worldwide to guide them in their practices.

Education

The inclusion of culture and comparative care in nursing curricula began in 1966 at the University of Colorado, where Leininger was a professor of nursing and anthropology. Awareness of the importance of culture care to nursing gradually began to appear in the late 1960s, but very few nurse-educators were adequately prepared to teach courses on transcultural nursing. Since the world's first masters and doctoral programs in transcultural nursing were approved and implemented in 1977 at the University of Utah, more nurses have been prepared specifically in transcultural nursing. Today, with the heightened public awareness of healthcare costs, different cultures, and human rights, there is a much greater demand for comprehensive, holistic, and transcultural people care to protect and provide quality-based care and to prevent legal suits related to improper client care. Leininger's demand[22,24,26] for culture-specific care based on theoretical insights has been critical to discover diverse and universal aspects of care. A critical need remains for nurses to be educated in transcultural nursing in undergraduate and graduate programs. There is also a need for well-qualified faculty prepared in transcultural nursing to teach and to guide research in nursing schools within the United States and in other countries.[22,26]

Since 1980, there has been an increasing number of nursing curricula emphasizing transcultural nursing and human care. One of the early programs to focus on care was at Cuestra College in California in the 1970s, where McDonald developed an undergraduate nursing program with care as a central curricula theme. Course titles included Caring Concepts I and II, Caring of Families, and Professional Self-Care.[6] In the late 1980s, four master and four doctoral programs in the United States offered transcultural nursing courses, research experiences, and guided field study experiences.[22] Leininger continues to receive numerous requests to give courses, lectures, and workshops on human care and transcultural nursing in the United States and other countries. The demand for transcultural nurses far exceeds available faculty, money, and other resources. Therefore in 1996, Leininger put out a call for schools of nursing to offer transcultural programs to meet the worldwide demand from many nurses and cultures.[20,21,26] These nursing programs are urgently needed for practice and preparation for certification of transcultural nurses. They are also needed for research and for worldwide consultation. At this time, there are still too few transcultural nursing research funds to study transcultural nursing education and practice. Although the societal demand for transcultural nurses is evident, the educational preparation remains weak and limited for many nurses worldwide. There are still a few graduate nursing programs and faculty members who do not understand transcultural nursing and the Theory of Culture Care and, consequently, will not permit students to study or research the phenomena, which causes great distress to nursing students.

Research

Many nurses today are using Leininger's Culture Care Theory worldwide. The theory is the only one in nursing focused specifically on culture care and with a research method (ethnonursing) to examine the theory.[16,22] Approximately 100 cultures and subcultures have been studied as of 1995 and more are in progress.[16,22,24] Funds to support transcultural nursing are meager and limited in most societies because biomedical and technical research funds head the priority list. Very few nursing schools receive federal support in the United States for nursing or transcultural nursing research unless they have a quantitative, objective (measurement) focus. Transcultural nurses and other nurses interested in transcultural nursing research are continuing their research despite limited or nonexisting funds. Nevertheless, these nurses are leaders in sharing their research at conferences and instructional programs related to transcultural nursing. They have been instrumental in opening doors to transcultural nursing in many organizations. Despite societal demands for culturally competent, sensitive, responsible care, national and international organizations only began to support transcultural nursing in the 1990s. Through persistent efforts and exacting competencies of transcultural nurse specialists, progress has been forthcoming. Transcultural nurses have stimulated many nurses to pursue research and to discover some entirely new knowledge in nursing. This knowledge will greatly reshape and transform nursing in the future.

FURTHER DEVELOPMENT

Leininger[5,22] predicts that all professional nurses in the world must be prepared in transcultural nursing and demonstrate competencies in transcultural nursing. Transcultural nursing must become an integral part of education and practice for nurses to be relevant in the twenty-first century. Currently, the demand for prepared transcultural nurses far exceeds the number of nurses, faculty, and clinical specialists in the world. Far more transcultural nurse theorists, researchers, and scholars are urgently needed to continue to develop a new body of transcultural knowledge and to transform nursing education and practice. By the year 2010 all nurses will need to have a basic knowledge about diverse cultures in the world and an in-depth knowledge of at least two or three cultures.[22,24] Leininger believes transcultural nursing research has already begun to

lead to some highly promising and different ways to advance nursing education and practice. All health disciplines, including medicine, pharmacy, and social work, will gradually incorporate transcultural health knowledge and practice into their programs of study in the near future. This trend will increase the demand for competent faculty in transcultural healthcare. Leininger[22] believes that the development of transcultural institutes will be essential to fill the growing need for transcultural nurses prepared to work with other disciplines.

Present and future theories and studies in transcultural nursing will be essential to meet the needs of culturally diverse people. The Theory of Culture Care will grow in importance worldwide. Both universal and diverse care knowledge will be extremely important to establish a substantive body of transcultural nursing knowledge and to make nursing a transcultural profession and discipline. Leininger's theory has already gained worldwide interest and use because it is holistic, relevant, and futuristic and deals with specific, yet abstract, care knowledge. The Sunrise Model remains invaluable as a dominant image and guide to study and assess people of diverse and similar cultural needs.

CRITIQUE
Simplicity

Transcultural nursing theory is really a broad, holistic, comprehensive perspective of human groups, populations, and species. This theory continues to generate many domains of inquiry for nurse researchers to pursue for scientific and humanistic knowledge. The theory challenges nurses to seek both universal and diverse culturally based care phenomena by diverse cultures, the culture of nursing, and the cultures of social unsteadiness worldwide. The theory is truly transcultural and global in scope; it is both complex and practical. It requires transcultural nursing knowledge and appropriate research methods to explicate the phenomena. Leininger's Culture Care Theory is relevant worldwide to help guide nurse researchers in conceptualizing the theory and research approaches and to guide practice. It is holistic and comprehensive in nature; therefore several concepts and constructs related to social structure, environment, and language are extremely important to discover and obtain culturally based knowledge or knowledge grounded in the people's world. The theory shows multiple interrelationships of concepts and diversity of key concepts and relationships, especially to social structure factors. It requires some basic anthropological knowledge, but also considerable transcultural nursing knowledge to be used accurately and scholarly. Once the theory has been fully conceptualized, Leininger finds that undergraduate and graduate nursing students are excited to use the theory and discover how practical, relevant, and useful it is in their work. The use of the Sunrise Model becomes imprinted on their minds as a way of knowing.

Generality

The transcultural nursing theory does demonstrate the criterion of generality because it is a qualitatively oriented theory that is broad, comprehensive, and worldwide in scope. In fact, transcultural nursing theory addresses nursing care from a multicultural and worldview perspective. It is useful and applicable to both groups and individuals with the goal of rendering culture-specific nursing care. The broad or generic concepts are well organized and defined for study in specific cultures. The research has led to a vast amount of expert knowledge largely unknown in the past. Many aspects of culture, care, and health are being identified because these factors have an impact on nursing. Even more research is needed for comparative purposes from both culture-specific data and some universal care knowledge. More of the world's cultural groups need to be studied and compared to validate the caring constructs in the future. The theory is most helpful as a guide for the study of any cultures and for the comparative study of several cultures. Findings from the theory are being used presently in client care in a variety of health and community settings worldwide to transform nursing education and service. It is being valued especially in developing a new and different approach to the traditional community nursing perspective.

Empirical Precision

The transcultural nursing theory is researchable and qualitative research has been the primary paradigm to discover largely unknown phenomena of care and health in diverse cultures. This qualitative approach differs from the traditional quantitative research method, which renders measurement the goal of research. However, the ethnoscience and ethnonursing research methods are extremely rigorous and linguistically exacting in nature and outcomes. One hundred thirty-five care constructs have been identified and more are being discovered each day with a wealth of other transcultural nursing knowledge. The important attribute is that accuracy of grounded data derived with the use of ethnomethods or from an emic or people's viewpoint is leading to high credibility, confirmability, and a wealth of empirical data. Ongoing and future research will lead to additional care and health findings and implications for ethnonursing practices and education to fit specific cultures and universal features. The qualitative criteria of credibility and confirmability from in-depth studies of informants and their contexts are becoming clearly evident. Unequivocally, a body of transcultural nursing knowledge has been established over the past decade that has a great impact on nursing and many healthcare systems.[22]

Derivable Consequences

Transcultural nursing theory has important outcomes for nursing. Rendering culture-specific care is a necessary and essential new goal in nursing. It places the transcultural nursing theory central to the domain of nursing knowledge acquisition and use. The theory is highly useful, applicable, and essential to nursing practice, education, and research. The concept of care as the primary focus of nursing and the base of nursing knowledge and practice is long overdue and essential to advance nursing knowledge and practices. Leininger notes that, although nursing has always made claims to the concept of care, rigorous research on care has been limited until the last three decades. This theory could be the means to establish a sound and defensible discipline and profession, guiding practice to meet a multicultural world, because it has a broad and multicultural focus.

CRITICAL THINKING *Activities*

1. Select four research studies reported in the *Journal of Transcultural Nursing* that used Leininger's Culture Care: Diversity and Universality Theory. Each of the studies selected should represent different cultures, different research settings, and cultures different from the student's culture.

    a. Analyze each of the studies and identify the relationship of the theory to domain of inquiry, purpose, assumptions, definitions, methods, research design, data analysis, nursing decisions, and conclusions.

    b. Provide evidence that the findings from the studies confirm the findings of the theory in relation to the domain of inquiry, theory tenets, and derivable consequences.

2. Discuss the usefulness of the Culture Care: Diversity and Universality Theory in the twenty-first century to discover nursing knowledge and provide culturally congruent care. Take into consideration the current trends of consumers of healthcare, cultural diversity factors, and changes in medical and nursing school curricula. Following are some examples of trends and changes you may want to consider in your discussion:

    a. The importance of transcultural nursing knowledge in an increasingly diverse world.

    b. An increase of lay support groups to provide information and sharing of experiences and support for patients and/or families experiencing chronic, terminal, or life-threatening illnesses or treatment modalities from diverse and similar (common) cultures.

    c. Use of cultural values, beliefs, health practices, and research knowledge in undergraduate and graduate nursing curricula across the life span.

    d. Inclusion of alternative or generic care in nursing curriculum, such as medicine men (Native-American healers and curers and herbalists in the Southwest) and the use of selected proven Chinese methods for the treatment of chronic diseases.

    e. Use of cultural caring research knowledge as the new and future direction of nursing in the twenty-first century.

    f. Increase in books, audiotapes, and videotapes published on health maintenance, alternative medicine, herbs, vitamins, minerals, and other over-the-counter medications, which demands a transcultural knowledge base.

    g. Spiraling health costs; forced use of health maintenance organizations; lack of health insurance; increased reliance on self-diagnoses, treatment, and care; and increased availability of diagnostic kits such as AIDS testing, glucose monitoring, cholesterol screening, and presence of occult blood in the stool.

    h. Problems related to cultural conflicts, stress, pain, and cultural imposition practices.

3. Arrange for several observation and interview experiences at a local university student health center or public health department with people of diverse cultures. Ascertain the following:

    a. Identify the cultures represented by the clientele with use of Leininger's theory and the Sunrise Model.

    b. What is the cultural mix of the staff (physicians, nurses, social workers, and clerical) of the center or health department? How does the cultural background of the staff differ from that of the clientele?

c. Arrange a conference with the nursing staff and ascertain their culture-based attitudes, values, and beliefs and those that are reflected in the clients using the center or department. Compare and contrast the values, attitudes, and beliefs of the staff with those of the clients. What are the cultural similarities and differences?

d. Arrange an interview with the director of the center or department and ascertain the economic, political, legal, and other factors from Leininger's Sunrise Model that affect the client's use of the center or department.

e. Survey the printed materials available in the waiting and examination rooms and classrooms and identify what cultures and languages are depicted by the visual aids, artifacts, and paintings.

f. On the basis of data obtained in exercises *a* through *e*, how can the Culture Care: Diversity and Universality Theory assist the organization in providing culturally sensitive and congruent care to the clients using the center or department and increasing the satisfaction with care received?

4. Discuss the type of prerequisite knowledge, experiences, attitudes, and skills needed to effectively use the Culture Care: Diversity and Universality Theory.

5. Discuss the relevancy of the Culture Care: Diversity and Universality Theory to nurses working in different practice settings and roles.

REFERENCES

1. Glasser, B.G. & Strauss, A.L. (1967). *The discovery of grounded theories: Strategies for qualitative research.* Chicago: Aldine.
2. Hofling, C.K. & Leininger, M. (1960). Basic psychiatric concepts in nursing. Philadelphia: J.B. Lippincott.
3. Leininger, M. (1970). *Nursing and anthropology: Two worlds to blend.* New York: John Wiley & Sons. (Reprinted in 1994 by Greyden Press, Columbus, OH.)
4. Leininger, M. (1978). *Transcultural nursing: Concepts, theories, and practice.* New York: John Wiley & Sons. (Reprinted in 1994 by Greyden Press, Columbus, OH.)
5. Leininger, M. (1981). *Caring: An essential human need.* Thorofare, NJ: Charles B. Slack. (Reprinted in 1988 by Wayne State University Press, Detroit.)
6. Leininger, M. (1984). *Care: The essence of nursing and health.* Thorofare, NJ: Charles B. Slack. (Reprinted in 1990 by Wayne State University Press, Detroit.)
7. Leininger, M. (1984). *Reference sources for transcultural health and nursing.* Thorofare, NJ: Charles B. Slack.
8. Leininger, M. (Ed.). (1988). *Care: Discovery and uses in clinical and community nursing.* Detroit: Wayne State University Press.
9. Leininger, M. (1985). *Qualitative research methods in nursing.* New York: Grune & Stratton.
10. Leininger, M. (1989). Transcultural nurse specialists and generalists: New practitioners in nursing. *Journal of Transcultural Nursing,* (1), 4-16.
11. Leininger, M. (1989). Transcultural nurse specialists: Imperative in today's world. *Nursing and Health Care,* 10(5), 250-256.
12. Leininger, M. (Ed.). (1990). *Ethical and moral dimensions of care. Chapters from conference on the ethics and morality of caring.* Detroit: Wayne State University Press.
13. Leininger, M. (1990). Ethnomethods: The philosophic and epistemic bases to explicate transcultural nursing knowledge. *Journal of Transcultural Nursing,* 1(2), 40-51.
14. Leininger, M. (1990). Issues, questions, and concerns related to the nursing diagnosis cultural movement from transcultural nursing perspective. *Journal of Transcultural Nursing,* 2(1), 23-32.
15. Leininger, M. (1991). Becoming aware of types of health practitioners and cultural imposition. *Journal of Transcultural Nursing,* 2(2), 32-39.
16. Leininger, M. (1991). *Culture care diversity and universality: A theory of nursing.* New York: National League for Nursing Press.
17. Leininger, M. (1991). The transcultural nurse specialist: Imperative in today's world. *Perspective in Family and Community Health,* 17, 137-144.
18. Leininger, M. (1994). Quality of life from a transcultural nursing perspective. *Nursing Science Quarterly,* 7(1), 22-28.
19. Leininger, M. (1994). Transcultural nursing education: A worldwide imperative. *Nursing and Health Care,* 15(5), 254-257.

20. Leininger, M. (1995). Culture care theory, research and practice. *Nursing Science Quarterly, 9*(20), 71-78.
21. Leininger, M. (1995). Editorial: Teaching transcultural nursing to transform nursing for the 21st century. *Journal of Transcultural Nursing, 6*(2), 2-3.
22. Leininger, M. (1995). *Transcultural nursing: Concepts, theories, and practice.* Columbus, OH: McGraw-Hill College Custom Series.
23. Leininger, M. (1996). Academic vitae and communication with contributing author.
24. Leininger, M. (1996). Major directions for transcultural nursing: A journey into the 21st century. *Journal of Transcultural Nursing, 7*(2), 37-40.
25. Leininger, M. (1996, Oct. 22). Personal interview.
26. Leininger, M. (1996, Nov./Dec.). Future directions for transcultural nursing in the 21st century. *International Nursing Review, 44*(1), 19-23.
27. Leininger, M. & Watson, J. (1990). *The caring imperative in education.* New York: National League for Nursing Press.

BIBLIOGRAPHY
Primary Sources
Books

Gaut, D. & Leininger, M. (1991). *Caring: The compassionate healer.* New York: National League for Nursing Press.

Hofling, C.F. & Leininger, M. (1960). *Basic psychiatric concepts in nursing.* Philadelphia: J.B. Lippincott.

Leininger, M. (1970). *Nursing and anthropology: Two worlds to blend.* New York: John Wiley & Sons.

Leininger, M. (1973). *Contemporary issues in mental health nursing.* Boston: Little, Brown.

Leininger, M. (Ed.). (1974). *Health care dimensions (Vol. 1): Health care issues.* Philadelphia: F.A. Davis.

Leininger, M. (Ed.). (1975). *Health care dimensions (Vol. 2): Barriers and facilitators to quality health care.* Philadelphia: F.A. Davis.

Leininger, M. (Ed.). (1976). *Health care dimensions (Vol. 3): Transcultural health care issues and conditions.* Philadelphia: F.A. Davis.

Leininger, M. (Ed.). (1976). *Transcultural nursing care of infants and children.* Salt Lake City: University of Utah College of Nursing.

Leininger, M. (Ed.). (1978). *Transcultural nursing care of the elderly.* Salt Lake City: University of Utah College of Nursing.

Leininger, M. (Ed.). (1978). *Transcultural nursing: Concepts, theories and practices.* New York: John Wiley & Sons.

Leininger, M. (Ed.). (1979). *Transcultural nursing care of the adolescent and middle age adult.* Salt Lake City: University of Utah College of Nursing.

Leininger, M. (Ed.). (1979). *Transcultural nursing: Proceedings from four transcultural nursing conferences.* New York: Masson.

Leininger, M. (Ed.). (1980). *Cultural change, ethics and the nursing care implications.* Salt Lake City: University of Utah College of Nursing.

Leininger, M. (Ed.). (1980). *Transcultural nursing: Teaching, practice, and research.* Salt Lake City: University of Utah College of Nursing.

Leininger, M. (Ed.). (1981). *Caring: An essential human need.* Thorofare, NJ: Charles B. Slack.

Leininger, M. (Ed.). (1984). *Care: The essence of nursing and health.* Thorofare, NJ: Charles B. Slack.

Leininger, M. (1984). *Reference sources for transcultural health and nursing: For teaching curriculum, research, and clinical-field practice.* Thorofare, NJ: Charles B. Slack.

Leininger, M. (Ed.). (1985). *Qualitative research methods in nursing.* New York: Grune & Stratton.

Leininger, M. (Ed.). (1988). *Care: Discovery and uses.* Detroit: Wayne State University Press.

Leininger, M. (Ed.). (1990). *Ethical and moral dimensions of care.* Detroit: Wayne State University Press.

Leininger, M. (1991). *Culture care diversity and universality: A theory of nursing.* New York: National League for Nursing Press.

Leininger, M. (1995). *Transcultural nursing: Concepts, theories, research, and practices* (2nd ed.). New York: McGraw-Hill.

Leininger, M. (1997). *Ethnonursing research method: Essential to advance Asian nursing knowledge* [Japanese translation]. New York: Igaku-Soin Medical Publishers.

Leininger, M. & Watson, J. (Eds.). (1990). *The caring imperative in education.* New York: National League for Nursing.

Smith, C.M., Wolf, V.C., & Leininger, M. (Eds.). (1973). *Nursing at the University of Washington, 1973-1975.* Seattle: University of Washington, Office of Publications and Department of Printing.

Book Chapters

Leininger, M. (1968). The research critique: Nature, function and art. In M. Batey (Ed.), *Communication nursing research: The research critique* (pp. 20-23). Boulder, CO: Western Interstate Commission on Higher Education.

Leininger, M. (1969). The young child's response to hospitalization: Separation anxiety or lack of mothering care? In M. Batey (Ed.), *Communicating nursing research* (pp. 26-39). Boulder, CO: Western Interstate Commission on Higher Education.

Leininger, M. (1970). Some cross-cultural universal and non-universal functions beliefs and practices of food. In J. Dupont (Ed.), *Dimensions of nutrition* (pp. 153-179). Proceedings of the Colorado Dietetic Association Conference held in Fort Collins, Colorado, 1969. Colorado Associated Universities Press.

Leininger, M. (1971). Anthropological approach to adaptation: Case studies from nursing. In J. Murphy (Ed.), *Theoretical issues in professional nursing* (pp. 72-102). New York: Appleton-Century-Crofts.

Leininger, M. (1973). Nursing in the context of social and cultural systems. In P. Mitchell (Ed.), *Concepts basic to nursing* (pp. 37-60). New York: McGraw-Hill.

Leininger, M. (1973). Primex. In M. Auld & L. Birum (Eds.), *The challenge of nursing: A book of readings* (pp. 237-242). St. Louis: Mosby.

Leininger, M. (1973). The culture concept and its relevance to nursing. In M. Auld & L. Birum (Eds.), *The challenge of nursing: A book of readings* (pp. 39-46). St. Louis: Mosby.

Leininger, M. (1974, Fall). Humanism, health and cultural values. In M. Leininger (Ed.), *Health care dimensions (Vol. 1): Health care issues* (pp. 37-60). Philadelphia: F.A. Davis.

Leininger, M. (1975, Spring). Health care delivery systems for tomorrow: Possibilities and guidelines. In M. Leininger (Ed.), *Health care dimensions (Vol. 2): Barriers and facilitators to quality health care* (pp. 83-95). Philadelphia: F.A. Davis.

Leininger, M. (1976). Transcultural nursing: A promising subfield of study for nurse educators and practitioners. In A. Reinhardt (Ed.), *Current practice in family centered community nursing* (pp. 36-50). St. Louis: Mosby.

Leininger, M. (1976, Spring). Conflict and conflict resolutions: Theories and processes relevant to the health professions. In M. Leininger (Ed.), *Health care dimensions (Vol. 3): Transcultural health care issues and conditions* (pp. 165-183). Philadelphia: F.A. Davis.

Leininger, M. (1976, Spring). Toward conceptualization of transcultural health care systems: Concepts and a model. In M. Leininger (Ed.), *Health care dimensions (Vol. 3): Transcultural health care issues and conditions* (pp. 3-22). Philadelphia: F.A. Davis.

Leininger, M. (1978). Futurology of nursing: Goals and challenges for tomorrow. In N. Chaska (Ed.), *Views through the mist: The nursing profession* (pp. 379-396). New York: McGraw-Hill.

Leininger, M. (1978). Professional, political, and ethnocentric role behaviors and their influence in multidisciplinary health education. In A. Hardy & M. Conway (Ed.), *Role theory: Perspectives for health professionals.* New York: Appleton-Century-Crofts.

Leininger, M. (1981). Transcultural nursing issues for the 1980's. In J. McCloskey & H. Grace (Ed.), *Current issues in nursing.* Boston: Blackwell Scientific Publications.

Leininger, M. (1983). Intercultural interviews, assessments, and therapy implications. In P. Pederson (Ed.), *Interviews and assessments.* Beverly Hills, CA: Sage.

Leininger, M. (1988). Cultural care and nursing administration. In B. Henry, C. Arndt, M. DiVincenti, & A. Marriner Tomey (Eds.), *Dimensions of nursing administration.* Boston: Blackwell Scientific Publications.

Leininger, M. (1990). Introduction. Care: The imperative of nursing education and service. In M. Leininger & J. Watson (Eds.), *The caring imperative in education.* New York: NLN Publication, Center for Human Caring.

Leininger, M. (1991). Culture care theory and uses in nursing administration. In M. Leininger (Ed.), *Culture care diversity and universality: A theory of nursing* (pp. 373-390). New York: National League for Nursing. (Rereleased 2000.)

Leininger, M. (1991). Ethnonursing: A research method with enablers to study the theory of culture care. In M. Leininger (Ed.), *Culture care diversity and universality: A theory of nursing* (pp. 73-118). New York: National League for Nursing. (Rereleased 2000.)

Leininger, M. (1992). Current issues, problems, and trends to advance qualitative paradigmatic research methods for the future. In J.M. Morse (Ed.), *Qualitative health research* (Vol. 2, pp. 392-415). Newbury Park, CA: Sage.

Leininger, M. (1992). Reflections on Nightingale with a focus on human care theory and leadership. In F. Nightingale & B.S. Barnum (Eds.), *Nightingale, notes on nursing: What it is, and what it is not.* Philadelphia: J.B. Lippincott.

Leininger, M. (1992). Theory of culture care and uses in clinical and community contexts. In M. Parker (Ed.), *Theories on nursing* (pp. 345-372). New York: National League for Nursing.

Leininger, M. (1992). Transcultural mental health nursing assessment of children and adolescents. In P. West & C. Sieloff Evans (Eds.), *Psychiatric and mental health nursing with children and adolescents* (pp. 53-58). Gaithersburg, MD: Aspen Publications.

Leininger, M. (1993). Culture care theory: The comparative global theory to advance human care nursing knowledge and practice. In D. Gaut (Ed.), *A global agenda for caring* (pp. 3-18). New York: National League for Nursing.

Leininger, M. (1993). Evaluation criteria and critique of qualitative research studies. In J. Morse (Ed.), *Qualitative nursing research: A contemporary dialogue* (pp. 393-414). Newbury Park, CA: Sage.

McFarland, G., Hall, B., Buckwalter, K., Dumas, R., Haack, M., Leininger, M., McBride, A., McKeon, K., Pender, N., & Tripp-Reimer, T. (1990). Group IV: Behavior problems/mental illness/addictions. In J.S. Stevens (Ed.), *Knowledge about care and caring: State of the art and future developments* (G-177, pp. 135-139). ANA Publication, American Academy of Nursing.

Journal and Other Articles

Brenner, P., Boyd, C., Thompson, T.C., Marz, M.S., Buerhaus, P., & Leininger, M.M. (1986). The care symposium: Considerations for nursing administrators. *Journal of Nursing Administration, 16*(1), 25-30.

Leininger, M. (1961, Oct.). Changes in psychiatric nursing. *Canadian Nurse, 57*, 938-948.

Leininger, M. (1964, June). A Gadsup village experiences its first election. *Journal of Polynesian Society, 73*, 29-34.

Leininger, M. (1967, Spring). Nursing care of a patient from another culture: Japanese-American patient. *Nursing Clinics of North America, 2*, 747-762.

Leininger, M. (1967, April). The culture concept and its relevance to nursing. *Journal of Nursing Education, 6*, 27-39.

Leininger, M. (1968, Sept./Oct.). The research critique: Nature, function, and art. *Nursing Research, 17*(5), 444-449.

Leininger, M. (1968, Nov.). Cultural differences among staff members and the impact on patient care. *Minnesota League for Nursing Bulletin, 16*, 5-9.

Leininger, M. (1968, Nov.). The significance of cultural concepts in nursing. *Minnesota League for Nursing Bulletin, 16*, 3-4.

Leininger, M. (1969, Jan.). Community psychiatric nursing: Trends, issues and problems. *Perspectives in Psychiatric Care, 7*, 10-20.

Leininger, M. (1969, Jan.). Ethnoscience: A new and promising research approach for the health sciences. *Image: Journal of Nursing Scholarship, 3*, 2-8.

Leininger, M. (1969, Sept./Oct.). Conference on the nature of science in nursing. Introduction: Nature of science in nursing. *Nursing Research, 18*, 388-389.

Leininger, M. (1970). Witchcraft practices and nursing therapy. *ANA Clinical Conferences*, p. 76.

Leininger, M. (1971, March). Anthropological issues related to community mental health programs in the United States. *Community Mental Health Journal, 7*, 50-62.

Leininger, M. (1971, Nov.). Dean proposes educational teamwork. *Health Science Review, 1*, 4.

Leininger, M. (1971, Dec.). This I believe . . . about interdisciplinary health education for the future. *Nursing Outlook, 19*, 787-791.

Leininger, M. (1972). Using cultural styles of people: Conflicts and changes in the subculture of nursing. *Psychiatric Nursing Bulletin*, pp. 43-61.

Leininger, M. (1972, July). This I believe . . . about interdisciplinary health education for the future. *AORN Journal, 16*(1), 89-104.

Leininger, M. (1973). *Becoming aware of types of health practitioners and cultural imposition. Speeches presented during the 48th convention.* Kansas City, MO: American Nurses Association.

Leininger, M. (1973, Spring). Witchcraft practices and psychocultural therapy with urban United States families. *Human Organization, 32*, 73-83.

Leininger, M. (1973, March). An open health care system model. *Nursing Outlook, 21*, 171-175.

Leininger, M. (1973, July). Primex: Its origins and significance. *American Journal of Nursing, 73*, 1274-1277.

Leininger, M. (1973, Aug.). Witchcraft practices and psychocultural therapy with U.S. urban families. *Mental Health Digest, 5*, 33-40.

Leininger, M. (1973, Fall). A new model: Working model for future nurse participation and utilization. *Washington State Journal of Nursing, 45*, 7-15.

Leininger, M. (1973, Winter). Health care delivery systems for tomorrow: Possibilities and guidelines. *Washington State Journal of Nursing, 45*, 10-16.

Leininger, M. (1974). *Leadership in nursing: Challenges, concerns, and effect. The challenge: Rational administration in nursing and health care services* (pp. 35-53). University of Arizona, Tucson.

Leininger, M. (1974, Spring). Scholars, scholarship and nursing scholarship. *Image: Journal of Nursing Scholarship, 6*, 1-14.

Leininger, M. (1974, March/April). The leadership crisis in nursing: A critical problem and challenge. *Journal of Nursing Administration, 4*, 28-34.

Leininger, M. (1974, Dec.). Conflict and conflict resolution: Theories and processes relevant to the health professions. *American Nurse, 6*, 17-21.

Leininger, M. (1975, Feb.). Conflict and conflict resolution. *American Journal of Nursing, 75*, 292-296.

Leininger, M. (1975, May). Transcultural nursing presents exciting challenge. *American Nurse, 5*, 4.

Leininger, M. (1976, Feb.). Caring: The essence and central focus of nursing. *American Nurses Foundations, 12*, 2-14.

Leininger, M. (1976, May/June). Doctoral programs for nurses: Trends, questions and projected plans. *Nursing Research, 25*, 201-210.

Leininger, M. (1976, Fall). Two strange health tribes: Gnisrun and Enicidem in the United States. *Human Organization, 35*, 253-261.

Leininger, M. (1977). Cultural diversities of health and nursing care. *Nursing Clinics of North America, 12*(1), 5-18.

Leininger, M. (1977). *Roles and directions in nursing and cancer nursing.* Proceedings of the Second National Conference of Cancer Nursing. Washington, DC: American Cancer Society.

Leininger, M. (1977). *Territoriality, power and creative leadership in administrative nursing contexts* (Publication No. 52-1675:6-18). New York: National League for Nursing.

Leininger, M. (1977, Nov.). Issues in nursing: A learning challenge. *Vital Signs, 2*, 3. (Publication of the Student Nurses' Association, University of Utah.)

Leininger, M. (1978, Spring). Political nursing: Essential for health and educational systems of tomorrow. *Nursing Administration Quarterly, 2*(3), 1-16.

Leininger, M. (1978, March). Changing foci in nursing education: Primary and transcultural care. *Journal of Advanced Nursing, 3*(2), 155-166.

Leininger, M. (1978, March). Nursing in the future: Some brief glimpses (Part I). *Vital Signs, 2,* 7. (Publication of the Student Nurses' Association, University of Utah.)

Leininger, M. (1978, April). Nursing in the future: Some brief glimpses (Part II). *Vital Signs, 2,* 8. (Publication of the Student Nurses' Association, University of Utah.)

Leininger, M. (1978, May). Nursing in the future: Some brief glimpses (Part III). *Vital Signs, 2,* 9. (Publication of the Student Nurses' Association, University of Utah.)

Leininger, M. (1978, Oct.). *Transcultural nursing: A new subfield to general nursing and health care knowledge.* Scholarly Lecture Series, University of Manitoba.

Leininger, M. (1978, Dec.). Creating and maintaining a nursing research support center. *Adelphi Report,* pp. 35-60.

Leininger, M. (1978, Dec.). Transcultural nursing for tomorrow's nurse. *Imprint, 25*(4), 44-47.

Leininger, M. (1979). *Consumer health care needs, nursing leadership and future directions.* Proceedings of the leadership conference. Seattle: University of Washington, School of Nursing.

Leininger, M. (1979). *Principles and guidelines to assist nurses in cross-cultural nursing and health practices. Hope conference report.* Millwood, VA: International Nursing Project, Hope Health Sciences Education Center.

Leininger, M. (1979, April). Health promotion and maintenance: An old transcultural challenge and a new emphasis for the health professions. *Health Promotion: In Health and Illness,* Monograph 4, Series 1978. Sigma Theta Tau.

Leininger, M. (1979, Oct.). *Sociocultural forces impacting upon health care and the nursing profession.* National Institutes of Health Annual Meeting of Nursing Departments. Washington, DC: National Institutes of Health.

Leininger, M. (1980, Aug.). Transcultural nursing: A new subfield. *Health Clinics International, 2,* 3-4.

Leininger, M. (1980, Oct.). Caring: A central focus for nursing and health care services. *Nursing and Health Care, 1,* 135-143, 176.

Leininger, M. (1980, Winter). University of Utah nursing clinics. *Western Journal of Nursing Research, 2,* 411.

Leininger, M. (1981, July/Aug.). Women's role in society in the 1980s. *Issues in Health Care of Women, 13*(4), 203-215.

Leininger, M. (1981, July/Aug.). Women's role in society in the 80's. *Issues of Health Care of Women, 3*(4), 203-215.

Leininger, M. (1981, Sept.). Transcultural nursing: Its progress and its future. *Nursing and Health Care, 2*(7), 365-371.

Leininger, M. (1982, Jan.). Creativity and challenges for nurse researchers in this economic recession. *Center for Health Research News, 1,* 1. (Publication of the College of Nursing, Wayne State University.)

Leininger, M. (1982, July/Aug.). Woman's role in society in the 1980s. *Issues in Health Care of Women, 3*(4), 203-215.

Leininger, M. (1982, Nov.). Getting to 'truths' or mastering numbers and research designs. *Center for Health Research News, 1,* 2. (Publication of the College of Nursing, Wayne State University.)

Leininger, M. (1983, March). Creativity and challenges for nurse researchers in this economic recession. *Journal of Nursing Administration, 13,* 21-22.

Leininger, M. (1983, May). Qualitative research methods: A new direction to document and discover nursing knowledge. *Center for Health Research News, 3,* 2. (Publication of the College of Nursing, Wayne State University.)

Leininger, M. (1983, Aug.). Cultural care: An essential goal for nursing and health care. *Journal of Nephrology Nursing, 10,* 11-17.

Leininger, M. (1983, Oct./Dec.). Community psychiatric nursing in community mental health: Trends, issues, and problems. *Perspective Psychiatric Care, 21*(4), 139-146.

Leininger, M. (1984). Transcultural nursing. *Canadian Nurse, 80*(11), 41-45.

Leininger, M. (1984, March/April). Transcultural nursing: An overview. *Nursing Outlook, 32*(2), 72-73.

Leininger, M. (1985, Feb.). Ethnoscience: A promising research approach to improve nursing practice [Translated from 'The best of image']. *Kango Tenbo, 37*(2), 113-123.

Leininger, M. (1985, April). Transcultural care diversity and universality: A theory of nursing. *Nursing and Health Care, 6*(4), 209-212.

Leininger, M. (1986). Care facilitation and resistance factors in the culture of nursing. *Topics in Clinical Nursing, 8*(2), 1-12.

Leininger, M. (1986). Care symposium: Resources on culture [Letter to the Editor]. *Journal of Nursing Administration, 16*(6), 35.

Leininger, M. (1986). Caring [Reply Letter]. *Journal of Nursing Administration, 16*(11), 4.

Leininger, M. (1987). A new generation of nurses discover transcultural nursing [Editorial]. *Nursing and Health Care, 8*(5), 263.

Leininger, M. (1987, Summer). Response to "Infant feeding practices of Vietnamese immigrants to the Northwest United States." *Scholarly Inquiry for Nursing Practice, 1*(2), 171-174.

Leininger, M. (1988, Nov.). Leininger's theory of nursing: Cultural care diversity and universality. *Nursing Science Quarterly, 1*(4), 152-160.

Leininger, M. (1992). Transcultural nursing care values, beliefs, and practices of American (USA) gypsies. *Journal of Transcultural Nursing, 4*(1), 17-28.

Leininger, M. (1994). Nursing's agenda of health care reform: Regressive or advanced—discipline status. *Nursing Science Quarterly, 7*(2), 93-94.

Leininger, M. (1994). Reflections: Culturally congruent care: Visible and invisible. *Journal of Transcultural Nursing,* 6(1), 23-25.

Leininger, M. (1995). Culture care theory, research and practice. *Nursing Science Quarterly,* 9(2), 71-78.

Leininger, M. (1995). Founder's focus: Nursing theories and cultures: Fit or misfit? *Journal of Transcultural Nursing,* 7(1), 41-42.

Leininger, M. (1996). Founder's focus: Transcultural nurses and consumers tell their stories. *Journal of Transcultural Nursing,* 7(2), 37-40.

Leininger, M. (1996). Transcultural nursing administration: What is it? *Journal of Transcultural Nursing,* 8(1), 28.

Leininger, M. & Cummings, S.H. (1996). Nursing's new paradigm is transcultural nursing: An interview with Madeleine Leininger. *Advanced Practice Nursing Quarterly,* 2(2), 62-70.

Leininger, M. & Shubin, S. (1980, June). Nursing patients from different cultures. *Nursing,* 80, 10.

Leininger, M.M. (1983). Creativity and challenges for nurse researchers in this economic recession part 2. *Nurse Educator,* 8(1), 13-14.

Leininger, M.M. (1984). Qualitative research methods—to document and discover nursing knowledge. *Western Journal of Nursing Research,* 6(2), 151-152.

Leininger, M.M. (1987). Importance and uses of ethnomethods: Ethnography and ethnonursing research. *Recent Advances in Nursing,* 17, 12-36.

Leininger, M.M. (1988). Leininger's theory of nursing: Cultural care diversity and universality. *Nursing Science Quarterly,* 1(4), 152-160.

Leininger, M.M. (1988). Transcultural eating patterns and nutrition: Transcultural nursing and anthropological perspectives. *Holistic Nursing Practice,* 3(1), 16-25.

Leininger, M.M. (1989). The Journal of Transcultural Nursing has become a reality. *Journal of Transcultural Nursing,* 1(1), 1-2.

Leininger, M.M. (1989). The transcultural nurse specialist: Imperative in today's world. *Nursing and Health Care,* 10(5), 250-256.

Leininger, M.M. (1989). Transcultural nurse specialists and generalists: New practitioners in nursing. *Journal of Transcultural Nursing,* 1(1), 4-16.

Leininger, M.M. (1989). Transcultural nursing: Quo vadis (where goeth the field?). *Journal of Transcultural Nursing,* 1(1), 33-45.

Leininger, M.M. (1990). A new and changing decade ahead: Are nurses prepared? *Journal of Transcultural Nursing,* 1(2), 1.

Leininger, M.M. (1990). Ethnomethods: The philosophic and epistemic bases to explicate transcultural nursing knowledge. *Journal of Transcultural Nursing,* 1(2), 40-51.

Leininger, M.M. (1990). Issues, questions, and concerns related to the nursing diagnosis cultural movement from a transcultural nursing perspective. *Journal of Transcultural Nursing,* 2(1), 23-32.

Leininger, M.M. (1990). The significance of cultural concepts in nursing. *Journal of Transcultural Nursing,* 2(1), 52-59.

Leininger, M.M. (1990, Nov./Dec.). Leininger clarifies transcultural nursing [Letter to the Editor]. *International Nursing Review,* 36(6), 356.

Leininger, M.M. (1991). Becoming aware of types of health practitioners and cultural imposition. *Journal of Transcultural Nursing,* 2(2), 32-39.

Leininger, M.M. (1991). Leininger's acculturation health care assessment tool for cultural patterns in traditional and non-traditional lifeways. *Journal of Transcultural Nursing,* 2(2), 40-42.

Leininger, M.M. (1991). Second reflection: Comparative care as central to transcultural nursing. *Journal of Transcultural Nursing,* 3(1), 2.

Leininger, M.M. (1991). Transcultural care principles, human rights, and ethical considerations. *Journal of Transcultural Nursing,* 3(1), 21-23.

Leininger, M.M. (1991). Transcultural nursing goals and challenges for 1991 and beyond. *Journal of Transcultural Nursing,* 2(2), 1-2.

Leininger, M.M. (1991). Transcultural nursing: The study and practice field. *Imprint,* 38(2), 55, 57, 59-63.

Book Prefaces and Forewords

Leininger, M. (1972). Introduction. In K. Leahy, M. Cobb, & M. Jones, *Community health nursing.* New York: McGraw-Hill.

Leininger, M. (1972). Introduction. In L. Schwartz & J. Schwartz, *Psychodynamic concepts of patient care.* Englewood Cliffs, NJ: Prentice-Hall.

Leininger, M. (1973, July). Foreword. In M. Disbrow (Ed.), *Meeting consumers' demands for maternity care.* Seattle: University of Washington Press.

Leininger, M. (1974, Fall). Preface. In M. Leininger (Ed.), *Health care issues: Health care dimensions. Second issue.* Philadelphia: F.A. Davis.

Leininger, M. (1975, Spring). Preface. In M. Leininger (Ed.), *Transcultural health care issues and conditions: Health care dimensions. Second issue.* Philadelphia: F.A. Davis.

Leininger, M. (1976, Spring). Preface. In M. Leininger (Ed.), *Transcultural health care issues and conditions: Health care dimensions. Third issue.* Philadelphia: F.A. Davis.

Leininger, M. (1978). Foreword. In J. Watson, *Nursing: The philosophy and science of caring.* Boston: Little, Brown.

Leininger, M. (1979). Foreword. In L.S. Bermosk & S.E. Porter, *Women's health and human wholeness.* New York: Appleton-Century-Crofts.

Leininger, M. (1979). Preface. In M. Leininger (Ed.), *Proceedings of the national transcultural nursing conferences.* New York: Masson.

Leininger, M. (1980). Foreword. In M. Leininger, *Transcultural nursing: Teaching, research, and practice.* Salt Lake City: University of Utah.

Leininger, M. (1981). Introduction. In M. Leininger (Ed.), *Six proceedings of the transcultural nursing conferences in 1976, 1977, 1978, 1979, 1980, 1981.* New York: Masson.

Leininger, M. (1981). Preface. In M. Leininger (Ed.), *Caring: An essential human need.* Thorofare, NJ: Charles B. Slack.

Leininger, M. (1981). Preface. In M. Leininger (Ed.), *Maternal child nursing in the 80's. Nursing perspective: A forum in honor of Katherine Kendall.* College Park, MD: University of Maryland, School of Nursing.

Leininger, M. (1983). Preface. In K. Vestal & C. McKenzie (Eds.), *High risk perinatal nursing.* Philadelphia: W.B. Saunders.

Leininger, M. (1983). Preface. In M. Leininger (Ed.), *Care: The essence of nursing and health.* Thorofare, NJ: Charles B. Slack.

Leininger, M. (1983). Preface. In M. Leininger, *Reference sources for transcultural health and nursing for teaching, curriculum, research, and clinical-field practice.* Thorofare, NJ: Charles B. Slack.

Secondary Sources

Journal Articles

Berry, A. (1999). Mexican American women's expressions of the meaning of culturally congruent prenatal care. *Journal of Transcultural Nursing, 10*(3), 203-212.

Bialoskurski, M., Cox, C.L., & Hayes, J.A. (1999). The nature of attachment in a neonatal intensive care unit. *Journal of Perinatal and Neonatal Nursing, 10*(3), 66-77.

Brooke, D. & Omeri, A. (1999). Beliefs about childhood immunisation among Lebanese Musilin immigrants in Australia. *Journal of Transcultural Nursing, 10*(3), 229-236.

George, T. (2000). Defining care in the culture of the chronically mentally ill living in the community. *Journal of Transcultural Nursing, 11*(2), 102-110.

Higgins, B. (2000). Puerto Rican cultural beliefs: Influence on infant feeding practices in western New York. *Journal of Transcultural Nursing, 11*(1), 19-30.

Lumberg, P. (2000). Cultural care of Thai immigrants in Uppsala: A study of transcultural nursing in Sweden. *Journal of Transcultural Nursing, 11*(4), 274-280.

Nahas, V. & Amasheh, N. (1999). Cultural care meanings and experiences of postpartum depression among Jordanian Australian women: A transcultural study. *Journal of Transcultural Nursing, 10*(1), 37-45.

Omeri, A. (1997). Cultural care of Iranian immigrants in New South Wales. Australia: Sharing transcultural nursing knowledge. *Journal of Transcultural Nursing,* 8(2), 5-16.

Sellers, S.C., Poduska, M.D., Propp, L.H., & White, S.I. (1999, Oct.). The health care meanings, values and practices of Anglo-American males in the rural midwest. *Journal of Transcultural Nursing, 10*(4), 320-330.

Dissertations Mentored by Leininger

Berry, A. (1995). *Culture care statements, meanings and experiences of pregnant Mexican-American women within Leininger's culture care theory.* Detroit: Wayne State University.

Cameron, C. (1990). *An ethnonursing study of health status of elderly Anglo-Canadian wives providing extended care giving to their disabled husbands.* Detroit: Wayne State University.

Curtis, M. (1997). *Cultural care by private practice APRNS in community contexts.* Detroit: Wayne State University.

Ehrmin, J. (1998). *Culture care meanings and statements, and experiences of care of African-American women residing in an inner city transitional home for substance abuse.* Detroit: Wayne State University.

Finn, J. (1993). *Professional nurse and generic care giving of child bearing women conceptualized with Leininger's theory of cultural care theory.* Detroit: Wayne State University.

Gates, M. (1988). *Care and care meanings, experiences and orientations of persons dying in hospitals and hospital settings.* Detroit: Wayne State University.

Gelazis, R. (1994). *Lithuanian care: Meanings and experiences with humor using Leininger's cultural care theory.* Detroit: Wayne State University.

George, T. (1998). *Meanings statements and experiences of care of chronically mentally ill in a day treatment center using Leininger's culture care theory.* Detroit: Wayne State University.

Horton, B. (1998). *Culture care by private practice APRN in community context.* Detroit: Wayne State University.

Lamp, J. (1998). *Generic and professional cultural care meanings and practices of Finnish women in birth within Leininger's theory of culture care diversity and universality.* Detroit: Wayne State University.

Luna, L. (1989). *Care and cultural context of Lebanese Muslims in an urban U.S. community within Leininger's cultural care theory.* Detroit: Wayne State University.

MacNeil, J. (1994). *Cultural care: Meanings, patterns, and expressions for Baganda women as AIDS caregivers within Leininger's theory.* Detroit: Wayne State University.

Miller, J.E. (1996). *Politics and care: A study of Czech Americans within Leininger's theory of culture care diversity and universality.* Detroit: Wayne State University.

Morgan, M. (1994). *African American neonatal care in northern and southern contexts using Leininger's culture care theory.* Detroit: Wayne State University.

Morris, E. (2001). *Culture care values, meanings experiences of African American adolescent gang members.* Detroit: Wayne State University.

Omeri, A.S. (1996). *Transcultural nursing care values, beliefs and practices of Iranian immigrants in New South Wales, Australia.* Sydney: University of Sydney.

Rosenbaum, J. (1990). *Cultural care, culture health and grief phenomena related to older Greek Canadian widows with Leininger's theory of culture care.* Detroit: Wayne State University.

Spangler, Z. (1991). *Nursing care values and practices of Philippine American and Anglo American nurses.* Detroit: Wayne State University.

Stitzlein, D. (1999). *The phenomenon of moral care/caring conceptualized within Leininger's theory of culture care diversity and universality.* Detroit: Wayne State University.

Thompson, T. (1990). *A qualitative investigation of rehabilitation nursing care in an inpatient rehabilitation unit using Leininger's theory.* Detroit: Wayne State University.

Villarruel, A. (1993). *Mexican American cultural meanings, expressions: Self-care and dependent care actions associated with experiences of pain.* Detroit: Wayne State University.

Welch, A. (1987). *Concepts of health, illness, caring, aging and problems of adjustment among elderly Filipinas residing in Hampton Roads, Virginia.* Salt Lake City: University of Utah.

Wenger, A.F. (1988). *The phenomenon of care of old order Amish: A high context culture.* Detroit: Wayne State University.

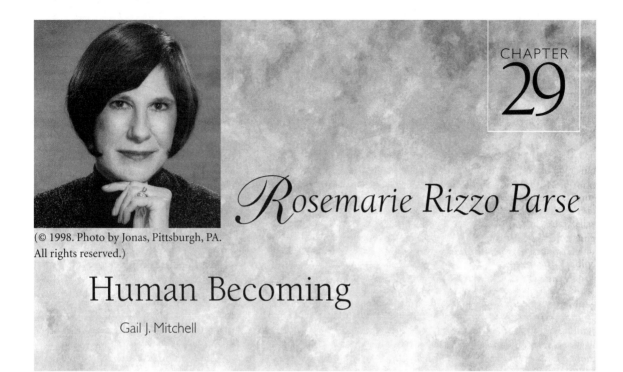

CHAPTER 29

Rosemarie Rizzo Parse

Human Becoming

Gail J. Mitchell

CREDENTIALS AND BACKGROUND OF THE THEORIST

Rosemarie Rizzo Parse is currently a professor and Niehoff Chair at the Marcella Niehoff School of Nursing, Loyola University Chicago. She is founder and editor of *Nursing Science Quarterly,* president of Discovery International Incorporated, which sponsors international nursing theory conferences, and founder of the Institute of Human Becoming, where she teaches the ontological, epistemological, and methodological aspects of the human becoming school of thought.[39] Parse has authored many articles and books including: *Nursing Fundamentals;*[32] *Man-Living-Health: A Theory of Nursing;*[33] *Nursing*

Previous authors: Kathleen D. Pickrell, Rickard E. Lee, Larry P. Schumacher, and Prudence Twigg.
The author wishes to thank Dr. Rosemarie Rizzo Parse for reviewing the chapter.

Science: Major Paradigms, Theories and Critiques;[34] *Qualitative Inquiry: The Path of Sciencing;*[44] *Illuminations: The Human Becoming Theory in Practice and Research;*[43] *The Human Becoming School of Thought: A Perspective for Nurses and Other Health Professionals;*[41] and *Hope: An International Human Becoming Perspective.*[42] Some of her works have been published in Danish, Finnish, French, German, Japanese, and Korean. In addition, *The Human Becoming School of Thought: A Perspective for Nurses and Other Health Professionals*[41] was selected for Sigma Theta Tau and Doody Publishing's Best Picks list in the nursing theory book category in 1998. *Hope: An International Human Becoming Perspective*[42] was selected for the same list in 1999.

Parse's multiple research projects and interests are focused on humanly lived experiences of health. She has developed basic and applied science research methodologies congruent with the ontology of human becoming and has conducted and published

527

numerous investigations on a wide variety of phenomena, including laughter, health, aging, quality of life, joy-sorrow, and hope. The hope study, for which she was the principle investigator, included participants and coinvestigators from nine countries.[42] Her current research projects include Parse method studies of the lived experiences of contentment, feeling very tired, and feeling confident.

Parse's research methodologies are used as methods of inquiry by nurse scholars in Australia, Canada, Denmark, Finland, Greece, Italy, Japan, South Korea, Sweden, the United Kingdom, and the United States; her theory is a guide for practice in healthcare settings in Canada, Finland, South Korea, Sweden, the United Kingdom, and the United States.[41] Human becoming is also used as a guide for nursing practice, education, administration, and regulation in several settings in North America.[13,25,36] Parse is a graduate of Duquesne University in Pittsburgh and received her masters and doctorate degrees from the University of Pittsburgh. She was a faculty member at the University of Pittsburgh, dean of the Nursing School at Duquesne University, and, from 1983 to 1993, she was professor and coordinator of the Center for Nursing Research at Hunter College of the City University of New York. She has consulted throughout the world with doctoral programs in nursing and with healthcare settings that have selected her theory as a guide to research, practice, administration, education, and regulation.

THEORETICAL SOURCES

The human becoming school of thought is grounded in the human sciences as espoused by Dilthey and others over the past century.[26,41] The human becoming school of thought is "consistent with Martha E. Rogers' principles and postulates about human beings and it is consistent with major tenets and concepts from existential-phenomenological thought, but it is a new product, a different conceptual system."[41:4,49] At the time she was developing her theory, Parse was working at Duquesne University in Pittsburgh. While she was there (during the 1960s and

1970s) Duquesne was regarded as the center of the existential-phenomenological movement in the United States. Dialogues she had with those in this school of thought, such as van Kaam and Giorgi, stimulated and focused her thinking on the lived experiences of human beings and their freedom and participation in life.

By synthesizing the science of unitary human beings, developed by Martha E. Rogers, and the fundamental tenets from existential-phenomenological thought, as articulated by Heidegger, Sartre, and Merleau-Ponty, Parse secured nursing's history as a human science.* Parse contends that humans cannot be reduced to constituent systems or parts and still be understood. Persons are living beings who are more than and different from any schemata that divides them. Parse challenges the traditional, medical view of nursing and distinguishes the discipline of nursing as a unique, basic science. Parse supports the notion that nurses require a unique knowledge base that informs their practice and research and this knowledge (of the human-universe-health process) is essential for nurses to fulfill their commitment to humankind.

In developing her theory, Parse was especially influenced by Rogers' principles of helicy, integrality, and resonancy and by her postulates (energy field, openness, pattern, and pandimensionality).[51,52] These ideas underpin Parse's notions about persons as open beings who relate at multiple realms with the universe and who are irreducible, ever changing, and recognized by patterns.

From existential-phenomenological thought, Parse drew on the tenets of intentionality and human subjectivity and the corresponding concepts of coconstitution, coexistence, and situated freedom. Parse uses the prefix *co* on many of her words to denote the participative nature of persons. *Co* means *together with* and for Parse, humans can never be separated from their relationships with the universe. Relationships with the universe include all the linkages humans have with other peo-

*References 26, 33, 34, 41, 51, 52.

ple and with ideas, projects, predecessors, history, and culture.

Intentionality means that "the human is open, knows, and is present with the world. To be human, then, is to be intentional and to be involved with the world through a fundamental nature of knowing, being present, and open."[41:14] Intentionality is about purpose and how persons choose direction and ways of acting toward projects and people. People choose attitudes and next actions.

The basic tenet, human subjectivity,

> posits that the human by nature is no thing but, rather, a unity of being with nonbeing—living what is and what is not-yet all-at-once. . . . In subjectivity the human is present with the world in a dialectical relationship, giving meaning to the projects that emerge in the process of becoming. Humans coparticipate with the world in the emergence of projects through choosing to live certain values.[41:15]

Every person, although inseparable from others, crafts a unique relationship with the universe. Human beings have a personal relationship with the universe that is open to new possibilities and directions. The personal relationship is the person's becoming and becoming is complex, multilayered, and full of explicit-implicit meanings.

Coconstitution

> refers to the idea that the meaning emerging in any situation is related to the particular constituents of that situation. The human is enabled and limited by the human-world dialectic through which situations come into being. The human is in mutual process with the various views of the world and others, and indeed cocreates these views by a personal presence.[41:17]

The term *coconstitution* links to the ways people create different meanings from the same situations. People change and are changed through their personal interpretations of life situations. Various ways of thinking and acting can both open and close doors as people proceed with crafting their unique realities.

The term *coexistence* means that

> the human is not alone in any dimension of becoming. The human, an emerging being, is with the world with others—predecessors, contemporaries, and successors; indeed, even the act of coming into the world is through others. The human knows becoming in the comprehension of dispersed concrete personal achievements and through the perspectives of others. Without others, one would not know that one is a being.[41:17]

Persons think about themselves in relation to how they are with others and how they might be with their plans and dreams. Coexistence links with the notion of mutual process and the unity of lived experience. There are no objective-subjective dualities or cause-effect relationships that can represent human becoming. Linked to the assumption of freedom, Parse describes an abiding respect for human change and possibility.

Finally, situated freedom means that "reflectively and prereflectively one participates in choosing the situations in which one finds oneself as well as one's attitude toward the situations."[41:17] Humans are always choosing. "In choosing ways of being with situations, one incarnates value priorities."[41:18] Persons decide what is important in their lives. Day to day living represents people choosing and acting on their value priorities. Sometimes being able to act on beliefs is as important as achieving the desired outcome. Personal integrity is intimately linked to the notion of situated freedom.

USE OF EMPIRICAL EVIDENCE

Research guided by the human becoming theory is meant to enhance the theoretical foundation or the description contained in the principles and concepts of the human becoming theory. Research is not used to test Parse's theory. Nurses do not set out to test the questions as to whether or not people have unique meanings or situated freedom, if they are unitary beings, if persons relate with others and the universe in paradoxical patterns, or if people choose their hopes and dreams. As noted, a nurse either has an attraction and commitment to these basic beliefs or not. The idea of a unitary human being in mutual process is an assumption that is either believable or not. Assumptions about human beings are theoretical creations. A student or nurse relates to one notion of human being or another. According to Parse, this is why there is a need for multiple paradigmatic views; the discipline of nursing can accommodate different views and different theories about the human-universe-health process. Parse[39:12] stated the following when discussing the issue of testing the human becoming theory:

> The human becoming theory does not lend itself to testing, since it is not a predictive theory and is not based on a cause-effect view of the human-universe process. The purpose of the research is not to verify the theory or test it but, rather, the focus is on uncovering the essences of lived phenomena to gain further understanding of universal human experiences. This understanding evolves from connecting the descriptions given by people to the theory, thus making more explicit the essences of being human.

Research with Parse's theory expands understanding about the human-universe-health process and inquiry builds new knowledge about human becoming. According to Parse,[41:59] "Scholarly research is formal inquiry leading to the discovery of new knowledge with the enhancement of theory." This idea of new knowledge with enhancement of theory requires additional attention to clarify the distinctions among different ways of thinking.

Research guided by the human becoming theory explores universal lived experiences with people as they live them in day-to-day life. Parse contends that there are universal human experiences, such as hope, joy, sorrow, grief, anticipation, fear, confidence, and contemplation. Further, persons experience the *what was,* the *what is,* and the *what will be* all at once. This means that research guided by human becoming theory explores lived experiences as people are living them in the moment. People live in the moment and what is remembered and what is hoped for are always viewed within the reality of the

now. Further, universal experiences cannot be reduced to linear time frames because lived experience is unitary and multidimensional. A nurse researcher conducting a Parse method study invites persons to speak about a particular universal experience. For instance, a researcher might invite a participant to talk about his or her experience of grieving. The researcher would not ask the participant to speak about grieving while in the hospital, for example. The researcher guided by human becoming knows that the person's reality encompasses the what was, is, and the will be as it is appearing in the moment. The researcher also assumes that the person knows his or her experience and can offer an account of the experience as he or she lives it.

In 1986, Parse[34] first developed a specific research method consistent with the human becoming theory; since then, the human becoming hermeneutic method has been articulated. A third method, an applied science method (qualitative descriptive preproject-process-postproject) has been articulated.[8,41] For details of all these methods, please see *The Human Becoming School of Thought: A Perspective for Nurses and Other Health Professionals.*[41] The Parse research method records accounts of personal experiences and systematically examines those accounts to identify the aspects of lived experiences that are shared across participants.[33] The Parse research method is described in several texts.[34,41,42,44] The core concepts, or ideas shared across all participants, form a structure of the phenomenon under study. The structure as defined by Parse[42:5] is the "paradoxical living of the remembered, the now-moment, and the not-yet, all-at-once." New knowledge is embedded in the core concepts and, once discovered, they enhance theory and understanding in ways that go beyond the particular study. The weaving of the new knowledge with the theoretical concepts expands the content of the human becoming theory and that is how the new knowledge with enhancement develops thinking and dialogue.

MAJOR CONCEPTS & DEFINITIONS

The three principles, which constitute the human becoming theory, flow from the themes.[41] Each principle contains three concepts that require thoughtful exploration to understand the depth of the human becoming theory. The principles are:

1. Structuring meaning multidimensionally is cocreating reality through the languaging of valuing and imaging.[41]
2. Cocreating rhythmical patterns of relating is living the paradoxical unity of revealing-concealing and enabling-limiting while connecting-separating.[41]
3. Cotranscending with the possibles is powering unique ways of originating in the process of transforming.[41]

The first principle proposes that persons structure, or choose, the meaning of their realities and this choosing happens at realms that are not always known explicitly. Sometimes questions are not answerable because people may not know why they think or feel one way or another. The first principle suggests that the way people see the world, their imaging of it, is their reality and they create this reality with others and they show or language their reality in the ways they speak and remain silent and in the ways they move and stay still. When people language their realities, they also language their value priorities and meanings (according to the first principle). The first principle has three concepts: (1) imaging, (2) valuing, and (3) languaging.

IMAGING

Imaging is an individual's view of reality. It is the "shaping of personal knowledge explicitly-tacitly."[41:36] For Parse, people are inherently curious and seek to find answers and figure things out. The answers to questions emerge as persons explore meaning in light of reality and their view of things. Imaging is a personal interpretation of meaning, possibility, and consequence. Nurses cannot completely know another's imaging, but they can explore, respect, and bear witness as people struggle with the processes of shaping, exploring, integrating, rejecting, and interpreting.

VALUING

Valuing is the second concept of the first principle. This concept is the "confirming-not confirming of cherished beliefs in light of a personal worldview."[41:38] Persons are continuously making choices about how to think, act, and feel and these choices may be consistent with prior choices or they may be radically different and require a shifting of value priorities. Sometimes people may think about anticipated choices and, once the choice arrives, they change their thinking and direction in life. Values reflect what is important in life to a person or a family. For Parse, living value priorities is how an individual expresses health and human becoming. Nurses learn about persons' perspectives by asking them what is most important.

LANGUAGING

Languaging is a concept that relates to how human beings symbolize and express their imaged realities and their value priorities. Languaging is visible in the way people speak and remain silent and in the way they move and remain still. Languaging is lived multidimensionally when people picture themselves in situations that have been or in situations that are only possibilities. When languaging is visible to others, it is often expressed in patterns that are shared with those who are close. Family members or close friends often share similar patterns, such as speaking, moving, and being quiet.[41] People disclose things about themselves when they language, even when they are silent and remain still. Nurses can witness some of the languaging that people show, but they cannot

Continued

know the meaning of the languaging. To understand languaging, nurses must ask people what their words, actions, and gestures mean. It is possible that the person does not yet know the meaning of their languaging, in which case the nurse respects the process of coming to understand the meaning of a situation. Explicating meaning can take time and people know when it is right to illuminate the meaning and significance of an event or happening.

The second principle of human becoming is "cocreating rhythmical patterns of relating is living the paradoxical unity of revealing-concealing and enabling-limiting while connecting-separating."[41:42] This principle means that human beings create patterns in day-to-day life and these patterns tell about personal meanings and values. In the patterns of relating that people create, there are many freedoms and restrictions that surface with choices; all patterns involve complex engagements and disengagements with people, ideas, and preferences. The second principle has three concepts: (1) revealing-concealing, (2) enabling-limiting, and (3) connecting-separating.

REVEALING-CONCEALING

"Revealing-concealing is disclosing-not disclosing all-at-once."[41:43] Parse identifies the notion of mystery as central to understanding this paradoxical concept. It is mysterious how people chose to give and withhold messages about who they are and what they think and know. Sometimes people know what they want to say and they deliver messages with great clarity and, at other times, people may surprise themselves with the messages they give. Mystery is also relevant because there is always more for people to know about themselves and others. Some layers of reality and experience remain concealed. People also reveal-conceal differently in different situations and with different people. Further, patterns of revealing-concealing are cocreated and inti-

mately linked to the mutual process of the moment and to the intentions of those persons present. In choosing how to be with others, nurses cocreate what happens in the nurse-person process.

ENABLING-LIMITING

Enabling-limiting represents the freedoms and opportunities that surface with the restrictions and obstacles of everyday living. Every choice, even those made at prereflective realms, surface opportunities and restrictions. It is not possible to know all the consequences of any given choice; therefore people make choices amid the reality of ambiguity. Every choice is pregnant with possibility in both opportunity and restriction; this is verified in practice daily when patients and families say things like, "This is the worst thing that could have happened to our family, but it has helped us in many ways." Enabling-limiting is about choosing from the possibilities and living with the consequences of those choices. Nurses can be helpful to others as they contemplate the options and anticipated consequences of difficult choices.

CONNECTING-SEPARATING

Connecting-separating is the third concept of the second principle. This concept has layers of paradoxical meaning. The concept relates to the ways persons create patterns of connecting and separating with people and projects. The patterns created reveal value priorities. Connecting-separating is about the paradox communion-aloneness and the ways people separate from some to join with others. Connecting-separating also explains the way two people can be very close and yet maintain separateness between the two. Sometimes there is connecting when people are separating because persons can dwell with an absent presence with great intimacy, especially when grieving another.[6,7,48] Nurses learn about persons' patterns

MAJOR CONCEPTS *&* DEFINITIONS—cont'd

of connecting-separating by asking about their important relationships and projects.

CONTRASCENDING

Contrascending is the third principle of human becoming theory. "Cotranscending with the possibles is powering unique ways of originating in the process of transforming."[41:46] The meaning of this principle is that persons are always engaging with and choosing from infinite possibilities. The choices reflect the persons' ways of moving and changing in the process of becoming. The three concepts of this principle are: (1) powering, (2) originating, and (3) transforming.

POWERING

Powering is a concept that conveys meaning about struggle and life and the will to go on despite hardship and threat. Parse[41:47] states that "powering is the pushing-resisting process of affirming-not affirming being in light of nonbeing." People constantly engage being and nonbeing. Nonbeing is about loss and the risk of death and rejection. Powering is the force exerted; that is, the pushing to act and live with purpose amid possibilities for affirming and holding what is cherished, while simultaneously living with loss and threat of nonbeing. There is always resistance with the pushing force of powering because persons live with others who are also powering toward different possibilities. Conflict, according to Parse,[41] presents opportunities to clarify meanings and values and nurses can enhance this process by being present with persons who are exploring issues, conflicts, and options.

ORIGINATING

Originating is a concept about human uniqueness and holds two paradoxes: (1) conforming-not conforming and (2) certainty-uncertainty. People strive to be like others and yet they also strive to be unique. Choices about originating occur with the reality of certainty-uncertainty. It is not possible to know all that may come from choosing to be different or from choosing to be like others. For some, there is greater danger in being too much like others; some may say the greater danger is in being different. Each person defines and lives originating in light of their worldview and values. Originating and creating anew is a pattern that coexists with constancy and conformity. Humans craft their unique patterns of originating as they engage the possibilities of everyday life. Nurses witness originating with persons who are in the process of choosing how they are going to be with their changing health patterns.

TRANSFORMING

Transforming, the third concept of the third principle, is about change and the shifting views that people have about their lives. People are always struggling to integrate the unfamiliar with the familiar in the living of everydayness. When new discoveries are made, people change their understanding and, sometimes, life patterns and worldviews can shift with the mystery of an insight that illuminates a familiar situation in a new light. Transforming is the ongoing change characteristic of mutual process and human ingenuity as people find ways to change in the direction of their cherished hopes and dreams. Nurses, in the way they are present with others, help or hinder persons' efforts to clarify their hopes, dreams, and desired directions.

MAJOR ASSUMPTIONS

Parse[41:19] synthesized "principles, tenets, and concepts from Rogers, Heidegger, Merleau-Ponty, and Sartre . . . in the creation of the assumptions about the human and becoming, underpinning a view of nursing grounded in the human sciences. Each assumption is unique and represents a synthesis of three of the postulates and concepts drawn from Rogers' work and from existential phenomenology"[41:19] This underscores just how firmly Parse's theoretical sources underpin her development of the human becoming school of thought. Parse draws upon the work of other theorists to build a solid foundation for a new nursing science. Accordingly, the assumptions underpinning the human becoming theory focus on beliefs about humans and about their becoming, which is health. Parse does not specify separate assumptions about the universe because her belief is that the universe is multidimensional and in mutual process with the human and not separate from the human. This is evident in the following assumptions about human beings and human becoming.

- The human is coexisting while coconstituting rhythmical patterns with the universe (coexistence, coconstitution, and pattern).
- The human is open, freely choosing meaning in situation, bearing responsibility for decisions (situated freedom, openness, and energy field).
- The human is unitary, continuously coconstituting patterns of relating (energy field, pattern, and coconstitution).
- The human is transcending multidimensionally with the possibles (pandimensionality, openness, and situated freedom).
- Becoming is unitary human-living-health (openness, situated freedom, and coconstitution).
- Becoming is a rhythmically coconstituting human-universe process (coconstitution, pattern, and pandimensionality).
- Becoming is the human's patterns of relating value priorities (situated freedom, pattern, and openness).
- Becoming is an intersubjective process of transcending with the possibles (openness, situated freedom, and coexistence).
- Becoming is unitary human's emerging (coexistence, energy field, and pandimensionality).[41:19-20,28]

Parse[38,40,41] synthesized the original nine assumptions about humans and becoming into three assumptions about human becoming:

1. Human becoming is freely choosing personal meaning in situation in the intersubjective process of living value priorities.
2. Human becoming is cocreating rhythmical patterns of relating in mutual process with the universe.
3. Human becoming is cotranscending multidimensionally with emerging possibles.[41:29]

There are three themes linked to the assumptions of the human becoming theory: (1) meaning, (2) rhythmicity, and (3) transcendence.[41] Meaning is borne in the messages individuals give and take with others in speaking, acting, silence, and stillness. Meaning indicates the significance of something and significance is chosen by people. Outsiders cannot decide the meaning or significance of something for another person. Nurses cannot know what it will mean for a family to hear news of an unexpected illness or change in health until they learn the meaning it holds from the family's perspective. Sometimes people may not know the significance of something until meaning is explored and possibilities are examined. Personal meanings are shared with others when people express their views, concerns, hopes, and dreams. According to Parse,[41:29] meaning "arises with the human-universe process and refers to ultimate meaning or purpose in life and the meaning moments of everyday living." Meaning is ever changing and expanding as persons live their becoming.

Rhythmicity is about patterns, paradox, and possibility. Parse[41] suggests that people live unrepeatable patterns that are their priorities and that these patterns are constantly changing as people engage new experiences and ideas. For Parse, people are recognized by their unique patterns that signify a consistency and change. People change their patterns when they integrate new priorities, ideas, and dreams.

Transcendence is the third major theme of the human becoming school of thought. Transcendence is about possibility; that is, the infinite possibility that is human becoming. "The possibilities arise with the human-universe process as options from which to choose personal ways of becoming."[41:30] To believe one thing or another, to go in one direction or another, to be persistent or to let go, to struggle or acquiesce, to hope or despair—all these options surface in day-to-day living. Considering and choosing from these options is cotranscending with the possibles.

Nursing

Consistent with her beliefs, Parse does not describe or write about nursing as a concept in the metaparadigm of the discipline. However, she has written extensively about her beliefs concerning nursing as a basic science. Parse[43:3] wrote, "It is the hope of many nurses that nursing as a discipline will enjoy the recognition of having a unique knowledge base and the profession will be sufficiently distinct from medicine that people will actually seek nurses for nursing care, not medical diagnoses." For more than 30 years, Parse has been advancing the belief that nursing is a basic science and that nurses require theories that are different from other disciplines. Parse believes that nursing is a unique service to humankind. This does not mean that nurses do not benefit from and employ knowledge from other disciplines and fields of study. It means that nurses rely on and value the knowledge of nursing in their practice and research activities. Parse[38:35] has clearly articulated that she believes "nursing is a science, the practice of which is a performing art." From this view, nursing is a learned discipline and nursing theories guide practice and research. The belief that nursing is a unique discipline requiring its own theories is not the predominant view and, hopefully, debates about this issue will continue to clarify the opportunities nurses have in the future of nursing science.

The practice of nursing is guided by a specific methodology that emerges directly from the human becoming ontology. The practice dimensions and processes are illuminating meaning through explicating, synchronizing rhythms through dwelling, and mobilizing transcendence through moving beyond. For details of practice methodology, see *The Human Becoming School of Thought: a Perspective for Nurses and Other Health Professionals.*[41] "Nurses who value the human becoming belief system live the theory in true presence with others."[39:12] Parse[39:12] describes practice in the following way:

> The nurse is in true presence with the individual (or family) as the individual (or family) uncovers the personal meaning of the situation and makes choices to move forward in the now moment with cherished hopes and dreams. The focus is on the meaning of the lived experience for the person (or family) unfolding 'there with' the presence of the nurse. . . . The living of the theory in practice is indeed what makes a difference to the people touched by it.

Nursing for Parse is a science and the performing art is practiced in relationships with persons (individuals, groups, and communities) in their processes of becoming. Parse offers a set of fundamentals that she believes are essential for practicing the art of nursing. Parse's list of fundamentals[35:111] follows:

- Know and use nursing frameworks and theories.
- Be available to others.
- Value the other as a human presence.
- Respect differences in view.
- Own what you believe and be accountable for your actions.
- Move on to the new and untested.
- Connect with others.
- Take pride in self.
- Like what you do.
- Recognize the moments of joy in the struggles of living.
- Appreciate mystery and be open to new discoveries.
- Be competent in your chosen area.
- Rest and begin anew.

Human-Universe-Health Process

Parse views the concepts human, universe, and health as inseparable and irreducible. Parse speaks of the human-universe-health process and, although each can be described, they are intimately linked in mutual process. For Parse, health is human becoming. Health is structuring meaning, cocreating rhythmical patterns of relating, and cotranscending with the possibles. Parse[37:136] also speaks of health as a personal commitment, which means "an individual's way of becoming is cocreated by that individual, incarnating his or her own value priorities." For Parse,[37] health is a flowing process, a personal creation, and a personal responsibility. As such, personal health can be changed by changing commitment, which "can include creative imagining, affirming self, and spontaneous glimpsing of the paradoxical."[37:138]

Human beings come into the world through others and live life in patterns of communion-aloneness. Persons change and are changed with the universe. Persons influence and are influenced by others. People become known and understood as they coexist with the universe through their patterns of relating with people, ideas, culture, history, meanings, and hopes. To understand human life and human beings an individual must start from the premise that all people are interconnected with predecessors, contemporaries, and even people who are not yet present in the world. Parents may imagine and have a relationship with a child long before the child is conceived and long after a child is lost

through death.[48] Experience has shown that many people with Alzheimer disease have relationships with their parents who are no longer in this world. These are examples of ways that people relate with the universe at multidimensional realms and these ways demonstrate the complex mutual process of human becoming.

THEORETICAL ASSERTIONS

Parse's principles are the assertions of the human becoming theory. Each principle interrelates nine concepts of human becoming: (1) languaging, (2) valuing, (3) imaging, (4) revealing-concealing, (5) enabling-limiting, (6) connecting-separating, (7) powering, (8) originating, and (9) transforming (Figure 29-1). Research projects generate structures that further specify relationships among the theoretical concepts. For example, Wang[57] studied hope for persons living with leprosy in Taiwan and she presented the following theoretical structure: the lived experience of hope is imaging the connecting-separating in originating valuing. Theoretical structures can be used to enhance understanding of specific phenomena as readers consider the detailed

Principle 1: Structuring meaning multidimensionally is cocreating reality through the languaging of valuing and imaging.

Principle 2: Cocreating rhythmical patterns of relating is living the paradoxical unity of revealing-concealing and enabling-limiting while connecting-separating.

Principle 3: Cotranscending with the possibles is powering unique ways of originating in the process of transforming.

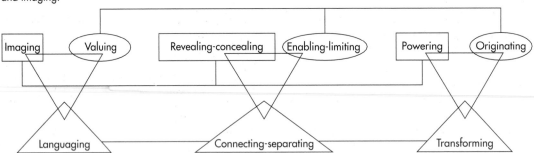

Relationship of the concepts in the squares: *Powering* is a way of *revealing and concealing imaging.*
Relationship of the concepts in the ovals: *Originating* is a manifestation of *enabling and limiting valuing.*
Relationship of the concepts in the triangles: *Transforming* unfolds in the *languaging of connecting and separating.*

Figure 29-1 Relationship of principles, concepts, and theoretical structures of the Human Becoming Theory. (From Parse, R.R. [1981]. *Man-living-health: A theory of nursing* [p. 69]. New York: John Wiley & Sons.)

participant descriptions that are linked to the concepts of human becoming theory.

LOGICAL FORM

The inductive-deductive process was central to the creation of the human becoming theory. The theory originated from Parse's personal experiences with her readings and in nursing practice. She deductively-inductively crafted major components of human becoming from Rogers' Science of Unitary Human Beings and existential-phenomenological thought. With her intuitive sense, Parse methodically derived the assumptions, concepts, principles, and practice and research methodologies of the human becoming school of thought.

ACCEPTANCE BY THE NURSING COMMUNITY

Practice

The following bibliography demonstrates the broad scope of acceptance by the nursing community. There is a strong and influential group of nursing scholars who are advancing human becoming in practice, research, and education. The theory has made a difference to nurses and to persons (patients) who experience human becoming practice.[25,58] A community-based health action model, for instance, has been developed and is receiving support from the local community and other funding agencies.[12] The theory of human becoming has also helped to generate controversy and dialogue about nursing as an evolving discipline and distinct human service.[14]

Education

In the text, *Man-Living-Health: A Theory of Nursing*,[33] Parse presented a sample masters-in-nursing curriculum that incorporated the assumptions, principles, concepts, and theoretical structures of human becoming theory. She outlined this process-based curriculum in detail, including course descriptions and course sequencing. The curriculum plan was updated in the 1998 text, *The*

Human Becoming School of Thought: a Perspective for Nurses and Other Health Professionals,[41] where Parse outlines a program philosophy and goals, a conceptual framework with themes for the curriculum, program indicators, course culture content, and the evaluation process and provides a sample curriculum plan consistent with human becoming.

A masters of nursing curriculum consistent with human becoming has been developed at Olivet Nazarene University in Kankakee, Illinois.[20] Many schools of nursing offer students some learning of human becoming theory. Most students who study the human becoming theory and who are guided by the theory in their practice and research activities are introduced to Parse's work at the master's level. This delay in introduction is unfortunate because many students who do not have the option to consider Parse's ideas and the human becoming theory in their undergraduate years have expressed frustration and disillusionment with programs that do not present an inclusive scope of nursing knowledge and practice and research methodologies.

Research

Human becoming theory has guided numerous research studies in many different countries. For instance, research findings have helped to promote understanding about how people experience hope, about how people create moments of respite when grieving a loss, and about how people with diabetes create quality amid the consequence of personal choice.*

Work with the human becoming theory will continue to evolve, as will the theory itself. An important development happened in 1998 when Parse extended thinking about human becoming beyond the notion of theory to the idea of the human becoming school of thought. Ongoing research will expand understanding and illuminate new relationships among theoretical concepts. As schools of nursing introduce and teach the human becoming school of

*References 6, 7, 23, 29, 42, 48.

thought, more nurses will try the theory in practice. Learning the theory requires formal study, a reverence for quiet contemplation, and creative synthesis.[45] As more nurses use the theory in practice and research, there will be more publications and more opportunities for thoughtful critique and scholarly discussion.

CRITIQUE

Human becoming is an abstract and complex theory. It is a theory, and not a model, because its concepts and interrelationships are defined in principles that are written at an abstract level of discourse—the language of science. Readers can study various critiques of human becoming that help clarify issues and the diversity of views that nurses hold.[11,27,46,55,59]

Simplicity

In keeping with the theoretical discourse, the major concepts of human becoming are defined in highly abstract and philosophical terms. The abstract language has been a source of comfort and discomfort for nurses.[25] The discomfort with the language is sometimes linked more with the unfamiliar beliefs and assumptions about human beings and how they relate with the universe than with the abstract concepts. Also, discomfiting for some are the nondirectional statements that do not specify causal or predictive relationships about the human-universe process.

The concepts of human becoming often resonate with people when considered at the level of lived experience. For instance, the concept of valuing when discussed at the level of lived experience focuses on the ways persons choose and act on what is important in their lives. This idea should be inherently familiar, as should the idea that people sometimes disclose intimate details about their lives and sometimes they keep secrets from others (revealing-concealing). Pickrell, Lee, Schumacher, and Twigg[47] noted that a first-time reader might be tempted to dismiss the concepts as too simple to convey the complexity inherent in the theory, but the authors

caution that to do so would be a mistake. Parse's principles describe a complex and realistic picture of human becoming and the picture provides a meaningful framework for understanding the human-universe-health interrelationship.

Generality

The human becoming school of thought has been chosen as a theoretical guide by nurses and other health professionals in many different settings, including acute care, long-term care, and community.* The theory has helped nurses be with individuals, families, and groups.[5,10,22,30,48] The theory has been evaluated in practice settings and it has been considered by patients.† Human becoming has helped leaders to create change in organizational culture and standards of care.[2,19,53]

The theory of human becoming changes what professionals see when they engage with persons in practice. The theory changes the thinking, acting, attitudes, and approaches that professionals rely on to fulfill their intentions with others. Indeed, the human becoming theory changes the intentions and purposes of professionals and there is no limit on how this learning can contribute to meaningful practices and approaches for all professional activities linked with research, education, and leadership.

Empirical Precision

Empirical precision, as discussed by Tomey,[56] relates to the testability, relevance, and usefulness of a theory. The questions asked are: Does evidence (taken here to mean *does reality*) support the theory?; Do the principles and concepts of the human becoming theory make sense to nurses when they are with people in practice?; Does the human becoming theory help nurses to be with persons in ways that are helpful and that make a difference from the patient's perspective?; Is the theory useful for administrators and researchers?; Do research findings expand knowledge and enhance the theo-

*References 1, 3, 4, 7, 9, 16, 17, 21, 24, 25, 28, 49, 50.

†References 15, 18, 25, 31, 54, 58.

retical base? The answer to these questions appears to be yes. The theory is useful because it provides a meaningful foundation that is helpful for nurses who want to live certain values in practice and research. Usefulness is a personal notion and each nurse must decide whether human becoming thought can enhance and direct practices with persons and families.

A nurse learning the theory might ask the following questions: What is the human becoming theory saying about people and do I believe in the ideas as they are presented?; Am I comfortable with the basic beliefs espoused in the human becoming theory? The answers to the initial questions about evidence or congruence with reality often lead to a decision to pursue the more difficult task of studying the theory. A commitment to learn more requires some attraction with the basic underlying values and assumptions Parse makes about the human-universe-health process. Additional questions that may be useful for nurses interested in the human becoming theory include the following: In my experience of reality, do different people have their own unique views about life and their health situations?; Do people speak about what things mean on a personal level?; Do people live their value priorities and pursue what is important to them?; Do people make their own choices?; Do people speak about paradoxical thoughts and feelings?; Have I ever heard a person say something like, "On the one hand I think this way, but on the other hand I think something else" or "I know I said I feel such and such, but as soon as I said it, I realized I also feel different than that"?; What is my experience of how people change?; Do I believe that people make choices that help them move in the direction of their own hopes and dreams?; How do people become who they want to be?

Derivable Consequences

Parse calls nursing a human science and, as such, it represents particular beliefs that have been around for more than 100 years. It is more than what was proposed before. The human becoming theory has taken human science beliefs into service and knowledge development in new and important ways. The human becoming research and practice methodologies are generating excitement and a renewed sense of professional purpose. Although not widely adopted, the theory is providing meaningful options for nursing in the twenty-first century. The consumer movement, technology, and the global transfer of knowledge on the Internet are happenings that invite new approaches in healthcare. People are recognizing that the human becoming theory is a fitting guide for practitioners who want to create respectful partnerships with people seeking healthcare.[25] More than a decade ago, Phillips suggested that Parse's work would transform the knowledge base and the practice of nursing from a unitary perspective.[46] Indeed, the human becoming theory is transforming practice in numerous settings and evaluations of the change are positive.[12,15,18,31,54] The human becoming theory directs attention to the persons' meanings of health and quality of life and to their wishes, needs, concerns, and preferences for information and care. The future of healthcare is based on the development of theories and practices that truly honor and respect people as partners and experts about life and health.

CRITICAL THINKING *Activities*

1. Mrs. Brown, a 48-year-old woman, is living with a diagnosis of breast cancer. She has not told her daughter about her diagnosis because she is afraid of how her daughter might react. Think about Parse's practice methodology and how you might act and speak with Mrs. Brown as she considers the meaning of her situation. How will you show respect for her concerns and fears? Describe how you will help her to clarify meaning and explore possibilities as she struggles with her issues.

2. Mr. Smith, an 88-year-old man, has been in the hospital for several days. Nursing staff reports that he fidgets, seems extremely

nervous, and calls out to his wife. Several of the nurses have asked the physician to prescribe a tranquilizer. Thinking about Parse's concepts and practice method, what might you add to the team's understanding about Mr. Smith? What is most important to understand given Parse's focus on how persons make decisions about how to act? How can nurses know what Mr. Smith finds helpful, given his situation?

REFERENCES

1. Baumann, S. (1997). Contrasting two approaches in a community-based nursing practice with older adults: The medical model and Parse's nursing theory. *Nursing Science Quarterly, 10,* 124-130.
2. Bournes, D.A. & Das Gupta, T.L. (1997). Professional practice leader: A transformational role that addresses human diversity. *Nursing Administration Quarterly, 21*(4), 61-68.
3. Bunkers, S.S. (1998). A nursing theory-guided model of health ministry: Human becoming in parish nursing. *Nursing Science Quarterly, 11,* 7-8.
4. Bunkers, S.S., Michaels, C., & Ethridge, P. (1997). Advanced practice nursing in community: Nursing's opportunity. *Advanced Practice Nursing Quarterly, 2*(4), 79-84.
5. Butler, M.J. (1988). Family transformation: Parse's theory in practice. *Nursing Science Quarterly, 1,* 68-74.
6. Cody, W.K. (1995a). The lived experience of grieving for families living with AIDS: Family-centered research using Parse's method. In R.R. Parse (Ed.), *Illuminations: The human becoming theory in practice and research* (pp. 197-242). New York: National League for Nursing Press.
7. Cody, W.K. (1995b). The meaning of grieving for families living with AIDS. *Nursing Science Quarterly, 8,* 104-114.
8. Cody, W.K. (1995c). Of life immense in passion, pulse, and power: Dialoguing with Whitman and Parse. A hermeneutic study. In R.R. Parse (Ed.), *Illuminations: The human becoming theory in practice and research* (pp. 269-308). New York: National League for Nursing Press.
9. Cody, W.K. (1995d). True presence with families living with HIV disease. In R.R. Parse (Ed.), *Illuminations: The human becoming theory in practice and research* (pp. 115-133). New York: National League for Nursing Press.
10. Cody, W.K., Hudepohl, J.H., & Brinkman, K.S. (1995). True presence with a child and his family. In R.R. Parse (Ed.), *Illuminations: The human becoming theory in practice and research* (pp. 135-146). New York National League for Nursing Press.
11. Cowling, W.R. (1989). Parse's theory of nursing. In J.J. Fitzpatrick & A.L. Whall (Eds.), *Conceptual models of nursing: Analysis and application* (2nd ed., pp. 385-399). Norwalk, CT: Appleton & Lange.
12. Crane, J., Josephson, D., & Letcher, D. (1999, Nov.). *The human becoming health action model in community.* Paper presented at The Seventh Annual International Colloquium on Human Becoming. Loyola University, Chicago.
13. Damgaard, G. & Bunkers, S.S. (1998). Nursing science-guided practice and education: A state board of nursing perspective. *Nursing Science Quarterly, 11,* 142-144.
14. Hall, B.A. (1993). Commentary: The inherent value of practice theories. *Nursing Science Quarterly, 6,* 10-11.
15. Jonas, C.M. (1995a). Evaluation of the human becoming theory in family practice. In R.R. Parse (Ed.), *Illuminations: The human becoming theory in practice and research* (pp. 347-366). New York: National League for Nursing Press.
16. Jonas, C.M. (1995b). True presence through music for persons living their dying. In R.R. Parse (Ed.), *Illuminations: The human becoming theory in practice* (pp. 97-104). New York: National League for Nursing Press.
17. Kelley, L.S. (1995). Parse's theory in practice with a group in the community. *Nursing Science Quarterly, 8,* 127-132.
18. Legault, F. & Ferguson-Paré, M. (1999). Advancing nursing practice: An evaluation study of Parse's theory of human becoming. *Canadian Journal of Nursing Leadership, 12*(1), 30-35.
19. Linscott, J., Spee, R., Flint, F., & Fisher, A. (1999). Creating a culture of patient-focused care through a learner-centered philosophy. *Canadian Journal of Nursing Leadership, 12*(4), 5-10.
20. Milton, C. (2000, July). Personal communication.
21. Mitchell, G.J. (1986). Utilizing Parse's theory of man-living-health in Mrs. M's neighborhood. *Perspectives, 10*(4), 5-7.
22. Mitchell, G.J. (1988). Man-living-health: The theory in practice. *Nursing Science Quarterly, 1,* 120-127.
23. Mitchell, G.J. (1998). Living with diabetes: How understanding expands theory for professional practice. *Canadian Journal of Diabetes Care, 22*(1), 30-37.
24. Mitchell, G.J., Bernardo, A., & Bournes, D. (1997). Nursing guided by Parse's theory: Patient views at Sunnybrook. *Nursing Science Quarterly, 10,* 55-56.
25. Mitchell, G.J., Closson, T., Coulis, N., Flint, F., & Gray, B. (2000). Patient-focused care and human becoming thought: Connecting the right stuff. *Nursing Science Quarterly, 13,* 216-224.

26. Mitchell, G.J. & Cody, W.K. (1992). Nursing knowledge and human science: Ontological and epistemological considerations. *Nursing Science Quarterly,* 5, 54-61.

27. Mitchell, G.J. & Cody, W.K. (1999). Human becoming theory: A complement to medical science. *Nursing Science Quarterly,* 12, 304-310.

28. Mitchell, G.J. & Copplestone, C. (1990). Applying Parse's theory to perioperative nursing: A nontraditional approach. *AORN Journal,* 51, 787-798.

29. Mitchell, G.J. & Lawton, C. (2000). Living with the consequences of personal choices for persons with diabetes: Implications for educators and practitioners. *Canadian Journal of Diabetes Care,* 24(2), 23-31.

30. Mitchell, G.J. & Pilkington, B. (1990). Theoretical approaches in nursing practice: A comparison of Roy and Parse. *Nursing Science Quarterly,* 3, 81-87.

31. Northrup, D.T. & Cody, W.K. (1998). Evaluation of the human becoming theory in practice in an acute care psychiatric setting. *Nursing Science Quarterly,* 11, 23-30.

32. Parse, R.R. (1974). *Nursing fundamentals.* Flushing, NY: Medical Examination.

33. Parse, R.R. (1981). *Man-living-health: A theory of nursing.* New York: Wiley.

34. Parse, R.R. (1987). *Nursing science: Major paradigms, theories, and critiques.* Philadelphia: W.B. Saunders.

35. Parse, R.R. (1989). Essentials for practicing the art of nursing. *Nursing Science Quarterly,* 2, 111.

36. Parse, R.R. (1989). Parse's man-living-health model and administration of nursing service. In B. Henry, C. Arndt, M. DiVincenti, & A. Marriner Tomey (Eds.), *Dimensions of nursing administration: Theory, research, education, and practice.* Cambridge, MA: Blackwell Scientific.

37. Parse, R.R. (1990). Health: A personal commitment. *Nursing Science Quarterly,* 3, 136-140.

38. Parse, R.R. (1992). Human becoming: Parse's theory of nursing. *Nursing Science Quarterly,* 5, 35-42.

39. Parse, R.R. (1993). Scholarly dialogue: Theory guides research and practice. *Nursing Science Quarterly,* 6, 12.[*]

40. Parse, R.R. (Ed.). (1995). *Illuminations: The human becoming theory in practice and research.* New York: National League for Nursing Press.

41. Parse, R.R. (1998). *The human becoming school of thought: A perspective for nurses and other health professionals.* Thousand Oaks, CA: Sage.[†]

42. Parse, R.R. (1999). *Hope: An international human becoming perspective.* Sudbury, MA: Jones and Bartlett Publishers, Inc.

43. Parse, R.R. (2000). Into the new millennium. *Nursing Science Quarterly,* 13, 3.

44. Parse, R.R. (2001). *Qualitative inquiry: The path of sciencing.* Boston: Jones & Bartlett.

45. Parse, R.R., Coyne, B., & Smith, M.J. (1985). *Nursing research: Qualitative methods.* Bowie, MD: Brady. (Coauthored.)

46. Phillips, J.R. (1987). A critique of Parse's man-living-health theory. In R.R. Parse (Ed.), *Nursing science: Major paradigms, theories, and critiques* (pp. 181-204). Philadelphia: W.B. Saunders.

47. Pickrell, K.D., Lee, R.E., Schumacher, L.P., & Twigg, P. (1998). Rosemarie Rizzo Parse: Human becoming. In A. Marriner Tomey & M.R. Alligood (Eds.), *Nursing theorists and their work* (4th ed., pp. 463-481). New York: Mosby.

48. Pilkington, F.B. (1993). The lived experience of grieving the loss of an important other. *Nursing Science Quarterly,* 6, 130-139.

49. Quiquero, A., Knights, D., & Meo, C.O. (1991). Theory as a guide to practice: Staff nurses choose Parse's theory. *Canadian Journal of Nursing Administration,* 4(1), 14-16.

50. Rasmusson, D.L., Jonas, C.M., & Mitchell, G.J. (1991). The eye of the beholder: Applying Parse's theory with homeless individuals. *Clinical Nurse Specialist Journal,* 5(3), 139-143.

51. Rogers, M.E. (1970). *An introduction to the theoretical basis of nursing.* Philadelphia: F.A. Davis.

52. Rogers, M. (1992). Nursing science and the space age. *Nursing Science Quarterly,* 5, 27-34.

53. Saltmarche, A., Kolodny, V., & Mitchell, G.J. (1998). An educational approach for patient-focused care: Shifting attitudes and practice. *Journal of Nursing Staff Development,* 14(2), 81-86.

54. Santopinto, M.D.A. & Smith, M.C. (1995). Evaluation of the human becoming theory in practice with adults and children. In R.R. Parse (Ed.), *Illuminations: The human becoming theory in practice and research* (pp. 309-346). New York: National League for Nursing Press.

55. Smith, M.C. & Hudepohl, J.H. (1988). Analysis and evaluation of Parse's theory of man-living-health. *The Canadian Journal of Nursing Research: Nursing Papers,* 20(4), 43-58.

56. (Marriner) Tomey, A.M. (1998). Introduction to analysis of nursing theories. In A.M. (Marriner) Tomey & M.R. Alligood (Eds.), *Nursing theorists and their work* (4th ed., pp. 3-15). St. Louis: Mosby.

57. Wang, C-E. (1999). He-bung: Hope for persons living with leprosy in Taiwan. In R.R. Parse (Ed.), *Hope: An international human becoming perspective* (pp. 143-162). Sudbury, MA: Jones and Bartlett Publishers, Inc.

58. Williamson, G.J. (2000). The test of a nursing theory: A personal view. *Nursing Science Quarterly,* 13, 124-128.

59. Winkler, S.J. (1983). Parse's theory of nursing. In J. Fitzpatrick & A. Whall (Eds.), *Conceptual models of nursing: Analysis and application* (pp. 275-294). Bowie, MD: Robert J. Brady.

BIBLIOGRAPHY
Primary Sources
Books

Parse, R.R. (1974). *Nursing fundamentals.* Flushing, NY: Medical Examination.

Parse, R.R. (1981). *Man-living-health: A theory of nursing.* New York: Wiley.

Parse, R.R. (1987). *Nursing science: Major paradigms, theories, and critiques.* Philadelphia: W.B. Saunders.

Parse, R.R. (Ed.). (1995). *Illuminations: The human becoming theory in practice and research.* New York: National League for Nursing Press.

Parse, R.R. (1998). *The human becoming school of thought: A perspective for nurses and other health professionals.* Thousand Oaks, CA: Sage.

Parse, R.R. (1999). *Hope: An international human becoming perspective.* Sudbury, MA: Jones and Bartlett Publishers, Inc.

Parse, R.R., Coyne, A.B., & Smith, M.J. (1985). *Nursing research: Qualitative methods.* Bowie, MD: Brady.

Doctoral Dissertation

Parse, R.R. (1969). An instructional model for the teaching of nursing, interrelating objectives and media. *Dissertation Abstracts International,* 31, 180A.

Book Chapters, Articles, and Editorials

Parse, R.R. (1967, Aug.). Advantages and disadvantages of associate degree nursing programs. *Journal of Nursing Education,* 6(15), 5-8.

Parse, R.R. (1978). Rights of medical patients. In C.T. Fischer & S.L. Brodsky (Eds.), *Client participation in human services.* New Brunswick, NJ: Transaction.

Parse, R.R. (1981). Caring from a human science perspective. In M.M. Leininger (Ed.), *Caring: An essential human need* (pp. 129-132). Thorofare, NJ: Slack.

Parse, R.R. (1988). Beginnings. *Nursing Science Quarterly,* 1(1), 1-2.

Parse, R.R. (1988). Creating traditions: The art of putting it together. *Nursing Science Quarterly,* 1(2), 45.

Parse, R.R. (1988). Scholarly dialogue: The fire of refinement. *Nursing Science Quarterly,* 1(4), 141.

Parse, R.R. (1988). The mainstream of science: Framing the issue. *Nursing Science Quarterly,* 1(3), 93.

Parse, R.R. (1989). Essentials for practicing the art of nursing. *Nursing Science Quarterly,* 2(3), 111.

Parse, R.R. (1989). Making more out of less. *Nursing Science Quarterly,* 2(4), 155.

Parse, R.R. (1989). Man-living-health: A theory of nursing. In J. Riehl-Sisca (Ed.), *Conceptual models for nursing practice* (3rd ed.). Norwalk, CT: Appleton & Lange.

Parse, R.R. (1989). Martha E. Rogers: A birthday celebration. *Nursing Science Quarterly,* 2(2), 55.

Parse, R.R. (1989). Parse's man-living-health model and administration of nursing service. In B. Henry, C. Arndt, M. DiVincenti, & A. Marriner Tomey (Eds.), *Dimensions of nursing administration: Theory, research, education, and practice.* Cambridge, MA: Blackwell Scientific.

Parse, R.R. (1989). Qualitative research: Publishing and funding. *Nursing Science Quarterly,* 2(1), 1-2.

Parse, R.R. (1989). The phenomenological research method: Its value for management science. In B. Henry, C. Arndt, M. DiVincenti, & A. Marriner Tomey (Eds.), *Dimensions of nursing administration: Theory, research, education, and practice.* Cambridge, MA: Blackwell Scientific.

Parse, R.R. (1990). A time for reflection and projection. *Nursing Science Quarterly,* 3(4), 143.

Parse, R.R. (1990). Health: A personal commitment. *Nursing Science Quarterly,* 3(3), 136-140.

Parse, R.R. (1990). Nurse theorist conference comes to Japan. *Japanese Journal of Nursing Research,* 23(3).

Parse, R.R. (1990). Nursing theory-based practice: A challenge for the 90s. *Nursing Science Quarterly,* 3(2), 53.

Parse, R.R. (1990). Parse's research methodology with an illustration of the lived experience of hope. *Nursing Science Quarterly,* 3(1), 9-17.

Parse, R.R. (1990). Promotion and prevention: Two distinct cosmologies. *Nursing Science Quarterly,* 3(3), 101.

Parse, R.R. (1991). Electronic publishing: Beyond browsing. *Nursing Science Quarterly,* 4(1), 1.

Parse, R.R. (1991). Growing the discipline of nursing. *Nursing Science Quarterly,* 4(4), 139.

Parse, R.R. (1991). Mysteries of health and healing: Two perspectives. *Nursing Science Quarterly,* 4(3), 93.

Parse, R.R. (1991). Parse's theory of human becoming. In I.E. Goertzen (Ed.), *Differentiating nursing practice: Into the twenty-first century* (pp. 51-53). Kansas City, MO: American Academy of Nursing.

Parse, R.R. (1991). Phenomenology and nursing. *Japanese Journal of Nursing,* 17(2), 261-269.

Parse, R.R. (1991). The right soil, the right stuff. *Nursing Science Quarterly,* 4(2), 47.

Parse, R.R. (1992). Human becoming: Parse's theory of nursing. *Nursing Science Quarterly,* 5(1), 35-42.

Parse, R.R. (1992). Moving beyond the barrier reef. *Nursing Science Quarterly,* 5(3), 97.

Parse, R.R. (1992). Nursing knowledge for the 21st century: An international commitment. *Nursing Science Quarterly,* 5(1), 8-12.

Parse, R.R. (1992). The performing art of nursing. *Nursing Science Quarterly,* 5(4), 147.

Parse, R.R. (1992). The unsung shapers of nursing science. *Nursing Science Quarterly,* 5(2), 47.

Parse, R.R. (1993). Cartoons: Glimpsing paradoxical moments. *Nursing Science Quarterly, 6*(1), 1.

Parse, R.R. (1993). Critical appraisal: Risking to challenge. *Nursing Science Quarterly, 6*(4), 163.

Parse, R.R. (1993). *Critique of critical phenomena of nursing science suggested by O'Brien, Reed, and Stevenson* (pp.71-81). Proceedings of the 1993 Annual Forum on Doctoral Nursing Education: A Call for Substance: Preparing Leaders for Global Health. St. Paul, MN: University of Minnesota School of Nursing.

Parse, R.R. (1993). Nursing and medicine: Two different disciplines. *Nursing Science Quarterly, 6*(3), 109.

Parse, R.R. (1993). Parse's human becoming theory: Its research and practice implications. In M.E. Parker (Ed.), *Patterns of nursing theories in practice* (pp. 49-61). New York: National League for Nursing Press.

Parse, R.R. (1993). Plant now; reap later. *Nursing Science Quarterly, 6*(2), 55.

Parse, R.R. (1993). Scholarly dialogue: Theory guides research and practice. *Nursing Science Quarterly, 6*(1), 12.

Parse, R.R. (1993). The experience of laughter: A phenomenological study. *Nursing Science Quarterly, 6*(1), 39-43.

Parse, R.R. (1994). Charley Potatoes or mashed potatoes? *Nursing Science Quarterly, 7*(3), 97.

Parse, R.R. (1994). Laughing and health: A study using Parse's research method. *Nursing Science Quarterly, 7*(2), 55-64.

Parse, R.R. (1994). Martha E. Rogers: Her voice will not be silenced. *Nursing Science Quarterly, 7*(2), 47.

Parse, R.R. (1994). Quality of life: Sciencing and living the art of human becoming. *Nursing Science Quarterly, 7*(1), 16-21.

Parse, R.R. (1994). Scholarship: Three essential processes. *Nursing Science Quarterly, 7*(4), 143.

Parse, R.R. (1995). Again: What is nursing? *Nursing Science Quarterly, 8*(4), 143.

Parse, R.R. (1995). Building the realm of nursing knowledge. *Nursing Science Quarterly, 8*(2), 51.

Parse, R.R. (1995). Commentary: Parse's theory of human becoming: An alternative to nursing practice for pediatric oncology nurses. *Journal of Pediatric Oncology Nursing, 12*(3), 128.

Parse, R.R. (1995). Foreword. In M.A. Frey & C.L. Sieloff (Eds.), *Advancing King's systems framework and theory of nursing.* Thousand Oaks, CA: Sage.

Parse, R.R. (1995). Man-living-health. A theory of nursing. In M. Mischo-Kelling & K. Wittneben (Eds.), *Auffassungen von pflege in theorie und praxis* (pp. 114-132). Munchen: Urban & Schwarzenberg.

Parse, R.R. (1995). Man-living-health. A theory of nursing. In M. Mischo-Kelling & K. Wittneben (Eds.), *Pflegebildung und pflegetheorien* (pp. 114-132). Munchen: Urban & Schwarzenberg.

Parse, R.R. (1995). Mensch(werden)-leben-gesundheit: Die pflegetheorie von Parse [Man-living-health: Parse's theory of nursing]. In M. Mischo-Kelling & K. Wit-

tneben (Eds.), *Pflegebildung und pflegetheorien* (pp.114-132). Mtinchen: Urban & Schwarzenberg.

Parse, R.R. (1995). Nursing theories and frameworks: The essence of advanced practice nursing. *Nursing Science Quarterly, 8*(1), 1.

Parse, R.R. (1995). Nursing theory based research and practice. A conference coming to Japan. Tokyo, Japan: Igacu Shoin. *Medical News Weekly.*

Parse, R.R. (1996). Building knowledge through qualitative research: The road less traveled. *Nursing Science Quarterly, 9*(1), 10-16.

Parse, R.R. (1996). Critical thinking: What is it? *Nursing Science Quarterly, 9*(3), 138.

Parse, R.R. (1996). Hear ye, hear ye: Novice and seasoned authors! *Nursing Science Quarterly, 9*(1), 1.

Parse, R.R. (1996). Nursing theories: An original path. *Nursing Science Quarterly, 9*(2), 85.

Parse, R.R. (1996). Quality of life for persons living with Alzheimer's disease: A human becoming perspective. *Nursing Science Quarterly, 9*(3), 126-133.

Parse, R.R. (1996). Reality: A seamless symphony of becoming. *Nursing Science Quarterly, 9*(4), 181-183.

Parse, R.R. (1996). [Review of the book *Martha E. Rogers: Her life and her work*]. *Visions: The Journal of Rogerian Science, 2,* 52-53.

Parse, R.R. (1996). The human becoming theory: Challenges in practice and research. *Nursing Science Quarterly, 9*(1), 55-60.

Parse, R.R. (1997). Concept inventing: Unitary creations. *Nursing Science Quarterly, 10*(2), 63-64.

Parse, R.R. (1997). Investing the legacy: Martha E. Rogers' voice will not be silenced. *Visions: The Journal of Rogerian Science, 5,* 7-11.

Parse, R.R. (1997). Joy-sorrow: A study using the Parse research method. *Nursing Science Quarterly, 10*(2), 80-87.

Parse, R.R. (1997). Leadership: The essentials. *Nursing Science Quarterly, 10*(3), 109.

Parse, R.R. (1997). New beginnings in a quiet revolution. *Nursing Science Quarterly, 10*(1), 1.

Parse, R.R. (1997). [Review of the book *Quality of life in behavioral medicine*]. *Women and Health, 25*(3), 83-86.

Parse, R.R. (1997). The human becoming theory and its research and practice methodologies. In J. Osterbrink (Ed.), *Pflegetheorien - eine zusammenfassung der 1st international conference.* Freiburg, Germany: Verlag Hans Huber.

Parse, R.R. (1997). The human becoming theory: The was, is, and will be. *Nursing Science Quarterly, 10*(1), 32-38.

Parse, R.R. (1997). The language of nursing knowledge: Saying what we mean. In J. Fawcett & I.M. King (Eds.), *The language of nursing theory and metatheory* (pp. 73-77). Indianapolis: Sigma Theta Tau Monograph.

Parse, R.R. (1997). Transforming research and practice with the human becoming theory. *Nursing Science Quarterly, 10*(4), 171-174.

Parse, R.R. (1998). Moving on. *Nursing Science Quarterly,* 11(4), 135.

Parse, R.R. (1998). The art of criticism. *Nursing Science Quarterly,* 11(2), 43.

Parse, R.R. (1998). Will nursing exist tomorrow? A reprise. *Nursing Science Quarterly,* 11(1), 1.

Parse, R.R. (1999). Authorship: Whose responsibility? *Nursing Science Quarterly,* 12(2), 99.

Parse, R.R. (1999). Community: An alternative view. *Nursing Science Quarterly,* 12(2), 119-124.

Parse, R.R. (1999). Expanding the vision: Tilling the field of nursing knowledge. *Nursing Science Quarterly,* 12(1), 3.

Parse, R.R. (1999). Integrity and the advancement of nursing knowledge. *Nursing Science Quarterly,* 12(3), 187.

Parse, R.R. (1999). Nursing Science: The transformation of practice. *Journal of Advanced Nursing,* 30(6), 1383-1387.

Parse, R.R. (1999). Nursing: The discipline and the profession. *Nursing Science Quarterly,* 12(4), 275.

Parse, R.R. (1999). The lived experience of hope for family members of persons living in a Canadian chronic care facility. In R.R. Parse (Ed.), *Hope: An international human becoming perspective* (pp. 63-77). Sudbury, MS: Jones and Bartlett.

Parse, R.R. (1999). Witnessing as true presence. *Illuminations: Newsletter for the International Consortium of Parse Scholars,* 8(3), 1.

Parse, R.R. (2000). Into the new millennium. *Nursing Science Quarterly,* 13(1), 3.

Parse, R.R. (2000). Language: Words reflect and cocreate meaning. *Nursing Science Quarterly,* 13(3), 187.

Parse, R.R. (2000). Obfuscating: The persistent practice of misnaming. *Nursing Science Quarterly,* 13(2), 91-92.

Parse, R.R. (2000). Paradigms: A reprise. *Nursing Science Quarterly,* 13(4), 275-276.

Parse, R.R. (2001). Contributions to the discipline. *Nursing Science Quarterly,* 14(1), 5.

Parse, R.R. (2001). Nursing: Still in the shadow of medicine. *Nursing Science Quarterly,* 14(3), 181.

Parse, R.R. (2001). The human becoming school of thought in research. In M. Parker (Ed.), *Nursing theories and nursing practice* (pp. 227-238). Philadelphia: F.A. Davis.

Parse, R.R. (2001). The universe is flat. *Nursing Science Quarterly,* 14(2), 93.

Parse, R.R. (2002, Jan.). Transforming healthcare with a unitary view of the human. Holistic nursing practice. Manuscript accepted for publication in *Nursing Science Quarterly,* 5(1).

Parse, R.R., Bournes, D. A., Barrett, E. A. M., Malinski, V. M., & Phillips, J. R. (1999). A better way: 10 things health professionals can do to move toward a more personal and meaningful system. On Call: A Magazine for Nurses and Healthcare Professionals, 2(8), 14-17.

Unpublished Manuscripts and Presentations

Parse, R.R. (1992). *Nursing knowledge-based practice: An ethical commitment.* Paper presented at European Nursing Congress 1992, Amsterdam, The Netherlands.

Parse, R.R. (1993). *The human becoming theory in practice and research.* Paper presented at Geneva, Switzerland.

Parse, R.R. (1993). *The human becoming theory in practice: A research study at Royal Ottawa Hospital.* Paper presented at Ottawa, Ontario, Canada.

Parse, R.R. (1993). *The human becoming theory: Its research and practice methodologies.* Paper presented at University of Illinois, Chicago, IL.

Parse, R.R. (1993). *True presence in languaging without words.* Paper presented at Immersion Weekend of International Consortium of Parse Scholars, McHenry, MD.

Parse, R.R. (1994). *Critique of the unitary field pattern profile portrait research method.* Paper presented at the 5th Annual Rogerian Conference at New York University, New York.

Parse, R.R. (1994). *Facing the mystery of being in true presence.* Presented at Immersion Weekend of International Consortium of Parse Scholars, Niagara-on-the-Lake, Ontario, Canada.

Parse, R.R. (1994). *Human becoming theory.* Paper presented at the O'Connor Chair for Nursing Lecture Series, Hartwick College, Oneonta, NY.

Parse, R.R. (1994). *Human becoming theory in practice and research* [Workshop]. Padoa, Italy.

Parse, R.R. (1994). *Knowledge building through qualitative research.* Paper presented at the Second Annual International Qualitative Nursing Research Colloquium, Loyola University Chicago.

Parse, R.R. (1994). *Quality of life: Ethics and values.* Paper presented at National Council for International Health Conference, Arlington, VA.

Parse, R.R. (1994). *The human becoming theory in practice.* Paper presented at International Congress, Aarau, Switzerland.

Parse, R.R. (1995, March). *Nursing science and the fine arts.* Paper presented at the D'Arcy Museum, Loyola University Chicago.

Parse, R.R. (1995, April). *Nursing theory-guided research.* Presented at the Midwest Nursing Research Society, Kansas City, MO.

Parse, R.R. (1995, Aug.). *The human becoming theory: Challenges in practice and research.* Paper presented at Discovery International, Inc., Biennial Nurse Theorist Conference, Tokyo, Japan.

Parse, R.R. (1995, Aug.). *The human becoming theory in research and practice.* Paper presented at Seoul, Korea.

Parse, R.R. (1995, Oct.). *Quality of life for persons living with Alzheimer's disease: A human becoming perspective.* Paper presented at "Quality of Life: Nursing's Commitment for the 21st Century" conference, Loyola University Chicago.

Parse, R.R. (1995, Nov.). *Research process on hope.* Paper presented at Immersion Weekend of International Consortium of Parse Scholars, Niagara-on-the-Lake, Ontario, Canada.

Parse, R.R. (1996, March). *Reality: The seamless symphony of becoming.* Paper presented at Sunnybrook Health Science Centre, Toronto, Ontario, Canada.

Parse, R.R. (1996, May). *Critical thinking in practice.* Paper presented at the University of Hami, Finland.

Parse, R.R. (1996, May). *Leadership from a human becoming perspective.* Paper presented at the University of Hami, Finland.

Parse, R.R. (1996, May). *The human becoming theory research and practice.* Paper presented at the University of Hami, Finland.

Parse, R.R. (1996, June). *Rogerian dialogue '96* [Informal discussion]. New York.

Parse, R.R. (1996, June). *The human becoming theory: A transformative theory.* Paper presented at the Discovery International Inc's Scandinavian Conference, Sweden.

Parse, R.R. (1996, June). *Transformation and practice through nursing theory.* Paper presented at the Discovery International Inc's Scandinavian Conference, Sweden.

Parse, R.R. (1996, July). *Human becoming theory workshop.* Paper presented at Institute of Human Becoming, Pittsburgh, PA.

Parse, R.R. (1996, Oct.). *Nursing knowledge-guided practice and the human becoming theory.* Paper presented to multidisciplinary groups at Rizzolo Research Institute, Bologna, Italy.

Parse, R.R. (1996, Nov.). *Notions on true presence and freedom-restriction at Checkpoint Charley.* Paper presented at Immersion Weekend of International Consortium of Parse Scholars, Niagara-on-the-Lake, Ontario, Canada.

Parse, R.R. (1996, Nov.). *Research process on hope.* Paper presented at Immersion Weekend of International Consortium of Parse Scholars, Niagara-on-the-Lake, Ontario, Canada.

Parse, R.R. (1996, Dec.). *Nursing theory-guided practice in the 21st century.* Paper presented to Parse scholars, New York.

Parse, R.R. (1997, April). *The human becoming theory in practice and research.* Paper presented at the International Nurse Theorists Conference, Nuemberg, Germany.

Parse, R.R. (1997, April). *Workshop on Parse's theory.* Paper presented at the International Nurse Theorists Conference, Nuemberg, Germany.

Parse, R.R. (1997, May). *Health as human becoming.* Paper presented to nurse faculty and nurses in practice, Sioux Falls, South Dakota.

Parse, R.R. (1997, May). *Human becoming as a guide to parish nursing.* Paper presented to nurse faculty and nurses in practice, Sioux Falls, South Dakota.

Parse, R.R. (1997, May). *Nursing science.* Paper presented to nurse faculty and nurses in practice, Sioux Falls, South Dakota.

Parse, R.R. (1997, May). *Rogerian dialogue 1997* [Informal discussion]. New York.

Parse, R.R. (1997, May). *The human becoming theory and the state board decision-making model.* Paper presented to nurse faculty and nurses in practice, Sioux Falls, South Dakota.

Parse, R.R. (1997, June). *The human becoming school of thought.* Paper presented to nurses in practice and students, University of Pittsburgh, Pittsburgh, PA.

Parse, R.R. (1997, Oct.). *Research-based knowledge and practice.* Paper presented at University of Hami, Finland.

Parse, R.R. (1997, Oct.). *Human becoming: A key to leadership.* Paper presented at University of Hami, Finland.

Parse, R.R. (1997, Oct.). *Human becoming practice in a variety of settings.* Paper presented at University of Hami, Finland.

Parse, R.R. (1997, Oct.). *Living human becoming in leadership.* Paper presented at University of Hami, Finland.

Parse, R.R. (1997, Oct.). *Research findings on human becoming theory guided practice.* Paper presented at University of Hami, Finland.

Parse, R.R. (1997, Oct.). *True presence and human interrelationships in nursing.* Paper presented at University of Hami, Finland.

Parse, R.R. (1997, Nov.). *Human becoming theory.* Paper presented at the Seventh Annual International Consortium of Parse Scholars, Niagara-on-the-Lake, Ontario, Canada.

Parse, R.R. (1997, Nov.). *Research on the 9-country 13 investigator-study on hope: A report.* Presented at the Seventh Annual International Consortium of Parse Scholars, Niagara-on-the-Lake, Ontario, Canada.

Parse, R.R. (1997, Dec.). *The international hope study.* A paper presented at Hunter College, New York.

Parse, R.R. (1998, May). *Community: A human becoming perspective.* Paper presented at the Nursing Theory Based Conference, Augustana College, Sioux Falls, South Dakota.

Parse, R.R. (1998, June). *Rogerian dialogue 1998* [Informal discussion]. New York.

Parse, R.R. (1998, June). *The human becoming school of thought: Ontology.* Paper presented at the Institute of Human Becoming, Pittsburgh, PA.

Parse, R.R. (1998, June). *The human becoming school of thought: Practice methodology.* Paper presented at the Institute of Human Becoming, Pittsburgh, PA.

Parse, R.R. (1998, July). *Challenges with translinguistic nursing research.* Paper presented at Sigma Theta Tau Congress, Utrecht, Netherlands.

Parse, R.R. (1998, Sept.). *Valuing lived experience: Human becoming as a guide to practice.* The Anne Marie Djupe Memorial Lecture, The 12th Annual Westburg Parish Nursing Symposium.

Parse, R.R. (1998, Nov.). *Human becoming theory.* Paper presented at the eighth meeting of the International Consortium of Parse Scholars, Niagara-on-the-Lake, Ontario, Canada.

Parse, R.R. (1999, April). *International research: Unfolding possibilities.* Paper presented at the International Consortium of Parse Scholars, Hunter College, New York.

Parse, R.R. (1999, June). *Research methodologies, the human becoming school of thought.* Workshop presented at the Institute of Human Becoming, Pittsburgh, PA.

Parse, R.R. (1999, June). *Rogerian dialogue* [Informal discussion]. New York.

Parse, R.R. (1999, Oct.). *Human becoming as a guide to practice.* Paper presented in Madrid, Valencia, and Barcelona, Spain.

Parse, R.R. (1999, Dec.). *The human becoming hermeneutic method.* Paper presented at the International Consortium of Parse Scholars, Hunter College, New York.

Parse, R.R. (2000, June). *Community: The human becoming perspective.* Workshop presented at the Institute of Human Becoming, Pittsburgh, PA.

Parse, R.R. (2000, June). *Enjoy your flight: Health in the new millennium.* Paper presented at the Rogerian Conference, New York.

Parse, R.R. (2000, June). *Human becoming: Assumptions and principles.* Workshop presented at the Institute of Human Becoming, Pittsburgh, PA.

Cassette Recordings

Parse, R.R. (Speaker). (1985). *Nursing education in the 21st century* (Cassette Recording No. DII-113). Louisville, KY: Meetings Internationale, Ltd.

Parse, R.R. (Speaker). (1985). *Presentation [at nurse theorist conference]* (Cassette Recording No. DII-105). Louisville, KY: Meetings Internationale, Ltd.

Parse, R.R. (Speaker). (1986). *An emerging research methodology unique to nursing* (Cassette Recording No. DII-303). Louisville, KY: Meetings Internationale, Ltd.

Parse, R.R. (Speaker). (1986). *Quantitative and qualitative methods in nursing research* (Cassette Recording No. DII-201). Louisville, KY: Meetings Internationale, Ltd.

Parse, R.R. (Speaker). (1986). *The ethnographic method* (Cassette Recording No. DII-204). Louisville, KY: Meetings Internationale, Ltd.

Parse, R.R. (Speaker). (1986). *The phenomenological method* (Cassette Recording No. DII-202 [A&B]). Louisville, KY: Meetings Internationale, Ltd.

Parse, R.R. (Speaker). (1987). *Parse theory* (Cassette Recording No. DII-403). Louisville, KY: Meetings Internationale, Ltd.

Parse, R.R. (Speaker). (1987). *Small group c* (Cassette Recording No. DII-411). Louisville, KY: Meetings Internationale, Ltd.

Parse, R.R. (Speaker). (1989). *Health as a personal commitment in Parse's theory* (Cassette Recording No. DII-503). Louisville, KY: Meetings Internationale, Ltd.

Parse, R.R. (Speaker). (1990). *Parse's research and practice methodologies* (Cassette Recording No. DII-601). Louisville, KY: Meetings Internationale, Ltd.

Parse, R.R. (Speaker). (1993). *Quality of life and human becoming* (Cassette Recording No. DII-701). Louisville, KY: Veranda Communications.

Parse, R.R., Cody, W.K., Beauchamp, C.J., Smith, M.C., Menke, E.M., Mitchell, G.J., & Santopinto, M.D.A. (Speakers). (1990). *Panel discussion/retrospective and evaluation* (Cassette Recording No. DII-605). Louisville, KY: Meetings Internationale, Ltd.

Parse, R.R., Leininger, M.M., Rogers, M.E., Peplau, H.E., & King, I.M. (Speakers). (1993). *Nursing and the next millennium [panel discussion with the theorists]* (Cassette Recording No. DII-708). Louisville, KY: Veranda Communications.

Parse, R.R., Meleis, A.I. Neuman, B.M., Rogers, M.E., Pender, N.J., & King, I.M. (Speakers). (1989). *Panel discussion with theorists* (Cassette Recording No. DII-507). Louisville, KY: Meetings Internationale, Ltd.

Parse, R.R., Orem, D.E., Roy, C., King, I.M., Rogers, M.E., & Peplau, H.E. (Speakers). (1985). *Panel discussion with nurse theorists* (Cassette Recording No. DII-112). Louisville, KY: Meetings Internationale, Ltd.

Parse, R.R., Peplau, H.E., King, I.M., Roy, C., Rogers, M.E., & Watson, J. (Speakers). (1987). *Panel discussion with theorists* (Cassette Recording No. DII-408). Louisville, KY: Meetings International, Ltd.

Parse, R.R. & Phillips, J.R. (Speakers). (1985). *Parse's man-living-health theory of nursing* (Cassette Recording No. DII-109). Louisville, KY: Meetings Internationale, Ltd.

Parse, R.R., Skiar, M., & Smith, M.J. (Speakers). (1986). *Panel discussion* (Cassette Recording No. DII-305). Louisville, KY: Meetings Internationale, Ltd.

Videotape Recordings

Parse, R.R. (Speaker). (1987). *Parse's theory* (Videotape Recording No. DII-V-403). Louisville, KY: Meetings Internationale, Ltd.

Parse, R.R. (Speaker). (1989). *Health as a personal commitment in Parse's theory* (Videotape Recording No. DIIV-503). Louisville, KY: Meetings Internationale, Ltd.

Parse, R.R. (Speaker). (1990). *A portrait in excellence* [Videotape]. Helene Fuld Health Trust. Oakland, CA: Studio Three Production.

Parse, R.R. (Speaker). (1993). *Quality of life and human becoming* (Videotape Recording No. DII-V-701). Louisville, KY: Veranda Communications.

Parse, R.R., Leininger, M.M., Rogers, M.E., Peplau, H.E., & King, I.M. (Speakers). (1993). *Nursing and the next millennium [panel discussion with the theorists]* (Videotape Recording No. DII-V-708). Louisville, KY: Veranda Communications.

Parse, R.R., Meleis, A.I., Neuman, B.M., Rogers, M.E., Pender, N.J., & King, I.M. (Speakers). (1989). *Panel discussion with theorists* (Videotape Recording No. DII-V-507). Louisville, KY: Meetings Internationale, Ltd.

Parse, R.R., Orem, D.E., Roy, C., King, I.M., Rogers, M.E., & Peplau, H.E. (Speakers). (1985). *Panel discussion with theorists* (Videotape Recording No. DII-V-112). Louisville, KY: Meetings Internationale, Ltd.

Parse, R.R., Peplau, H.E., King, I.M., Roy, C., Rogers, M.E., Watson, J., & Leininger, M. (Speakers). (1987). *Panel discussion with theorists* (Videotape Recording No. DII-V-408). Louisville, KY: Meetings Internationale, Ltd.

Secondary Sources
Reviews on Parse's Books

Clarke, P.N. (1996). [Review of the book *Illuminations: The human becoming theory in practice and research*]. *Nursing Science Quarterly, 9*(2), 81-82.

Fawcett, J. (1996). [Review of the book *Illuminations: The human becoming theory in practice and research*]. *Nursing Science Quarterly, 9*(2), 82-83.

Fawcett, J. & Phillips, J.R. (1999). [Review of the book *The human becoming school of thought: A perspective for nurses and other health professionals*]. *Nursing Science Quarterly, 12*(1), 85-89.

Jacobs-Kramer, M.K., Levine, M.E., & Menke, E.M. (1988). Three perspectives on a scholarly work [Review of the book *Nursing science: Major paradigms, theories, and critiques*]. *Nursing Science Quarterly, 1*(4), 182-186.

Limandri, B.J. (1982). [Review of the book *Man-living-health: A theory of nursing*]. *Western Journal of Nursing Research, 4*(1), 105-106.

Rawnsley, M.M. (1988). Quest for quality: A comparative review [Review of the book *Nursing research: Qualitative methods*]. *Nursing Science Quarterly, 1*(1), 40-41.

[Review of the book *Man-living-health: A theory of nursing*]. (1981). *International Journal of Rehabilitation Research, 4*, 449.

[Review of the book *Nursing fundamentals*]. (1975). *Australian Nurses Journal, 5*(37).

Articles and Chapters About Parse's Theory

Allchin-Petardi, L. (1998). Weathering the storm: Persevering through a difficult time. *Nursing Science Quarterly, 11*(4), 172-177.

Allchin-Petardi, L. (1999). Hope for American women with children. In R.R. Parse (Ed.), *Hope: An international human becoming perspective* (pp. 273-285). Sudbury, MS: Jones and Bartlett.

Andrus, K. (1995). Parse's nursing theory and the practice of perioperative nursing. *Canadian Operating Room Nursing Journal, 13*(3), 19-22.

Arndt, M.J. (1995). Parse's theory of human becoming in practice with hospitalized adolescents. *Nursing Science Quarterly, 8*(2), 86-90.

Banonis, B.C. (1989). The lived experience of recovering from addiction: A phenomenological study. *Nursing Science Quarterly, 2*(1), 37-43.

Banonis, B.C. (1995). Metaphors in the practice of the human becoming theory. In R.R. Parse (Ed.), *Illuminations: The human becoming theory in practice and research* (pp. 87-95). New York: National League for Nursing Press.

Baumann, S. (1994). No place of their own: An exploratory study. *Nursing Science Quarterly, 7*(4), 162-169.

Baumann, S. (1995). Two views of children's art: Psychoanalysis and Parse's human becoming theory. *Nursing Science Quarterly, 8*(2), 65-70.

Baumann, S. (1996). Feeling uncomfortable: Children in families with no place of their own. *Nursing Science Quarterly, 9*(4), 152-159.

Baumann, S. (1996). Parse's research methodology and the nurse-researcher-child process. *Nursing Science Quarterly, 9*(1), 27-32.

Baumann, S. (1997). Contrasting two approaches in a community-based nursing practice with older adults: The medical model and Parse's nursing theory. *Nursing Science Quarterly, 10*(3), 124-130.

Baumann, S. & Braddick, M. (1999). Out of their element: Fathers of children who are "not the same." *Journal of Pediatric Nursing, 14*(6), 269-278.

Baumann, S.L. (1997). Qualitative research with children as participants. *Nursing Science Quarterly, 10*(2), 68-69.

Baumann, S.L. (1999). The lived experience of hope: Children in families struggling to make a home. In R.R. Parse (Ed.), *Hope: An international human becoming perspective* (pp. 191-210). Sudbury, MS: Jones and Bartlett.

Benedict, L.L., Bunkers, S.S., Damgaard, G.A., Duffy, C.E., Hohman, M.L., & Vander Woude, D.L. (2000). The South Dakota board of nursing theory-based regulatory decisioning model. *Nursing Science Quarterly, 13*(2), 167-171.

Bernardo, A. (1998). Technology and true presence in nursing. *Holistic Nursing Practice, 12*(4), 40-49.

Bournes, D.A. (2000). A commitment to honoring people's choices. *Nursing Science Quarterly, 13*(1), 18-23.

Bournes, D.A. (2000). Concept inventing: A process for creating a unitary definition of having courage. *Nursing Science Quarterly, 13*(2), 143-149.

Bournes, D.A. & Das Gupta, T.L. (1997). Professional practice leader: A transformational role that addresses human diversity. *Nursing Administration Quarterly, 21*(4), 61-68.

Bournes, D.A. & Linscott, J. (1998). Patient-focused care: A process of discovery. *Theoria, 7*(4), 3-5.

Butler, M.J. (1988). Family transformation: Parse's theory in practice. *Nursing Science Quarterly, 1*(2), 68-74.

Butler, M.J. & Snodgrass, F.G. (1991). Beyond abuse: Parse's theory in practice. *Nursing Science Quarterly, 4*(2), 76-82.

Bunkers, S.S. (1998). A nursing theory-guided model of health ministry: Human becoming in parish nursing. *Nursing Science Quarterly,* 11(1), 7-8.

Bunkers, S.S. (1998). Considering tomorrow: Parse's theory-guided research. *Nursing Science Quarterly,* 11(2), 56-63.

Bunkers, S.S. (1999). Commentary on Parse's view of community. *Nursing Science Quarterly,* 12(2), 121-124.

Bunkers, S.S. (1999). Emerging discoveries and possibilities in nursing. *Nursing Science Quarterly,* 12(1), 26-29.

Bunkers, S.S. (1999). Learning to be still. *Nursing Science Quarterly,* 12, 172-173.

Bunkers, S.S. (1999). The lived experience of hope for those working with homeless persons. In R.R. Parse (Ed.), *Hope: An international human becoming perspective* (pp. 227-250). Sudbury, MS: Jones and Bartlett.

Bunkers, S.S. (1999). The meaning of new age: The judging and misjudging of values and beliefs. *Nursing Science Quarterly,* 12(2), 100-105.

Bunkers, S.S. (1999). The teaching-learning process and the theory of human becoming. *Nursing Science Quarterly,* 12(3), 227-232.

Bunkers, S.S. (1999). Translating nursing conceptual frameworks and theory for nursing practice. In A. Solari-Twadell & M.A. McDermott (Eds.), *Parish nursing: Promoting whole person health within faith communities* (pp. 205-214). Thousand Oaks, CA: Sage.

Bunkers, S.S. & Daly, J. (1999). The lived experience of hope for Australian families living with coronary disease. In R.R. Parse (Ed.), *Hope: An international human becoming perspective* (pp. 45-61). Sudbury, MS: Jones and Bartlett.

Bunkers, S.S., Michaels, C., & Ethridge, P. (1997). Advanced practice nursing in community: Nursing's opportunity. *Advanced Practice Nursing Quarterly,* 2(4), 79-84.

Carson, M.G. & Mitchell, G.J. (1998). The experience of living with persistent pain. *Journal of Advanced Nursing,* 28(6), 1242-1248.

Cody, W.K. (1991). Grieving a personal loss. *Nursing Science Quarterly,* 4, 61-68.

Cody, W.K. (1991). Multidimensionality: Its meaning and significance. *Nursing Science Quarterly,* 4, 140-141.

Cody, W.K. (1995). Of life immense in passion, pulse, and power: Dialoguing with Whitman and Parse. A hermeneutic study. In R.R. Parse (Ed.), *Illuminations: The human becoming theory in practice and research* (pp. 269-307). New York: National League for Nursing Press.

Cody, W.K. (1995). The lived experience of grieving for families living with AIDS: Family-centered research using Parse's method. In R.R. Parse (Ed.), *Illuminations: The human becoming theory in practice and research* (pp. 197-242). New York: National League for Nursing Press.

Cody, W.K. (1995). The meaning of grieving for families living with AIDS. *Nursing Science Quarterly,* 8(3), 104-114.

Cody, W.K. (1995). The view of the family within the human becoming theory. In R.R. Parse (Ed.), *Illuminations: The human becoming theory in practice and research* (pp. 9-26). New York: National League for Nursing Press.

Cody, W.K. (1995). True presence with families living with HIV disease. In R.R. Parse (Ed.), *Illuminations: The human becoming theory in practice and research* (pp. 115-133). New York: National League for Nursing Press.

Cody, W.K. (1996). Drowning in eclecticism. *Nursing Science Quarterly,* 9, 86-88.

Cody, W.K. (1996). Occult reductionism in the discourse of theory development. *Nursing Science Quarterly,* 9(4), 140-142.

Cody, W.K. & Filler, J.E. (1999). The lived experience of hope for women residing in a shelter. In R.R. Parse (Ed.), *Hope: An international human becoming perspective* (pp. 211-225). Sudbury, MS: Jones and Bartlett.

Cody, W.K., Hudepohl, J.H., & Brinkman, K.S. (1995). True presence with a child and his family. In R.R. Parse (Ed.), *Illuminations: The human becoming theory in practice and research* (pp. 135-146). New York: National League for Nursing Press.

Cody, W.K. & Mitchell, G.J. (1992). Parse's theory as a model for practice: The cutting edge. *Advances in Nursing Science,* 15(2), 52-65.

Costello-Nickitas, D.M. (1994). Choosing life goals: A phenomenological study. *Nursing Science Quarterly,* 7(2), 87-92.

Daly, J. (1995). The lived experience of suffering. In R.R. Parse (Ed.), *Illuminations: The human becoming theory in practice and research* (pp. 253-268). New York: National League for Nursing Press.

Daly, J. (1995). The view of suffering within the human becoming theory. In R.R. Parse (Ed.), *Illuminations: The human becoming theory in practice and research* (pp. 45-59). New York: National League for Nursing Press.

Daly, J., Mitchell, G.J., & Jonas-Simpson, C.M. (1996). Quality of life and the human becoming theory: Exploring discipline-specific contributions. *Nursing Science Quarterly,* 9(4), 170-174.

Daly, J. & Watson, J. (1996). Parse's human becoming theory of nursing. In J. Greenwood (Ed.), *Nursing theory in Australia: Development and application* (pp. 177-200). Pymble, NSW, Australia: Harper Educational Publishers.

Damgaard, G. & Bunkers, S.S. (1998). Nursing science-guided practice and education: A state board of nursing perspective. *Nursing Science Quarterly,* 11(4), 142-144.

Davis, C. & Cannava, E. (1995). The meaning of retirement for communally-living retired performing artists. *Nursing Science Quarterly,* 8(1), 8-16.

Fisher, M.A. & Mitchell, G.J. (1998). Patients' views of quality of life: Transforming the knowledge base of nursing. *Clinical Nurse Specialist,* 12(3), 99-105.

Futrell, M., Wondolowski, C., & Mitchell, G.J. (1994). Aging in the oldest old living in Scotland: A phenomenological study. *Nursing Science Quarterly,* 6(4), 189-194.

Gates, K.M. (2000). The experience of caring for a loved one: A phenomenological study. *Nursing Science Quarterly,* 13(1), 54-59.

Hamalis, P. (1999). Reaching out. *Nursing Science Quarterly,* 12(4), 346.

Heine, C. (1991). Development of gerontological nursing theory: Applying man-living-health theory of nursing. *Nursing and Health Care,* 12, 184-188.

International Consortium of Parse Scholars. (1999). A nursing position on global healthcare: Our commitment to humankind. *Nursing Science Quarterly,* 12(4), 347.

Jacono, B.J. & Jacono, J.J. (1996). The benefits of Newman and Parse in helping nurse teachers determine methods to enhance student creativity. *Nursing Education Today,* 16, 356-362.

Janes, N.M. & Wells, D.L. (1997). Elderly patients' experiences with nurses guided by Parse's theory of human becoming. *Clinical Nursing Research,* 6, 205-224.

Jonas, C.M. (1995). Evaluation of the human becoming theory in family practice. In R.R. Parse (Ed.), *Illuminations: The human becoming theory in practice and research* (pp. 347-366). New York: National League for Nursing Press.

Jonas, C.M. (1992). The meaning of being an elder in Nepal. *Nursing Science Quarterly,* 5(4), 171-175.

Jonas, C.M. (1995). True presence through music for persons living their dying. In R.R. Parse (Ed.), *Illuminations: The human becoming theory in practice* (pp. 97-104). New York: National League for Nursing Press.

Jonas-Simpson, C.M. (1996). The patient focused care journey: Where patients and families guide the way. *Nursing Science Quarterly,* 9(4), 145-146.

Jonas-Simpson, C. (1997). Living the art of the human becoming theory. *Nursing Science Quarterly,* 10(4), 175-179.

Jonas-Simpson, C.M. (1997). The Parse research method through music. *Nursing Science Quarterly,* 10(3), 112-114.

Kelley, L.S. (1991). Struggling with going along when you do not believe. *Nursing Science Quarterly,* 4(3), 123-129.

Kelley, L.S. (1995). Parse's theory in practice with a group in the community. *Nursing Science Quarterly,* 8(3), 127-132.

Kelley, L.S. (1995). The house-garden-wilderness metaphor: Caring frameworks and the human becoming theory. In R.R. Parse (Ed.), *Illuminations: The human becoming theory in practice and research* (pp. 61-76). New York: National League for Nursing Press.

Kelley, L.S. (1999). Evaluating change in quality of life from the perspective of the person: Advanced practice nursing and Parse's goal of nursing. *Holistic Nursing Practice,* 13(4), 61-70.

Kelley, L.S. (1999). Hope as lived by native Americans. In R.R. Parse (Ed.), *Hope: An international human becoming perspective* (pp. 251-272). Sudbury, MS: Jones and Bartlett.

Kim, M.S., Shin, K.R., & Shin, S.R. (1998). Korean adolescents' experiences of smoking cessation: A prelude to research with the human becoming perspective. *Nursing Science Quarterly,* 11(3), 105-109.

Kruse, B.G. (1999). The lived experience of serenity: Using Parse's research method. *Nursing Science Quarterly,* 12(2), 143-150.

Lee, O.J. & Pilkington, F.B. (1999). Practice with persons living their dying: A human becoming perspective. *Nursing Science Quarterly,* 12(4), 324-328.

Legault, F. & Ferguson-Paré, M. (1999). Advancing nursing practice: An evaluation study of Parse's theory of human becoming. *Canadian Journal of Nursing Leadership,* 12(1), 30-35.

Liehr, P.R. (1989). The core of true presence: A loving center. *Nursing Science Quarterly,* 2(1), 7-8.

Linscott, J., Spee, R., Flint, F., & Fisher, A. (1999). Creating a culture of patient-focused care through a learner-centered philosophy. *Canadian Journal of Nursing Leadership,* 12(4), 5-10.

Liu, S.L. (1994). The lived experience of health for hospitalized older women in Taiwan. *Journal of National Taipei College of Nursing,* 1, 1-84.

Markovic, M. (1997). From theory to perioperative practice with Parse. *Canadian Operating Room Nursing Journal,* 15(1), 13-16.

Mattice, M. (1991). Parse's theory of nursing in practice: A manager's perspective. *Canadian Journal of Nursing Administration,* 4(1), 11-13.

Mattice, M. & Mitchell, G.J. (1990). Caring for confused elders. *The Canadian Nurse,* 86(11), 16-18.

Milton, C.L. (2000). Befeficience: Honoring the commitment. *Nursing Science Quarterly,* 13(2), 111-115.

Mitchell, G.J. (1986). Utilizing Parse's theory of man-living-health in Mrs. M's neighborhood. *Perspectives,* 10(4), 5-7.

Mitchell, G.J. (1988). Man-living-health: The theory in practice. *Nursing Science Quarterly,* 1(3), 120-127.

Mitchell, G.J. (1990). Struggling in change: From the traditional approach to Parse's theory-based practice. *Nursing Science Quarterly,* 3(4), 170-176.

Mitchell, G.J. (1990). The lived experience of taking life day-by-day in later life: Research guided by Parse's emergent method. *Nursing Science Quarterly,* 3(1), 29-36.

Mitchell, G.J. (1991). Diagnosis: Clarifying or obscuring the nature of nursing. *Nursing Science Quarterly,* 4(2), 52-53.

Mitchell, G.J. (1991). Distinguishing practice with Parse's theory. In I.E. Goertzen (Ed.), *Differentiating nursing practice into the twenty-first century* (pp. 55-58). New York: American Nurses Association Publication.

Mitchell, G.J. (1991). Human subjectivity: The cocreation of self. *Nursing Science Quarterly,* 4(3), 144-145.

Mitchell, G.J. (1991). Nursing diagnosis: An ethical analysis. *Image: Journal of Nursing Scholarship,* 23(2), 99-103.

Mitchell, G.J. (1992). Parse's theory and the multidisciplinary team: Clarifying scientific values. *Nursing Science Quarterly,* 5(3), 104-106.

Mitchell, G.J. (1993). Living paradox in Parse's theory. *Nursing Science Quarterly,* 6(1), 44-51.

Mitchell, G.J. (1993). Parse's theory in practice. In M.E. Parker (Ed.), *Patterns of nursing theories in practice* (pp. 62-80). New York: National League for Nursing Press.

Mitchell, G.J. (1993). The same-thing-yet-different phenomenon: A way of coming to know—or not? *Nursing Science Quarterly,* 6(2), 61-62.

Mitchell, G.J. (1993). Time and a waning moon: Seniors describe the meaning to later life. *The Canadian Journal of Nursing Research,* 25(1), 51-66.

Mitchell, G.J. (1994). The meaning of being a senior: A phenomenological study and interpretation with Parse's theory of nursing. *Nursing Science Quarterly,* 7, 70-79.

Mitchell, G.J. (1995). Evaluation of the human becoming theory in practice in an acute care setting. In R.R. Parse (Ed.), *Illuminations: The human becoming theory in practice and research* (pp. 367-399). New York: National League for Nursing Press.

Mitchell, G.J. (1995). The lived experience of restriction-freedom in later life. In R.R. Parse (Ed.), *Illuminations: The human becoming theory in practice and research* (pp. 159-195). New York: National League for Nursing Press.

Mitchell, G.J. (1995). The view of freedom within the human becoming theory. In R.R. Parse (Ed.), *Illumination: The human becoming theory in practice and research* (pp. 27-43). New York: National League for Nursing Press.

Mitchell, G.J. (1996). Clarifying contributions of qualitative research findings. *Nursing Science Quarterly,* 9(4), 143-144.

Mitchell, G.J. (1996). Pretending: A way to get through the day. *Nursing Science Quarterly,* 9(2), 92-93.

Mitchell, G.J. (1997). Retrospective and prospective of practice applications: Views in the fog. *Nursing Science Quarterly,* 10(1), 8-9.

Mitchell, G.J. (1998). Living with diabetes: How understanding expands theory for professional practice. *Canadian Journal of Diabetes Care,* 22(1), 30-37.

Mitchell, G.J., Bernardo, A., & Bournes, D. (1997). Nursing guided by Parse's theory: Patient views at Sunnybrook. *Nursing Science Quarterly,* 10(1), 55-56.

Mitchell, G.J. & Cody, W.K. (1999). Human becoming theory: A complement to medical science. *Nursing Science Quarterly,* 12(4), 304-310.

Mitchell, G.J. & Cody, W.K. (1992). Nursing knowledge and human science: Ontological and epistemological considerations. *Nursing Science Quarterly,* 5(2), 54-61.

Mitchell, G.J. & Copplestone, C. (1990). Applying Parse's theory to perioperative nursing: A nontraditional approach. *AORN Journal,* 51(3), 787-798.

Mitchell, G. J. & Heidt, P. (1994). The lived experience of wanting to help another. *Nursing Science Quarterly,* 7(3), 119-127.

Mitchell, G.J. & Lawton, C. (2000). Living with the consequences of personal choices for person with diabetes: Implications for educators and practitioners. *Canadian Journal of Diabetes Care,* 24(2), 23-31.

Mitchell, G.J. & Pilkington, F.B. (1990). Theoretical approaches in nursing practice: A comparison of Roy and Parse. *Nursing Science Quarterly,* 3(2), 81-87.

Mitchell, G.J. & Pilkington, F.B. (2000). Comfort-discomfort with ambiguity: Flight and freedom in nursing practice. *Nursing Science Quarterly,* 13(1), 31-36.

Mitchell, G.J. & Santopinto, M.D.A. (1988). An alternative to nursing diagnosis. *The Canadian Nurse,* 84(10), 25-28.

Mitchell, G.J. & Santopinto, M.D.A. (1988). The expanded role nurse: A dissenting viewpoint. *Canadian Journal of Nursing Administration,* 4(1), 8-14.

Nokes, K.M. & Carver, K. (1991). The meaning of living with AIDS: A study using Parse's theory of man- living-health. *Nursing Science Quarterly,* 4(4), 175-179.

Northrup, D.T. & Cody, W.K. (1998). Evaluation of the human becoming theory in practice in an acute care psychiatric setting. *Nursing Science Quarterly,* 11(1), 23-30.

Pickrell, K.D., Lee, R.E., Schumacher, L.P., & Twigg, P. (1998). Rosemarie Rizzo Parse: Human becoming. In A. Marriner Tomey & M.R. Alligood (Eds.). *Nursing theorists and their work* (4th ed.). St. Louis: Mosby.

Pilkington, F.B. (1993). The lived experience of grieving the loss of an important other. *Nursing Science Quarterly,* 6(3), 130-139.

Pilkington, F.B. (1999). An ethical framework for nursing practice: Parse's human becoming theory. *Nursing Science Quarterly,* 12(1), 21-25.

Pilkington, F.B. (1999). A qualitative study of life after stroke. *Journal of Neuroscience Nursing,* 31(6), 336-347.

Pilkington, F.B. (2000). A unitary view of persistence-change. *Nursing Science Quarterly,* 13(1), 5-11.

Pilkington, F.B. & Millar, B. (1999). The lived experience of hope with persons from Wales, UK. In R.R. Parse (Ed.), *Hope: An international human becoming perspective* (pp. 163-189). Sudbury, MS: Jones and Bartlett.

Quiquero, A., Knights, D., & Meo, C.O. (1991). Theory as a guide to practice: Staff nurses choose Parse's theory. *Canadian Journal of Nursing Administration,* 4(1), 14-16.

Rasmusson, D.L. (1995). True presence with homeless persons. In R.R. Parse (Ed.), *Illuminations: The human becoming theory in practice and research* (pp. 105-113). New York: National League for Nursing Press.

Rasmusson, D.L., Jonas, C.M., & Mitchell, G.J. (1991). The eye of the beholder: Applying Parse's theory with homeless individuals. *Clinical Nurse Specialist Journal,* 5(3), 139-143.

Rendon, D.C., Sales, R., Leal, I., & Pique, J. (1995). The lived experience of aging in community-dwelling elders in Valencia, Spain: A phenomenological study. *Nursing Science Quarterly,* 8(4), 152-157.

Saltmarche, A., Kolodny, V., & Mitchell, G.J. (1998). An educational approach for patient-focused care: Shifting attitudes and practice. *Journal of Nursing Staff Development,* 14(2), 81-86.

Santopinto, M.D.A. (1989). The relentless drive to be ever thinner: A study using the phenomenological method. *Nursing Science Quarterly,* 2(1), 29-36.

Santopinto, M.D.A. & Smith, M.C. (1995). Evaluation of the human becoming theory in practice with adults and children. In R.R. Parse (Ed.), *Illuminations: The human becoming theory in practice and research* (pp. 309-346). New York: National League for Nursing Press.

Smith, M.C. (1990). Struggling through a difficult time for unemployed persons. *Nursing Science Quarterly,* 3(1), 18-28.

Smith, M.J. (1989). Research and practice application related to man-living-health. In J. Riehl-Sisca (Ed.), *Conceptual models for nursing practice* (3rd ed., pp. 267-276). Norwalk, CT: Appleton & Lange.

Spenceley, S.M. (1995). The CNS in multidisciplinary pulmonary rehabilitation: A nursing science perspective. *Clinical Nurse Specialist,* 9, 192-198.

Takahashi, T. (1999). Kibou: Hope for persons in Japan. In R.R. Parse (Ed.), *Hope: An international human becoming perspective* (pp. 115-128). Sudbury, MS: Jones and Bartlett.

Toikkanen, T. & Muurinen, E. (1999). Toivo: Hope for persons in Finland. In R.R. Parse (Ed.), *Hope: An international human becoming perspective* (pp. 79-96). Sudbury, MS: Jones and Bartlett.

Vander Woude, D. (1998). Nursing theory-based regulatory decisioning model in South Dakota. *Issues,* 19(3), 14.

Walker, C.A. (1996). Coalescing the theories of two nurse visionaries: Parse and Watson. *Journal of Advanced Nursing,* 24, 988-996.

Wang, C-E.H. (1999). He-Bung: Hope for persons living with leprosy in Taiwan. In R.R. Parse (Ed.), *Hope: An international human becoming perspective* (pp. 45-61). Sudbury, MS: Jones and Bartlett.

Wang, C.H. (1997). Quality of life and health for persons living with leprosy. *Nursing Science Quarterly,* 10(3), 144-145.

Williamson, G.J. (2000). The test of a nursing theory: A personal view. *Nursing Science Quarterly,* 13(2), 124-128.

Willman, A. (1999). Hopp: The lived experience for Swedish elders. In R.R. Parse (Ed.), *Hope: An international human becoming perspective* (pp. 129-142). Sudbury, MS: Jones and Bartlett.

Wimpenny, P. (1993). The paradox of Parse's theory. *Senior Nurse,* 13(5), 10-13.

Wing, D.M. (1999). The aesthetics of caring: Where folk healers and nurse theorists converge. *Nursing Science Quarterly,* 12(13), 256-262.

Wondolowski, C. & Davis, D.K. (1988). The lived experience of aging in the oldest old: A phenomenological study. *The American Journal of Psychoanalysis,* 48, 261-270.

Wondolowski, C. & Davis, D.K. (1991). The lived experience of health in the oldest old: A phenomenological study. *Nursing Science Quarterly,* 4(3), 113-118.

Zanotti, R. & Bournes, D.A. (1999). Speranza: A study of the lived experience of hope with persons from Italy. In R.R. Parse (Ed.), *Hope: An international human becoming perspective* (pp. 97-114). Sudbury, MS: Jones and Bartlett.

Books and Articles Mentioning Parse's Theory

Abelsohn, J. (1999). Music as healer. *Registered Nurse Journal,* 11(4), 7-8.

Allen, M.N., Hayne, Y., Hodgins, M.J., Kikuchi, J., Letourneau, N.L., McQueen, M., Myrick, F., Romyn, D.M., Simmons, H., Blissitt, P.A., & Cody, W.K. (1998). Is eclecticism a threat to the discipline of nursing? Commentary and response. *Nursing Science Quarterly,* 11(3), 99-104.

Barrett, E.A.M. (1998). Unique nursing methods: The diversity chant of pioneers. *Nursing Science Quarterly,* 11(3), 94-96.

Baumann, S.L. (1998). Nursing: The missing ingredient in nurse practitioner education. *Nursing Science Quarterly,* 11, 89-90.

Baumann, S.L. (1999). Art as a path of inquiry. *Nursing Science Quarterly,* 12(2), 106-110.

Bernat, S.H. (1993). *Contraceptive decision-making: A phenomenological approach.* Unpublished doctoral Dissertation, State University of New York at Buffalo.

Bowers, R. & Moore, K.N. (1997). Bakhtin. Nursing narratives, and dialogical consciousness. *Advances in Nursing Science,* 19(3), 70-77.

Bunkers, S.S. (1995). Stories. The tour. *Nursing Forum,* 30(3), 33-35.

Bunkers, S.S. (1999). A frigid climate. *Nursing Science Quarterly,* 12(1), 83-84.

Bunkers, S.S. (2000). The nurse scholar of the 21st century. *Nursing Science Quarterly,* 13, 116-123.

Bunkers, S.S. & Mitchell, G.J. (1997). Weaver women. *Nursing Science Quarterly,* 10(3), 146-148.

Chapman, J.S., Mitchell, G.J., & Forchuk, C. (1994). A glimpse of nursing theory-based practice in Canada. *Nursing Science Quarterly,* 7(3), 104-112.

Chinn, P.L. & Jacobs, M.K. (1987). *Theory and nursing: A systematic approach* (2nd ed.). St. Louis: Mosby.

Cody, W.K. (1993). Norms and nursing science: A question of values. *Nursing Science Quarterly,* 6(3), 110-112.

Cody, W.K. (1994). Meaning and mystery in nursing science and art. *Nursing Science Quarterly,* 7(2), 48-51.

Cody, W.K. (1994). Nursing theory-guided practice: What it is and what it is not. *Nursing Science Quarterly,* 7(4), 144-145.

Cody, W.K. (1994). Radical health care reform: The person as case manager. *Nursing Science Quarterly,* 7(4), 180-182.

Cody, W.K. (1995). All those paradigms: Many in the universe, two in nursing. *Nursing Science Quarterly,* 8(4), 144-147.

Cody, W.K. (1997). The many faces of change: Discomfort with the new. *Nursing Science Quarterly,* 10(2), 65-67.

Cody, W.K. (1998). Critical theory and nursing science: Freedom in theory and practice. *Nursing Science Quarterly,* 11(2), 44-46.

Cody, W.K. (1999). Affirming reflection. *Nursing Science Quarterly,* 12(1), 4-6.

Cody, W.K. (1999). Middle-range theories: Do they foster the development of nursing science? *Nursing Science Quarterly,* 12(1), 9-14.

Cody, W.K. (2000). Paradigm shift or paradigm drift? A meditation on commitment and transcendence. *Nursing Science Quarterly,* 13(2), 93-102.

Cody, W.K. (2000). The challenge of unitary conceptualizations: An exemplar. *Nursing Science Quarterly,* 13(1), 4.

Daiski, I. (1996). Staff nurses' perspectives of hospital power structures. *The Canadian Nurse,* 92, 26-30.

Daiski, I. (2000). The road to professionalism in nursing: Case management or practice based in nursing theory? *Nursing Science Quarterly,* 13(1), 74-79.

Daly, J. & Jackson, D. (1999). On the use of nursing theory in nursing education, nursing practice, and nursing research in Australia. *Nursing Science Quarterly,* 12(4), 342-345.

Edwards, S.D. (1999). The idea of nursing science. *Journal of Advanced Nursing,* 29, 563-569.

Elwood, K.H. & Lewson. B. (1999). Art therapy and audiology: Joining hands to hear the story of a resident in long term care. *Perspectives,* 23(4), 18-23.

Fawcett, J. (1993). *Analysis and evaluation of nursing theories.* Philadelphia: Davis.

Fite, S., Frank, D.I., & Curtin, J. (1996). The relationship of social support to women's obtaining mammography screening. *Journal of the American Academy of Nurse Practitioners,* 8, 565-569.

Fitzpatrick, J.J. & Whall, A.L. (1989). *Conceptual models of nursing: Analysis and application* (2nd ed.). Norwalk, CT: Appleton & Lange.

Fraser, C. (1999). The experience of transition for a daughter caregiver of a stroke survivor. *Journal of Neuroscience Nursing,* 31(1), 9-16.

Freshwater, D. (1998). From acorn to oak tree: A neoplatonic perspective of reflection and caring. *Australian Journal of Holistic Nursing,* 5(2), 14-19.

Gilje, F.L. (1993). *A phenomenological study of patients' experiences of the nurse's presence.* Unpublished doctoral dissertation, University of Colorado Health Sciences Center.

George, J. (1990). *Nursing theories: The base for professional nursing practice* (3rd ed.). New York: Prentice Hall.

Heise, J.L. (1993). The valuing process: A vehicle for creating reality. *Journal of Holistic Nursing,* 11(1), 56-63.

Henderson, E. & Duggleby, W. (1995). Dr. Gail Mitchell: An interview. *AARN Newsletter,* 51(11), 12-13.

Hodnicki, D.R., Horner, S.D., & Simmons, S.J. (1993). The sea of life: A metaphorical vehicle for theory explication. *Nursing Science Quarterly,* 6(1), 25-27.

Huch, M.H. (1999). International perspectives: Welcome and introduction. *Nursing Science Quarterly,* 12(1), 80-83.

Kieffel, D. (1991). Rethinking the environment as a domain of nursing knowledge. *Advances in Nursing Science,* 14(1), 40-51.

Koithan, M.Z. (1994). *The dance of human becoming: A philosophic inquiry into health promotion and healing within the unitary-transformative paradigm.* Unpublished doctoral dissertation, University of Colorado Health Sciences Center.

Langford, D.R. & Hardin, S. (1999). Distance learning: Issues emerging as the paradigm shifts. *Nursing Science Quarterly,* 12(3), 191-196.

Marriner Tomey, A. (1989). *Nursing theorists and their work* (2nd ed.). St. Louis: Mosby.

Martin, M.L., Forchuk, C., Santopinto, M., & Butcher, H.K. (1992). Alternative approaches to nursing practice: Application of Peplau, Rogers, and Parse. *Nursing Science Quarterly,* 5(2), 80-85.

Martsolf, D.S. & Mickley, J.R. (1998). The concept of spirituality in nursing theories: Differing world-views and extent of focus. *Journal of Advanced Nursing,* 27(2), 294-303.

McMahon, S. (1991). The quest for synthesis: Human-companion animal relationships and nursing theories. *Holistic Nursing Practice,* 5(2), 1-5.

Meleis, A.I. (1985). *Theoretical nursing: Development and progress.* Philadelphia: Lippincott.

Miklaucich, M. (1998). Limitations on life: Women's lived experiences of angina. *Journal of Advanced Nursing,* 28, 1207-1215.

Milton, C.L. (1999). Ethical codes and principles: The link to nursing theory. *Nursing Science Quarterly,* 12(4), 290-291.

Minicucci, D.S. (1998). A review and synthesis of the literature: The use of presence in the nursing care of families. *Journal of the New York State Nurses Association,* 29(3/4), 9-15.

Mitchell, G.J. (1991). Nursing diagnosis: An ethical analysis. *Image: Journal of Nursing Scholarship,* 23, 99-103.

Mitchell, G.J. (1992). Specifying the knowledge base of theory in practice. *Nursing Science Quarterly,* 5(1), 6-7.

Mitchell, G.J. (1994). Discipline-specific inquiry: The hermeneutics of theory-guided nursing research. *Nursing Outlook,* 42(5), 224-228.

Mitchell, G.J. (1994). The dignity of risk and the right to failure: One profile of patient-focused care. *Perspectives,* 18(3), 10.

Mitchell, G.J. (1997). Have the disciplines fallen? *Nursing Science Quarterly,* 10(3), 110-111.

Mitchell, G.J. (1997). Reengineered healthcare: Why nurses matter. *Nursing Science Quarterly,* 10(2), 70-71.

Mitchell, G.J. (1997). Theory and practice in long term care: The acorn doesn't fall far from the tree. *Long Term Care,* 7(4), 31-34.

Mitchell, G.J. (1998). Standards of nursing and the winds of change. *Nursing Science Quarterly,* 11(3), 97-98.

Mitchell, G.J. (1998). The colour of nursing practice. *Hospital News: Canada's Health Care Newspaper,* 11(6), 12.

Mitchell, G.J. (1999). Evidence-based practice: Critique and alternative view. *Nursing Science Quarterly,* 12(1), 30-35.

Mitchell, G.J. & Cody, W.K. (1993). The role of theory in qualitative research. *Nursing Science Quarterly,* 6(4), 170-178.

Mitchell, G.J. & Pilkington, F.B. (1999). A dialogue on the comparability of research paradigms—and other theoretical things. *Nursing Science Quarterly,* 12(4), 283-289.

Mitchell, G.J. & Santopinto, M.D. (1988). The expanded role nurse: A dissenting viewpoint. *Canadian Journal of Nursing Administration,* 4(1), 8-14.

Nagle, L., Mitchell, G.J., Koziol-McLain, J., & Maeve, M.K. (1994). Nursing theory in perspective. *Nursing Outlook,* 42(3), 141-142.

Nagle, L.M. & Mitchell, G.J. (1991). Theoretic diversity: Evolving paradigmatic issues in research and practice. *Advances in Nursing Science,* 14, 17-25.

Newman, M.A., Sime, A.M., & Corcoran-Perry, S.A. (1991). The focus of the discipline of nursing. *Advances in Nursing Science,* 14, 1-6.

Plank, D.M.P. (1994). Framing treatment options: A method to enhance informed consent. . .addressing treatment options that are important to the client. *Clinical Nurse Specialist,* 8(4), 174-178.

Profile: Rosemarie Rizzo Parse. (1991). *The Japanese Journal of Nursing,* 55(8), 744.

Randell, B.P. (1992). Nursing theory: The 21st century. *Nursing Science Quarterly,* 5(4), 176-185.

Relf, M.V. (1997). Illuminating meaning and transforming issues of spirituality in HIV disease and AIDS: An application of Parse's theory of human becoming. *Holistic Nursing Practice,* 12(1), 1-8.

Ross, J.R.L. (1997). A paradigm shift: What a difference a day makes. *Perspectives,* 21, 4 2-6.

Spee, R., Watson, C., & Krock, M. (1998). Integrating RAI into patient focused care planning. *Canadian Journal of Quality in Health Care,* 14(4), 10-14.

Takahashi, T. (1992). Perspectives on nursing knowledge. *Nursing Science Quarterly,* 5(2), 86-91.

Thorne, S.E. (1999). Are egalitarian relationships a desirable ideal in nursing? *Western Journal of Nursing Research,* 21(1), 16-34.

Wall, L.M. (1999). Exercise: A unitary concept. *Nursing Science Quarterly,* 12(1), 68-72.

Book Chapters and Articles by Others Critiquing Parse's Theory

Cowling, W.R. (1989). Parse's theory of nursing. In J.J. Fitzpatrick & A.L. Whall (Eds.), *Conceptual models of nursing: Analysis and application* (2nd ed., pp. 385-399). Norwalk, CT: Appleton & Lange.

Hickman, J.S. (1990). Rosemarie Rizzo Parse. In J.B. George (Ed.), *Nursing theories: The base for professional nursing practice* (3rd ed., pp. 311-332). Norwalk, CT: Appleton & Lange.

Lee, R.E. & Schumacher, L.P. (1989). Rosemarie Rizzo Parse: Man-living-health. In A. Marriner Tomey (Ed.), *Nurse theorists and their work* (2nd ed., pp. 174-186). St. Louis: Mosby.

Phillips, J. (1987). A critique of Parse's man-living-health theory. In R.R. Parse (Ed.), *Nursing science: Major paradigms, theories, and critiques* (pp. 181-204). Philadelphia: W.B. Saunders.

Pugliese, L. (1989). The theory of man-living-health: An analysis. In J. Riehl-Sisca (Ed.), *Conceptual models for nursing practice* (3rd ed., pp. 259-265). Norwalk, CT: Appleton & Lange.

Smith, M.C. & Hudepohl, J.H. (1988). Analysis and evaluation of Parse's theory of man-living-health. *The Canadian Journal of Nursing Research: Nursing Papers,* 20(4), 43-58.

Winkler, S.J. (1983). Parse's theory of nursing. In J.J. Fitzpatrick & A.L. Whall (Eds.), *Conceptual models of nursing: Analysis and application* (pp. 275-294). Bowie, MD: Brady.

Authors Citing Parse's Works

Batra, C. (1987). Nursing theory for undergraduates. *Nursing Outlook,* 35(4), 189-192.

Boyd, C.O. (1989). Dialogue on a research issue: Phenomenological research in nursing- response. *Nursing Science Quarterly,* 2(1), 16-19.

Boyd, C.O. (1990). Critical appraisal of developing nursing research methods. *Nursing Science Quarterly,* 3(1), 42-43.

Bunkers, S.S. (1996). Storyteller and the tall man. *Nursing Science Quarterly,* 9(1), 42-43.

Bunkers, S.S. (1998). Considering tomorrow: Parse's theory guides research. *Nursing Science Quarterly,* 11(2), 56-63.

Bunkers, S.S., Petardi, L.A., Pilkington, F.B., & Walls, P.A. (1996). Challenging the myths surrounding qualitative research in practice. *Nursing Science Quarterly,* 9(1), 33-37.

Campbell, J. (1986). A survivor group for battered women. *Advances in Nursing Science,* 8(2), 13-20.

Cohen, M.Z. (1987). A historical overview of the phenomenological movement. *Image: Journal of Nursing Scholarship,* 19(1), 31-34.

Counts, M.M. & Boyle, J.S. (1987). Nursing, health, and policy within a community context. *Advances in Nursing Science,* 9(3), 12-23.

Cull-Wiliby, B.L. & Pepin, J.I. (1987). Toward a co-existence of paradigms in nursing knowledge development. *Journal of Advanced Nursing,* 12(4), 515-521.

DeFeo, D.J. (1990). Change: A central concern in nursing. *Nursing Science Quarterly,* 3(2), 88-94.

Drew, N. & Dahlberg, K. (1995). Challenging a reductionistic paradigm as a foundation for nursing. *Journal of Holistic Nursing,* 13(4), 332-345.

Duffy, M.E. (1986). Qualitative research: An approach whose time has come. *Nursing and Health Care,* 7(5), 237-239.

Duldt, B.W. (1995). Integrating nursing theory and ethics. *Perspectives in Psychiatric Care,* 31(2), 4-10.

Gortner, S.R. & Schultz, P.R. (1988). Approaches to nursing science methods. *Image: Journal of Nursing Scholarship,* 20(1), 22-24.

Haase, J.E. (1987). Components of courage in chronically ill adolescents: A phenomenological study. *Advances in Nursing Science,* 9(2), 64-80.

Huch, M.H. (1995). Nursing science as a basis for advanced practice. *Nursing Science Quarterly,* 8(1), 6-7.

Kidd, P. & Morrison, E.F. (1988). The progression of knowledge in nursing: A search for meaning. *Image: Journal of Nursing Scholarship,* 20(4), 222-224.

Kohl, T. (1995). Interpretative approaches in nursing research: The influence of Husserl and Heidegger. *Journal of Advanced Nursing,* 21(5), 827-836.

Malinski, V.M. (1990). Three perspectives on a scholarly issue. *Nursing Science Quarterly,* 3(1), 49-50.

May, C. (1995). Patient autonomy and the politics of professional relationships. *Journal of Advanced Nursing,* 21(1), 83-87.

Mitchell, G.J. (1992) Is nursing pot-bound? *Nursing Science Quarterly,* 5(4), 152-153.

Mitchell, G.J. (1996). A reflective moment with false cheerfulness. *Nursing Science Quarterly,* 9, 53-54.

Moch, S.D. & Diemert, C.A. (1987). Health promotion within the nursing environment. *Nursing Administration Quarterly,* 11(3), 9-12.

Moody, L. (1990). *Advancing nursing science through research* (Vol. 1 & 2). Newbury Park, CA: Sage.

Page, N.E. & Arena, D.M. (1994). Rethinking the merger of the clinical nurse specialist and the nurse practitioner roles. *Image: Journal of Nursing Scholarship,* 26(4), 315-318.

Pearson, B.D. (1987). Pain control: An experiment with imagery. *Geriatric Nursing,* 8(1), 28-30.

Perry, J. (1985). Has the discipline of nursing developed to the stage where nurses do think nursing? *Journal of Advanced Nursing,* 10(1), 31-37.

Phillips, J.R. (1989). Qualitative research: A process of discovery. *Nursing Science Quarterly,* 2(1), 5-6.

Phillips, J.R. (1990). Guest editorial: New methods of research: Beyond the shadows of nursing science. *Nursing Science Quarterly,* 3(1), 1-2.

Ray, M.A. (1987). Technological caring: A new model in critical care. *Dimensions of Critical Care Nursing,* 6(3), 166-173.

Ray, M.A. (1990). Critical reflective analysis of Parse's and Newman's research methodologies. *Nursing Science Quarterly,* 3(1), 44-46.

Reed, P.G. (1986). Religiousness among terminally ill and healthy adults. *Research in Nursing and Health,* 9(1), 35-41.

Reed, P.G. (1987). Constructing a conceptual framework for psychosocial nursing. *Journal of Psychosocial Nursing and Mental Health Services,* 25(2), 24-28.

Ruffingrahal, M.A. (1985). Qualitative methods in community analysis. *Public Health Nursing,* 2, 130-137.

Sarter, B. (1987). Evolutionary idealism: A philosophical foundation for holistic nursing theory. *Advances in Nursing Science,* 9, 1-9.

Sarter, B. (1988). Philosophical sources of nursing theory. *Nursing Science Quarterly,* 1(2), 52-59.

Smith, M.C. (1990). Nursing's unique focus on health promotion. *Nursing Science Quarterly,* 3(3), 105-106.

Smith, M.C. (1990). Pattern in nursing practice. *Nursing Science Quarterly,* 3(2), 57-59.

Smith, M.J. (1984). Transformation: A key to shaping nursing. *Image: Journal of Nursing Scholarship,* 16(1), 28-30.

Thompson, J.L. (1985). Practical discourse in nursing: Going beyond empiricism and historocism. *Advances in Nursing Science,* 7(4), 59-71.

Uys, L.R. (1987). Foundational studies in nursing. *Journal of Advanced Nursing,* 12(3), 275-280.

Vander Woude, D.L. & Hutcherson, C. (1999). Health policy and regulatory decisioning based on nursing theory. *Nursing Science Quarterly,* 12(3), 209-213.

Watson, J. (1995). Advanced nursing practice . . . and what might be. *Nursing and Health Care: Perspectives on Community, 16*(2), 78-83.

Willman, A. (1996). *Health is living: A theoretical and empirical analysis of the concept of health with examples from geriatric care.* Unpublished doctoral dissertation. The University of Lund, Stockholm, Sweden.

Wilson, T.L. (1995). Applying critical social theory in nursing education to bridge the gap between theory, research and practice. *Journal of Advanced Nursing, 21*(3), 568-575.

Unpublished Manuscripts

Beauchamp, C.J. (1990). *The lived experience of struggling with making a decision in a critical life situation.* Paper presented at Discovery International, Inc., Nursing Science Seminar, Research and Practice Related to Parse's Theory of Nursing, Cincinnati, OH.

Bernardo, A. & Bournes, D.A. (1996, June). *Shifting patterns and purposes in nursing education.* Paper presented at the Practical Nurse Executive Interest Group Networking '96 Conference, Toronto, Canada.

Bournes, D.A. (1996, Nov.). *The human becoming theory and patient focused care.* Paper presented to graduate students at Loyola University Chicago, Chicago, Illinois.

Bournes, D.A. (1997, April). *Patient-focused care: The human becoming theory in practice.* Paper presented at the First International Nursing Theories Conference held April 10-12, 1997, in Nuremberg, Germany.

Bournes, D.A. (1997, June). *Caring and reflective practice: What it is and what it is not.* Panel discussion on Reflective Nursing Practice and Caring at the Caring and Reflective Practice Workshop, Kempenfelt Bay. Sponsored by Georgian College.

Bournes, D.A. (1998, May). *Nursing theory-based practice.* Presentation to a BScN Leadership Class, Loyola University Chicago.

Bournes, D.A. (1998, Sept.). *Remembering "nursing" in the development and implementation of professional practice models.* Presentation to the Professional Practice Model Task Force for Catholic Health Partners. Held at St. Joseph's Hospital, Chicago, Illinois.

Bournes, D.A. (1998, Nov.). *Human becoming in practice: A synthesis of what we know from the findings of six evaluation studies.* Participant in a panel discussion on the "so what" of the Human Becoming Research Methodologies. The Sixth Annual Qualitative Nursing Research Colloquium: The Human Becoming School of Thought. Loyola University Chicago, Chicago, Illinois.

Bournes, D.A. & Beitel-Wardrop, J. (1997, May). *Operationalizing the paradigm shift to patient focused care.* Paper presented at the 1st Annual Conference: Celebrate Nursing into the Next Millennium; Changing Boundaries: Creating Healing Environments, Expert Practice and New Visions for Care, Toronto, Canada, May 22-23, 1997.

Bournes, D.A. & Bernardo, A. (1996, May). *Implementing patient focused care: Our experiences so far.* Paper presented at a meeting of the Toronto Chapter of the International Consortium of Parse Scholars, Toronto, Canada.

Bournes, D.A. & Bernardo, A. (1996, Dec.). *Caring moments: Nursing's contribution to patient focused care.* Paper presented at Creative Connections: Human Caring in Action, Vaughan Estate, Toronto, Ontario. Conference sponsored by The Canadian Centers for Human Caring Consortium.

Bournes, D.A. & Bernardo, A. (1997, Feb.). *An introduction to patient focused care: The human becoming perspective.* Presentations to undergraduate students, Ryerson Polytechnical University, Toronto, Canada.

Bournes, D.A. & Bernardo, A. (1997, April). *Patient-focused care and shared governance: Shifting patterns and purposes in professional collaboration.* Presentation to staff and administrators at Staffordshire National Health Services Trust, Stafford, UK.

Bournes, D.A. & Bernardo, A. (1997, April). *Patient-focused care: The human becoming perspective.* Presentation/workshop for undergraduate and graduate students at the School of Nursing Studies, University of Wales College of Medicine, Cardiff, Wales.

Bournes, D.A. & Carroll, K. (1998, Nov.). *Bringing order to the whole.* Paper presented at the Parse Scholars Seminar Weekend, Niagara-on-the-Lake, Ontario, Canada.

Bournes, D.A. & Carroll, K. (1998, Nov.). *Human becoming: A blank canvas.* Paper presented at the Parse Scholars Seminar Weekend, Niagara-on-the-Lake, Ontario, Canada.

Bournes, D.A. & Das Gupta, T.L. (1997, June). *Professional practice leaders: Inspiring a shared vision for patient focused care.* Paper presented at International Council of Nurses 21st Quadrennial Congress, Vancouver, Canada, June 15-20, 1997.

Bournes, D.A. & Hollett, J. (1996, Nov.). *The human becoming theory and patient focused care.* Paper presented at the annual seminar weekend of the International Consortium of Parse Scholars at the Queen's Landing Inn, Niagara-on-the-Lake, Ontario.

Cody, W.K. (1990). *Parse's theory in practice with a grieving family.* Paper presented at Sigma Theta Tau, Alpha Phi Chapter, Annual Research Day, Hunter-Bellevue School of Nursing, City University of New York, NY.

Cody, W.K. (1991). *A hermeneutical reading of Whitman's Leaves of Grass in light of the theory of human becoming.* International Parse Interest Group First Annual Weekend Seminar, Killington, VT, Oct. 20, International.

Cody, W.K. (1992). *Grieving as becoming: Theory, research, and practice.* Paper presented at Nursing Research: Road to Excellence Annual Nursing Research Conference, Nashville, TN. Sponsored by Vanderbilt School of Nursing, Sigma Theta Tau, and Nashville Veterans Administration.

Cody, W.K. (1996). *Critique of Goudy's study "Feeling alone while with others."* The Fourth Annual International Qualitative Nursing Research Colloquium: Research Related to the Human Becoming Theory, Niehoff School of Nursing, Loyola University Chicago, Nov. 7, International.

Cody, W.K. (1998). *The human becoming hermeneutic method.* Presented at the Sixth Annual International Qualitative Nursing Research Colloquium: The Human Becoming School of Thought, Loyola University Chicago, Nov. 4., International.

Cody, W.K. & Pilkington, F.B. (1995). *Research workshop.* Presented at the 5th Annual Parse Scholar Weekend, Niagara-on-the-Lake, Canada, Nov. 17.

Cody, W.K. & Pilkington, F.B. (1996). *Research workshop.* Presented at the 6th Annual Parse Scholar Weekend, Niagara-on-the-Lake, Canada, Nov. 1.

Jonas, C.M. (1989). *Parse's theory in practice with older people.* Paper presented at St. Michael's Hospital, Toronto, Canada.

Jonas, C.M. (1989). *Parse's theory: Research and practice.* Paper presented at the University of Toronto, School of Nursing, Canada.

Jonas, C.M. (1990). *Practicing Parse's theory with groups of individuals in the community.* Paper presented at The Queen Elizabeth Hospital, Toronto, Ontario.

Jonas, C.M. (1994, March). *Quality of life for older persons living their dying.* Presentation given at Telemedicine Canada, Toronto, Canada.

Jonas, C.M. (1994, April). *Parse's theory of nursing in practice, education and research.* Paper presentations given at Lahti College of Health Professionals, Lahti, Finland.

Jonas, C.M. & Mitchell, G.J. (1995, June). *Practice innovations with Parse's theory: When patient's lead the way.* Paper presentation given at the Nursing Scholarship and Practice Conference, Reykjavik, Iceland.

Jonas, C.M. & Mitchell, G.J. (1995, July/Aug.). *Quality of life: The Patient's perspective.* Paper presentations given at The Queen Elizabeth Hospital, Toronto, Ontario.

Jonas-Simpson, C. (1995, Oct.). *Human science: A metaphorical explication.* Paper presented at the second annual Qualitative Research Colloquium, Loyola University, Chicago, Illinois.

Jonas-Simpson, C. (1996, June). *Living the human becoming theory through music.* Paper presented at the First European Nursing Theory Conference in Scandinavia. Malmo, Sweden.

Jonas-Simpson, C. (1996, June). *Quality of life: Enhancing freedoms amid restrictions.* Paper presented at The Queen Elizabeth Hospital Foundation luncheon, Toronto, Canada.

Jonas-Simpson, C. (1996, Oct.). *Taking the road less traveled: The qualitative research journey.* Paper presentation at the annual Qualitative Research Colloquium, Loyola University, Chicago, Illinois.

Jonas-Simpson, C. (1997, May). *The human becoming theory in practice, research and education.* Paper presentations given at Lahti College of Health Professionals, Lahti, Finland.

Jonas-Simpson, C. (1997, Oct.). *Feeling understood: A melody of human becoming.* Paper presented at the annual Qualitative Research Colloquium, Loyola University, Chicago, Illinois.

Jonas-Simpson, C. (1997, Nov.). *Quality of life: Enhancing understanding of human becoming.* Paper presented at the annual Parse Scholar Weekend, Niagara-on-the-lake, Ontario.

Jonas-Simpson, C. & Pilkington, F.B. (1997, Nov.). *Human sciences: Moving nursing to the new millennium.* Paper presented to the Collaborative Research Program at the Rehabilitation Institute of Toronto, Ontario.

Liehr, P.R. (1988, Dec.). *A study of the experience of "living on the edge."* Research study presented at the Southern Council on Collegiate Education for Nursing, Atlanta, GA.

Mattice, M. (1990). *Evaluating Parse's theory in practice.* Paper presented at The Queen Elizabeth Hospital, Toronto, Ontario.

Menke, E.M. (1990). *Critique of the research studies and the research methodology.* Paper presented at Discovery International, Inc., Nursing Science Seminar, Research and Practice Related to Parse's Theory of Nursing, Cincinnati, OH.

Misselwitz, S.K. (1989). *A phenomenological study of getting through the day for women who are homeless.* Research study presented at conference sponsored by Barry University School of Nursing Honor Society, Sigma Theta Tau, Beta Tau Chapter, University of Miami, and South Florida Nursing Research Society.

Mitchell, G.J. (1987). *Man-living-health in practice with the elderly.* Paper presented at Gerontological Society meeting, Washington, DC.

Mitchell, G.J. (1988). *Man-living-health in practice.* Paper presented at Wayne State University Summer Research Symposium, Detroit.

Mitchell, G.J. (1990). *An evaluation study of Parse's theory of nursing in an acute care setting.* Paper presented at St. Michael's Hospital, Nursing Department, Toronto, Canada.

Mitchell, G.J. (1990). *A dialogue with nurse theorists: A basis for differentiating nursing practice—Parse in practice.* Paper presented at American Academy of Nursing Conference, Charleston, SC.

Mitchell, G.J. (1990). *From traditional nursing to Parse's theory.* Paper presented at The Queen Elizabeth Hospital, Toronto, Ontario.

Mitchell, G.J. (1990). *Nursing practice guided by Parse's theory.* Paper presented at North Shore Medical Center, Miami, FL.

Mitchell, G.J. (1990). *Parse in practice.* Paper presented at UCLA National Nursing Theory Conference, Los Angeles, CA.

Mitchell, G.J. (1990). *Parse's theory as a guide to practice.* Paper presented at Discovery International, Inc., Nursing Science Seminar, Research and Practice Related to Parse's Theory of Nursing, Cincinnati, OH.

Mitchell, G.J. & Bournes, D.A. (1997, Nov.). *The human becoming theory: A focus on practice.* Workshop conducted at the Parse Scholars Seminar Weekend, November 7-9, 1997, Niagara-on-the-Lake, Ontario, Canada. Sponsored by the International Consortium of Parse Scholars.

Mitchell, G.J., Bournes, D.A., MacMaster, L., & McGrath, P. (1997, April). *Clarifying nursing's unique contribution to health care: Opportunities and dangers.* Telemedicine presentation. Sponsored by the faculty of Medicine, University of Toronto and The Toronto Hospital, Toronto, Canada.

Mitchell, G.J. & Pilkington, F.B. (1998, April). *Alternative paradigms for human science: To what end in nursing?* Workshop presented at Research Utilization: Preparing for the New Millennium, sponsored by the Faculty of Nursing, University of Toronto.

Pilkington, F.B. (1990). *Research guided by Parse's theory.* Paper presented at The Queen Elizabeth Hospital, Toronto, Ontario.

Pilkington, F.B. (1994, Oct.). *Practicing the human becoming theory with families grieving losses through childbirth.* Paper presented at the 4th Annual International Parse Scholar Seminar Weekend, Killington, Vermont.

Pilkington, F.B. (1994, Nov.). *Persisting in a situation while wanting to change.* Paper presented at the Second Annual International Nursing Research Colloquium, Marcella Niehoff School of Nursing, Loyola University Chicago.

Pilkington, F.B. (1994, Nov.). *The myth that "you don't need nursing theories to guide nursing science development."* Paper presented at the Second Annual International Nursing Research Colloquium, Marcella Niehoff School of Nursing, Loyola University Chicago.

Pilkington, F.B. (1994, Dec.). *Persisting while wanting to change.* Paper presented at the Nursing Theory Symposium, cosponsored by Alpha Beta Chapter, Sigma Theta Tau, and Marcella Niehoff School of Nursing, Loyola University Chicago.

Pilkington, F.B. (1995, Oct.). *The human science tradition and qualitative research.* Paper presented at the Third Annual International Nursing Research Colloquium, Marcella Niehoff School of Nursing, Loyola University Chicago.

Pilkington, F.B. (1996, Nov.). *Persisting while wanting to change: Research guided by Parse's theory.* Paper presented at the Fourth Annual International Qualitative Research Colloquium, Marcella Niehoff School of Nursing, Loyola University Chicago.

Pilkington, F.B. (1996, Nov.). *Persisting while wanting to change: Research guided by Parse's theory.* Poster presented at the Sixth Annual Parse Scholars Seminar Weekend, Niagara-on-the-Lake, Ontario.

Pilkington, F.B. (1997, April). *Persisting while wanting to change: The lived experience.* Paper presented at Research '97, Cosponsored by the Faculty of Nursing, University of Toronto Alumnae Association and Lambda Pi Chapter, Sigma Theta Tau, Toronto, Canada.

Pilkington, F.B. (1997, April). *The human becoming theory in practice: Experiences in diverse settings.* Paper presented at the First International Conference on Nursing Theories. Nürnberg, Germany.

Pilkington, F.B. (1997, Nov.). *The lived experience of persisting while wanting to change.* Paper presented at 7th Annual Parse Scholars Seminar Weekend, Niagara-on-the-Lake, Ontario.

Pilkington, F.B. (1997, Dec.). *Life after a stroke: Persons' experiences over time.* Paper presented at Focus on the Patient: Care, Satisfaction and Quality of Life Conference, cosponsored by Sunnybrook Health Science Centre, Hospital Management Research Unit and Faculty of Medicine, University of Toronto.

Pilkington, F.B. (1998, Jan.). *What life is like after a stroke.* Poster presented at Research Day, Sunnybrook Health Science Centre, Toronto, Canada.

Pilkington, F.B. (1998, May). *Persisting while wanting to change: The lived experience.* Paper presented at Qualitatives '98: Reflecting Social Life: Analysis and Interpretation in Qualitative Research, Ontario Institute for Studies in Education.

Pilkington, F.B. (1998, July). *Persisting while wanting to change: The lived experience.* Paper presented at the 10th International Nursing Research Congress, Sigma Theta Tau International, Utrecht, The Netherlands.

Pilkington, F.B. & Jonas-Simpson, C. (1997, Nov.). *Research workshop.* Presented at the 7th Annual Parse Scholar Weekend. Niagara-on-the-Lake, Ontario, Canada.

Santopinto, M.D.A. (1987). *Parse's theory of nursing as a base for innovative practice.* Paper presented at Hamilton Psychiatric Hospital, Hamilton, Ontario.

Santopinto, M.D.A. (1988). *A qualitative evaluation study of Parse's theory in practice: What happens when theory is implemented?* Research study presented at Eighth Annual Southern Council on Collegiate Education for Nursing Research Conference, Emory University, Atlanta, Georgia.

Santopinto, M.D.A. (1988). *A test of Parse's theory in a gerontological setting: An evaluation study.* Research study presented at Ryerson Theory Congress, Toronto, Ontario.

Santopinto, M.D.A. (1988). *Close encounters of the theoretical kind: Three theory-based approaches.* Paper presented at Tenth Southeastern Conference of Specialists in Psychiatric-Mental Health Nursing, Asheville, North Carolina.

Santopinto, M.D.A. (1989). *An emergent methodology study of caring about self for individuals who exercise relentlessly.* Research study presented at the Scientific Sessions of the Sigma Theta Tau Research Conference, Taipei, Taiwan.

Santopinto, M.D.A. (1989). *An evaluation study of Parse's practice methodology in a chronic care setting.* Research study presented at 19th Quadrennial Congress of the International Council of Nurses, Seoul, Korea.

Santopinto, M.D.A. (1990). *An evaluation of Parse's theory.* Paper presented at UCLA National Nursing Theory Conference, Los Angeles, CA.

Santopinto, M.D.A. (1990). *An evaluation study of Parse's theory in practice.* Paper presented at Discovery International, Inc., Nursing Science Seminar, Research and Practice Related to Parse's Theory of Nursing, Cincinnati, OH.

Santopinto, M.D.A. (1990). *An evaluation study of Parse's theory in practice in a chronic long-term setting.* Paper presented at Battle Creek Veteran's Administration Medical Center Conference, Kalamazoo, MI.

Smith, M.C. (1990). *Speculation on Parse in nursing education.* Paper presented at The Queen Elizabeth Hospital, Toronto, Ontario.

Smith, M.C. (1990). *The lived experience of hope in families of critically ill persons.* Paper presented at UCLA National Nursing Theory Conference, Los Angeles, CA.

Spee, R. (1995). *The client: The cry, the call, and the commitment.* Paper presented at the fourth National Conference of Canadian Clinical Nurse Specialists, Vancouver, British Colombia.

Spee, R. (1997). *The lived experience of feeling at home.* Paper presented at the Parse Scholars Seminar Weekend, Niagara-on-the-Lake, Ontario, Canada.

Spee, R. & Beitel, J. (1996). *Patient focused care: Advancing nursing practice.* Poster presented at the Parse Scholars Seminar Weekend, Niagara-on-the-Lake, Ontario, Canada.

Cassette Recordings

Beauchamp, C.J. (Speaker). (1990). *The lived experience of struggling with making a decision in a critical life situation* (Cassette Recording No. DII-602). Louisville, KY: Meetings Internationale, Ltd.

Cody, W.K. (Speaker). (1990). *The lived experience of grieving a personal loss* (Cassette Recording No. DII-602). Louisville, KY: Meetings Internationale, Ltd.

Menke, E.M. (Speaker). (1990). *Critique of the research studies and the research methodology* (Cassette Recording No. DII-603). Louisville, KY: Meetings Internationale, Ltd.

Menke, E.M. (Moderator). (1990). *Panel discussion/retrospective and evaluation* (Cassette Recording No. DII-605). Louisville, KY: Meetings Internationale, Ltd.

Mitchell, G.J. (Speaker). (1990). *Parse's theory as a guide to practice* (Cassette Recording No. DII-604). Louisville, KY: Meetings Internationale, Ltd.

Santopinto, M.D.A. (Speaker). (1990). *An evaluation study of Parse's theory in practice* (Cassette Recording No. DII-604). Louisville, KY: Meetings Internationale, Ltd.

Skiar, M. (Speaker). (1986). *The experience of living in a three generational family constellation: A case study* (Cassette Recording No. DII-302). Louisville, KY: Meetings Internationale, Ltd.

Smith, M.J. (Moderator). (1986). *Panel discussion of research related to man-living-health: Evaluation* (Cassette Recording No. DII-305). Louisville, KY: Meetings Internationale, Ltd.

Smith, M.J. (Speaker). (1986). *The experience of being confined: A study using the emerging method* (Cassette Recording No. DII-304). Louisville, KY: Meetings Internationale, Ltd.

Smith, M.C. (Speaker). (1990). *The lived experience of struggling through difficult times* (Cassette Recording No. DII-603). Louisville, KY: Meetings Internationale, Ltd.

Theses and Dissertations Using Parse's Theory

Beauchamp, C. (1990). *The lived experience of struggling with making a decision in a critical life situation.* Unpublished doctoral dissertation, University of Miami, FL.

Blanchard, D. (1996). *Intimacy as a lived experience of health.* Unpublished doctoral dissertation, Wayne State University, Detroit, MI.

Bournes, D.A. (1997). *Quality of life: Exploring the perspective of patients with congestive heart failure.* Unpublished master's thesis, University of Toronto, Toronto, Canada.

Bournes, D.A. (2000). *Having courage: A lived experience of human becoming.* Unpublished doctoral dissertation, Loyola University Chicago.

Brunsman, C.S. (1988). *A phenomenological study of the lived experience of hope in families with chronically ill children.* Unpublished master's thesis, Michigan State University, Lansing, MI.

Bunkers, S. (1995). *Considering tomorrow: Parse's theory-guided research.* Unpublished doctoral dissertation, Loyola University, Chicago, IL.

Cody, W.K. (1989). *Grieving a personal loss: A preliminary investigation of Parse's man-living-health methodology.* Unpublished master's thesis, Hunter College, The City University of New York, NY.

Cody, W.K. (1992). The meaning of grieving for families living with AIDS. *Dissertation Abstracts International-B,* 53/11, 5640. (University Microfilms International No. 9307924)

Costello-Nickitas, D.M. (1989). The lived experience of choosing among life goals: A phenomenological study. *Dissertation Abstracts International-B,* 50/09, 3916. (University Microfilms International No.9004353)

Daly, J. (1994). *Lived experience of suffering.* Unpublished doctoral dissertation, Southern Cross University, New South Wales, Australia.

Dowling, T.C. (1987). *Sharing who you really are with another: A phenomenological inquiry.* Unpublished master's thesis, Hunter College, The City University of New York, NY.

Felblinger, D.M. (1994). Responsibility: The lived experience of women who have taken illegal drugs during pregnancy. *Dissertation Abstracts International-B,* 55/09, 3813. (University Microfilms International No. 9502556)

Gouty, C.A. (1996). *Feeling alone while with others.* Unpublished doctoral dissertation, Loyola University, Chicago, IL.

Huckshorn, K.A. (1988) *The lived experience of creating a new way of being.* Unpublished master's thesis, Florida State University, Tallahassee, FL.

Jonas-Simpson, C. (1998). *Feeling understood: A melody of human becoming.* Unpublished doctoral dissertation, Loyola University Chicago, Chicago, IL.

Lavenia-Anderson, J.T. (1991). The lived experience of the spouse whose husband has cancer. *Masters Abstracts International,* 30/01, 96. (University Microfilms International No. 1345023)

Liu, S.L. (1993). *The meaning of health in hospitalized older women in Taiwan.* Unpublished doctoral dissertation, University of Colorado Health Sciences Center, Denver, CO.

Milton, C. (1998). *Making a promise.* Unpublished doctoral dissertation, Loyola University Chicago.

Mitchell, G.J. (1992). *Exploring the paradoxical experience of restriction-freedom in later life: Parse's theory guided research.* Unpublished doctoral dissertation, University of South Carolina, Columbia, SC.

Montgomery, C.A. (1994). The experience of conjugal loss from a cancer death in young to middle-aged persons. *Masters Abstracts International,* 33/03, 873. (University Microfilms International No. 1359274)

Norris, J.R. (1998). *One-to-one apprenticeship as a means for nurses teaching and learning Parse's theory of human becoming.* Unpublished doctoral dissertation, University of Toronto, Ontario, Canada.

Northrup, D. (1995). Exploring the experience of time passing for persons with HIV disease: Parse's theory guided research. *Dissertation Abstracts International,* 56/06, 3129. (University Microfilms International No. 9534912)

Petardi, L.A. (1995). *Weathering the storm: Persevering through a difficult time.* Unpublished doctoral dissertation, Loyola University, Chicago, IL.

Petras, E.M. (1986). *The lived experience of sharing a painful moment with someone close: A phenomenological study.* Unpublished master's thesis, Hunter College, The City University of New York, NY.

Pilkington, F.B. (1997). *Persisting while wanting to change: Research guided by Parse's theory.* Unpublished doctoral dissertation, Loyola University Chicago, Chicago, IL

Porteous, E.A. (1994). Preoperative education in a preadmission assessment clinic: Its effects on anxiety levels. *Masters Abstracts International,* 33/02, 518. (University Microfilms International No. 1358089)

Santopinto, M.D.A. (1987). *The relentless drive to be ever thinner: A phenomenological study.* Unpublished master's thesis, The University of Western Ontario, London, Ontario.

Sklar, M.B. (1985). *Qualitative investigation of the health patterns lived in an intergenerational family lifestyle.* Unpublished master's thesis, Hunter College, The City University of New York, NY.

Tambini, D. (1993). *Attentive presence: A phenomenological study.* Unpublished master's thesis, Hunter College, The City University of New York, NY.

Thornburg, P.D. (1993). The meaning of hope in parents whose infants died from sudden infant death syndrome. *Dissertation Abstracts International-B,* 54/06, 3000. (University Microfilms International No.9329939)

Wang, C.E. (1997). *Mending a torn fish net: A metaphor for hope.* Unpublished doctoral dissertation, Loyola University Chicago, Chicago, IL.

Directories and Biographical Sources

AAN directory: Fellows of the American academy of nursing. (1989). Kansas City, MO: American Academy of Nursing.

Directory of nurse researchers (2nd ed.). (1987). Indianapolis: Sigma Theta Tau.

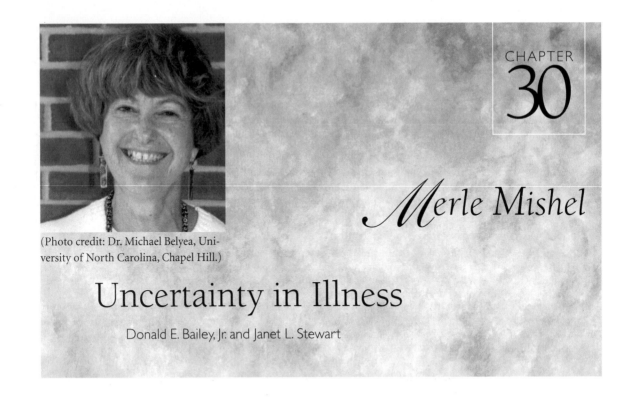

(Photo credit: Dr. Michael Belyea, University of North Carolina, Chapel Hill.)

Merle Mishel

Uncertainty in Illness

Donald E. Bailey, Jr. and Janet L. Stewart

CREDENTIALS AND BACKGROUND OF THE THEORIST

Merle H. Mishel was born in Boston, Massachusetts. She graduated from Boston University with a B.A. in 1961 and received her M.S. in psychiatric nursing from the University of California in 1966. Mishel completed her M.A. and Ph.D. in social psychology at the Claremont Graduate School, Claremont California in 1976 and 1980, respectively. Her dissertation research, supported by an individual National Research Service Award, was the development and testing of the Perceived Ambiguity in Illness Scale, later renamed the Mishel Uncertainty in Illness Scale (MUIS-A). The original scale has been used as the basis for three additional scales: (1) a community version (MUIS-C) for chronically ill individuals who are not hospitalized or receiving active medical care, (2) a mea-

The authors wish to thank Dr. Merle Mishel for her review and input for this chapter.

sure of parent's perception of uncertainty (PPUS) with regards to their child's illness experience, and (3) a measure of uncertainty in spouses or other family members when another member of the family is acutely ill (PPUS-FM).

Early in her professional career, Mishel practiced as a psychiatric nurse in acute care and community settings. While perusing her doctorate, she was on faculty in the Department of Nursing at the California State University at Los Angeles, rising from assistant to full professor. In addition, she practiced as a nurse therapist in both community and private practice settings from 1973 to 1979. After completing her doctorate in social psychology, she relocated to the University of Arizona College of Nursing in 1981 as an associate professor and was promoted to professor in 1988. She served as Division Head of Mental Health Nursing from 1984 to 1991. While at the University of Arizona, Mishel received numerous intramural and extramural research grants, which supported the continued development of the theoretical framework of uncertainty in illness. During this period, she continued practicing as a nurse therapist, working with the Heart Transplant Program at the University Medical Center. She was inducted as a Fellow in the American Academy of Nursing in 1990.

Mishel returned to the East Coast in 1991, joined the faculty as a professor in the School of Nursing at the University of North Carolina at Chapel Hill, and was awarded the endowed Kenan Professor of Nursing Chair in 1994. Friends of the National Institute of Nursing Research (NINR) presented her with a Research Merit Award in 1997. She was invited by the Friends of the NINR to present her research as an exemplar of federally funded nursing intervention studies at a Congressional Breakfast in 1999. In addition, she is the Director of the T-32 Institutional National Research Service Award Training Grant, Interventions for Preventing and Managing Chronic Illness, and a Core Director of the P-30 Center Grant, Preventing and Managing Chronic Illness in Vulnerable People. The T-32 awards predoctoral and postdoctoral fellowships to nurses interested in developing interventions for a variety of underserved chronically ill patients. The P-30 is a center grant designed to stimulate multidisciplinary research with the chronically ill. Mishel also maintains a prolific program of nursing intervention research with several different cancer populations. Since 1984, Mishel's research program has been continually funded by the National Institutes of Health (NIH), such that each research grant has built upon findings from previous studies to move systematically toward theoretically derived, scientifically tested nursing interventions.

In addition to the awards previously identified, Mishel was the recipient of a Sigma Theta Tau International-Sigma Xi Chapter Nurse Research Predoctoral Fellowship from 1977 to 1979 and received the Mary Opal Wolanin Research Award in 1986. In 1987, Mishel was first alternate to the Fulbright Award. She has been a visiting scholar at many institutions throughout North America, including University of Nebraska, University of Texas at Houston, University of Tennessee at Knoxville, University of South Carolina, University of Rochester, Yale University, and McGill University. She has also served as doctoral program consultant for the University of Cincinnati, College of Nursing from 1991 to 1992 and for Rutgers University, School of Nursing in 1993. Over the last 10 years, Mishel has presented more than 50 invited addresses at schools of nursing throughout the United States and Canada.

Mishel is a member of a number of professional organizations. They include the American Academy of Nursing, Sigma Theta Tau International, American Psychological Association, American Nurses' Association, Society of Behavioral Medicine, Oncology Nursing Society, Southern Nursing Research Society, and the Society for Education and Research in Psychiatric Nursing. She has served as a grant reviewer for the National Cancer Institute, National Center for Nursing Research, and National Institute on Aging and was a charter member of the study section on human immunodeficiency virus (HIV) at the National Institute of Mental Health. Mishel serves as a manuscript reviewer for *Research in Nursing and Health, Western Journal of Nursing Research, Heart and Lung, Scholarly Inquiry for Nursing Practice,* and *Sage Press* and is a collaborative editor for *Annals of Behavioral Medicine.*

THEORETICAL SOURCES

When Mishel began her research into uncertainty, the concept had not been applied previously in the health and illness context. Her Uncertainty in Illness Theory (Figure 30-1) drew from existing information processing models[56] and personality research[7] from the psychology discipline, which characterized uncertainty as a cognitive state resulting from insufficient cues with which to form a cognitive schema, or internal representation of a situation or event. Mishel attributes the underlying stress/appraisal/coping/adaptation framework in the original theory to the work of Lazarus and Folkman.[25] What was unique was her application of this framework to uncertainty as a stressor in the context of illness, which made the framework particularly meaningful for nursing.

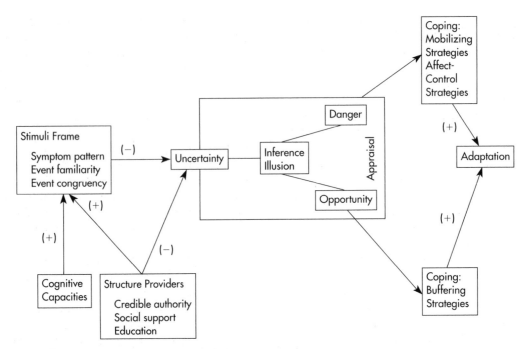

Figure 30-1 Model of perceived uncertainty in illness. (From Mishel, M.H. [1998, Winter]. Uncertainty in illness. *Image: Journal of Nursing Scholarship,* 20, 225-232.)

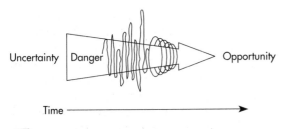

Figure 30-2 Reconceptualized model of uncertainty in chronic illness. (Reprinted with permission of M.H. Mishel.)

With the reconceptualization of the theory (Figure 30-2), Mishel[32] recognized that the Western approach to science supported a mechanistic view in its emphasis on control and predictability. By using critical social theory, Mishel recognized the bias inherent in the original theory, an orientation toward certainty and adaptation. Mishel then incorporated tenets from Chaos Theory, which, because it focused on open systems, allowed for a more accurate representation of how chronic illness creates disequilibrium and how people can ultimately incorporate continual uncertainty to find new meaning in illness.

USE OF EMPIRICAL EVIDENCE

The Uncertainty in Illness Theory grew out of Mishel's dissertation research with hospitalized patients, for which she used both qualitative and quantitative findings to generate the first conceptualization of uncertainty in the context of illness. Beginning with the publication of Mishel's Uncertainty in Illness Scale,[30] there has been extensive research into adults' experiences with uncertainty related to chronic and life-threatening illnesses. Considerable empirical evidence has accumulated to support Mishel's theoretical model in adults. Several recent integrative reviews of uncertainty research have comprehensively summarized and critiqued the current state of the science.[28,33,35,42,52] This chapter includes studies that directly support the elements of Mishel's uncertainty model.

The majority of empirical studies have focused predominantly on two of the antecedents of uncertainty: (1) *stimuli frame* and (2) *structure providers,* and the relationship between uncertainty and psychological outcomes. Mishel[36,40,41] tested other elements of the model, such as the mediating roles of appraisal and coping early in her program of research, but these model elements, with cognitive capacity as an antecedent to uncertainty, have generated less research attention.

Several studies have shown that objective or subjective indicators of the severity of life threat and/or illness symptoms were positively associated with uncertainty.[4,16,20,21,53] Across a sustained illness trajectory, unpredictability in symptom onset, duration, and intensity have been related to perceived uncertainty.[3,6,22,37,42] Similarly, the ambiguous nature of illness symptoms and the consequent difficulty in determining the significance of physical sensations have frequently been identified as sources of uncertainty.[10,11,17,43,57]

Mishel and Braden[37] found that social support had a direct impact on uncertainty by reducing perceived complexity and an indirect impact through its effect on the predictability of symptom pattern. The perception of stigma associated with some conditions, particularly HIV infection[48,57] and Down syndrome,[55] served to create uncertainty when families were unsure about how others would respond to the diagnosis. Family members have been consistently shown to experience high levels of uncertainty also, which may further reduce the amount of support experienced by the patient.[6,19,59] In addition, uncertainty was heightened by interactions with healthcare providers in which patients and family members received unclear information or simplistic explanations that did not fit their experience, or perceived that care providers were not expert or responsive enough to help them manage the intricacies of the illness.[3,11,26,51]

Numerous studies have reported the negative impact of uncertainty on psychological outcomes, characterized variously as anxiety, depression, hopelessness, and psychological distress.* Uncertainty has also been shown to negatively impact quality of life,[4,46] satisfaction with family relationships,[59] satisfaction with healthcare services,[15,54] and family caregivers' maintenance of their own self-care activities.[5,24,45]

Mishel reconceptualized the Uncertainty Theory in 1990 to accommodate responses to uncertainty over time in people with chronic conditions. The original theory was expanded to include the idea that uncertainty may not be resolved, but may become part of an individual's reality. In this context, uncertainty is reappraised as an opportunity and prompts the formation of a new, probabilistic view of life. To adopt this new view of life, the patient must be able to rely on social resources and healthcare providers who themselves accept the idea of probabilistic thinking.[32] If uncertainty can be framed as a normal part of life, it can become a positive force for multiple opportunities with resulting positive mood states.[14,32]

Support for the reconceptualized Uncertainty in Illness Theory has been found in predominantly qualitative studies of people with a variety of chronic and life-threatening illnesses. The process of formulating a new view of life has been described by women with breast cancer and cardiac disease as a revised life perspective,[17] new life goals,[8] new ways of being in the world,[27,43] growth through uncertainty,[47] and new levels of self-organization.[13] In studies of predominantly men with chronic illness or their caregivers, the process has been described as transformed self-identity and new goals for living,[6] a more positive perspective on life,[23] reevaluating what is worthwhile,[44] contemplation and self-appraisal,[9] uncertainty viewed as opportunity,[1] and redefining normal and building new dreams.[39]

*References 12, 16, 22, 29, 41, 50, 58.

MAJOR CONCEPTS & DEFINITIONS

UNCERTAINTY

Uncertainty is the inability to determine the meaning of illness-related events that occur when the decision maker is unable to assign definite value to objects or events and/or is unable to predict outcomes accurately.[31]

COGNITIVE SCHEMA

Cognitive schema is a person's subjective interpretation of illness, treatment, and hospitalization.[31]

STIMULI FRAME

Stimuli frame is the form, composition, and structure of the stimuli that a person perceives, which are then structured into a cognitive schema.[31]

Symptom Pattern

Symptom pattern is the degree to which symptoms present with sufficient consistency to be perceived as having a pattern or configuration.[31]

Event Familiarity

Event familiarity is the degree to which a situation is habitual, repetitive, or contains recognized cues.[31]

Event Congruence

Event congruence refers to the consistency between the expected and the experienced in illness-related events.[31]

STRUCTURE PROVIDERS

Structure providers are the resources available to assist the person in the interpretation of the stimuli frame.[31]

Credible Authority

Credible authority is the degree of trust and confidence a person has in his or her healthcare providers.[31]

Social Supports

Social supports influence uncertainty by assisting the individual to interpret the meaning of events.[31]

COGNITIVE CAPACITIES

Cognitive capacities are the information-processing abilities of a person, reflecting both innate capabilities and situational constraints.[31]

INFERENCE

Inference refers to the evaluation of uncertainty using related, recalled experiences.[31]

ILLUSION

Illusion refers to beliefs constructed from uncertainty.[31]

ADAPTATION

Adaptation reflects biopsychosocial behavior occurring within persons' individually defined range of usual behavior.[31]

NEW VIEW OF LIFE

New view of life refers to the formulation of a new sense of order, resulting from the integration of continual uncertainty into self-structure, in which uncertainty is accepted as the natural rhythm of life.[32]

PROBABILISTIC THINKING

Probabilistic thinking refers to a belief in a conditional world in which the expectation of continual certainty and predictability is abandoned.[32]

MAJOR ASSUMPTIONS

Mishel's original Uncertainty in Illness Theory, first published in 1988,[31] included several major assumptions. The first two reflect how uncertainty was originally conceptualized within the psychology discipline's information processing models.[31]

1. Uncertainty is a *cognitive* state, representing the inadequacy of an existing cognitive schema to support the interpretation of illness-related events.
2. Uncertainty is an inherently *neutral* experience, neither desirable nor aversive until it is appraised as such.

The next two assumptions reflect the uncertainty theory's roots in traditional stress and coping models, which posit a linear stress → coping → adaptation relationship.

3. Adaptation represents the continuity of an individual's usual biopsychosocial behavior and is the desired outcome of coping efforts to either reduce uncertainty appraised as danger or maintain uncertainty appraised as opportunity.
4. The relationships between illness events, uncertainty, appraisal, coping, and adaptation are linear and unidirectional, moving from situations promoting uncertainty towards adaptation.

Mishel herself challenged these last two assumptions in her reconceptualization of the theory, published in 1990.[32] The reconceptualization came about as a result of contradictory findings when the theory was applied to people with chronic illnesses. The original formulation of the theory held that uncertainty is typically appraised as an opportunity only in conditions that represent a known downward trajectory; in other words, uncertainty is appraised as opportunity when it is the alternative to negative certainty. Mishel and others found that people also appraised uncertainty as an opportunity in situations without a certain downward trajectory, particularly in long-term chronic illnesses, and that people often developed a new view of life in this context.

Dissatisfied with the traditional linear models that informed the original theory, Mishel turned to the more dynamic Chaos Theory to explain how prolonged uncertainty could function as a catalyst to change a person's perspective on life and illness. Chaos Theory contributed two theoretical assumptions, which replace the linear stress → coping → adaptation outcome portion of the model.[32]

1. People, as biopsychosocial systems, typically function in far-from-equilibrium states.
2. Major fluctuations in a far-from-equilibrium system enhance the system's receptivity to change.
3. Fluctuations result in repatterning, which is repeated at each level of the system.

In Mishel's reconceptualized model, neither the antecedents to uncertainty nor the process of cognitive appraisal of uncertainty as danger or opportunity change. However, uncertainty over time, associated with a serious illness, functions as a catalyst for fluctuation in the system by threatening preexisting cognitive models of life as predictable and controllable. Uncertainty pervades nearly every aspect of a person's life; therefore its effects become concentrated and ultimately challenge the stability of the system. In response to the confusion and disorganization created by continued uncertainty, the system must ultimately change to survive.

Ideally, under conditions of chronic uncertainty, a person gradually moves away from an evaluation of uncertainty as aversive to adopt a new view of life that accepts uncertainty as a part of reality. Therefore uncertainty, especially in chronic and/or life-threatening illness, can result in a new level of organization and a new perspective on life, incorporating the growth and change that can result from uncertain experiences.

THEORETICAL ASSERTIONS

1. Uncertainty occurs when a person cannot adequately structure or categorize an illness-related event because there is a lack of sufficient cues.
2. Uncertainty can take the form of ambiguity, complexity, lack of or inconsistent information, and/or unpredictability.
3. As symptom pattern, event familiarity, and event congruence (stimuli frame) increase, uncertainty decreases.

4. Structure providers (credible authority, social support, and education) decrease uncertainty directly by promoting interpretation of events and indirectly by strengthening the stimuli frame.

5. Uncertainty appraised as danger prompts coping efforts directed at reducing the uncertainty and managing the emotional arousal generated by it.

6. Uncertainty appraised as opportunity prompts coping efforts directed at maintaining the uncertainty.

7. The influence of uncertainty on psychological outcomes is mediated by the effectiveness of coping efforts to reduce uncertainty appraised as danger or to maintain uncertainty appraised as opportunity.

8. When uncertainty appraised as danger cannot be effectively reduced, coping strategies can be employed to manage the emotional response.

9. The longer uncertainty continues in the illness context, the more unstable the individual's previously accepted mode of functioning becomes.

10. Under conditions of enduring uncertainty, individuals may develop a new, probabilistic perspective on life, which accepts uncertainty as a natural part of life.

11. The process of integrating continual uncertainty into a new view of life can be blocked or prolonged by structure providers who do not support probabilistic thinking.

12. Prolonged exposure to uncertainty appraised as danger can lead to intrusive thoughts, avoidance, and severe emotional distress.[31,32]

LOGICAL FORM

As a midrange theory both derived from and applicable to clinical practice, Mishel's Uncertainty in Illness Theory is a classic example of the multiple steps required to develop theory with both heuristic and practical value. Neither purely inductive nor deductive, Mishel's theoretical work initially arose from her asking questions about the nature of an important clinical problem, followed by systematic qualitative and quantitative inquiry, and the careful application of theoretical models borrowed from other disciplines. With the publication of the original theory in 1988, Mishel and others have carried out numerous empirical tests of the relationships among the major constructs in the model, applying and largely confirming the theory in many illness contexts. Mishel's reconceptualization of the theory in 1990 was deductive; it was generated from principles of Chaos Theory and was confirmed by empirical evidence from multiple qualitative studies that suggested people's responses to uncertainty changed over time within the context of serious chronic illnesses. Mishel's theory represents the bidirectional process by which theory both informs and is shaped by research.

ACCEPTANCE BY THE NURSING COMMUNITY

Practice

Mishel's theory describes a phenomenon experienced by acute and chronically ill individuals and their families. The theory has its beginning in Mishel's own experience with her father's battle with cancer. During his illness, he began to focus on events that seemed unimportant to those around him. When asked why he had chosen to focus on such events, he replied that when these activities were being done, he understood what was happening to him. Mishel believed this was her father's way of taking control and making sense out of an overwhelming situation. She knew early in the development of her concept and theory that nurses could identify the phenomenon from their experiences in caring for patients.

Recent clinical publications have moved the theory from research to practice. Writing for an audience of critical care nurses, Hilton[18] applies the theory in prescribing how to assess and intervene with patients experiencing uncertainty. Using examples of patients recovering from a cardiac event, Hilton explains how patients who misinterpret unclear physical symptoms may overprotect themselves by limiting physical activity that could be essential to their recovery. She further delineates how uncertainty can activate different types of coping to manage the situation and describes appropriate nursing interventions based on a thorough assessment of uncertainty in the patient or family member.

Wurzbach,[60] writing for medical-surgical nurses, exemplifies the experience of a woman hospitalized with a lump in her breast. The woman had a family history of breast cancer and no previous experience with hospitalization; therefore Wurzbach counsels nurses to assess for certainty and uncertainty. Based on this assessment, management strategies in the form of nursing interventions are prescribed. Wurzbach cautions nurses that intervention may not be appropriate in situations where the patient experiences a moderate or optimal level of certainty or uncertainty. In these circumstances, patients may feel hopeful and not require nursing intervention.

Mishel's Uncertainty in Illness Theory has also been applied to the practice of enterostomal (ET) nursing. Righter[49] describes how trust in the ET nurse's knowledge and experiences helps patients develop a cognitive schema for the ostomy experience. Functioning as a credible authority, an antecedent of uncertainty, ET nurses are able to intervene with patients to promote effective coping strategies.

Based on review of the database of the Managing Uncertainty in Illness Scale users,[34] many are masters-prepared clinicians seeking to understand the experience of uncertainty in a variety of clinical settings with different patient populations. The scale and theory have also been used by clinicians in eight countries outside the United States.

Education

The Theory of Uncertainty in Illness has been widely used by graduate students both nationally and internationally as the framework for theses and dissertations, as the topic of concept analysis, and for the critique of midrange nursing theory. Mishel also uses the theory as an exemplar of how theory guides the development of nursing interventions in her doctoral level courses. Frequently, Mishel is an invited guest at schools of nursing seminars and symposia throughout the country, presenting both her empirical findings and the process of theory development for audiences of faculty and students.

Research

As described above, a large body of knowledge has been generated by researchers using the Uncertainty in Illness Theory and scales. With her colleagues at the University of Arizona, Mishel tested and confirmed the major components of the theoretical model, predominantly in samples of women with cancer. Currently, her program of research encompasses the testing of psychoeducational nursing interventions derived from the theoretical model in samples of adults with breast and prostate cancer. The scales and theory have been used by nurse researchers and scientists from other disciplines to describe and explain the psychological responses of people experiencing uncertainty from illness. The scales have been successfully translated into 12 languages and applied in research throughout the world. Mishel[33,35] has reviewed the research conducted on uncertainty in both acute and chronic illness. However, she notes that although many investigators have used one of the scales derived from the theory, most studies have not used the uncertainty in illness framework to guide their research.

FURTHER DEVELOPMENT

Mishel and her colleagues have used the original theory as the framework for five federally funded nursing intervention studies. The intervention has proven effective in increasing cancer knowledge, reducing symptom burden, and improving quality of life in Mexican-American women, Caucasian women, and African-American women with breast cancer and in African-American men and Caucasian men with localized prostate cancer and their family members. The intervention study currently underway extends the intervention to African-American men and Caucasian men with advanced or recurrent prostate cancer and their primary support persons. The applicability of the theory to the experience of children facing serious illness is currently being tested by J.L. Stewart in her dissertation research with children undergoing treatment for cancer.

From qualitative data supporting the reconceptualized theory, Mishel and Fleury[38] developed the Growth Through Uncertainty Scale (GTUS) to measure the new view of life that can emerge from continual uncertainty. The reconceptualized theory has also been used by researchers to understand the uncertainty experience of long-term breast cancer survivors[27] and individuals with schizophrenia and their family members.[1] The reconceptualized theory serves as the foundation for Mishel and colleagues' most recent nursing intervention study with women facing the enduring uncertainties inherent in surviving breast cancer. Bailey and Mishel[2] have used the theory, with data from qualitative interviews with older men electing watchful waiting as treatment for their prostate cancer, to develop a nursing intervention helping men integrate uncertainty into their lives, view their lives in a positive perspective, and improve their quality of life. The first trial of this new intervention is the dissertation research of D.E. Bailey.[2]

Mishel believes the most important product of her research program is the return of knowledge to practice. Towards that end, plans are underway to move the theoretically derived intervention into current practice, allowing nurses responsible for different types of patient populations to incorporate uncertainty assessment and intervention into their plan of care.

CRITIQUE
Clarity

Clarity refers to how well the theory is understood and how consistently the concepts are presented and conceptualized. Uncertainty is the primary concept of this theory and is defined as a cognitive state in which individuals are unable to determine the meaning of illness-related events.[31] The original theory postulates that managing uncertainty is critical to adaptation during illness and it explains how individuals cognitively process illness-associated events and construct meaning from them.

The original theory's concepts are organized in a linear model around three major themes: (1) an-

tecedents of uncertainty, (2) the process of uncertainty appraisal, and (3) coping with uncertainty. The framework is easy to follow and is clear in all sections of the model. The antecedents of uncertainty include the stimuli frame, cognitive capacities, and structure providers. In the linear model, these antecedent variables have both a direct and indirect inverse relationship with uncertainty.

The second conceptual component of the model is appraisal. Uncertainty is seen as a neutral state, neither positive nor negative, until it has been appraised by the individual. Appraisal of uncertainty involves two processes: (1) inference and (2) illusion. Inference is constructed from the individual's personality disposition and includes learned resourcefulness, mastery, and locus of control. They refer to the individual's belief that they have the ability to handle life events. Illusion is defined as a belief constructed from uncertainty that considers the favorable aspects of a situation. Based on the appraisal process, uncertainty is viewed as either a danger or an opportunity. Uncertainty viewed as a danger results when the individual considers the possibility of a negative outcome. Uncertainty is viewed as an opportunity primarily through the use of illusion, but inference can also lead to the individual appraising the situation as having a positive outcome. In this situation, uncertainty is preferred and the individual remains hopeful.

Coping is the third theme contained in the original model of uncertainty. Coping occurs in two forms with the end result of adaptation. If uncertainty is appraised as a danger, then coping includes direct action, vigilance, seeking information from mobilizing strategies, affect management using faith, disengagement, and cognitive support. If uncertainty is appraised as an opportunity, coping offers a buffer to maintain the uncertainty.

The original theory was reconceptualized in 1990 to incorporate the idea that chronic illness unfolds over time (possibly years) and with that, uncertainty is reappraised. The person is viewed as an open system exchanging energy within his or her environment. Rather than seek a return to a stable state, chronically ill individuals may move toward a complex world orientation, forming a new meaning for their lives. If uncertainty can be framed as a normal view of life, it can become a positive force for multiple opportunities with resulting positive mood states. To do so, the individual must develop probabilistic thinking, which allows the individual to examine a variety of possibilities and to consider numerous ways of achieving them. The individual envisions a variety of responses to situations and realizes that life can change from day to day.

Mishel described this process as a new view of life in which uncertainty shifts from being seen as a danger to being viewed as an opportunity. To adopt this new view of life, the patient must be able to rely on social resources and healthcare providers who themselves accept the idea of probabilistic thinking. The relationship between the healthcare provider and the patient must focus on recognizing continual uncertainty and teaching the patient how to use the uncertainty to generate different explanations for events. Therefore the importance of structure providers, introduced in the original theory, is maintained in the reconceptualized model.

Despite the complexity and dimensionality of the two models, they are clearly presented and comprehensively conceptualized. Mishel published her measurement model in 1981, her original theoretical model in 1988, and her reconceptualized theory in 1990 and these publications fully explicate the model so it is easily applied in clinical and research contexts.

Simplicity

The two uncertainty in illness models contain multiple concepts whose relationships range from simple to complex and direct to indirect. There are 11 major concepts found in the three themes of the original theory and several new concepts are introduced in the reconceptualized model. The antecedents of uncertainty are concise and their definitions are clear and simple. The appraisal component is complex because it considers cognitive processes with beliefs and values held by the individual. The coping phase of the theory is also complex because it is dependent on the appraisal

portion of the model and again involves different kinds of strategies targeted toward adaptation. The outcome portion of the model is differentiated in two conceptualizations of the theory: (1) relating to patients with acute illness and (2) representing an expansion of the model to accommodate patients with chronic illness. Although the models are not simple, overall, the concept definitions and relationships are well operationalized and easily understood.

Generality

The theories explain how individuals construct meaning from illness-related events. They are broad and generalizable and can be used with individuals experiencing their own illness to spouses and parents of people experiencing illness-related uncertainty. The concept of credible authority can be applied to physicians, nurses, and other healthcare workers. The theories can be applied to many areas of nursing practice and have been used by clinicians for acute and chronic illnesses such as cancer, cardiac disease, and multiple sclerosis.

Empirical Precision

Mishel derived both theoretical models from her own program of research and the research of others. Many of the concepts, assumptions, and relationships among variables draw support from empirical investigation. The concepts are well described and their relationships are precisely constructed; operational definitions have been written and tested. Testing of the theories has occurred in both research and clinical settings. The theories have allowed for the development and testing of nursing interventions to manage uncertainty.

Derivable Consequences

Derivable consequences are determined by examining whether a theory guides research, informs practice, generates new ideas, and differentiates the focus of nursing from other professions. Mishel's work represents an exemplar of midrange theory, which informs clinical practice within the encompassing context of acute and chronic illness. The theories have generated considerable empirical research in adults dealing with their own illness or that of their family member and the theories continue to stimulate new research directions, such as uncertainty in ill children, in older men electing *watchful waiting* as their treatment for prostate cancer, and in healthcare providers informing patients of treatment choices in conditions with uncertain prognoses. Mishel believes that by defining and conceptualizing an important clinical problem, her work supports and enriches nursing practice. The Uncertainty in Illness Theory and its reconceptualization represent frameworks derived from and for practice, a process that is essential to nursing as a practice discipline.

CRITICAL THINKING *Activities*

1. Imagine you are interviewing a patient new to your practice. Think about the questions you would ask to assess the patient's level of uncertainty about their health issue. What would you want to know about their perceptions of their current situation? Their supportive relationships? Their previous experiences with health and illness?

2. You are working with a young woman who has been living with multiple sclerosis for the last six years. During an exacerbation of her MS, she focuses not on her symptoms, but on her plans for going to law school. One of your colleagues suggests that she may be in denial about the severity of her illness. How might you use the reconceptualized Uncertainty in Illness Theory to propose an alternative interpretation of her perspective?

REFERENCES

1. Baier, M. (1995). Uncertainty of illness for persons with schizophrenia. *Issues in Mental Health Nursing,* 16, 201-212.
2. Bailey, D.E. & Mishel, M.H. (1997). *Uncertainty and watchful waiting in men with prostate cancer: Findings from qualitative interviews.* Paper presented at the 11th Annual Meeting of the Southern Nursing Research Society, April 10-12, 1997, Norfolk, VA.
3. Becker, G., Jason-Bjerklie, S., Benner, P., Slobin, K., & Ferketich, S. (1993). The dilemma of seeking urgent care: Asthma episodes and emergency service use. *Social Science and Medicine,* 37, 305-313.
4. Braden, C.J. (1990). A test of the self-help model: Learned response to chronic illness experience. *Nursing Research,* 39, 42-47.
5. Brett, K.M. & Davies, E.M.B. (1988). "What does it mean?" Sibling and parental appraisals of childhood leukemia. *Cancer Nursing,* 11, 329-338.
6. Brown, M.A. & Powell-Cope, G.M. (1991). AIDS family caregiving: Transitions through uncertainty. *Nursing Research,* 40, 338-345.
7. Budner, S. (1962). Intolerance of ambiguity as a personality variable. *Journal of Personality,* 30, 29-50.
8. Carter, B.J. (1993). Long-term survivors of breast cancer. *Cancer Nursing,* 16(5), 354-361.
9. Charmaz, K. (1995). Identity dilemmas of chronically ill men. In D. Sobo & D.F. Gordon (Eds.), *Men's health and illness: Gender, power, and the body* (pp. 266-291). Thousand Oaks, CA: Sage.
10. Cohen, M.H. (1993). The unknown and the unknowable—Managing sustained uncertainty. *Western Journal of Nursing Research,* 15, 77-96.
11. Comaroff, J. & Maguire, P. (1981). Ambiguity and the search for meaning: Childhood leukaemia in the modern clinical context. *Social Science and Medicine,* 15B, 115-123.
12. Failla, S., Kuper, B.C., Nick, T.G., & Lee, F.A. (1996). Adjustment of women with systemic lupus erthematosus. *Applied Nursing Research,* 9, 87-96.
13. Fleury, J., Kimbrell, L.C. & Kruszewski, C. (1995). Life after cardiac event: Women's experience in healing. *Heart and Lung,* 24, 474-482.
14. Gelatt, H.B. (1989). Positive uncertainty: A new decision-making framework for counseling. *Journal of Consulting and Clinical Psychology,* 36, 252-256.
15. Green, J.M. & Murton, F.E. (1996). Diagnosis of Duchenne muscular dystrophy: Parents' experiences and satisfaction. *Child: Care, Health, and Development,* 22, 113-128.
16. Grootenhuis, M.A. & Last, B.L. (1997). Parents' emotional reactions related to different prospects for the survival of their children with cancer. *Journal of Psychosocial Oncology,* 15, 43-61.
17. Hilton, B.A. (1988). The phenomenon of uncertainty in women with breast cancer. *Issues in Mental Health Nursing,* 9, 217-238.
18. Hilton, B.A. (1992). Perceptions of uncertainty: Its relevance to life-threatening and chronic illness. *Critical Care Nurse,* 12, 70-73.

19. Hilton, B.A. (1996). Getting back to normal: The family experience during early stage breast cancer. *Oncology Nursing Forum, 23,* 605-614.

20. Hinds, P.S., Birenbaum, L.K., Clarke-Steffen, L., Quargnenti, A., Kreissman, S., Kazak, A., Meyer, W., Mulhern, R., Pratt, C., & Wilimas, J. (1996). Coming to terms: Parents' response to a first cancer recurrence in their child. *Nursing Research, 45,* 148-153.

21. Janson-Bjerklie, S., Ferketich, S., & Benner, P. (1993). Predicting the outcomes of living with asthma. *Research in Nursing and Health, 16,* 241-250.

22. Jessop, D.J. & Stein, R.E.K. (1985). Uncertainty and its relation to the psychological and social correlates of chronic illness in children. *Social Science and Medicine, 20,* 993-999.

23. Katz, A. (1996). Gaining a new perspective of life as a consequence of uncertainty in HIV infection. *Journal of the Association of Nurses in AIDS Care, 7,* 51-60.

24. Lang, A. (1987). Nursing of families with an infant who requires home apnea monitoring. *Issues in Comprehensive Pediatric Nursing, 10,* 123-133.

25. Lazarus, R.S. & Folkman, S. (1984). *Stress, appraisal, and coping.* New York: Springer Publishing.

26. Mason, C. (1985). The production and effects of uncertainty with special reference to diabetes mellitus. *Social Science and Medicine, 21,* 1329-1334.

27. Mast, M.E. (1998). Survivors of breast cancer: Illness uncertainty, positive reappraisal, and emotional distress. *Oncology Nursing Forum, 25,* 555-562.

28. Mast, M.E. (1995). Adult uncertainty in illness: A critical review of the literature. *Scholarly Inquiry for Nursing Practice, 9,* 3-24.

29. Miles, M.S., Funk, S.G., & Kasper, M.A. (1992). The stress response of mothers and fathers of preterm infants. *Research in Nursing and Health, 15,* 261-269.

30. Mishel, M.H. (1981). The measurement of uncertainty in illness. *Nursing Research, 30,* 258-263.

31. Mishel, M.H. (1988). Uncertainty in illness. *Image: Journal of Nursing Scholarship, 20,* 225-231.

32. Mishel, M.H. (1990). Reconceptualization of the uncertainty in illness theory. *Image: Journal of Nursing Scholarship, 22,* 256-262.

33. Mishel, M.H. (1997a). Uncertainty in acute illness. *Annual Review of Nursing Research, 15,* 57-80.

34. Mishel, M.H. (1997b). Uncertainty in Illness scales manual. Available upon request from the author.

35. Mishel, M.H. (1999). Uncertainty in chronic illness. *Annual Review of Nursing Research, 17,* 269-294.

36. Mishel, M.H. & Braden, C.J. (1987). Uncertainty: A mediator between support and adjustment. *Western Journal of Nursing Research, 9,* 43-57.

37. Mishel, M.H. & Braden, C.J. (1988). Finding meaning: Antecedents of uncertainty in illness. *Nursing Research, 37,* 98-103.

38. Mishel, M.H. & Fleury, J. (1994). *Psychometric testing of the growth through uncertainty scale.* Unpublished data.

39. Mishel, M.H. & Murdaugh, C.L. (1987). Family adjustment to heart transplantation: Redesigning the dream. *Nursing Research, 36,* 332-338.

40. Mishel, M.H., Padilla, G., Grant, M., & Sorenson, D.S. (1991). Uncertainty in illness theory: A replication of the mediating effects of mastery and coping. *Nursing Research, 40,* 236-240.

41. Mishel, M.H. & Sorenson, D.S. (1991). Coping with uncertainty in gynecological cancer: A test of the mediating function of mastery and coping. *Nursing Research, 40,* 167-171.

42. Murray, J. (1993). Coping with the uncertainty of uncontrolled epilepsy. *Seizure, 2,* 167-178.

43. Nelson, J.P. (1996). Struggling to gain meaning: Living with the uncertainty of breast cancer. *Advances in Nursing Science, 18*(3), 59-76.

44. Nyhlin, K.T. (1990). Diabetic patients facing long-term complications: Coping with uncertainty. *Journal of Advanced Nursing, 15,* 1021-1029.

45. O'Brien, R.A., Wineman, N.M., & Nealon, N.R. (1995). Correlates of the caregiving process in multiple sclerosis. *Scholarly Inquiry for Nursing Practice, 9,* 323-342.

46. Padilla, G.V., Mishel, M.H., & Grant, M.M. (1992). Uncertainty, appraisal, and quality of life. *Quality of Life Research, 1,* 155-165.

47. Pelusi, J. (1997). The lived experience of surviving breast cancer. *Oncology Nursing Forum, 24,* 1343-1353.

48. Regan-Kubinski, M.J., Sharts-Hopko, N. (1995). Illness cognition of HIV-infected mothers. *Issues in Mental Health Nursing, 16,* 327-344.

49. Righter, B.M. (1995). Ostomy care: Uncertainty and the role of the credible authority during an ostomy experience. *Journal of Wound, Ostomy, and Continence Nurses Society, 22,* 100-104.

50. Schepp, K.G. (1991). Factors influencing the coping effort of mothers of hospitalized children. *Nursing Research, 40,* 42-46.

51. Sharkey, T. (1995). The effects of uncertainty in families with children who are chronically ill. *Home Healthcare Nurse, 13*(4), 37-42.

52. Stewart, J.L. & Mishel, M.H. (2000). Uncertainty in childhood illness: A synthesis of the parent and child literature. *Scholarly Inquiry for Nursing Practice, 14,* 299-320.

53. Tomlinson, P.S., Kirschbaum, M., Harbaugh, B., & Anderson, K.H. (1996). The influence of illness severity and family resources on maternal uncertainty during critical pediatric hospitalization. *American Journal of Critical Care, 5,* 140-146.

54. Turner, M.A., Tomlinson, P.S., & Harbaugh, B.L. (1990). Parental uncertainty in critical care hospitalization of children. *Maternal-Child Nursing Journal,* 19, 45-62.

55. Van Riper, M. & Selder, F.E. (1989). Parental responses to the birth of a child with Down syndrome. *Loss, Grief, and Care,* 3(3-4), 59-76.

56. Warburton, D.M. (1979). Physiological aspects of information processing and stress. In V. Hamilton & D.M. Warburton (Eds.), *Human stress and cognition: An information processing approach* (pp. 33-65). New York: John Wiley & Sons.

57. Weitz, R. (1989). Uncertainty and the lives of persons with AIDS. *Journal of Health and Social Behavior,* 30, 270-281.

58. Wineman, N. (1990). Adaptation to multiple sclerosis: The role of social support, functional disability, and perceived uncertainty. *Nursing Research,* 39, 294-299.

59. Wineman, N.M., O'Brien, R.A., Nealon, N.R., & Kaskel, B. (1993). Congruence in uncertainty between individuals with multiple sclerosis and their spouses. *Journal of Neuroscience Nursing,* 25, 356-361.

60. Wurzbach, M.E. (1992). Assessment and intervention for certainty and uncertainty. *Nursing Forum,* 27, 29-35.

BIBLIOGRAPHY
Primary Sources
Book Chapters

Allen, C., McHenry, J., Mishel, M.H., & Braden, C.J. (1993). Uncertainty management for women receiving treatment for breast cancer. In S. Funk, E. Tornquist, M. Champagne, & R.A. Wiese (Eds.), *Key aspects of caring for the chronically ill: Hospital and home* (pp. 170-177). New York: Springer Publishing Company.

Kay, R., Mishel, M.H., & DeZapien, J. (1994). Intervention for change: A support group for Mexican-American widows. In M. Sotomayer (Ed.), *Triple jeopardy: Aged Hispanic women: Insights and experiences* (pp. 59-73). Washington, DC: National Hispanic Council on Aging.

Mishel, M.H. (1993) Living with chronic illness. In S. Funk, E. Tornquist, M. Champagne, & R.A. Wiese (Eds.), *Key aspects of caring for the chronically ill: Hospital and home* (pp. 46-58.) New York: Springer Publishing Company.

Mishel, M.H. (1998). Methodological studies: Instrument development. In P. Brink & M. Woods (Eds.), *Advanced design in nursing research* (2nd ed., pp. 235-282). Beverly Hills, CA: Sage Press.

Journal Articles

Badger, T.A., Braden, C.J., Longman, A.J., Mishel, M.H. (1999). Depression burden, self-help interventions, and social support in women receiving treatment for breast cancer. *Journal of Psychosocial Oncology,* 17(2), 17-35.

Badger, T.A., Braden, C.J., & Mischel, M.H. (2001). Depression burden, self-help interventions, and side effect experience in women receiving treatment for breast cancer. *Oncology Nursing Forum,* 28, 567-574.

Badger, T.A., Cardea, J.M., Biocca, L.J. & Mishel, M.H. (1990). Assessment and management of depression: An imperative for community-based practice. *Archives of Psychiatric Nursing,* 4(4), 235-241.

Badger, T.A., Mishel, M.H., Cardea, J.M., & Biocca, L.J. (1991). Depression assessment and management: Evaluating a community-based mental health training program. *Public Health Nursing,* 8(3), 170-176.

Braden, C.J., Mishel, M.H., Longman, A., & Burns, L.R. (1990). A self-help intervention (SHIP) in breast cancer treatment. *Innovations in Oncology Nursing,* 6(2) 1, 8, 19.

Braden, C.J., Mishel, M.H., Longman, A.J., & Burns, L.R. (1998). Self-help intervention project: Women receiving treatment for breast cancer. *Cancer Practice,* 6(2), 87-98.

Germino, B.B., Mishel, M.H., Belyea, M., Harris, L., Ware, A., & Mohler, J. (1998). Uncertainty in prostate cancer: Ethnic and family patterns. *Cancer Practice,* 6(2), 107-113.

Longman, A., Braden, C.J., & Mishel, M.H. (1997). Pattern of association over time of side-effects burden, self-help and self-care in women with breast cancer. *Oncology Nursing Forum,* 24(9), 1555-1560.

Mishel, M.H. (1978). Assertion training with handicapped persons. *Journal of Counseling Psychology,* 25(3), 238-241.

Mishel, M.H. (1981). The measurement of uncertainty in illness. *Nursing Research,* 30(5), 258-263.

Mishel, M.H. (1983). Adjusting the fit: Development of uncertainty scales for specific clinical populations. *Western Journal of Nursing Research,* 5(4), 355-370.

Mishel, M.H. (1983). Parents' perception of uncertainty concerning their hospitalized child: Reliability and validity of a scale. *Nursing Research,* 32(6), 324-330.

Mishel, M.H. (1984). Perceived uncertainty and stress in medical patients. *Research in Nursing and Health,* 7, 163-171.

Mishel, M.H. (1986). Try the alternative! *Heart and Lung,* 16(3), 321-322.

Mishel, M.H. (1988). Commentary on "Patterns of self-care in patients with breast cancer." *Western Journal of Nursing Research,* 10(1), 20-21.

Mishel, M.H. (1988). Commentary on "Perceived uncertainty and coping post myocardial infarction: A pilot study." *Western Journal of Nursing Research,* 10(4), 396-398.

Mishel, M.H. (1988). Uncertainty in illness. *Image: Journal of Nursing Scholarship,* 20(4), 225-232.

Mishel, M.H. (1989). Response to "The relationship among background characteristics, purpose in life, and caregiving demands on perceived health of spouse caregivers." *Scholarly Inquiry for Nursing Practice: An International Journal,* 3(2), 155-159.

Mishel, M.H. (1990). Reconceptualization of the uncertainty in illness theory. *Image: Journal of Nursing Scholarship,* 22(4), 256-262.

Mishel, M.H. (1991). Response to "Validation of a Swedish version of the Mishel Uncertainty in Illness Scale." *Scholarly Inquiry for Nursing Practice,* 5(1), 67-70.

Mishel, M.H. (1995). Response to "Adult uncertainty in illness: A critical review of research." *Scholarly Inquiry for Nursing Practice,* 9, 25-29.

Mishel, M.H. (1996). Commentary on "Uncertainty and coping in fathers of children with cancer." *Journal of Pediatric Oncology Nursing,* 13, 89-91.

Mishel, M.H. (1997). Uncertainty in acute illness. *Annual Review of Nursing Research,* 15, 57-80.

Mishel, M.H. (1999). Uncertainty in chronic illness. *Annual Review of Nursing Research,* 17, 269-294.

Mishel, M.H. & Braden, C.J. (1987). Uncertainty as a mediator in the relationship between social support and adjustment. *Western Journal of Nursing Research,* 9, 43-57.

Mishel, M.H. & Braden, C.J. (1988). Finding meaning: Antecedents of uncertainty in women receiving treatment for gynecological cancer. *Nursing Research,* 37(2), 98-103.

Mishel, M.H., Hostetter, T., King, B. and Graham, V. (1984). Predictors of psychosocial adjustment in patients newly diagnosed with gynecological cancer. *Cancer Nursing,* 1(4), 291-299.

Mishel, M.H. & Kreulen, G. (1992). Evaluation of nurse case manager effectiveness. *Oncology Nursing Forum,* 19(2), 308.

Mishel, M.H. & Murdaugh, C. (1987). Redesigning the dream: Family adjustment to heart transplantation. *Nursing Research,* 36(6), 332-338.

Mishel, M.H., Padilla, G., Grant, M., Sorenson, D.S. (1991). Uncertainty in illness theory: A replication of the mediating effects of mastery and coping. *Nursing Research,* 40(4), 236-240.

Mishel, M.H. & Sorenson, D.S. (1991). Coping with uncertainty in gynecological cancer: A test of the mediating function of mastery and coping. *Nursing Research,* 40(3), 167-171.

Mishel, M.H. & Sorenson, D. (1993) Revision of the ways of coping scale for a clinical population. *Western Journal of Nursing Research,* 15(1), 59-74.

Padilla, G.V., Mishel, M.H., & Grant, M.M. (1992) Uncertainty, appraisal and quality of life. *Quality of Life Research,* 1, 155-165.

Stewart, J.L. & Mishel, M.H. (2000). Uncertainty in childhood illness: A synthesis of the parent and child literature. *Scholarly Inquiry for Nursing Practice,* 14, 299-320.

Conference Proceedings

Badger, T., Mishel, M.H., Biocca, L., and Cardea, J. (1989). *Depression awareness: A community-based training program for nurses at the WHO.* Netherlands Institute of Primary Health Care, International Community Health Nursing Conference, The Netherlands, The Hague.

Bailey, D.E. Jr., Mishel, M.H., Germino, B.B., & Stewart, J.L. (2001). Intervention efficacy in men treated for prostate cancer: Moderator effects. In M.H. Mishel (Chair), *How to improve who benefits from an intervention: The use of moderator effects.* Symposium conducted at the meeting of the Southern Nursing Research Society, Baltimore, MD.

Belyea, M.J., Mishel, M.M., & Germino, B.B. (2001). Testing and interpreting moderator effects. In M.H. Mischel (Chair), *How to improve who benefits from an intervention: The use of moderator effects.* Symposium conducted at the meeting of the Southern Nursing Research Society, Baltimore, MD.

Braden, C.J. & Mishel, M.H. (1992). Intervention effectiveness research: Older women with breast cancer [Abstract]. *Communicating Nursing Research Conference,* 25, 388.

Braden, C.J., Mishel, M.H., & Germino, B.B. (2001). Older Mexican-American women with breast cancer: Moderators of treatment effect. In M.H. Mischel (Chair), *How to improve who benefits from an intervention: The use of moderator effects.* Symposium conducted at the meeting of the Southern Nursing Research Society, Baltimore, MD.

Braden, C.J., Mishel, M.H., & Longman, A. (1992). Demographic, diagnosis, treatment differences: Breast cancer in older women [Abstract]. *Communicating Nursing Research,* 25, 389.

Braden, C.J., Mishel, M.H., & Longman, A. (1995). *Efficacy of the self-help course/uncertainty management intervention for women receiving treatment for breast cancer.* 28th Annual Communicating Nursing Research Conference, "Innovation and collaboration: responses to health care needs," Western Society for Research in Nursing of the Western Institute of Nursing, San Diego, CA.

Braden, C.J., Mishel, M.H., Longman, A., & Burns, L.R. (1995). Efficacy of a self-help course/uncertainty management intervention [Abstract]. *Communicating Nursing Research,* 28, 225.

Braden, C.J., Mishel, M.H., Longman, A., & Burns, R. (1995). *Ethnicity as a factor in breast cancer treatment experience.* The Second International and Interdisciplinary Health Research Symposium, School of Nursing, West Virginia University, Morgantown, WV.

Brookes, A., Braden, C.J., & Mishel, M.H. (1992). Evaluating the efficacy of nursing interventions for women over age 65 [Abstract]. *Communicating Nursing Research,* 25, 391.

Germino, B.B., Mischel, M.H., & Belyea, M.J. (2001). Moderators of an uncertainty management intervention for family care providers of men with early stage prostate cancer. In M.H. Mischel (Chair), *How to improve who benefits from an intervention: The use of moderator effects.* Symposium conducted at the meeting of the Southern Nursing Research Society, Baltimore, MD.

Kay, R. & Mischel, M.H. (1990). *Evaluation of treatment efficacy from the viewpoints of different disciplines.* Meeting of the Society for Applied Anthropology, York, England.

McHenry, J., Braden, C.J., & Mischel, M.H. (1992). Self-help activities rated most helpful by older women with breast cancer [Abstract]. *Communicating Nursing Research,* 25, 392.

Mischel, M.H. (1983). Adjusting the fit: Method and issues to consider in developing a clinical tool from a research instrument [Abstract]. *Communicating Nursing Research,* 16, 43.

Mischel, M.H. (1983). Parents' perception of uncertainty concerning their hospitalized child [Abstract]. *Communicating Nursing Research,* 16, 44.

Mischel, M.H. (1983). *Parents' perceptions of their child's illness: Measurement of uncertainty.* Annual Meeting of the American Psychological Association, Anaheim, CA.

Mischel, M.H. (1984). *Antecedents of uncertainty: Alternative models.* Research for Clinical Nursing: Its Strategies and Findings, Twelfth Annual Nursing Research Conference, Tucson, AZ.

Mischel, M.H. (1984). *Mediators of adjustment to treatment in gynecological cancer patients.* Annual Meeting of the American Psychological Association, Toronto, Canada.

Mischel, M.H. (1985). *Coping with uncertainty in systemic lupus erythematosus.* Annual Meeting of the American Psychological Association, Los Angeles, CA.

Mischel, M.H. (1985). *Predictors of psychosocial adjustment during the stabilization phase in women with gynecological cancer.* Research for Clinical Nursing: Its Strategies and Findings, Thirteenth Annual Nursing Research Conference, Tucson, AZ.

Mischel, M.H. (1985). *The nature of uncertainty in women with gynecological cancer.* National Symposium of Nursing Research, San Francisco, CA.

Mischel, M.H. (1985). Uncertainty: A mediator in the relationship between social support and adjustment [Abstract]. *Communicating Nursing Research,* 18, 148.

Mischel, M.H. (1986). The theory of uncertainty in illness [Abstract]. *Communicating Nursing Research,* 19, 180.

Mischel, M.H. (1986). Theory testing research: Testing the uncertainty theory [Abstract]. *Communicating Nursing Research,* 19, 178.

Mischel, M.H. (1987). *Conducting qualitative research: Lessons learned along the way* [Abstract]. *Communicating Nursing Research,* 20, 150.

Mischel, M.H. (1987). *Response: Adjusting for initial differences.* Strengthening Causal Interpretations of Non-Experimental Data, National Center for Health Services Research and Health Care Technology Assessment. Tucson, AZ.

Mischel, M.H. (1987). *The existence of uncertainty after treatment ends.* Nursing Advances in Health: Models, Methods and Applications, ANA Council of Nurse Researchers 1987 International Nursing Research Conference, Washington, DC.

Mischel, M.H. (1988). *Coping with uncertainty in gynecological cancer. Uncertainty and coping: Measurement and conceptual update.* Research for Clinical Nursing: Its Strategies and Findings, The Sixteenth Annual Nursing Research Conference, University of Arizona, Tucson, AZ.

Mischel, M.H. (1988). *Coping with uncertainty in illness.* Stress, Coping Processes and Health Outcomes: New Directions for Theory Development and Research, University of Rochester, Rochester, NY.

Mischel, M.H. (1989). *A reconceptualization of uncertainty in illness.* Symposium on middle range theory development: Three models, Unity in Diversity, ANA Council of Nurse Researcher 1989 National Nursing Research Conference, Chicago, IL.

Mischel, M.H. (1989). Issues in conducting experimental studies with Mexican Americans [Abstract]. *Communicating Nursing Research,* 22, 172.

Mischel, M.H. (1989). *Psychosocial instrumentation.* Clinical Research: Biophysical and Psychosocial Instrumentation, The 17th Annual Nursing Research Conference, College of Nursing, University of Arizona, Tucson, AZ.

Mischel, M.H. (1989). Testing the efficacy of the intervention [Abstract]. *Communicating Nursing Research,* 22, 179.

Mischel, M.H. (1990). *Ethical issues in creating behavior change cross culture.* Women's Worlds: Realities and Choices: Fourth International Interdisciplinary Congress on Women, New York.

Mischel, M.H. (1990) *Response: The family's functioning with breast cancer in the mother: Test of an explanatory model with both acute and long-term illness.* Oncology Nursing Society Congress, Washington, DC.

Mischel, M.H. (1990). *Spouses as care providers for Alzheimer's disease victims.* The Fourth International Congress on Women's Health Issues, Massey University, North Palmersten, New Zealand.

Mischel, M.H. (1990). *The uncertainty in illness theory applied to primary care.* Primary Health Care Conference, Massey University, North Palmersten, New Zealand.

Mischel, M.H. (1991). *Issues in the development and use of disease-specific scales.* Instrumentation in Oncology Nursing Research Instructional Session, Annual Congress of the Oncology Nursing Society, San Antonio, TX.

Mishel, M.H. (1992). *Theory-driven treatment: Uncertainty management intervention.* Sixth Annual Research Conference, Southern Nursing Research Society, Nashville, TN.

Mishel, M.H. (1993). *Nursing interventions to promote self-help response to cancer.* Conference of the Society for Behavioral Medicine Convention, San Francisco.

Mishel, M.H. (1996). *Interventions sensitive to regional and cultural issues.* Symposium on issues in the design and implementation of nursing interventions for underserved cancer patients, 10th Annual Conference, Southern Nursing Research Society, Miami, FL.

Mischel, M.H. (2001). *How to improve who benefits from an intervention: The use of moderator effects.* Symposium conducted at the meeting of the Southern Nursing Research Society, Baltimore, MD.

Mishel, M.H., Allen, C., & McHenry, J. (1991). *Managing the uncertainty of the cancer experience.* Annual Congress of the Oncology Nursing Society Congress, San Antonio, TX.

Mishel, M.H. & Braden, C.J. (1992). Perceptions of breast cancer treatment experience: Older and younger women [Abstract]. *Communicating Nursing Research, 25, 390.*

Mishel, M.H., Braden, C.J., & Hostetter, T. (1985). *Social support: A method of uncertainty reduction in women with gynecological cancer.* Meeting of the Rocky Mountain Psychological Association, Tucson, AZ.

Mishel, M.H. & Epstein, D.R. (1991). *Normative data from the Mishel uncertainty in illness scale.* Nursing Research: Global Health Perspectives, ANA Council of Nurse Researchers 1991 International Nursing Research Conference, Los Angeles, CA.

Mishel, M.H., Germino, B., Belyea, M., & Braden, C.J. (1999). *Cultural beliefs of older African-American and Caucasian men treated for breast cancer.* 5th National Cancer Nursing Research Conference, Newport Beach, CA.

Mishel, M.H., Germino, B., Belyea, M., & Braden, C.J. (1999). *Cultural health beliefs of older African American and Caucasian women treated for breast cancer.* Pan American Congress of Psychosocial and Behavioral Oncology, New York.

Mishel, M.H., Germino, B., Belyea, M., Hamilton-Spruill, J., & Bailey, D. (1998). *Efficacy of an uncertainty management intervention on psychosocial outcomes in men treated for localized prostate cancer.* 4th International Congress of Psycho-oncology, Hamburg, Germany.

Mishel, M.H., Germino, B., Belyea, M., Hamilton-Spruill, J., & Bailey, D. (1999). *Efficacy and moderators of efficacy of an uncertainty management intervention in men treated for localized prostate cancer.* Conference on Key Aspects of Interventions for the Prevention and Management of Chronic Illness, Chapel Hill, NC.

Mishel, M.H., Germino, B., Belyea, M., Hamilton-Spruill, J., & Bailey, D. (1999). *Efficacy of an uncertainty management intervention in men treated for localized prostate cancer.* 13th Annual Conference of the Southern Nursing Research Society, Charleston, SC.

Mishel, M.H., Germino, B., Harris, L., Hamilton-Spruill, J., & Ware, A. (1997). *Developing culturally sensitive nursing intervention research.* 11th Annual Conference of the Southern Nursing Research Society, Norfolk, VA.

Mishel, M.H. & Hostetter, T. (1983). *Predictors of psychological adjustment in newly-diagnosed cancer patients.* Annual Convention of the Western Psychological Association Annual Convention, San Francisco, CA.

Mishel, M.H. & Hostetter, T. (1983). *Psychosocial adjustment in patients with gynecological cancer: The impact of uncertainty and optimism during the diagnosis and treatment phase.* Research for Clinical Nursing, Its Strategies and Findings, 11th Annual Nursing Research Conference, Tucson, AZ.

Mishel, M.H. & Hostetter, T. (1983). *The impact of uncertainty and optimism upon adjustment after receiving diagnosis of gynecological cancer.* Third Conference on Cancer Nursing Research, Portland, OR.

Mishel, M.H. & Hostetter, T. (1984). Mediators of adjustment in patients with gynecological cancer: Diagnosis to treatment phase [Abstract]. *Communicating Nursing Research, 17, 26.*

Mishel, M.H. & Murdaugh, C. (1985). *Family experiences with heart transplantation: Stages and issues.* Sixth Annual Scientific Sessions, The Society of Behavioral Medicine, New Orleans, LA.

Mischel, M.H. & Murdaugh, C. (1987). Use of groups in qualitative research [Abstract]. *Communicating Nursing Research, 20, 151.*

Mishel, M.H. & Murdaugh, C. (1993). *Life after heart transplantation: Views of patients.* Annual Conference of the Southern Nursing Research Society, Birmingham, AL.

Mishel, M.H. & Portillo, C. (1991). *Use of debriefing strategy to verify the integrity of an intervention.* Conference on Qualitative Health Research, University of Alberta, Edmonton, Alberta.

Mishel, M.H. & Sorenson, D. (1990). Coping with uncertainty: A test of the uncertainty theory [Abstract]. *Communicating Nursing Research, 23, 154.*

Murdaugh, C. & Mishel, M.H. (1986). *An analysis of stages and themes in families following organ transplantation.* Second International Intensive Care Nursing Conference, The Hague, Netherlands.

Murdaugh, C. & Mishel, M.H. (1987). Generating quantitative measures from qualitatively induced concepts [Abstract]. *Communicating Nursing Research, 20, 153.*

Stewart, J.L., Mishel, M.H., Germino, B.B., Belyea, M.J., & Braden, C.J. (2001). Determining who benefits most: Looking beyond ethnicity. In M.H. Mischel (Chair),

How to improve who benefits from an intervention: The use of moderator effects. Symposium conducted at the meeting of the Southern Nursing Research Society, Baltimore, MD.

Williams, M., Mishel, M.H., & Murdaugh, C. (1987). *Substantive nursing theory: Redesigning the dream.* 20th Annual Communicating Nursing Research Conference, Western Society for Research in Nursing, Tempe, AZ.

Monographs

Mishel, M.H. (1965). Crisis theory and crisis therapy applied in a nurse-patient situation (pp. 39-46). In ANA Regional Clinical Conferences, *Exploring progress in psychiatric nursing practice* (Serial #4). New York: American Nurses Association.

Mishel, M.H. (1976). *Patient problems in self-esteem and nursing intervention.* Los Angeles: Trident Shop, California State University at Los Angeles.

Mishel, M.H. (1990). Confounding variables. In L. Sechrest, E. Perrin, & J. Bunker (Eds.), *Research methodology: Strengthening causal interpretations of nonexperimental data* (pp. 115-118). Rockville, MD: Agency for Health Care Policy and Research, Public Health Service, US Department of Health and Human Services.

Book Reviews

Mishel, M.H. (1987). [Review of the book *Annual review of nursing research* (Vol. 4)]. *Research in Nursing and Health,* 10(6), 405-406.

Mishel, M.H. (1991). [Review of the book *Multimethod research*]. *Research in Nursing and Health,* 14(2), 162-176.

Correspondence

Mishel. M.H. (2000, July). Curriculum vitae.

Research Grant Awards

Braden, C.J. (Principal Investigator) & Mishel, M.H. (Co-Principal Investigator). (1987/1988). *Antecedents of uncertainty, uncertainty appraisal and coping in patients with multiple sclerosis.* Biomedical Research Support Grant from Department of Health and Human Services, Division of Nursing, University of Arizona.

Braden, C.J. (Principal Investigator) & Mishel, M.H. (Co-investigator). (1989, May/1994, June). *Nurse interventions promoting self help response to cancer* (R01 CA48450-01A1). Grant from National Institute of Health, National Cancer Institute.

Braden, C.J. (Principal Investigator) & Mishel, M.H. (Site Principal Investigator). (1994, Sept./1998, Sept.). *Self-help in underserved women* (R01 CA64706-02). Grant from National Institutes of Health, National Cancer Institute.

Kay, M. (Principal Investigator) & Mishel, M.H. (Co-Principal Investigator). (1987, April/1990, Aug.). *Efficacy of support groups for Mexican-American widows* (R01 MH41978-01A1). Grant from National Institute of Health, National Institute of Mental Health.

Mishel, M.H. (Project Director). (1972/1973). *Integration of a nursing curriculum utilizing extended role and external degree concepts* (HEW Grant #0347823). Grant from Division of Nursing, Nursing Department, California State University at Los Angeles.

Mishel, M.H. (Principal Investigator). (1982/1983). *Analysis of the reliability and validity of the parents' perception of uncertainty in illness scale.* Dean's Research Award from College of Nursing, University of Arizona.

Mishel, M.H. (Principal Investigator). (1982/1983). *The impact of uncertainty and optimism upon adjustment in patients with gynecological cancer.* Institutional Research Grant from University of Arizona, American Cancer Society.

Mishel, M.H. (Principal Investigator). (1983/1984). *Living with uncertainty in systemic lupus erythematosus.* Grant from American Lupus Society.

Mishel, M.H. (Principal Investigator). (1983/1984, Fall). *A longitudinal investigation of psycho-social adjustment in patients with gynecological cancer.* Nurse Research Emphasis Grant from Department of Health and Human Services, Division of Nursing.

Mishel, M.H. (Principal Investigator). (1984/1985). *The impact of cognitive style on perception of and response to uncertainty during a diagnostic procedure.* Dean's Research Award from College of Nursing, University of Arizona.

Mishel, M.H. (Principal Investigator). (1984, Aug./1988, May). *Coping with uncertainty in gynecological cancer* (R01 NU/CA01103-01). Grant from National Institute of Health Center for Nursing Research.

Mishel, M.H. (Principal Investigator). (1985/1986). *Maintaining hope and managing unpredictability: Scale development and testing.* Biomedical Research Support Grant from Department of Health and Human Services, Division of Nursing, University of Arizona.

Mishel, M.H. (Principal Investigator). (1987, Oct./1988, Sept.). *Depression awareness: A training program for nurses* (1T15MH18874-01). Grant from National Institute of Health, National Institute of Mental Health.

Mishel, M.H. (Principal Investigator). (1993, Sept./1997, March). *Managing uncertainty in stage B prostate cancer* (R01 NR03782-01). Grant from National Institutes of Health, National Institute of Nursing Research/National Cancer Institute.

Mishel, M.H. (Principal Investigator). (1993, Sept./1997, Aug.). *Managing uncertainty: Self help in breast cancer* (R01 CA57764-01A2). Grant from National Institute of Health, National Cancer Institute.

Mishel, M.H. (Principal Investigator). (1994, Aug./1995, July). *Managing uncertainty: Self help in breast cancer* [Supplement] (R01 CA55164). Grant from National Institute of Health, National Cancer Institute.

Mishel, M.H. (Principal Investigator). (1995, Oct./1996, Sept.). *Supplement: Managing uncertainty in stage B prostate cancer* (R01 NR/CA03781-03). Grant from National Institutes of Health Office for Research on Minority Health.

Mishel, M.H. (Principal Investigator). (1996, Sept./2002, Aug.). *Interventions for preventing and managing chronic illness* (T32 NR07091-01). Grant from National Institutes of Health, National Institute of Nursing Research.

Mishel, M.H. (Principal Investigator). (1998, March/2002, Aug.). *Managing uncertainty in advanced prostate cancer* (R01 NR03782-05). Grant from National Institutes of Health, National Institute of Nursing Research.

Mishel, M.H. (Principal Investigator). (1999, May/2004, Feb.). *Managing uncertainty in older breast cancer survivors* (R01 CA78955-02). Grant from National Institutes of Health, National Cancer Institute.

Mishel, M.H. (Center Investigator and Core Director) & Harrell, J.S. (Principal Investigator). (1994, Sept./2004, Sept.). *Preventing/managing chronic illness in vulnerable people* (P30 NR03692). Grant from National Institutes of Health, National Institute of Nursing Research.

Mishel, M.H., Murdaugh, C., & Pergrin, J. (Co-Principal Investigators). (1983/1984). *The impact of stress on caregivers of Alzheimer's disease victims.* Dean's Research Award from College of Nursing, University of Arizona.

Mishel, M.H., Murdaugh, C., & Pergrin, J. (Recipients). (1986, Fall). *Mary Opal Wolanin award for excellence in clinical research.* Grant from University of Arizona.

Murdaugh, C. & Mishel, M.H. (Co-Principal Investigators). (1988, April/1990, Aug.). *Predictors of quality of life in heart transplantation* (R01 NR01559). Grant from National Institute of Health Center for Nursing Research.

Secondary Sources

Selected Publications Citing Mishel's Work

Acton, G.J., Irvin, B.L., & Hopkins, B.A. (1991). Theory testing research—Building the science. *Advances in Nursing Science,* 14(1), 52-61.

Admi, H. (1997). Nursing students' stress during the initial clinical experience. *Journal of Nursing Education,* 36(7), 323-327.

Affleck, G., Tennen, H., Pfeiffer, C., & Fifield, J. (1987). Appraisal of control and predictability in adapting to chronic disease. *Journal of Personality and Social Psychology,* 53(2), 273-279.

Affleck, G., Tennen, H., Pfeiffer, C., & Fifield, J. (1987). Attributional processes in rheumatoid arthritis patients. *Arthritis and Rheumatism,* 39(8), 927-931.

Afifi, W.A. & Burgoon, J.K. (1998). "We never talk about that": A comparison of cross-sex friendships and dating relationships on uncertainty and topic avoidance. *Personal Relationships,* 5(3), 255-272.

Akkasilpa, S., Minor, M., Goldman, D., Magder, L.S., & Petri, M. (2000). Association of coping responses with fibromyalgia tender points in patients with systemic lupus erythematosus. *Journal of Rheumatology,* 27(3), 671-674.

Allison, P.J., Locker, D., & Feine, J.S. (1997). Quality of life: A dynamic construct. *Science and Medicine,* 45(2), 221-230.

Alonzo, A.A. & Reynolds, N.R. (1995). Stigma, HIV and AIDS—An exploration and elaboration of a stigma trajectory. *Social Science and Medicine,* 41(3), 303-315.

Alonzo, A.A. & Reynolds, N.R. (1997). Responding to symptoms and signs of acute myocardial infarction—How do you educate the public? A social-psychologic approach to intervention. *Heart and Lung,* 26(4), 263-272.

Alonzo, A.A. & Reynolds, N.R. (1998). The structure of emotions during acute myocardial infarction: A model of coping. *Social Science and Medicine,* 46(9), 1099-1110.

Babrow, A.S. (1995). Communication and problematic integration—Kunderas, Milan lost-letters in the book of laughter and forgetting. *Communication Monographs,* 62(4), 283-300.

Babrow, A.S., Kasch, C.R., & Ford, L.A. (1998). The many meanings of uncertainty in illness: Toward a systematic accounting. *Health Communication,* 10(1), 1-23.

Badger, T.A. (1996). Family members' experiences living with members with depression. *Western Journal of Nursing Research,* 18(2), 149-171.

Barroso, J. (1997). Reconstructing my life: Becoming a long-term survivor of AIDS. *Qualitative Health Research,* 7(1), 57-74.

Barroso, J. (1997). Social support and long-term survivors of AIDS. *Western Journal of Nursing Research,* 19(5), 554-573.

Bar-Tal, Y. (1994). Monitoring, blunting, and the ability to achieve cognitive structure. *Anxiety Stress and Coping,* 6(4), 265-274.

Bar-Tal, Y. (1994). Uncertainty and the perception of sufficiency of social support, control, and information. *Psychological Record,* 44(1), 13-24.

Bar-Tal, Y., Raviv, A., & Spitzer, A. (1999). The need and ability to achieve cognitive structuring: Individual differences that moderate the effect of stress on information processing. *Journal of Personality and Social Psychology,* 77(1), 33-51.

Bennett, S.J. (1993). Relationships among selected antecedent variables and coping effectiveness in post myocardial infarction patients. *Research in Nursing and Health,* 16(2), 131-139.

Bertero, C., Eriksson, B.E., & Ek, A.C. (1997). Explaining different profiles in quality of life experiences in acute and chronic leukemia. *Cancer Nursing,* 20(2), 100-104.

Blanchard, C.G., Albrecht, T.L., Ruckdeschel, J.C., Grant, C.H., & Hemmick, R.M. (1995). The role of social support in adaptation to cancer and to survival. *Journal of Psychosocial Oncology,* 13(1-2), 75-95.

Bogart, L.M. & Helgeson, V.S. (2000). Social comparisons among women with breast cancer: A longitudinal investigation. *Journal of Applied Social Psychology,* 30(3), 547-575.

Boter, H., Mistiaen, P., & Groenewegen, I. (2000). A randomized trial of a telephone reassurance programme for patients recently discharged from an ophthalmic unit. *Journal of Clinical Nursing,* 9(2), 199-206.

Botsford, A.L. (1995). Review of literature on heart transplant recipients return to work—Predictors of outcomes. *Social Work Health Care,* 21(2), 19-39.

Braden, C.J. (1991). Learned response to chronic illness—Disability payment recipients vs. non-recipients. *Rehabilitation Psychology,* 36(4), 265-277.

Bramwell, L. & Whall, A.L. (1986). Effect of role clarity and empathy on support role performance and anxiety. *Nursing Research,* 35(5), 282-287.

Brashers, D.E., Haas, S.M., & Neidig, J.L. (1999). The patient self-advocacy scale: Measuring patient involvement in health care decision-making interactions. *Health Communication,* 11(2), 97-121.

Brashers, D.E., Neidig, J.L., Cardillo, L.W., Dobbs, L.K., Russell, J.A., & Haas, S.M. (1999). 'In an important way, I did die': Uncertainty and revival in persons living with HIV or AIDS. *AIDS Care-Psychological and Socio-Medical Aspects of AIDS/HIV,* 11(2), 201-219.

Brashers, D.E., Neidig, J.L., Haas, S.M., Dobbs, L.K., Cardillo, L.W., & Russell, J.A. (2000). Communication in the management of uncertainty: The case of persons living with HIV or AIDS. *Communication Monographs,* 67(1), 63-84.

Brown, M.A. & Powell-Cope, G.M. (1991). Aids family caregiving—Transitions through uncertainty. *Nursing Research,* 40(6), 338-345.

Browne, G.B, Byrne, C., Roberts, J., Streiner, D., Fitch, M., Corey, P., & Arpin, K. (1988). The meaning of illness questionnaire—Reliability and validity. *Nursing Research,* 37(6), 368-373.

Browne, G., Roberts, J., Gafni, A., Byrne, C., Weir, R., Majumdar, B., & Watt, S. (1999). Economic evaluations of community-based care: Lessons from twelve studies in Ontario. *Journal of Evaluation in Clinical Practice,* 5(4), 367-385.

Bunzel, B., Laederach-Hofmann, K., & Schubert, M.T. (1999). Patients benefit—Partners suffer? The impact of heart transplantation on the partner relationship. *Transplant International,* 12(1), 33-41.

Burman, M.E. (1996). Daily symptoms and responses in adults: A review. *Public Health Nursing,* 13(4), 294-301.

Callery, P. & Smith, L. (1991). A study of role negotiation between nurses and the parents of hospitalized children. *Journal of Advanced Nursing,* 16(7), 772-781.

Canning, R.D., Dew, M.A., & Davidson, S. (1996). Psychological distress among caregivers to heart transplant recipients. *Social Science and Medicine,* 42(4), 599-608.

Carlsson, M.E. & Strang, P.M. (1998). Educational support programme for gynaecological cancer patients and their families. *Acta Oncologica,* 37(3), 269-275.

Carroll, D.L., Hamilton, G.A., & McGovern, B.A. (1999). Changes in health status and quality of life and the impact of uncertainty in patients who survive life-threatening arrhythmias. *Heart and Lung,* 28(4), 251-260.

Cella, D.F., Mahon, S.M., & Donovan, M.I. (1990). Cancer recurrence as a traumatic event. *Behavioral Medicine,* 16(1), 15-22.

Cella, D.F., McCain, N.L., Peterman, A.H., Mo, F., & Wolen, D. (1996). Development and validation of the functional assessment of human immunodeficiency virus infection (FAHI) quality of life instrument. *Quality of Life Research,* 5(4), 450-463.

Christman, N.J. (1990). Uncertainty and adjustment during radiotherapy. Nursing Research, 39(1), 17-20.

Christman, N.J., McConnell, E.A., Pfeiffer, C., Webster, K.K., Schmitt, M., & Ries, J. (1988). Uncertainty, coping, and distress following myocardial infarction—Transition from hospital to home. *Research in Nursing and Health,* 11(2), 71-82.

Clark, M.S. & Smith, D.S. (1999). Changes in family functioning for stroke rehabilitation patients and their families. *International Journal of Rehabilitation Research,* 22(3), 171-179.

Clements, H. & Melby, V. (1998). An investigation into the information obtained by patients undergoing gastroscopy investigations. *Journal of Clinical Nursing,* 7(4), 333-342.

Collins, E.G., White-Williams, C., & Jalowiec, A. (1996). Impact of the heart transplant waiting process on spouses. *Journal of Heart and Lung Transplantation,* 15(6), 623-630.

Collins, E.G., White-Williams, C., & Jalowiec, A. (1996). Spouse stressors while awaiting heart transplantation. *Heart and Lung,* 25(1), 4-13.

Conger, C.O. & Marshall, E.S. (1998). Recreating life: Toward a theory of relationship development in acute home care. *Qualitative Health Research,* 8(4), 526-546.

Cormier-Daigle, M. & Stewart, M. (1997). Support and coping of male hemodialysis-dependent patients. *International Journal of Nursing Studies,* 34(6), 420-430.

Cox, K. (1998). Investigating psychosocial aspects of participation in early anti-cancer drug trials: Towards a choice of methodology. *Journal of Advanced Nursing,* 27(3), 488-496.

Craven, J.L., Bright, J., & Dear, C.L. (1990). Psychiatric, psychosocial, and rehabilitative aspects of lung transplantation. *Clinics in Chest Medicine,* 11(2), 247-257.

Crigger, N.J. (1996). Testing an uncertainty model for women with multiple sclerosis. *Advances in Nursing Science,* 18(3), 37-47.

Deane, K.A. & Degner, L.F. (1998). Information needs, uncertainty, and anxiety in women who had a breast biopsy with benign outcome. *Cancer Nursing,* 21(2), 117-126.

Delude, D., Wright, J., & Belanger, C. (2000). The effects of pregnancy complications on the parental adaptation process. *Journal of Reproductive and Infant Psychology,* 18(1), 5-20.

Dew, M.A., Roth, L.H., Schulberg, H.C. Simmons, R.G., Kormos, R.L. Trzepacz, P., & Griffith, B.P. (1996). Prevalence and predictors of depression and anxiety-related disorders during the year after heart transplantation. *General Hospital Psychiatry,* 18(6, Suppl), 48S-61S.

Dew, M.A., Simmons, R.G., Schulber, H.C., Armitage, J.M., & Griffith, B.P. (1994). Psychosocial predictors of vulnerability to distress in the year following heart transplantation. *Psychological Medicine,* 24(4), 929-945.

Dias, L. & Lobel, M. (1997). Social comparison in medically high-risk pregnant women. *Journal of Applied Psychology,* 27(18), 1629-1649.

DiIorio, C., Faherty, B., & Manteuffel, B. (1991). Cognitive perceptual factors associated with antiepileptic medication compliance. *Research in Nursing and Health,* 14(5), 329-338.

Dikken, C. & Sitzia, J. (1998). Patients' experiences of chemotherapy: Side-effects associated with 5-fluorouracil plus folinic acid in the treatment of colorectal cancer. *Journal of Clinical Nursing,* 7(4), 371-379.

Dluhy, N.M. (1995). Mapping knowledge in chronic illness. *Journal of Advanced Nursing,* 21(6), 1051-1058.

Dougherty, C.M. & Shaver, J.F. (1995). Psychological responses after sudden cardiac arrest during hospitalization. *Applied Nursing Research,* 8(4), 160-168.

Edwards, J.R. & O'Neill, R.M. (1998). The construct validity of scores on the ways of coping questionnaire: Confirmatory analysis of alternative factor structures. *Educational and Psychological Measurement,* 58(6), 955-983.

Ell, K. (1996). Social networks, social support and coping with serious illness: The family connection. *Social Science and Medicine,* 42(2), 173-183.

Failla, S., Kuper, B.C., Nick, T.G., & Lee, F.A. (1996). Adjustment of women with systemic lupus erythematosus. *Applied Nursing Research,* 9(2), 87-93.

Floyd, J.A., Falahee, M.L., & Fhobir, R.H. (1999). The use of the arcs software system to store and examine sleep research results. *Computers in Nursing,* 17(6), 259-268.

Ford, L.A., Babrow, A.S., & Stohl, C. (1996). Social support messages and the management of uncertainty in the experience of breast cancer: An application of problematic integration theory. *Communication Monographs,* 63(3), 189-207.

Ford, L.A. & Ellis, B.H. (1998). A preliminary analysis of memorable support and nonsupport messages received by nurses in acute care settings. *Health Communication,* 10(1), 37-63.

Fukui, S., Kamiya, M., Koike, M., Kugaya, A., Okamura, H., Nakanishi, T., Imoto, S., Kanagawa, K., & Uchitomi, Y. (2000). Applicability of a western-developed psychosocial group intervention for Japanese patients with primary breast cancer. *Psycho-Oncology,* 9(2), 169-177.

Galbraith, M.E. (1995). What kind of social support do cancer patients get from nurses. *Cancer Nursing,* 18(5), 362-367.

Galloway, S.C. & Graydon, J.E. (1996). Uncertainty, symptom distress, and information needs after surgery for cancer of the colon. *Cancer Nursing,* 19(2), 112-117.

Galloway, S., Graydon, J., Harrison, D., Evans-Boyden, B., Palmer-Wickham, S., Burlein-Hall, S., Richvander-Bij, L., West, P., & Blair, A. (1997). Informational needs of women with a recent diagnosis of breast cancer: Development and initial testing of a tool. *Journal of Advanced Nursing,* 25(6), 1175-1183.

Gambrill, E., Florain, V., & Splaver, G. (1986). Assertion, loneliness, and perceived control among students with and without physical disabilities. *Rehabilitation Counseling Bulletin,* 30(1), 4-12.

Glueckauf, R.L. & Quittner, A.L. (1992). Assertiveness training for disabled adults in wheelchairs—Self-report, role-play, and activity patterns outcomes. *Journal of Consulting and Clinical Psychology,* 60(3), 419-425.

Good, M. & Moore, S.M. (1996). Clinical practice guidelines as a new source of middle-range theory: Focus on acute pain. *Nursing Outlook,* 44(2), 74-79.

Gortner, S.R. (2000). Knowledge development in nursing: Our historical roots and future opportunities. *Nursing Outlook,* 48(2), 60-67.

Gross, S.M., Ireys, H.T., & Kinsman, S.L. (2000). Young women with physical disabilities: Risk factors for symptoms of eating disorders. *Journal of Developmental and Behavioral Pediatrics,* 21(2), 87-96.

Gulanick, M., Bliley, A., Perino, B., & Keough, V. (1998). Recovery patterns and lifestyle changes after coronary angioplasty: The patient's perspective. *Heart and Lung,* 27(4), 253-262.

Haase, J.E., Heiney, S.P., Ruccione, K.S., & Stutzer, C. (1999). Research triangulation to derive meaning-based quality-of-life theory: Adolescent Resilience Model and instrument development. *International Journal of Cancer,* 12(Suppl), 125-131.

Harvey, J. (1996). Achieving the indeterminate: Accomplishing degrees of certainty in life and death situations. *Sociological Review,* 44(1), 78-98.

Harvey, S. (1993). The genesis of a phenomenological approach to advanced nursing practice. *Journal of Advanced Nursing,* 18(4), 526-530.

Hawley, G. (1998). Facing uncertainty and possible death: The Christian patients' experience. *Journal of Clinical Nursing,* 7(5), 467-478.

Hays, B.J., Norris, J., Martin, K.S., & Androwich, I. (1994). Informatics issues for nursing future. *Advances in Nursing Science,* 16(4), 71-81.

Helgeson, V.S., Cohen, S., Schulz, R., & Yasko, J. (1999). Education and peer discussion group interventions and adjustment to breast cancer. *Archives of General Psychiatry,* 56(4), 340-347.

Helgeson, V.S., Cohen, S., Schulz, R., & Yasko, J. (2000). Group support interventions for women with breast cancer: Who benefits from what? *Health Psychology,* 19(2), 107-114.

Hicks, F.D., Larson, J.L., & Ferrans, C.E. (1992). Quality of life after liver transplant. *Research in Nursing and Health,* 15(2), 111-119.

Hilton, B.A. (1989). The relationship of uncertainty, control, commitment, and threat of recurrence to coping strategies used by women diagnosed with breast cancer. *Journal of Behavioral Medicine,* 12(1), 39-54.

Holmes, B.C. (1987). Psychological evaluation and preparation of the patient and family. *Cancer,* 60(8), 2021-2024.

Holmes, S. (1997). The maintenance of health during radiotherapy: a nursing perspective. *Journal of the Royal Society of Health,* 117(6), 393-399.

Horner, S.D. (1997). Uncertainty in mothers' care for their ill children. *Journal of Advanced Nursing,* 26(4), 658-663.

Horstman, L. & Erdman, R.A.M. (1990). Psychological aspects of heart transplantation—An exploration. *Gedrag and Gezondheid,* 18(1), 5-13.

Hughes, K.K. (1993). Psychosocial and functional status of breast cancer patients—The influence of diagnosis and treatment choice. *Cancer Nursing,* 16(3), 222-229.

Janson-Bjerklie, S., Ferketich, S., & Benner, P. (1993). Predicting the outcomes of living with asthma. *Research in Nursing and Health,* 16(4), 241-250.

Joiner, J.G., Lovett, P.S., & Goodwin, L.K. (1989). Positive assertion and acceptance among person with disabilities. *Journal of Rehabilitation,* 55(3), 22-29.

Jonsen, E., Athlin, E., & Suhr, O.B. (1999). Waiting for a liver transplant: The experience of patients with familial amyloidotic polyneuropathy. *Journal of Clinical Nursing,* 9(1), 63-70.

Katz, P.P. (1998). The stresses of rheumatoid arthritis: Appraisals of perceived impact and coping efficacy. *Arthritis Care and Research,* 11(1), 9-22.

Kavanagh, T., Yacoub, M.H., Kennedy, J., & Austin, P.C. (1999). Return to work after heart transplantation: 12-year follow-up. *Journal of Heart and Lung Transplantation,* 18(9), 846-851.

Kendall, E. & Terry, D.J. (1996). Psychosocial adjustment following closed head injury: A model for understanding individual differences and predicting outcome. *Neuropsychological Rehabilitation,* 6(2), 101-132.

Kessler, T.A. (1998). The cognitive appraisal of health scale: Development and psychometric evaluation. *Research in Nursing and Health,* 21(1), 73-82.

King, F.E., Figge, J., & Harman, P. (1986). The elderly coping at home—A study of continuity of nursing care. *Journal of Advanced Nursing,* 11(1), 41-46.

Kirk, K. (1992). Confidence as a factor in chronic illness care. *Journal of Advanced Nursing,* 17(10), 1238-1242.

Knafl, K.A. & Howard, M.J. (1984). Interpreting and reporting qualitative research. *Research in Nursing and Health,* 7(1), 17-24.

Konstam, V., Surman, O., Hizzazi, K.H., Fierstein, J., Konstam, M., Turbett, A., Dec, G.W., Keck, S., Mudge, G., Flavell, C., McCormack, M., & Hurley, L. (1998). Marital adjustment in heart transplantation patients and their spouses: A longitudinal perspective. *American Journal of Family Therapy,* 26(2), 147-158.

Kristensson-Hallstrom, I., Elander, G., & Malmfors, G. (1997). Increased parental participation in a paediatric surgical day-care unit. *Journal of Clinical Nursing,* 6(4), 297-302.

Kristensson-Hallstrom, I. & Nilstun, T. (1997). The parent between the child and the professional—Some ethical implications. *Child Care Health and Development,* 23(6), 447-455.

Kroencke, D.C. & Denney, D.R. (1999). Stress and coping in multiple sclerosis: Exacerbation, remission and chronic subgroups. *Multiple Sclerosis,* 5(2), 89-93.

Kroenke, K., Taylor-Vaisey, A., Dietrich, A.J., & Oxman, T.E. (2000). Interventions to improve provider diagnosis and treatment of mental disorders in primary care—A critical review of the literature. *Psychomatics,* 41(1), 39-52.

Kulbok, P.A., Baldwin, J.H., Cox, C.L., & Duffy, R. (1997). Advancing discourse on health promotion: Beyond mainstream thinking. *Advances in Nursing Science,* 29(1), 12-20.

Lamb, G.S. & Stempel, J.E. (1994). Nurse case-management from the clients view—Growing as insider-expert. *Nursing Outlook,* 42(1), 7-13.

Latimer, E.J., Crabb, M.R., Roberts, J.G., Ewen, M., & Roberts, J. (1998). the patient care travelling record (c) in palliative care: Effectiveness and efficiency. *Journal of Pain and Symptom Management,* 16(1), 41-51.

Lauver, D.R., Kruse, K., & Baggot, A. (1999). Women's uncertainties, coping, and moods regarding abnormal papanicolaou results. *Journal of Women's Health and Gender-Based Medicine,* 8(8), 1103-1112.

LeFort, S.M., Gray-Donald, K., Rowat, K.M., & Jeans, M.E. (1998). Randomized controlled trial of a community-based psychoeducation program for the self-management of chronic pain. *Pain,* 74(2-3), 297-306.

Leidy, N.K., Rentz, A.M., & Zyczynski, T.M. (1999). Evaluating health-related quality-of-life outcomes in patients with congestive heart failure—A review of recent randomized controlled trials. *Pharmacoeconomics,* 15(1), 19-46.

Leith, B.A. (1999). Patients' and family members' perceptions of transfer from intensive care. *Heart and Lung,* 28(3), 210-218.

Lemaire, G.S. & Lenz, E.R. (1995). Perceived uncertainty about menopause in women attending an educational program. *International Journal of Nursing Studies,* 32(1), 39-48.

Lenz, E.R., Suppe, F., Gift, A.G., Pugh, L.C., & Milligan, R.A. (1995). Collaborative development of middle-range nursing theories—Toward a theory of unpleasant symptoms. *Advances in Nursing Science,* 17(3), 1-13.

Lev, E.L., Paul, D., & Owen, S.V. (1999). Age, self-efficacy, and change in patients' adjustment to cancer. *Cancer Practice,* 7(4) 170-176.

Lewis, F.M. (1997). Behavioral research to enhance adjustment and quality of life among adults with cancer. *Preventive Medicine,* 26(5), S19-S29.

Liehr, P. & Smith, M.J. (1999). Middle range theory: Spinning research and practice to create knowledge for the new millennium. *Advances in Nursing Science,* 21(4), 81-91.

Lin, L.C., Snyder, M., & Egan, E.C. (1996). The development of Taiwanese elderly stressor inventory. *International Journal of Nursing Studies,* 33(1), 29-36.

Livneh, H. (2000). Psychosocial adaptation to cancer: The role of coping strategies. *Journal Rehabilitation,* 16(2), 40-49.

LoBiondo-Wood, G., Williams, L., Wood, R.P., & Shaw, B.W. (1997). Impact of liver transplantation on quality of life: A longitudinal perspective. *Applied Nursing Research,* 10(1), 27-32.

Lok, P. (1996). Stressors, coping mechanisms and quality of life among dialysis patients in Australia. *Journal of Advanced Nursing,* 23(5), 873-881.

Lyle, C.M. & Wells, D.L. (1997). Description of a self-care instrument for elders. *Western Journal of Nursing Research,* 19(5), 637-653.

Manninen, E. (1998). Changes in nursing students' perceptions of nursing as they progress through their education. *Journal of Advanced Nursing,* 27(2), 390-398.

Manninen, E. (1999). Longitudinal study of Finnish nursing students' preferences for knowledge in nursing practice. *Scandinavian Journal of Caring Sciences,* 13(2), 83-90.

Margalith, I. & Shapiro, A. (1997). Anxiety and patient participation in clinical decision-making: The case of patients with ureteral calculi. *Social Science and Medicine,* 45(3), 419-427.

Mason, P.J., Olson, R.A., Myers, J.G., Huszti, H.C., & Kenning, M. (1989). AIDS and hemophilia—Implications for interventions with families. *Journal of Pediatric Psychology,* 14(3), 341-355.

Mast, M.E. (1998). Correlates of fatigue in survivors of breast cancer. *Cancer Nursing,* 21(2), 136-142.

Mast, M.E. (1998). Survivors of breast cancer: Illness uncertainty, positive reappraisal, and emotional distress. *Oncology Nursing Forum,* 25, 555-562.

Mathews, R.M. & Seekins, T. (1987). An interactional model of independence. *Rehabilitation Psychology,* 32(3), 165-172.

McCain, N.L. & Cella, D.F. (1995). Correlates of stress in HIV disease. *Western Journal of Nursing Research,* 17(2), 141-155.

McCain, N.L., Zeller, J.M., Cella, D.F., Urbanski, P.A., & Novak, R.M. (1996). The influence of stress management training in HIV disease. *Nursing Research,* 45(4), 246-253.

Meyer, E.C., DeMaso, D.R., & Koocher, G.P. (1996). Mental health consultation in the pediatric intensive care unit. *Profession Psychology-Research and Practice,* 27(2), 130-136.

Miles, M.S., Funk, S.G., & Kasper, M.A. (1992). The stress response of mothers and fathers of pre-term infants. *Research in Nursing and Health,* 15(4), 261-269.

Milliken, P.J. & Northcott, H.C. (1996). Seeking validation: Hypothyroidism and the chronic illness trajectory. *Qualitative Health Research,* 6(2), 202-223.

Mills, M.E. & Sullivan, K. (1999). The importance of information giving for patients newly diagnosed with cancer: A review of the literature. *Journal of Clinical Nursing,* 8(6), 631-642.

Morse, J.M. (1997). Responding to threats to integrity of self. *Advances in Nursing Science,* 19(4), 21-36.

Moser, D.K., Clements, P.J., Brecht, M.L., & Weiner, S.R. (1993). Predictors of psychosocial adjustment in systemic sclerosis—The influence of formal education level, functional ability, hardiness, uncertainty, and social support. *Arthritis and Rheumatism,* 36(10), 1398-1405.

Moser, D.K., Dracup, K.A., & Marsden, C. (1993). Needs of recovering cardiac patients and their spouses—Compared views. *International Journal of Nursing Studies,* 30(2), 105-114.

Mu, P.F. & Tomlinson, P. (1997). Parental experience and meaning construction during a pediatric health crisis. *Western Journal of Nursing Research,* 19(5), 608-628.

Mullins, L.L., Chaney, J.M., Pace, T.M., & Hartman, V.L. (1997). Illness uncertainty, attributional style, and psychological adjustment in older adolescents and young adults with asthma. *Journal of Pediatric Psychology,* 22(6), 871-880.

Murdach, A.D. (1995). Decision-making situations in health-care. *Health and Social Work,* 29(3), 187-191.

Mushlin, A.I., Mooney, C., Grow, V., & Phelps, C.E. (1994). The value of diagnostic information to patients with suspected multiple sclerosis. *Archives of Neurology,* 51(1), 67-72.

Nelson, J.P. (1996). Struggling to gain meaning: Living with the uncertainty of breast cancer. *Advances in Nursing Science,* 18(3), 59-76.

Nimbocks, M.J.A., Webb, L., & Connell, J.R. (1987). Communication and the terminally ill—A theoretical model. *Death Studies,* 11(5), 323-344.

Northouse, L.L. (1988). Social support in patients and husbands adjustment to breast cancer. *Nursing Research,* 37(2), 91-95.

Northouse, L.L., Dorris, G., & Charronmoore, C. (1995). Factors affecting couples adjustment to recurrent breast cancer. *Social Science and Medicine,* 41(1), 69-76.

Northouse, L.L., Jeffs, M., Cracchiolo-Caraway, A., Lampman, L., & Dorris, G. (1995). Emotional distress reported by women and husbands prior to a breast biopsy. *Nursing Research,* 44(4), 196-201.

Northouse, L.L., Laten, D., & Reddy, P. (1995). Adjustment of women and their husbands to recurrent breast cancer. *Research in Nursing and Health,* 18(6), 515-524.

Northouse, L.L., Mood, D., Templin, T., Mellon, S., & George, T. (2000). Couples' patterns of adjustment to colon cancer. *Social Science and Medicine,* 50(2), 271-284.

Northouse, L.L., Templin, T., Mood, D., & Oberst, M. (1998). Couples' adjustment to breast cancer and benign breast disease: A longitudinal analysis. *Psycho-Oncology,* 7(1), 37-48.

Nussbaum, P.D. & Goldstein, G. (1992). Neuropsychological sequelae of heart transplantation—A preliminary review. *Clinical Psychology Review,* 12(5), 475-483.

O'Conner, P., Detsky, A.S., Tansey, C., & Kucharczyk, W. (1994). Effect of diagnostic testing for multiple sclerosis on patient health perceptions. *Archives in Neurology,* 51(1), 46-51.

Onega, L.L. (1991). A theoretical framework for psychiatric nursing practice. *Journal of Advanced Nursing,* 16(1), 68-73.

Penticuff, J.H. (1991). Conceptual issues in nursing ethics research. *Journal of Medicine and Philosophy,* 16(3), 235-258.

Poole, K. (1997). The emergence of the 'waiting game': A critical examination of the psychosocial issues in diagnosing breast cancer. *Journal of Advanced Nursing,* 25(2), 273-281.

Powell-Cope, G.M. (1995). The experiences of gay couples affected by HIV- infection. *Qualitative Health Research,* 5(1), 36-62.

Rendle, K. (1997). Survivorship and breast cancer: The psychosocial issues. *Journal of Clinical Issues,* 6(5), 403-410.

Richardson, J.L., Marks, G., Johnson, C.A., Grahm, J.W., Chan, K.K., Selser, J.N., Kisbaugh, C., Barranday, Y., & Levine, A. (1987). Path model of multidimensional compliance with cancer therapy. *Health Psychology,* 6(3), 183-207.

Rimer, B., Keintz, M.K., & Glassman, B. (1985). Cancer patient education—Reality and potential. *Preventive Medicine,* 14(6), 801-818.

Ronayne, R. (1985). Feelings and attitudes during early convalescence following vascular surgery. *Journal of Advanced Nursing,* 10(5), 435-441.

Rowat, K.M. & Knafl, K.A. (1985). Living with chronic pain—The spouses perspective. *Pain,* 23(3), 259-271.

Ryan, K.A. (1993). Mothers of adult children with schizophrenia—An ethnographic study. *Schizophrenia Research,* 11(1), 21-31.

Sandelowski, M. (1993). Toward a theory of technology dependency. *Nursing Outlook,* 41(1), 36-42.

Schepp, K.G. (1991). Factors influencing the coping effort of mothers of hospitalized children. *Nursing Research,* 40(1), 42-46.

Serovich, J.M. & Mosack, K.E. (2000). Training issues for supervisors of marriage and family therapists working with persons living with HIV. *Journal of Marital and Family Therapy,* 26(1), 103-111.

Siegel, D. & Morse, J.M. (1994). Tolerating reality—The experience of parents of HIV positive sons. *Social Science and Medicine,* 38(7), 959-971.

Siegel, K., Dean, L., & Schrimshaw, E.W. (1999). Symptom ambiguity among late-middle-aged and older adults with HIV. *Research on Aging,* 21(4), 595-618.

Sitzia, J. (1999). How valid and reliable are patient satisfaction data? An analysis of 195 studies. *International Journal for Quality in Health Care,* 11(4), 319-328.

Sitzia, J. & Huggins, L. (1998). Side effects of cyclophosphamide, methotrexate, and 5- fluorouracil (CMF) chemotherapy for breast cancer. *Cancer Practice,* 6(1),13-21.

Sitzia, J., North, C., Stanley, J., & Winterberg, N. (1997). Side effects of CHOP in the treatment of non-Hodgkin's lymphoma. *Cancer Nursing,* 20(6), 430-439.

Small, S.P. & Graydon, J.E. (1993). Uncertainty in hospitalized patients with chronic obstructive pulmonary disease. *International Journal of Nursing Studies,* 30(3), 239-246.

Smyth, K. & Yarandi, H.N. (1996). Factor analysis of the ways of coping questionnaire for African American women. *Nursing Research,* 45(1), 25-29.

Spearman, S.A., Duldt, B.W. & Brown, S. (1993). Research testing theory—A selective review of Orem self-care theory, 1986-1991. *Journal of Advanced Nursing,* 18(10), 1626-1631.

Spitzer, A., Bartal, Y., & Golander, H. (1995). Social support—How does it really work. *Journal of Advanced Nursing, 22*(5), 850-854.

Sprangers, M.A.G. & Schwartz, C.E. (1999). Integrating response shift into health-related quality of life research: A theoretical model. *Social Science and Medicine, 48*(11), 1507-1515.

Steele, R.G., Tripp, G., Kotchick, B.A., Summers, P., & Forehand, R. (1997). Family members' uncertainty about parental chronic illness: The relationship of hemophilia and HIV infection to child functioning. *Journal of Pediatric Psychology, 22*(4), 577-591.

Stephenson, C. (1991). The concept of hope revisited for nursing. *Journal of Advanced Nursing, 16*(12), 1456-1461.

Stetz, K.M., Lewis, F.M., & Houck, G.M. (1994). Family goals as indicants of adaptation during chronic illness. *Public Health Nursing, 11*(6), 385-391.

Stewart, M.J., Hart, G., & Mann, K.V. (1995). Living with hemophilia and HIV/AIDS—Support and coping. *Journal of Advanced Nursing, 22*(6), 1101-1111.

Stull, D.E., Starling, R., Haas, G., & Young, J.B. Becoming a patient with heart failure. *Heart and Lung, 28*(4), 284-292.

Suominen, T. (1993). How do nurses assess the information received by breast cancer patients. *Journal of Advanced Nursing, 18*(1), 64-68.

Suominen, T., Leinokilpi, H., & Laippala, P. (1994). Nurses role in informing breast cancer patients—A comparison between patient and nurses opinions. *Journal of Advanced Nursing, 19*(1), 6-11.

Sweet, L., Savoie, J.A., & Lemyre, L. (1999). Appraisals, coping, and stress in breast cancer screening: A longitudinal investigation of causal structure. *Canadian Journal of Behavioural Science-Revue Canadienne des Sciences du Comportement, 31*(4), 240-253.

Thomas, M.L. (1998). Quality of life and psychosocial adjustment in patients with myelodysplastic syndromes. *Leukemia Research, 22,* S41-S47.

Thorne, S.E. (1999). The science of meaning in chronic illness. *International Journal of Nursing Studies, 36*(5), 397-404.

Tollett, J.H. & Thomas, S.P. (1995). A theory-based nursing intervention to instill hope in homeless veterans. *Advances in Nursing Science, 18*(2), 76-90.

Tope, D.M., Ahles, T.A., & Silberfarb, P.M. (1993). Psychooncology-psychological well-being as one component of quality of life. *Psychotherapy and Psychosomatics, 60*(3-4), 129-147.

Verran, J.A., Mark, B.A., & Lamb, G. (1992). Focus on psychometrics—Psychometric examination of instruments using aggregated data. *Research in Nursing and Health, 15*(3), 237-240.

Webster, D.C. (1996). Sex, lies, and stereotypes: Women and interstitial cystitis. *Journal of Sex Research, 33*(3), 197-203.

Weinstein, C.L. (1985). Assertiveness, anxiety, and interpersonal discomfort among amputees—Implications for assertiveness training. *Archives of Physical Medicine and Rehabilitation, 66*(10), 687-689.

Weitz, R. (1989). Uncertainty and the lives of persons with AIDS. *Journal of Health and Social Behavior, 30*(3), 270-281.

Wineman, N.M. (1990). Adaptation to multiple sclerosis—The role of social support, functional disability, and perceived uncertainty. *Nursing Research, 39*(5), 294-299.

Wineman, N.M., Durand, E.J., & McCullouch, B.J. (1994). Examination of the factor structure of the ways of coping questionnaire with clinical populations. *Nursing Research, 43*(5), 268-273.

Wineman, N.M., Durand, E.J., & Steiner, R.P. (1994). A comparative analysis of coping behaviors in persons with multiple sclerosis or a spinal cord injury. *Research in Nursing and Health, 17*(3), 185-194.

Wineman, N.M., Schwetz, K.M., Goodkin, D.E., Rudick, R.A. (1996). Relationships among illness uncertainty, stress, coping, and emotional well-being at entry into a clinical drug trial. *Applied Nursing Research, 9*(2), 53-60.

Winslow, B. & Obrien, R. (1992). Use of formal community resources by spouse caregivers of chronically ill adults. *Public Health Nursing, 9*(2), 128-132.

Wong, C.A. & Bramwell, L. (1992). Uncertainty and anxiety after mastectomy for breast cancer. *Cancer Nursing, 15*(5), 363-371.

Younger, J.B. (1991). A theory of mastery. *Advances in Nursing Science, 14*(1), 76-89.

Younger, J.B. (1993). Development and testing of the mastery of stress instrument. *Nursing Research, 42*(2), 68-73.

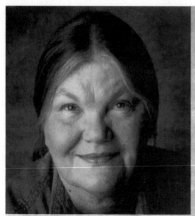

CHAPTER

31

*M*argaret A. Newman

(Photo credit: Marc Norberg, Minneapolis, Minnesota.)

Model of Health

Janet M. Witucki

CREDENTIALS AND BACKGROUND OF THE THEORIST

Margaret A. Newman was born on October 10, 1933 in Memphis, Tennessee.[80] She earned her first bachelor's degree in home economics and English from Baylor University in Waco, Texas in 1954 and she earned her second bachelor's degree in nursing from the University of Tennessee in Memphis in 1962.[47]

Newman received her master's degree in medical-surgical nursing and teaching from the University of California, San Francisco in 1964. She earned her Ph.D. in nursing science and rehabilitation nursing in 1971 from New York University in New York City.

Newman progressed through the academic ranks at the University of Tennessee, New York University, and Pennsylvania State University and was a professor at the University of Minnesota in Minneapolis until her retirement in 1996. She has been Professor Emeritus at the University of Minnesota since 1996.[53] In addition, she has been the director of nursing for the Clinical Research Center at the University of Tennessee, the acting director of the Ph.D. program in the Division of Nursing at New York University, and Professor-in-Charge of the Graduate Program and Research at Pennsylvania State University.

Newman was admitted to the American Academy of Nursing in 1976. She received the Outstanding Alumnus Award from the University of Tennessee College of Nursing in Memphis in 1975, the Distinguished Alumnus Award from the Division of Nursing at New York University in 1984, and she was admitted to the Hall of Fame at the University of Mississippi School of Nursing in 1988.[53] She was a Latin-American Teaching Fellow in 1976 and 1977

Previous authors: Snehlata Desai, M. Jan Keffer, DeAnn M. Hensley, Kimberly A. Kilgore-Keever, Jill Vass Langfitt, and LaPhyllis Peterson.
The author wishes to thank Margaret A. Newman for reviewing the chapter.

and an *American Journal of Nursing* Scholar in 1979. She was Distinguished Faculty at the Seventh International Conference on Human Functioning at Wichita, Kansas in 1983, she received the E. Louis Grant Award for Nursing Excellence from the University of Minnesota in 1996, and she is listed in *Who's Who in American Women, Who's Who in America,* and *Who's Who in American Nursing.*[80,81] Newman was included as one of the featured nursing theorists in the videotape series sponsored by Helene Fuld Health Trust in 1990.[53] She was a Distinguished Resident at Westminster College in Salt Lake City, Utah in 1991; she received the Distinguished Scholar in Nursing, New York University Division of Nursing in 1992, the Sigma Theta Tau Founders Elizabeth McWilliams Miller Award for Excellence in Research in 1993, and the Nurse Scholar Award at Saint Xavier University School of Nursing in 1994.[48,53]

In 1978, Newman presented her ideas on a theory of health for the first time at a conference on nursing theory in New York. During that time, she was also pursuing research on the relationship of movement, time, and consciousness and was expanding development of the Theory of Health as Expanding Consciousness.

In 1985, as a Traveling Research Fellow, Newman[35] conducted workshops in four locations throughout New Zealand. At the University of Tampere, Finland in 1985, Newman[35] was the major speaker for a week-long conference on the Theory of Consciousness as it related to nursing.

Newman has presented many papers on topics pertaining to her Theory of Health as Expanding Consciousness. She published *Theory Development in Nursing*[29] in 1979, *Health as Expanding Consciousness* in 1986[32] and 1994,[43] and *A Developing Discipline: Selected Works of Margaret Newman*[44] in 1995. She has written numerous articles in journals and book chapters. In 1986, she did a case-study analysis of practice in three sites within the Minneapolis-St. Paul area in which she discussed the background of the healthcare system, findings within each site, and conclusions concerning the changes necessary for hospital nursing practice.[56] From 1986 to 1997, Newman[46,59] investigated sequential patterns of per-

sons with heart disease and cancer. Her more recent publications reflect her passion for integration of nursing theory, practice, and research. Her evolving viewpoints on trends in philosophy of nursing, analysis of theoretical models of nursing practice, and nursing research are noteworthy.[42,51,52]

During 1989 and 1990, Newman was the principal investigator of a project that explored the theory and structure of a professional model of nursing practice. This research was conducted at Carondelet St. Mary's Community Hospitals and Health Centers in Tucson, Arizona.[39,58]

In addition to her research and teaching, Newman is sought for consultation regarding the expansion her theory of health in over 40 states and Australia, Brazil, Canada, Finland, Germany, Japan, New Zealand, and the United Kingdom.[41] Newman has served on several editorial boards, including *Nursing Research, Western Journal of Nursing Research, Nursing and Health Care, Advances in Nursing Science,* and *Nursing Science Quarterly.*[41] She also participated as a member of the nurse-theorist task force from 1978 to 1982 with the North American Nursing Diagnosis Association (NANDA).

RELATIONSHIP TO METAPARADIGM CONCEPTS

Nursing's metaparadigm concepts of nursing, person, health, and environment were not explicitly defined in the 1986[32] or 1994[43] editions of *Health as Expanding Consciousness.* Newman[50,51,52] has since elaborated on some of the metaparadigm concepts, particularly nursing and health, in subsequent works. In the following paragraphs, implicit definitions from Newman's earlier works, plus material from Newman's later works, are used to discuss the four nursing components.

Nursing

From the Newman perspective, nursing is the study of "caring in the human health experience."[60:3] The role of the nurse in this experience is to help clients recognize their own patterns.[37] Intervention is a form of *nonintervention* whereby the nurse's presence assists clients to recognize their own patterns of interacting with the environment.[55] Insight into these patterns provides clients with illumination of action possibilities, which then opens the way for transformation to occur.[37]

The nurse facilitates pattern recognition in clients by forming relationships with clients at critical points in their lives and rhythmically connecting with them in an authentic way. The nurse-client relationship is characterized by "a rhythmic coming together and moving apart as clients encounter disruption of their organized, predictable state and moving through disorganization and unpredictability to a higher, organized state."[52:228] The nurse comes together with clients at these critical choice points in their lives and participates with them in the process of expanding consciousness. The relationship is one of rhythmicity and timing with the nurse letting go of the need to direct the relationship or *fix* things. As the nurse relinquishes the need to manipulate or control, there is a greater ability to enter into this fluctuating, rhythmic partnership with the client.[52]

Nurses are seen as partners in the process of expanding consciousness. The nurse can connect with the person when an understanding of changing circumstances is sought.[55] As a facilitator, the nurse helps an individual, family, or community focus on his or her pattern.[32] The nursing process is one of pattern recognition.

Newman's early suggestion[45] was that the NANDA health assessment framework, based on unitary person-environment patterns of interaction, be used to facilitate clients' pattern recognition. These nine patterns of interaction consist of dimensions of (1) choosing, (2) communicating, (3) exchanging, (4) feeling, (5) knowing, (6) moving, (7) perceiving, (8) relating, and (9) valuing.[67] At the time, the patterns were intended to guide nurses to make holistic observations of "person-environment behaviors that together depict a very specific pattern of the whole for each person."[45:261] Newman[55] has since emphasized concentrating on what is most meaningful to clients in their own stories and patterns of relating. Descriptions of the evolving pattern

of the person are presented as sequential patterns over time.[38]

"Pattern recognition comes from within the observer."[34:38] The nurse perceives the patterns of the set of data or sequence of events and the pattern of the individual changes with the new information. The process of pattern recognition first involves an attempt to view the pattern of a person as "sequential patterns over time."[34:38] Follow-up interviews are conducted next to share the nurse researcher's perspective with the client. The nurse can use this process to identify the client's pattern and point individuals towards action possibilities.[34]

Person

Throughout Newman's work, the terms *client, patient, person, individual,* and *human being* are used interchangeably. Person is defined as *consciousness.* Persons as individuals are identified by their individual patterns of consciousness.[32] Persons are further defined as "centers of consciousness within an overall pattern of expanding consciousness."[32:31] The definition of persons has also been expanded to include family and community.[32,43]

Environment

Environment is not explicitly defined, but it is described as being the larger whole, which is beyond the consciousness of the individual. The pattern of consciousness that is the person interacts within the pattern of consciousness that is the family and within the pattern of community interactions.[32] A major assumption is that "consciousness is coextensive in the universe and resides in all matter."[32:33]

Newman identifies interactions between person and environment as a key process that creates unique configurations for each individual. Patterns of person-environment evolve to higher levels of consciousness of the self. The assumption is that all matter in the universe-environment possesses consciousness, but at different levels. Interpretation of Newman's view clarifies that it is the interaction pattern of a person with the environment. Disease

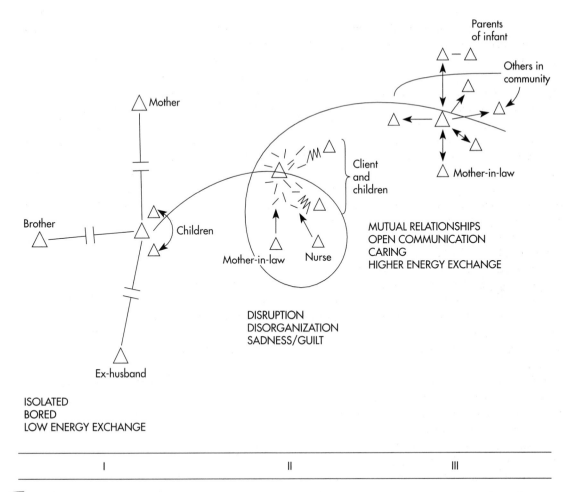

Figure **31-1** Sequential patterns of person-environment relations. (From Newman, M.A. [1987]. Nursing's emerging paradigm: The diagnosis of pattern. In A.M. McLane [Ed.], *Classification of nursing diagnoses: Proceedings of the seventh conference.* St. Louis: Mosby.)

in a human energy field is a manifestation of a unique pattern of person-environment interaction (Figure 31-1).

Health

Health is the major concept of Newman's Theory of Expanding Consciousness. A fusion of disease and nondisease creates a synthesis that is regarded as health.[28,29] Disease and nondisease are each reflections of the larger whole; therefore a new concept, "pattern of the whole," is formed.[32:12] Newman[52:228] has further elaborated her view of health by stating that "health is the pattern of the whole, and wholeness *is*. One cannot lose or gain it." Within this perspective, becoming ill does not diminish wholeness, but wholeness takes on a different form. Newman[32:13] has stated that the "essence of the emerging paradigm of health is pattern recognition." Further, "Manifest health, encompassing disease and non-disease can be regarded as the explication of the underlying pattern of person-environment."[43:11] Therefore health and the evolving pattern of consciousness are the same.[43]

THEORETICAL SOURCES

Central to Newman's assumptions[29:56] was the philosopher Hegel's "dialectical process of the fusion of opposites." Newman used many fields of inquiry as sources for theory development. The rationale for drawing broad conclusions from the use of a limited number of concepts came from Capra, a physicist. Capra held that many phenomena can be explained in terms of a few. Newman[29] drew from Capra in general, and Bentov[2] in particular, for her position on the importance of health as expanding consciousness. Newman[44] credited Johnson during her undergraduate studies and Rogers, in a more extensive way, during her graduate study as the nurse theorists who were most influential on her thinking.

Bohm's Theory of Implicate Order supports Newman's postulate that disease is a manifestation of the pattern of health. Newman[43:xxvi] stated she began to comprehend "the underlying, unseen pattern that manifests itself in varying forms, including disease, and the interconnectedness and omnipresence of all that there is." Young's Theory of Human Evolution pinpointed the role of pattern recognition for Newman[43:xxvi] and "was the impetus for . . . efforts to integrate the basic concepts of my theory—movement, space, time, and consciousness—into a dynamic portrayal of life and health." Moss' experience[25] of love as the highest level of consciousness "provided affirmation and elaboration of my intuition regarding the nature of health."[43:xxvi] Prigogine, a chemist and winner of the Nobel Prize for his Theory of Dissipative Structures, described the pattern of harmony and disharmony as part of a rhythmic process.[43] Newman incorporated Prigogine's theory into her own theory.[32,40] Although Newman[50:23] acknowledges the contributions of

these theories to her theory, she has stated that her theory "was enriched by them, but was not based on them," emphasizing that her theory emerged from a new science of unitary human beings.

USE OF EMPIRICAL EVIDENCE

Evidence for the Theory of Health emanated from Newman's early personal family experiences. Her mother's struggle with amyotrophic lateral sclerosis, a chronic illness, and her dependence on Newman, then a young college graduate, sparked an interest in nursing. From that experience evolved the idea that "illness reflected the life patterns of the person and that what was needed was the recognition of that pattern and acceptance of it for what it meant to that person."[32:3]

Throughout Newman's writing,[32] terms are used such as *call to nursing, growing conscience-like feeling, fear, power, meaning of life and health, belief of life after death, rituals of health,* and *love.* The terms provide a clue concerning Newman's endeavors to make a disturbing life experience logical. The life experience triggered her beginning maturation toward theory development in nursing. Within her philosophical framework, Newman began to develop a synthesis of disease-nondisease-health as recognition of the total patterning of a person.

Research has been conducted on the theoretical sources.[33] In 1979, Newman[29:23] wrote that "in order for nursing research to have meaning in terms of theory development, it must (1) have as its purpose the testing of theory, (2) make explicit the theoretical framework upon which the testing relies, and (3) reexamine the theoretical underpinnings in light of the findings." She believed that if health is considered an individual personal process, research should focus on studies that explore changes and similarities in personal meaning and patterns.

MAJOR CONCEPTS & DEFINITIONS

HEALTH

Health encompasses disease and nondisease. Health can be regarded as the evolving pattern of the person and the environment.[32] Health is viewed as a process of developing awareness of self and environment together with an increasing ability to perceive alternatives and respond in a variety of ways.[28] Health is viewed as the "pattern of the whole" of a person and is further described as including disease as a meaningful manifestation of the pattern of the whole, based on the premise that life is an ongoing process of expanding consciousness.[32:12,39]

Using Hegel's dialectical fusion of opposites, Newman explained how the concept disease fuses with its opposite, nondisease or absence of disease, to create a new concept, health. She explained that this new paradigm of health is relational and is "patterned, emergent, unpredictable, unitary, intuitive, and innovative"; whereas the traditional paradigm is linear, "causal, predictive, dichotomous, rational, and controlling."[43:13] However, she appears to take the characteristics of the old paradigm of health as special cases of the new holistic paradigm to find patterns and new meaning. To her, health and the evolving pattern of consciousness are the same. The essence of the emerging paradigm of health is recognition of pattern. Newman[43] sees the life process as a progression toward higher levels of consciousness.

PATTERN

Pattern is "information that depicts the whole, understanding of the meaning and relationships at once. It is a fundamental attribute of all there is and gives unity in diversity."[32:13] Pattern is what identifies an individual as a particular person. Examples of explicit manifestations of the underlying pattern of a person would be the genetic pattern that contains information that directs becoming, the voice pattern, and the movement pattern.[32] Characteristics of pattern include movement, diversity, and rhythm. Pattern is "somehow intimately involved in energy exchange and transformation."[32:14] According to Newman[34:37] "*Whatever* manifests itself in a person's life is the explication of the underlying implicate pattern . . . the phenomenon we call health is the manifestation of that evolving pattern."

In *Health as Expanding Consciousness,*[32,43] Newman developed pattern as a major concept that was used to understand the individual as a whole being. Newman described a paradigm shift that was occurring in the field of healthcare. The shift was from treatment of symptoms of a disease to the search for patterns and the meaning of those patterns. Newman[32] stated that the patterns of interaction of person-environment constitute health. Embedded within the concepts of movement, time, and space is the idea that an event such as a disease occurrence is part of a larger process. By interacting with the event, no matter how destructive the force might seem to be, its energy augments the person's own energy and enhances his or her own power in the situation. To see this, it is necessary to grasp the pattern of the whole.[32]

CONSCIOUSNESS

Consciousness is defined as the "informational capacity of the system: the ability of the system to interact with its environment."[32:33] Newman asserts that an understanding of her definition of consciousness is essential to understanding the theory. Consciousness includes not only cognitive and affective awareness, but also the "interconnectedness of the entire living system which includes physicochemical maintenance and growth processes as well as the immune system."[37:38] In 1978, three correlates of consciousness (time, movement, and space) were cited as explanations for the changing pattern of the whole and major concepts in the theory of health.

The life process was seen as a progression toward higher levels of consciousness.[26] Newman

Continued

viewed the expansion of consciousness as what life, and therefore health, was all about.[26] Newman referred to the sense of time as a factor altered in the changing level of consciousness. The perception of time was seen as an indicator of humankind's health status.[26]

Bentov[2:67] defined absolute consciousness as "a state in which contrasting concepts become reconciled and fused. Movement and rest fuse into one." The last stage of absolute consciousness is equated with love, where all opposites are reconciled and all experiences are accepted equally and unconditionally, such as love and hate, pain and pleasure, and disease and nondisease.

Reed[65] concurred that Newman's theory described the phase of evolutionary development at which the person moves beyond a focus on self as limited by time, space, and physical concerns. To Newman, transcendence is a process through which the person reaches the highest level of consciousness.

MOVEMENT

"Movement is the means whereby one perceives reality and, therefore, is a means of becoming aware of self."[31:165] Newman[28:23] emphasized that "movement through space is integral to the development of a concept of time in man and is utilized by man as a measure of time." She maintained that "movement brings about change, without which there is no manifest reality."[29:61] To further explain this concept, Newman[29] used the example of a person, restricted in mobility by structural or psychological pathology, who must adapt to an altered rate of movement.

TIME AND SPACE

Time and space have a complementary relationship.[29] "The concept of space is inextricably linked to the concept of time. . . . When one's life space is decreased, as by either physical or social immobility, one's time is increased."[29:61]

Time in Newman's model includes a sense of time perspective (orientation to past, present, and future), but it centers primarily on time as perceived duration. Perceived duration is used synonymously with subjective time as defined by Bentov.[2] Newman used Bentov's conceptualization of time as an index of consciousness to demonstrate expanding consciousness across life span. Time is also not merely conceptualized as either subjective or objective, but is also viewed in a holographic sense. According to Newman,[43:62] "Each moment has an explicate order and also enfolds all others, meaning that each moment of our lives contains all others of all time."

MAJOR ASSUMPTIONS

The foundation for Newman's assumptions[55] is her definition of health, which is grounded in Rogers' 1970 model for nursing, specifically the focus on wholeness, pattern, and unidirectionality. From this, Newman[29:57-58] developed the following assumptions:

"1. Health encompasses conditions heretofore described as illness or, in medical terms, pathology . . .

2. These 'pathological' conditions can be considered a manifestation of the total pattern of the individual . . .

3. The pattern of the individual that eventually manifests itself as pathology is primary and exists prior to structural or functional changes . . .

4. Removal of the pathology in itself will not change the pattern of the individual . . .

5. If becoming 'ill' is the only way an individual's pattern can manifest itself, then that is health for that person . . .

6. Health is the expansion of consciousness . . ."

Newman's implicit assumptions about human nature[55] include being unitary, being an open energy system, being in continuous interconnectedness with the open system of the universe, and being continuously engaged in an evolving pattern of the whole.

Newman[26:58] developed her central premise and assumption, "Health is the expansion of consciousness." Unfolding consciousness is a process that will occur regardless of what actions nurses perform. Nurses can assist clients in getting in touch with what is going on and, in that way, facilitate the process.[43]

THEORETICAL ASSERTIONS

Early development of the theory focused heavily on the concepts of movement, space, time, and consciousness. In *Theory Development in Nursing*,[29] Newman delineated the relationships between movement, space, time, and consciousness. "Time and space have a complementary relationship."[29:60,31:165] Newman gave examples of this relationship at the macrocosmic, microcosmic, and humanistic (everyday) levels. She stated that, at the humanistic level, "the highly mobile individual lives in a world of expanded space and compartmentalized time. When one's life space is decreased, as by either physical or social immobility, one's time is increased."[29:61]

"Movement is a means whereby space and time become a reality."[29:60,31:165] Humankind is in a constant state of motion and is constantly changing. This occurs both internally (at the cellular level) and externally (through body movement and interaction with the environment). This movement through time and space is what gives humankind a unique perception of reality. Movement brings change and enables the individual to experience the world.[29]

"Movement is a reflection of consciousness."[29:60,31:165] Movement is the means of experiencing reality and also the means by which an individual expresses thoughts and feelings about the reality of experiences. An individual conveys his or her awareness of self through the movement in-volved in language, posture, and body movement.[29] "The rhythm and pattern which are reflected in movement are an indication of the internal organization of the person and his perception of the world. Movement provides a means of communication beyond that which language can convey."[29:63]

"Time is a function of movement."[29:60] This assertion is supported by Newman's previous studies[27] regarding the experience of time as related to movement and gait tempo. Newman's research showed that the slower an individual walks, the less subjective time he or she experiences. However, when compared with clock time, time seems to *fly*. Although the individual who is moving quickly subjectively feels that he or she is *beating the clock,* the individual finds that time seems to be dragging when checking a clock.[26,29]

"Time is a measure of consciousness."[29:60] Bentov,[2] who measured consciousness with a ratio of subjective to objective time, first proposed this assertion in 1977. Newman applied this measure of consciousness to the subjective and objective data compiled in her research. She found that the consciousness index increased with age. Some of her research has also supported the finding of "increasing consciousness with age."[30:293] Newman cited this evidence as support for her position that the life process evolves toward consciousness expansion. "However, certain moods, such as depression, may be accompanied by a diminished sense of time."[57:139]

As the theory evolved, time in the Theory of Health as Expanding Consciousness was not merely conceptualized as either subjective or objective, but was also viewed in a holographic sense.[55] According to Newman[43:62] "Each moment has an explicate order and also enfolds all others, meaning that each moment of our lives contains all others of all time."

Excellent examples were used by Newman[32:56] to illustrate the centrality of space-time, one of which is included here:

> Mrs. V. made repeated attempts to *move* away from her husband and to *move* into an educational program to become more independent. She felt she

had no *space* for herself, and she tried to distance herself (space) from her husband. She felt she had no *time* for leisure (self), was overworked, and was constantly meeting other people's needs. She was submissive to the demands and criticism of her husband.

Space, time, and movement later became linked as Newman[32:49] stated "the intersection of movement-space-time represents the person as a center of consciousness and varies from person to person, place to place, and time to time." Newman[32:48] stated that the crucial task "is to be able to see the concepts of movement-space-time in relation to each other, all at once, as patterns of evolving consciousness."

In *Health as Expanding Consciousness*,[32,43] Newman drew heavily on the theoretical work of Young's *The Reflexive Universe: Evolution of Consciousness*.[85] "The central theme of Young's theory is that a self, or a universe, is of the same nature. The essential nature is undefinable, but the beginning and the end are characterized by complete freedom, unrestricted choice."[32:43]

Newman established a corollary between her model of health as expanding consciousness and Young's conception of the evolution of human beings (Figure 31-2). "We come into being from a state of consciousness, are bound in time, find our identity in space, and through movement learn the 'law' of the way things work and make choices that ultimately take us beyond space and time to a state of absolute consciousness."[32:46]

Newman[32:46] stated that "restrictions in movement-space-time force an awareness that extends beyond the physical self." When natural movement is altered, space and time are also altered. When movement is restricted (physical or social), it is necessary for an individual to move beyond self, thereby making movement an important choice point in the process of evolving human consciousness.[43] She assumed that the awareness corresponded to the "inward, self-generated reformation

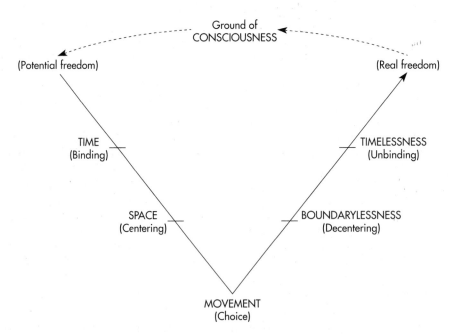

Figure 31-2 Parallel between Newman's Theory of Expanding Consciousness and Young's stages of human evolution. (From Newman, M.A. [1990]. Newman's theory of health as praxis. *Nursing Science Quarterly*, 3[1], 37-41. Reprinted with permission.)

that Young [spoke] of as the turning point of the process."[43:46] "Progression to the sixth state (timelessness) involves increasing freedom from time."[32:46] Finally, the last stage is absolute consciousness, "which has been equated with love."[32:47]

Newman[51] has described the evolution of the theory as it moved from linear explication and testing of concepts of time, space, and movement to an elaboration of interacting patterns as manifestations of expanding consciousness. Illumination of the Theory of Health as Expanding Consciousness as a process of evolving, in conjunction with the research, progressed through several stages.[50,51] These stages included testing the relationships of the concepts of movement, space, and time; identifying sequential person-environment patterns; and recognizing of the centrality of nurse-client relationships or dialogue in the clients' evolving insight and accompanying potential for action. The process actually became cyclical as the original concepts of movement-space-time emerged as dimensions in the unitary evolving process of consciousness.[50]

LOGICAL FORM

In the early development of the theory, Newman used both inductive and deductive logic. Inductive logic is based on observing particular instances and then relating those instances to form a whole. Newman's theory development was derived from her earlier research on time perception and gait tempo. Time and movement, with space and consciousness, are used subsequently as central components in her conceptual framework. These concepts help explain "the phenomena of the life process and therefore of health."[29:59]

Although Newman[50:23] started with a rational, empirical approach that was both inductive and deductive, she found it restrictive and "not consistent with the paradigm from which the theory was drawn." Little by little, she relinquished some of the experimental control and her work evolved to a more interactive, integrative approach that continued to be objective and controlled. When that still did not work, she gave up the research paradigm with its objectivity and control and allowed the

principles of her theoretical paradigm to guide her research. Then she began to see the core of pattern and process as nursing practice. She saw the evolving pattern as meaning in process that required an approach of mutual process, not just objective observation. Patterns showed that expanding consciousness was related to quality and connectedness of relationships. The nurse-researcher's creative presence was important to the participant's insight. Newman[35] concludes that individuals experience a theory in living it. She labels her research as hermeneutic dialectic.

ACCEPTANCE BY THE NURSING COMMUNITY
Practice

In Newman's view,[43] the responsibility of professional nursing practice is to establish a primary relationship with the client for the purpose of identifying healthcare needs and facilitating the client's action potential and decision-making ability. Communication and collaboration with other nurses, associates, and healthcare professionals are essential. Maintenance of a direct, ongoing relationship so long as nursing consultation and services are required, is the structure of the practice. Such primary care providers focusing directly and completely relates to her view of the role of professional nursing, which Newman[58] refers to as nursing clinician/case manager, which is the sine qua non of the integrative model.

Relating her Theory of Health as Expanding Consciousness and acknowledging the contemporary and radical shift in philosophy of nursing that views health as a unitary human field dynamic embedded in a larger unitary field, Newman[29:67] believes that "the goal of nursing is not to make people well, or to prevent their getting sick, but to assist people to utilize the power that is within them as they evolve toward higher levels of consciousness." She states that the task of nursing is not to try to change the pattern of another person, but to recognize it as information that depicts the whole and relate to it as it unfolds.[43]

Newman's more recent works have elaborated on the role of nursing practice in the theory. From the

Newman perspective,[60:3] nursing is the study of "caring in the human health experience." Within this framework, the role of the nurse in this experience is to help clients recognize their own patterns, which results in the illumination of action possibilities that open the way for transformation to occur.[37]

At first, Newman's Model of Health was useful in the practice of nursing because it contained concepts used by the nursing profession. Movement and time are an intrinsic part of nursing intervention, such as range-of-motion and ambulation.[33] During the 1980s, Doberneck[4] used Newman's model to work with caregivers of chronically ill people. Doberneck[4] believed Newman's model addressed issues intrinsic to caring that other theories omit, such as unconditionally being with another person and noncommitment to specific predetermined outcomes.

Also during the 1980s, Marchione[22] used Newman's model to investigate and report the meaning of disabling events in families. She presented a case study in which an additional person became part of the nuclear family for an extended period. The addition was a disruptive event for the family and created disturbances in time, space, movement, and consciousness. Analysis of the case study of the family suggested that Newman's work with patterns could be used to understand family interactions.[21,22] Marchione[21] has also advocated application of the theory to practice with communities.

Kalb applied Newman's Theory of Health in the clinical management of pregnant women hospitalized for complications of maternal-fetal health. The pregnant woman is the conduit through which care can be delivered to the unborn child; therefore she becomes the choice maker for the care of the child.[15]

Gustafson[10] found that practice as a parish nurse supported Newman's Theory of Health as demonstration of pattern recognition. Patient needs were based on effective communication and quality nursing decisions and actions by the development of pattern recognition.[10]

The theory has also been used in practice with various client populations. Endo[5] has studied pattern recognition as nursing intervention with adults with cancer. Litchfield[18] described the patterning of nurse-client relationships in families with frequent

illnesses and in the hospitalization of toddlers. Additionally, Magan, Gibbon, and Mrozek[20] reported on implementation of the theory, as one of several theories, in the care of the mentally ill. More recently, Weingourt[79] reported on use of Newman's Theory of Health with elderly nursing home residents.

Quinn's reconceptualization of therapeutic touch[64] described a shared consciousness. Schubert[74] viewed the nurse-client relationship as progressing from trusting through joining to bonding and Lamb and Stempel[16] described the role of the nurse as an insider-expert. Newman, Lamb, and Michaels[58] described the role of the nurse case manager at St. Mary's as emanating from a philosophical and theoretical base agreeing with the unitary-transformative paradigm and exemplifying an integrated stage of professional nursing. Finally, Flanagan and colleagues[7] reported on the use of the theory in development of a Preadmission Nursing Practice Model (PNPM) and its use at Massachusetts General Hospital.

From the inception of Newman's theory in 1971 until the present, numerous nurse-practitioners and scientists have used the theory either to incorporate the concepts in their nursing practice or to elaborate the theory in research. Newman[32] did not advocate one model as the sole basis for curriculum because students should have the opportunity to study various approaches to health and nursing and to choose what is relevant to them in their practice and research.

Newman has consulted with faculty and students from numerous universities. Graduate students at various institutions continue to conduct research based on her theory.

Newman's Theory of Pattern Recognition provides the basis for the process of nurse-client interaction. Newman[32:71] suggested that the task in intervention is pattern recognition accomplished by the health professional becoming aware of the pattern of the other person by becoming "in touch with one's own pattern." Newman[32:70] suggested that the professional should focus on the pattern of the other person, acting as the "reference beam in a hologram." The holographic model of intervention is described by "imagining the emanating waves that appear when two pebbles are thrown into water. As the

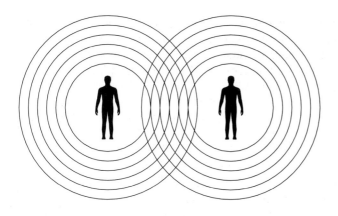

Figure 31-3 Interaction pattern of two persons—A holographic model of intervention. (From Newman, M. *Health as expanding consciousness* [2nd ed., p. 106]. 1994: National League for Nursing Press, New York, NY/Jones and Bartlett Publishers, Sudbury, MA. *www.jbpub.com.* Reprinted with permission.)

waves radiate . . . they meet and interact . . . [forming] an interference pattern"[32:70] (Figure 31-3).

Education

Newman stated that a new role is needed for the nurse to function in the paradigm of the evolving consciousness of the whole. "Nurses need to be free to relate to patients in an ongoing partnership that is not limited to a particular place or time."[32:89] Nursing education would revolve around the "concept of pattern: pattern as substance, pattern as process, and pattern as method."[32:89] Education by this method would enable nursing to be an important resource for the continued development of healthcare. Newman[32:90] stated that nursing is at the intersection of the focus of the healthcare industry; therefore "nursing is in position to bring about the fluctuation within the system that will shift the system to a new higher order of functioning."

Examining pragmatic adequacy of Newman's theory in relation to nursing education reveals that teaching the research method associated with the theory also teaches the students a practice method that is congruent with the theory. Newman sees the theory, the practice, and the research as a process rather than a separate domain of nursing discipline. Teaching the Theory of Health as Expanding Consciousness would necessitate a shift in thinking from the existing view of health to a newer and synthesized view that accepts disease as a manifestation of health. Not only that, learning to let go of the professional's control and respecting the client's choices

are an integral part of practice within this framework. Students and practicing nurses who plan to use Newman's theory will face personal transformation in learning to recognize pattern by acting as a participant-observer of phenomena related to health. An individual's personal experience will be the core of not just teaching and practice, but research as well. Newman[43] explains that the nurse would need to sense into her own pattern of relating as an indication of the nurse-client interacting pattern. There needs to be a study or sense of the process of the relationship with clients from within, giving attention to the "we" in the nurse-client relationship.[51]

Newman's theory has also been used in nursing education to provide some content into a model called the Healing Web. This model was designed to integrate nursing education and nursing service together with private and public education programs for baccalaureate and associate nursing degree programs in South Dakota.[3] Additionally, Jacono and Jacono[12] suggested that student creativity could be enhanced if nursing faculty apply the theory by recognizing that all experience has the potential for expanding the creativity (consciousness) of individuals.

Research

Research has a dual role; that is, to test theory and establish a scientific knowledge base from which to practice professional nursing. Early research on the theory manipulated the basic theory conc space, time, and movement. In addition to Newman, several researchers have undertaken research about time, space, or movement. Newman and Gaudiano[57] focused on the occurrence of depression in the elderly and decreased subjective time. Mentzer and Schorr[23] used Newman's model of duration of time as an index to consciousness in a study of institutionalized elderly. Engle[6] addressed the relationship between movement, time, and assessment of health. Schorr and Schroeder[71] studied differences in consciousness with regard to time and movement, with results supporting the concept of expanding consciousness. In another study by Schorr and Schroeder,[70] relationships among type A behavior, temporal orientation, and death anxiety were examined as manifestations of consciousness, with mixed results.

However, with evolution of the theory, research was also viewed as practice having a function of assisting clients in pattern recognition.[37] Schorr and others[70] investigated the health patterns in 60 aging women using the Theory of Health as the theoretical framework. The phenomenon of powerlessness was assumed to be operative for the subjects, but was rejected in favor of high levels of perceived situational control or powerfulness. The results supported Newman's Model of Health as Expanding Consciousness.[69] Fryback's dissertation[8] revealed that persons with acquired immunodeficiency syndrome (AIDS) and human immunodeficiency syndrome (HIV) infection did describe health within physical, health promotion, and spiritual domains and was congruent with Newman's theory.

Other studies investigating patterns of expanding consciousness included Smith's work[76] with the health of rural African-American women and Yamashita's work[83,84] with Japanese and Canadian family caregivers. Further examples of research with the theory focusing on pattern include the conceptualization of breast cancer as a meaningful part of 'th[14,24,66,78] and the recognition of patterns in patients,[5,46] life patterns of persons with heart disease,[59] patterns of persons with bstructive pulmonary disease,[13,61] and expanding consciousness in persons IDS.[17] Additional research includes

exploring health patterning in persons with multiple sclerosis,[9] recognizing help-seeking patterns in older wife caregivers of husbands with dementia,[82] recognizing patterns in adolescent males incarcerated for murder,[62] and giving and receiving social support by spouse caregivers and their spouses.[68] Newman's research as praxis has been used to describe the lived experience of life passing in middle-adolescent females;[75] to describe patterns of expanding consciousness in midlife women;[63] to explore pain reduction with music therapy,[69] with pattern recognition of high-risk pregnant women,[73] and low-risk pregnant women;[1] and to explore the nature of nursing practice with families of young children[19] and patterns of families of medically fragile children.[77]

Newman states that her research over time assisted not only clients who participated, but also her and fellow researchers in gaining a better understanding of self as a nurse-researcher and understanding the limitations of previous methods used. Newman[32:94] further stated that research should center around "participatory investigations in which subjects (clients) are our partners, our core-searchers, in our search for health patterns." This method of inquiry is called cooperative inquiry or interactive, integrative participation. Newman[36,37] has developed a method to describe pattern as unfolding and evolving over time. She used the method of interviewing a subject in different time frames to establish a pattern for that subject.[34] Newman[37:37] stated that during the development of a methodology to test the theory of health, "sharing our (researcher's) perception of the person's pattern with the person was meaningful to the participants and stimulated new insights regarding their lives." The process made a difference in the researchers' lives and the participants' lives. Newman[37] asserted that the research process took on the form of nursing practice. More recently, she has stipulated a protocol for the research and has labeled it *hermeneutic dialectic*. This method allows the pattern of person-environment to reveal itself without disturbing the unity of the pattern.[54] A website is maintained at the University of Minnesota for disseminating research information pertaining to the theory.[11]

FURTHER DEVELOPMENT

Newman reported that operationalization of the model of health as expanding consciousness has been approached in two ways: (1) by research methods designed to describe and test the relationships between the major concepts of movement, time, space, and consciousness and (2) by attempts to describe evolving patterns of consciousness in terms of the integration of movement-space-time.[32]

Previously discussed research studies have supported the model of health as expanding consciousness, verifying the relationships between the major concepts, and more recently, illuminating the importance of pattern recognition in the process of expanding consciousness. The theory has been used extensively in exploring and understanding the experience of health within illness, supporting a basic premise of the theory that crisis situations may provide a catalytic effect and facilitate movement to higher levels of consciousness. Newman's work has evolved from the testing of time, movement, and consciousness through identification of sequential patterns of person-environment to recognition of the integrality of nurse-client dialogue in the client's evolving insight and actions. Once again, the original concepts of movement-time-space are seen as dimensions in the unitary patterns of consciousness as the theory development continues.

CRITIQUE
Clarity

Semantic clarity is evident in the definitions, descriptions, and dimensions of the concepts of the theory. Clarity is needed regarding movement as a concept or dimension.

Simplicity

In Newman's Theory Development in Nursing, the concepts of movement, time, space, and consciousness, with the five resulting relationship statements, represented the evolution of the theory at that time. In *Health as Expanding Consciousness*,[32,43] pattern became a major concept included for the purpose of understanding consciousness. According to Newman,[39:132] the addition of the concept of pattern of the whole was essential because "pattern as an identification of the wholeness of a person is basic to the theory" unifies the theory and prevents oversimplification. The theory is unitary in terms of pattern.

The deeper meaning of the Theory of Health as Expanding Consciousness is complex. The theory as a whole must be understood, not just the isolated concepts. If an individual wanted to use a positivist approach, Newman's original propositions would serve as guides for hypothesis development. However, researchers who have tried that approach have concluded that it is inadequate to study the theory. As Newman has advocated in the 1994 edition of her book, Health As Expanding Consciousness,[43] the holistic approach of the hermeneutic dialectic method is consistent with the theory and requires a high level of understanding of the theory on the part of the researcher to extend the theory in praxis research.[49]

Generality

The concepts in Newman's theory are broad in scope because they all relate to health. This renders her theory generalizable. The broad scope provides a focus for future theory development.

Empirical Precision

In the early stages of development, aspects of the theory have been operationalized and tested within a traditional scientific mode. However, quantitative methods are inadequate in capturing the dynamic, changing nature of this model. A hermeneutic dialectic approach is being developed for a full explication of its meaning and application.

Derivable Consequences

The focus of Newman's Theory of Health as Expanding Consciousness provides an evolving guide for all health-related disciplines. In the quest for understanding the phenomenon of health, this unique view of health challenges nurses to make a difference in nursing practice by the application of this theory.

CRITICAL THINKING *Activities*

1. What is the worldview of nursing? What is the nurse-scientist view of nursing?

2. How does that worldview dictate or direct knowledge development for nursing?

3. What dictates the change in paradigms of health, healthcare practice, and nursing practice? Examine Newman's view about it.

4. How is the process of health as expanding consciousness different from the process of self-actualization? Compare and contrast the characteristics of both processes and phenomena.

5. Where and how does Newman accept or depart from the Rogerian Unitary Man Theory?

6. How does Newman relate her Theory of Health with contemporary and future nursing practice, education, and research?

7. How do you agree or disagree with her claims and explanations regarding relatedness of her theory with the pragmatic expectations of the nursing profession?

REFERENCES

1. Batty, M.L.E. (1999). *Pattern identification and expanding consciousness during the transition of "low risk" pregnancy.* Unpublished master's thesis. The University of New Brunswick, Fredrickton.
2. Bentov, I. (1977). *Stalking the wild pendulum.* New York: E.P. Dutton.
3. Bunkers, S.S., Bendtro, M., Holmes, P.K., Howell, J., Johnson, S., Koerner, J., Larson, J., Nelson, J., & Weaver, R. (1992). The healing web: A transformative model for nursing. *Nursing and Health Care,* 13, 68-73.
4. Doberneck, B. (1985). Telephone interview.
5. Endo, E. (1998). Pattern recognition as a nursing intervention with Japanese women with ovarian cancer. *Advances in Nursing Science,* 20(4), 49-61.
6. Engle, V. (1986). The relationship of movement and time to older adults' functional health. *Research in Nursing and Health,* 9, 123-129.
7. Flanagan, J., Farrell, C., Zelano, P., Morrison, H., Quigley, J.D., & Braccio, J. (2000). *The nursing theory and practice link: Creating a healing environment.* Proceedings of the International Conference on Emerging Nursing Knowledge Boston, Massachusetts.
8. Fryback, P.B. (1991). Perceptions of health by persons with a terminal disease: Implications for nursing. *Dissertation Abstracts International,* 52-04B, 1951.
9. Gulick, E.E. & Bugg, A. (1992). Holistic health patterning in multiple sclerosis. *Research in Nursing and Health,* 15, 175-185.
10. Gustafson, W. (1990). Application of Newman's theory of health: Pattern recognition as nursing practice. In M. Parker (Ed.), *Nursing theories in practice* (pp. 141-161). New York: National League for Nursing.
11. Hoyman, K. (2000). *Health as expanding consciousness* [Online]. Available: http://hoym0003@tc.umn.edu.
12. Jacono, B.J. & Jacono, J.J. (1996). The benefits of Newman and Parse in helping nurse teachers determine methods to enhance student creativity. *Nurse Education Today,* 16, 356-362.
13. Jonsdottir, H. (1998). Life patterns of people with chronic obstructive pulmonary disease: Isolation and being closed in. *Nursing Science Quarterly,* 11, 160-166.
14. Kaiser Larsen, N.K. (1999). Life patterns of Native American women experiencing breast cancer. *Dissertation Abstracts International,* 60-05B, 2062.
15. Kalb, K.A. (1990). The gift: Applying Newman's theory of health in nursing practice. In M. Parker (Ed.), *Nursing theories in practice* (pp. 163-186). New York: National League for Nursing.
16. Lamb, G.S. & Stempel, J.E. (1994). Nurse case management from the client's view: Growing as insider-expert. *Nursing Outlook,* 42, 7-13.
17. Lamendola, F.P. & Newman, M.A. (1994). The paradox of HIV/AIDS as expanding consciousness. *Advances in Nursing Science,* 16(3), 13-21.
18. Litchfield, M.C. (1993). *The process of health patterning in families with young children who have been repeatedly hospitalized.* Unpublished master's thesis, University of Minnesota, Rochester.
19. Litchfield, M.C. (1997). The process of nursing partnership in family health. *Dissertation Abstracts International,* 59-04B, 1802.
20. Magan, S.J., Gibbon, E.J., & Mrozek, R. (1990). Nursing theory application: A practice model. *Issues in Mental Health Nursing,* 11, 297-312.
21. Marchione, J. (1985). Telephone interview.
22. Marchione, J.M. (1986). Pattern as methodology for assessing family health: Newman's theory of health. In P. Winstead-Fry (Ed.), *Case studies in nursing theory.* New York: National League for Nursing.

23. Mentzer, C. & Schorr, J.A. (1986). Perceived situational control and perceived duration of time: Expressions of life patterns. *Advances in Nursing Science,* 9(1), 13-20.

24. Moch, S.D. (1990). Health within the experience of breast cancer. *Journal of Advanced Nursing,* 15, 1426-1435.

25. Moss, R. (1981). *The i that is we.* Millbrae, CA: Celestial Arts.

26. Newman, M.A. (1971). *An investigation of the relationship between gait tempo and time perception.* Unpublished doctoral dissertation, New York University, New York.

27. Newman, M.A. (1972). Time estimation in relation to gait tempo. *Perceptual and Motor Skills,* 34, 359-366.

28. Newman, M.A. (1978). *Second annual nurse educator's conference* [Audiotape]. Available: Teach 'em, Inc., 160 E. Illinois Street, Chicago, IL, 60611. New York: Teach 'em, Inc.

29. Newman, M.A. (1979). *Theory development in nursing.* Philadelphia: F.A. Davis.

30. Newman, M.A. (1982). Time as an index of expanding consciousness with age. *Nursing Research,* 31, 290-293.

31. Newman, M.A. (1983). Newman's health theory. In I.W. Clements & F.B. Roberts (Eds.), *Family health: A theoretical approach to nursing care.* New York: John Wiley & Sons.

32. Newman, M.A. (1986). *Health as expanding consciousness.* St. Louis: Mosby.

33. Newman, M.A. (1987). Aging as increasing complexity. *Journal of Gerontological Nursing,* 13(9), 16-18.

34. Newman, M.A. (1987). Patterning. In M. Duffy & N.J. Pender (Eds.), *Conceptual issues in health promotion, a report of proceedings of a wingspread conference, Racine, WI, April 13-15, 1987.* Indianapolis: Sigma Theta Tau.

35. Newman, M.A. (1988). Personal correspondence.

36. Newman, M.A. (1989). The spirit of nursing. *Holistic Nursing Practice,* 3(3), 1-6.

37. Newman, M.A. (1990). Newman's theory of health as praxis. *Nursing Science Quarterly,* 3, 37-41.

38. Newman, M.A. (1990). Nursing paradigms and realities. In N.L. Chaska (Ed.), *The nursing profession: Turning points* (pp. 230-235). St Louis: Mosby.

39. Newman, M.A. (1990). Shifting to higher consciousness. In M. Parker (Ed.), *Nursing theories in practice* (pp. 129-139). New York: National League for Nursing.

40. Newman, M.A. (1991). Health conceptualizations. In J.J. Fitzpatrick, R.L. Taunton, & A.K. Jacox (Eds.), *Annual review of nursing research* (Vol. 9). New York: Springer.

41. Newman, M.A. (1992). Curriculum vitae.

42. Newman, M.A. (1992). Nightingale's vision of nursing theory and health. In Nightingale, F., *Notes on nursing: What it is, and what it is not* (Commemorative Edition, pp. 44-47). Philadelphia: Lippincott. (Original work published in 1958.)

43. Newman, M.A. (1994). *Health as expanding consciousness.* New York: National League for Nursing Press.

44. Newman, M.A. (1995). *A developing discipline: Selected works of Margaret Newman.* New York: National League for Nursing Press.

45. Newman, M.A. (1995). Dialogue: Margaret Newman and the rhetoric of nursing theory. *Image: Journal of Nursing Scholarship,* 27, 261.

46. Newman, M.A. (1995). Recognizing a pattern of expanding consciousness in persons with cancer. In M.A. Newman (Ed.), *A developing discipline: Selected works of Margaret Newman* (pp. 159-171). New York: National League for Nursing Press.

47. Newman, M.A. (1996). Curriculum vitae.

48. Newman, M.A. (1996). Personal correspondence.

49. Newman, M.A. (1996). Telephone interviews.

50. Newman, M.A. (1997). Evolution of the theory of health as expanding consciousness. *Nursing Science Quarterly,* 10, 22-25.

51. Newman, M.A. (1997). Experiencing the whole. *Advances in Nursing Science,* 20, 34-39.

52. Newman, M.A. (1999). The rhythm of relating in a paradigm of wholeness. *Image: Journal of Nursing Scholarship,* 31, 227-230.

53. Newman, M.A. (2000). Curriculum vitae.

54. Newman, M.A. (2000, May 17). Personal correspondence.

55. Newman, M.A. (2000). Telephone interview.

56. Newman, M.A. & Autio, S. (1986). *Nursing in a prospective payment system health care environment.* Minneapolis: University of Minnesota.

57. Newman, M.A. & Gaudiano, J.K. (1984). Depression as an explanation for decreased subjective time in the elderly. *Nursing Research,* 33, 137-139.

58. Newman, M.A., Lamb, G.S., & Michaels, C. (1991). Nurse case management: The coming together of theory and practice. *Nursing and Health Care,* 12, 404-408.

59. Newman, M.A. & Moch, S.D. (1991). Life patterns of persons with coronary heart disease. *Nursing Science Quarterly,* 4, 161-167.

60. Newman, M.A., Sime, M.A., & Corcoran-Perry, S.A. (1991). The focus of the discipline of nursing. *Advances in Nursing Science,* 14, 1-6.

61. Noveletsky-Rosenthal, H.T. (1996). Pattern recognition in older adults living with chronic illness. *Dissertation Abstracts International,* 57-10B, 6180.

62. Pharris, M.D. (1999). *The process of pattern recognition as a nursing intervention with adolescent males incarcerated for murder.* Unpublished Doctoral dissertation, University of Minnesota.

63. Picard, C.A. (2000). Pattern of expanding consciousness in mid-life women: Creative movement and the narrative as modes of expression. *Nursing Science Quarterly,* 13, 150-158.

64. Quinn, J.F. (1992). Holding sacred space: The nurse as healing environment. *Holistic Nursing Practice,* 6(4), 26-36.

65. Reed, P.G. (1996). Transcendence: Formulating nursing perspectives. *Nursing Science Quarterly,* 9(1), 2-4.

66. Roux, G.M. (1994). *Phenomenologic study: Inner strength in women with breast cancer.* Unpublished doctoral dissertation, Texas Women's University, Denton.

67. Roy, C., Rogers, M.C., Fitzpatrick, J.J., Neuman, M., & Orem, D.E. (1982). Nursing diagnosis and nursing theory. In M.J. King & D.A. Moritz (Eds.), *Classification of nursing diagnosis* (pp. 215-231). New York: McGraw Hill.

68. Schmitt, N. (1991). *Caregiving couples: The experience of giving and receiving social support.* Unpublished doctoral dissertation, University of Minnesota, Rochester.

69. Schorr, J.A. (1993). Music and pattern change in chronic pain. *Advances in Nursing Science,* 15(4), 27-36.

70. Schorr, J.A., Farnham, R.C., & Ervin, S.M. (1991). Health patterns in aging women as expanding consciousness. *Advances in Nursing Science,* 13(4), 52-63.

71. Schorr, J.A. & Schroeder, C.A. (1989). Consciousness as a dissipative structure: An extension of the Newman model. *Nursing Science Quarterly,* 2, 183-193.

72. Schorr, J.A. & Schroeder, C.A. (1991). Movement and time: Exertion and perceived duration. *Nursing Science Quarterly,* 4, 104-112.

73. Schroeder, C.A. (1993) Perceived duration of time and bedrest in high risk pregnancy: An exploration of the Newman Model. *Dissertation Abstracts International,* 54-04B, 1894.

74. Schubert, P.E. (1989). *Mutual connectedness: Holistic nursing practice under varying conditions of intimacy.* Unpublished doctoral dissertation, University of California, San Francisco.

75. Shanahan, S.M. (1993). The lived experience of lifepassing in middle adolescent females. *Masters Abstracts International,* 32-05, 1376.

76. Smith, C.A. (1995). The lived experience of staying healthy in rural African American families. *Nursing Science Quarterly,* 8, 17-21.

77. Tommet, P.A. (1997). Nurse-parent dialogue: Illuminating the pattern of families with children who are medically fragile. *Dissertation Abstracts International,* 58-05B, 2359.

78. Utley, R. (1999). The evolving meaning of cancer for long-term survivors of breast cancer. *Oncology Nursing Forum,* 26, 1519-1523.

79. Weingourt, R. (1998). Using Margaret A. Newman's theory of health with elderly nursing home residents. *Perspectives in Psychiatric Care,* 34(3), 25-30.

80. *Who's Who in American Nursing.* (1996/1997). New Providence, NJ: Marquis.

81. *Who's Who of American Women.* (1983/1984). Chicago: Marquis.

82. Witucki, J. (2000). *Help-seeking by older wife caregivers of demented husbands: A grounded theory approach.* Unpublished doctoral dissertation, University of Tennessee, Knoxville.

83. Yamashita, M. (1995). *Family coping with mental illness: An application of Newman's research as praxis.* Paper presented at the Midwest Nursing Research Society 19th Annual Conference, Kansas City, MO.

84. Yamashita, M. (1999). Newman's theory of health applied to family caregiving in Canada. *Nursing Science Quarterly,* 12, 73-79.

85. Young, A.M. (1976). *The reflexive universe: Evolution of consciousness.* San Francisco: Robert Briggs.

BIBLIOGRAPHY
Primary Sources
Books

Downs, F.S. & Newman, M.A. (Eds.). (1973). *A source book of nursing research.* Philadelphia: F.A. Davis.

Downs, F.S. & Newman, M.A. (Eds.). (1977). *A source book of nursing research* (2nd ed.). Philadelphia: F.A. Davis.

Newman, M.A. (1979). *Theory development in nursing.* Philadelphia: F.A. Davis. (Japanese rights assigned to Gendasha Publishing Company, Tokyo, 1986.)

Newman, M.A. (1986). *Health as expanding consciousness.* St. Louis: Mosby. (Japanese translation, 1995; Korean translation, 1996.)

Newman, M.A. (1994). *Health as expanding consciousness* (2nd ed.). New York: National League for Nursing Press. (Japanese translation, 1995; Korean translation, 1996.)

Newman, M.A. (1995). *A developing discipline: Selected work of Margaret Newman.* New York: National League for Nursing Press.

Newman, M.A. & Autio, S. (1986). *Nursing in a prospective payment system health care environment.* Minneapolis: University of Minnesota.

Book Chapters

Downs, F.S. & Newman, M.A. (1977). Elements of a research critique. In F.S. Downs & M.A. Newman (Eds.), *A source book of nursing research* (2nd ed., pp. 1-12). Philadelphia: F.A. Davis.

Field, L. & Newman, M.A. (1982). Clinical application of the unitary man framework: Case study analysis. In M.J. Kim & D.A. Morita (Eds.), *Classification of nursing diagnosis* (pp. 249-263). New York: McGraw-Hill.

Newman, M.A. (1973). Identifying patient needs in short-span nurse-patient relationships. In M.E. Auld & L.H. Birum (Eds.), *The challenge of nursing* (pp. 98-103). St. Louis: Mosby.

Newman, M.A. (1981). The meaning of health. In G.E. Laskar (Ed.), *Applied systems research and cybernetics: Vol. 4. Systems research in health care, biocybernetics and ecology* (pp. 1739-1743). New York: Pergamon.

Newman, M.A. (1983). Newman's health theory. In I. Clements & F. Roberts (Eds.), *Family health: A theoretical approach to nursing care* (pp. 161-175). New York: John Wiley & Sons.

Newman, M.A. (1983). Nursing's theoretical evolution. In T.A. Duespohol (Ed.), *Nursing in transition* (pp. 15-24). Rockville, MD: Aspen Systems.

Newman, M.A. (1983). The continuing revolution: A history of nursing science. In N.L. Chaska (Ed.), *The nursing profession: A time to speak* (pp. 385-393). New York: McGraw-Hill.

Newman, M.A. (1986). Nursing's theoretical evolution. In L.H. Nicoll (Ed.), *Perspectives on nursing theory* (pp. 72-78). Boston: Little, Brown.

Newman, M.A. (1987). Nursing's emerging paradigm: The diagnosis of pattern. In A.M. McLane (Ed.), *Classification of nursing diagnoses. Proceedings of the seventh conference, North American nursing diagnosis association* (pp. 53-60). St. Louis: Mosby.

Newman, M.A. (1987). Patterning. In M. Duffy & N.J. Pender (Eds.), *Conceptual issues in health promotion: A report of proceedings of a wingspread conference, Racine, WI* (pp. 36-50). Indianapolis: Sigma Theta Tau.

Newman, M.A. (1990). Nursing paradigms and realities. In N.L. Chaska (Ed.), *The nursing profession: Turning points* (pp. 230-235). St. Louis: Mosby.

Newman, M.A. (1990). Professionalism: Myth or reality. In N.L. Chaska (Ed.), *The nursing profession: Turning points* (pp. 49-52). St. Louis: Mosby.

Newman, M.A. (1990). Shifting to higher consciousness. In M. Parker (Ed.), *Nursing theories in practice* (pp. 129-139). New York: National League for Nursing.

Newman, M.A. (1992). Nightingale's vision of nursing theory and health. In F. Nightingale, *Notes on nursing: What it is, and what it is not* (Commemorative Edition, pp. 44-47). Philadelphia: Lippincott. (Original work published in 1958.)

Newman, M.A. (1992). Nursing's theoretical evolution. In L.H. Nicoll (Ed.), *Perspectives in nursing theory* (pp. 77-84). Philadelphia: Lippincott.

Newman, M.A. (1995). Recognizing a pattern of expanding consciousness in persons with cancer. In M.A. Newman (Ed.), *A developing discipline: Selected works of Margaret Newman* (pp. 159-171). New York: National League for Nursing Press.

Newman, M.A. (1996). Prevailing paradigms in nursing. In J.W. Kenney (Ed.), *Philosophical and theoretical perspectives for advanced nursing practice* (pp. 302-307). Sudbury, MA: Jones and Bartlett.

Newman, M.A. (1996). Theory of the nurse-client partnership. In E. Cohen (Ed.), *Nurse case management in the 21st century* (pp. 119-123). St. Louis: Mosby.

Newman, M.A. (1997). A dialogue with Martha Rogers and David Bohm about the science of unitary human beings. In M. Madrid (Ed.), *Patterns of Rogerian knowing* (pp. 3-10). New York: National League for Nursing Press.

Newman, M.A., Sime, A.M., & Corcoran-Perry, S.A. (1996). The focus of the discipline of nursing. In J.W. Kenney (Ed.), *Philosophical and theoretical perspectives for advanced nursing practice* (pp. 297-301). Sudbury, MA: Jones and Bartlett.

Roy, C., Rogers, M.E., Fitzpatrick, J.J., Newman, M., & Orem, D.E. (1982). Nursing diagnosis and nursing theory. In M.J. Kim & D.A. Moritz (Eds.), *Classification of nursing diagnosis* (pp. 215-231). New York: McGraw-Hill.

Journal Articles

Allender, C.D., Egan, E.C., & Newman, M.A. (1995). An instrument for measuring differentiated nursing practice. *Nursing Management, 26*(4), 42-44.

Butrin, J. & Newman, M.A. (1986). Health promotion in Zaire: Time perspective and cerebral hemispheric dominance as relevant factors. *Public Health Nursing, 3,* 183-191.

Lamendola, F. & Newman, M.A. (1994). The paradox of HIV/AIDS as expanding consciousness. *Advances in Nursing Science, 16*(3), 13-21.

Newman, M.A. (1966). Identifying and meeting patients' needs in short-span nurse-patient relationships. *Nursing Forum, 5,* 76-86.

Newman, M.A. (1972). Nursing's theoretical evolution. *Nursing Outlook, 20,* 449-453.

Newman, M.A. (1972). Time estimation in relation to gait tempo. *Perceptual and Motor Skills, 34,* 359-366.

Newman, M.A. (1975). The professional doctorate in nursing: A position paper. *Nursing Outlook, 23,* 704-706.

Newman, M.A. (1976). Movement, tempo, and the experience of time. *Nursing Research, 25,* 273-279.

Newman, M.A. (1982). Time as an index of expanding consciousness with age. *Nursing Research, 31,* 290-293.

Newman, M.A. (1982). What differentiates clinical research? *Image: Journal of Nursing Scholarship, 14,* 86-88.

Newman, M.A. (1983). Editorial. *Advances in Nursing Science, 5*(2), x-xi.

Newman, M.A. (1984). Nursing diagnosis: Looking at the whole. *American Journal of Nursing, 84,* 1496-1499.

Newman, M.A. (1987). Aging as increasing complexity. *Journal of Gerontological Nursing, 13*(9), 16-18.

Newman, M.A. (1987). Commentary: Perception of time among Japanese inpatients. *Western Journal of Nursing Research, 9,* 299-300.

Newman, M.A. (1989). The spirit of nursing. *Holistic Nursing Practice, 3*(3), 1-6.

Newman, M.A. (1990). Newman's theory of health as praxis. *Nursing Science Quarterly, 3,* 37-41.

Newman, M.A. (1990). Toward an integrative model of professional practice. *Journal of Professional Practice, 6,* 167-173.

Newman, M.A. (1991). Commentary: Research as practice. *Nursing Science Quarterly, 4,* 100-101.

Newman, M.A. (1991). Health conceptualizations. *Annual Review of Nursing Research, 9,* 221-243.

Newman, M.A. (1992). Prevailing paradigms in nursing. *Nursing Outlook, 40,* 10-13, 32.

Newman, M.A. (1994). Into the 21st century. *Nursing Science Quarterly, 7,* 44-46.

Newman, M.A. (1994). Theory for nursing practice. *Nursing Science Quarterly, 7,* 153-157.

Newman, M. A. (1995). Dialogue: Margaret Newman and the rhetoric of nursing theory. *Image: Journal of Nursing Scholarship, 27,* 261.

Newman, M.A. (1997). Evolution of the theory of health as expanding consciousness. *Nursing Science Quarterly, 10,* 22-25.

Newman, M.A. (1997). Experiencing the whole. *Advances in Nursing Science, 20,* 34-39.

Newman, M.A. (1997). The professional doctorate in nursing: A position paper. *Image: Journal of Nursing Scholarship, 29,* 361-362.

Newman, M.A. (1999). Letters to the editor . . . A commentary on Newman's theory of health as expanding consciousness (ANS 21:1). *Advances in Nursing Science, 21*(3), viii-ix.

Newman, M.A. (1999). The rhythm of relating in a paradigm of wholeness. *Image: Journal of Nursing Scholarship, 31,* 227-230.

Newman, M.A. & Gaudiano, J.K. (1984). Depression as an explanation for decreased subjective time in the elderly. *Nursing Research, 33,* 137-139.

Newman, M.A., Lamb, G.S., & Michaels, C. (1991). Nurse case management: The coming together of theory and practice. *Nursing and Health Care, 12,* 404-408.

Newman, M.A. & Moch, S.D. (1991). Life patterns of persons with coronary heart disease. *Nursing Science Quarterly, 4,* 161-167.

Newman, M.A. & O'Brien, R.A. (1978). Experiencing the research process via computer simulation. *Image: Journal of Nursing Scholarship, 10,* 5-9.

Newman, M.A., Sime, A.M., & Corcoran-Perry, S.A. (1991). The focus of the discipline of nursing. *Advances in Nursing Science, 14,* 1-6.

Portonova, M., Young, E., & Newman, M.A. (1984). Elderly women's attitudes toward sexual activity among their peers. *Health Care for Women, International, 5,* 289-298.

Dissertation

Newman, M.A. (1971). *An investigation of the relationship between gait tempo and time perception.* Unpublished doctoral dissertation, New York University, School of Education.

Reports

Newman, M.A. (1977). *Nursing course content in doctoral education.* Proceedings of National Conference on Doctoral Education in Nursing. Philadelphia: University of Pennsylvania.

Newman, M.A. (1982). *What differentiates clinical research?* Proceedings of the Second Phyllis J. Verhonick Nursing Research Course. Washington, DC: Nursing Research Service, Walter Reed Army Medical Center.

Newman, M.A. (1984). *Health as expanding consciousness.* Proceedings of the Third Phyllis J. Verhonick Nursing Research Course. Washington, DC: Nursing Research Service, Walter Reed Army Medical Center.

Newman, M.A. (1985). *Health as expanding consciousness.* Proceedings of Ninth National Forum of Doctoral Education in Nursing. Birmingham, AL: University of Alabama School of Nursing.

Newman, M. & Autio, S. (1986). Nursing in the world of DRGs and prospective payment. *CURA Reporter* (Published by University of Minnesota Center for Urban and Regional Affairs), 16(5), 1-7.

Newman, M.A., Tompkins, E.S., Isenberg, M.A., Fitzpatrick, J.J., & Scott, D.W. (1980). Movement, time and consciousness: Parameters of health [Symposium]. *Proceedings of Western Society for Research in Nursing Research, 13,* 45-49.

Reviews

Newman, M.A. (1984). [Review of the book *Annual review of nursing research, Vol I*]. *American Journal of Nursing, 84,* 1437-1438.

Newman, M.A. (1987). Commentary [Review of the article Perception of time among Japanese inpatients]. *Western Journal of Nursing Research, 9,* 299-300.

Newman, M.A. (1991). [Review of the article Caring and responsibility: The crossroads between holistic practice and traditional medicine]. *Journal of Professional Nursing, 7,* 319-320.

Newman, M.A. (1991). [Review of the article Visions of Rogers' science-based nursing]. *Nursing Science Quarterly, 4,* 41-42.

Other Media

Margaret Newman, nurse theorists: Portraits of excellence [Videotape]. (1990). Produced by Helene Fuld Health Trust. Oakland, CA: Studio Three Production.

Newman, M.A. (1978, Dec.). *Toward a theory of health* [Audiotape]. Paper presented at Second Annual Conference, New York City. Available: Teach 'em Inc., 160 E. Illinois Street, Chicago, IL 60611.

Newman, M.A. (1984, May). *A theory of health* [Audiotape]. Paper presented at Nursing Theory Conference, Boyle, Letourneau Conference, Edmonton, Canada. Available: Ed Kennedy, Kennedy Recording, R.R. 5, Edmonton, Alberta, Canada T5P 4B7, (403) 470-0013.

Newman, M.A. (1997). *Margaret Newman: Health as expanding consciousness* [CD-ROM]. Available: Fuld Institute for Technology in Nursing Education, Inc., 5 Depot Street, Athens, OH 45701, (800) 691-8480.

Newman, M.A., Koerner, J., Bunkers, S., Cocoran-Perry, S., & Nelson, M. (1992, Feb.). *Differentiated practice: Implications for practice and education* [Videotape]. Interactive video conference linked to nursing leaders in New Zealand, sponsored by Telecom, New Zealand.

Selected Paper Presentations from 1990 to 2000

Newman, M.A. (1990, Feb.). *Theory of health: Expanding consciousness.* Paper presented at Sigma Theta Tau, Beta Mu Chapter, University of Arizona, Tucson.

Newman, M.A. (1990, March). *Historical review of nursing theory development.* Paper presented at Edmonton Board of Health, Edmonton, Alberta, Canada.

Newman, M.A. (1990, March). *The Newman model: Health as expanding consciousness.* Public lecture presented at University of Alberta, Edmonton.

Newman, M.A. (1990, April). *The conceptualization and measurement of health-related research.* Keynote address presented at the Sigma Theta Tau Research Day, Delta Xi and Iota Psi Epsilon Chapters, Kent, Ohio.

Newman, M.A. (1990, April). *Theoretical framework of Newman theory of health.* Paper presented at Second South Florida Nursing Theorist Conference, Miami.

Newman, M.A. (1990, April). *The quest for knowledge in nursing.* Linnea Henderson Lectureship, Kent State University School of Nursing, Kent, Ohio.

Newman, M.A. (1991, March). *Nursing theory and its application to long-term care.* Paper presented at Minnesota Association of Homes for the Aging 1991 Institute, Minneapolis.

Newman, M.A. (1991, April). *Nursing's essential questions.* Paper presented at Sigma Theta Tau Induction Program, Iota Iota Chapter, Salt Lake City, Utah.

Newman, M.A. (1991, June). *Differentiated nursing practice: Implications and applications.* Keynote speaker, Presbyterian Hospital, New York City.

Newman, M.A. (1991, June). *Nursing theory for the future.* Paper presented at School of Nursing, Wayne State University, Detroit.

Newman, M.A. (1991, June). *Prevailing paradigms in nursing.* National Forum on Doctoral Education, Amelia Island, Florida.

Newman, M.A. (1992, April). *Development of the discipline.* Viana McCowan Lecture, College of Nursing, University of South Carolina, Columbia, SC.

Newman, M.A. (1992, Oct.). *Theory for nursing practice.* Keynote address, Symposium 3, Developing Knowledge for Nursing Practice: Research and Practice Linkages Within Four Philosophical Perspectives, University of Rhode Island College of Nursing, Newport, RI.

Newman, M.A. (1993, April). *Into the 21st century.* Keynote speaker, 25th Anniversary Celebration, School of Nursing, The Pennsylvania State University, Harrisburg.

Newman, M.A. (1993, Sept.). *The paradoxes of nursing practice.* Keynote address, 7th Annual Granger Westberg Symposium, Chicago, IL.

Newman, M.A. (1994, May). *Perspectives of differentiated practice.* Paper presented at Seventh Annual Nurse Scholar Lecture, Saint Xavier University School of Nursing, Chicago, IL.

Newman, M.A. (1994, Nov.). *Theory underlying case management.* Paper presented at United Health Care Systems, Oswego, NY.

Newman, M.A. (1995, Oct.). *Dialogue on theory underlying practice.* Paper presented at First National Healing Web Partners Conference, Park City, UT.

Newman, M.A. (1996, June). *A dialogue with Martha Rogers and David Bohm.* Paper presented at Society of Rogerian Scholars, New York.

Newman, M.A. (1996, June). *The rhythm of relating.* Paper presented at American Holistic Nurses Association, St. Louis.

Newman, M.A. (1996, Oct.). *Process as content.* Paper presented at Knowledge Conference 1996: Developing Knowledge for Nursing Practice, Boston College of Nursing and Eastern Nursing Research Society Theory Interest Group, Boston.

Newman, M.A. (1998, April). *Dialogue with Margaret Newman: Health, nursing theory and research as praxis.* Paper presented at Keynote address, Ann Berdahl Lecture Series and Zeta Zeta Research Day, Augustana College, Sioux Fall, SD.

Newman, M.A. (1998, May). *Dialogue with Margaret Newman and panel.* Paper presented at Sixth Nurse Theorist Conference, Augsburg College, Minneapolis.

Newman, M.A. (1999, May). *The science of nursing practice: Philosophy in the nurse's world.* Paper presented at

Pursuit of Nursing Science: Contemporary Issues and Controversies, Institute for Philosophical Nursing Research, University of Alberta, The Banff Centre, Banff Alberta, Canada.

Correspondence

Newman, M.A. (1984). Personal correspondence.
Newman, M.A. (1985). Personal correspondence.
Newman, M.A. (1988). Personal correspondence.
Newman, M.A. (1992). Personal correspondence.
Newman, M.A. (1996). Personal correspondence.
Newman, M.A. (2000). Personal correspondence.

Interviews

Newman, M.A. (1985). Telephone interview.
Newman, M.A. (1996). Telephone interview.
Newman, M.A. (2000, April). Telephone interview.

Secondary Sources

Book Reviews

Cowling, W.R., Pearson, B.D., & Silva, M.C. (1988). [Review of the book *Health as expanding consciousness*]. *Nursing Science Quarterly, 1*(3), 133-135.
Gold, C.R. (1996). [Review of the book *Health as expanding consciousness*]. *Nursing Science Quarterly, 9*(3), 136-137.
Matas, K.E. (1995). [Review of the book *Health as expanding consciousness*]. *Image: Journal of Nursing Scholarship, 27*(2), 163.
[Review of the book *Health as expanding consciousness*]. (1995, Feb.). *Journal of Advanced Nursing, 21*(2), 407-408.
[Review of the book *Health as expanding consciousness*]. (1995, Summer). *Image: Journal of Nursing Scholarship, 27*(2), 163.
[Review of the book *Theory development in nursing*]. (1979, Nov./Dec.). *Continuing Education in Nursing, 2*, 8.
[Review of the book *Theory development in nursing*]. (1980, March). *Nursing Leadership, 3*, 38.
[Review of the book *Theory development in nursing*]. (1980, Spring). *Nursing Administration Quarterly, 4*, 81-82.
[Review of the book *Theory development in nursing*]. (1980, Spring). *Western Journal of Nursing Research, 2*, 250-251.
[Review of the book *Theory development in nursing*]. (1980, Sept./Oct.). *Nursing Research, 29*, 311.
Watson, J. (1987). [Review of the book *Health as expanding consciousness*]. *Journal of Professional Nursing, 3*(5), 315.
Yamashita, M. (1997). [Review of the book *A developing discipline*]. *Image: Journal of Nursing Scholarship, 29*(4), 391.

Books

Chinn, P.L. & Kramer, M.K. (1995). *Theory and nursing: A systematic approach* (4th ed.). St. Louis: Mosby.

Kim, H.S. (1983). *The nature of theoretical thinking in nursing.* Norwalk, CT: Appleton-Century-Crofts.
Marchione, J. (1993). *Margaret Newman: Health as expanding consciousness.* Newbury Park, CA: Sage.
Meleis, A.J. (1991). *Theoretical nursing: Development and progress* (2nd ed.). Philadelphia: Lippincott.

Listings

Who's Who of American Women. (1983-1985). New Providence, NJ: Reed Reference Publishing Co.
Who's Who in America. (1996). New Providence, NJ: Reed Reference Publishing Co.
Who's Who in American Nursing. (1996-2000). New Providence, NJ: Reed Reference Publishing Co.

Book Chapters

Burd, C. (1985). Appendix D. Newman's nursing theory of health. In B.W. Duldt & K. Geffin (Eds.), *Theoretical perspectives for nursing.* Boston: Little, Brown.
Chinn, P.L. (1983). Nursing theory development: Where we have been and where we are going. In N.L. Chaska (Ed.), *The nursing profession: A time to speak.* New York: McGraw-Hill.
Desai, S.M., Keffer, J., Hensley, D.M., Kilgore-Keever, K.A., Langfitt, J.V., & Peterson, L. (1998). Margaret A. Newman: Model of health. In A. Marriner Tomey & M.R. Alligood (Eds.), *Nursing theorists and their work* (4th ed.). St Louis: Mosby.
Engle, V. (1983). Newman's model of health. In J.J. Fitzpatrick & A.L. Whall (Eds.), *Conceptual models of nursing: Analysis and application* (pp. 263-273). Bowie, MD: Robert J. Brady.
Fawcett, J. (1993). Newman's theory of health as expanding consciousness. In J. Fawcett (Ed.), *Analysis and evaluation of nursing theories* (pp. 89-114). Philadelphia: F.A. Davis.
George, J.B. (1990). Other extant theory. In J.B. George (Ed.), *Nursing theories* (3rd ed., pp. 373-379). Norwalk, CT: Appleton & Lange.
Gustafson, W. (1990). Application of Newman's theory of health: Pattern recognition as nursing practice. In M. Parker (Ed.), *Nursing theories in practice* (pp. 141-161). New York: National League for Nursing.
Hichman, J.S. (1995). An introduction to nursing theory. In J.B. George (Ed.), *Nursing theories. The base for professional nursing practice* (4th ed., pp. 1-12). Norwalk, CT: Appleton & Lange.
Kalb, K.A. (1990). The gift: Applying Newman's theory of health in nursing practice. In M. Parker (Ed.), *Nursing theories in practice* (pp. 163-186). New York: National League for Nursing.
Marchione, J.M. (1986). Pattern as methodology for assessing family health: Newman's theory of health. In P. Winstead-Fry (Ed.), *Case studies in nursing theory.* New York: National League for Nursing.

Witucki, J. (2000). Newman's theory of health and nursing practice. In M.R. Alligood & A. Marriner Tomey (Eds.), *Nursing theory: Utilization and application* (2nd ed.). St. Louis: Mosby.

Journal Articles

Ammende, M. (1996). Change of paradigm in nursing. Part 1: Theory of Martha Rogers [German]. *Pflege, 9,* 5-11.

Ammende, M. (1996). Change of paradigm in nursing. Part 2: Elizabeth Barrett's "Theory of power" [German]. *Pflege, 9,* 98-104.

Batra, C. (1987). Nursing theory for undergraduates. *Nursing Outlook, 35,* 189-192.

Boyd, C.O. (1990). Critical appraisal of developing nursing research methods. *Nursing Science Quarterly, 3,* 42-43.

Bramlett, M.H., Gueldner, S.H., & Sowell, R.L. (1990). Consumer-centric advocacy: Its connection to nursing frameworks. *Nursing Science Quarterly, 3,* 156-161.

Bunkers, S.S., Brendtro, M., Holmes, P.K., Howell, J., Johnson, S., Koerner, J., Larson, J., Nelson, J., & Weaver, R. (1992). The healing web: A transformative model for nursing. *Nursing and Health Care, 13,* 68-73.

Bunkers, S.S., Michaels, C., & Ethridge, P. (1997) Advanced practice nursing in community: Nursing's opportunity. *Advanced Practice Nursing Quarterly, 2(4),* 79-84.

Butrin, J.E. (1992). Cultural diversity in the nurse-client encounter. *Clinical Nursing Research, 1,* 238-251.

Capasso, V.A. (1998). The theory is the practice: An exemplar. *Clinical Nurse Specialist, 12,* 226-229.

Connor, M.J. (1998). Expanding the dialogue on praxis in nursing research and practice. *Nursing Science Quarterly, 11,* 51-55.

Cull-Wilby, B.L. & Pepin, J.I. (1987). Towards a coexistence of paradigms in nursing knowledge development. *Journal of Advanced Nursing, 12,* 515-521.

DeGrott, H.A., Ferketich, S.L., & Larson, P.J. (1987). Theory development in a non-university service setting. *Journal of Nursing Administration, 17(4),* 38-44.

Doherty, W.J. (1985). Family interventions in health care. *Family Relations, 34,* 129-137.

Endo, E. (1998). Pattern recognition as a nursing intervention with Japanese women with ovarian cancer. *Advances in Nursing Science, 20(4),* 49-61.

Endo, E. (1999). Letters to the editor . . . A commentary on Newman's theory of health as expanding consciousness. *Advances in Nursing Science, 21(3),* vii-viii.

Engle, V.F. (1984). Newman's conceptual framework and the measurement of older adults' health. *Advances in Nursing Science, 7,* 24-36.

Engle, V.F. (1986). The relationship of movement and time to older adults' functional health. *Research in Nursing and Health, 9,* 123-129.

Engle, V.F. & Graney, M.J. (1985/1986). Self-assessed and functional health of older women. *International Journal of Aging and Human Development, 22,* 301-313.

Ethridge, P. (1991). A nursing HMO: Carondolet St. Mary's experience. *Nursing Management, 22(7),* 22-27.

Ford-Gilboe, M.V. (1994). A comparison of two nursing models: Allen's developmental health model and Newman's theory of health as expanding consciousness. *Nursing Science Quarterly, 7,* 113-118.

Freshwater, D. (1999). Polarity and unity in caring: The healing power of symptoms. *Complementary Therapies in Nursing and Midwifery, 5,* 136-139.

Fryback, P.B. (1993). Health for people with a terminal diagnosis. *Nursing Science Quarterly, 6,* 147-159.

Gulick, E.E. & Bugg, A. (1992). Holistic health patterning in multiple sclerosis. *Research in Nursing and Health, 15,* 175-185.

Gupta, S. & Cummings, L.L. (1986). Perceived speed of time and task affect. *Perceptual and Motor Skills, 63,* 971-980.

Haggman, L.A. (1997). Health as an individual's way of existence. *Journal of Advanced Nursing, 25,* 45-53.

Hall, E.O.C. (1996). Husserlian phenomenology and nursing in a unitary-transformative paradigm. Vard I. Norden. *Nursing Science and Research in the Nordic Countries, 16(3),* 4-8.

Holmes, C.A. (1993). Praxis: A case study in the depoliticization of methods in nursing research . . . including commentary by Thompson, J.L. *Scholarly Inquiry for Nursing Practice, 7,* 3-15.

Jacono, B.J. & Jacono, J.J. (1996). The benefits of Newman and Parse in helping nurse teachers determine methods to enhance student creativity. *Nurse Education Today, 16,* 356-362.

Jan, R. & Smith, C.A. (1998). Staying healthy in immigrant Pakistani families living in the United States. *Image: Journal of Nursing Scholarship, 30,* 157-159.

Jennings, B.M. (1987). Nursing theory development: Successes and challenges. *Journal of Advanced Nursing, 12,* 63-69.

Jonsdottir, H. (1998). Life patterns of people with chronic obstructive pulmonary disease: Isolation and being closed in. *Nursing Science Quarterly, 11,* 160-166.

Karian, V.E., Jankowski, S.M., & Beal, J.A. (1998). Exploring the lived-experience of childhood cancer survivors. *Journal of Pediatric Oncology Nursing, 15,* 153-162.

Keene, L. (1985). Nursing as a partnership. *New Zealand Nursing Journal, 78(12),* 10-11.

Kendall, J. (1996). Human association as a factor influencing wellness in homosexual men with human immunodeficiency virus disease. *Applied Nursing Research, 9,* 195-203.

Koerner, J.G. & Bunkers, S.S. (1994) The healing web: An expansion of consciousness. *Journal of Holistic Nursing, 12,* 51-63.

Litchfield, M. (1999). Practice wisdom. *Advances in Nursing Science, 22,* 62-73.

Magen, S.J., Gibbon, E.J., & Mrozek, R. (1990). Nursing theory application: A practice model. *Issues in Mental Health Nursing,* 11, 297-312.

Martsolf, D.S. & Mickley, J.R. (1998). The concept of spirituality in nursing theories: Differing world-views and extent of focus. *Journal of Advanced Nursing, 27,* 294-303.

Meleis, A.I. (1990). Being and becoming healthy: The core of nursing knowledge. *Nursing Science Quarterly, 3,* 107-114.

Mentzer, C.A. & Schorr, J.A. (1986). Perceived situational control and perceived duration of time: Expressions of life patterns. *Advances in Nursing Science,* 9, 12-20.

Michaels, C. (1992). Carondolet St. Mary's nursing enterprise. *Nursing Clinics of North America,* 27, 77-85.

Michaels, C. (2000). Becoming a Bard: A journey to self. *Nursing Science Quarterly,* 13, 28-30.

Mitchell, G.J. & Cody, W.K. (1992). Nursing knowledge and human science: Ontological and epistemological considerations. *Nursing Science Quarterly,* 5, 54-61.

Moccia, P. (1985). A further investigation of "dialectical thinking as a means of understanding systems-in-development: Relevance to Rogers's principles." *Advances in Nursing Science,* 7(4), 33-38.

Moch, S.D. (1990). Health within the experience of breast cancer. *Journal of Advanced Nursing,* 15, 1426-1435.

Moch, S.D. (1991). Using health models for promoting organizational health in nursing. *Journal of Holistic Nursing,* 9(2), 22-30.

Moch, S.D. (1998). Health-within-illness: Concept development through research and practice. *Journal of Advanced Nursing,* 28, 305-310.

Overman, B. (1994). Lessons from the Tao for birthing practice. *Journal of Holistic Nursing,* 12, 142-147.

Peplau, H.E. (1988). The art and science of nursing: Similarities, differences, and relations. *Nursing Science Quarterly,* 1, 8-15.

Picard, C. (1997). Embodied soul: The focus for nursing praxis. *Journal of Holistic Nursing,* 15, 41-53.

Picard, C. (2000). Pattern of expanding consciousness in mid-life women: Creative movement and the narrative as modes of expression. *Nursing Science Quarterly,* 13, 150-158.

Picard, C., Sickul, C., & Natale, S. (1998). Healing reflections: The transformative mirror. *International Journal for Human Caring,* 2(3), 29-47.

Pridham, K.F. & Hansen, M.F. (1985). Nursing and medicine: Complementary modes of thought and action. *Public Health Nursing,* 2, 195-201.

Ray, M.A. (1990). Critical reflective analysis of Parse's and Newman's research methodologies. *Nursing Science Quarterly,* 3, 44-46.

Reed, P.G. (1986). Developmental resources and depression in the elderly. *Nursing Research,* 35, 368-374.

Reed, P.G. (1996). Theoretical concerns. Transcendence: Formulating nursing perspectives. *Nursing Science Quarterly,* 9, 2-4.

Rosenbaum, J.N. (1986). Comparison of two theorists on care: Orem and Leininger. *Journal of Advanced Nursing,* 11, 409-419.

Roy, C. (1979). Relating nursing theory to education: A new era. *Nurse Educator,* 29, 16-21.

Sanders, S.A. (1986). Development of a tool to measure subjective time experience. *Nursing Research,* 35, 178-182.

Sarter, B. (1987). Evolutionary idealism: A philosophical foundation for holistic nursing theory. *Advances in Nursing Science,* 9(2), 1-9.

Sarter, B. (1988). Philosophical sources of nursing theory. *Nursing Science Quarterly,* 1, 52-60.

Schlotzhauser, M. & Farnham, R. (1997). Newman's theory and insulin dependent diabetes mellitus in adolescence. *Journal of School Nursing,* 13(3), 20-23.

Schorr, J.A. (1993). Music and pattern change in chronic pain. *Advances in Nursing Science,* 15(4), 27-36.

Schorr, J.A., Farnham, R.C., & Ervin, S.M. (1991). Health patterns in aging women as expanding consciousness. *Advances in Nursing Science,* 13(4), 52-63.

Schorr, J.A. & Schroeder, C.A. (1989). Consciousness as a dissipative structure: An extension of the Newman model. *Nursing Science Quarterly,* 2, 183-193.

Schorr, J.A. & Schroeder, C.A. (1991). Movement and time: Exertion and perceived duration. *Nursing Science Quarterly,* 4, 104-112.

Silva, M.C. (1986). Research testing nursing theory: State of the art. *Advances in Nursing Science,* 9, 1-11.

Silva, M.C. & Rothbart, D. (1984). An analysis of changing trends in philosophies of science on nursing theory development and testing. *Advances in Nursing Science,* 6, 1-13.

Smith, C.A. (1995). The lived experience of staying healthy in rural African American families. *Nursing Science Quarterly,* 8, 17-21.

Smith, M.J. (1984). Temporal experience and bed rest: Replication and refinement. *Nursing Research,* 33, 298-302.

Smith, S.K. (1997). Women's experience of victimizing sexualization, part I: Responses related to abuse and home and family environment. *Issues in Mental Health Nursing,* 18, 395-416.

Smith, S.K. (1997). Women's experience of victimizing sexualization, part II: Community and longer term personal impacts. *Issues in Mental Health Nursing,* 18, 417-435.

Sohl-Krieger, R., Lagaard, M.W., & Scherrer, J. (1996). Nursing case management—Relationships as a strategy to improve care. *Clinical Nurse Specialist,* 10, 107-113.

Solari-Twadell, P., Bunkers, S., Wang, C., & Snyder, D. (1995). The pinwheel model of bereavement. *Image: Journal of Nursing Scholarship,* 27, 323-326.

Tompkins, E. (1980). Effect of restricted mobility and dominance in perceived duration. *Nursing Research, 29,* 333-338.

Utley, R. (1999). The evolving meaning of cancer for long-term survivors of breast cancer. *Oncology Nursing Forum, 26,* 1519-1523.

Wade, G.H. (1998). A concept analysis of personal transformation. *Journal of Advanced Nursing, 28,* 713-719.

Weingourt, R. (1998). Using Margaret A. Newman's theory of health with elderly nursing home residents. *Perspectives in Psychiatric Care, Journal of Nurse Psychotherapists, 34*(3), 25-30.

Wendler, M.C. (1996). Understanding healing: A conceptual analysis. *Journal of Advanced Nursing, 24,* 836-842.

Whall, A.L. (1986). The family as the unit of care in nursing: A historical review. *Public Health Nursing, 3,* 240-249.

Yamashita, M. (1997). Family caregiving: Application of Newman's and Peplau's theories. *Journal of Psychiatric and Mental Health Nursing, 4,* 401-405.

Yamashita, M. (1998). Family coping with mental illness: A comparative study. *Journal of Psychiatric and Mental Health Nursing, 5,* 515-523.

Yamashita, M. (1998). Newman's theory of health as expanding consciousness: Research on family caregiving in mental illness in Japan. *Nursing Science Quarterly, 11,* 110-115.

Yamashita, M. (1999). Newman's theory of health applied in family caregiving in Canada. *Nursing Science Quarterly, 12,* 73-79.

Yamashita, M. & Forsyth, D.M. (1998). Family coping with mental illness: An aggregate from two studies, Canada and the United States. *Journal of the American Psychiatric Nurses Association, 4,* 1-8.

Yamashita, M., Jensen, E., & Tall, F. (1998). Therapeutic touch: Applying Newman's theoretic approach. *Nursing Science Quarterly, 11*(2), 49-50.

Yamashita, M. & Tall, F.D. (1998). A commentary on Newman's theory of health as expanding consciousness. *Advances in Nursing Science, 21,* 65-75.

Yamashita, M. & Tall, F.D. (1999). Letters to the editor . . . A commentary on Newman: Theory of health as expanding consciousness. *Advances in Nursing Science, 22*(1), vi-viii.

News Releases

Brown, N.M. (1983, Nov.). The body is not a machine. *Research/Penn State, 4*(4), 19-20.

M.A. Newman appointed as full tenured professor at University of Minnesota School of Nursing. (1984, March). *Nursing Outlook, 32,* 2.

Abstract

Newman, M.A. (1981). *Relationship of age to perceived duration. Abstracts of ANF funded research 1979-1980.* Kansas City: American Nurses' Foundation.

Dissertations

Brenner, P.S. (1987). Temporal perspective, professional identity, and perceived well-being. *Dissertation Abstracts International, 47*-12B, 4821.

Butrin, J.E. (1990). The experience of culturally diverse nurse-client encounters. *Dissertation Abstracts International, 51*-06B, 2815.

DeBrun, K.T. (1989). An investigation of the relationships among standing, sitting, recumbent postures, judgment of time duration and preferred personal space in adult females. *Dissertation Abstracts International, 50,* 122B.

Endo, E. (1996). Pattern recognition as a nursing intervention with adults with cancer. *Dissertation Abstracts International, 57*-06B, 3653.

Engle, V.F. (1981). A study of the relationship between self-assessment of health, function, personal tempo, and time perception in elderly women. *Dissertation Abstracts International, 42*-03B, 0967.

Fryback, P.B. (1991). Perceptions of health by persons with a terminal disease: Implications for nursing. *Dissertation Abstracts International, 52*-04B, 1951.

Geddes, N.J. (1999). The experience of personal transformation in healing touch (HT) practitioners: A heuristic inquiry. *Dissertation Abstracts International, 60*-06B, 2607.

Gross, S.W. (1995). The impact of a nursing intervention of relaxation with guided imagery on breast cancer patients' stress and health as expanding consciousness. *Dissertation Abstracts International , 56*-10B, 5416.

Jonsdottir, H. (1994). Life patterns of people with chronic obstructive pulmonary disease: Isolation and being closed in. *Dissertation Abstracts International, 56*-03B, 1346.

Kelley, F.J. (1990). Spatial temporal experiences and self-assessed health in the older adult. *Dissertation Abstracts International, 51,* 1194B.

Kiser Larsen, N.K. (1999). Life patterns of Native American women experiencing breast cancer. *Dissertation Abstracts International, 60*-05B, 2062.

Koither, M.Z. (1994). The dance of human becoming: A philosophic inquiry into health promotion and healing within the unitary-transformative paradigm. *Dissertation Abstracts International, 55*-10B, 4322.

Krejci, J.W. (1992). An exploration of synchrony in nursing. *Dissertation Abstracts International, 53*-05B, 2247.

Lamendola, F.P. (1998). Patterns of the caregiving experience of selected nurses in hospice and HIV/AIDS care. *Dissertation Abstracts International, 59*-03B, 1048.

Leners, D.W. (1990). The deep connection: an echo of transpersonal caring. *Dissertation Abstracts International, 51,* 2818B.

Litchfield, M.C. (1997). The process of nursing partnership in family health. *Dissertation Abstracts International, 59*-04B, 1802.

Moch, S.D. (1989). Health in illness: Experiences with breast cancer. *Dissertation Abstracts International, 50-02B*, 0497.

Muscari, M.E. (1992). Binge/purge behaviors and attitudes as a manifestation of relational patternings in a woman with bulimia nervosa. *Dissertation Abstracts International, 53-11B,* 5647.

Noveletsky-Rosenthal, H.T. (1996). Pattern recognition in older adults living with chronic illness. *Dissertation Abstracts International, 57-10B,* 6180.

Page, G. (1989). An exploration of the relationship between daily patterning and weight loss maintenance. *Dissertation Abstracts International, 50,* 497B.

Picard, C.A. (1998). Uncovering pattern of expanding consciousness in mid-life women: Creative movement and the narrative as modes of expression. *Dissertation Abstracts International, 59-03B,* 1049.

Roux, G.M. (1994). Phenomenologic study: Inner strength in women with breast cancer. *UMI Dissertation Services,* No. 9417377.

Schmitt, N.A. (1992). Caregiving couples: The experience of giving and receiving social support. *Dissertation Abstracts International, 52,* 5761B.

Schroeder, C.A. (1993). Perceived duration of time and bedrest in high risk pregnancy: An exploration of the Newman Model. *Dissertation Abstracts International, 54-04B,* 1894.

Sipple, J.E.A. (1989). A model for curriculum change based on retrospective analysis. *Dissertation Abstracts International, 50,* 1927A.

Smith, C.A. (1990). The lived experience of staying healthy in rural black families. *Dissertation Abstracts International, 50,* 3925B.

Smith, S.K. (1995). Women's experiences of victimizing sexualization. *Dissertation Abstracts International, 57-06B,* 3659.

Tennyson, M.G. (1992). Becoming pregnant: Perceptions of black adolescents. *Dissertation Abstracts International, 52,* 5196B.

Tommet, P.A. (1997). Nurse-parent dialogue: Illuminating the pattern of families with children who are medically fragile. *Dissertation Abstracts International, 58-05B,* 2359.

Utley, R. (1997). Life patterns of older women who have survived breast cancer. *Dissertation Abstracts International, 58-11B,* 5892.

Van Nostrand, J.A. (1992). The process of perspective transformation: Instrument development and testing in smokers and exsmokers. *Dissertation Abstracts International, 53-11B,* 5649.

Witucki, J. (2000). *Help-seeking by older wife caregivers of demented husbands: A grounded theory approach.* Unpublished Doctoral dissertation, University of Tennessee, Knoxville.

Theses

Allender, C. (1993). *An instrument to measure Newman's trilevel model of differentiated nursing practice.* Unpublished master's thesis, University of Minnesota.

Batty, M.L.E. (1999). *Pattern identification and expanding consciousness during the transition of "low risk" pregnancy.* Unpublished master's thesis, The University of New Brunswick.

Bruce-Barrett, C.A. (1998). Patterns of health and healing: Peer support and prostate cancer. *Masters Abstracts International, 37-01,* 0233.

Butrin, J. (1983). *Differences in time perspective and hemisphericity between educated and noneducated Zairians.* Unpublished master's thesis, Pennsylvania State University.

Casper, S.A. (1999). Psychosocial adaptation as a dimension of health as expanding consciousness: Effectiveness of burn survivors support groups. *Masters Abstracts International, 37-05,* 1433.

Griscabage, D. (1982). *Relationships among state anxiety time estimation, body movement, and repression-sensitization in preoperative patients.* Unpublished master's thesis, Pennsylvania State University.

Jonsdottir, H. (1988). *Health patterns of clients with chronic obstructive pulmonary disease.* Unpublished master's thesis, University of Minnesota.

Kuhn, M.E. (1989). Comparison of health beliefs of adolescents with diabetes and those of their mothers. *Masters Abstracts International, 28,* 412.

Litchfield, M.C. (1993). *The process of health patterning in families with young children who have been repeatedly hospitalized.* Unpublished master's thesis, University of Minnesota.

Mentzer, C. (1985). An investigation into the conceptual system proposed by Margaret Newman. The relationship between perceived situational control and perceived duration of time among institutionalized elderly. *Masters Abstracts International, 24-02,* 0136.

Pollard, M. (1981). *Emotional expressiveness in cancer and noncancer patients.* Unpublished master's thesis, Pennsylvania State University.

Pollock, D. (1983). *The relationship of sleep deprivation to cerebral hemisphericity and temporal orientation.* Unpublished master's thesis, Pennsylvania State University.

Polych, C.F. (1993). Nurses' responses to abuse of nurses at work. *Masters Abstracts International, 32-01,* 0230.

Shanahan, S.M. (1993). The lived experience of life-passing in middle adolescent females. *Masters Abstracts International, 32-05,* 1376.

Terhaar, N.C. (1989). Blood sugar and cognition patterns in the elderly. *Masters Abstracts International, 28,* 116.

Zack, C. (1983). *Hospitalized patients' personal space preferences in relation to female and male nurses.* Unpublished master's thesis, Pennsylvania State University.

Other

Acton, H.B. (1967). George Wilhelm Freidrich Hegel 1770-1831. In P. Edwards (Ed.), *The encyclopedia of philosophy* (Vols. 3 & 4). New York: Macmillan & Free Press.

Barnard, R. (1973). *Field-dependent-independence and selected motor abilities*. Unpublished doctoral dissertation, New York University.

Bentov, I. (1977). *Stalking the wild pendulum*. New York: E.P. Dutton.

Bentov, I. (1978, Nov.). *The mechanics of consciousness*. Paper presented at the symposium on New Dimensions of Consciousness, sponsored by Sufi Order in the West, New York.

Bohm, D. (1980). *Wholeness and the implicate order*. London: Routledge and Kegan Paul.

Capra, F. (1975). *The tao of physics*. Boulder, CO: Thambhala Publications.

Chapman, J. (1978). The relationship between auditory stimulation and gross motor activity of short-gestation infants. *Research in Nursing and Health, 1*, 29-36.

de Chardin, T. (1971). *Activation of energy*. New York: Harcourt, Brace, & Jovanovich.

Downs, F. & Fitzpatrick, J. (1976). Preliminary investigation of the reliability and validity of a tool for the assessment of body position and motor activity. *Nursing Research, 25*, 404-408.

Engle, V. (1981). *A study of the relationship between self-assessment of health, function, personal tempo and time perception in elderly women*. Unpublished doctoral dissertation, Wayne State University.

Fitzpatrick, J. & Donovan, M. (1978). Temporal experience and motor behavior among the aging. *Research in Nursing and Health, 1*, 60-68.

Gendlin, E.T. (1978). *Focusing*. New York: Everest.

Goldberg, W. & Fitzpatrick, J. (1980). Movement therapy and the aged. *Nursing Research, 29*, 339-346.

Marcuse, H. (1954). *Reason and revolution: Hegel and the rise of social theory* (2nd ed.). New York: Beacon.

Moss, R. (1981). *The i that is we*. Millbrae, CA: Celestial Arts.

Prigogine, I. (1976). Order through fluctuation: Self-organization and social system. In E. Jantsch & C.H. Waddington (Eds.), *Evolution and consciousness* (pp. 93-133). Reading, MA: Addison-Wesley.

Prigogine, I., Allen, P.M., & Herman, R. (1977). Long term trends and the evolution of complexity. In E. Laszlo & J. Bierman (Eds.), *Goals in a global community: The original background papers for goals for mankind* (Vol. 1, pp. 1-63). New York: Pergamon.

Rogers, M.E. (1970). *An introduction to the theoretical basis of nursing*. Philadelphia: F.A. Davis.

Rogers, M.E. (1980). Nursing, a science of unitary man. In J.P. Riehl & C. Roy (Eds.), *Conceptual models for nursing practice*. New York: Appleton-Century-Crofts.

Smith, M. (1979). Duration experience for bed-confined subjects: A replication and refinement. *Nursing Research, 28*, 139-144.

Tompkins, E. (1980). Effect of restricted mobility and dominance in perceived duration. *Nursing Research, 29*, 333-338.

Whyte, L.L. (1974). *The universe of experience*. New York: Harper & Row.

Young, A.M. (1976). *The reflexive universe: Evolution of consciousness*. San Francisco: Robert Briggs.

Interviews and Correspondence

Doberneck, B. (1985). Telephone interview.

Marchione, J. (1985). Telephone interview.

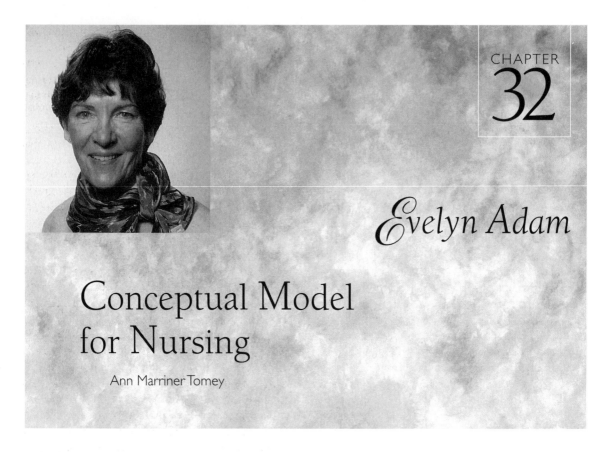

Evelyn Adam

Conceptual Model for Nursing

Ann Marriner Tomey

CREDENTIALS AND BACKGROUND OF THE THEORIST

Evelyn Adam was born April 9, 1929 in Lanark, Ontario, Canada. She graduated from Hotel Dieu Hospital in Kingston, Ontario in 1950 with a diploma in nursing. She received a B.Sc. degree from the University of Montreal in 1966 and an M.N. degree from the University of California, Los Angeles in 1971. There she met Dorothy Johnson, who she believes has "definitely been the most important influence" on her professional life.[12]

Previous authors: Linda S. Harbour, Terri Creekmur, Janet DeFelice, Marilyn Sue Doub, Anne Hodel, Ann Marriner Tomey, and Cheryl Y. Petty.
The author wishes to thank Evelyn Adam for reviewing the chapter and Steve Hardin, reference librarian, for assistance in locating obscure information.

In 1979, Adam published her first book, *Être Infirmière*,[3] and published the second edition in 1983[9] and the third edition in 1991.[17] In 1980, she wrote the English version of *To Be a Nurse*[4] and published the second edition in 1991.[18] Since then, *To Be a Nurse* has been translated into Dutch,[7] Spanish,[8] Italian,[19] Portuguese,[20] and Japanese.[22] Adam authored several chapters and was coeditor of *La personne âgée et ses besoins: Interventions infirmières.*[28] This book, published in 1996, presents the nursing care of the aged based on Henderson's model for nursing care. Adam has also written numerous articles on conceptual models for nursing and has coauthored several others. Professional journals publishing her articles include *L'infirmière Canadienne,*[2,6,13,25] *Canadian Nurse,*[1,5] *Journal of Advanced Nursing,*[10] *Canadian Journal of Nursing Research,*[23] *Nursing Papers: Perspectives in Nursing,*[11] and *Journal of Nursing Education.*[14]

Adam has been a visiting professor at several universities. She has functioned as a resource person and speaker for various professional corporations, clinical and educational settings, and national and international conventions. From 1983 to 1989, she was a member of the review board for *Nursing Papers: Perspectives in Nursing.* She taught at both undergraduate and graduate levels at the Faculty of Nursing of the University of Montreal. She was faculty secretary from 1982 until her retirement in 1989, at which time the university named her Professor Emeritus. She has been in *Who's Who in the World* since its eighth edition in 1987/1988. In 1992, Laval University in Quebec City awarded her an honorary doctorate. In 1995, the Order of Nurses of Quebec awarded her its highest distinction, the Order of Merit, in recognition of her important contributions to nursing. She does volunteer work in her church parish and continues to write, speak, and do consulting work. She is writing a book about her childhood and early nursing experiences.[21,24]

Although nursing care of the elderly is a recent professional interest, promoting conceptual models for nursing has predominated since 1970. She strongly feels that "nursing practice, education, and research must be based on an explicit frame of reference specific to nursing."[12]

Adam's work makes an important distinction between a conceptual model and a theory. "A [conceptual] model is usually based on, or derived from, a theory. . . . A model, emerging from a theory, may become the basis for a new theory."[1:40] "A conceptual model, for whatever discipline, is not reality; it is a mental image of reality or a way of conceptualizing reality. A conceptual model for nursing is therefore a conception of nursing."[10:42]

Adam[11,12] accepts Roy and Roberts' definition[29:5] of a theory as "a system of interrelated propositions used to describe, predict, explain, understand, and control a part of the empirical world."

Therefore a theory is useful to more than one discipline. A conceptual model for a discipline is useful only to that particular discipline. Adam[14] believes that some day, nursing theory will be as useful to related disciplines as existing theories, developed in other fields, are useful to nursing.

Adam[4:5] writes that "a conceptual model is an abstraction, a way of looking at something, an invention of the mind." Further, she states that "a conceptual model for a discipline is a very broad perspective, a global way of looking at a discipline. Most of the conceptual models for nursing that we know have come from two sources: one, a theory, chosen by the author, and the other, her professional experience."[12]

A conceptual model is the precursor of a theory. The model specifies the discipline's focus of inquiry, identifies those phenomena of particular interest to nursing, and provides a broad perspective for nursing research, practice, and education. The study of phenomena that concern nursing (nursing research) may lead to theories that will describe, explain, or predict those phenomena. Such theories will not be theories of nursing, but theories of the phenomena that are nursing's focus of inquiry.[11]

Many nurses are unable to communicate their conception of the service they offer to society clearly and explicitly. Adam contends that this is not because they do not have a conception of nursing, but because their conceptual base is not clear. If the nurse's mental image of nursing is vague or blurred, it will therefore be difficult to put into words. The nurse will then be unable to articulate his or her particular role in healthcare and may find that professional activities are based on a perspective borrowed from another discipline.

Adam[1:41] states that "a model indicates the goal of our [nursing] profession—an ideal and limited goal, because it gives us direction for nursing practice, nursing education, and nursing research." Nurses who have a clear, concise conceptual base specific to nursing will be able to identify areas for theory development, prepare future practitioners of nursing, and demonstrate nursing's contribution to healthcare in their own practice. In this way, healthcare will improve and the nursing profession will grow.

Although it is not necessary for every nurse to adopt the same conceptual model, it is essential that every nurse have a concise and explicit framework on which to base his or her work. The conceptual model is the conceptual departure point for teaching, research, or nursing care. Speaking figuratively, Adam places the conceptual model in the nurse's occipital lobe, known also as the visual lobe. The nurse uses a great deal of scientific knowledge, experience, intuition, and creativity. In drawing on this knowledge, the nurse is guided by the conceptual model; that is, the mental image of nursing.[14]

Through the nursing process, the abstraction that is the conceptual model is linked to the reality that is nursing practice.[4] The data nurses collect depend on their conceptual base. The way nurses interpret the data, the plan they develop, the nursing action they choose, and the evaluation of their intervention also depend on their model. The number of steps in the nursing process is not significant because the difference is the conceptual base.[12]

In addition to the conceptual model and the nursing process, the nurse must also establish, with the client, what will be perceived to be a helping relationship. Adam considers this perhaps the most important component of being a nurse. It is the climate of empathy, warmth, mutual respect, caring, and acceptance that determines the effectiveness of nursing care.[4,14]

Adam feels that three components constitute nursing practice: (1) the client, (2) the nurse (with his or her conceptual model as a base for the nursing process), and (3) the relationship between the client and the nurse. She has created a pictorial representation of nursing practice in her books (Figure 32-1).[4,14]

Adam insists that the helping relationship and the systematic process (that nurses have, perhaps wrongly, labeled the *nursing* process) are important to all health professionals. Nursing fits into the whole of healthcare as an integral component of the interdisciplinary health team. Each discipline makes a unique contribution to the promotion and preservation of health and to the prevention of health problems. Although some services overlap within this interdisciplinary health team, each discipline is present because it has a distinct and specific contribution to health.

This relationship can be illustrated with a schematic flower (Figure 32-2). Each petal represents a distinct health discipline; for example, nursing, medicine, physical therapy, speech therapy, or nutrition. The center of the flower indicates the shared functions. A part of each petal is separate and distinct from the others and the largest part of each petal represents the unique contribution of each discipline. Nurses' conceptual model clarifies and makes nursing's *petal* explicit.

Nurses currently have several conceptual models from which to choose. The decision to adopt one of the conceptual models for (not of) nursing is often made by considering the eventual evaluation of that particular model. Adam insists that conceptual models must be evaluated by criteria different from those used to evaluate theories. Adam notes the three criteria established by Johnson:[27]

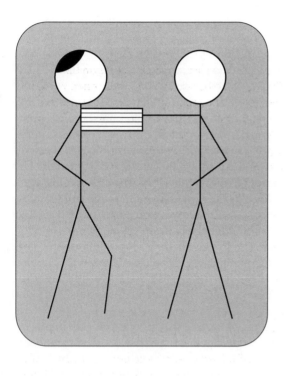

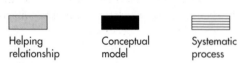

| Helping relationship | Conceptual model | Systematic process |

Figure **32-1** Pictoral representation of nursing practice. (From Adam, E. [1991]. *To be a nurse* [2nd ed.]. Toronto: W.B. Saunders.)

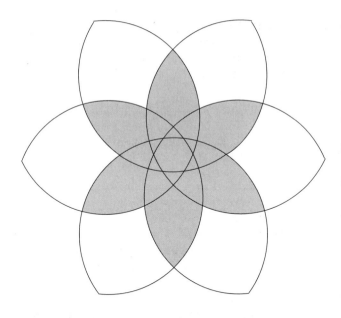

Figure 32-2 Interdisciplinary health team illustrated with schematic flower. (From Adam, E. [1991]. *To be a nurse* [2nd ed.]. Toronto: W.B. Saunders.)

1. *Social significance.* Clients would be asked whether the service (nursing) was significant to their health.
2. *Social congruence.* Clients would be asked whether the service (nursing) was congruent with their expectations.
3. *Social utility.* Nurses would be asked whether the conceptual model provided useful direction for education, practice, and research.

Such criteria are extrinsic to the model itself. However, for these criteria to be used, the conceptual model in question must already have been adopted in practice, education, and research settings. A vicious cycle may develop because some nurses may hesitate to adopt a model until it has been evaluated and it cannot be evaluated until it has been adopted.[9-11,14]

Adam recognizes that a model can be evaluated intrinsically for clarity, logic, and other criteria that will help nurses choose one model rather than another. However, the social decisions (extrinsic criteria) constitute the definitive evaluation of the conceptual base of a service profession.[9,16]

Adam's conviction that every nurse should have a conceptual base specific to nursing rather than one borrowed from another discipline has led her to publish many articles and books, to speak at profes-

sional meetings, and to teach courses on this subject. She feels that the existing models are often viewed as being too abstract or too complex and therefore beyond the understanding of many nurses. Adam published *Être Infirmière*[3] and *To Be a Nurse*[4] to help nurses understand the writings of Virginia Henderson. She accomplished this by placing Henderson's concept of nursing within the structure of a conceptual model and by developing and refining the subconcepts identified by Henderson.

This chapter evaluates the conceptual model Adam developed in her book. The model is not a theory, but it does suggest areas for theory development.

SUMMARY OF THE CONCEPTUAL MODEL FOR NURSING

In *To Be a Nurse,*[4] Adam explains the essential elements of a conceptual model as presented by Johnson. She then develops Henderson's concepts within the structure of a conceptual model.*

*The following summary material is reprinted with permission from Adam, E. (1980). *To be a nurse* (pp. 13-15). Toronto: W.B. Saunders.

Assumptions

The assumptions that form the theoretical foundation of Henderson's vision of nursing are drawn in part from the works of Thorndike, an American psychologist, and in part from Henderson's experience in rehabilitation. There are three assumptions:

1. Every individual strives for and desires independence.
2. Every individual is a complex whole, made up of fundamental needs.
3. When a need is not satisfied, it follows that the individual is not complete, whole, or independent.

Values

Henderson's conception of nursing is also composed of three beliefs:

1. The nurse has a unique function, although he or she shares certain functions with other professionals.
2. When the nurse takes over the physician's role, the nurse delegates his or her primary function to inadequately prepared personnel.
3. Society wants and expects this service (nursing) from the nurse and no other worker is as able, or willing, to give it.

Major Units

The following are major units of Henderson's model:[26]

1. The goal of nursing is to maintain or restore the client's independence in the satisfaction of his or her fundamental needs.
2. The client or beneficiary of the nurse's service is a whole being made up of 14 fundamental needs:

> "[a] Breathe normally.
> [b] Eat and drink adequately.
> [c] Eliminate body wastes.
> [d] Move and maintain desirable postures.
> [e] Sleep and rest.
> [f] Select suitable clothes—dress and undress.
> [g] Maintain body temperature within normal range by adjusting clothing and modifying the environment.

> [h] Keep the body clean and well groomed and protect the integument.
> [i] Avoid dangers in the environment and avoid injuring others.
> [j] Communicate with others in expressing emotions, needs, fears, or opinions.
> [k] Worship according to individual faith.
> [l] Work in such a way that brings a sense of accomplishment.
> [m] Play, or participate in various forms of recreation.
> [n] Learn, discover, or satisfy the curiosity that leads to normal development and health and use the available health facilities."[26:66]

3. The role of the nurse is a complementary-supplementary one.
4. The source of difficulty or the probable origin of those problems known as nursing problems is an insufficiency of either knowledge, will, and/or strength.
5. The intervention: the focus, or center of attention, of the nurse's action is the client's resources (knowledge, will, and strength).
6. The desired consequences are need satisfaction, independence in need satisfaction, or, in some cases, a peaceful death.

THEORETICAL SOURCES

Adam[12] states that she chose to work with Henderson's concept of nursing for two reasons. First, she felt that Henderson's work was partly known but badly known; that is, incompletely known or understood, although many nurses were acquainted with it. She hoped that her own publications would contribute to the recognition of Henderson's work as a useful conceptual base for nursing practice, research, and education. Second, she felt that Henderson's work was more immediately accessible than other works because the language was already familiar to nurses. Adam[12] "is not saying that Henderson's frame of reference is any better, or more useful, or more significant or more congruent than others. Such an evaluation has not yet been done . . . but it seems more immediately accessible."

Adam's concern for the need of an explicit conceptual model for nursing was developed when she was Johnson's student. Through Johnson, Adam also became familiar with the structure of a concep-tual model: assumptions, values, and major units. Adam[6,12] believes that Johnson was the first nurse to avail herself of that structure, which was already being used in fields such as sociology, psychology, and mathematics.

USE OF EMPIRICAL EVIDENCE

In choosing Henderson's writings as the basis of the conceptual model, Adam accepted the scientific principles on which Henderson based her work. The chapter on Henderson discusses the contribution of Bernard's principle of physiological balance and Maslow's hierarchy of needs. Adam did not change the basic content, but merely developed it further; therefore this empirical foundation also is unchanged.

In the previous section of this chapter, the source of the structure (assumptions, values, and six major units) was identified as sociology, mathematics, and other sciences. This structure has been used extensively in several sciences; it has good reliability.

MAJOR CONCEPTS & DEFINITIONS

ASSESSMENT TOOL

Instrument that the professional uses in collecting information about the beneficiary, the nursing history tool, and the data collection tool.

ASSUMPTION

The theoretical or scientific basis of a conceptual model; the premises that support the major units of the model.

BENEFICIARY

The second major unit of a conceptual model; the person or group of persons toward whom the professional directs his or her activities; the client; the patient.

CHANGE

A substitution of one thing in place of another (an alteration).

COLLECTION OF DATA

The first step of the nursing process; the collecting of information about the client and the client's nursing history.

CONCEPT

An idea, a mental image, or a generalization formed and developed in the mind.

CONCEPTION

A way of conceptualizing a reality, an invention of the mind, or a mental image. Depending on its level of abstraction, a conception may be a philosophy, a theory, or a conceptual model.

CONCEPTUAL MODEL

An abstraction or a way of conceptualizing a reality; a theoretical frame of reference sufficiently explicit so as to provide direction for a particular discipline; a conception made up of assumptions, values, and major units.

CONCEPTUAL MODEL FOR NURSING

A mental representation, concept, or conception of nursing that is sufficiently complete and explicit so as to provide direction for all fields of activity of the nursing profession.

CONSEQUENCES

The sixth major unit of a conceptual model; the results of the professional's efforts to attain the ideal and limited goal.

GOAL OF THE PROFESSION

The first major unit of a conceptual model; the end that the members of the profession strive to achieve.

Continued

MAJOR CONCEPTS & DEFINITIONS—cont'd

HELPING RELATIONSHIP

The interaction between the beneficiary (the helpee) and the professional (the helper) that aids the helpee to live more fully; the interpersonal exchange in which the helper illustrates such facilitating qualities as empathy and respect, among others.

INTERVENTION

The fifth major unit of a conceptual model, the focus and modes of the professional's intervention. (In the context of the nursing process, the intervention is the fourth step [implementation of the plan of action or the nursing action itself.])

INTERVENTION FOCUS

Part of the fifth major unit of a model; the focus, or center, of the professional's attention at the moment he or she intervenes with a client.

INTERVENTION MODES

Part of the fifth major unit, the means or ways of intervening at the professional's disposal.

MAJOR UNITS

The six essential components of a complete and explicit conception.

NEED

A requirement or necessity.

NEED, FUNDAMENTAL

A requirement common to all human beings, either well or ill.

NEED, INDIVIDUAL

A specific, particular, or personal requirement that derives from a fundamental need.

NURSING CARE PLAN

A written plan of action; the written communication that comes from the second and third steps of the nursing process; a plan to be followed; a projection of what is to be done.

NURSING PROCESS

A methodical, systematic way of proceeding toward an action; a dynamic and logical method; a five-step process.

PRACTICE

One of the three fields of activity of a service profession (the other two being education and research); the field of activity of the administrator and the practitioner of the service.

PROBLEM

A difficulty to be reduced or removed.

PROBLEM-SOLVING METHOD

The scientific process of solving problems; the systematic manner of proceeding used to solve problems.

ROLE

The third major unit of a conceptual model; the part played by the professional; the societal function of the professional.

SOURCE OF DIFFICULTY

The fourth major unit of a conceptual model; the probable origin of the client difficulty with which the professional is prepared to cope.

VALUES

The value system underlying a conceptual model.

Reprinted with permission from Adam, E. (1980). *To be a nurse* (pp. 116-118). Toronto: W.B. Saunders.

MAJOR ASSUMPTIONS

In developing Henderson's work into a conceptual model, Adam[4,16] described the goal of nursing as maintaining or restoring the client's independence in the satisfaction of the 14 fundamental needs. The nurse plays a complementary-supplementary role, complementing and supplementing the client's resources (strength, knowledge, and will).

Although the nurse shares certain functions with other health professionals, the nurse has a unique province. Society wants and expects the nurse to provide unique service. In this model, the person is portrayed as a complex whole, made up of 14 fundamental needs and the resources to satisfy them. Each need has biological, physiological, and psychosociocultural dimensions. When a need is not satisfied, the person is not complete, whole, or independent. The nurse's client may also be a family or a group.[3] The concept of environment is specifically addressed in only one of the fundamental needs. However, environment is implicit in all the fundamental needs because the sociocultural dimension is integral to each need.

Health is not defined separately in *To Be a Nurse*,[4] but Adam uses this term in discussing the goal of nursing. She states, "The goal of nursing is to maintain or to restore the client's independence in the satisfaction of his fundamental needs. This goal, congruent with the goal common to the entire health team, makes clear the nurse's specific contribution to the preservation and improvement of health."[4:14] An entirely satisfactory definition of health is still a subject of debate; therefore it behooves each health discipline to make its particular contribution to health explicit.[3]

THEORETICAL ASSERTIONS

In the description of the conceptual model's major units, the relationships among the basic concepts can be seen in the elements that Adam has labeled beliefs and values. She believes these constitute the why of the model and must be shared by all who use the model. Values are not subject to the criteria of truths, but must reflect the values of the larger society nursing wishes to serve.

1. "The nurse has a unique function, although she shares certain functions with other professionals."[4:13] The nurse must have a conceptual model to have a distinct professional identity and to assert himself or herself as a colleague of the other health-team members.
2. "When the nurse takes over the physician's role, she delegates her primary function to inadequately prepared personnel."[4:13] The nurse who strives to assume the physician's role will relinquish the nurse's role to some other care provider who may not have the skills and the knowledge base required for nursing.
3. "Society wants and expects this service (nursing) from the nurse and no other worker is as able, or willing to give it."[4:14] Nursing owes its existence to the fact that it fulfills a societal need, as does any service profession.

LOGICAL FORM

Adam has used the structure of a conceptual model that was useful in various other sciences before being introduced into nursing. The essential elements of a model for a helping or service profession follow.

Assumptions

The assumptions are "the suppositions that are taken for granted by those who wish to use the model; they are the 'how' of the model, its foundation."[4:6]

Beliefs and Values

"The beliefs and values constitute the 'why' of the model and are not subject to the criteria of truth. They must however reflect the value system of the larger society that the profession wishes to serve [and] . . . be shared by the members of the profession who wish to use the model."[4:7]

Major Units

"The major units are the what of the conceptual model. They . . . make clear what nursing is in any setting and at any time."[4:7]

Ideal and limited goal. The ideal and limited goal of the profession is "'ideal' because it represents the ideal that all members of the profession would like to achieve and 'limited' because it delineates the parameters of the profession."[4:7]

Beneficiary. The beneficiary of the professional service is "that person or group of persons towards whom the professional directs his attention . . . . The nurse must have a clear mental image of her client, whether he is well or ill."[4:8]

Role of the professional. The role of the professional is "the role in society played by the members of the discipline."[4:8]

Source of difficulty of the beneficiary. The source of difficulty of the beneficiary "refers to the probable origin of the client's difficulty; one with professional, because of his education and experience, is prepared to cope."[3:8] "The probable origin of those client problems which the nurse is prepared to solve must be made explicit."[4:9]

Intervention

Intervention focus. The focus or center of the intervention is "the focus of the professional's attention at the moment he intervenes with the client. The patient or beneficiary is perceived as an extremely complex individual however within that complexity only one aspect can receive all the professional's attention at any given moment. . . . No one person can do everything at the same time."[4:9]

Intervention modes. The modes of intervention "are the means the professional has at his disposal to intervene. . . . A conceptual model for nursing will indicate what means are at the nurse's disposal when she intervenes as a health professional."[4:9]

Consequences. The consequences "are the desired results of the professional activities and must be congruent with the ideal goal."[4:9-10]

Adam has developed Henderson's concept of nursing into a conceptual model for nursing by placing Henderson's writings in the structure of a model. She has supplied the logical form that was less apparent in Henderson's work. Through the logical form of the resulting conceptual model, clear direction is provided to nursing practitioners, educators, and researchers.

Through the use of the structure that comprises a conceptual model and Henderson's writings, it may be said that Adam used the deductive form of logical reasoning.

ACCEPTANCE BY THE NURSING COMMUNITY

Practice

Basing practice on this conceptual model, the nurse is seen in a complementary-supplementary role and the goal is client independence in the satisfaction of his or her needs. The model serves as a guide for using the nursing process and the problem-solving method. Guided by the 14 fundamental needs, the practitioner, in whatever setting, will assess the independence of the client in need satisfaction. The nurse will then identify the client's specific needs; determine the source of difficulty; and plan the intervention to complement client strength, will, or knowledge. After the care is given, it is evaluated in reference to the client's objectives; for example, have the specific needs been satisfied and has the client's independence been increased? A nursing problem (a client's health problem requiring a nurse's intervention) is a dependency problem in need satisfaction.[4] A nursing diagnosis is a specific need that is unsatisfied because there is insufficient strength, will, or knowledge. Criteria for identifying specific needs have been developed.[4] According to Adam,[4:66] the nurse "carries out the social mission of contributing to the public's improved health by working toward greater client independence."

Education

Adam discusses the educational objectives and goals and the program content in *To Be a Nurse*.[4] She states, "Following Henderson's concept of nursing, the nursing curriculum is planned to prepare a health worker capable of maintaining and restoring the client's independence in the satisfaction of his fundamental needs."[4:57] With this concept, a student learns the complementary-supplementary role.

Adam divides the program into official and unofficial content, both of equal importance. Unofficial content "covers everything that is learned in an educational program without being taught."[4:58] Official content "is formally recognized and actually taught."[4:58] Official content is further divided into nursing and nonnursing.

According to Henderson's frame of reference, nursing content includes:

1. The goal of nursing, which is to preserve or reestablish the client's independence in the satisfaction of his or her basic needs.
2. The detailed description of the 14 fundamental needs, each with its biological, physiological, psychological, social, and cultural dimensions.
3. The individual variations in fundamental needs.
4. The various problems of dependence originating from a lack of strength, will, or knowledge.
5. The explanation of the complementary-supplementary role.
6. The description of the various needs of intervention.
7. The study of the desired consequences: continued or increased independence and, in certain circumstances, a peaceful death.
8. The study of the systematic process and the problem-solving method as applied to nursing.[4]

Essential subject matters, regardless of the conceptual model for nursing, are "the helping relationship, . . . the concept of health, . . . and the history of nursing."[4:59]

The theoretical courses, in the nonnursing content, include anatomy, physiology, pathology, psychology, sociology, and anthropology. In relation to Henderson's model, the first three relate to the biophysiological dimension and the last three to the psychosociocultural aspect of the fundamental needs.

Subject matter derived from the conceptual model's assumptions is "1. The concepts of independence and dependence. 2. The concepts of universal and individual human needs, hierarchy of human needs, and need satisfaction. 3. The concept of wholeness."[4:60]

The practical aspect of nursing content consists of technical procedures and clinical experiences.

Techniques are important in the complementary-supplementary role because the nurse is assisting the client in those activities that cannot be completed because there is insufficient strength, will, or knowledge. Techniques help pursue the goal of client independence in the satisfaction of his or her needs. Adam[4:62] believes that "the goal of clinical experiences is to provide the student with opportunities to help a client recover his independence in the satisfaction of his basic needs."

Although the level of education may increase, the model remains the conceptual base. Baccalaureate students' formal education will help them identify complex and subtle specific needs, find new ways of complementing and supplementing, and form and continue a helping relationship. Master's level students learn to be specialists in independence nursing or in the teaching and administration of independence nursing. Doctoral students may use the concept of independence in need satisfaction as a basis of research for theory development.

Research

Adam[4:66-67] posed 12 questions from the conceptual model for research development. These include:

"1. How can client independence be measured?

2. How can his degree of dependence be quantified?

3. What dependency problems are solved by what nursing interventions?

4. At what point must the intervention be discontinued if independence is to be promoted?

5. How can certain interventions be made more easily acceptable?

6. How can the nurse determine how much intervention is enough?

7. What dependency problems are most often encountered among selected groups (cancer patients, the aged, the mentally confused)?

8. How does pain and anxiety affect independence?

9. How can linguistic barriers be overcome?

10. How can the nurse help certain ethnic or socioeconomic groups to be independent?

11. How can the nurse increase client participation in healthcare?

12. Is the conceptual model socially useful, significant, and congruent?"

Adam[11] states that various clinical and educational settings in Canada are at varying stages of basing nursing care and teaching on Henderson's model and that the research for a small number of master's theses has been based on this model. Correspondence received from Canada, the United States, and abroad indicates her books have received very favorable reviews.

FURTHER DEVELOPMENT

Although no empirical evidence has been collected for theories deriving from this model, Adam[15] believes that the model could be the basis for theory development. As with other conceptual models for nursing, this one specifies nursing's focus of inquiry. From Henderson's conceptual departure point of independence in need satisfaction, descriptive and experimental studies could be carried out to result in the identification of descriptive terms particular to the concept under scrutiny. The identification of descriptive terms is the first step in theory development. Possible developments might be a theory of need satisfaction or a theory of complementing knowledge or supplementing motivation in specific client populations. Such theories would not be theories of nursing, but theories of the phenomena that concern nursing.[11]

"Nurse theorists will of course look at phenomena that interest other disciplines as well. They must, however, study them from a nursing perspective if they want to develop nursing theory."[15:9] "For example, if pain were studied from Henderson's perspective, it would be examined as a phenomenon that interferes with client independence in need satisfaction."[15:10]

In a letter of February 16, 1988, Adam[16] states, "Some Ontario colleges and clinical settings are showing increasing interest in basing their practice and teaching on Henderson's model as I presented it. It is still popular in Quebec and in the Atlantic provinces. Graduate students often quote it as their conceptual departure point, i.e., to justify

their research project. They seldom seek to develop it."

CRITIQUE
Simplicity

The essential elements Adam listed give the appearance of a simple conceptual model. However, on closer inspection, the number of subconcepts produces a complex picture. The interrelatedness of the components necessary for the care of the whole client also adds to the complexity of the model. The concepts presented are clearly defined and easy to follow.

Generality

The assumptions, values, and major units involve nursing and clients in all aspects of society. They are not limited to age, medical diagnosis, or healthcare setting. Each of the 14 basic needs has biophysiological and psychosociocultural aspects.

Empirical Precision

Although testing of the model is unavailable at this time, it appears to have the potential for a high degree of empirical precision. This is related to its reality base and designated subconcepts.

Derivable Consequences

The empirically based concepts and broad scope of the model make it potentially applicable to nursing practice, education, and research.

CONCLUSION

Adam's work in developing the conceptual model is unique in that she has taken Henderson's previously existing concept of nursing and presented it within the previously existing structure of a model. The result is something more than the sum of the two. It is a complete, concise, explicit conceptual model. Adam then clarified the interrelatedness of the model, the process, and the client-nurse relationship. Making a clear distinction between model and theory, Adam explained the impact of the model on nursing research, practice, and education.

Adam[12] states that "the adoption of a conceptual model will not solve all of nursing's problems." A conceptual model makes nursing's particular contribution to healthcare explicit and provides nurses with a professional identity and a conceptual point of departure.

It would seem that every nurse who adopts a concise and explicit conceptual model is a potential nursing theorist. A nurse who is able to articulate the scope of nursing practice would be more likely to identify areas for nursing theory development and nursing research. Imagine that the majority of nurses have an explicit conceptual model (a conceptual departure point for theory development) and are able and willing to provide written documentation that would become the basis for empirical evidence. This opens the door to a marked increase in nursing theory and knowledge.

CRITICAL THINKING *Activities*

1. Adam states that all nurses have a conceptual model for nursing practice, but it is often difficult to communicate. From the perspective that the nurse needs a clear conceptual model of nursing as a basis for the nursing process, identify components of the theorist's development of Henderson's concept of nursing that you could use in implementing the nursing process.

2. Analyze the components of Henderson's model as developed by Adam and identify those that you think are significant in clarifying nursing's unique contribution to healthcare. State the rationale for your response.

3. Review Adam's three theoretical assertions (beliefs and values). Do you think that these theoretical assertions reflect values of today's society that nursing serves?

4. Analyze your practice from the perspective of Adam's development of Henderson's

concept of nursing. Is this conceptual model appropriate for adoption, implementation, and evaluation in your practice? State the rationale for your response.

REFERENCES

1. Adam, E. (1975, Sept.). A conceptual model for nursing. *Canadian Nurse,* 71(9), 40-41.
2. Adam, E. (1975, Sept.). Un modèle conceptuel: à quoi bon? *L'infirmière Canadienne,* 19(9), 22-23.
3. Adam, E. (1979). *Être infirmière.* Montréal: Editions Holt, Rinehart, & Winston Ltée.
4. Adam, E. (1980). *To be a nurse.* Toronto: W.B. Saunders.
5. Adam, E. (1981, Sept.). CNA's standards for nursing practice: An interpretation. *Canadian Nurse,* 77(8), 32-33.
6. Adam, E. (1981, Sept.). Les normes de la pratique infirmière de l'A.I.I.C.: Une interprétation. *L'Infirmière Canadienne,* 23(9), 28-29.
7. Adam, E. (1981). *To be a nurse* (Dutch translation). Holland: De Tỹdstroom.
8. Adam, E. (1982). *To be a nurse* (Spanish translation). Madrid: Editora Inportecnica.
9. Adam, E. (1983). *Être infirmière* (2nd ed.). Montréal: Editions Holt, Rinehart, & Winston Ltée.
10. Adam, E. (1983). Frontiers of nursing in the 21st century: Development of models and theories on the concept of nursing. *Journal of Advanced Nursing,* 8, 41-45.
11. Adam, E. (1983). Modèles conceptuels. *Nursing Papers: Perspectives in Nursing,* 15(2), 10-21.
12. Adam, E. (1984, Dec. 4). Personal interview [Videotape].
13. Adam, E. (1984). Questions et réponses relatives au schème conceptuel de Virginia Henderson. *L'Infirmière Canadienne,* 26(3), 27-31.
14. Adam, E. (1985, April). Toward more clarity in terminology: Frameworks, theories and models. *Journal of Nursing Education,* 24(4), 151-155.
15. Adam, E. (1987). Nursing theory: What it is and what it is not. *Nursing Papers: Perspectives in Nursing,* 19(2), 5-14.
16. Adam, E. (1988, Feb. 16). Personal correspondence.
17. Adam, E. (1991). *Être infirmière* (3rd ed.). Montréal: Êtudes Vivantes.
18. Adam, E. (1991). *To be a nurse* (2nd ed.). Toronto: W.B. Saunders.
19. Adam, E. (1992). *To be a nurse* (Italian translation). Milan: Catholic University of Milan.
20. Adam, E. (1993). *To be a nurse* (Portuguese translation). Lisbon: Instituto Piaget.
21. Adam, E. (1996, Nov. 1). Telephone interview.

22. Adam, E. (1996). *To be a nurse* (Japanese translation). Tokyo: Igaku-Shoin.
23. Adam, E. (1999, March). Conceptual models. *Canadian Journal of Nursing Research,* 30(4), 103-114.
24. Adam, E. (2000, May). E-mail correspondence.
25. Guyonnet, M., Adam, E. (1992). L'infirmière dans l'equipe pluridisciplinaire. *Canadian Nurse/L'infirmière Canadienne,* 88(10), 41-44.
26. Henderson, V. (1964, Aug.). The nature of nursing. *American Journal of Nursing,* 64(8), 63-68.
27. Johnson, D. (1974, Sept./Oct.). Development of theory: A requisite for nursing as a primary health profession. *Nursing Research,* 23(5), 372-377.
28. Lauzon, S. & Adam, E. (Eds.). (1996). *La personne âgée et ses besoins: Interventions infirmières.* Montreal: Editions du Renouveau Pédagogique.
29. Roy, C. & Roberts, S.L. (1981). *Theory construction in nursing: An adaptation model.* Englewood Cliffs, NJ: Prentice-Hall.

BIBLIOGRAPHY
Primary Sources
Books

Adam, E. (1979). *Être infirmière.* Montréal: Editions Holt, Rinehart, & Winston Ltée.
Adam, E. (1980). *To be a nurse.* Toronto: W.B. Saunders.
Adam, E. (1981). *To be a nurse* (Dutch translation). Holland: De Tÿdstroom.
Adam, E. (1982). *To be a nurse* (Spanish translation). Madrid: Editora Inportecnica.
Adam, E. (1983). *Être infirmière* (2nd ed.). Montréal: Editions Holt, Rinehart, & Winston Ltée.
Adam, E. (1991). *Être infirmière* (3rd ed.). Montréal: Êtudes Vivantes.
Adam, E. (1991). *To be a nurse* (2nd ed.). Toronto: W.B. Saunders.
Adam, E. (1992). *To be a nurse* (Italian translation). Milan: Catholic University of Milan.
Adam, E. (1993). *To be a nurse* (Portuguese translation). Lisbon: Instituto Piaget.
Adam, E. (1996). *To be a nurse* (Japanese translation). Tokyo: Igaku-Shoin.
Lauzon, S. & Adam, E. (Eds.). (1996). *La personne âgée et ses besoins: Interventions infirmières.* Montreal: Editions du Renouveau Pédagogique.

Book Chapters

Adam, E. (1983). Development of models and theories on the concept of nursing. In *Health care for all: Challenge for nursing* (17th quadrennial Congress, International Council for Nurses 1981). Geneva: International Council for Nurses.
Adam, E. (1983). The shape of the nursing world to come: The nursing process. In *Health care for all: Challenge for nursing* (17th quadrennial Congress, International Council for Nurses 1981). Geneva: International Council for Nurses.
Adam, E. (1984). Modèles conceptuels. In M. McGee (Ed.), *Theoretical pluralism in nursing science.* Ottawa: University of Ottawa Press.
Adam, E. (1990). Levels of abstraction in nursing content development. In *Proceedings of the first and second Rosemary Ellis scholars' retreat* (pp. 229-261). Cleveland, OH: Case Western Reserve University.
Adam, E. (1992). Contemporary conceptualizations of nursing. In J.F. Kikuchi & H. Simmons (Eds.), *Philosophic inquiry in nursing* (pp. 55-63). Newbury Park, CA: Sage.

Journal Articles

Adam, E. (1975, Sept.). A conceptual model for nursing. *Canadian Nurse,* 71(9), 40-41.
Adam, E. (1975, Sept.). Un modèle conceptuel: à quoi bon? *L'infirmière Canadienne,* 19(9), 22-23.
Adam, E. (1981, Sept.). CNA's standards for nursing practice: An interpretation. *Canadian Nurse,* 77(8), 32-33.
Adam, E. (1981, Sept.). Les normes de la pratique infirmière de l'A.I.I.C.: Une interprétation. *L'Infirmière Canadienne,* 23(9), 28-29.
Adam, E. (1983). Frontiers of nursing in the 21st century: Development of models and theories on the concept of nursing. *Journal of Advanced Nursing,* 8, 41-45.
Adam, E. (1983). Modèles conceptuels. *Nursing Papers: Perspectives in Nursing,* 15(2), 10-21.
Adam, E. (1984). Questions et réponses relatives au schème conceptuel de Virginia Henderson. *L'Infirmière Canadienne,* 26(3), 27-31.
Adam, E. (1985, April). Toward more clarity in terminology: Frameworks, theories, and models. *Journal of Nursing Education,* 24(4), 151-155.
Adam, E. (1987). Nursing theory: What it is and what it is not. *Nursing Papers: Perspectives in Nursing,* 19(2), 5-14.
Adam, E. (1999, March). Conceptual models. *Canadian Journal of Nursing Research,* 30(4), 103-114.
Guyonnet, M., Adam, E. (1992). L'infirmière dans l'equipe pluridisciplinaire. *Canadian Nurse/L'infirmière Canadienne,* 88(10), 41-44.

Reports

Adam, E. (1980). Implementing the curriculum based on a nursing model. In G. Zilm (Ed.), *Back to basics* (pp. 22-28). Ottawa: Association des Infirmieres et Infirmiers du Canada.
Adam, E. (1980). *Normes de la pratique infirmière.* Ottawa: Association des Infirmieres et Infirmiers du Canada.
Adam, E. (1980). Programmes s'inspirant d'un modèle nursing. In *Retour aux sources* (pp. 27-33). Ottawa: Association des Infirmieres et Infirmiers du Canada.

Adam, E. (1980). *Standards for nursing practice.* Ottawa: Association des Infirmieres et Infirmiers du Canada.

Adam, E. (1980). The case for a nursing model. In *Nursing explorations: Proceedings September 26, 1980.* Montreal, Quebec: McGill University.

Adam, E. (1981). L'application d'un model conceptuel au programme de'ètudes collegial. Dans *Rapport du-colloque des techniques infirmières. Partie I* (pp. 49-55). Montreal, Quebec: Gouvernement du Québec.

Adam, E. (1981). Leadership in nursing: The case for a conceptual model. In *Report of annual meeting* (pp. 1-15). Saskatoon, Saskatchewan: The Canadian Association of University Schools of Nursing, Western Region, University of Saskatchewan.

Correspondence

Adam, E. (1984, Oct. 2). Personal correspondence.

Adam, E. (1984, Nov. 1). Telephone interview.

Adam, E. (1984, Nov. 4). Telephone interview.

Adam, E. (1984, Nov. 6). Personal correspondence.

Adam, E. (1984, Nov. 12). Telephone interview.

Adam, E. (1984, Nov. 26). Telephone interview.

Adam, E. (1984, Dec. 4). Personal interview [Videotape].

Adam, E. (1988, Feb. 16). Personal correspondence.

Adam, E. (1988, April 2). Telephone interview.

Adam, E. (1993). Personal correspondence.

Secondary Sources

Books

Chinn, P. & Kramer, M. (1995). *Theory and nursing: A systematic approach* (4th ed.). St. Louis: Mosby.

Henderson, V. (1966). *The nature of nursing.* New York: Macmillan.

Journal Articles

Henderson, V. (1964). The nature of nursing. *American Journal of Nursing, 64,* 62-68.

Henderson, V. (1982). The nursing process: Is the title right? *Journal of Advanced Nursing, 7,* 103-109.

Winkler, J. (1983). Conceptual models (a response to "Modèles conceptuels," by E. Adam). *Nursing Papers: Perspectives in Nursing, 15*(4), 69-70.

Book Reviews

[Review of the book *Être infirmière*]. (1979, March). *Le Devoir (daily newspaper, Montreal),* p. 15.

[Review of the book *Être infirmière*]. (1979, April). *Infirmière Canadienne, 21,* 46.

[Review of the book *Être infirmière*]. (1979, June). *Infirmière Canadienne, 21,* 10.

[Review of the book *Être infirmière*]. (1979, June). *Revue de l'infirmière (Paris), 6,* 75.

[Review of the book *Être infirmière*]. (1979, Oct.). *Revue de l'infirmière (Paris), 8,* 8-9.

[Review of the book *Être infirmière*]. (1980, Feb.). *Infirmière enseiqnante (Paris), 10,* 11.

[Review of the book *To be a nurse*]. (1981, March). *Canadian Nurse, 77,* 50.

[Review of the book *To be a nurse*]. (1981, June). *Nursing Times, 77,* 1041.

[Review of the book *To be a nurse*]. (1981, Oct.). *Australian Nurses Journal, 11,* 28.

[Review of the book *To be a nurse*]. (1981, Nov./Dec.). *Continuing Education in Nursing, 12,* 39.

Other

Riehl, J.P. & Roy, C. (1974). *Conceptual models for nursing practice.* New York: Appleton-Century-Crofts.

Riehl, J.P. & Roy, C. (1980). *Conceptual models for nursing practice* (2nd ed.). New York: Appleton-Century-Crofts.

Roy, C. & Roberts, S.L. (1981). *Theory construction in nursing: An adaptation model.* Englewood Cliffs, NJ: Prentice-Hall.

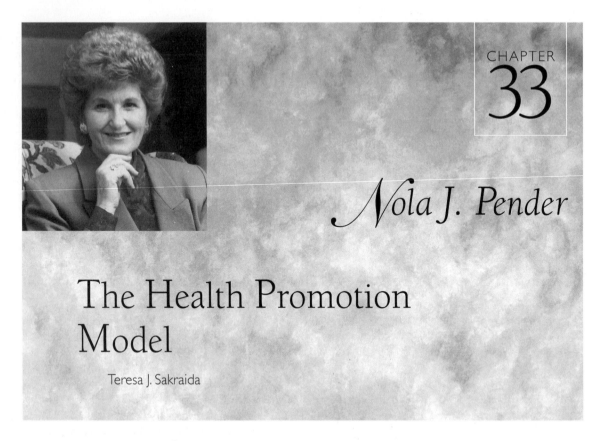

$\mathcal{N}$ola J. Pender

The Health Promotion Model

Teresa J. Sakraida

CREDENTIALS AND BACKGROUND OF THE THEORIST

Nola J. Pender's first encounter with professional nursing occurred at the age of seven when she observed the nursing care given to her hospitalized aunt. This experience and her subsequent education instilled a desire to care for others in her and influenced her belief that the goal of nursing was to help people care for themselves. Pender contributes to nursing knowledge of health promotion through her research, teaching, presentations, and writings.

Pender was born in 1941 in Lansing, Michigan. She was the only child of parents who were advocates of education for women. Family encouragement for her goal of becoming a registered nurse led her to attend the School of Nursing at West Suburban Hospital in

Previous author: Lucy Anne Tillett.

The author wishes to express appreciation to Nola J. Pender for reviewing the chapter.

Oak Park, Illinois. This school was chosen for its ties with Wheaton College and its strong Christian foundation. She received her nursing diploma in 1962 and began working on a medical-surgical unit and subsequently in a pediatric unit in a Michigan hospital.

In 1964, Pender completed her B.S.N. at Michigan State University in East Lansing. She credits Helen Penhale, the assistant to the dean, for helping to streamline her program and foster her options for further education. As was common in the 1960s, Pender changed her major from nursing as she pursued her graduate degrees. She earned her M.A. in human growth and development from Michigan State University in 1965. She completed her Ph.D. in psychology and education in 1969 at Northwestern Univer-sity in Evanston, Illinois. Pender's dissertation[7] investigated developmental changes in encoding processes of short-term memory in children. Several years later, she completed master's level work in community health nursing at Rush University in Chicago.[17]

After earning her Ph.D., Pender notes a shift in her thinking toward defining the goal of nursing care as the optimal health of the individual. A series of conversations with Dr. Beverly McElmurry at Northern Illinois University and reading *High-Level Wellness*[3] by Halpert Dunn inspired expanded notions of health and nursing. Her marriage to Albert Pender, an associate professor of business and economics who has collaborated with his wife in writing about the economics of healthcare, and the birth of a son and daughter provided increased personal motivation to learn more about optimizing human health.

In 1975, Pender published "A Conceptual Model for Preventive Health Behavior,"[8] which was a basis for studying how individuals made decisions about their own healthcare in a nursing context. This article identified factors that were found in earlier research to influence decision making and actions of individuals in preventing disease. The original Health Promotion Model (HPM) was presented in the first edition of the text *Health Promotion in Nursing Practice,* published in 1982.[9] Based on subsequent research, the HPM was revised and is presented in the second edition, published in 1987,[10] and in the third edition, published in 1996.[11] A fourth edition of the *Health Promotion in Nursing Practice,*[19] jointly authored by Pender with Murdaugh and Parsons, will publish in 2002.

A six-year study funded by the National Institutes of Health was conducted at Northern Illinois University in DeKalb by Pender and her colleagues Susan Walker (Ed.D.), Karen Sechrist (Ph.D.), and Marilyn Frank-Stromborg (Ed.D.). The study tested the validity of the HPM.[20] An instrument, the Health Promoting Lifestyle Profile, was developed by the research team to study the health-promoting behavior of working adults, older adults, cardiac rehabilitation patients, and ambulatory cancer patients.[22] Published results from these studies support the HPM.[11] Subsequently, over 50 studies have tested the predictive capability of the model for health-promoting lifestyle, exercise, nutrition practices, use of hearing protection, and avoidance of exposure to environmental tobacco smoke.[19,15]

Pender has provided important leadership in the development of nursing research in the United States. Her work in support of the National Center for Nursing Research in the National Institutes of Health was instrumental to its formation in 1981. She has promoted scholarly activity in nursing through her involvement with Sigma Theta Tau International, as a past president of the Midwest Nursing Research Society (1985 to 1987), and as Chair of the Cabinet on Nursing Research of the American Nurse's Association. Inducted as a Fellow of the American Academy of Nursing in 1981, she served as President of the Academy from 1991 until 1993.[17] In 1998, she was appointed to a four-year term on the U.S. Preventative Services Task Force, an independent panel charged to evaluate scientific evidence and make age-specific and risk-specific recommendations for clinical preventative services.[17]

A recipient of many awards and honors, Pender has served as a distinguished scholar at a number of universities. She received an honorary doctoral degree from Widener University in 1992. In 1988, she received the Distinguished Research Award from the Midwest Nursing Research Society for her contributions to research and research leadership and in 1997, she received the American Psychological Association Award for outstanding contributions to nursing and health psychology. In 1998, the University of Michigan School of Nursing honored Pender[16] with the Mae Edna Doyle Award for excellence in teaching.

As Professor and Associate Dean for Research at the University of Michigan School of Nursing since 1990, she promotes nursing science. In her current position, Pender[16] facilitates external funding of faculty research, supports emerging centers of research excellence in the School of Nursing, promotes interdisciplinary research, supports translating research into science-based practice, and links nursing research to the formulation of health policy. A child and adolescent health behavior research center initiated at the University of Michigan in 1991 represents Pender's efforts[14] to build a large interdisciplinary research team to study and influence the health-promoting behaviors of individuals by understanding how these behaviors are first established in youth. Her current and future program of research has two major foci: (1) understanding how self-efficacy affects the exertion and affective (activity-related affect) responses of adolescent girls to the physical activity challenge and (2) developing an interactive computer program as an intervention to increase physical activity among adolescent girls.[15]

Pender[16] has published numerous articles on exercise, behavior change, and relaxation training as aspects of health promotion and has served as an editor for journals and books. Pender is recognized as a scholar, presenter, and consultant on health-promotion topics. She has consulted with nurse scientists in Japan, Korea, Mexico, Thailand, the Do-minican Republic, Jamaica, England, New Zealand, and Chile.[15,16] Her book is now available in the Japanese and Korean languages.[12,13]

THEORETICAL SOURCES

Pender's background in nursing, human development, experimental psychology, and education led her to use a holistic nursing perspective, social psychology, and learning theory as the foundations for the HPM. The HPM (Figure 33-1) integrates several constructs. Central to the HPM is the Social Learning

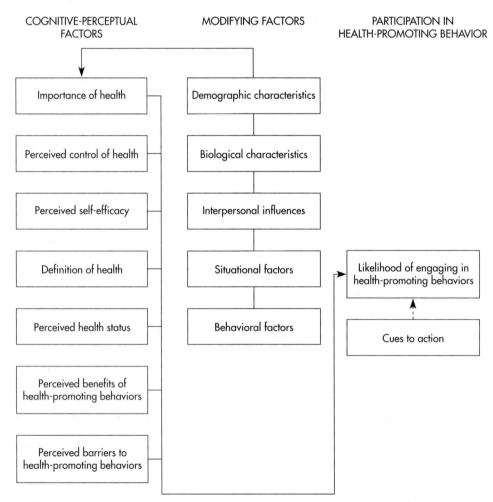

Figure **33-1 Health Promotion Model.** (From Pender, N.J. [1987]. *Health promotion in nursing practice* [2nd ed., p. 58]. New York: Appleton & Lange. ©Reprinted by permission of Pearson Education, Inc., Upper Saddle River, NJ.)

Theory of Albert Bandura,[1] which postulates the importance of cognitive processes in the changing of behavior. Social Learning Theory, now titled Social Cognitive Theory, includes the following self-beliefs: self-attribution, self-evaluation, and self-efficacy. Self-efficacy is a central construct of the HPM.[11] In addition, the Expectancy-Value Model of Human Motivation that Feather[4] described, which supports that behavior is rational and economical, is important to the model's development.

The HPM is similar in construction to the Health Belief Model,[2] but is not limited to explaining disease-prevention behavior. The HPM differs from the Health Belief Model because the HPM does not include fear or threat as a source of motivation for health behavior.[11] For this reason, the HPM expands to encompass behaviors for enhancing health and potentially applies across the life span.[11]

USE OF EMPIRICAL EVIDENCE

The HPM, as depicted in Figure 33-1, has served as a framework for research aimed at predicting overall health-promoting lifestyles and specific behaviors such as exercise and use of hearing protection.[11] Pender and colleagues have conducted a program of research funded by the National Institute of Nursing Research to evaluate the HPM in four populations: (1) working adults, (2) older community-dwelling adults, (3) ambulatory cancer patients, and (4) cardiac rehabilitation patients. The studies tested the validity of the HPM.[20] A summary of findings from earlier studies is listed in the 1996 edition of *Health Promotion in Nursing Practice.*[11] Additional studies testing the model will be presented in the fourth edition of *Health Promotion in Nursing Practice.*[19]

The rationale for revision of the HPM stemmed from the analyses of research studies. The process of refining the HPM, as published in 1987, led to several changes (see Figure 33-1).[10] First, importance of health, perceived control of health, and cues for action were deleted from the model. Second, definition of health, perceived health status, and demographic and biological characteristics were repositioned in the category of personal factors as noted in the 1996 revision of the HPM[11] (Figure 33-2). Last, the revised HPM (see Figure 33-2) adds three new variables that

serve to influence the individual to engage in health-promoting behaviors: (1) activity-related affect, (2) commitment to a plan of action, and (3) immediate competing demand and preferences.[11]

The HPM (see Figure 33-2) has been refined to focus on 10 categories of determinants of health-promoting behavior. Currently being tested empirically, the revised model identifies concepts relevant to health-promoting behaviors and facilitates the generation of testable hypotheses.[19]

The HPM provides a paradigm for the development of instruments. The Health Promoting Lifestyle Profile and the Exercise Benefits/Barriers Scale (EBBS) are two examples.* Both of these instruments serve to test the model and further model development.

The purpose of the Health Promoting Lifestyle Profile instrument is to measure health-promoting lifestyle.[20] The Health Promotion Lifestyle Profile II (HPLP-II), a revision of the original instrument, is used in research.† The 52-item, four-point, Likert-styled instrument consists of six subscales: (1) health responsibility, (2) physical activity, (3) nutrition, (4) interpersonal relations, (5) spiritual growth, and (6) stress management. Means can be derived for each subscale or a total mean signifying overall health-promoting lifestyle.[20] The instrument provides an assessment of health-promoting lifestyle of individuals that is useful to nurses clinically in patient support and education.

The HPM identifies cognitive and perceptual factors as major determinants of health-promoting behavior. The EBBS measures the cognitive and perceptual factors of perceived benefits and perceived barriers to exercise.[21] The 43-item, four-point, Likert-styled instrument consists of a 29-item benefits scale and a 14-item barriers scale that may be scored separately or as a whole. The higher the overall score on the 43-item instrument, the more positively the individual perceives the benefits to exercise in relation to barriers to exercise.[21] The EBBS provides a clinically useful means for evaluating exercise perceptions.

---

*The EBBS can be obtained from the Health Promotion Research Program, Social Science Research Institute, Northern Illinois University, DeKalb, Illinois, 60115.
†The HPLP-II can be obtained from Dr. Susan Noble Walker, University of Nebraska Medical Center, College of Nursing, 600 South 42nd Street, Omaha, Nebraska, 68198-5330.

INDIVIDUAL
CHARACTERISTICS
AND EXPERIENCES

BEHAVIOR-SPECIFIC
COGNITIONS
AND AFFECT

BEHAVIORAL
OUTCOME

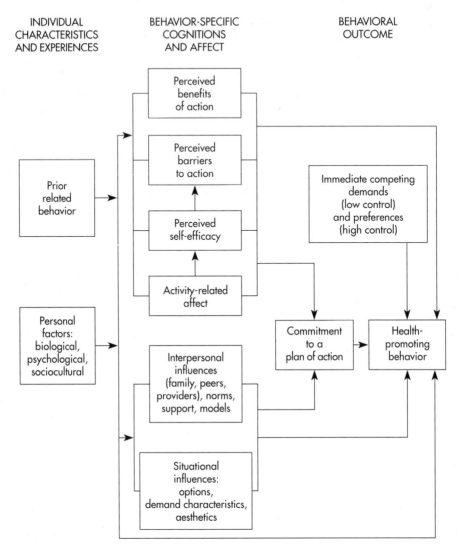

Figure **33-2 Revised Health Promotion Model.** (From Pender, N.J. [1996]. *Health promotion in nursing practice* [3rd ed., p. 67]. Stamford, CT: Appleton & Lange. ©Reprinted by permission of Pearson Education, Inc., Upper Saddle River, NJ.)

MAJOR CONCEPTS & DEFINITIONS

The major concepts and definitions presented are found in the revised HPM.[1] The following are individual characteristics and experiences that affect subsequent health actions:[11]

PRIOR RELATED BEHAVIOR

Frequency of the same or similar behavior in the past. Direct and indirect effects on the likelihood of engaging in health-promoting behaviors.

PERSONAL FACTORS

Categorized as biological, psychological, and sociocultural. These factors are predictive of a given behavior and shaped by the nature of the target behavior being considered.

Personal Biological Factors

Include variables such as age, gender, body mass index, pubertal status, menopausal status, aerobic capacity, strength, agility, or balance.

Personal Psychological Factors

Include variables such as self-esteem, self-motivation, personal competence, perceived health status, and definition of health.

Personal Sociocultural Factors

Include variables such as race, ethnicity, acculturation, education, and socioeconomic status.

The following are behavioral-specific cognitions and affect that are considered of major motivational significance and these variables are modifiable through nursing actions:[11]

PERCEIVED BENEFITS OF ACTION

Anticipated positive outcomes that will occur from health behavior.

PERCEIVED BARRIERS TO ACTION

Anticipated, imagined, or real blocks and personal costs of undertaking a given behavior.

PERCEIVED SELF-EFFICACY

Judgment of personal capability to organize and execute a health-promoting behavior. Perceived self-efficacy influences perceived barriers to action so higher efficacy results in lowered perceptions of barriers to the performance of the behavior.

ACTIVITY-RELATED EFFECT

Subjective positive or negative feelings that occur before, during, and following behavior based on the stimulus properties of the behavior itself.

Activity-related affect influences perceived self-efficacy, which means the more positive the subjective feeling, the greater the feeling of efficacy. In turn, increased feelings of efficacy can generate further positive affect.

INTERPERSONAL INFLUENCES

Cognitions concerning behaviors, beliefs, or attitudes of others. Interpersonal influences include: norms (expectations of significant others), social support (instrumental and emotional encouragement), and modeling (vicarious learning through observing others engaged in a particular behavior). Primary sources of interpersonal influences are families, peers, and healthcare providers.

SITUATIONAL INFLUENCES

Personal perceptions and cognitions of any given situation or context that can facilitate or impede behavior. Includes perceptions of options available, demand characteristics, and aesthetic features of the environment in which given health-promoting behavior is proposed to take place. Situational influences may have direct or indirect influences on health behavior.

The following are immediate antecedents of behavior or behavioral outcomes. A behavioral event is initiated by a commitment to action unless there is a competing demand that cannot be avoided or a competing preference that cannot be resisted:[11]

COMMITMENT TO A PLAN OF ACTION

The concept of intention and identification of a planned strategy leads to implementation of health behavior.

IMMEDIATE COMPETING DEMANDS AND PREFERENCES

Competing demands are those alternative behaviors over which individuals have low control because there are environmental contingencies such as work or family care responsibilities. Competing

Continued

MAJOR CONCEPTS & DEFINITIONS—cont'd

preferences are alternative behaviors over which individuals exert relatively high control, such as choice of ice cream or an apple for a snack.

HEALTH-PROMOTING BEHAVIOR

Endpoint or action outcome directed toward attaining positive health outcomes such as optimal

well being, personal fulfillment, and productive living. Examples of health-promoting behavior are eating a healthy diet, exercising regularly, managing stress, gaining adequate rest and spiritual growth, and building positive relationships.

MAJOR ASSUMPTIONS

The assumptions reflect the behavioral science perspective and emphasize the active role of the patient for managing health behaviors by modifying the environmental context. In the third edition of her book, *Health Promotion in Nursing Practice,* Pender[11:54-55] states the major assumptions of The HPM:

"1. Persons seek to create conditions of living through which they can express their unique human health potential.
2. Persons have the capacity for reflective self-awareness, including assessment of their own competencies.
3. Persons value growth in directions viewed as positive and attempt to achieve a personally acceptable balance between change and stability.
4. Individuals seek to actively regulate their own behavior.
5. Individuals in all their biopsychosocial complexity interact with the environment, progressively transforming the environment and being transformed over time.
6. Health professionals constitute a part of the interpersonal environment, which exerts influence on persons throughout their life span.
7. Self-initiated reconfiguration of person-environment interactive patterns is essential to behavior change."

THEORETICAL ASSERTIONS

The model is an attempt to depict the multifaceted nature of persons interacting with the environment as they pursue health. Unlike avoidance-oriented

models that rely upon fear or threat to health as motivation for health behavior, the HPM has a competence or approach-oriented focus.[11] Health promotion is motivated by the desire to increase well being and actualize human potential.[11] In her first book, *Health Promotion in Nursing Practice,*[9] Pender asserts that there are complex biopsychosocial processes that motivate individuals to engage in behaviors directed toward the enhancement of health. Fourteen theoretical assertions derived from the model appear in the fourth edition of the book, *Health Promotion in Nursing Practice,*[19:63-64] which are listed below:

"1. Prior behavior and inherited and acquired characteristics influence beliefs, affect, and enactment of health-promoting behavior.
2. Persons commit to engaging in behaviors from which they anticipate deriving personally valued benefits.
3. Perceived barriers can constrain commitment to action, mediator of behavior, and actual behavior.
4. Perceived competence or self-efficacy to execute a given behavior increases the likelihood of commitment to action and actual performance of behavior.
5. Greater perceived self-efficacy results in fewer perceived barriers to specific health behavior.
6. Positive affect toward a behavior results in greater perceived self-efficacy, which can, in turn, result in increased positive affect.
7. When positive emotions or affect are associated with a behavior, the probability of commitment and action are increased.
8. Persons are more likely to commit to and engage in health-promoting behaviors when sig-

nificant others model the behavior, expect the behavior to occur, and provide assistance and support to enable the behavior.

9. Families, peers, and healthcare providers are important sources of interpersonal influence that can increase or decrease commitment to and engagement in health-promoting behavior.

10. Situational influences in the external environment can increase or decrease commitment to or participation in health-promoting behavior.

11. The greater the commitment to a specific plan of action, the more likely health-promoting behaviors are to be maintained over time.

12. Commitment to a plan of action is less likely to result in the desired behavior when competing demands over which persons have little control require immediate attention.

13. Commitment to a plan of action is less likely to result in the desired behavior when other actions are more attractive and thus preferred over the target behavior.

14. Persons can modify cognitions, affect, and the interpersonal and physical environments to create incentives for health actions."

LOGICAL FORM

The HPM has been formulated through induction by use of existing research to form a pattern of knowledge about health behavior. Middle-range theories are commonly generated through this approach. The HPM is a conceptual model that was formulated with the goal of integrating what is known about health-promoting behavior to generate questions for further testing. This model provides a framework for seeing how the results of previous research fit together more clearly and how concepts can be manipulated for further study.

ACCEPTANCE BY THE NURSING COMMUNITY

Practice

Wellness as a nursing specialty has grown in prominence in the past decade. Current state-of-the-art clinical practice includes health-promotion education. Nursing professionals find the HPM very relevant because it applies across the life span and is useful in a variety of settings.[11]

The clinical interest in health behaviors represents a philosophical shift that emphasizes the quality of lives alongside the saving of lives. In addition, there are financial, human, and environmental burdens upon society when individuals do not engage in prevention and health promotion. The HPM contributes a nursing solution to health policy and healthcare reform by providing a means for understanding how consumers can be motivated to attain personal health. Future empirical findings will be of increasing importance to nurse planners of healthcare delivery and those who provide the care.

Education

The HPM is widely used in graduate education and it is increasingly being used in undergraduate nursing education in the United States.[14] In the past, health promotion was being placed behind illness care as clinical education was conducted primarily in acute care settings.[18] Increasingly, the HPM is incorporated in nursing curricula as an aspect of health assessment, community health nursing, and wellness-focused courses.[14] There are growing international efforts across a number of countries to integrate the HPM into nursing curricula.[15]

Research

The HPM is a tool for research. Pender's research agenda and other researchers test the empirical precision of the model. Many research reports use the model as a frame of reference. The Health Promoting Lifestyle Profile, derived from the model, often serves as the operational definition for health-promoting behaviors. The model has implications for application by emphasizing the importance of individual assessment of the factors believed to influence health behavior changes.

FURTHER DEVELOPMENT

The model continues to be refined and tested for its power to explain the relationships among the factors believed to influence changes in a wide array of health behaviors. Sufficient empirical support for model variables now exists for some behaviors to warrant design and conduct of intervention studies to test model-based nursing interventions. Lusk and colleagues[5,6] used important predictors of construction workers' use of hearing protection from the HPM (self-efficacy, barriers, interpersonal influences, and situational influences) to develop an interactive, video-based program to increase construction workers' use of hearing protection. This large, multisite intervention study found that the intervention increased use of workers' hearing protection by 20% compared with the group without intervention, a statistically significant improvement from baseline.[5] Further intervention studies represent the next step in the use of the model to build nursing science.

CRITIQUE
Simplicity

The HPM is simple to understand. The conceptual definitions provide clarity and lead to greater understanding of the complexity of health behavior phenomena. The various factors in each set are logically linked. The relationships are clarified in the theoretical assertions. The sets of factors, which are direct or indirect influences, are clearly set out in a visually simple diagram that displays their association. Factors are seen as independent, but the sets have an interactive effect that results in action.

Generality

The model is middle range in scope. It is highly generalizable to adult populations. The research used to derive the model was based on male, female, young, old, well, and ill samples. The research agenda includes application in a variety of settings. Applicability of the model to children aged 10 to 16 years is currently being tested.[14]

Empirical Precision

The model has been supported through testing by Pender and others as a framework for explaining

health promotion. The model continues to evolve through planned programs of research. Continued empirical research, especially intervention studies, will further refine the model. The Health Promoting Lifestyle Profile has emerged as an instrument to assess health-promoting behaviors.[11]

Derivable Consequences

Pender has identified health promotion as a goal for the twenty-first century, just as disease prevention was a task of the twentieth century. The model can potentially influence the interaction between the nurse and the consumer. Pender has responded to the political, social, and personal environment of her time to clarify nursing's role in delivering health-promotion services to persons of all ages.

CRITICAL THINKING *Activities*

1. Choose one health-promoting behavior in which you do not engage. Identify your own factors, as defined in the HPM, which contribute to your decision not to participate. Include immediate competing alternatives.

2. Analyze the factors present in your life that contribute to your participation in any health-promoting activity in which you currently engage. Place each factor under the appropriate label from the HPM.

3. Prepare your own description of wellness. Ask three friends, three family members, and three co-workers to describe what wellness means to them. Compare the descriptions given by individuals with different ages and backgrounds. How are they alike? Is absence of disease more prominent than positive, active statements of health?

4. Anticipate the health-promoting behaviors important at various stages of development across the life span. In light of the nurse as a health educator, what health-promotion topics would you include in your practice?

5. Consider the changes made in healthcare delivery in the last century related to advances in disease prevention and cure. What changes can you predict for the nurse of 2050 if health promotion becomes the primary focus of healthcare? Include the potential locations for the work of nursing, possible new tools, and how the shift in emphasis would affect the demand for nurses.

REFERENCES

1. Bandura, A. (1977). Self-efficacy: Toward a unifying theory of behavioral change. *Psychology Review,* 84(2), 191-215.
2. Becker, M.H. (1974). *The health belief model and personal behavior.* Thorofare, NJ: Charles B. Slack.
3. Dunn, H.L. (1961). *High-level wellness.* Arlington, VA: Beatty.
4. Feather, N.T. (1982). *Expectations and actions: Expectancy-value models in psychology.* Hillsdale, NJ: Lawrence Erlbaum Associates, Inc.
5. Lusk, S.L., Hong, O.S., Ronis, S.L., Eakin, B.L., Kerr, M.J., & Early, M.R. (1999). Effectiveness of an intervention to increase construction worker's use of hearing protection. *Human Factors,* 41(3), 487-494.
6. Lusk, S.L., Kwee, M.J., Ronis, D.L., & Eakin, B.L. (1999). Applying the health promotion model to development of a worksite intervention. *American Journal of Health Promotion,* 13(4), 219-226.
7. Pender, N.J. (1970). A developmental study of conceptual, semantic differential, and acoustical dimensions as encoding categories in short-term memory. *Dissertation Abstracts International,* A, 30(10), 4283.
8. Pender, N.J. (1975). A conceptual model for preventive health behavior. *Nursing Outlook,* 23(6), 385-390.
9. Pender, N.J. (1982). *Health promotion in nursing practice.* New York: Appleton-Century-Crofts.
10. Pender, N.J. (1987). *Health promotion in nursing practice* (2nd ed.). New York: Appleton & Lange.
11. Pender, N.J. (1996). *Health promotion in nursing practice* (3rd ed.). Stamford, CT: Appleton & Lange.
12. Pender, N.J. (1997). *Health promotion in nursing practice* (3rd ed.). Stamford, CT: Appleton & Lange. (Japanese Translation.)
13. Pender, N.J. (1997). *Health promotion in nursing practice* (3rd ed.). Stamford, CT: Appleton & Lange. (Korean Translation.)
14. Pender, N.J. (2000, May 24). Personal interview.
15. Pender, N.J. (2000, July 19). Personal interview.
16. Pender, N.J. (2000). *Biographic sketch* [Online]. Available: http://www.umich.edu/%7Enursing/faculty/pender_bio.html.
17. Pender, N.J. (2000). Curriculum vitae.
18. Pender, N.J., Baraukas, V.H., Hayman, L., Rice, V.H., & Anderson, E.T. (1992). Health promotion and disease prevention: Toward excellence in nursing practice and education. *Nursing Outlook,* 40(3), 106-120.
19. Pender, N.J., Murdaugh, C.L., & Parsons, M.A. (2002). *Health promotion in nursing practice* (4th ed.). Upper Saddle River, NJ: Prentice-Hall.
20. Pender, N.J., Walker, S.N., Sechrist, K.R., & Stromborg, M.F. (1988). Development and testing of the health promotion model. *Cardiovascular Nursing,* 24(6), 41-43.
21. Sechrist, K.R., Walker, S.N., & Pender, N.J. (1987). Development and psychometric evaluation of the exercise/barriers scale. *Research in Nursing and Health,* 10, 357-365.
22. Walker, S.N., Sechrist, K.R., & Pender, N.J. (1987). The health-promoting lifestyle profile: Development and psychometric characteristics. *Nursing Research,* 36(2), 76-80.

BIBLIOGRAPHY
Primary Sources
Books

Pender, N.J. (1982). *Health promotion in nursing practice.* New York: Appleton-Century-Crofts.
Pender, N.J. (1987). *Health promotion in nursing practice* (2nd ed.). New York: Appleton & Lange.
Pender, N.J. (1996). *Health promotion in nursing practice* (3rd ed.). Stamford, CT: Appleton & Lange.

Book Chapters

Pender, N.J. (1984). Health promotion and illness prevention. In H. Werley & J. Fitzpatrick (Eds.), *Annual review of nursing research* (pp. 83-105). New York: Springer.
Pender, N.J. (1985). Self modification. In G. Bulechek & J. McCloskey (Eds.), *Interventions: Treatments for nursing diagnosis* (pp. 80-91). Philadelphia: Saunders.
Pender, N.J. (1986). Health promotion: Implementing strategies. In B. Logan & C. Dawkins (Eds.), *Family-centered nursing in the community* (pp. 295-334). Menlo Park, CA: Addison-Wesley.
Pender, N.J. (1987). Health and health promotion: The conceptual dilemmas. In M.E. Duffy & N.J. Pender (Eds.), *Conceptual issues in health promotion: Report of proceedings of a wingspread conference* (pp. 7-23). Indianapolis: Sigma Theta Tau International.
Pender, N.J. (1989). Languaging a health perspective for NANDA taxonomy on research and theory. In R.M. Carroll-Johnson (Ed.), *Classification of nursing diagnoses* (pp. 31-36). Philadelphia: Lippincott.
Pender, N.J. (1989). The pursuit of happiness, stress, and health. In S. Wald (Ed.), *Community health nursing:*

Issues and topics (pp. 145-175). Englewood Cliffs, NJ: Prentice-Hall.

Pender, N.J. (1998). Motivation for physical activity among children and adolescents. In J. Fitzpatrick & J.S. Stevenson (Eds.), *Annual review of nursing research* (Vol. 16, pp. 139-172). New York: Springer.

Pender, N.J. & Pender, A.R. (1989). Attitudes, subjective norms, and intentions to engage in health behaviors. In C.A. Tanner (Ed.), *Using nursing research* (NLN Publication No. 15-2232, pp. 466-472). National League for Nursing Publications.

Pender, N.J. & Sallis, J. (1995). Exercise counseling by health professionals. In R. Dishman (Ed.), *Exercise adherence* (2nd ed.). Champaign, IL: Human Kinetics.

Journal Articles

Brimmer, P.F., Skoner, M., Pender, N.J., Williams, C.A., Fleming, J.W., & Werley, H.H. (1983). Nurses with doctoral degrees: Education and employment characteristics. *Research in Nursing and Health*, 6, 157-165.

Frank-Stromborg, M., Pender, N.J., Walker, S.N., & Sechrist, K.R. (1990). Determinants of health-promoting lifestyle in ambulatory cancer patients. *Social Science and Medicine*, 31(10), 1159-1168.

Garcia, A.W., Broda, M.A.N., Frenn, M., Coviak, C., Pender, N.J., & Ronis, D.L. (1995). Gender and developmental differences in exercise beliefs among youth and prediction of their exercise behavior. *Journal of School Health*, 65(6), 213-219.

Garcia, A.W., Broda, M.A.N., Frenn, M., Coviak, C., Pender, N.J., & Ronis, D.L. (1997). Gender differences: Exercise beliefs among youth. *Reflections*, 23(1), 21-22.

Garcia, A.W., Pender, N.J., Antonakos, C.L., Ronis, D.L. (1998). Changes in physical activity beliefs and behaviors of boys and girls across the transition to junior high school. *Journal of Adolescent Health*, 5, 394-402.

Pender, N.J. (1967). The debate as a teaching and learning tool. *Nursing Outlook*, 15, 42-43.

Pender, N.J. (1970). A developmental study of conceptual, semantic differential, and acoustical dimensions as encoding categories in short term memory. *Dissertation Abstracts International*, A, 30(10), 4283.

Pender, N.J. (1971). Students who choose nursing: Are they success oriented? *Nursing Forum*, 16(1), 64-71.

Pender, N.J. (1974). Patient identification of health information received during hospitalization. *Nursing Research*, 23(3), 262-267.

Pender, N.J. (1975). A conceptual model for preventive health behavior. *Nursing Outlook*, 23(6), 385-390.

Pender, N.J. (1984). Physiologic responses of clients with essential hypertension to progressive muscle relaxation training. *Research in Nursing and Health*, 7, 197-203.

Pender, N.J. (1985). Effects of progressive muscle relaxation training on anxiety and health locus of control among hypertensive adults. *Research in Nursing and Health*, 8, 67-72.

Pender, N.J. (1987). Interview: James Michael McGinnis, MD, MPP. *Family and Community Health*, 10(2), 59-65.

Pender, N.J. (1988). Research agenda: Identifying research ideas and priorities. *American Journal of Health Promotion*, 2(4), 42-51.

Pender, N.J. (1988). Research agenda: The influences of health policy on an evolving research agenda. *American Journal of Health Promotion*, 2(3), 51-54.

Pender, N.J. (1990). Expressing health through lifestyle patterns. *Nursing Science Quarterly*, 3(3), 115-122.

Pender, N.J. (1990). Research agenda: A revised research agenda model. *American Journal of Health Promotion*, 4(3), 220-222.

Pender, N.J. (1992). Making a difference in health policy . . . from AAN president. *Nursing Outlook*, 40(3), 104-105.

Pender, N.J. (1992). Reforming health care: Future direction . . . from AAN president. *Nursing Outlook*, 40(1), 8-9.

Pender, N.J. (1992). The NIH strategic plan: How will it affect the future of nursing science and practice? *Nursing Outlook*, 40(2), 55-56.

Pender, N.J. (1993). Creating change through partnerships . . . from AAN president. *Nursing Outlook*, 41(1), 8-9.

Pender, N.J. (1993). Health care reform: One view of the future . . . from AAN president. *Nursing Outlook*, 41(2), 56-57.

Pender, N.J. (1993). Reaching out . . . from AAN president. *Nursing Outlook*, 41(3), 103-104.

Pender, N.J., Barkaukas, V.H., Hayman, L., Rice, V.H., & Anderson, E.T. (1992). Health promotion and disease prevention: Toward excellence in nursing practice and education. *Nursing Outlook*, 40(3), 106-12, 120.

Pender, N.J. & Pender, A.R. (1980). Illness prevention and health promotion services provided by nurse practitioners: Predicting potential consumers. *American Journal of Public Health*, 70(8), 798-803.

Pender, N.J. & Pender, A.R. (1986). Attitudes, subjective norms, and intentions to engage in health behaviors. *Nursing Research*, 35(1), 15-18.

Pender, N.J., Sechrist, K.R., Stromborg, M., & Walker, S.N. (1987). Collaboration in developing a research program grant. *Image: Journal of Nursing Scholarship*, 19(2), 75-77.

Pender, N.J., Smith, L.C., & Vernof, J.A. (1987). Building better workers. *American Association of Occupational Health Nurses Journal*, 35(9), 386-390.

Pender, N.J., Walker, S.N., Sechrist, K.R., & Frank-Stromborg, M. (1988). Development and testing of the health promotion model. *Cardiovascular Nursing*, 24(6), 41-43.

Pender, N.J., Walker, S.N., Stromborg, M.F., & Sechrist, K.R. (1990). Predicting health-promoting lifestyles in the workplace. *Nursing Research*, 39(6), 326-332.

Porter, C.P., Pender, N.J., Hayman, L.L., Armstrong, M.L., Riesch, S.K., & Lewis, M.A. (1997). Educating APHs for implementing the guidelines for adolescents in bright futures: Guidelines of health supervision of infants, children, and adolescents. *Nursing Outlook,* 45(6), 252-257.

Sechrist, K.R., Walker, S.N., & Pender, N.J. (1987). Development and psychometric evaluation of the exercise benefits/barriers scale. *Research in Nursing and Health,* 10, 357-365.

Walker, S.N., Ken, M.J., Pender, N.J., & Sechrist, K.R. (1990). A Spanish language version of the health promoting lifestyle profile. *Nursing Research,* 39(5), 268-273.

Walker, S.N., Sechrist, K.R., & Pender, N.J. (1987). The health-promoting lifestyle profile: Development and psychometric characteristics. *Nursing Research,* 36(2), 76-81.

Walker, S.N., Volkan, K., Sechrist, K.R., & Pender, N.J. (1988). Health-promoting life styles of older adults: Comparisons with young and middle-aged adults, correlates and patterns. *Advances in Nursing Science,* 11(1), 76-90.

International Journal Articles

Garcia, A.W., Broda, M.A., Frenn, M., Coviak, C., Pender, N.J., & Ronis, D.L. (1997). Gender and developmental differences in exercise beliefs among youth and prediction of their exercise behavior (Japanese translation). *The Japanese Journal of Nursing Research,* 30(3), 51-61.

Garcia, A.W., George, T.R., Coviack, C., & Pender, N.J. (1997). Development of the child/adolescent activity log: A comprehensive and feasible measure of leisure-time physical activity. *International Journal of Behavioral Medicine,* 4(4), 323-338.

Reports

Pender, N.J., Walker, S.N., Frank-Stromberg, M., & Sechrist, K.R.. (1990). *The health promotion model: Refinement and validation.* Final report to the National Center for Nursing Research, National Institutes of Health (Grant No. NR01121). DeKalb, IL: Northern Illinois University Press.

Secondary Sources
Authors Citing Pender's Work

Bonin, J. (1999). Psychosocial determinants for lithium compliance in bipolar disorder [French]. *Canadian Journal of Nursing Research,* 31(2), 25-40.

Burns, C.M. (1998). A retrospective theoretical model of the pathway to chemical dependency in nurses. *Archives of Psychiatric Nursing,* 12(1), 59-65.

Campbell, J. & Kreidler, M. (1994). Older adults' perceptions about wellness. *Journal of Holistic Nursing,* 12(4), 437-447.

Capik, L.K. (1998). The health promotion model applied to family-centered perinatal education. *Journal of Perinatal Education,* 7(1), 9-17.

Clement, M., Bouchard, L., Jankowski, L.W., & Perreault, M. (1995). Health promotion behaviors in first-year undergraduate nursing students: A pilot study [French]. *Canadian Journal of Nursing Research,* 27(4), 111-131.

Coppens, M.N. & McCabe, B.M. (1995). Promoting children's use of bicycle helmets. *Journal of Pediatric Health Care,* 9(2), 51-58.

Duffy, M.E. (1988). Determinants of health promotion in midlife women. *Nursing Research,* 37(6), 358-362.

Duffy, M.E. (1988). Health promotion in the family: Current findings and directives for nursing research. *Journal of Advanced Nursing,* 13(1), 109-117.

Duffy, M.E. (1989). Determinants of health status in employed women. *Health Values: Achieving High Level Wellness,* 13(2), 50-57.

Duffy, M.E. (1993). Determinants of health-promoting lifestyles of older persons. *Image: Journal of Nursing Scholarship,* 25(1), 23-28.

Duffy, M.E. (1997). Determinants of reported health promotion behaviors in employed Mexican American women. *Health Care For Women International,* 18(2), 149-163.

Felton, G.M. (1996). Female adolescent contraceptive use or nonuse at first and most recent coitus. *Public Health Nursing,* 13(3), 223-230.

Flowers, J.S. & McLean, J.E. (1996). Psychometric studies of the Flowers midlife questionnaire (FMHQ) for women. *Journal of Nursing Science,* 1(3/4), 115-126.

Foster, M.F. (1992). Health promotion and life satisfaction in elderly Black adults . . . including commentary by Hess, P., Foxall, M.J., Roberson, M.H.B., and author response. *Western Journal of Nursing Research,* 14(4), 444-463.

Gillis, A. & Perry, A. (1991). The relationships between physical activity and health-promoting behaviours in mid-life women. *Journal of Advanced Nursing,* 16(3), 299-310.

Gillis, A.J. (1993). Determinants of a health-promoting lifestyle: An integrative review. *Journal of Advanced Nursing,* 18(3), 345-353.

Gillis, A.J. (1994). Determinants of health-promoting lifestyles in adolescent females. *Canadian Journal of Nursing Research,* 26(2), 13-28.

Haddad, L.G, Al-Ma'aitah, R.M., Cameron, S.J., & Armstrong-Stassen, M. (1998). An Arabic language version of the health promotion lifestyle profile. *Public Health Nursing,* 15(2), 74-81.

Harrison, L.L. (1990). A health promotion model for wellness education. *American Journal of Maternal/Child Nursing,* 15(3), 191.

Jackson, C.P. (1995). The association between childbirth education, infant birthweight, and health promotion behaviors. *Journal of Perinatal Education,* 4(1), 27-33.

Johnson, J.L., Ratner, P.A., Botteroff, J.L., & Hayduk, L.A. (1993). An exploration of Pender's health promotion model using LISREL. *Nursing Research,* 42(3), 132-138.

Jones, M. & Nies, M.A. (1996). The relationship of perceived benefits of and barriers to reported exercise in older African American women. *Public Health Nursing,* 13(2), 151-158.

Lannon, S.L. (1997). Using a health promotion model to enhance medication compliance. *Journal of Neuroscience Nursing,* 29(3), 170-178.

Lookinland, S. & Harms, J. (1996). Comparison of health-promotive behaviours among seniors: Exercisers versus nonexercisers. *Social Sciences in Health: International Journal of Research and Practice,* 2(3), 147-161.

Lusk, S.L., Hong, O.S., Ronis, S.L., Eakin, B.L., Kerr, M.J., & Early, M.R. (1999). Effectiveness of an intervention to increase construction worker's use of hearing protection. *Human Factors,* 41(3), 487-494.

Lusk, S.L. & Kelemen, M.J. (1993). Predicting use of hearing protection: A preliminary study. *Public Health Nursing,* 10(3), 189-196.

Lusk, S.L., Kwee, M.J., Ronis, D.L., & Eakin, B.L. (1999). Applying the health promotion model to development of a worksite intervention. *American Journal of Health Promotion,* 13(4), 219-226.

Lusk, S.L., Ronis, D.L., & Baer, L.M. (1997). Gender differences in blue collar worker's use of hearing protection. *Women and Health,* 25(4), 69-89.

Lusk, S.L., Ronis, D.L., & Hogan, M.M. (1997). Test of the health promotion model as a causal model of construction worker's use of hearing protection. *Research in Nursing and Health,* 20(3), 183-194.

Lusk, S.L., Ronis, D.L., Kerr, M.J., & Atwood, J.R. (1994). Test of the health promotion model as a causal model of worker's use of hearing protection. *Nursing Research,* 43(3), 151-157.

MacDonald, M.B., Laing, G.B., & Faulkner, R.A. (1994). The relationship of health-promoting behaviour to health locus of control: Analysis of one baccalaureate nursing class. *Canadian Journal of Cardiovascular Nursing,* 5(2), 11-18.

Martinelli, A.M. (1999). An explanatory model of variables influencing health promotion behaviors in smoking and nonsmoking college students. *Public Health Nursing,* 16(4), 263-269.

McCabe, B.W., Walker, S.N., & Clark, K.A. (1997). Health promotion in long term care facilities. *Journal of Nursing Science,* 2(1-6), 153-167.

McCleary-Jones, V. (1996). Health promotion practices of smoking and non-smoking black women. *Association of Black Nursing Faculty Journal,* 7(1), 7-10.

Moylan, J.P. (1993). The achievement of dietary goals in patients with documented CAD: A test of Nola Pender's health promotion model. *Nursing Scan in Research,* 6(6), 3-4.

Neuberger, G.B., Kasal, S., Smith, K.V., Hassanein, R., & DeViney, S. (1994). Determinants of exercise and aerobic fitness in outpatients with arthritis. *Nursing Research,* 43(1), 11-17.

O'Quinn, J.L. (1995). Worksite wellness programs and lifestyle behaviors. *Journal of Holistic Nursing,* 13(4), 346-360.

Padula, C.A. (1997). Predictors of participation in health promotion activities by elderly couples. *Journal of Family Nursing,* 3(1), 88-106.

Palank, C.L. (1991). Determinants of health-promotive behavior: A review of current research. *Nursing Clinics of North America,* 26(4), 815-832.

Ratner, P.A., Bottorff, J.L., Johnson, J.L., & Hayduk, L.A. (1994). The interaction effects of gender within the health promotion model. *Research in Nursing and Health,* 17(5), 341-350.

Ratner, P.A., Bottorff, J.L., Johnson, J.L., & Hayduk, L.A. (1996). Using multiple indicators to test the dimensionality of concepts in the health promotion model. *Research in Nursing and Health,* 19(3), 237-247.

Riffle, K.L., Yoho, J., & Sams, J. (1989). Health-promoting behaviors, perceived social support, and self-reported health of Appalachian elderly. *Public Health Nursing,* 6(4), 204-211.

Sisk, R.J. (2000). Caregiver burden and health promotion. *International Journal of Nursing Studies,* 37(1), 37-43.

Speake, D.L., Cowart, M.E., & Pellet, K. (1989). Health perceptions and lifestyles of the elderly. *Research in Nursing and Health,* 12(2), 93-100.

Speake, D.L., Cowart, M.E., & Stephens, R. (1991). Healthy lifestyle practices of rural and urban elderly. *Health Values: Achieving High Level Wellness,* 15(1), 45-51.

Stegbauer, C.C. (1995). Smoking cessation in women: Findings from qualitative research. *Nurse Practitioner: American Journal of Primary Health Care,* 20(11), 80,83-86.

Stuifbergen, A.K. & Becker, H.A. (1994). Predictors of health-promoting lifestyles in persons with disabilities. *Research in Nursing and Health,* 17(1), 3-13.

Telleen, T.M. (1993). Health promotion practices of pregnant and nonpregnant women. *Journal of Holistic Nursing,* 11(3), 237-245.

Volden, C., Langemo, D., Adamson, M., & Oechsle, L. (1990). The relationship of age, gender, and exercise practices to measures of health, lifestyle, and self-esteem. *Applied Nursing Research,* 3(1), 20-26.

Wang, H. (1999). Predictors of health promotion lifestyle among three ethnic groups of elderly rural women in Taiwan. *Public Health Nursing,* 16(5), 321-328.

Weitzel, M.H. (1989). A test of the health promotion model with blue collar workers. *Nursing Research*, 38(2), 99-104.

Dissertations and Theses

Al-Obeisat, S.M. (1999). Prenatal care utilization among Jordanian women (health care utilization, health Promotion Model). *Dissertations Abstracts International*, 60-04B, 1525.

Anthony, J.S. (1999). Mental health correlates of self-advocacy in health care decision-making among elderly African-Americans. *Dissertations Abstracts International*, 59-12B, 6259.

Bagwell, M.M. (1988). *Wellness in two developmental phases of employed adults*. Unpublished doctoral dissertation, Texas Woman's University, Houston.

Barnett, F.C. (1989). *The relationship of selected cognitive-perceptual factors to health-promoting behaviors of adolescents*. Unpublished doctoral dissertation, University of Texas, Austin.

Beunting, J.A. (1990). *Psychosocial variables and gender as factors in wellness promotion*. Unpublished doctoral dissertation, State University of New York at Buffalo.

Bilderback, L.K. (1990). Health-promoting behaviors and perceived health status of rural families: A descriptive-correlational study. *Masters Abstracts International*, 29-01, 0089.

Bolio, S.M. (1999). Reported health-promoting behaviors of incarcerated males (prisoner health, family support). *Dissertations Abstracts International*, 60-02B, 0575.

Bond-Kinkade, M.A. (1999). The relationship of locus of control and participation in health-promoting behaviors among kidney transplant recipients. *Masters Abstracts International*, 37-06, 1815.

Butler, M.R. (1995). *Self-esteem and health-promoting lifestyle as predictors of health-risk behavior among older adolescents*. Unpublished doctoral dissertation, Texas Woman's University, Houston.

Carroll, S.A. (1995). The relationship of choice of infant feeding method and influencing factors among Hispanic mothers of the permian basin. *Masters Abstracts International*, 34-03, 1147.

Carter, L.M. (1990). *Functional wellness among older adults: The interface of motivation, lifestyle, and capability*. Unpublished doctoral dissertation, Texas Woman's University, Houston.

Chandrasekhar, R. (1999). Cues to action which influence engagement in health-promoting behaviors among nursing students. *Masters Abstracts International*, 37-02, 0587.

Chen, C. (1995). *Physical exercise and sense of well-being among Chinese elderly in Taiwan*. Unpublished doctoral dissertation, The University of Texas at Austin.

Cunningham, G.D. (1989). Health promoting self care behaviors in an older adult community. *Dissertations Abstracts International*, 50-11B, 4968.

Dunham, K.L. (1992). Health promoting lifestyles of nursing faculty. *Masters Abstracts International*, 31-02, 0760.

Ellis, J.R. (1990). *Health status, health behavior, multidimensional health locus-of-control and factors in the development of personal control in individuals with rheumatoid arthritis*. Unpublished doctoral dissertation, The University of Texas at Austin.

Fehir, J.S. (1988). Motivation, and selected demographics as determinants of health-promoting lifestyle behavior in men 35 to 64 years old: A nursing investigation. *Dissertations Abstracts International*, 50-05B, 1851.

Gasalberti, D. (1999). Early detection of breast cancer by self-examination: The influence of perceived barriers and health conception (cancer detection). *Dissertations Abstracts International*, 60-01B, 0129.

Gava, M.Z. (1996). *The AIDS crisis: Examining factors that influence use of condoms by young adult Zimbabwean males*. Unpublished doctoral dissertation, University of Michigan, Ann Arbor.

Gerard, M.S. (1993). *Factors related to long-term physical activity following coronary artery bypass graft surgery*. Unpublished doctoral dissertation, Rush University College of Nursing, Chicago.

Gillis, A.J. (1993). *The relationship of definition of health, perceived health status, self-efficacy, parental health-promoting lifestyle, and selected demographics to health-promoting lifestyle in adolescent females*. Unpublished doctoral dissertation, The University of Texas at Austin.

Grabowski, B.J. (1997). Determinants of health promotion behavior in active duty air force personnel. *Masters Abstracts International*, 36-01, 0156.

Harms, J.M. (1995). Health-promoting behaviors in exercising and nonexercising seniors: A comparison. *Masters Abstracts International*, 34-02, 0719.

Harrison, R.L. (1993). *The relationship among hope, perceived health status, and health-promoting lifestyle among HIV seropositive men*. Unpublished doctoral dissertation, New York University, New York.

Hatmaker, D.D. (1993). *The effects of individual factors and health promotion during pregnancy on maternal-child health*. Unpublished doctoral dissertation, Medical College of Georgia, Augusta.

Hemstron, M.M. (1993). *Relationships and differences in definition of health, perceived personal competence, perceived health status and health-promoting lifestyle profile in three elderly cohorts*. Unpublished doctoral dissertation, Rush University College of Nursing, Chicago.

Hubbard, D. (1987). The patterns of family interaction that promote positive child health behaviors. *Masters Abstracts International*, 26-04, 0419.

Hudak, J.W. (1988). A comparative study of the health beliefs and health-promoting behaviors of normal weight and overweight male Army personnel. *Dissertations Abstracts International*, 50-06B, 2337.

Jones, C.J. (1991). *Relationship of participation in health promotion behaviors to health-related hardiness and other selected factors in older adults.* Unpublished doctoral dissertation, Texas Woman's University, Houston.

Kerr, M.J. (1994). Factors related to Mexican-American workers' use of hearing protection (noise). *Dissertations Abstracts International,* 50-08B, 3238.

Kurtz, A.C. (1996). *Correlates of health-promoting lifestyles among women with rheumatoid arthritis.* Unpublished doctoral dissertation, Columbia University Teachers College, New York.

Lee, N. (1987). Health knowledge and health-promoting behavior in Chinese students. *Masters Abstracts International,* 27-01, 0086.

Lewallen, L.P. (1995). *Barriers to prenatal care in low-income women.* Unpublished doctoral dissertation, The University of North Carolina at Chapel Hill.

Martinelli, A.M. (1996). *A study of health locus of control, self-efficacy, health promotion behaviors, and environmental factors related to the self-report of the avoidance of environmental smoke in young adults.* Unpublished doctoral dissertation, The Catholic University of America, Washington, DC.

McKeon, F.M. (1997). Health-promoting behaviors: Predictors of early vs. late initiation to prenatal care. *Masters Abstracts International,* 35-05, 1390.

Medcalf, P.L. (1988). Value placed on health and number of health promoting behaviors of adults. *Masters Abstracts International,* 27-04, 0492.

Merren, V.A. (1991). Determinants of health promotion in the elderly. *Masters Abstracts International,* 29-04, 0648.

Mitchell, M.L. (1993). *Effects of a self-efficacy intervention on adherence to antihypertensive regimens.* Unpublished doctoral dissertation, The University of Rochester.

Moore, E.J. (1992). *The relationship among self-efficacy, health knowledge, self-rated health status, and selected demographics as determinants of health promoting behavior of older adults.* Unpublished doctoral dissertation, The University of Akron.

Oh, H. (1993). Health promoting behaviors and quality of life of Korean women with arthritis. *Dissertations Abstracts International,* 54-08B, 4083.

Phillips, P.S. (1993). Health promoting behaviors of adults attending a worksite health fair. *Masters Abstracts International,* 32-05, 1375.

Rothschild, S.L. (1996). *Mental health representations of attachment: implications for health-promoting behavior and perceived stress.* Unpublished doctoral dissertation, Ohio State University, Columbus.

Rummel, C.B. (1991). *The relationship of health value and hardiness to health-promoting behavior in nurses.* Unpublished doctoral dissertation, New York University, New York.

Sallee, A.M. (1996). The relationship of health locus of control and participation in health-promoting behaviors among older hypertensive persons. *Masters Abstracts International,* 34-18, 2349.

Smith Hendricks, C.K. (1992). *Perceptual determinants of early adolescent health promoting behaviors in one Alabama black belt country.* Unpublished doctoral dissertation, Boston College.

Stone, S.A. (1990). The relationship between self-esteem and health promoting behaviors in working women. *Masters Abstracts International,* 30-04, 1326.

Stutts, W.C. (1997). *Use of the health promotion model to predict physical activity in adults.* Unpublished doctoral dissertation, University of North Carolina at Chapel Hill.

Suwonnaroop, N. (1999). Health-promoting behaviors in older adults: The effect of social support, perceived health status, and personal factors. *Dissertations Abstracts International,* 60-08B, 3854.

Tapler, D.A. (1996). *The relationship between health value, self-efficacy, health barriers, and health behavior practices in mothers.* Unpublished doctoral dissertation, Texas Woman's University, Houston.

Tashiro, J. (1996). Health promoting lifestyle behaviors of college women in Japan: An exploratory study. *Dissertations Abstracts International,* 57-04B, 2486.

Thompson, E.M. (1995). *A descriptive study of women who successfully quit smoking.* Unpublished doctoral dissertation, Georgia State University, Atlanta.

Turner, S.J. (1989). Health protective behavior and the elderly: Hemoccult testing for early colorectal cancer detection. *Masters Abstracts International,* 28-02, 0277.

Vines, W.R. (1991). *Psychological stress reaction, coping strategies, and health promotion lifestyles among hospital nurses.* Unpublished doctoral dissertation, University of Alabama at Birmingham.

Warren, M.T. (1993). *The relationships of self-motivation and perceived personal competence to engaging in a health-promoting lifestyle for men in cardiac rehabilitation programs.* Unpublished doctoral dissertation, New York University, New York.

White, D.A. (1994). The relationship of intrinsic motivation and health beliefs on positive health behavior in pregnant adolescents. *Masters Abstracts International,* 34-02, 0730.

White, J.L. (1996). *Outcomes of an individualized health promotion program for homebound older community residents.* Unpublished doctoral dissertation, Texas Woman's University, Houston.

Wilson, A.H. (1991). Health promoting behaviors among married and unmarried mothers. *Dissertations Abstracts International,* 52-06B, 2999.

Wisnewski, C.A. (1996). *A study of the health-promoting behavioral effects of an exercise educational intervention in adult diabetics.* Unpublished doctoral dissertation, Texas Woman's University, Houston.

Yue, S.P. Assessing the needs if the post-cardiac event population in a rural southeastern New Mexico community. *Masters Abstracts International, 36-06,* 1594.

Yuhos, J.L. (1997). Health patterns of nurses who smoke. *Masters Abstracts International, 36-01,* 0166.

Videotapes

Pender, N.J. (1986, Oct.). *Enhancing wellness through nursing research* [Videotape]. Recorded at the Nursing Conference October 16-17. Available: University of Tennessee Memphis School of Nursing, Memphis, TN.

Pender, N.J. (1989, May). *Expressing health through beliefs and actions* [Videotape]. Recorded live at Discovery International, Inc.'s Nurse Theorist Conference at the Hyatt Pittsburgh, May 11-12, Pittsburgh, PA. Available: Meetings Internationale, Louisville, KY.

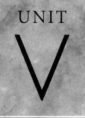

UNIT

V

Future of Nursing Theory

- *Theoretical systems are active and give direction to future research studies and administrative, educational, and practice applications.*

- *The theoretical works developed in a discipline affect the nature of the questions asked, the methods used to answer the questions, and the scope of knowledge addressed.*

- *Nursing models and theories exhibit characteristics of Kuhn's criteria for normal science; that is, research based on scientific achievements that a scientific community uses as the foundation of practice.*

- *The expansion of the philosophy of nursing science has increased the use of qualitative theory development in addition to quantitative methods and has increased the development of middle-range theories.*

- *A global community of nurse scholars has emerged as a result of the communication possibilities using the Internet.*

The State of the Art and Science of Nursing Theory

Martha Raile Alligood

From studying this text, it becomes obvious that the theoretical systems are active and growing and that they point the way to future research studies, educational and administrative uses, and practice applications. Reviews of the fourth edition of this text have been given careful consideration in the production of this fifth edition.[7,21,29] For example, middle-range theories are discussed and new middle-range theories have been added to the theoretical works included. As Burns[7:263] commented, "the more recent interest in middle-range theories is seen as the result of an evolving understanding of theoretic thought and the growing recognition of the potential impact of theory on nursing practice." She suggested that middle-range theory be acknowledged, such as those with qualitative research approaches that are emerging in the nursing literature. Her suggestion contributed to our inclusion of new chapters of that nature in this edition, such as Kolcaba's work on comfort in Chapter 24 and Mishel's work on uncertainty in Chapter 30.

The references have been recognized consistently as a strong point of this text in its earlier editions.

Malinski[21:265] notes that "they provide a valuable resource for students." With each edition, the references and the chapters are updated, reflecting that more and more nurses are coming to a working understanding of theory-based nursing for professional practice. Although theories are interesting as individuals learn the unique ways that nursing is presented, they are not just something to contemplate. Rather, they are vital for nurses to know and apply in nursing practice.[4] In this fifth edition, each chapter has been updated and particular attention has been given to the growing number of references, which is evidence of nursing science growth.

Reed[29:268] has noted that "the book supports the momentum building within nursing to transcend the tired debate about the relevance of nursing models and to apply this field of knowledge as a basis for understanding the substance and scholarship of nursing." Effort has been given to clarify the relevance of nursing theoretical works, recognizing them as the systematic presentations of nursing substance and tools for continuing contributions to nursing scholarship and nursing science.

Nursing theory continues to grow and stimulate scholarly guidance for nursing practice, nursing research, education, and nursing administration. The theoretical works developed in a discipline affect the nature of the questions that are asked by the discipline, the methods of research used to answer the questions, and the scope of the knowledge the questions address. How might nurses explore the state of the art and science of nursing theory? The evidence to answer that question is found in the nursing literature that documents the use of nursing theoretical works around the world.

This chapter addresses the continuing growth of nursing theory using Kuhn's philosophy of normal science.[19] This is followed with a discussion of the shift in the philosophy of nursing science that has led to the development of theory using qualitative approaches and quantitative methods. This chapter discusses the relevance of nursing theory when postmodern philosophy leads professional nurses to consider things from the past, such as early theoretical works, in a new light. Finally, this chapter addresses the global future, pointing to the growing bodies of communities of scholars, identifying important theoretical websites, and calling attention to the vital nature of theory use and application for professional nursing practice.

THE NATURE OF NORMAL SCIENCE

Many of the nursing models and some of the theories included in this text have developed to the point in which they exhibit characteristics of Kuhn's criteria for normal science.[19] Increasingly over the past 20 years, the conceptual models of nursing and nursing theories critiqued by Fawcett,[10,11,12,13,14] Fitzpatrick and Whall,[15,16,17] Meleis,[26,27,28] Marriner Tomey,[22,23,24] and Marriner Tomey and Alligood,[25] among others, have led to paradigm-based education, administration, research, and practice. The communities of scholars continue to grow in membership numbers, to become more formally organized as groups, and to address more difficult questions. Nursing models and theories provide a perspective of the main concepts of the discipline (metaparadigm),[14] they generate scholarship in the

form of theoretical guidance for research and practice, and they lead to the development of new research instruments unique to the perspective. This is carried out by a community of scholars who ascribe to the particular paradigm. Kuhn[19:15] states, "History suggests that the road to a firm research consensus is extraordinarily arduous." Conceptual models of nursing or "paradigms gain their status by being more successful than their competitors in solving a few problems that the group of practitioners have come to recognize as acute"[19:23]

Kuhn[19:10] defines normal science as "research firmly based upon one or more past scientific achievements, achievements that some particular scientific community acknowledges for a time as supplying the foundation for its further practice." Therefore the characteristics of paradigms that give evidence of their nature and lead to normal science include a community of scholars who base their research and practice on the paradigm, the formation of specialized journals, the foundation of specialists' societies, and the claim for a special place in curricula.[19] Each of the conceptual models of nursing included in this text have met these criteria. Some have made more progress than others in one or more of the criteria. For example, Rogers' Science of Unitary Human Beings (see Chapter 15) has generated many research studies, 13 research instruments, and 12 nursing process clinical tools for use in nursing practice.[14] In the mid1980s, an organized community of scholars formed an organization known as The Society of Rogerian Scholars. The organization supports a quarterly newsletter and a refereed journal, *Visions: The Journal of Rogerian Nursing Science*, to facilitate communication among the membership and foster the development of the science. There are numerous Rogerian texts and Rogerian science has been used to structure curricula used to teach students in many undergraduate nursing programs and graduate nursing programs. Other conceptual models of nursing that have experienced similar growth are Orem's Self-Care Deficit Theory (see Chapter 13), the Neuman Systems Model (see Chapter 18), Roy's Adaptation Model (see Chapter 17), and King's Interacting Systems Framework (see Chapter 19). There are nursing theories that also exhibit some characteristics of normal science, such as Erickson, Tomlin, and Swain's Theory of Modeling and Role-Modeling (see Chapter 25); Leininger's Theory of Cultural Diversity and Universality (see Chapter 28); Parse's Theory of Human Becoming (see Chapter 29); and Margaret Newman's Theory of Health as Expanding Consciousness (see Chapter 31). Not only are the number of societies of nursing scholars increasing, but the volume of articles published by the communities of scholars who use nursing models or theories for their practice and research is growing exponentially (Table 34-1).

EXPANSION OF THEORY DEVELOPMENT

In the last decade of the twentieth century, nursing experienced phenomenal growth in its science.[9] Nursing as a discipline eagerly embraced qualitative research approaches to explore questions that quantitative research could not answer and this expansion in the philosophy of nursing science has led to qualitative theory development.[30] Concomitantly, the continued use of conceptual models of nursing and nursing theories has led to a greater understanding of the nature of middle-range or practice

Table **34-1**

Nursing Theorist Names, Chapters of Their Theoretical Work, and Number of Publications in CINAHL Database		
NURSING THEORETICAL WORK RANKED BY NUMBER OF PUBLICATION*	**NURSING THEORIST'S CHAPTER IN THIS TEXTBOOK**	**NUMBER OF PUBLICATIONS IN CINAHL (1982 TO 2000)**
1. Orem	13	606
2. Rogers	15	400
3. Roy	17	366
4. Neuman	18	232
5. Parse	29	189
6. Leininger	28	188
7. Watson	11	142
8. Benner	12	141
9. King	19	137
10. Pender	33	135
11. Peplau	21	120
12. Newman	31	93
13. Johnson	16	42
14. Henderson	8	40
15. Roper, Logan, and Tierney	20	40
16. Levine	14	36
17. Mishel	30	30
18. Orlando	22	20
19. Nightingale	6	10
20. Wiedenbach	7	1

Note: Created October 27, 2000 using the Cumulative Index of Nursing and Allied Health Literature (CINAHL) Database, Information Systems, Glendale, CA.
*1 being the highest number of publications.

theory.[31] In addition, contemporary postmodern philosophy has led to considerations of the wealth of knowledge in the early theoretical writings by nursing scholars who interpret them in a new light.[3,8] These early writings are rich resources for new theory; for example, the theory of nursing empathy discovered in King's Interacting Systems Framework.[5]

Middle-range theory has been defined as the "least abstract set of related concepts that propose a truth specific to the details of nursing practice."[4:224] Most of the recent growth in the area of theory development has been in nursing theories and middle-range theories. This development clarifies the elusive practice theory that nurses have sought for so long.[2] Liehr and Smith[20] explored the nature of middle-range theories in the nursing literature from 1988 to 1998 and identified 24 middle-range theories. They noted that the theory-generating approaches used to develop the 24 middle-range theories were both quantitative and qualitative methods.[20]

Although there is dialogue in the nursing literature about the myriad of ways scholars classify nursing theoretical works, it is important to remember that each theoretical work is unique and therefore any attempt to classify the works is arbitrary and dependent upon the knowledge and judgment of the person doing the classification. Rather than emphasizing that the works be classified correctly, a more important and vital emphasis would be on *knowing* the individual works and *using* them to improve the professional practice of nursing.

The prevalence of middle-range theories is encouraging for the profession of nursing, whether developed using quantitative methods or qualitative approaches, because they are at the level of abstraction for application in nursing practice.[30] There is a need to explore the relationship of the theories from all of these methods and approaches.[31] Although they address different kinds of questions, all of the questions, whether studied with quantitative methods or qualitative approaches, are specific to nursing and generate knowledge for nursing. Consideration of nursing theoretical works in relation to a generic structure of knowledge reveals that theory from the hypothetico-deductive method and qualitative ap-

proaches eventually meet as they each reach the level of abstraction of middle-range theory. They just arrive there in different ways (Figure 34-1). Perhaps considering nursing knowledge in this generic structure will help move the discipline forward beyond research method debates and theory classification disagreements. It is important to understand that middle-range theories are at various levels of abstraction within that category, just as all of the theoretical works in the other classifications (philosophies, models, grand theories, and theories) have differences and similarities. Middle-range theories generally include practice specifics, such as the situation or health condition, patient population or age group, location or area of practice, and action of the nurse or the intervention and proposed outcome.[1] Middle-range theories may also be developed by exploring and interpreting some aspect of the lived experience of persons with a goal of under-

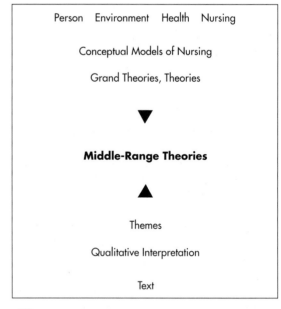

Figure **34-1** Middle-range theory in a generic structure of nursing knowledge from quantitative research methods and qualitative research approaches. (Reference: Fawcett, J. [2000]. *Contemporary nursing knowledge: Nursing models and theories.* Philadelphia: F.A. Davis.)

standing the meaning of life events related to health and nursing.

GLOBAL COMMUNITIES OF NURSING SCHOLARS AND WEBSITE RESOURCES

In addition to the growth stimulated by a broader philosophy of nursing science, expansion of research methods and approaches, and the emergence of middle-range theories, another contributor to the current state of the art and science of nursing theory is the global nature of communities of nurse scholars and communication and information possibilities via the Internet. Most of the communities of scholars organized around the conceptual models of nursing have international memberships. For example, the organization for Orem scholars is The International Orem Society. It was founded in 1990 and sponsors biannual conferences in the United States and in other countries. The sixth conference was held in Bankok, Thailand in February 2000. Similarly, the theme for the Eighth International Biennial Neuman Systems Model Symposia in March 2001 was organized with the theme, "Neuman Systems Model: Local to Global Connections." This has come about through the communication possibilities with colleagues around the world on the Internet, the increase of worldwide travel, and the publication of nursing theory textbooks in other languages. Nurses around the world are interested in nursing theory. For example, the second edition of *Nursing Theorists and Their Work*[23] has been translated into Italian, German, Finnish, and Japanese; the third edition[24] has been translated into Italian and Japanese; and the fourth edition[25] has been translated into Spanish. This text is also distributed widely in English-speaking countries such as Canada, the United Kingdom, Australia, and New Zealand. Our other textbook, *Nursing Theory: Utilization and Application,*[4] has been translated into classical Chinese, which is Taiwanese. Both texts have had consistent international circulations.

In consideration of this topic of global interest in conceptual models of nursing and nursing theory, reviewing the Cumulative Index of Nursing and Allied Health Literature (CINAHL) references for nursing theory articles in Spanish, French, and German verified the international use of nursing models and theories originating in the United States and identified theory development using contributions from other countries using both quantitative and qualitative approaches. For example, the German publications numbered 33 between 1995 and 2000 and included articles based on the use of Rogers, Orem, King, Leininger, and Erickson, Tomlin, and Swain. There is reference to a nursing model, developed by Kappeli[18] of the Department of Health of the State of Zurich in Switzerland, which has been introduced in five Swiss hospitals.[6] Kappeli[18] presented a paper at the symposium on Nursing Science at the University of Basel examining the requirements for nursing science for the nursing service of a university hospital and she concluded that nursing science is compatible with the ethos and goals of the nursing profession. The Spanish literature included 10 nursing theory articles with Orem, Peplau, and Henderson studies. The French literature included the use of Orem and Pender. These are only a few examples of the global use of nursing theory. We have included the theoretical work of Evelyn Adam, who is Canadian, (see Chapter 32) since the first edition of this text and we added the work of Roper, Logan, and Tierney (see Chapter 20), who are nurses from Scotland, with the nursing conceptual models in the fourth edition.

As the Internet leads to increased communication with nurses around the world, not only will more nurses embrace the scientific knowledge of the discipline of nursing from the United States, but American nurses will also be able to embrace more of the nursing theoretical works from other countries. For example, American nurses are publishing in a new peer-reviewed journal in Sweden, *Theoria, Journal of Nursing Theory.* It is published in English and is sponsored by the Swedish Society for Nursing Theories in Practice, Education, and Research. Similarly, *Nursing Science Quarterly* has reflected increasing global contributions from many countries.

There are several general nursing theory websites such as the Nursing Theory Page offered by Valdosta State University, College of Nursing; the Nursing

Theory Link Page maintained by Clayton College and State University Department of Nursing; and the Nursing Theory Page designed and maintained by Dr. Judy Norris, nursing faculty at the University of Alberta in Canada. Her site links to homepages or websites for many of the nursing theorists and their work (see appendix).

In conclusion, the state of the art and science of nursing theory is one of continuing growth. First, it has been noted that nursing theoretical works are used by communities of scholars who are support groups for the development of nursing science using a particular paradigm and the nursing science they are producing exhibits the characteristics of normal science.[19] Second, theory development has expanded with a broadened philosophy of nursing science and the introduction of new research approaches that address unanswered nursing questions. Perhaps one of the most exciting developments in the past decade has been the recognition of the usefulness of middle-range theory with an understanding that it is the level of theory that guides nursing practice, whether developed using quantitative methods or qualitative approaches. Third, the fact that global communities of nursing scholars are forming around the use of most of the conceptual models of nursing and nursing theories, the possibilities for further developments of nursing knowledge are tremendous. Using the Internet, the nurses of the world can share ideas and knowledge, carrying on the work begun by the nursing theorists, and continue the growth and the development of new nursing knowledge. It is vital that nursing knowledge is learned, used, and applied in theory-based practice for the profession and the continued development of nursing as an academic discipline.

REFERENCES

1. Alligood, M.R. (1997). Areas for further development of theory-based nursing practice. In M. Alligood & A. Marriner Tomey (Eds.), *Nursing theory: Utilization and application* (pp. 203-210). St. Louis: Mosby.
2. Alligood, M.R. (1997). The nature of knowledge needed for nursing practice. In M. Alligood & A. Marriner Tomey (Eds.), *Nursing theory: Utilization and application* (pp. 3-13). St. Louis: Mosby.
3. Alligood, M.R. & Fawcett, J. (1999). Acceptance of the invitation to dialogue: Examination of an interpretive approach for the science of unitary human beings. *Visions: The Journal of Rogerian Nursing Science,* 7(1), 5-13.
4. Alligood, M.R. & Marriner Tomey, A. (1997). *Nursing theory: Utilization and application.* St. Louis: Mosby.
5. Alligood, M.R. & May, B.A. (2000). A nursing theory of personal system empathy: Interpreting a conceptualization of empathy in King's interacting systems. *Nursing Science Quarterly,* 13(3), 243-247.
6. Anderregg-Tschudin, H. (1999). The complex interrelations between nursing diagnostic and nursing management [German]. *Pflege,* 12(4), 216-222.
7. Burns, N. (1999). [Review of the book *Nursing theorists and their work* (4th ed.)]. *Nursing Science Quarterly,* 12(3), 263-264.
8. Butcher, H.K. (1999). Rogerian ethics: An ethical inquiry into Rogers' life and science. *Nursing Science Quarterly,* 12(2), 111-118.
9. Cody, W. (1999). Affirming reflection. *Nursing Science Quarterly,* 12(1), 4-8.
10. Fawcett, J. (1984). *Analysis and evaluation of conceptual models of nursing.* Philadelphia: F.A. Davis.
11. Fawcett, J. (1989). *Analysis and evaluation of conceptual models of nursing* (2nd ed.). Philadelphia: F.A. Davis.
12. Fawcett, J. (1993). *Analysis and evaluation of nursing theories.* Philadelphia: F.A. Davis.
13. Fawcett, J. (1995). *Analysis and evaluation of conceptual models of nursing* (3rd ed.). Philadelphia: F.A. Davis.
14. Fawcett, J. (2000). *Analysis and evaluation of contemporary nursing knowledge: Nursing models and theories.* Philadelphia: F.A. Davis.
15. Fitzpatrick, J.J. & Whall, A.L. (1984). *Conceptual models of nursing: Analysis and application.* Norwalk, CT: Appleton & Lange.
16. Fitzpatrick, J.J. & Whall, A.L. (1989). *Conceptual models of nursing: Analysis and application* (2nd ed.). Norwalk, CT: Appleton & Lange.
17. Fitzpatrick, J.J. & Whall, A.L. (1996). *Conceptual models of nursing: Analysis and application* (3rd ed.). Stamford, CT: Appleton & Lange.
18. Kappeli, S. (1999). What sort of science does nursing require? [German]. *Pflege,* 12(3), 153-157.
19. Kuhn, T.S. (1970). *The structure of scientific revolutions* (2nd ed.). Chicago: The University of Chicago Press.
20. Liehr, P. & Smith, M.J. (1999). Middle range theory: Spinning research and practice to create knowledge for the new millennium. *Advances in Nursing Science,* 21(4), 81-91.

21. Malinski, V. (1999). [Review of the book *Nursing theorists and their work* (4th ed.)]. *Nursing Science Quarterly,* 12(3), 264-266.
22. Marriner Tomey, A. (1986). *Nursing theorists and their work.* St. Louis: Mosby.
23. Marriner Tomey, A. (1989). *Nursing theorists and their work* (2nd ed.). St. Louis: Mosby.
24. Marriner Tomey, A. (1994). *Nursing theorists and their work* (3rd ed.). St. Louis: Mosby.
25. Marriner Tomey, A. & Alligood, M. (1998). *Nursing theorists and their work* (4th ed.). St. Louis: Mosby.
26. Meleis, A.I. (1985). *Theoretical nursing: Development and progress.* Philadelphia: Lippincott.
27. Meleis, A.I. (1991). *Theoretical nursing: Development and progress* (2nd ed.). Philadelphia: Lippincott.
28. Meleis, A.I. (1997). *Theoretical nursing: Development and progress* (3rd ed.). Philadelphia: Lippincott.
29. Reed, P.G. (1999). [Review of the book *Nursing theorists and their work* (4th ed.)]. *Nursing Science Quarterly,* 12(3), 266-268.
30. Thorne, S., Kirkham, S.R., & MacDonald-Emes, J. (1997). Interpretive description: A noncategorical qualitative alternative for developing nursing knowledge. *Research in Nursing and Health,* 20, 169-177.
31. Whall, A. (1996). The structure of nursing knowledge: Analysis and evaluation of practice, middle range, and grand theory. In J.J. Fitzpatrick & A.L. Whall (Eds.), *Conceptual models of nursing: Analysis and application.* Stamford, CT: Appleton & Lange.

$\mathscr{R}$elated Websites

General Sites

NURSING THEORY PAGE, VALDOSTA STATE UNIVERSITY, COLLEGE OF NURSING:
http://www.valdosta.edu/nursing/history_theory/theory.html

NURSING THEORY LINK PAGE, CLAYTON COLLEGE AND STATE UNIVERSITY DEPARTMENT OF NURSING:
http://www.healthsci.clayton.edu/eichelberger/nursing.htm

NURSING THEORY PAGE, DESIGNED AND MAINTAINED BY DR. JUDY NORRIS, NURSING FACULTY AT THE UNIVERSITY OF ALBERTA, CANADA:
http://www.ualberta.ca/~jrnorris/nt/theory.html
(includes helpful links, such as Searching Bibliographic Databases for Nursing Theory by Margaret Allen, MLS-AHIP)

OMVÅRDNADSTEORETIKER:
http://www.omv.lu.se/bibl/Lankar/omvteor.htm
Memorial University of Newfoundland:
http://www.courses.mun.ca/nurs2700/weblinks.html

Nursing Theorist Sites

Abdellah
NURSING THEORY LINK PAGE, CLAYTON COLLEGE AND STATE UNIVERSITY DEPARTMENT OF NURSING:
http://www.healthsci.clayton.edu/eichelberger/nursing.htm

Barnard
UNIVERSITY OF WASHINGTON:
http://www.depts.Washington.edu/chdd/MRDDRC/biomedbehav/barnard.html

Benner
BENNER ASSOCIATES:
http://www.home.earthlink.net/~bennerassoc/index.html

Erickson, et al.
UNIVERSITY OF ALBERTA, CANADA:
http://www.ualberta.ca/~jrnorris/nt/theory.html#MRM

Hall
UNIVERSITY OF ALBERTA, CANADA:
http://www.ualberta.ca/~jrnorris/nt/theory.html#Hall

Henderson
UNIVERSITY OF ALBERTA, CANADA:
http://www.ualberta.ca/~jrnorris/nt/henderson.htm

Kolcaba
THE COMFORT LINE:
http://www.uakron.edu/comfort

Leininger
TRANSCULTURAL NURSING SOCIETY:
http://www.tcns.org

Mercer
UNIVERSITY OF ALBERTA, CANADA:
http://www.ualberta.ca/~jrnorris/nt/mercer.htm

Neuman
DEMON WORLD WIDE WEB:
http://www.lemmus.demon.co.uk/neuman.html

Newman
UNIVERSITY OF MINNESOTA:
http://www.tc.umn.edu/~hoym0003/bio.html

Orlando
UNIVERSITY OF SOUTH CAROLINA:
http://www.sc.edu/library/pubserv/herman/nurs700orlando2.htm

Parse
INTERNATIONAL CONSORTIUM OF PARSE SCHOLARS:
http://humanbecoming.org

Pender
UNIVERSITY OF MICHIGAN SCHOOL OF NURSING:
http://www.umich.edu/%7Enursing/faculty/pender_nola.html

Peplau
UNIVERSITY OF ALBERTA, CANADA:
http://www.ualberta.ca/~jrnorris/nt/theory.html#Peplau

Rogers
UNIVERSITY OF WALES COLLEGE OF MEDICINE, CARDIFF:
http://www.uwcm.ac.uk.uwcm/ns/martha/homepage.html

Roper, et al.
UNIVERSITY OF ALBERTA, CANADA:
http://www.ualberta.ca/~jrnorris/nt/theory.html#Roper

Watson
UNIVERSITY OF COLORADO HEALTH SCIENCES CENTER:
http://son.uchsc.edu/son/clinic/watson

Wiedenbach
UNIVERSITY OF ALBERTA, CANADA:
http://www.ualberta.ca/~jrnorris/nt/theory.html#Wiedenbach

$\mathcal{I}$ndex